# Essential Cardiology

## PRINCIPLES AND PRACTICE

*Edited By*

## Clive Rosendorff, MD, PhD, FRCP

Professor of Medicine
Associate Chairman, Department of Medicine
The Mount Sinai Medical Center
New York, New York

Chief, Medical Service
VA Medical Center
Bronx, New York

**W.B. SAUNDERS COMPANY**
*A Harcourt Health Sciences*
Philadelphia London New York St. Louis Sydney Toronto

**W.B. SAUNDERS COMPANY**
*A Harcourt Health Sciences Company*

The Curtis Center
Independence Square West
Philadelphia, Pennsylvania 19106

**Library of Congress Cataloging-in-Publication Data**

Essential cardiology / [edited by] Clive Rosendorff.—1st ed.

p.    cm.

Includes bibliographical references and index.

ISBN 0–7216–8144–1

1. Heart—Diseases.    2. Cardiology.    I. Rosendorff, Clive.
   [DNLM: 1. Heart Diseases—Outlines.    2. Cardiovascular
   Physiology—Outlines.    WG 18.2 E78 2001]

RC681.E85 2001     616.1′2—dc21

DNLM/DLC                                                      99–089412

*Editor:*   Richard Zorab
*Designer:*   Jonel Sofian
*Project Manager:*   Tina K. Rebane
*Production Manager:*   Frank Polizzano
*Illustration Coordinator:*   Lisa Lambert

ESSENTIAL CARDIOLOGY                                    ISBN 0–7216–8144–1

Printed in the United States of America.

Last digit is the print number:     9    8    7    6    5    4    3    2    1

# CONTRIBUTORS

**JONATHAN ABRAMS, MD**
Professor of Medicine, University of
New Mexico, and Professor of
Medicine, University Hospital,
Albuquerque, New Mexico
*Physical Examination of the Heart and
Circulation*

**KENNETH L. BAUGHMAN, MD**
Professor of Medicine and Director,
Division of Cardiology, The Johns
Hopkins School of Medicine; Chief of
Cardiology, The Johns Hopkins
Hospital, Baltimore, Maryland
*Myocarditis and Cardiomyopathies*

**NIRAT BEOHAR, MD**
Instructor in Medicine, Northwestern
University Medical School; Attending
Physician, Northwestern Memorial
Hospital, Chicago, Illinois
*Cardiac Catheterization and Coronary
Angiography*

**ROBERT W.W. BIEDERMAN, MD**
Associate in Cardiology, Department
of Medicine, Division of
Cardiovascular Disease, Center for
Nuclear Magnetic Research and
Development, University of Alabama
at Birmingham, Birmingham, Alabama
*Cardiovascular Magnetic Resonance
and X-Ray Computed Tomography*

**DANIEL G. BLANCHARD, MD**
Associate Professor of Medicine,
Division of Cardiovascular Medicine,
University of California, San Diego,
School of Medicine; Director, Cardiac
Noninvasive Laboratories, University
of California, San Diego, Medical
Center, San Diego, California
*Echocardiography*

**E.A.W. BRICE, MBChB, PhD, FCP(SA)**
Lecturer, Department of Medicine,
University of Cape Town, Senior
Registrar, Cardiac Clinic, Groote
Schuur Hospital, Observatory, Cape
Town, South Africa
*Rheumatic Fever and Valvular Heart
Disease*

**JAMES F. BURKE, MD**
Director, Cardiology Fellowship
Program, Lankenau Hospital,
Wynnewood, Pennsylvania
*Electrocardiography*

**CHRISTOPHER P. CANNON, MD**
Assistant Professor of Medicine,
Harvard Medical School; Associate
Physician, Cardiovascular Division,
Department of Medicine, Brigham and
Women's Hospital, Boston,
Massachusetts
*Acute Myocardial Infarction*

**SIMON CHAKKO, MD**
Professor of Medicine, University of
Miami; Chief, Cardiology Section,
Veterans Affairs Medical Center,
Miami, Florida
*Cardiovascular Complications in
Patients with Renal Disease*

**DAVID J. CHRISTINI, PhD**
Instructor in Medicine, Weill Medical
College of Cornell University, New
York, New York
*Electrophysiology of Cardiac
Arrhythmias*

**JACK M. COLMAN, MD, FRCP(C)**
Assistant Professor (Medicine),
University of Toronto; Staff

Cardiologist, University of Toronto Congenital Cardiac Centre for Adults, University Health Network and Mount Sinai Hospital, Toronto, Ontario, Canada
*Pregnancy and Cardiovascular Disease*

**P.J. COMMERFORD, MBChB, FCP(SA)**
Helen and Morris Mauerberger Professor of Cardiology, Department of Medicine, University of Cape Town; Head, Cardiac Clinic, Groote Schuur Hospital, Cape Town, South Africa
*Rheumatic Fever and Valvular Heart Disease*

**CHARLES J. DAVIDSON, MD**
Associate Professor of Medicine, Northwestern University Medical School; Attending Physician, Northwestern Memorial Hospital, Chicago, Illinois
*Cardiac Catheterization and Coronary Angiography*

**ROBIN L. DAVISSON, PhD**
Assistant Professor of Anatomy and Cell Biology, Department of Anatomy and Cell Biology, The University of Iowa College of Medicine, Iowa City, Iowa
*Choosing Appropriate Imaging Techniques*

**ANTHONY N. DeMARIA, MD**
Professor of Medicine and Chief, Division of Cardiovascular Medicine, University of California, San Diego, School of Medicine; Chief, Division of Cardiovascular Medicine, University of California, San Diego, Medical Center, San Diego, California
*Echocardiography*

**MARK DOYLE, PhD**
Associate Professor of Medicine, Department of Medicine, Division of Cardiovascular Diseases, University of Alabama at Birmingham, Birmingham, Alabama
*Cardiovascular Magnetic Resonance and X-Ray Computed Tomography*

**VICTOR J. DZAU, MD**
Hersey Professor of the Theory and Practice of Medicine, Harvard Medical School; Physician in Chief, Department of Medicine, Brigham and Women's Hospital, Boston, Massachusetts
*Myocardial and Vascular Gene Therapy*

**AFSHIN EHSAN, MD**
Fellow, Cardiovascular Medicine, Brigham and Women's Hospital, Boston, Massachusetts
*Myocardial and Vascular Gene Therapy*

**MURRAY EPSTEIN, MD**
Professor of Medicine, University of Miami School of Medicine; Attending Physician, University of Miami/ Jackson Medical Center and Miami Veterans Affairs Medical Center, Miami, Florida
*Cardiovascular Complications in Patients with Renal Disease*

**JOHN FARMER, MD**
Associate Professor, Sections of Cardiology and Atherosclerosis, Department of Medicine, Baylor College of Medicine, Chief of Cardiology, Ben Taub General Hospital, Houston, Texas
*Risk Factors and Prevention, Including Hyperlipidemias*

**LEE A. FLEISHER, MD**
Associate Professor of Anesthesiology, Medicine (Cardiology), and Health Policy and Management, The Johns Hopkins University School of Medicine; Clinical Director of the Operating Rooms, The Johns Hopkins Hospital, Baltimore, Maryland
*Assessment of Patients with Heart Disease for Fitness for Noncardiac Surgery*

**VICTOR F. FROELICHER, MD**
Professor of Medicine, Stanford University School of Medicine; Director, ECG and Exercise Lab, Palo

Alto VA Medical Center, Palo Alto, California
*Exercise Testing*

## SEAN P. GAINE, MD, PhD
Assistant Professor of Medicine, The Johns Hopkins University; Director, Pulmonary Hypertension Center, The Johns Hopkins Hospital, Baltimore, Maryland
*Disorders of the Pulmonary Circulation*

## MICHAEL H. GOLLOB, MD
Cardiology Fellow, Baylor College of Medicine, Houston, Texas
*Chronic Coronary Artery Disease: Stable and Unstable Angina*

## J. ANTHONY GOMES, MD, FACC
Professor, Department of Medicine, Mount Sinai School of Medicine of New York University; Director, Section of Electrophysiology and Electrocardiography, The Mount Sinai Medical Center, New York, New York
*Treatment of Cardiac Arrhythmias*

## STEPHEN S. GOTTLIEB, MD
Associate Professor of Medicine, University of Maryland School of Medicine; Director, Heart Failure Service, and Director, Cardiac Care Unit, University of Maryland Hospital, Baltimore, Maryland
*Treatment of Congestive Heart Failure*

## ANTONIO M. GOTTO, Jr., MD, DPhil
The Stephen and Suzanne Weiss Dean Professor of Medicine, Weill Medical College of Cornell University, New York, New York
*Risk Factors and Prevention, Including Hyperlipidemias*

## JONATHAN L. HALPERIN, MD
Robert and Harriet Heilbrunn Professor of Medicine (Cardiology), Mount Sinai School of Medicine; Director, Cardiology Clinical Services, The Zena and Michael A. Wiener Cardiovascular Institute, The Mount

Sinai Medical Center, New York, New York
*Peripheral Vascular Disease*

## ROBERT J. HENNING, MD, FACP, FCCP, FACC
Professor of Medicine, University of South Florida College of Medicine; Attending, James A. Haley Hospital, Moffitt Hospital, and Tampa General Hospital, Tampa, Florida
*Coronary Blood Flow and Myocardial Ischemia*

## JULIEN I.E. HOFFMAN, MD
Professor of Pediatrics (Emeritus), University of California, San Francisco; Attending Pediatric Cardiologist, Moffitt/Long Hospitals, University of California Medical Center, San Francisco, California
*Congenital Heart Disease*

## ERIC M. ISSELBACHER, MD
Instructor in Medicine, Harvard Medical School; Assistant in Medicine, Massachusetts General Hospital, Boston, Massachusetts
*Diseases of the Aorta*

## ALEXANDER IVANOV, MD
Fellow in Cardiology, Lankenau Hospital, Wynnewood, Pennsylvania
*Electrocardiography*

## DIWAKAR JAIN, MD, FACC
Associate Professor of Medicine, Section of Cardiovascular Medicine, Yale University School of Medicine; Attending Physician, Yale–New Haven Hospital, New Haven, Connecticut
*Nuclear Imaging in Cardiovascular Medicine*

## WILLIAM B. KANNEL, MD, MPH
Professor of Medicine and Public Health, Boston University School of Medicine, Boston; Head, Visiting Scientist Program, Framingham Heart Study, Framingham, Massachusetts
*Multivariate Evaluation of Persons at Risk for Cardiovascular Disease*

**NORMAN M. KAPLAN, MD**
Clinical Professor of Medicine,
University of Texas Southwestern
Medical School, Dallas, Texas
*Hypertension Therapy*

**WISHWA N. KAPOOR, MD, MPH**
Falk Professor of Medicine, and Vice-
Chairman, Department of Medicine,
University of Pittsburgh School of
Medicine; Chief, Division of General
Internal Medicine, University of
Pittsburgh Medical Center Health
System, Pittsburgh, Pennsylvania
*Syncope*

**ADOLF W. KARCHMER, MD**
Professor of Medicine, Harvard
Medical School; Chief, Division of
Infectious Diseases, Beth Israel
Deaconess Medical Center, Boston,
Massachusetts
*Infective Endocarditis*

**NEAL S. KLEIMAN, MD**
Associate Professor of Medicine,
Baylor College of Medicine; Assistant
Director, Cardiac Catheterization
Laboratories, The Methodist Hospital,
Houston, Texas
*Chronic Coronary Artery Disease:
Stable and Unstable Angina*

**PETER R. KOWEY, MD**
Professor of Medicine, Jefferson
Medical College, Philadelphia; Chief,
Cardiovascular Diseases Division,
Lankenau Hospital and Main Line
Health, Wynnewood, Pennsylvania
*Electrocardiography*

**JAMES A. de LEMOS, MD**
Instructor in Medicine, Harvard
Medical School; Associate Physician,
Brigham and Women's Hospital,
Boston, Massachusetts
*Acute Myocardial Infarction*

**BRUCE B. LERMAN, MD**
H. Altschul Mestor Professor of
Medicine; Chief, Division of
Cardiology; and Director, Cardiac

Electrophysiology Laboratory, Weill
Medical College of Cornell University,
and New York Hospital, New York,
New York
*Electrophysiology of Cardiac
Arrhythmias*

**MICHAEL J. MANN, MD**
Instructor, Cardiovascular Medicine,
Harvard Medical School; Instructor,
Cardiovascular Medicine, Brigham and
Women's Hospital, Boston,
Massachusetts
*Myocardial and Vascular Gene
Therapy*

**STEVEN M. MARKOWITZ, MD**
Assistant Professor of Medicine, Weill
Medical College of Cornell University,
New York, New York
*Electrophysiology of Cardiac
Arrhythmias*

**ANDREW R. MARKS, MD**
Clyde and Helen Wu Professor of
Molecular Cardiology, Professor of
Medicine, and Professor of
Pharmacology, and Director of the
Center for Molecular Cardiology,
College of Physicians and Surgeons of
Columbia University, New York, New
York
*Cardiac Contraction and Relaxation:
Molecular and Cellular Physiology*

**STEVEN O. MARX, MD**
Assistant Professor of Medicine,
Columbia University College of
Physicians and Surgeons; Assistant
Attending, New York Presbyterian
Hospital, New York, New York
*Cardiac Contraction and Relaxation:
Molecular and Cellular Physiology*

**DAVENDRA MEHTA, MD, MRCP, PhD**
Associate Professor, Department of
Medicine, Mount Sinai School of
Medicine of New York University;
Director, Electrophysiology Laboratory,
The Mount Sinai Medical Center, New
York, New York
*Treatment of Cardiac Arrhythmias*

**MICHAEL MILLER, MD, FACC**
Associate Professor of Medicine,
University of Maryland School of
Medicine; Director, Center for
Preventive Cardiology, University of
Maryland Medical System, Baltimore,
Maryland
*Preventive Cardiology*

**SUNEET MITTAL, MD**
Assistant Professor of Medicine, Weill
Medical College of Cornell University,
New York, New York
*Electrophysiology of Cardiac
Arrhythmias*

**YALE NEMERSON, MD**
Phillip J. and Harriet L. Goodhart
Professor of Medicine and Chief,
Division of Thrombosis, Department
of Medicine, The Mount Sinai Medical
Center, New York, New York
*Thrombosis*

**RAY A. OLSSON, MD**
Professor of Medicine, University of
South Florida College of Medicine;
Attending, James A. Haley Hospital,
Tampa, Florida
*Coronary Blood Flow and Myocardial
Ischemia*

**LIONEL H. OPIE, MD, DPhil, FRCP**
Professor of Medicine, University of
Cape Town, Medical School; Director,
Heart Research Unit, and Co-Director,
Medical Research Council Inter-
University Heart Research Group,
Cape Heart Centre, University of Cape
Town Medical School, Cape Town,
South Africa
*Ventricular Function*

**JOSEPH P. ORNATO, MD, FACC,
FACEP**
Professor and Chairman, Department
of Emergency Medicine, Virginia
Commonwealth University's Medical
College of Virginia, Richmond,
Virginia
*Cardiopulmonary Resuscitation*

**FREDRIC J. PASHKOW, MD**
Professor of Medicine, University of
Hawaii School of Medicine, and
Medical Director, The Heart Institute
Queens Medical Center, Honolulu,
Hawaii; Adjunct Staff, Cleveland
Clinic Foundation, Cleveland, Ohio
*Rehabilitation after Acute Myocardial
Infarction*

**GERALD M. POHOST, MD**
Professor of Medicine and Radiology
and Mary Gertrude Waters Professor
of Cardiovascular Medicine,
University of Alabama at Birmingham,
Birmingham, Alabama
*Cardiovascular Magnetic Resonance
and X-Ray Computed Tomography*

**PHILIP A. POOLE-WILSON, MD, FRCP,
FACC, FESC**
Professor of Cardiology, Department
of Cardiac Medicine, Imperial College
School of Medicine at the National
Heart and Lung Institute, London,
United Kingdom
*Pathophysiology of Heart Failure*

**RICHARD A. PRESTON, MD, MBA**
Associate Professor of Clinical
Medicine and Chief, Division of
Clinical Pharmacology, University of
Miami School of Medicine, Miami,
Florida
*Cardiovascular Complications in
Patients with Renal Disease*

**IAN F. PURCELL, BSc, MB, ChB,
MRCP, MD**
British Heart Foundation Clinical
Research Fellow, Department of
Cardiac Medicine, Imperial College
School of Medicine at the National
Heart and Lung Institute; Honorary
Specialist Registrar in Cardiology,
Royal Brompton Hospital, London,
United Kingdom
*Pathophysiology of Heart Failure*

**GAUTHAM P. REDDY, MD, MPH**
Assistant Professor of Radiology,
University of California, San Francisco,
San Francisco, California
*Radiology of the Heart*

**MARK J. RICCIARDI, MD**
Assistant Professor of Medicine,
Northwestern University Medical
School; Attending Physician,
Northwestern Memorial Hospital,
Chicago, Illinois
*Cardiac Catheterization and Coronary
Angiography*

**MICHAEL W. RICH, MD**
Associate Professor of Medicine,
Washington University School of
Medicine; Director, Cardiac Rapid
Evaluation Unit, Barnes-Jewish
Hospital, St. Louis, Missouri
*Heart Disease in the Elderly*

**CLIVE ROSENDORFF, MD, PhD, FRCP**
Professor of Medicine, and Associate
Chairman, Department of Medicine,
The Mount Sinai Medical Center, New
York; Chief, Medical Service, VA
Medical Center, Bronx, New York
*Vascular Function; Hypertension:
Mechanisms and Diagnosis*

**MARC SCHEINER, MD**
Fellow in Cardiology, Weill Medical
College of Cornell University, New
York, New York
*Electrophysiology of Cardiac
Arrhythmias*

**PREDIMAN K. SHAH, MD, FACC**
Professor of Medicine, University of
California, Los Angeles, School of
Medicine; Director, Division of
Cardiology and Atherosclerosis
Research Center, and Shapell and
Webb Chair in Cardiology, Cedars-
Sinai Medical Center, Los Angeles,
California
*Pathogenesis of Atherosclerosis*

**SAMUEL C. SIU, MD, SM, FRCPC,
FACC**
Assistant Professor of Medicine,
University of Toronto; Director of
Research, University of Toronto
Congenital Cardiac Centre for Adults,

Toronto General Hospital; Director of
Echocardiography, University Health
Network and Mount Sinai Hospital,
Toronto, Ontario, Canada
*Pregnancy and Cardiovascular Disease*

**DAVID J. SKORTON, MD**
Professor of Medicine, Electrical and
Computer Engineering, and
Biomedical Engineering, Colleges of
Medicine and Engineering, and Vice
President for Research, the University
of Iowa, Iowa City, Iowa
*Choosing Appropriate Imaging
Techniques*

**DAVID J. SLOTWINER, MD**
Assistant Professor of Medicine, Weill
Medical College of Cornell University,
New York, New York
*Electrophysiology of Cardiac
Arrhythmias*

**DAVID H. SPODICK, MD, DSc, FACC,
MD, DSC**
Professor of Medicine, University of
Massachusetts Medical School;
Director of Clinical Cardiology and
Director of Cardiovascular Fellowship
Training, Worcester Medical Center,
Worcester, Massachusetts
*Pericardial Disease*

**KENNETH M. STEIN, MD**
Assistant Professor of Medicine, Weill
Medical College of Cornell University,
New York, New York
*Electrophysiology of Cardiac
Arrhythmias*

**ROBERT M. STEINER, MD**
Professor of Radiology, Weill Medical
College of Cornell University, New
York; Chairman, Department of
Radiology, New York Methodist
Hospital, Brooklyn; Associate
Chairman, Department of Radiology,
New York/Presbyterian Medical
Center, New York, New York
*Radiology of the Heart*

**PETER H. STONE, MD**
Associate Professor of Medicine,
Harvard Medical School; Co-Director,
Samuel A. Levine Cardiac Unit;
Director, Clinical Trials Center,
Brigham and Women's Hospital,
Boston, Massachusetts
*Acute Myocardial Infarction*


**H.J.C. SWAN, MD, PhD**
Professor of Medicine (Emeritus),
University of California, Los Angeles,
School of Medicine; Director
(Emeritus), Division of Cardiology,
Cedars Sinai Medical Center, Los
Angeles, California
*The Medical History and Symptoms of
Heart Disease*


**MARK B. TAUBMAN, MD**
Irene and Arthur Fishberg Professor of
Medicine and Director of Cardiology
Fellowship and MD/PhD Programs,
The Mount Sinai Medical Center, New
York, New York
*Thrombosis*


**BARRY L. ZARET, MD, FACC**
Robert W. Berliner Professor of
Medicine; Professor of Medicine, and
Chief, Section of Cardiovascular
Medicine; Associate Chair, Department
of Medicine, Yale University School of
Medicine; Attending Physician, Yale
New Haven Hospital, New Haven,
Connecticut
*Nuclear Imaging in Cardiovascular
Medicine*

# PREFACE

"A big book," said Callimachus, the Alexandrian poet, "is a big evil!" Not always. There are some excellent, very big encyclopedias of cardiology, wonderful as works of reference. There are also many small books of cardiology, "handbooks" or "manuals," which serve a different purpose, to summarize, list, or simplify. This book is designed to fill a large gap between these extremes, to provide a textbook that is both substantial and readable, compact and reasonably comprehensive, and to provide an intelligent blend of molecular, cellular, and physiologic concepts with current clinical practice.

A word about the title. "Essential" is used here not in the sense of indispensable or absolutely required in all circumstances, for there is much more here than the generalist needs in order to practice good medicine, especially if there is easy access to a cardiology consultant. Rather, the word as used here denotes the *essence* or distillation or fundamentals of the mechanisms and practice of cardiology. The "Principles and Practice" subtitle affirms the idea that theory without a practical context may be academically satisfying but lacks usefulness, and practice without theory is plumbing. Good doctors understand the basic science foundation of what they do with patients, and great doctors are those who, as researchers or as teachers, see new connections between the basic sciences and clinical medicine.

I have been very fortunate to be able to assemble together a team of great doctors, who are outstanding physicians and scientists, most of them internationally recognized for their leadership position in their areas of specialization. They represent a careful blend of brillance and experience, and, most of all, they all write with the authority of undoubted experts in their fields. They have all been asked to write up-to-date reviews of their respective areas of expertise, at a level which will be intelligible to non-cardiologists as well as cardiologists, to medical students, internal medicine residents, general internists, and cardiology fellows. I believe that they have succeeded brilliantly, and I know that they are all very proud to have participated as authors in this project, the first textbook of cardiology of the new millenium. I am deeply grateful to all of them for the care and enthusiasm with which they carried out this task.

The general organization of this book follows fairly standard principles. After a review of the epidemiology of cardiovascular disease, with emphasis on risk stratification, there is a section on physiology, with chapters on the molecular and cellular basis of cardiac contraction, on ventricular and vascular function, and on thrombosis and fibrinolysis. A section of the examination and investigation of the patient focuses on diagnostic skills and tools, with chapters on history taking, the physical examination of the cardiovascular system, electrocardiography, echocardiography, exercise testing, radiology of the heart, cardiac catheterization and coronary angiography, nuclear cardiology, magnetic resonance, and x-ray tomographic imaging, with a review of the appropriate choice of imaging techniques. The section on disorders of rhythm and conduction includes chapters on the electrophysiology and the treatment of cardiac arrhythmias, and syncope. A heart failure section addresses the pathophysiology and the management of heart failure, followed by a chapter on congenital heart disease in the adult. The section on coronary artery disease has chapters on pathogenesis, coronary blood flow and ischemia, risk factors and prevention, acute myocardial infarction, chronic coronary artery disease (stable and unstable angina), cardiopulmonary resuscitation, and rehabilitation after myocardial infarction. Rheumatic valve disease and infective endocarditis are discussed in the section on valvular heart disease, and there are chapters on the mechanisms and diagnosis and therapy of hypertension. Other conditions affecting the heart are described in chapters on cardiomyopathies and myocarditis, pericardial disease, disorders of the pulmonary circulation (pulmonary embolism, primary pulmonary hypertension), and diseases of the aorta. A "miscellaneous" section includes chapters on pregnancy and cardiovascular disease, heart disease in the elderly, the heart in patients with renal disease, the assessment of patients with heart disease for general anesthesia, gene therapy, preventive cardiology, and peripheral vascular disease.

This organization reflects pretty much the key issues that concern cardiologists and other internists at present; I have no doubt that the field will develop and change in time so that many of the modes of diagnosis and therapy described here will become much more prominent (such as gene therapy), while others may diminish or even disappear. This is what second or later editions of textbooks are for.

I wish to thank, also, Richard Zorab, Jennifer Shreiner, Shelly Hampton, Frank Polizzano, Lisa Lambert, and Jonel Sofian of the W.B. Saunders Company for their encouragement and hard work, and my assistants, Maria Anthony and Anitra Collins.

CLIVE ROSENDORFF, MD, PhD, FRCP

# CONTENTS

*Color figures follow page xvi.*

## VIII. VALVULAR HEART DISEASE

## IX. HYPERTENSION

## X. OTHER CONDITIONS THAT AFFECT THE HEART

## XI. MISCELLANEOUS

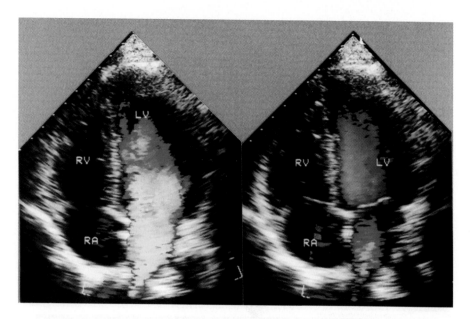

**Color Figure 9–5** ▪ Apical four-chamber images with color-flow Doppler during diastole *(left)* and systole *(right)*. Red flow indicates movement toward the transducer (diastolic filling); blue flow indicates movement away from the transducer (systolic ejection). RA, right atrium; RV, right ventricle; LV, left ventricle. (From DeMaria AN, Blanchard DG: The echocardiogram. *In* Schlant RC, Alexander RW, Fuster V [eds]: Hurst's The Heart, 9th ed. New York: McGraw-Hill, 1998:415–517, with permission.)

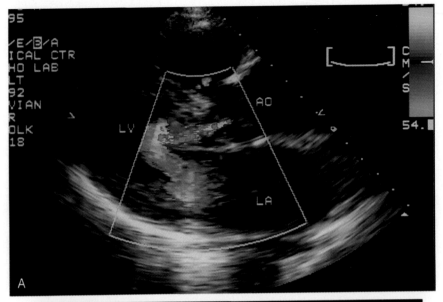

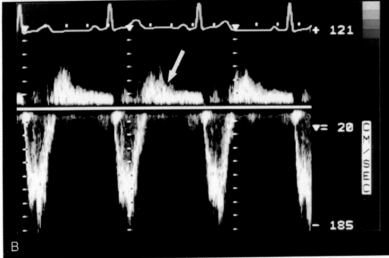

**Color Figure 9–11** ▪ *(A)* Parasternal long-axis image showing a multicolored jet (indicating turbulent flow) of aortic regurgitation in the left ventricular outflow tract. The jet is narrow in width, suggesting mild regurgitation. *(B)* Pulsed-wave Doppler tracing (from the suprasternal transducer position) in a case of severe aortic regurgitation. The sample volume is in the descending thoracic aorta, and holodiastolic flow reversal *(arrow)* is present. AO, aorta; LA, left atrium; LV, left ventricle. (From DeMaria AN, Blanchard DG: The echocardiogram. *In* Schlant RC, Alexander RW, Fuster V [eds]: Hurst's The Heart, 9th ed. New York: McGraw-Hill, 1998:415–517, with permission.)

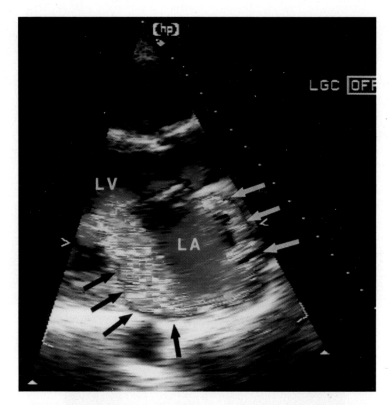

**Color Figure 9-13** ▪ Parasternal long-axis view in a case of severe mitral regurgitation. The color Doppler jet is directed posteriorly and is eccentric *(black arrows)*. The jet "hugs" the wall of the left atrium (LA) and wraps around all the way to the aortic root *(white arrows)*. LV, left ventricle. (From DeMaria AN, Blanchard DG: The echocardiogram. *In* Schlant RC, Alexander RW, Fuster V [eds]: Hurst's The Heart, 9th ed. New York: McGraw-Hill, 1998:415–517, with permission.)

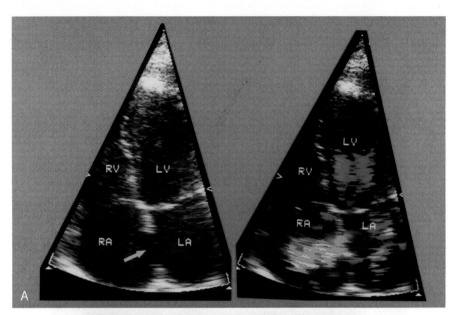

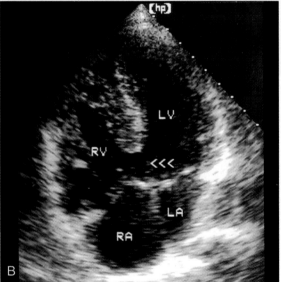

**Color Figure 9–22** ■ *(A)* Apical four-chamber view of an ostium secundum atrial septal defect. On the left, a defect in the mid-atrial septum is present *(arrow)*. On the right, there is color flow through the shunt. RA, right atrium; RV, right ventricle; LA, left atrium; LV, left ventricle. *(B)* Apical four-chamber image of an inlet ventricular septal defect. RV, right ventricle; RA, right atrium; LA, left atrium; LV, left ventricle. (From DeMaria AN, Blanchard DG; The echocardiogram. *In* Schlant RC, Alexander RW, Fuster V [eds]: Hurst's The Heart, 9th ed. New York: McGraw-Hill, 1998:415–517, with permission.)

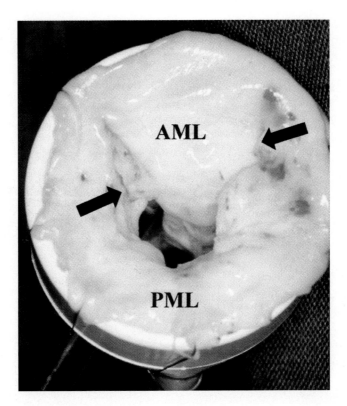

**Color Figure 29–1** ▪ Stenosed mitral valve excised at the time of mitral valve replacement (atrial view). Fusion of the commissures *(arrows)* between the anterior mitral leaflet (AML) and posterior mitral leaflet (PML) is evident.

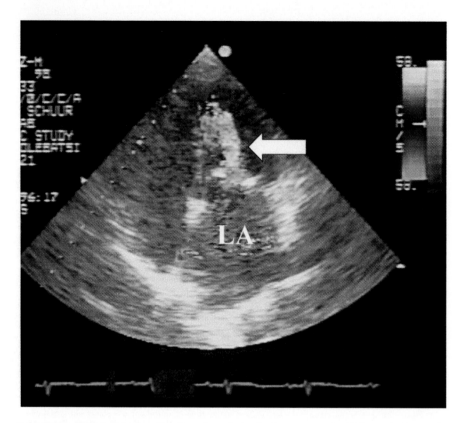

**Color Figure 29–5** ▪ Color-flow Doppler echocardiography demonstrates the high-velocity jet entering the left ventricle *(arrow)*. LA, left atrium.

# EPIDEMIOLOGY

*Chapter* 1

# Multivariate Evaluation of Persons at Risk for Cardiovascular Disease

*W.B. Kannel*

A preventive approach to management of cardiovascular disease is needed, because, once the disease appears, it is often immediately lethal and those fortunate enough to survive usually cannot be restored to full function. Prevention of the major atherosclerotic cardiovascular events is now feasible because several modifiable predisposing risk factors have been identified that, when corrected, can reduce the likelihood of such events.[1, 2] Multivariate risk formulations for estimating the probability that a cardiovascular event will occur that rely on the number of specified risk factors have been produced to facilitate evaluation of candidates for cardiovascular disease.[3–6]

The risk factor concept has become an integral feature of clinical assessment of candidates for initial or recurrent cardiovascular events. These risk factors may or may not be causal. Most risk factors associated with an initial cardiovascular event are also predictive of recurrent episodes, but the risk of a recurrence is usually dominated by indicators of the severity of the first event, such as the number of arteries occluded or the amount of ventricular dysfunction. Risk factors that are not modifiable (e.g., a strong family history) may nevertheless assist in risk estimation and indicate the need for greater urgency for correction of modifiable risk factors.

Observational studies can provide support for a causal link between risk factors and cardiovascular disease. Strong associations are more likely to indicate a causal relationship, particularly if the exposure to the risk factor antedates the onset of disease. Likewise, a causal relationship is likely if the association is dose dependent, consistently demonstrated, and biologically plausible.

Four decades of epidemiologic research identified a number of major modifiable cardiovascular risk factors that have strong dose-dependent and independent relationships to the rate of development of the major atherosclerotic cardiovascular diseases.[2] Importantly, these can be readily evaluated by ordinary office procedures. Epidemiologic data collected by the Framingham Study over four decades of biennial follow-up of a cohort of 5209 men and women make it possible to compare the cardiovascular risk profiles, which are composed of multiple risk factors for each of the atherosclerotic cardiovascular events. This information has implications for prevention of these diseases.

Framingham Study epidemiologic research has documented several classes of risk factors, such as atherogenic personal traits, lifestyles that promote them, signs of organ damage, and innate susceptibility. Most of the relevant risk factors are easy to assess during an office visit—systolic blood pressure, blood lipids, glucose tolerance, cigarette smoking, and left ventricular hypertrophy on electrocardiography (ECG).[2, 7]

## ■ AGE-, SEX-, AND CARDIOVASCULAR DISEASE–SPECIFIC EFFECTS

All of the major cardiovascular risk factors contribute powerfully and independently to the development of coronary disease in all its clinical manifestations (Table 1–1). For atherothrombotic brain infarction, hypertension and ECG-demonstrated left ventricular hypertrophy predominate and lipids appear to play a lesser role (Table 1–2). For peripheral arterial disease, glucose intolerance, left ventricular hypertrophy, and cigarette smoking are paramount, whereas cholesterol is less important (Table 1–3). For heart failure, hypertension, diabetes, and ECG demonstrated–left ventricular hypertrophy are all important, whereas total cholesterol appears to be unrelated (unless expressed as the ratio of total to high-density lipoprotein [HDL] cholesterol) (Table 1–4).

The standard risk factors also affect cardiovascular rates differently in men and women. Diabetes affects women more to the extent that it eliminates their cardiovascular disease advantage over men.[1, 8] Left ventricular hypertrophy is more ominous in women than in men.[9] Some of the standard risk factors tend to have lower risk ratios in advanced age, but this reduced relative risk is offset by a high absolute incidence of disease in advanced age, making the standard risk factors very relevant in elderly persons.

Table 1–1

**Risk of Coronary Heart Disease According to Standard Risk Factors: Framingham Heart Study 36-Year Follow-up**

| | Age 35–64 yr | | | | Age 65–94 yr | | | |
|---|---|---|---|---|---|---|---|---|
| | Age-Adjusted Biennial Rate per 1000 | | Age-Adjusted Relative Risk† | | Age-Adjusted Biennial Rate per 1000 | | Age-Adjusted Relative Risk† | |
| Factors | *Men* | *Women* | *Men* | *Women* | *Men* | *Women* | *Men* | *Women* |
| High cholesterol (>240 mg/dl) | 34 | 15 | 1.9*** | 1.8** | 59 | 39 | 1.2* | 2.0*** |
| Hypertension (>140/90 mm Hg) | 45 | 21 | 2.0*** | 2.2*** | 73 | 44 | 1.6*** | 1.9*** |
| Diabetes | 39 | 42 | 1.5*** | 3.7*** | 79 | 62 | 1.6** | 2.1*** |
| Electrocardiographic left ventricular hypertrophy | 79 | 55 | 3.0*** | 4.6*** | 134 | 94 | 2.7*** | 3.0*** |
| Smoking | 33 | 13 | 1.5** | 1.1 | 53 | 38 | 1.0 | 1.2 |

Key: *.01 < *p* < .05; **.001 < *p* < .01; ***p* < .001.
†Relative risk for persons with a given trait versus those without it. For cholesterol >240 mg/dl compared to <200 mg/dl.

Table 1–2

**Risk of Atherothrombotic Brain Infarction According to Standard Risk Factors: Framingham Heart Study 36-Year Follow-up**

| | Age 35–64 yr | | | | Age 65–94 yr | | | |
|---|---|---|---|---|---|---|---|---|
| | Age-Adjusted Biennial Rate per 1000 | | Age-Adjusted Relative Risk† | | Age-Adjusted Biennial Rate per 1000 | | Age-Adjusted Relative Risk† | |
| Factors | Men | Women | Men | Women | Men | Women | Men | Women |
| High cholesterol (>240 mg/dl) | 3 | 2 | 1.0 | 1.1 | 10 | 12 | 1.0 | 1.0 |
| Hypertension (>140/90 mm Hg) | 7 | 4 | 5.7*** | 4.0*** | 20 | 17 | 2.0*** | 2.6*** |
| Diabetes | 7 | 4 | 3.0** | 2.4* | 20 | 28 | 1.6 | 2.9*** |
| Electrocardiographic left ventricular hypertrophy | 13 | 13 | 5.1*** | 8.1*** | 44 | 51 | 3.6*** | 5.0*** |
| Smoking | 4 | 1 | 2.5** | 1.0 | 17 | 20 | 1.4 | 1.9*** |

Key: *.01 < $p$ < .05; **.001 < $p$ < .01; ***$p$ < .001.
†Relative risk for persons with a given trait versus those without it. For cholesterol >240 mg/dl compared to <200 mg/dl.

## Refinements in the Standard Risk Factors

The atherogenic potential of the serum total cholesterol derives from its low-density lipoprotein (LDL)–cholesterol fraction, whereas its HDL component is protective and its level inversely related to the development of coronary disease.[10, 11] The strength of the relation of total cholesterol to coronary disease declines after age 60 years, but the total-to-HDL ratio continues to predict events reliably in

Table 1–3

**Risk of Peripheral Artery Disease According to Standard Risk Factors: Framingham Heart Study 36-Year Follow-up**

| | Age 35–64 yr | | | | Age 65–94 yr | | | |
|---|---|---|---|---|---|---|---|---|
| | Age-Adjusted Biennial Rate per 1000 | | Age-Adjusted Relative Risk† | | Age-Adjusted Biennial Rate per 1000 | | Age-Adjusted Relative Risk† | |
| Factors | Men | Women | Men | Women | Men | Women | Men | Women |
| High cholesterol (>240 mg/dl) | 8 | 4 | 2.0** | 1.9 | 18 | 8 | 1.4 | 1.0 |
| Hypertension (>140/90 mm Hg) | 10 | 7 | 2.0*** | 3.7*** | 17 | 10 | 1.6* | 2.0** |
| Diabetes | 18 | 18 | 3.4** | 6.4*** | 21 | 16 | 9.7* | 2.6** |
| Electrocardiographic left ventricular hypertrophy | 16 | 17 | 2.7 | 5.3*** | 36 | 14 | 23.7** | 2.2 |
| Smoking | 9 | 5 | 2.5*** | 2.0** | 18 | 18 | 8.5** | 1.8* |

Key: *.01 < $p$ < .05; **.001 < $p$ < .01; ***$p$ < .001.
†Relative risk for persons with a given trait versus those without it. For cholesterol >240 mg/dl compared to <200 mg/dl.

Table 1–4

**Risk of Cardiac Failure According to Standard Risk Factors:
Framingham Heart Study 36-Year Follow-up**

| | Age 35–64 yr | | | | Age 65–94 yr | | | |
| --- | --- | --- | --- | --- | --- | --- | --- | --- |
| | Age-Adjusted Biennial Rate per 1000 | | Age-Adjusted Relative Risk† | | Age-Adjusted Biennial Rate per 1000 | | Age-Adjusted Relative Risk† | |
| Factors | *Men* | *Women* | *Men* | *Women* | *Men* | *Women* | *Men* | *Women* |
| High cholesterol (>240 mg/dl) | 7 | 4 | 1.2 | 1.1 | 21 | 18 | 1.0 | 1.0 |
| Hypertension (>140/90 mm Hg) | 14 | 6 | 4.0*** | 3.0*** | 33 | 24 | 1.9*** | 1.9*** |
| Diabetes | 23 | 21 | 4.4** | 8.0*** | 40 | 51 | 2.0*** | 3.6*** |
| Electrocardiographic left ventricular hypertrophy | 71 | 36 | 15.0*** | 13.0*** | 99 | 84 | 4.9*** | 5.4*** |
| Smoking | 7 | 3 | 1.5*** | 1.1 | 23 | 22 | 1.0 | 1.3* |

Key: $*.01 < p < .05$; $**.001 < p < .01$; $***p < .001$.

elderly persons (Table 1–5). This ratio has been found to be one of the most efficient lipid profiles for predicting cardiovascular events.[12, 13]

Evaluation of hypertension is now inclined to place more emphasis on the systolic blood pressure component and to recognize isolated systolic hypertension as a hazard for development of cardiovascular disease. For persons of any age or sex, for all the atherosclerotic cardiovascular disease outcomes, systolic blood pressure has been shown to have a greater impact than diastolic pressure.[14]

Diabetes and obesity are now conceptualized as components of an insulin resistance syndrome that includes abdominal obesity, elevated blood pressure, dyslipidemia, hyperinsulinemia, glucose intolerance, and abnormal lipoprotein lipase levels.[15]

## Risk Factors in Women

Cardiovascular risk factors are very prevalent in middle-aged and elderly women. Two thirds of such women have at least one major risk factor. The national burden of atherosclerotic cardiovascular disease is expected to increase substantially as elderly women constitute a progressively greater proportion of the U.S. popula-

Table 1–5

**Risk Ratio for Development of Coronary Heart Disease by Total/HDL Cholesterol Ratio
According to Age: Framingham Study 16-Year Follow-up**

| Age (yr) | Total/HDL Ratio Quintile 5/Quintile 1 | | | Total Cholesterol (≥240 vs <200 mg/dl) | |
| --- | --- | --- | --- | --- | --- |
| | 49–59 | 60–69 | 70–81 | 35–64 | 65–94 |
| Men | 3.4* | 2.9* | 2.3* | 1.9*** | 1.2 |
| Women | 3.7* | 6.7* | 3.3* | 1.8** | 2.0*** |

Key: $*.01 < p < .05$; $**.001 < p < .01$; $***p < .001$.

tion. Women and men share the same cardiovascular risk factors, but some are more prevalent or more powerful in women than in men. Others are unique to women. With the exception of diabetes, the absolute risk for most risk factors is lower for women than for men. Because of the lower incidence of cardiovascular disease in women, the most cost-effective preventive approach requires evaluating high-risk women for preventive measures. Most vulnerable are elderly women, black women, and those of lower socioeconomic status. High total-HDL cholesterol ratios, ECG–left ventricular hypertrophy, and diabetes markedly reduce women's coronary disease advantage.[9]

Diabetes is clearly a greater cardiovascular hazard for women than for men, eliminating their advantage over men for coronary disease, heart failure, and peripheral artery disease (Table 1–6). Women with diabetes require intensive screening to detect the elevated triglycerides, reduced HDL cholesterol, hypertension, and abdominal obesity usually associated with it. Minority women and those with gestational diabetes who are prone to develop an adverse coronary risk profile deserve particular attention.

Reduced HDL cholesterol predicts coronary disease even better in women than in men. Throughout life, women, on average, have HDL-cholesterol values that are 10 mg/dl greater than those of men, so that it seems more appropriate to characterize "low" HDL cholesterol as 45 mg/dl rather than 35 mg/dl as recommended in Adult Treatment Panel II guidelines. Hypertriglyceridemia remains controversial as an independent risk factor for women as it does for men, but the combination of low HDL and high triglycerides carries increased risk.

The majority of elderly women have hypertension, and isolated systolic hypertension is more prevalent in women than in men. Its concordance with obesity, dyslipidemia, and insulin resistance should be noted.

Risk factors unique to women include early menopause and bilateral oophorectomy. Estrogen replacement therapy can virtually eliminate the more than twofold increase in risk of coronary disease in this subgroup of women. Women who experience menopause early and do not use estrogen replacement therapy require close surveillance for the development of an adverse cardiovascular risk profile.

## The Elderly

The strength of risk factors associated with cardiovascular disease diminishes with advancing age, but this lower risk is invariably offset by higher absolute risk. This makes risk factor control in the elderly at least as cost-effective as it is in

Table 1–6

**Risk of Cardiovascular Events in Diabetics 36-Year Follow-up: Framingham Study Persons Aged 35–64 Years**

| Cardiovascular Events | Age-Adjusted Biennial Rate per 1000 | | Age-Adjusted Risk Ratio | | Excess Risk Per 1000 | |
|---|---|---|---|---|---|---|
| | Men | Women | Men | Women | Men | Women |
| Coronary heart disease | 39 | 21 | 1.5** | 2.2*** | 12 | 12 |
| Stroke | 15 | 6 | 2.9*** | 2.6*** | 10 | 4 |
| Peripheral arterial disease | 18 | 18 | 3.4*** | 6.4*** | 13 | 15 |
| Cardiac failure | 23 | 21 | 4.4*** | 7.8*** | 18 | 18 |
| Cardiovascular events | 76 | 65 | 2.2*** | 3.7*** | 42 | 47 |

Key: **$p < .001$; ***$p < .0001$.

middle-aged persons. Epidemiologic research has quantified the impact of the major cardiovascular risk factors on elders.[16] Dyslipidemia, hypertension, glucose intolerance, and cigarette smoking all have smaller hazard ratios in advanced age, but these are offset by higher absolute and attributable risks. Diabetes operates substantially more strongly in elderly women than in elderly men, eliminating their waning advantage over men in advanced age (see Tables 1–1 through 1–4). Insulin resistance, promoted by development of abdominal obesity in advanced age, is an important feature of the cardiovascular hazard of diabetes in elderly persons.

Hypertension is very prevalent in the elderly, particularly the isolated systolic variety, which has been shown to be a distinct and safely modifiable hazard. Dyslipidemia remains a major risk factor in old age, particularly the total cholesterol–HDL ratio, which, in contrast to total cholesterol, continues to be highly predictive in advanced age (see Table 1–5). Left ventricular hypertrophy remains an ominous harbinger of cardiovascular disease in the elderly, indicating urgent need for attention to associated hypertension, diabetes, obesity, myocardial ischemia, or valve disease. High normal fibrinogen and leukocyte counts in the elderly may indicate the presence of unstable atherosclerotic lesions. As in middle-aged persons, all the major risk factors in the elderly tend to cluster in individual persons so that the hazard of each is powerfully influenced by the associated burden of the others. Multivariate risk assessment can quantify the concurrent effect of risk factors, making it possible to more efficiently target elderly candidates for cardiovascular disease for preventive measures.[3–6]

A substantial proportion of the elderly warrant preventive measures because they remain active in their retirement years. Also, because of the aging of the general population, it will be necessary for more of the elderly to remain in the workforce. Because of the high average risk of cardiovascular events in the elderly, there is actually great potential benefit from preventive measures, but to avoid overtreatment it is important to assess multivariate risk and to take into account their general heath status. There is little justification for pessimism about the efficacy of preventive measures in elderly persons. The major risk factors can safely be modified without inducing intolerable side effects or adversely affecting the quality of the last years of life. The major risk factors remain very relevant in the elderly, not only for primary prevention but for secondary prevention as well.

## ■ ATHEROSCLEROTIC COMORBIDITY

Atherosclerotic cardiovascular disease is a diffuse process involving the heart, brain, and peripheral arteries. The presence of one clinical manifestation substantially increases the likelihood of having or developing others.[17] The major risk factors tend to affect all arterial territories, and clinical atherosclerosis affecting the heart may also directly predispose to strokes and heart failure. Measures taken to prevent coronary disease should have an additional benefit in preventing atherosclerotic peripheral artery and stroke events and heart failure.

The prevalence of other cardiovascular diseases accompanying coronary disease is substantial.[18] The Framingham Study found that, in men and women, respectively, an initial myocardial infarction is accompanied by intermittent claudication 9% and 10% of the time, by strokes or transient ischemic attacks 5% and 8% of the time, and by heart failure 3% and 10% of the time.[18] Persons in the Framingham Study with intermittent claudication had two to three times greater risk of developing coronary disease. Over 10 years, 45% did so. After an initial myocardial infarction, the 10-year probability of a stroke or transient ischemic attack was 16% in men and 24% in women, rates three to four times those for the general population. Heart failure occurred in about 30% of patients who had experienced a myocardial infarction. After sustaining an atherothrombotic stroke, 25% to 45% developed coronary disease, a twofold increase in risk over that of persons without a stroke. After a myocardial infarction, coexistence of intermittent claudication increased age-adjusted coronary mortality 1.7 times in men and 1.5 times in women.[18]

## ■ NOVEL RISK FACTORS

Because many coronary events occur in persons whose risk factors are considered acceptable or average, novel risk factors are being sought. Among these are lipoprotein(a), homocysteine, fibrinogen, small dense LDL, insulin resistance, fibrinolytic function assessed by tissue plasminogen activator (t-PA) and plasminogen activator inhibitor (PAI-1) antigens, and inflammatory parameters such as C-reactive protein.

Evidence from several large observational epidemiologic studies implicates a number of hemostatic risk factors in the development of myocardial infarction and stroke. Early markers of a procoagulatory tendency that have been identified prospectively include elevated fibrinogen, factor VII, PAI-1 activity, and decreased t-PA.

### Fibrinogen

With data from at least 10 major prospective epidemiologic investigations, meta-analysis indicates a 2.3-fold increased risk for persons whose fibrinogen values fall in the top tertile as compared with those in the bottom tertile.[19] The strength and consistency of the association, its biologic plausibility, and its independent contribution to risk suggest a causal relationship, and there is some evidence that assessment of the fibrinogen adds to our ability to predict cardiovascular events. The high prevalence of elevated values and the substantial hazard ratio confer substantial attributable risk, which rivals that of cholesterol.

### Factor VII

The evidence linking factor VII to cardiovascular disease is less consistent. The Northwick Park Heart study reported an independent association with nonfatal ischemic events (risk ratio 1.55).[20] The Prospective Cardiovascular Munster (PROCAM) study reported only a trend toward higher factor VII values (p = .06) for fatal events.[21] The Atherosclerosis Risk in Communities (ARIC) study, on the other hand, found no association.[22]

### Platelets

Platelets play a major role in atherogenesis and in thrombotic clinical events, but clinically valid tests to identify persons at increased risk because of increased platelet activity are lacking. One study of healthy middle-aged men showed an association between platelet count and rapid platelet aggregability and excessive prevalence of fatal coronary events,[23] and another linked spontaneous platelet aggregation with recurrent coronary events.[24]

### PAI-1 and t-PA

The intravascular fibrinolytic system is regulated by a balance between t-PA and its PAI-1 inhibitor. Higher PAI-1 values have been reported in postinfarction patients as compared with matched controls[25] and have been shown to be associated with increased risk of reinfarctions.[26] In the Physicians' Health Study, concentrations of t-PA were found to be higher in cases than in controls.[26] Comparing the highest with the lowest quintile of t-PA values, and adjusting for other risk factors, indicated a 1.56:1 risk ratio, a figure that was not statistically significant. In the Northwick Park Heart Study, fibrinolytic activity measured by blood clot lysis time was found to be related to initial coronary events in men aged 45 to 54 years but not in older ones.[27] The European Concerted Action on Thrombosis and Disabilities (ECAT) cohort had t-PA antigen, t-PA activity, and PAI-1 activity simultaneously measured in patients with angina pectoris and found that all these variables were positively associated with myocardial infarction and sudden coronary death, after adjustments were made for age and sex.[28] The associations of PAI-1 and t-PA with risk of these events disappeared after adjustment for variables reflecting insulin resistance (body mass index, triglycerides, and HDL cholesterol).

## Lipoprotein(a)

Owing to the structural similarity of apolipoprotein(a) to plasminogen, Lp(a) interferes with fibrinolysis by competing with plasminogen. The association of Lp(a) with coronary disease was examined in 10 prospective studies and was found to be positive in those that examined large samples of subjects who at baseline were free of atherosclerotic disease and who were not taking aspirin.[29] A recent 14-year, large, prospective study of 9936 men and women who were at the outset free of coronary disease found Lp(a) to be a significant predictor of coronary events in both genders.[30] Lp(a) appears to be an important determinant of coronary disease, but the lack of standardized methods for measuring it has made assessment of its impact and clinical application difficult.

## C-Reactive Protein

C-reactive protein, a sensitive marker of acute phase response, has been shown to be strongly and independently related to subsequent coronary events in patients with angina pectoris[31] and in healthy participants in the Physicians' Health Study.[32] Although no currently available therapies alter C-reactive protein levels, it is interesting that the efficacy of low-dose aspirin and statin therapy in preventing coronary disease may be greater in persons with underlying inflammation signified by high-sensitivity C-reactive protein.[32]

## Homocysteine

More than 25 epidemiologic studies have demonstrated that homocysteine independently predicts myocardial infarctions with an odds ratio of 1.7:1. In a recent metaanalysis, it was estimated that 10% of the risk of coronary disease might be attributable to elevated homocysteine.[33] Although severe elevations of homocysteine are rare, mild hyperhomocysteinemia occurs in about 5% to 7% of the general population.[34, 35] Abundant convincing epidemiologic evidence indicates that mild hyperhomocysteinemia independently predisposes to coronary, cerebral, and peripheral atherosclerotic disease.[36] Normal total plasma homocysteine appears to range from 5 to 15 nmol/l. Elevations of plasma homocysteine are caused by genetic defects in the enzymes involved in homocysteine metabolism or by deficiencies in vitamin cofactors. Nutritional vitamin deficiencies in folate, $B_{12}$, and $B_6$, required for homocysteine metabolism, promote elevated homocysteine levels.

Inadequate intake of these B vitamins contributes to about two thirds of all cases of hyperhomocysteinemia.[37] Vitamin supplementation can normalize homocysteine levels, but whether this can reduce the risk of cardiovascular events remains to be determined. A graded response has been demonstrated between plasma homocysteine and the risk of coronary disease and strokes.[36] Elevated plasma homocysteine has been shown to confer an independent risk of vascular disease of an order of magnitude similar to that of smoking or hypercholesterolemia and has also been shown to increase risk for cigarette smokers and hypertensive persons.[38] Boushey and coworkers,[33] in a recent metaanalysis, estimated that an increase of 5 nmol/l of homocysteine raises the risk of coronary disease as much as does an increase in cholesterol of 20 mg/dl. The current folate food fortification program is reducing the level of plasma homocysteine throughout the population, and it will be interesting to determine whether this will affect the prevalence of coronary disease in the general population.

The novel risk factors under consideration must be characterized as emerging risk factors, because information about their relevance is still incomplete. There is no consensus about sensitive and specific diagnostic tests for many of these risk factors, so it is difficult to make recommendations for screening to detect persons at high risk. For some risk factors there is lack of consistent prospective epidemiologic evidence indicating that the novel marker can be detected in healthy persons prior to the onset of an initial cardiovascular event. Fibrinogen, Lp(a), C-reactive protein, and homocysteine sometimes increase after a myocardial infarction, an effect that makes interpretation of retrospective data speculative. To date, consistent prospective data are available for fibrinogen, C-reactive protein, t-PA, and PAI-1. Findings of prospective studies for Lp(a) and homocysteine have been both positive and negative. It is also not clear whether these novel risk factors enhance our ability to predict events over and above what is achievable using established cardiovascular risk factors. Only the inflammatory parameters, such as fibrinogen and C-reactive protein, have been shown to improve multivariate prediction. Whether some novel risk factors are modifiable and whether such modifications reduce the risk of cardiovascular events is not known for certain. Interest and enthusiasm for screening for these emerging risk factors must be tempered by common sense and should not supersede the need to deal more effectively with the established risk factors where there are widely available methods of measurement, a prevalence of high risk, a consistent prospective connection with the rate of development of cardiovascular disease, and demonstrated benefits of correction, in terms of reduced morbidity and mortality. Assessment of these risk factors should at present be reserved for persons who, despite a benign risk profile, have a premature myocardial infarction, those who have high LDL cholesterol values, and those who, for other reasons, are at very high risk. Our failure to deal optimally with the standard risk factors and to implement proven preventive measures testifies to the need to improve our performance while keeping informed about new developments.

## ■ MULTIVARIATE RISK STRATIFICATION

Atherosclerotic cardiovascular events can be efficiently predicted from risk factors that are readily evaluated through routine office procedures and laboratory tests.[3-6] Optimal risk predictions require quantitative synthesis of the various contributing risk factors into a composite estimate. For this purpose, multivariate risk formulations are employed to quantify the combined effect of these interrelated risk factors. This concept takes into account the multifarious nature of cardiovascular risk and the continuous gradient of response. This allows us to identify persons at high overall risk for some coronary event, because of multiple mild to moderate abnormalities in individual risk factors. Categorical assessment of risk by arbitrarily assigning values to designate the point at which any "continuous risk variable" is to be considered a "risk factor" has some practical utility, as the cardiovascular risk increased with the number of categorically defined risk factors. This approach is inefficient, however, because it overlooks the high-risk segment of the population who have multiple marginal abnormalities. Multivariate risk assessment is also essential, because the major risk factors tend to cluster together at four to five times the rate expected by chance, so that the physician whose patient has any particular risk factor is obliged to seek out the others. Multivariate risk formulations, incorporating the major risk factors for coronary disease, can quantify the multivariate risk based on the actual risk factor values over a wide range. For office use, scoring systems based on Framingham Study multivariate risk formulations have been devised that provide an estimate of global risk for any combination of risk factors. The standard risk factors to be determined are total and HDL cholesterol, systolic blood pressure, cigarette smoking, diabetic status, and age. From the estimated rate of disease, for the risk factor makeup of the patient, and in comparison to the average rate for persons of the same age, the urgency for instituting treatment can be estimated without needlessly alarming patients who have only one risk factor in isolation or falsely reassuring those at high risk because of multiple marginal abnormalities.

These risk formulations have been shown to accurately predict disease in a variety of population samples.[39–41] Other risk factor information important in implementing therapy includes triglycerides, weight, physical activity, and family history, but having such data does not enhance estimation of risk.

## Coronary Risk Profile

Because coronary disease is the most common and also the most lethal of the atherosclerotic sequelae of the standard risk factors, prevention deserves the highest priority (Fig. 1–1). Multivariate coronary risk assessment formulations have been based on continuous variable risk factor relationships to this outcome, and, more recently, integrating categorical approaches that have become part of the framework of blood pressure (Sixth Report of the Joint National Committee on Prevention, Detection, Evaluation and Treatment of High Blood Pressure [JNC-VI]) and cholesterol (National Cholesterol Education Program [NCEP]) prevention programs in the United States.[42] This enables physicians to pull together all the relevant risk factor

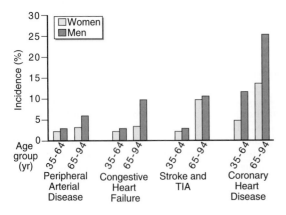

**Figure 1–1** ▪ Incidence of cardiovascular events by age and sex: Framingham Heart Study 36-year follow-up. TIA, transient ischemic attack.

information to derive a composite estimate of the risk of a coronary event and to compare this to the average or optimal risk for persons of the same age and sex (Tables 1–7, 1–8). The risk of coronary disease associated with any particular factor varies much, depending on the burden of other risk factors (Fig. 1–2).

## Stroke Risk Profile

Propensity to stroke, the most feared of the atherosclerotic diseases of the elderly, can also be risk stratified using the standard risk factors plus knowledge of the presence of coronary disease, heart failure, or atrial fibrillation (Table 1–9).[4] The chief risk factor for a stroke is hypertension, but the risk of elevated blood pressure can increase tenfold depending on whether other risk factors that commonly accompany hypertension are operating (Fig. 1–3). Using the stroke risk profile table, it is possible to estimate the combined effect of any of the major predisposing factors in terms of absolute and of relative risk.

## Heart Failure Profile

Heart failure is a lethal terminal stage of cardiac disease whose survival experience resembles that of cancer.[43] Substantial reduction in heart failure incidence and mortality can be achieved only by early identification of persons prone to left ventricular dysfunction so that it can be corrected before overt failure ensues. Candidates at high risk for heart failure must be cost-effectively targeted for echocardiographic evaluation for such left ventricular dysfunction. The Framingham Study has identified and quantified major contributing risk factors for the development of heart failure.[44] Using these, multivariable risk profiles have been developed that efficiently provide risk estimates of heart failure in persons who have major predisposing conditions such as hypertension, coronary disease, and valvular heart disease.[6] The ingredients of the profile consist of ECG-left ventricular

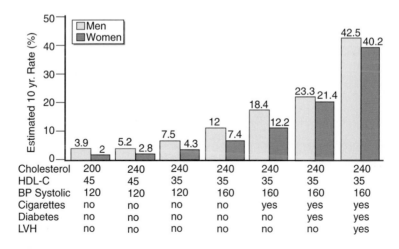

**Figure 1–2** ▪ Incidence of coronary heart disease: Framingham Heart Study 1972–1984, 42-year-old adults. (Kannel WB: Epidemiologic contributions to preventive cardiology and challenges for the 21st century. *In* Wong, Black, Gardin [eds]: Practical Strategies in Preventing Heart Disease. New York: McGraw Hill, 2000, pp 3–20).

Table 1–7

## Coronary Heart Disease Score Sheet for Men Using TC or LDC-C Categories*

**Step 1 — Age**

| Years | LDL Pts | Chol Pts |
|-------|---------|----------|
| 30-34 | −1 | (−1) |
| 35-39 | 0 | (0) |
| 40-44 | 1 | (1) |
| 45-49 | 2 | (2) |
| 50-54 | 3 | (3) |
| 55-59 | 4 | (4) |
| 60-64 | 5 | (5) |
| 65-69 | 6 | (6) |
| 70-74 | 7 | (7) |

**Step 2 — LDL-C**

| (mg/dl) | (mmol/L) | LDL Pts |
|---------|----------|---------|
| <100 | <2.59 | -3 |
| 100-129 | 2.60-3.36 | 0 |
| 130-159 | 3.37-4.14 | 0 |
| 160-190 | 4.15-4.92 | 1 |
| ≥190 | ≥4.92 | 2 |

Cholesterol

| (mg/dl) | (mmol/L) | Chol Pts |
|---------|----------|----------|
| <160 | <4.14 | (-3) |
| 160-199 | 4.15-5.17 | (0) |
| 200-239 | 5.18-6.21 | (1) |
| 240-279 | 6.22-7.24 | (2) |
| ≥280 | ≥7.25 | (3) |

**Step 3 — HDL-C**

| (mg/dl) | (mmol/L) | LDL Pts | Chol Pts |
|---------|----------|---------|----------|
| <35 | <0.90 | 2 | (2) |
| 35-44 | 0.91-1.16 | 1 | (1) |
| 45-49 | 1.17-1.29 | 0 | (0) |
| 50-59 | 1.30-1.55 | 0 | (0) |
| ≥60 | ≥1.56 | -1 | (-2) |

**Key**

Relative risk
- Very low
- Low
- Moderate
- High
- Very high

**Step 4 — Blood Pressure**

| Systolic (mm Hg) | Diastolic (mm Hg) <80 | 80-84 | 85-89 | 90-99 | ≥100 |
|------------------|------|------|------|-------|------|
| <120 | 0 (0) pts | | | | |
| 120-129 | | 0 (0) pts | | | |
| 130-139 | | | 1 (1) pts | | |
| 140-159 | | | | 2 (2) pts | |
| ≥160 | | | | | 3 (3) pts |

+ Note: When systolic and diastolic pressures provide different
estimates for point scores, use the higher number

**Step 5 — Diabetes**

| | LDL Pts | Chol Pts |
|---|---------|----------|
| No | 0 | (0) |
| Yes | 2 | (2) |

**Step 6 — Smoker**

| | LDL Pts | Chol Pts |
|---|---------|----------|
| No | 0 | (0) |
| Yes | 2 | (2) |

**Step 7 — Adding up the points**

| | |
|---|---|
| Age | — |
| LDL-C or Chol | — |
| HDL-C | — |
| Blood Pressure | — |
| Diabetes | — |
| Smoker | — |
| Point total | — |

(sum from steps 1-6)

**Step 8 — CHD Risk**

| LDL Pts Total | 10 Yr CHD Risk | Chol Pts Total | 10 Yr CHD Risk |
|---------------|----------------|----------------|----------------|
| <-3 | 1% | | |
| -2 | 2% | | |
| -1 | 2% | (<-1) | (2%) |
| 0 | 3% | (0) | (3%) |
| 1 | 4% | (1) | (3%) |
| 2 | 4% | (2) | (4%) |
| 3 | 6% | (3) | (5%) |
| 4 | 7% | (4) | (7%) |
| 5 | 9% | (5) | (8%) |
| 6 | 11% | (6) | (10%) |
| 7 | 14% | (7) | (13%) |
| 8 | 18% | (8) | (16%) |
| 9 | 22% | (9) | (20%) |
| 10 | 27% | (10) | (25%) |
| 11 | 33% | (11) | (31%) |
| 12 | 40% | (12) | (37%) |
| 13 | 47% | (13) | (45%) |
| ≥14 | ≥56% | (≥14) | (≥53%) |

(determine CHD risk from point total)

**Step 9 — Comparative Risk**

| Age (years) | Average 10 Yr CHD Risk | Average 10 Yr Hard* CHD Risk | Low** 10 Yr CHD Risk |
|-------------|------------------------|------------------------------|----------------------|
| 30-34 | 3% | 1% | 2% |
| 35-39 | 5% | 4% | 3% |
| 40-44 | 7% | 4% | 4% |
| 45-49 | 11% | 8% | 4% |
| 50-54 | 14% | 10% | 6% |
| 55-59 | 16% | 13% | 7% |
| 60-64 | 21% | 20% | 9% |
| 65-69 | 25% | 22% | 11% |
| 70-74 | 30% | 25% | 14% |

(compare to average person your age)

Risk estimates were derived from the experience of the Framingham Heart Study, a predominantly Caucasian population in Massachusetts, USA

* Hard CHD events exclude angina pectoris

** Low risk was calculated for a person the same age, optimal blood pressure, LDL-C 100-129 mg/dL or cholesterol 160-199 mg/dL, HDL-C 45 mg/dL for men or 55 mg/dL for women, non-smoker, no diabetes

*The scoring uses age, TC (or LDL-C), HDL-C, blood pressure, diabetes, and smoking and estimates risk for CHD over a period of 10 years based on Framingham experience in men 30 to 74 years old at baseline. Average risk estimates are based on typical Framingham subjects, and estimates of idealized risk are based on optimal blood pressure, TC 160 to 199 mg/dl (or LDL 100 to 129 mg/dl), HDL-C of 45 mg/dl in men, no diabetes, and no smoking. Use of the LDL-C categories is appropriate when fasting LDL-C measurements are available. Pts indicates points. (TCA, total cholesterol; LDL-C, low-density lipoprotein cholesterol; HDL-C, high-density lipoprotein cholesterol; CHD, coronary heart disease.)

Wilson PW, D'Agostino RB, Levy D, et al: Prediction of coronary heart disease. Circulation 1998; 97:1837.

Table 1–8

## Coronary Heart Disease Score Sheet for Women Using TC or LDL-C Categories*

| Step 1 | Age | | | Step 2 | LDL-C | | | Step 3 | HDL-C | | |
|---|---|---|---|---|---|---|---|---|---|---|---|
| Years | LDL Pts | Chol Pts | | (mg/dl) | (mmol/L) | LDL Pts | | (mg/dl) | (mmol/L) | LDL Pts | Chol Pts |
| 30-34 | −9 | (−9) | | <100 | <2.59 | -2 | | <35 | <0.90 | 5 | (5) |
| 35-39 | −4 | (−4) | | 100-129 | 2.60-3.36 | 0 | | 35-44 | 0.91-1.16 | 2 | (2) |
| 40-44 | 0 | (0) | | 130-159 | 3.37-4.14 | 0 | | 45-49 | 1.17-1.29 | 1 | (1) |
| 45-49 | 3 | (3) | | 160-190 | 4.15-4.92 | 2 | | 50-59 | 1.30-1.55 | 0 | (0) |
| 50-54 | 6 | (6) | | ≥190 | ≥4.92 | 2 | | ≥60 | ≥1.56 | -2 | (-3) |
| 55-59 | 7 | (7) | | | | | | | | | |
| 60-64 | 8 | (8) | | | Cholesterol | | | | | | |

| (mg/dl) | (mmol/L) | Chol Pts |
|---|---|---|
| <160 | <4.14 | (-2) |
| 160-199 | 4.15-5.17 | (0) |
| 200-239 | 5.18-6.21 | (1) |
| 240-279 | 6.22-7.24 | (1) |
| ≥280 | ≥7.25 | (3) |

65-69 | 8 | (8)
70-74 | 8 | (8)

**Key**

Relative risk

| | Very low | | High |
| | Low | | Very high |
| | Moderate | | |

| Step 4 | | Blood Pressure | | | | |
|---|---|---|---|---|---|---|
| Systolic (mm Hg) | <80 | Diastolic (mm Hg) | | 90-99 | ≥100 | |
| | | 80-84 | 85-89 | | | |
| <120 | -3 (-3) pts | | | | | |
| 120-129 | | 0 (0) pts | | | | |
| 130-139 | | | 0 (0) pts | | | |
| 140-159 | | | | 2 (2) pts | | |
| ≥ 160 | | | | | 3 (3) pts | |

+ Note: When systolic and diastolic pressures provide different estimates for point scores, use the higher number

**Step 5  Diabetes**

| | LDL Pts | Chol Pts |
|---|---|---|
| No | 0 | (0) |
| Yes | 4 | (4) |

**Step 6  Smoker**

| | LDL Pts | Chol Pts |
|---|---|---|
| No | 0 | (0) |
| Yes | 2 | (2) |

**Step 7  Adding up the points**

| | |
|---|---|
| Age | _____ |
| LDL-C or Chol | _____ |
| HDL-C | _____ |
| Blood Pressure | _____ |
| Diabetes | _____ |
| Smoker | _____ |
| Point total | _____ |

(sum from steps 1-6)

**Step 8  CHD Risk**

| LDL Pts Total | 10 Yr CHD Risk | Chol Pts Total | 10 Yr CHD Risk |
|---|---|---|---|
| ≤-2 | 1% | (≤-2) | (1%) |
| -1 | 2% | (-1) | (2%) |
| 0 | 2% | (0) | (2%) |
| 1 | 2% | (1) | (2%) |
| 2 | 3% | (2) | (3%) |
| 3 | 3% | (3) | (3%) |
| 4 | 4% | (4) | (4%) |
| 5 | 5% | (5) | (4%) |
| 6 | 6% | (6) | (5%) |
| 7 | 7% | (7) | (6%) |
| 8 | 8% | (8) | (7%) |
| 9 | 9% | (9) | (8%) |
| 10 | 11% | (10) | (10%) |
| 11 | 13% | (11) | (11%) |
| 12 | 15% | (12) | (13%) |
| 13 | 17% | (13) | (15%) |
| 14 | 20% | (14) | (18%) |
| 15 | 24% | (15) | (20%) |
| 16 | 27% | (16) | (24%) |
| ≥17 | ≥32% | (≥17) | (≥27%) |

(determine CHD risk from point total)

**Step 9  Comparative Risk**

| Age (years) | Average 10 Yr CHD Risk | Average 10 Yr Hard* CHD Risk | Low** 10 Yr CHD Risk |
|---|---|---|---|
| 30-34 | <1% | <1% | <1% |
| 35-39 | <1% | <1% | 1% |
| 40-44 | 2% | 1% | 2% |
| 45-49 | 5% | 2% | 3% |
| 50-54 | 8% | 3% | 5% |
| 55-59 | 12% | 7% | 7% |
| 60-64 | 12% | 8% | 8% |
| 65-69 | 13% | 8% | 8% |
| 70-74 | 14% | 11% | 8% |

(compare to average person your age)

Risk estimates were derived from the experience of the Framingham Heart Study, a predominantly Caucasian population in Massachusetts, USA

* Hard CHD events exclude angina pectoris

** Low risk was calculated for a person the same age, optimal blood pressure, LDL-C 100-129 mg/dL or cholesterol 160-199 mg/dL, HDL-C 45 mg/dL for men or 55 mg/dL for women, non-smoker, no diabetes

*Scoring uses age, TC, HDL-C, blood pressure, diabetes, and smoking and estimates risk for CHD over a period of 10 years based on Framingham experience in women 30 to 74 years old at baseline. Average risk estimates are based on typical Framingham subjects, and estimates of idealized risk are based on optimal blood pressure, TC 160 to 199 mg/dl (or LDL 100 to 129 mg/dl), HDL-C of 55 mg/dl in women, no diabetes, and no smoking. Use of the LDL-C categories is appropriate when fasting LDL-C measurements are available. Pts indicates points. (TCA, total cholesterol; LDL-C, low-density lipoprotein cholesterol; HDL-C, high-density lipoprotein cholesterol; CHD, coronary heart disease.)

Wilson PW, D'Agostino RB, Levy D, et al: Prediction of coronary heart disease. Circulation 1998; 97:1837.

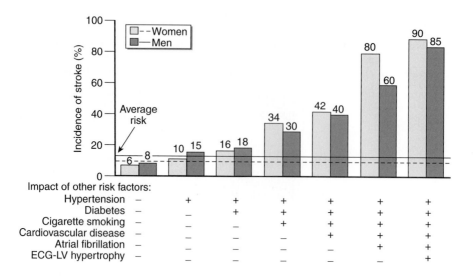

**Figure 1–3** ■ The Framingham Heart Study: 10-year probability of stroke, subjects aged 70 years, systemic blood presure 160 mm Hg. ECG-LV, Electrocardiographic left ventricular. (Wilson PW, D'Agostino RB, Levy D, et al: Prediction of coronary heart disease. Circulation 1998;97:1837.)

hypertrophy, cardiomegaly on chest film, reduced vital capacity, increased heart rate, presence of heart murmurs, systolic blood pressure, and diabetes (Tables 1–10, 1–11). Using this risk assessment, it should be possible to identify persons at high risk for heart failure who are in turn high-yield candidates for positive echocardiographic findings. Such persons stand to benefit from vigorous preventive measures such as therapy with angiotensin-converting enzyme (ACE) inhibitors, cardiac revascularization, or valve surgery.

## Profile for Peripheral Artery Disease

Using 38 years of follow-up data from the Framingham Study, investigators developed a profile to identify persons at high risk for intermittent claudication.[5] The variables are age, sex, serum cholesterol, blood pressure, cigarette smoking status, and diabetes and coronary disease status (Table 1–12). This risk profile allows physicians to educate such patients about modifying their cardiovascular risk factors. Identifying persons at risk of intermittent claudication is important, not only because the condition limits mobility and can lead to limb loss but also because it is associated with a twofold to fourfold increased mortality, predominantly from cardiovascular disease. Physicians can readily determine the probability of developing peripheral artery disease using a point score based on risk factor data on a routine examination (see Table 1–12).

## Risk Stratification of Existing Coronary Disease

Based on Framingham Study data, risk formulations have been developed for predicting another coronary event, a stroke, or a death from cerebrovascular disease in persons who have already experienced a coronary event.[45] The 2-year probability

# Table 1-9

## Stroke Risk Factor Prediction Chart: Framingham Heart Study

### 1. Find Points for Each Risk Factor

**Men**

| Age | SBP | HYP RX | Diabetes | Cigs | CVD | AF | LVH |
|---|---|---|---|---|---|---|---|
| 54–56 = 0 | 95–105 = 0 | No = 0 | No = 0 | No = 0 | No = 0 | No = 0 | No = 0 |
| 57–59 = 1 | 106–116 = 1 | Yes = 2 | Yes = 2 | Yes = 3 | Yes = 3 | Yes = 4 | Yes = 6 |
| 60–62 = 2 | 117–126 = 2 | | | | | | |
| 63–65 = 3 | 127–137 = 3 | | | | | | |
| 66–68 = 4 | 138–148 = 4 | | | | | | |
| 69–71 = 5 | 149–159 = 5 | | | | | | |
| 72–74 = 6 | 160–170 = 6 | | | | | | |
| 75–77 = 7 | 171–181 = 7 | | | | | | |
| 78–80 = 8 | 182–191 = 8 | | | | | | |
| 81–83 = 9 | 192–202 = 9 | | | | | | |
| 84–86 = 10 | 203–213 = 10 | | | | | | |

**Women**

| Age | SBP | HYP RX | Diabetes | Cigs | CVD | AF | LVH |
|---|---|---|---|---|---|---|---|
| 54–56 = 0 | 95–104 = 0 | No = 0 | No = 0 | No = 0 | No = 0 | No = 0 | No = 0 |
| 57–59 = 1 | 105–114 = 1 | If Yes see below | Yes = 3 | Yes = 3 | Yes = 2 | Yes = 6 | Yes = 4 |
| 60–62 = 2 | 115–124 = 2 | | | | | | |
| 63–65 = 3 | 125–134 = 3 | | | | | | |
| 66–68 = 4 | 135–144 = 4 | | | | | | |
| 69–71 = 5 | 145–154 = 5 | | | | | | |
| 72–74 = 6 | 155–164 = 6 | | | | | | |
| 75–77 = 7 | 165–174 = 7 | | | | | | |
| 78–80 = 8 | 175–184 = 8 | | | | | | |
| 81–83 = 9 | 185–194 = 9 | | | | | | |
| 84–86 = 10 | 196–204 = 10 | | | | | | |

If Currently Under Anti-Hypertensive Therapy Add The Following Points Depending On SBP Level

| SBP | 95–104 | 105–114 | 115–124 | 125–134 | 135–144 | 145–154 |
|---|---|---|---|---|---|---|
| Points | 6 | 5 | 5 | 4 | 3 | 3 |

| SBP | 155–164 | 165–174 | 175–184 | 185–194 | 195–204 |
|---|---|---|---|---|---|
| Points | 2 | 1 | 1 | 0 | 0 |

### 2. Sum Points for All Risk Factors

Age \_\_\_ + SBP \_\_\_ + HYP RX \_\_\_ + Diabetes \_\_\_ + Cigs \_\_\_ + CVD \_\_\_ + AF \_\_\_ + LVH \_\_\_ = \_\_\_ Point Total

### 3. Look Up Risk Corresponding to Point Total

**Men 10 Yr.**

| Pts. | Prob. | Pts. | Prob. | Pts. | Prob. |
|---|---|---|---|---|---|
| 1 | 2.6% | 11 | 11.2% | 21 | 41.7% |
| 2 | 3.0% | 12 | 12.9% | 22 | 46.6% |
| 3 | 3.5% | 13 | 14.8% | 23 | 51.8% |
| 4 | 4.0% | 14 | 17.0% | 24 | 57.3% |
| 5 | 4.7% | 15 | 19.5% | 25 | 62.8% |
| 6 | 5.4% | 16 | 22.4% | 26 | 68.4% |
| 7 | 6.3% | 17 | 25.5% | 27 | 73.8% |
| 8 | 7.3% | 18 | 29.0% | 28 | 79.0% |
| 9 | 8.4% | 19 | 32.9% | 29 | 83.7% |
| 10 | 9.7% | 20 | 37.1% | 30 | 87.9% |

**Women 10 Yr.**

| Pts. | Prob. | Pts. | Prob. | Pts. | Prob. |
|---|---|---|---|---|---|
| 1 | 1.1% | 11 | 7.6% | 21 | 43.4% |
| 2 | 1.3% | 12 | 9.2% | 22 | 50.0% |
| 3 | 1.6% | 13 | 11.1% | 23 | 57.0% |
| 4 | 2.0% | 14 | 13.3% | 24 | 64.2% |
| 5 | 2.4% | 15 | 16.0% | 25 | 71.4% |
| 6 | 2.9% | 16 | 19.1% | 26 | 78.2% |
| 7 | 3.5% | 17 | 22.8% | 27 | 84.4% |
| 8 | 4.3% | 18 | 27.0% | | |
| 9 | 5.2% | 19 | 31.9% | | |
| 10 | 6.3% | 20 | 37.3% | | |

### 4. Compare To Average 10-Year Risk

Avg. 10 Yr. Prob. By Age

| Men | | Women | |
|---|---|---|---|
| 55–59 | 5.9% | 55–59 | 3.0% |
| 60–64 | 7.8% | 60–64 | 4.7% |
| 65–69 | 11.0% | 65–69 | 7.2% |
| 70–74 | 13.7% | 70–74 | 10.9% |
| 75–79 | 18.0% | 75–79 | 15.5% |
| 80–84 | 22.3% | 80–84 | 23.9% |

Key For Symbols:
SBP, systolic blood pressure
HYP RX, under anti-hypertensive therapy?
Diabetes, history of diabetes?
Cigs, smokes cigarettes?
CVD, history of myocardial infarction, angina pectoris, coronary insufficiency, intermittent claudication, or congestive heart failure?
AF, History of atrial fibrillation?
LVH, Left ventricular hypertrophy on ECG?

Wolf PA, et al: Probability of stroke: A risk profile from the Framingham Study. Stroke 1991;3:312–318. Copyright American Heart Association.

Table 1–10

**Probability of CHF within 4 Years for Women Ages 45–94 with Either Coronary Disease, Hypertension, or Valvular Disease**

| Points | 0 | +1 | +2 | +3 | +4 | +5 | +6 | +7 | +8 | +9 |
|---|---|---|---|---|---|---|---|---|---|---|
| Age | 45–49 | 50–59 | 60–69 | 70–79 | 80–89 | 90–94 | | | | |
| Forced vital capacity | >299 | 250–299 | 200–249 | 150–199 | <150 | | | | | |
| Systolic BP | <130 | 130–189 | >189 | | | | | | | |
| Heart rate | <55 | 55–79 | 80–99 | >99 | | | | | | |
| LVH on ECG | No | | | | | Yes | | | | |
| Coronary disease | No | | | | | | | | Yes | |
| Cardiomegaly | No | | Yes | | | | | | | |
| If no valve disease | No | | | | | | | | | |
| Diabetes* | No | | | | | | Yes | | | |
| If has valve disease | | | | | | | | | | |
| Diabetes† | No | | Yes | | | | | | | |

| Points | 4-yr Prob | Points | 4-yr Prob | Points | 4-yr Prob | Points | 4-yr Prob |
|---|---|---|---|---|---|---|---|
| 5 | <1% | 18 | 4% | 26 | 18% | 31 | 37% |
| 10 | 1% | 20 | 6% | 27 | 21% | 32 | 42% |
| 12 | 1% | 22 | 9% | 28 | 24% | 33 | 46% |
| 14 | 2% | 24 | 13% | 29 | 28% | 34 | 51% |
| 16 | 3% | 25 | 15% | 30 | 32% | 35 | 56% |

*Points for diabetes when you do not have valve disease.
†Points for diabetes when you have valve disease.
Kannel WB, et al: Profile for estimating risk of heart failure. Arch Intern Med 1999;159:1197–1204. Copyright 1999, American Medical Association.

Table 1–11

**Probability of CHF within 4 Years: Women Ages 45–94 with Either Coronary Disease, Hypertension, or Valvular Disease\***

| Points | 0 | +1 | +2 | +3 | +4 | +5 | +6 | +7 | +8 | +9 |
|---|---|---|---|---|---|---|---|---|---|---|
| Age | 45–49 | 50–54 | 55–59 | 60–64 | 65–69 | 70–74 | 75–79 | 80–84 | 85–89 | 90–94 |
| BMI | >21 | 21–25 | 26–29 | >29 | | | | | | |
| Systolic BP | <140 | 140–209 | >209 | | | | | | | |
| Heart rate | <59 | 60–79 | 80–104 | >104 | | | | | | |
| LVH on ECG | No | | | | | Yes | | | | |
| Coronary disease | No | | | | | | Yes | | | |
| If no valve disease† | No | | | | | | | | | |
| Diabetes | No | | | | | | Yes | | | |
| If has valve disease‡ | | | | | | | | | | |
| Diabetes | No | | Yes | | | | | | | |

| Points | 4-yr Prob | Points | 4-yr Prob | Points | 4-yr Prob | Points | 4-yr Prob |
|---|---|---|---|---|---|---|---|
| 5 | <1% | 14 | 4% | 19 | 14% | 24 | 36% |
| 10 | 2% | 15 | 5% | 20 | 17% | 25 | 42% |
| 11 | 2% | 16 | 7% | 21 | 21% | 26 | 48% |
| 12 | 3% | 17 | 9% | 22 | 25% | 27 | 54% |
| 13 | 3% | 18 | 11% | 23 | 30% | 28 | 60% |

*Note: excludes forced vital capacity and cardiomegaly.
†Points for diabetes when you do not have valve disease.
‡Points for diabetes when you have valve disease.
Kannel WB, et al: Profile for estimating risk of heart failure. Arch Intern Med 1999;159:1197–1204. Copyright 1999, American Medical Association.

Table 1–12

**Four-Year Probability of Intermittent Claudication for Persons Aged 45–84 Years: Framingham Heart Study**

| Risk Factor | Risk Factor Points | | | | | | | | Line Score | Points | 4-Year Probability |
|---|---|---|---|---|---|---|---|---|---|---|---|
| | 0 | +1 | +2 | +3 | +4 | +5 | +6 | +7 | | <10 | <1% |
| Age, yr | 45–49 | 50–54 | 55–59 | 60–64 | 65–69 | 70–74 | 75–79 | 80–84 | | 10–12 | 1% |
| Sex | Female | | Male | | | | | | | 13–15 | 2% |
| Cholesterol, mg/dl | <170 | 170–209 | 210–249 | 250–289 | >289 | | | | | 16–17 | 3% |
| Blood pressure | Normal | High normal | Stage 1 | | Stage 2+ | | | | | 18 | 4% |
| Cigarettes/d, n | 0 | 1–5 | 6–10 | 11–20 | >20 | | | | | 19 | 5% |
| Diabetes | No | | | | | Yes | | | | 20 | 6% |
| CHD | No | | | | | Yes | | | | 21 | 7% |
| | | | | | | | Point total | | | 22 | 8% |

| 4-Year Rates of Intermittent Claudication by Age and Sex: Framingham Heart Study, 38-Year Follow-up | | | Points | 4-Year Probability |
|---|---|---|---|---|
| Age Group, yr | Men | Women | 23 | 10% |
| | | | 24 | 11% |
| 45–54 | 0.9% | 0.4% | 25 | 13% |
| 55–64 | 2.1% | 1.2% | 26 | 16% |
| 65–74 | 2.5% | 1.5% | 27 | 18% |
| 75–84 | 1.9% | 1.1% | 28 | 21% |
| | | | 29 | 24% |
| | | | 30 | 28% |

Murabito JM, et al: Intermittent claudication: A risk profile from the Framingham Study. Circulation 1997;96:44–49.

of these adverse outcomes, compared to average, in men and women can be estimated from the joint effects of age, diabetic status, total and HDL cholesterol, and systolic blood pressure (Tables 1–13, 1–14).

## ■ PREVENTIVE IMPLICATIONS

The risk profiles for the various atherosclerotic cardiovascular diseases strongly suggest that correcting any particular set of risk factors confers a bonus in preventing all the outcomes. Reliance on single risk factor detection and treatment may be justified on a population basis but is shortsighted on an individual basis. The goal of treating hypertension or dyslipidemia is not simply to correct these abnormalities but to prevent the cardiovascular sequelae that would surely develop. Persons being evaluated should be targeted for treatment from a multivariate risk profile, and the goal of treatment should be to improve the global risk. Because of the tendency of all of the major risk factors to cluster, physicians confronted with any particular risk factor should seek out the others and take these into account in evaluating the patient's risk and formulating treatment.

Controlled trials have provided consistent evidence of the benefit of reducing elevated blood pressure and correcting dyslipidemia.[46, 47] Lowering LDL and raising

Table 1–13

**Risk of Coronary Artery Disease Event, Stroke or Cerebrovascular Disease Death in Men with Existing Coronary Artery Disease**

| Age (yr) | Points | Total-C (mg/dl) | \- Points by HDL-C (mg dl) - | | | | | | | | | SBP (mm Hg) | Points |
|---|---|---|---|---|---|---|---|---|---|---|---|---|---|
| | | | 25 | 30 | 35 | 40 | 45 | 50 | 60 | 70 | 80 | | |
| 35 | 0 | 160 | 6 | 5 | 4 | 4 | 3 | 2 | 1 | 1 | 1 | 100 | 0 |
| 40 | 1 | 170 | 6 | 5 | 5 | 4 | 3 | 3 | 2 | 1 | 1 | 110 | 1 |
| 45 | 1 | 180 | 7 | 6 | 5 | 4 | 4 | 3 | 2 | 1 | 1 | 120 | 1 |
| 50 | 2 | 190 | 7 | 6 | 5 | 4 | 4 | 3 | 2 | 2 | 1 | 130 | 2 |
| 55 | 2 | 200 | 7 | 6 | 5 | 5 | 4 | 4 | 3 | 2 | 1 | 140 | 2 |
| 60 | 3 | 210 | 7 | 6 | 6 | 5 | 4 | 4 | 3 | 2 | 1 | 150 | 3 |
| 65 | 3 | 220 | 8 | 7 | 6 | 5 | 5 | 4 | 3 | 2 | 2 | 160 | 3 |
| 70 | 4 | 230 | 8 | 7 | 6 | 5 | 5 | 4 | 3 | 3 | 2 | 170 | 4 |
| 75 | 4 | 240 | 8 | 7 | 6 | 6 | 5 | 4 | 4 | 3 | 2 | 180 | 4 |
| | | 250 | 8 | 7 | 6 | 6 | 5 | 5 | 4 | 3 | 2 | 190 | 4 |
| | | 260 | 8 | 7 | 7 | 6 | 5 | 5 | 4 | 3 | 2 | 200 | 5 |
| | | 270 | 9 | 8 | 7 | 6 | 6 | 5 | 4 | 3 | 3 | 210 | 5 |
| Other | Pts | 280 | 9 | 8 | 7 | 6 | 6 | 5 | 4 | 4 | 3 | 220 | 5 |
| Diabetes | 1 | 290 | 9 | 8 | 7 | 7 | 6 | 5 | 4 | 4 | 3 | 230 | 6 |
| | | 300 | 9 | 8 | 7 | 7 | 6 | 6 | 5 | 4 | 3 | 240 | 6 |
| | | | | | | | | | | | | 250 | 6 |

| Total Points | 2-yr Probability (%) | Average 2-yr Risk in Men with CVD | |
|---|---|---|---|
| | | Age (yr) | Probability (%) |
| 0 | 2 | 35–39 | 1 |
| 2 | 2 | 40–44 | 8 |
| 4 | 3 | 45–49 | 10 |
| 6 | 5 | 50–54 | 11 |
| 8 | 7 | 55–59 | 12 |
| 10 | 10 | 60–64 | 12 |
| 12 | 14 | 65–69 | 14 |
| 14 | 20 | 70–74 | 14 |
| 16 | 28 | | |
| 18 | 37 | | |
| 20 | 49 | | |
| 22 | 63 | | |
| 24 | 77 | | |

CVD, cerebrovascular disease.
From Califf RM, Armstrong PW, Carver JR, et al: Stratification of patients into high, medium and low risk subgroups for purposes of risk factor management. Reprinted with permission from the American College of Cardiology (Journal of the American College of Cardiology, 1996, Vol. 27, pp 964–1047).

HDL cholesterol have been shown to slow progression of atherosclerosis.[46–48] Primary prevention trials have shown consistent benefit in reducing LDL and raising HDL cholesterol, even in persons with only average lipid values.[49, 50] Metaanalysis of hypertension trials indicates treatment benefits for overall vascular mortality, stroke morbidity and mortality, and fatal and nonfatal coronary events.[51] It appears necessary to sustain therapy for many years to achieve the expected 25% reduction in coronary events predicted by epidemiologic data.[52] Recent trials demonstrate the benefits on risk of stroke, coronary disease, and heart failure of treating isolated systolic hypertension in elderly persons.[53, 54] Current recommendations for diabetes focus on correcting the metabolically linked dyslipidemia and hypertension that usually accompany it. Weight control is an important preventive measure against atherosclerotic cardiovascular disease, but there is as yet no direct evidence that weight reduction reduces the risk of clinical cardiovascular events. There is, how-

Table 1–14

**Risk of Coronary Artery Disease Event, Stroke or Cerebrovascular Disease Death in Women with Existing Coronary Artery Disease**

| Age (yr) | Points | Total-C (mg/dl) | Points by HDL-C (mg dl) | | | | | | | | | SBP (mm Hg) | Points |
|---|---|---|---|---|---|---|---|---|---|---|---|---|---|
| | | | 25 | 30 | 35 | 40 | 45 | 50 | 60 | 70 | 80 | | |
| 35 | 0 | 160 | 4 | 3 | 3 | 2 | 2 | 1 | 1 | 0 | 0 | 100 | 0 |
| 40 | 1 | 170 | 4 | 3 | 3 | 2 | 2 | 2 | 1 | 1 | 0 | 110 | 0 |
| 45 | 2 | 180 | 4 | 3 | 3 | 2 | 2 | 2 | 1 | 1 | 0 | 120 | 1 |
| 50 | 3 | 190 | 4 | 4 | 3 | 3 | 2 | 2 | 1 | 1 | 1 | 130 | 1 |
| 55 | 4 | 200 | 4 | 4 | 3 | 3 | 2 | 2 | 2 | 1 | 1 | 140 | 2 |
| 60 | 5 | 210 | 4 | 4 | 3 | 3 | 3 | 2 | 2 | 1 | 1 | 150 | 2 |
| 65 | 6 | 220 | 5 | 4 | 4 | 3 | 3 | 2 | 2 | 1 | 1 | 160 | 2 |
| 70 | 7 | 230 | 5 | 4 | 4 | 3 | 3 | 3 | 2 | 2 | 1 | 170 | 3 |
| 75 | 7 | 240 | 5 | 4 | 4 | 3 | 3 | 3 | 2 | 2 | 1 | 180 | 3 |
| | | 250 | 5 | 4 | 4 | 4 | 3 | 3 | 2 | 2 | 1 | 190 | 3 |
| | | 260 | 5 | 5 | 4 | 4 | 3 | 3 | 2 | 2 | 1 | 200 | 3 |
| | | 270 | 5 | 5 | 4 | 4 | 3 | 3 | 2 | 2 | 2 | 210 | 4 |
| Other | Pts | 280 | 5 | 5 | 4 | 4 | 3 | 3 | 3 | 2 | 2 | 220 | 4 |
| Diabetes | 3 | 290 | 5 | 5 | 4 | 4 | 4 | 3 | 3 | 2 | 2 | 230 | 4 |
| Smoking | 3 | 300 | 6 | 5 | 4 | 4 | 4 | 3 | 3 | 2 | 2 | 240 | 4 |
| | | | | | | | | | | | | 250 | 4 |

| Total Points | 2-yr Probability (%) | Average 2-yr Risk in Women with CVD | |
|---|---|---|---|
| | | Age (yr) | Probability (%) |
| 0 | 0 | 35–39 | <1 |
| 2 | 1 | 40–44 | <1 |
| 4 | 1 | 45–49 | <1 |
| 6 | 1 | 50–54 | 4 |
| 8 | 2 | 55–59 | 6 |
| 10 | 4 | 60–64 | 8 |
| 12 | 6 | 65–69 | 12 |
| 14 | 10 | 70–74 | 12 |
| 16 | 15 | | |
| 18 | 23 | | |
| 20 | 35 | | |
| 22 | 51 | | |
| 24 | 68 | | |
| 26 | 85 | | |

From Califf RM, Armstrong PW, Carver JR, et al: Stratification of patients into high, medium and low risk subgroups for purposes of risk factor management. Reprinted with permission from the American College of Cardiology (Journal of the American College of Cardiology, 1996, Vol. 27, pp 964–1047).

ever, convincing evidence that slimming improves a person's entire cardiovascular risk profile. Persons who maintain optimal weight have 35% to 60% lower risk of developing cardiovascular disease than those who become obese.[47, 55]

A metaanalysis of the benefits of physical activity for coronary disease estimates a 50% reduction in risk attributable to exercise.[56] Even moderate exercise appears to improve both the predisposing risk factors and the risk of developing coronary disease.[57] Although controlled trial data are lacking, observational data indicate that, after cessation of smoking, coronary disease risk declines rapidly to half that of persons who continue to smoke, without regard for the amount smoked or the duration of smoking.[58] Quitting smoking deserves high priority in cardiovascular disease prevention, because it ranks as a leading preventable cause of the disease.

It is claimed that antioxidant vitamins E and C and carotene may reduce cardiovascular risk, although randomized trials of antioxidant vitamin supplements have produced contradictory results.[59] Metaanalysis of randomized trials conducted in persons with clinical vascular disease has shown that low-dose aspirin can reduce the incidence of subsequent myocardial infarction, stroke, or cardiovascular mortality by about 25%. In primary prevention trials, initial myocardial infarctions were reduced by 33%. As a result, aspirin has been recommended for primary prevention in men who are at high risk for coronary disease.[60]

Coronary heart disease and stroke *mortality* have declined over the past several decades, but the incidence of new events has not. The result is a growing pool of persons who have coronary disease, strokes, and heart failure. Implementation of comprehensive preventive programs using global risk stratification is a specific challenge for the future. The occurrence of an overt cardiovascular event should come to be regarded as a medical failure rather than the first indication for treatment.

# ■ REFERENCES

1. Manson JE, Tosteson H, Ridker PM, et al: The primary prevention of myocardial infarction. N Engl J Med 1992;326:1406–1416.
2. Kannel WB: Contribution of the Framingham Study to preventive cardiology. J Am Coll Cardiol 1990;15:206–211.
3. Anderson KM, Wilson PWF, Odell PM, et al: An updated coronary risk profile: A statement for health professionals. Circulation 1991;83:357–363.
4. Wolf PA, D'Agostino RB, Belanger AJ, et al: Probability of stroke: A risk profile from the Framingham Study. Stroke 1991;3:312–318.
5. Murabito JM, D'Agostino RB, Silbershatz H, Wilson PWF: Intermittent claudication: A risk profile from the Framingham Study. Circulation 1997;96:44–49.
6. Kannel WB, D'Agostino RB, Silbershatz H, et al: Profile for estimating risk of heart failure. Arch Intern Med 1999;159:1197–1204.
7. Kannel WB, Sytkowski PA: Atherosclerosis risk factors. Pharmacol Ther 1987;32:207–235.
8. Kannel WB, McGee DL: Diabetes and glucose tolerance as risk factors for cardiovascular disease: The Framingham Study. Diabetes Care 1979;2:120–126.
9. Kannel WB, Wilson PWF: Risk factors that attenuate the female coronary disease advantage. Arch Intern Med 1995;155:57–91.
10. NIH Consensus Development Panel: Triglyceride, high-density lipoprotein and coronary heart disease. JAMA 1993;269:505–510.
11. Kannel WB: High-density lipoproteins: Epidemiologic profile and risks of coronary artery disease. Am J Cardiol 1983;52:9B–12B.
12. Wilson PWF, Kannel WB: Hypercholesterolemia and coronary risk in the elderly: The Framingham Study. Am J Geriat Cardiol 1993;2:52–56.
13. Corti MC, Guralnic JM, Salive ME, et al: HDL cholesterol predicts coronary heart disease mortality in older persons. JAMA 1995;274:539–544.
14. Kannel WB, Dawber TR, McGee DL, et al: Perspectives on systolic blood hypertension: The Framingham Study. Circulation 1980;61:1179–1182.
15. Reaven GM: Banting Lecture 1988: Role of insulin resistance in human disease. Diabetes 1988;37;1595–1607.
16. Castelli WP, Wilson PWF, Levy D, Anderson K: Cardiovascular risk factors in the elderly. Am J Cardiol 1989;63:12H–19H.
17. Kannel WB: Epidemiologic relationship of disease among the different vascular territories. *In* Fuster V, Ross R, Topol EJ (eds): Atherosclerosis and Coronary Artery Disease. Philadelphia: Lippincott-Raven, 1996:II:1591–1599.
18. Cupples LA, Gagnon DR, Wong ND, et al: Preexisting cardiovascular conditions and long-term prognosis after initial myocardial infarction. The Framingham Study. Am Heart J 1993;125:863–872.
19. Koenig W: Haemostatic risk factors for cardiovascular disease. Eur Heart J 1998;19(Suppl C):C39–C43.
20. Meade TW, Mellows S, Brozovic M, et al: Haemostatic function and ischaemic heart disease: Principal results of the Northwick Park Heart Study. Lancet 1986;ii:533–537.
21. Heinrich J, Balleisen L, Schulte H, et al: Fibrinogen and factor VII in the prediction of coronary risk. Results from the PROCAM Study in healthy men. Arterioscler Thromb 1994;14:54–59.
22. Folsom AR, Wu KK, Rosamond WD, et al: Prospective study of hemostatic factors and incidence of coronary heart disease. The ARIC Study. Circulation 1997;96:1102–1108.

23. Thaulow E, Erikssen J, Sandvik L, et al: Blood platelet count and function are related to total and cardiovascular death in apparently healthy men. Circulation 1991;84:613–617.
24. Trip MD, Cats VM, van Capelle FJL, Vreeken J: Platelet hyperreactivity and prognosis in survivors of myocardial infarction. N Engl J Med 1990;322:1549–1554.
25. Hamsten A, Walldus G, Szamosi A, et al: Plasminogen activator inhibitor in plasma: Risk factor for recurrent myocardial infarction. Lancet 1993;ii:3–9.
26. Ridker PM, Vaughan DE, Stampfer MJ, et al: Endogenous tissue-type plasminogen activator and risk of myocardial infarction. Lancet 1993;341:1165–1168.
27. Meade TW, Ruddock V, Stirling Y, et al: Fibrinolytic activity, clotting factors and long-term incidence of ischaemic heart disease in the Northwick Park Heart Study. Lancet 1993;342:1076–1079.
28. Juhan-Vague I, Pyke SDM, Alessi MC, et al: Fibrinolytic factors and the risk of myocardial infarction or sudden death in patients with angina pectoris. Circulation 1996;94:2057–2063.
29. Stein JH, Rosenson RS: Lipoprotein Lp(a) excess and coronary heart disease. Arch Intern Med 1997;157:1170–1176.
30. Nguyen TT, Ellefson RD, Hodge DO, et al: Predictive value of electrophoretically detected lipoprotein(a) for coronary heart disease and cerebrovascular disease in a community-based cohort of 9936 men and women. Circulation 1997;96:1390–1397.
31. Haverkate F, Thompson SG, Pyke SDM, et al: Production of C-reactive protein and risk of coronary events in stable and unstable angina. Lancet 1997;349:462–466.
32. Ridker PM, Cushman M, Stampfer MJ, et al: Inflammation, aspirin and the risk of cardiovascular disease. N Engl J Med 1997;336:973–979.
33. Boushey CJ, Beresford SAA, Omenn GS, Motulski AG: A quantitative assessment of plasma homocysteine as a risk factor for cardiovascular disease. JAMA 1995;274:1049–1057.
34. Ueland PM, Refsum H: Plasma homocysteine a risk factor for vascular disease: Plasma levels in health, disease and drug therapy. J Lab Clin Med 1989;114:473–501.
35. Mcully KS: Homocysteine and vascular disease. Nat Med 1996;2:386–389.
36. Welch GN, Loscalzo J: Homocysteine and atherothrombosis. N Engl J Med 1998;338:1042–1050.
37. Selhub J, Jacqes PF, Wilson PW, et al: Vitamin status and intake as primary determinants of homocysteinemia in an elderly population. JAMA 1993;270:2693–2698.
38. Graham IM, Daly LE, Refsum HM, et al: Plasma homocysteine as a risk factor for vascular disease: The European Concerted Action Project. JAMA 1997;277:1775–1781.
39. Leaverton PE, Sorlie PD, Kleinman JC, et al: Representativeness of the Framingham risk model for coronary heart disease mortality: A comparison with a national cohort study. J Chronic Dis 1987;40:775–784.
40. Brand RJ, Rosenmann RH, Sholtz RI, et al: Multivariate prediction of coronary heart disease in the Western Collaborative Group Study compared to the findings of the Framingham Study. Circulation 1976;53:348–355.
41. Schulte H, Assmann G: CHD risk equations obtained from the Framingham Heart Study applied to PROCAM Study. Cardiovasc Risk Factors 1991;1:126–133.
42. Wilson PWF, D'Agostino RB, Levy D, et al: Prediction of coronary heart disease using risk factor categories. Circulation 1998;97:1837–1847.
43. Ho KL, Anderson KM, Grossman W, Levy D: Survival after onset of congestive heart failure in the Framingham Study. Circulation 1993;88:107–115.
44. Kannel WB, Belanger AJ: Epidemiology of heart failure. Am Heart J 1994;121:951–957.
45. Califf RM, Armstrong PW, Carver JR, et al: Stratification of patients into high, medium and low risk subgroups for purposes of risk factor management. J Am Coll Cardiol 1996;27(5):1007–1019.
46. Manson JE, Tosteson H, Ridker PM, et al: The primary prevention of myocardial infarction. N Engl J Med 1992;326:1406–1416.
47. Rich-Edwards JW, Manson JE, Hennekens CH, et al: The primary prevention of coronary heart disease in women. N Engl J Med 1995;332:1758–1766.
48. Kane JP, Malloy MJ, Ports TA, et al: Regression of coronary atherosclerosis during treatment of familial hypercholesterolemia with combined drug regimens. JAMA 1990;264:3007–3012.
49. Sacks FM, Pfeffer MA, Moye LA, et al: The effect of pravastatin on coronary events after myocardial infarction in patients with average cholesterol levels. N Engl J Med 1996;335:1001–1009.
50. Downs JR, Clearfield M, Weis S, et al: For the AFCAPS/TexCAPS Research Group. Primary prevention of acute coronary events with lovastatin in men and women with average cholesterol levels: Results of AFCAPS/TexCAPS. JAMA 1998;279:1615–1622.
51. Collins R, Peto R, MacMahon S, et al: Blood pressure, stroke and coronary heart disease: II. Short-term reductions in blood pressure: Overview of randomized drug trials in their epidemiologic context. Lancet 1990;335:827–838.
52. McMahon S, Peto R, Cutler J, et al: Blood pressure, stroke and coronary heart disease: I Prolonged differences in blood pressure: Prospective observational studies corrected for regression dilution bias. Lancet 1990;335:765–774.
53. Systolic Hypertension in the Elderly Program Cooperative Research Group: Prevention of stroke by antihypertensive drug treatment in older persons with isolated systolic hypertension: Final results of the Systolic Hypertension in the Elderly Program (SHE). JAMA 1991;265:3255–3264.
54. Stassen JA, Fagard R, Thijs L, et al: Randomized double-blind comparison of placebo and active

treatment for older patients with isolated systolic hypertension. The Systolic Hypertension in Europe (Syst-Eur) Trial investigators. Lancet 1997;350:757–764.

55. Hubert HB, Feinleib M, McNamara PM, et al: Obesity as an independent risk factor for cardiovascular disease: A 26 year follow-up of participants in the Framingham Study. Circulation 1983;67:968–977.

56. Berlin JA, Colditz JA: A meta-analysis of physical activity in the prevention of coronary heart disease. Am J Epidemiol 1990;132:612–628.

57. Blair SN, Kohl HW III, Paffenbarger RS Jr, et al: Physical fitness and all-cause mortality: A prospective study of healthy men and women. JAMA 1989;262:2395–2401.

58. Rosenberg L, Pakmer JR, Shapiro S: Decline in the risk of myocardial infarction among women who stop smoking. N Engl J Med 1990;322:213–217.

59. Hennekens CH, Buring JE, Peto R: Antioxidant vitamins: Benefits not yet proved (Editorial). N Engl J Med 1994;330:1080–1081.

60. Fuster V, Dyken ML, Vokonas PS, et al: Aspirin as a therapeutic agent in cardiovascular disease. Circulation 1993;87:659–675.

# ■ RECOMMENDED READING

Califf RM, Armstrong PW, Carver JR, et al: Stratification of patients into high, medium and low risk subgroups for purposes of risk factor management. J Am Coll Cardiol 1996;27(5):1007–1019.

Kannel WB: Contribution of the Framingham Study to preventive cardiology. J Am Coll Cardiol 1990;15:206–211.

Kannel WB, Sytkowski PA: Atherosclerosis risk factors. Pharmacol Ther 1987;32:207–235.

Koenig W: Haemostatic risk factors for cardiovascular disease. Eur Heart J 1998;19(Suppl C):C39–C43.

Murabito JM, D'Agostino RB, Silbershatz H, Wilson PWF: Intermittent claudication: A risk profile from the Framingham Study. Circulation 1997;96:44–49.

Wilson PWF, D'Agostino RB, Levy D, et al: Prediction of coronary heart disease using risk factor categories. Circulation 1998;97:1837–1847.

*Chapter* **2**

# Cardiac Contraction and Relaxation: Molecular and Cellular Physiology

*Andrew R. Marks* ■ *Steven O. Marx*

## ■ MOLECULAR BIOLOGY OF EXCITATION-CONTRACTION COUPLING

Proper function of the circulatory system requires the highly controlled regulation of calcium concentration inside cardiomyocytes. Calcium is the second messenger that signals muscle contraction via a process referred to as *excitation-contraction (EC) coupling.* The "calcium cycle" is integral to the regulation of cardiac contractility, which in turn determines circulatory function. The calcium cycle involves the controlled release of intracellular calcium, which raises the concentration of calcium within cardiac muscle cells and triggers contraction, followed by reuptake of calcium into the sarcoplasmic reticulum (SR). Perturbations of either the release (systolic) phase of the cycle or the reuptake (diastolic) phase can contribute to heart failure and sudden cardiac death (SCD).

The initial signal for contraction is an electrical one, the depolarization of the muscle cell membrane, triggered by the cardiac action potential. The translation of this electrical signal to a mechanical one is the basis for the term *EC coupling.*[1] The electrical signal travels into the heart muscle via specialized membranes known as the *transverse (T) tubule* system (Fig. 2–1). These membranes contain the voltage-dependent calcium channel or dihydropyridine receptor (DHPR); (Fig. 2–2). The DHPR/calcium channel is the molecular target for the widely used calcium channel blockers. The DHPR contains positively charged amino acids in specialized transmembrane segments (S4 regions) that serve as voltage sensors and are involved in activating the channel in response to depolarization of the muscle membrane (Fig. 2–3). Once the DHPR is activated, a small amount of calcium enters the heart muscle cell; however, the amount of calcium entering via the DHPR is insufficient to raise the concentration of calcium inside the heart muscle cell enough to trigger contraction. This small calcium influx is, however, sufficient to activate much larger intracellular calcium release channels on the SR membrane within the cardiac muscle cells (Fig. 2–4). These intracellular calcium release channels are known as *ryanodine receptors* (RyR; Fig. 2–5). They are the largest ion channels described to

*Text continued on page 28*

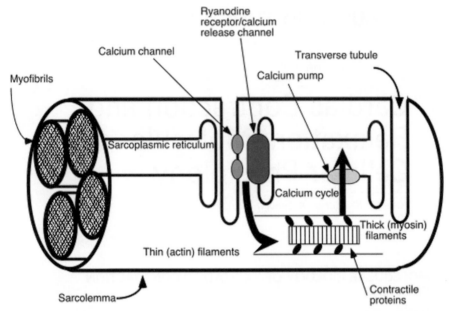

**Figure 2–1** ■ Model of cardiac excitation-contraction coupling. The model depicts the molecular basis of the "calcium cycle" that regulates cardiac contractility. The fundamental unit of contraction is the sarcomere. These units make up the functional components of each myofibril and the myofibrils are in turn bundled together to form a muscle fiber. The components of the sarcomere include the sarcoplasmic reticulum, which surrounds the contractile proteins and contains the large intracellular store of calcium, which serves as the trigger for muscle contraction. With each heartbeat, the action potential depolarizes the cardiac muscle cell membrane (sarcolemma). This electrical signal travels into the myofibril via a specialized invagination of the sarcolemma known as the transverse (T) tubule. The T tubule membrane contains voltage-dependent (gated) calcium channels (VDCC) or dihydropyridine receptors (DHPR). When these calcium channels are activated, they allow a small amount of extracellular calcium to enter the heart muscle cell and activate the much larger intracellular calcium release channels (ryanodine receptors). The calcium release channels open and release a large amount of calcium very rapidly into the cytoplasm of the heart muscle cell. This calcium binds to and activates the contractile proteins. The released calcium is then pumped back into the sarcoplasmic reticulum via the calcium (ATPase) pump.

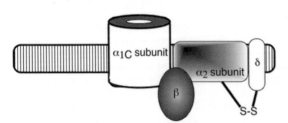

**Figure 2–2** ■ The subunit structure of the cardiac calcium channel. The cardiac calcium channel (VDCC, or DHPRC) in the sarcolemma or plasma membrane is comprised of four subunits. The $\alpha_{1C}$ subunit forms the actual calcium channel pore through which calcium enters the heart muscle cell to trigger muscle contraction.

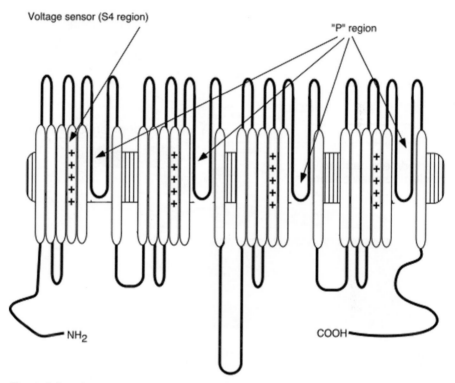

**Figure 2-3** ■ The molecular structure of the cardiac calcium channel. The $\alpha_{1C}$ subunit of the cardiac calcium channel comprises 24 transmembrane segments and four P regions that form the calcium channel pore through the sarcolemma. The fourth transmembrane segment (S4) in each grouping of six contains positively charged amino acid residues that serve as voltage sensors that allow the calcium channel to be activated by the action potential depolarization.

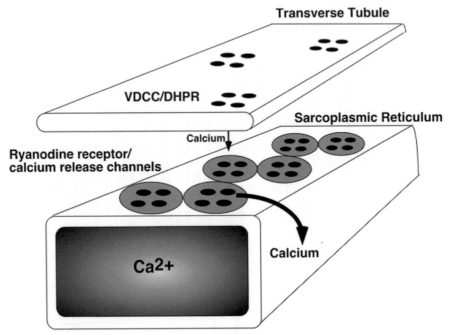

**Figure 2–4** ▪ Membranes involved in cardiac excitation-contraction coupling. The top membrane, the transverse tubule, contains the voltage-dependent calcium channel (VDCC) or dihydropyridine receptor (DHPR). A small amount of calcium flowing in via the VDCC activates the ryanodine receptor/calcium release channels to release intracellular stores of calcium from the sarcoplasmic reticulum. The released calcium activates contractile proteins in the heart.

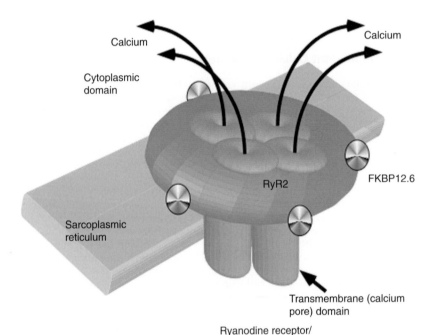

**Figure 2–5** ■ The molecular structure of the calcium release channel/ryanodine receptor. The ryanodine receptor is the largest ion channel identified to date and is comprised of four ~600-kd subunits, resulting in a single channel with a molecular mass of ~2,400 kd (more than 10 times the size of the next largest ion channel). The channel has two domains, the transmembrane calcium pore–containing domain that provides the pathway for calcium release through the sarcoplasmic reticulum membrane and the much larger cytoplasmic domain that is required for regulation of channel activity.

date and conduct approximately 10 times as much calcium via their pores as the much smaller DHPR calcium channels on the T tubule.

The calcium released via the RyR binds in turn to calcium-binding proteins inside the heart muscle cell, including troponin C. When calcium binds troponin C it undergoes a conformational change that permits actin and myosin to form crossbridges and cause contraction of the heart muscle cells (Fig. 2–6). During the relaxation phase, when the heart cell membrane is repolarized, calcium pumps (adenosine triphosphatases, ATPases) in the SR membrane pump the calcium back into the SR (Fig. 2–7). When the calcium concentration in the cytosol of the muscle cell falls, calcium no longer binds to troponin C (which then returns to a conformation that prohibits actin-myosin crossbridging) and relaxation occurs (see Fig. 2–6).

## Voltage-Dependent Calcium Channels

The voltage-dependent calcium channels (VDCC) or DHPR in the heart are composed of four subunits, $\alpha_1$, $\alpha_2$, $\beta$, and $\delta$. These subunits are encoded by three separate genes, one for the $\alpha_1$ subunit, which contains the pore that forms the calcium channel, one for the $\beta$ subunit, and one for the $\alpha_2$ and $\delta$ subunits, both of which are encoded by a single gene and are subsequently processed as two separate polypeptides linked by disulfide bridges (see Fig. 2–2). The binding sites for the clinically useful calcium channel blockers are encoded by the $\alpha_1$ subunit. The $\alpha_1$ subunit is expressed in a tissue-specific manner so that distinct genes encode different isoforms of the $\alpha_1$ subunit in each type of tissue (e.g., cardiac, skeletal, and smooth muscle). Thus, in each of these tissues, the calcium channels are slightly different in structure, although they all share highly conserved structural motifs present in voltage-gated ion channels (including sodium and potassium channels).

As noted above, the $\alpha_1$ subunit of the VDCC contains the calcium pore and the voltage sensors of the channel. The VDCC is activated by membrane depolarization that occurs during the action potential. Activation of the VDCC allows a small amount of calcium to enter the cell due to the large chemical gradient for calcium across the plasma membrane. The calcium concentration in the extracellular space is millimolar compared to nanomolar calcium inside the heart muscle cell. This huge gradient in the calcium concentration drives calcium into the cell when the VDCC is activated.

It has been proposed that the small amount of calcium that enters the cardiac muscle cell via the activated VDCC in turn triggers the activation of the much larger intracellular calcium release channel known as the RyR (Fig. 2–8). This process has been termed *calcium-induced calcium release*.[2, 3] It is well-documented that, in contrast to skeletal muscle, cardiac muscle requires calcium influx from the extracellular space for EC coupling, although the entering calcium clearly is not sufficient by itself to trigger muscle contraction. Therefore, the bulk of the calcium signal required for muscle contraction in the heart (and in skeletal muscle) is generated by the release of intracellular calcium stores from the SR (see Fig. 2–1). This fact has important implications for disease states such as heart failure and sudden cardiac death, because defects in the regulation of intracellular calcium release are believed to play a role in the associated altered calcium homeostasis.

Activation of the VDCC creates an inward calcium current that contributes to the depolarization of the cardiac muscle cells during the action potential. Thus, the VDCC is both activated by and contributes to the cardiac action potential. The VDCC are also referred to as *L-type calcium channels*. This terminology is based on physiologic measurements of calcium currents that were performed before a calcium channel structure was identified after its cDNA was cloned in 1987. The *L*

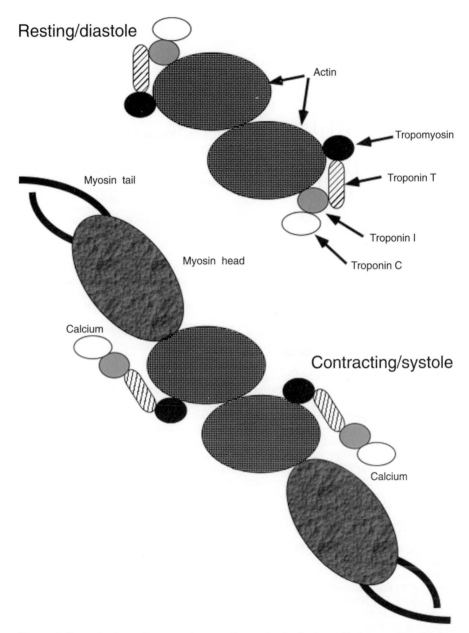

Resting/diastole

Actin

Tropomyosin

Myosin tail

Troponin T

Myosin head

Troponin I

Troponin C

Calcium

Contracting/systole

Calcium

**Figure 2–6** ■ Molecular architecture of contractile proteins in the heart. During rest (diastole) the tropomyosin-actin complex assumes a conformation that blocks actin-myosin crossbridge formation. When calcium binds to troponin C, a conformational change occurs that permits actin-myosin crossbridge formation and contraction (systole).

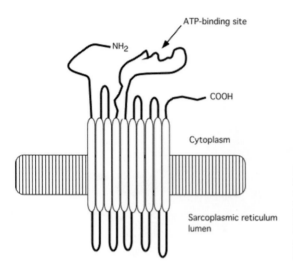

**Figure 2–7** ▪ Molecular structure of the calcium (ATPase) pump. The calcium (ATPase) pump in the sarcoplasmic reticulum pumps calcium back into the sarcoplasmic reticulum during diastole, when the heart relaxes. The pump comprises 10 transmembrane regions. An ATP-binding site is located in the cytoplasmic domain.

(for long-lasting) denotes the fact that the DHPR/VDCC current is activated rapidly but inactivated slowly. Other types of calcium currents, some of which are present in the heart, have been termed the T, N, P, Q, and R currents of channels; however, the DHPR/VDCC/L–type channel accounts for the major calcium influx current in cardiac muscle cells.

## Intracellular Calcium Release Channels

Most calcium-dependent signaling systems have evolved to depend principally on the release of intracellular calcium rather than on calcium influx to provide the second messenger calcium signal. EC coupling is an example of such a calcium-dependent signaling system. This type of calcium-dependent signaling is similar to signals in many other types of cells that couple external stimuli to intracellular functions. Other examples include stimulation-secretion coupling, hormonal and growth factor activation of cells, and antigen-specific T lymphocyte activation, to mention just a few. All of these processes share with EC coupling the basic principle of exciting a cell with an extracellular stimulus which is then converted to an intracellular response. In the case of EC coupling, the extracellular stimulus is electrical depolarization of the plasma membrane of the cell.

The immediate intracellular response to the depolarization-induced activation of the VDCC/DHPR is activation of a specialized form of intracellular calcium release channel, the RyR. RyRs and inositol 1,4,5-trisphosphate (IP3) receptors (see Fig. 2–8) form a unique class of ion channels that have no similarities to the voltage-gated ion channels discussed earlier. The intracellular calcium release channels are roughly 10 times the size of the VDCC and conduct much larger currents through their pores. The IP3 receptors are found in all types of cells, including heart muscle, whereas the RyR are less widely distributed. It is likely that RyR evolved from IP3 receptors as more specialized functions such as muscle contraction evolved. RyR have three forms and type 2 RyR (RyR2) are the ones found in heart muscle cells, where they are required for EC coupling. The RyR in the heart muscle is activated by the small amount of calcium that enters via the VDCC; thus, the term *calcium-induced calcium release*. When the RyR is activated, calcium stored at high concentrations in the SR (about 2 mM) is released into the cytoplasm of the heart muscle cell

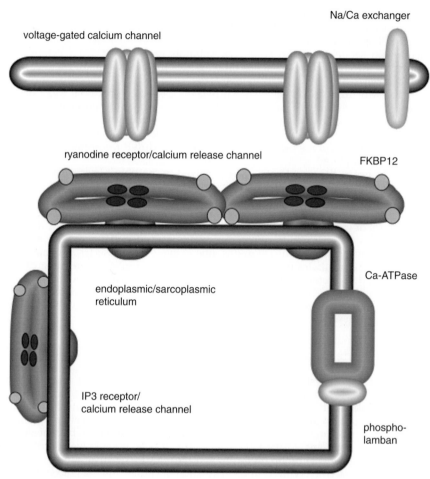

**Figure 2–8** ▪ Molecules involved in regulating cardiac calcium homeostasis. On the plasma membrane are the voltage-dependent (gated) calcium channel and the sodium-calcium exchanger. The ryanodine receptor, the major calcium release channel in the heart, is on the sarcoplasmic reticulum membrane along with the calcium (ATPase) pump, phospholamban (which regulates the calcium pump), and the IP3 receptor (a second form of calcium release channel in the heart). Each ryanodine receptor/calcium release channel has four molecules of FKBP12 bound tightly to the channel. FKBP12 is required for normal physiologic function of the calcium release channel.

because of the high concentration gradient between the lumen of the SR and the cytoplasm of the heart muscle cell, where the calcium concentration is about 100 nmol/l when the cell is at rest (during diastole). Much of the calcium inside the SR is bound to calcium-binding proteins, including calsequestrin, a 45-kd protein, and calreticulin (44-kd).

The RyR are the largest ion channels described to date (more than 2.4 million daltons), and single RyR channels can readily be seen with electron microscopy. These tetrameric structures are comprised of four large, equivalent subunits, each of which contributes a quarter of the transmembrane segments that form the pore of the channel through the sarcoplasmic reticulum. Bound tightly to each of these four large subunits is a small regulatory subunit of the channel known as the *FK506-binding protein* or FKBP12 (so called because it binds the immunosuppressant drug FK506). FKBP12 is required for normal function of the RyR channel. Most of the protein sequence of the large RyR subunits comprises a giant cytoplasmic domain of the channel that contains binding sites for modulators of channel function (see Fig. 2–5).

Ultrastructural studies have shown that the association between RyR2 on the SR and the DHPR on the T tubule in cardiac muscle is not as uniform as in skeletal muscle, suggesting that some of the RyR2, particularly in the atria, may be activated without a direct association with DHPR. This would be consistent with a lack of direct protein-protein interactions between DHPR and RyR in cardiac compared to skeletal EC coupling.

In the heart, IP3 receptors may be involved in the physiologic modulation of cardiac contractility in response to drugs and hormones, but it is generally agreed that they do not play a major role in excitation-contraction coupling in cardiac muscle. IP3R levels are about 50 times lower than those of RyR2 in the heart,[4] and the kinetics of calcium release from IP3R are too slow, as compared with RyR2, to contribute to the calcium transient during EC coupling. IP3 receptors are also present in larger numbers in (1) Purkinje fibers[5] that conduct electrical signals from the atria to the ventricles (suggesting that it may play a role in generating cardiac rhythms) and (2) in the intercalated disks,[6] where it may have a role in cell-to-cell communication. IP3 receptors may also play a role in signaling necessary for cell death and for activation of gene transcription in the heart, as they have been shown to do in other types of cells such as T lymphocytes.[7-9]

## Cardiomyocyte Relaxation

Four transport systems can compete for cytoplasmic calcium during relaxation in cardiac muscle: (1) the calcium reuptake pump on the sarcoplasmic reticulum, (2) the sarcolemmal sodium-calcium (Na-Ca) exchanger, (3) the sarcolemmal calcium pump, and (4) the mitochondrial calcium uniport system. Calcium uptake by the SR is the most important factor in relaxation, but relaxation can be achieved by the other three systems. In the normal human ventricle, the relative contributions of the calcium reuptake pump on the SR and the Na-Ca exchanger are close to 2:1.[1]

The key molecule involved in the regulation of cardiac muscle relaxation is the sarcoplasmic (endoplasmic) reticulum Ca-ATPase (SERCA). The form in heart muscle, SERCA2a, is a member of a family of Ca-ATPases that share a common structure having 10 transmembrane segments and a cytosolic domain that develops energy required for calcium reuptake (against its chemical gradient) into the SR by hydrolizing ATP (see Fig. 2–7). In heart muscle Ca-ATPases are also present on the plasma membrane, and they pump calcium out of the cell into the extracellular space. SERCA2a is tonically inhibited by the regulatory protein phospholamban (see Fig. 2–8). When phospholamban is phosphorylated, its tonic inhibition of SERCA2a is released and the uptake of calcium into the SR is enhanced. A major pathway that leads to the phosphorylation of SERCA2a is the adrenergic signaling system that results in cyclic AMP–mediated phosphorylation of SERCA2a by protein kinase A. Thus, adrenergic stimulation by catecholamines binding to β-adrenergic receptors on the heart muscle cells can enhance relaxation of the heart. In the failing heart, SERCA2a levels decrease and sodium-calcium exchange may become more important.

The sodium-calcium exchanger also transports calcium out of the cell against its chemical gradient (see Fig. 2–8). The exchanger uses osmotic energy of the sodium gradient across the plasma membrane rather than hydrolysis of ATP to move calcium out of the cell. One calcium ion is moved out of the cardiac muscle cell for every three sodium ions that enter. The sodium pump (sodium-potassium ATPase, N-K-ATPase) is responsible for generating the sodium gradient across the plasma membrane and thus indirectly provides the energy that drives the sodium-calcium exchanger. The sodium-calcium exchanger is comprised of 12 transmembrane segments.

The sodium pump or Na-K-ATPase is responsible for maintaining the intracellular concentrations of sodium and potassium. Utilizing energy derived from ATP hydrolysis, the Na-K-ATPase pumps out three sodium ions for every two potassium ions that enter the cardiac muscle cell. The Na-K-ATPase is the molecular target for digitalis. A small amount of total cellular calcium is sequestered within mitochondria.

## Actions of Calcium in Cardiac Muscle Cells

Cardiac muscle cells, cardiomyocytes, contain contractile proteins organized as myofibrils. The contractile proteins within the myofibrils are the basis for the striations observed by light microscopy that are characteristic of both cardiac and skeletal muscles, which are known as striated muscles. Crossbridges link thick (myosin) and thin (actin) filaments. Via a calcium-activated energy-dependent process, the myosin crossbridges interact with the thin actin filaments and "pull" them toward the center of the sarcomere (myofibrillar unit), producing contraction of the muscle cell (myocyte; see Fig. 2–6). The calcium dependence of this contractile function is mediated by calcium-activated enzymes that are integral components of the myofibril. These calcium-activated proteins include troponin C, which contains high-affinity calcium-binding sites; troponin T, which binds the troponin C; and troponin I (an inhibitory regulator) to tropomyosin, which in turn regulates the interaction between myosin and actin. The signal that initiates contraction, therefore, is the rise in cytosolic calcium, which causes troponin C to bind calcium and initiates conformational changes in the troponin-tropomyosin complex that enable myosin to crossbridge to actin. The subsequent lowering of cytosolic calcium concentration (during diastole in the heart) causes release of calcium from troponin C, resulting in reversal of the conformational changes that permitted myosin-actin interaction. This process leads to relaxation. Myosin-actin crossbridging requires ATP hydrolysis (as does calcium reuptake into the sarcoplasmic reticulum); thus, both contraction and relaxation in the heart require energy.

## ■ MOLECULAR PHYSIOLOGY OF PERTURBATIONS OF CALCIUM HOMEOSTASIS THAT ALTER CIRCULATORY FUNCTION

### Heart Failure

Regardless of the initial insult, the progression from normal cardiac function to heart failure is marked by ventricular remodeling. Features of remodeling include hypertrophy, disruption of the extracellular matrix, and left ventricular (LV) dilatation. Structural and functional remodeling of the heart are accompanied by molecular changes that affect multiple signaling pathways, including calcium signaling, adrenergic signaling, and cell growth. One key question still to be answered is whether functional deterioration of the heart is caused by a defect in the function of individual cardiomyocytes, a defect in extracellular matrix, or a combination of the two. On the basis of Laplace's law, the increased chamber diameter in a dilated heart places cardiomyocytes at a mechanical disadvantage so that the force generated by each contracting myocyte is less efficiently transduced into LV pressure and flow.[10] Thus, structural remodeling of the heart alone, even in the absence of a defect in the function of the individual myocyte, leads to a loss of efficiency and increased work (because of greater wall tension). Hypertrophy may occur in response to signals generated by increased wall tension that are transmitted to intracellular signaling pathways. Current therapies for congestive heart failure are designed to counteract or arrest changes induced by remodeling. Recent data from patients with end-stage heart failure treated with a LV assist device (LVAD) as a bridge to cardiac transplantation suggest that even the remodeling observed in end-stage cardiomyopathies (once thought to be irreversible) is reversible.

Remodeling of the heart that occurs during the progression to heart failure is associated with changes in the expression of calcium-handling molecules. Whether these changes in the levels of calcium-handling molecules translate into alterations in calcium homeostasis has been controversial. For example, most agree that there is a reduction in the level of SERCA2 which pumps calcium back into the SR after each contraction. The calcium uptake rate measured using the radiolabeled tracer calcium 45 in cardiac biopsy homogenates was significantly decreased in cardiomyopathic hearts (3.3 nmol/mg/min versus 6.5 nmol/mg/min in controls).[11] Isolated ventricular myocytes from failing hearts loaded with fura 2 showed high resting intracellular calcium concentration ($[Ca]_i$) ($165 \pm 61$ nmol/l versus $96 \pm 47$ nmol/l in controls), and low peak $[Ca]_i$ ($367 \pm 109$ nmol/l versus $746 \pm 249$ nmol/l in controls).[12] Furthermore, intracellular calcium transients recorded with aequorin in myopathic trabeculae carnae showed a slower rise and decline of luminescence as compared with control tissue.[13, 14] Abnormalities in postrest potentiation and in the force-frequency relationship in cardiomyopathic human hearts have also been reported.[15] These data indicate that in human cardiomyopathy both calcium release and sequestration can be impaired. Other studies using purified left ventricular SR vesicles, however, reported no differences between normal and cardiomyopathic hearts with regard to maximal calcium uptake rate, $[Ca]_i$ at half-maximal calcium uptake, the Hill coefficient, and phospholamban-stimulated calcium uptake.[16] Moreover, recordings of single calcium release channel behavior using SR vesicles isolated from failing hearts and incorporated into lipid bilayers were essentially the same as those from normal hearts.[17] These discrepancies may be due to differences in methods or models (e.g., intact fibers or whole-muscle homogenates versus isolated SR vesicles). An additional confounding issue is the role of phosphorylation in the regulation of both the voltage-gated calcium channels and RyR2 and whether a defect in phosphorylation or dephosphorylation of the channels plays a role in the pathogenesis of heart failure.[18]

In support of functional data showing abnormal calcium homeostasis in cardiomyopathy, previous human studies have demonstrated downregulation of the mRNA encoding the EC-coupling calcium channels in myopathic left ventricular tissue. We and others have shown that the mRNA level of SR Ca-ATPase is reduced by 35% to 55% in end-stage heart failure.[19–21] We also found that DHPR mRNA expression was decreased in myopathic left ventricles by 47%.[21] Our group and others have shown that RyR2 mRNA in the left ventricle was decreased in cardiomyopathic patients by 28% to 37%.[19, 22, 23] More recently, we investigated the possibility that the levels of the RYR2 and IP3R calcium release channels, each activated by different pathways, might be regulated differently during human heart failure. RyR2 and IP3R mRNA levels in myocardium from 32 cardiac transplant recipients and six normal controls were determined using Northern and slot blot analyses. Interestingly, the two cardiac intracellular calcium release channels were regulated in opposite directions. RyR2 expression was decreased by 31% ($P > .025$) while IP3R expression was increased by 123% ($P > .005$) in myopathic left ventricle as compared with controls; similar findings were observed in the right ventricle and septum.[24] [$^3$H]-ryanodine and [$^3$H]-IP3 binding, as well as enzyme-linked immuno-sorbent assay (ELISA) using monoclonal antibodies to SR Ca-ATPase, showed that protein levels were regulated in parallel with the mRNAs.[24] However, other groups have reported either no changes in mRNA levels for RyR2 and DHPR[25] or normal protein levels despite decreased mRNA levels.[26–28]

In addition to a potential for an alteration in the function of the sarcolemmal calcium channel that provides the trigger for calcium release within the myocyte, there is an accumulating body of evidence that suggests that the cycling of calcium in myocytes or diseased tissue like that from failing or hypertrophic hearts is altered.[12, 13, 18, 29–34]

## Sudden Cardiac Death

There are two pathways by which calcium can enter the cytoplasm and cause an elevation in cytosolic calcium: (1) Calcium release from intracellular pools contained in the SR and endoplasmic reticulum (ER) via intracellular calcium release channels (RyR2 and IP3R2); and (2) calcium influx via channels and ex-changers in the plasma membrane (primarily the L-type, voltage-gated calcium channel, or dihydropyridine receptor [DHPR]). EC coupling in cardiomyocytes is activated by a small calcium influx via the L-type calcium channel (formed by the $\alpha_1$ subunit of the DHPR), which initiates release of much more intracellular calcium via the RyR2, a process referred to as *calcium-induced calcium release*.[2, 3] In addition to this highly regulated and absolutely critical process of repeated elevations of cytosolic calcium concentration in cardiomyocytes that is required for muscle con-traction, it has been proposed that aberrant calcium fluxes occur and may be involved in triggering certain types of ventricular arrhythmias. These aberrant calcium fluxes have been attributed to both inappropriate SR calcium release during diastole when the calcium release channel (RyR2) is supposed to be closed and from excessive calcium influx via the L-type calcium channel. SR calcium overload has been proposed as a predisposing factor for aberrant calcium fluxes due to SR calcium release, and action potential duration (APD) prolongation has been pro-posed as a predisposing factor for aberrant calcium fluxes due to calcium influx via the L-type calcium channel. The possible role of the IP3R2 in the generation of abnormal SR calcium release signals in cardiomyocytes has not been confirmed. Indeed, the levels of IP3R2 are elevated in at least one condition associated with increased risk of SCD, in heart failure.[23] Moreover, IP3R2 is activated via pathways that activate phospholipase C (PLC), including α-adrenergic receptors and angioten-sin receptors. Blockers of pathways that activate these receptors or of the receptors themselves (e.g., captopril and carvedilol) have been shown to reduce the preva-lence of sudden cardiac death in large clinical trials that generally involve patients with decreased LV function.[35] Clearly, these studies did not address possible mecha-nisms, but they suggested that receptors coupled to activation of PLC may be involved in generating signals (possibly involving activation of IP3R2) that increase the risk of sudden cardiac death.

Both the aberrant release of SR calcium during diastole and excessive calcium influx via the L-type calcium channel during late systole (when the action potential is repolarizing) can initiate depolarizations.[36] SR calcium release activates inward depolarizing currents principally by activating an inward (depolarizing) current via the sodium-calcium exchanger, and calcium influx via the L-type channel is itself a depolarizing current. These aberrant depolarizations have been termed *afterdepolar-izations*.[36] Early afterdepolarizations occur during the repolarization phase of the action potential, and delayed afterdepolarizations when the action potential has completed or nearly completed its repolarization during diastole.[36] Depolarizations initiated by SR calcium release can in turn generate extrasystoles in cardiomyocytes. When these extrasystoles are conducted via intercellular communications throughout the heart they result in premature ventricular contraction. These premature contractions can generate fatal ventricular arrhythmias when they occur in bursts or are sustained at a high frequency referred to as *ventricular tachycardia* (e.g., more than 200 beats per minute). These calcium-dependent ventricular arrhythmias have been termed *triggered activity*.[37] Furthermore, it has been proposed that alterations in intracellular calcium cycling play a role in T-wave alternans.[38] Further studies have suggested that T-wave alternans in ventricular fibers is controlled by [Ca]$_i$ and that SR calcium release plays an important role in T-wave alternans.[39]

# ■ REFERENCES

1. Bers DM: Excitation-Contraction Coupling and Cardiac Contractile Force. Boston: Kluwer, 1991.
2. Fabiato A: Calcium-induced release of calcium from the cardiac sarcoplasmic reticulum. Am J Physiol 1983;245:C1–C14.
3. Fabiato A, Fabiato F: Calcium and cardiac excitation-contraction coupling. Annu Rev Physiol 1984;41:743.
4. Moschella MC, Marks AR: Inositol 1,4,5-trisphosphate receptor expression in cardiac myocytes. J Cell Biol 1993;120:1137–1146.
5. Gorza L, Schiaffino S, Volpe P: Inositol 1,4,5-trisphosphate receptor in heart: Evidence for its concentration in Purkinje myocytes of the conduction system. J Cell Biol 1993;121:345–353.
6. Kijima Y, Saito A, Jetton T, et al: Different intracellular localization of inositol 1,4,5-trisphosphate and ryanodine receptors in cardiomyocytes. J Biol Chem 1993;268:3499–3506.
7. Jayaraman T, Ondriasova E, Ondrias K, et al: The inositol 1,4,5-trisphosphate receptor is essential for T cell receptor signaling. Proc Natl Acad Sci USA 1995;92:6007–6011.
8. Jayaraman T, Marks AR: T cells deficient in inositol 1,4,5-trisphosphate receptor are resistant to apoptosis. Molec Cell Biol 1997;17:3005–3012.
9. Marks AR: Intracellular calcium release channels: Regulators of cell life and death. Am J Physiol 1997;41:H597–H605.
10. Katz AM: Physiology of the Heart. New York: Raven, 1992.
11. Limas C, Spier S, Kahlon J: Enhanced calcium transport by sarcoplasmic reticulum in mild cardiac hypertrophy. J Molec Cell Cardiol 1980;12:1103–1116.
12. Beuckelmann D, Nabauer M, Erdmann E: Intracellular calcium handling in isolated ventricular myocytes from patients with terminal heart failure. Circulation 1992;85:1046–1055.
13. Gwathmey JK, et al: Abnormal intracellular calcium handling in myocardium from patients with end-stage heart failure. Circ Res 1987;61:70–76.
14. Morgan J, Erny R, Allen P, et al: Abnormal intracellular calcium handling: A major cause of systolic and diastolic dysfunction in ventricular myocardium from patients with end-stage heart failure. Circulation 1990;81(Suppl III):III21–III32.
15. Pieske B et al: Diminished post-rest potentiation of contractile force in human dilated cardiomyopathy. Functional evidence for alterations in intracellular Ca$^{2+}$ handling. J Clin Invest 1996;98,764–776.
16. Movsesian M, Colyer J, Wang J, Krall J: Phospholamban-mediated stimulation of Ca$^{2+}$ uptake in sarcoplasmic reticulum from normal and failing hearts. J Clin Invest 1990;85:1698–1702.
17. Holmberg S, Williams A: The calcium-release channel from cardiac sarcoplasmic reticulum: Function in the failing and acutely ischemic heart. Basic Res Cardiol 1992;87(Suppl I):255–268.
18. Gomez AM et al: Defective excitation-contraction coupling in experimental cardiac hypertrophy and heart failure [see Comments]. Science 1997;276:800–806.
19. Brillantes A, Allen P, Takahasi T, et al: Differences in cardiac calcium release channel (ryanodine receptor) expression in myocardium from patients with end-stage heart failure caused by ischemic versus dilated cardiomyopathy. Circ Res 1992;71:18–26.
20. Mercardier J, et al: Altered sarcoplasmic reticulum Ca$^{2+}$-ATPase gene expression in the human ventricle during end-stage heart failure. J Clin Invest 1990;85:305–309.
21. Takahashi T, et al: Expression of dihydropyridine receptor (Ca$^{2+}$ channel) and calsequestrin genes in the myocardium of patients with end-stage heart failure. J Clin Invest 1992;90:927–935.
22. Arai M, Alpert N, MacLennan D, et al: Alterations in sarcoplasmic reticulum gene expression in human heart failure: A possible mechanism for alterations in systolic and diastolic properties of the failing myocardium. Circ Res 1993;72:463–469.
23. Go LO, et al: Differential regulation of two types of intracellular calcium release channels during end-stage heart failure. J Clin Invest 1995;95:888–894.
24. Go LO, et al: Chamber specific regulation of the sarcoplasmic reticulum Ca$^{2+}$ ATPase pump in human heart failure [Abstr]. J Am Coll Cardiol 1995;283A.

25. Meyer M, et al: Alterations of sarcoplasmic reticulum proteins in failing human dilated cardiomyopathy. Circulation 1995;92:778–784.
26. Movsesian M, Bristow M, Krall J: Ca$^{2+}$ uptake by cardiac sarcoplasmic reticulum from patients with idiopathic cardiomyopathy. Circ Res 1989;65:1141–1144.
27. Movsesian M, Karimi M, Green K, Jones L: Ca$^{2+}$-transporting ATPase, phospholamban and calsequestrin levels in nonfailing and failing human myocardium. Clin Res 1994;42(2):166-A.
28. Hasenfuss G, et al: Calcium handling proteins in the failing human heart. Basic Res Cardiol 1997;92(Suppl 1):87–93.
29. Siri F, Krueger J, Nordin C, et al: Depressed intracellular calcium transients and contraction in myocytes from hypertrophied and failing guinea pig hearts. Am J Physiol 1991;261:H514–H530.
30. Bailey BA, Houser SA: Calcium transients in feline left ventricular myocytes with hypertrophy induced by slow progressive pressure overload. J Molec Cell Cardiol 1992;24:365–373.
31. Beuckelmann DJ, Nabauer M, Kruger C, Erdmann E: Altered diastolic Ca handling in human ventricular myocytes from patients with terminal heart failure. Am Heart J 1995;129:684–689.
32. Gwathmey JK, Morgan JP: Altered calcium handling in experimental pressure overload in the ferret. Circ Res 1985;57:836–843.
33. Bing OHL, et al: Intracellular calcium transients in myocardium from spontaneously hypertensive rats during the transition to heart failure. 1991;68:1390–1400.
34. Delbridge LM, et al: Cardiac myocyte volume, Ca$^{2+}$ fluxes, and sarcoplasmic reticulum loading in pressure-overload hypertrophy. Am J Physiol 1997;272:H2425–2435.
35. Lechat P, et al: Clinical effects of α-adrenergic blockade in chronic heart failure. A meta-analysis of double-blind, placebo-controlled, randomized trials. Circulation 1998;98:1184–1191.
36. Fozzard HA: Afterdepolarizations and triggered activity. Basic Res Cardiol 1992;87:105–113.
37. Wit AL, Rosen MR: Pathophysiologic mechanisms of cardiac arrhythmias. Am Heart J 1983;106:798–811.
38. Hirayama Y, Saitoh H, Atarashi H, Hayakawa H: Electrical and mechanical alternans in canine myocardium in vivo. Dependence on intracellular calcium cycling. Circulation 1993;88:2894–2902.
39. Saitoh H, Bailey JC, Surawicz B: Action potential duration alternans in dog Purkinje and ventricular muscle fibers. Further evidence in support of two different mechanisms. Circulation 1989;80:1421–1431.

## ■ RECOMMENDED READING

Bers DM: Excitation-Contraction Coupling and Cardiac Contractile Force. Boston: Kluwer, 1991.
Brillantes A, Allen P, Takahasi T, et al: Differences in cardiac calcium release channel (ryanodine receptor) expression in myocardium from patients with end-stage heart failure caused by ischemic versus dilated cardiomyopathy. Circ Res 1992;71:18–26.
Go LO, et al: Differential regulation of two types of intracellular calcium release channels during end-stage heart failure. J Clin Invest 1995;95:888–894.
Katz AM: Physiology of the Heart. New York: Raven, 1992.
Marks AR: Intracellular calcium release channels: Regulators of cell life and death. Am J Physiol 1997;41:H597–H605.
Moschella MC, Marks AR: Inositol 1,4,5-trisphosphate receptor expression in cardiac myocytes. J Cell Biol 1993;120:1137–1146.
Wit AL, Rosen MR: Pathophysiologic mechanisms of cardiac arrhythmias. Am Heart J 1983;106:798–811.

# Chapter 3

# Ventricular Function

*Lionel H. Opie*

## ■ SYSTOLE AND DIASTOLE

### Contraction Phases

The basic events of the cardiac cycle can be represented by the Wiggers diagram (Fig. 3–1) as follows: (1) left ventricular (LV) contraction, (2) LV relaxation, and (3) LV filling. A natural starting point is the arrival of calcium ions at the contractile protein that initiates actin-myosin interaction and LV contraction. During the initial phase of contraction, the LV pressure builds up until it exceeds that in the left atrium (normally 10 to 15 mm Hg), whereupon the mitral valve closes. Now, with two valves (aortic and mitral) both shut, the LV volume cannot change and contraction must be *isovolumic* (from *isos*, equal) until the aortic valve is forced open as the LV pressure exceeds that in the aorta. Once the aortic valve is open, blood is vigorously ejected from the LV into the aorta during the phase of *maximal* or *rapid ejection*. The speed of ejection of blood is determined both by the pressure gradient across the aortic valve and by the elastic properties of the aorta.

### Ventricular Relaxation

After the LV pressure rises to a peak it starts to fall. As the cytosolic calcium is taken up into the sarcoplasmic reticulum (SR) under the influence of active phospholamban, more and more myofibers enter the state of relaxation. As a result, the rate of ejection of blood from the aorta falls *(phase of reduced ejection)*. Although the LV pressure is falling, blood flow is maintained by recoil of the aorta that had expanded during the phase of rapid ejection. Next, the aortic valve closes as the pressure in the aorta exceeds the falling pressure in the LV. Now the ventricular volume is once again sealed, because both aortic and mitral valves are closed. The left ventricle therefore relaxes without changing its volume *(isovolumic relaxation)*. Thereafter, the filling phase of the cardiac cycle restarts as the LV pressure falls below that in the left atrium, whereupon the mitral valve opens and ventricular filling proceeds.

### Ventricular Filling Phases

The *first phase of rapid or early filling,* starting very soon after mitral valve opening, accounts for most of ventricular filling. In addition, early filling may also be aided by active diastolic relaxation of the ventricle *(ventricular suction)*. The next phase is *diastasis* (i.e., separation), during which pressures in the atrium and ventricle equalize so that LV filling temporarily stops. Thereafter, atrial contraction *(atrial systole or the left atrial booster)* increases the pressure gradient across the open mitral valve to complete ventricular filling.

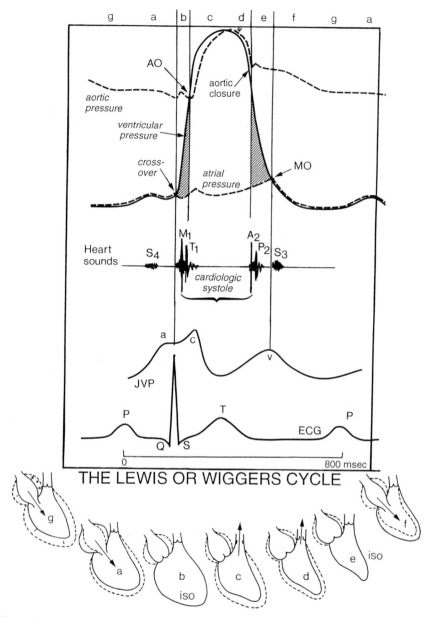

**Figure 3–1** ▪ The cardiac cycle, first assembled by Lewis in 1920 although conceived by Wiggers.[19] Note that mitral valve closure occurs after the crossover point of atrial and ventricular pressures at the start of systole. The 'a' and 'c' waves of JVP (jugular venous pressure) coincide with small 'a' and 'c' in the bottom panel. (Visual phases of the ventricular cycle are modified from Shepherd and Vanhoutte: The Human Cardiovascular System, New York, Raven Press, 1979, p 68.) Phases a to g in bottom panel should be related to the corresponding letters at the top of figure. ECG, electrocardiogram; JVP, jugular venous pressure; M₁, mitral component of the first sound at time of mitral valve closure; T₁, tricuspid valve closure, second component of first heart sound; AO, aortic valve opening, normally inaudible; A₂, aortic valve closure, aortic component of second sound; P₂, pulmonary component of second sound, pulmonary valve closure; MO, mitral valve opening, sometimes audible in mitral stenosis as the opening snap; S₃, third heart sound; S₄, fourth heart sound; a, wave produced by right atrial contraction; c, carotid wave artifact during rapid LV ejection phase; v, venous return wave, which causes pressure to rise while tricuspid valve is closed. Cycle length of 800 msec for 75 bpm.

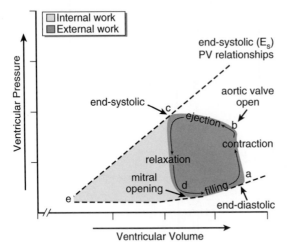

**Figure 3–2** ■ Pressure-volume loops. Normal left ventricular pressure-volume relationship. The aortic valve opens at b and closes at c. The mitral valve opens at d and closes at a. External work is defined by a, b, c, and d and internal work by e, d, and c. The pressure-volume area is the sum of external and internal work.

## Physiologic and Cardiologic Definitions of Systole and Diastole

In Greek, *systole* means *contraction* and *diastole* means to *send apart*. The start of systole can be regarded as either (1) the beginning of isovolumic contraction when LV pressure exceeds the atrial pressure or (2) mitral valve closure ($M_1$). The former is physiologic systole; the latter, cardiologic systole. These correspond reasonably well, because mitral valve closure actually occurs only about 20 msec after the crossover point of the pressures. Thus, in practice the term *isovolumic contraction* often also includes this brief period of early systolic contraction even before the mitral valve shuts, when the heart volume does not change substantially.

Physiologically, end systole is just before the ventricle starts to relax, a concept that fits well with the standard pressure-volume curve.[1] Physiologic diastole commences as calcium ions are taken up into the SR, so that myocyte relaxation dominates over contraction and the LV pressure starts to fall as shown on the pressure-volume curve (Fig. 3–2). In contrast, cardiologic systole is demarcated by the interval between the first and second heart sounds, lasting from the first heart sound ($M_1$) to the closure of the aortic valve ($A_2$). The remainder of the cardiac cycle automatically becomes cardiologic diastole. Thus, cardiologic systole, demarcated by heart sounds rather than physiologic events, starts fractionally later than physiologic systole and ends significantly later.

In contrast stands another physiologic concept, one promulgated by Brutsaert and colleagues, who argue that diastole starts much later, only when the whole of the contraction-relaxation cycle is over. According to this view, diastole would occupy only a small portion of the pressure-volume cycle (see Fig. 3–1).[2] This definition of diastole, although seldom used in cardiology practice, does remind us that abnormalities of LV contraction often underlie defective relaxation.

## ■ CONTRACTILITY AND LOAD

*Contractility is the inherent capacity of the myocardium to contract independently of changes in preload or afterload.* It is a key word in the language of cardiology. Increased contractility means a greater rate of contraction, to reach a greater peak force. Often, increased contractility is associated with enhanced rates of relaxation, called the *lusitropic effect*. Alternate names for contractility are the *inotropic state* (*ino*, fiber; *tropos*, to move) and the *contractile* state. Contractility is an important regulator of myocardial oxygen uptake. Factors that increase contractility include adrenergic stimulation, digitalis, and other inotropic agents. At a molecular level, an increased inotropic state can be explained by enhanced interaction between calcium ions and the contractile proteins. Such an interaction could result from either increased calcium transients or from increased sensitivity of the contractile proteins to a given level of cytosolic calcium. The new calcium-sensitizing drugs act by the latter mechanism, and conventional inotropes such as digitalis and sympathomimetics through an increase in internal calcium.

## Preload and Afterload

It is important to stress that any change in the contractile state must occur independently of the loading conditions. The two types of load are preload and the afterload (the latter is discussed later). The *preload* is the load present before contraction has started, at the end of diastole. The preload reflects the venous filling pressure that fills the left atrium, which in turn fills the left ventricle during diastole. When the preload increases, the left ventricle distends during diastole and the stroke volume rises according to Starling's Law (see later). The heart rate also increases by stimulation of the atrial mechanoreceptors that enhance the rate of discharge of the sinoatrial node. Thus, the cardiac output (the product of stroke volume and heart rate) rises.

## Venous Filling Pressure and Heart Volume: Starling's Law of the Heart

Starling[3] related the venous pressure in the right atrium to the heart volume in dog heart-lung preparations (Fig. 3–3). His initial observation, "The output of the heart is equal to and determined by the amount of blood flowing into the heart," he explained as follows:

Within physiological limits, the larger the volume of the heart, the greater the energy of its contraction and the amount of chemical change at each contraction.

Of note, Starling also stated that increased heart volume meant increased fiber length, so, "The energy of contraction is a function of the length of the muscle fiber." This observation holds in normal, compliant hearts.

One modern version of Starling's law is that stroke volume is related to the end-diastolic volume. The LV volume can now be measured directly with two-dimensional echocardiography. Yet the value derived depends on a number of simplifying assumptions, such as a spherical LV shape, and neglects the confounding influence of the complex anatomy of the LV. In practice, therefore, LV volume is not often measured.

The LV diastolic *filling pressure* (the difference between the left atrial pressure and the LV diastolic pressure) is easier to measure and in diseased, noncompliant hearts, may be taken as a surrogate for heart volume. This is important because the venous filling pressure can be measured in humans, albeit indirectly, by the technique of Swan-Ganz catheterization (Fig. 3–4), as can the stroke volume. The LV pressure and volume are not linearly related because of variations in the compliance of the myocardium. Therefore, a jump from pressure to volume is required to apply the Starling concept to the hemodynamic management of critically ill persons who have received a Swan-Ganz catheter.

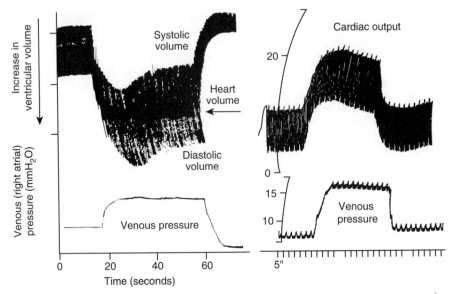

**Figure 3–3** ■ Starling's law of the heart as applied to the preload (venous filling pressure). As the preload increases (*bottom* in both figures), the heart volume increases (*left top*), as does the cardiac output (*right top*). Starling's explanation was, "*The output of the heart is a function of its filling; the energy of contraction depends on the state of dilatation of the heart's cavities.*"

## Frank and Isovolumic Contraction

Thus, according to Starling, in a healthy heart, a larger heart volume would lead to an increase in the initial length of the muscle fiber, to increase the stroke volume and thus the cardiac output. This sequence suggests, but does not prove, that diastolic stretch of the LV actually increases contractility. In fact, Starling's German predecessor, Frank, had already reported in 1895 that the greater the initial volume, the more rapid was the rate of rise, the greater the peak pressure, and the faster the rate of relaxation (Fig. 3–5).[3] He described both a positive inotropic effect and an increased lusitropic effect. These complementary findings of Frank and Starling are often combined into the Frank-Starling law. The beauty of this dual name is that, between them, they could account for two of the mechanisms underlying the increased stroke volume of exercise; namely, both the increased inotropic state[4] and the increased diastolic filling.[4]

## Afterload

The *afterload* is the systolic load on the LV after it has started to contract. Starling found that, within limits, "It seems to be immaterial to the heart" whether it has to contract against high or low resistance: "It puts out as much blood as it receives, so that the total outflow remains constant." In other words, in nonfailing hearts, the LV can overcome any physiologic acute increase in load. Over the long term, however, the LV must hypertrophy to overcome sustained arterial hypertension or significant aortic stenosis.

In clinical practice, arterial blood pressure is often taken to be synonymous with afterload, an assumption that ignores *aortic compliance*, the extent to which the

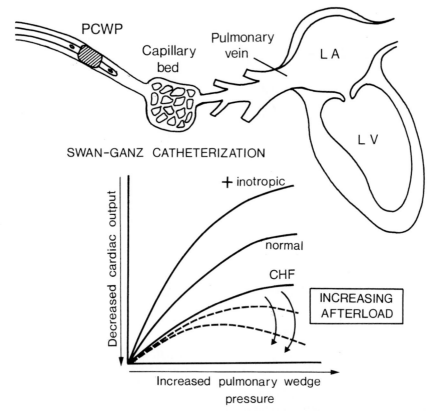

**Figure 3–4** ▪ A family of Starling curves with relevance to Swan-Ganz catheterization. Each curve relates the filling pressure (PCPW, pulmonary capillary wedge pressure) to the left ventricular (LV) stroke output and to the cardiac output. Note that the depressed inotropic state of the myocardium causes an abnormally low curve and that the downward limb can be related to increased afterload. Clinically, the measurements relating filling pressure to cardiac output are obtained by Swan-Ganz catheterization (a procedure undertaken less frequently today than before). Note the close association between LV diastolic dysfunction and pulmonary congestion. LA, left atrium; CHF, congestive heart failure.

aorta can "yield" during systole. A stiff aorta, like that associated with isolated systolic hypertension of elderly persons, increases the afterload. *Aortic impedance* is an index of the afterload and is derived by dividing the aortic pressure by the aortic flow at that time, so that the afterload varies during each phase of the contraction cycle.

### Preload and Afterload are Interlinked

The distinctions just described between preload and afterload do not encompass situations when the two change concurrently. By the Frank-Starling law, increased LV volume leads to increased contractility, which in turn increases the systolic blood pressure and, thus, the afterload. Nonetheless, in general, the preload is related to the degree to which the myocardial fibers are stretched at the end of diastole, and the afterload is related to the wall stress generated by those fibers during systole.

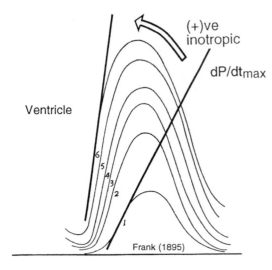

**Figure 3–5** ■ Frank related heart volume to contractility. Each curve was obtained at a greater initial filling of the left ventricle by an increased left atrial filling pressure. Then, valves were shut to produce isovolumic conditions. Curve 6 has a greater velocity of shortening, reflecting greater contractility. Thus, the initial fiber length (volume of ventricle) can affect contractility. This effect of initial fiber length on contractility has recently been rediscovered. Contractility is the maximal rate of change of the intraventricular pressure ($dP/dt_{max}$) as indicated by the two tangential lines showing the steepest parts of the curves of the original figure of Frank.

## ■ CELLULAR BASIS OF CONTRACTILITY AND STARLING'S LAW

### Length-Dependent Activation

How could increased end-diastolic muscle length increase the force and rate of muscle contraction? Previously, this effect of increased muscle length was ascribed to a more "optimal" overlap between actin and myosin. Intuitively, however, if actin and myosin are stretched farther apart, there would be less overlap rather than more. Another earlier proposal—that there is a length sensor residing in troponin C, one of the contractile proteins—is no longer favored. A more current view is that there is a complex interplay between anatomic and regulatory factors[5] whereby increased sarcomere length leads to greater sensitivity of the contractile apparatus to the prevailing cytosolic calcium. The major mechanism for this regulatory change, although not yet clarified, may reside in the interfilament spacing.[6] At short sarcomere lengths, as the lattice spacing increases, the number of strong crossbridges decreases.[7] Conversely, as the heart muscle is stretched, the interfilament distance decreases (Fig. 3–6), and, hypothetically, the rate of transition from the weak to the strong binding state increases. Thus, the stretched fibers are more sensitive to an unchanged cytosolic calcium ion concentration.

### Beta-Adrenergic Stimulation, Contractility, and Calcium

Beta-adrenergic stimulation mediates the major component of its inotropic effect by increasing the cytosolic calcium transient and the factors that control it (Fig. 3–7). The following are all enhanced: the rate of entry of calcium ions through the sarcolemmal L-type channels, the rate of calcium uptake under the influence of phospholamban into the SR, and the rate of calcium release from the ryanodine receptor on the SR in response to calcium entry, which in turn follows depolarization (see Chapter 2). Of all these factors, phosphorylation of phospholamban may be the most important,[8] as it acts on the calcium uptake pump of the SR to increase the rate of uptake of calcium during diastole. Thus, the SR is preloaded with increased $Ca^{2+}$ so that more can be liberated during ensuing depolarizations.

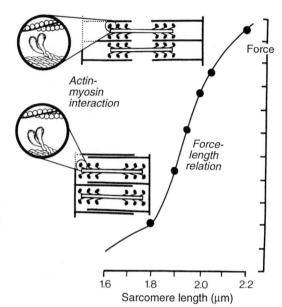

**Figure 3–6** ■ The force-length relationship of the cardiac sarcomere, derived from Fuchs.[5] This corresponds to the Frank-Starling relationship for the whole heart. Note the greater proximity of myosin heads to actin when the sarcomere is stretched. Increased sensitization of troponin C to calcium during stretch is another proposed explanation for the effect of stretch.

Conversely, contractility is decreased whenever calcium transients are depressed, as when β-adrenergic blockade decreases calcium entry through the L-type calcium channel. Alternatively, there may be faulty control of the uptake and release of calcium ions by the SR, as when the SR is damaged by congestive heart failure. Anoxia or ischemia depletes the calcium uptake pump of the SR of the adenosine triphosphate (ATP) required for calcium uptake, so that the contraction-relaxation cycle is inhibited.

## Problems with the Contractility Concept

The concept of contractility has serious defects. First, there is no ideal noninvasive index that can be measured in situ and is free of significant criticism. Second, it is impossible to separate the cellular mechanisms of contractility changes from those of load or heart rate. For example, increased heart rate increases the force of contraction by the Bowditch, or treppe, phenomenon (mechanism for increased cytosolic calcium discussed later). Another example is that increased afterload may indirectly, through stimulation of stretch-sensitive channels, increase cytosolic calcium. Thus, in relation to the underlying cellular mechanisms, there is clearly overlap between contractility, which should be independent of load or heart rate, and the effects of myocyte stretch and heart rate, which have some effects that simulate an increase in contractility. Because muscle length can influence contractility, the traditional separation of length and inotropic state into two independent regulators of cardiac muscle performance is no longer true if the end result is considered.

In clinical terms, it is still important to separate the effects of a primary increase in load or heart rate, on the one hand, from a primary increase in contractility on the other. This distinction is especially relevant in congestive heart failure, when decreased contractility could indirectly or directly increase afterload, preload, and heart rate, all of which could then predispose to a further decrease in myocardial

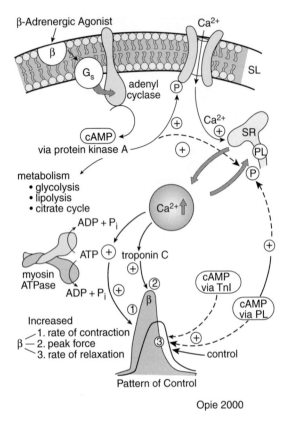

**Figure 3–7** ■ Beta-adrenergic signal systems involved in positive inotropic and lusitropic (enhanced relaxation) effects. When the β-adrenergic agonist interacts with the β receptor, the stimulatory G protein activates adenylate cyclase to produce the adrenergic second messenger, cyclic AMP (cAMP). The latter acts via protein kinase A to stimulate metabolism and to phosphorylate the calcium channel protein, thus increasing the opening probability of this channel. More $Ca^{2+}$ ions enter through the sarcolemma (SL) channel, to release more $Ca^{2+}$ from the sarcoplasmic reticulum (SR). Thus, the cytosolic $Ca^{2+}$ increases and more troponin C is activated. $Ca^{2+}$ ions also increase the rate of breakdown of adenosine triphosphate (ATP) to adenosine diphosphate (ADP) and inorganic phosphate ($P_i$). Enhanced myosin ATPase activity explains the increased rate of contraction, with increased activation of troponin C explaining increased peak force development. An increased rate of relaxation (lusitropic effect) is explained by phosphorylation of the protein phospholamban (PL), situated on the membrane of the SR, that controls the rate of uptake of calcium into the SR. (© *LH Opie, 2000.*)

performance. Despite all these reservations, it remains true that β-adrenergic stimulation has a calcium-dependent positive inotropic effect that is independent of loading conditions, which is, therefore, truly a positive inotropic effect.

## ■ CARDIAC OUTPUT

*Cardiac output* is the product of the stroke volume (SV) and the heart rate (HR):

$$\text{Cardiac output (l/min)} = \text{SV (l/beat)} \times \text{HR (bpm)}$$

The normal value is about 6 to 8 l/min, but it doubles or sometimes even triples during peak aerobic exercise. The stroke volume is determined by the preload, the afterload, and the contractile state. The heart rate is also one of the major determinants of myocardial oxygen uptake. The heart rate responds to a large variety of stimuli that indirectly alter myocardial oxygen uptake. Three physiologic factors that consistently increase the heart rate are exercise, awakening in the morning, and emotional stress.

### Heart Rate and Heart Work

Each cycle of contraction and relaxation performs a certain amount of work and takes up a certain amount of oxygen. The faster the heart rate, the higher are the cardiac output and the oxygen uptake. When the heart rate is extremely fast, however, as it can be during paroxysmal tachycardia, time for diastolic filling is inadequate so that cardiac output decreases. Another exception is in coronary artery disease when tachycardia of lesser degrees can decrease the stroke volume because of ischemic failure of the LV.

## Force-Frequency Relation

An increased heart rate progressively increases the force of ventricular contraction, even in an isolated papillary muscle preparation (Bowditch or treppe [staircase] phenomenon). In isolated human ventricular strips, increasing the stimulation rate from 60 to about 160 per minute, stimulates force development. In strips from failing hearts there is no such increase.[9] In the human heart in situ, pacing rates of up to 150 per minute can be tolerated, whereas higher rates cause atrioventricular (AV) block. Yet, during exercise, a maximal heart rate of 170 bpm causes no block, presumably because of concurrent adrenergic stimulation of the AV node. Thus, an excessive heart rate decreases, rather than increases, cardiac contraction and cardiac output. Recently, *tachycardia-induced cardiomyopathy* has been recognized, which is the result of excessive and prolonged tachycardia.[10]

## Sodium Pump Lag

To explain the staircase effect during rapid stimulation, the proposal is that each wave of depolarization brings more sodium ions into the myocardial cells than the sodium pump can eject. Sodium overload leads to an increase of cytosolic calcium by the sodium-calcium exchanger, with increased force of contraction. Too rapid stimulation causes the force of contraction to decrease by limiting the duration of ventricular filling—and probably by calcium overload.

## Loading Conditions and Cardiac Output

In general, when afterload decreases, cardiac output increases. Physiologic examples of this principle exist during peripheral vasodilatation induced by a hot bath or sauna or by a meal. In these conditions, however, tachycardia is also associated, as during drug-induced vasodilatation. Conversely, when the afterload increases, initially there is a compensatory mechanism, as described by Starling (see earlier). The proposal is that an increased end-diastolic fiber stretch increases contractility (see Fig. 3–5) and maintains the stroke volume. If the afterload keeps rising, compensatory mechanisms cannot adapt and the stroke volume eventually drops. In exercise, although the peripheral vascular resistance decreases, systolic blood pressure rises, so that afterload increases. Thus, at really high rates of upright exercise, stroke volume falls even though cardiac output continues to rise, the latter as a result of heart rate increases.[11] The LV in congestive heart failure reaches the critical point at which stroke volume (and thus cardiac output) starts to fall in response to exercise much sooner than does a normal LV.

## Contractility and Cardiac Output

During β-adrenergic stimulation or exercise, the contractile state is enhanced to contribute to the increased cardiac output. Conversely, during congestive heart failure or therapy with β-adrenergic blockade, decreased contractility means decreased stroke volume.

## ▪ CARDIAC OUTPUT DURING EXERCISE

During dynamic exercise cardiac output can increase severalfold (Fig. 3–8). There are three possible explanations: increased heart rate, increased contractility, and increased venous return. In humans, increased heart rate provides most of the increased cardiac output, and the Starling mechanism and increased contractility play less prominent roles.[11]

### Heart Rate During Exercise

The mechanism of the increase in heart rate during exercise is a combination of withdrawal of inhibitory vagal tone and increased β-adrenergic stimulation. The signals for these changes come from the vasomotor center in the brain stem, which coordinates two types of input: one is from the cerebral cortex (e.g., the runner's "readiness to go" at the start of exercise), and the second is the Bainbridge reflex, which is stimulated by atrial distention following increased venous return during exercise. Tachycardia, whatever the cause, can further induce a positive inotropic effect by the Bowditch (treppe) effect.

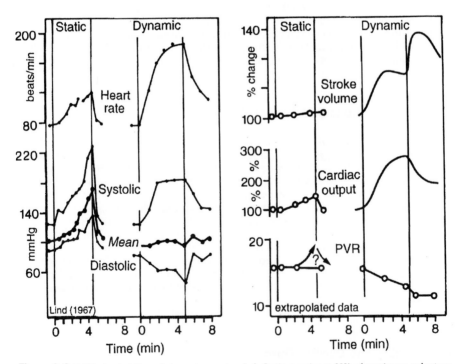

**Figure 3–8** ▪ Effects of static and dynamic exercise. *Left,* Static exercise at 30% of maximum voluntary contraction causes a much larger rise in mean blood pressure than does dynamic exercise, at comparable values of oxygen consumption. Conversely, dynamic exercise increases heart rate much more. For original data, see Lind and McNicol.[20] *Right,* Cardiac output increases much more with dynamic than with static exercise. Stroke volume increases only with dynamic exercise.[11] Peripheral vascular resistance (PVR) data for 0 to 2 min based on Waldrop et al.[21] and for 2 to 4 min on Lind and McNicol.[20]

### Venous Return During Exercise

Starling postulated (but did not measure) events at the start of exercise as follows: "If a man starts to run, his muscular movements pump more blood into the heart, so increasing the venous filling."[4] Because cardiac output must equal venous return, the increase in cardiac output during exercise must reflect an equal increase in venous return. This increase does not, however, necessarily prove the operation of the Starling mechanism, which requires increased venous filling pressure. If contractility were increased by β-adrenergic stimulation during exercise, then the venous filling pressure could actually fall, despite the increase in venous return. To be sure of the events at the start of exercise in humans, we would need to measure simultaneously venous return, venous filling pressure, and heart volume. Such data are missing. Nonetheless, the combination of increased venous return and enhanced sympathetic stimulation provides satisfactory explanations.

Increased venous return and filling pressure could explain the increased diastolic heart volume during exercise documented in radionuclide studies.[12, 13] This is not cardiac failure, because the end-systolic volume decreases and the stroke volume increases. The Starling mechanism appears to operate in both supine and upright postures when low-level exercise is compared with rest.[12] This effect is not inviolate: it may be altered by posture,[14] by exercise training,[15] or by increased contractility. Thus, at the start of exercise, there is an increase in venous return, which increases the venous filling pressure. This increase usually (but not invariably) elicits a Starling response, because concurrent sympathetic stimulation with increased heart rate and contractility contribute importantly. Once exercise has been initiated, the venous return stays high and equals the cardiac output. The exercise-induced decrease in the systemic vascular resistance helps to keep the cardiac output and venous return high. The end result is that the increased venous return and increased cardiac output will have achieved a new enhanced equilibrium.

### Static Exercise

Major hemodynamic features of static exercise, as compared with dynamic exercise, are (1) a smaller rise in heart rate; (2) a greater rise in blood pressure; and (3) no increase in stroke volume. Thus the cardiac output rises only in relation to the heart rate (see Fig. 3–8).

### ■ WALL STRESS

Myocardial wall stress, or *wall tension*, increases when the myofilaments slide over each other during cardiac contraction as they are squeezing blood out of the ventricles into the circulation. An analogy is the human effort required to squeeze a ball in the palm of the hand. A small rubber ball can be compressed easily. A rubber ball the size of a tennis ball is compressed less readily, and two large rubber balls or one really large ball can be compressed only with the greatest difficulty. As the size of the object in the hand increases, so does the force required to compress it. Intuitively, we know that the stress on the hand increases as the ball increases in diameter. But what is wall stress?

At this point, it is appropriate to digress briefly into a description of force, tension, and wall stress. *Force* is a term frequently used in studies of muscle mechanics. Strictly speaking,

$$Force = Mass \times Acceleration$$

Thus, when a load is suspended from one end of a muscle as the muscle contracts, it is exerting force against the mass of that load. In many cases, it is not possible to define force with such exactitude, but, in general, force has the following properties. First, force is always applied by one object (such as muscle) to another object (such as a load). Second, force is characterized both by the direction in which it acts and its magnitude. Thus, it is a vector, and the effect of a combination of forces can be established by the principle of vectors. Third, each object exerts a force on the other, so that force and counterforce are equal and opposite (Newton's third law of motion).

*Tension* exists when the two forces are applied to an object so that the forces tend to pull the object apart. When a spring is pulled by a force, tension is exerted; when more force is applied, the spring stretches and the tension increases.

*Stress* develops when tension is applied to a cross-sectional area; it is expressed as force per unit of area. According to the Laplace law,

$$\text{Wall stress} = \frac{\text{Pressure} \times \text{Radius}}{\text{Wall thickness} \times 2}$$

In ventricular hypertrophy associated with arterial hypertension or LV outflow obstruction, the increased wall thickness balances the increased pressure, so wall stress remains constant during the phase of compensatory hypertrophy. In congestive heart failure, the dilated heart has a larger radius, which elevates wall stress. Furthermore, because ejection of blood is inadequate, the radius stays large throughout the contractile cycle, so that both end-diastolic and end-systolic tensions are higher.

## Wall Stress and Myocardial Oxygen Demand

At a fixed heart rate, myocardial wall stress is the major determinant of myocardial oxygen consumption that ultimately reflects the rate of mitochondrial metabolism and ATP production. Thus, any increase of ATP requirement will be met by increased oxygen uptake. It is not only external work that determines the requirement for ATP. Rather, tension development (increased wall stress) requires oxygen even when no external work is being done. The difference between external work and tension developed can be characterized by comparing a man standing and holding a heavy suitcase, doing no external work yet becoming very tired, with a man lifting a much lighter suitcase, doing external work yet not tiring. The greater the left ventricular cavity size, the greater is the radius and the greater the wall stress. Thus, ejection of a given stroke volume from a large LV against a given blood pressure will produce as much external work as ejection of the same stroke volume by a normal-sized LV. Yet there would be much greater wall stress in the larger ventricle. Therefore, more oxygen would be required. In clinical terms, in a patient with angina and an enlarged LV, the appropriate therapy to reduce LV size will also reduce the myocardial oxygen demand, so that clinical improvement should result.

The overall concept of wall stress includes afterload, because increased afterload generates increased systolic wall stress. Wall stress is also determined by the preload, which generates diastolic wall stress. Wall stress increases in proportion to the pressure generated and to the radius of the LV cavity, factors that are responsive to increases in afterload and preload, respectively. The concept of wall stress allows for energy required for generation of muscle contraction that does not result in external work. Furthermore, in states of enhanced contractility, wall stress is increased. Thus, thinking in terms of wall stress provides a comprehensive approach to the problem of myocardial oxygen consumption. Apart from a metabolic component (usually small but prominent when circulating free fatty acids are abnormally high), *changes in heart rate and wall stress account for most of the clinically relevant changes in myocardial oxygen uptake.*

## External and Internal Work and Oxygen Demand

Bearing in mind that the major factor in cardiac work is the product of pressure and volume, it follows that external work can be quantified by the integrated pressure-volume area that represents the product of the systolic pressure and the stroke volume. To relate work to oxygen consumption, account must be taken of both the *external work* (the area enclosed by *a, b, c, d* in Fig. 3–2) and *internal work,* the volume-pressure triangle joining the end-systolic and mitral opening volume-pressure points to the origin (the area enclosed by *c, d, e* assuming that *e* represents the theoretical origin when pressure equals zero).

## Pressure and Volume Work and Oxygen Demand

In analyzing the difference between oxygen cost of pressure work and volume work, the established clinical observation is that the myocardium can tolerate a chronic volume load better than a pressure load. Thus, when cardiac work is chronically increased by augmenting the afterload, as during severe hypertension or narrowing of the aortic valve by aortic stenosis, the peak systolic pressure in the LV must increase and pressure power increases. Because of the complex way in which the muscle fibers of the myocardium run, however, a greater proportion of the work is opposed by the internal resistance. The result is that efficiency falls. An extreme example of the loss of efficiency during pressure work would be if the aorta were completely occluded so that none of the work would be external and all would be internal. Internal work is done against the noncontractile elements of the myocardium and is not useful work, in terms of calculating efficiency.

When the heart is subjected to a chronic volume load, as in mitral regurgitation, the increased work that the heart must perform is met by increased end-diastolic volume. The myofibers stretch, and length-dependent activation occurs. The primary adaptation to increased heart volume is increased fiber length and not increased pressure development, so that more external work is done but that against the internal resistance is unchanged, so that the efficiency of work rises. (The efficiency of work relates the amount of work performed to myocardial oxygen consumption.)

## ■ LEFT VENTRICULAR FUNCTION

### Maximal Rate of Left Ventricular Pressure Generation

During the early period of isovolumic contraction, preload and afterload are constant, and the maximal rate of pressure generation becomes an index of the inotropic state:

$$\text{Inotropic index} = dP/dt_{max},$$

where $P$ is LV pressure, $t$ is time, and $d$ indicates rate of change. Unfortunately, this index, which has stood the test of years, is not fully load independent, because, as Frank showed, increasing preload enhances the contractile state even during the isovolumic period (see Fig. 3–5). In humans, the measurements required for $dP/dt$ can be obtained only by LV catheterization, except with mitral regurgitation, when Doppler echocardiography can show changes in the LV-atrial pressure gradient.

## Ejection Phase Indices of Contractile State

These indices of function are, by definition, afterload dependent, because the LV is contracting against the afterload. This problem, is especially serious in failing myocardium, which must work against increases in afterload.[16] The initial fiber length helps to determine contractility, which in turn influences the afterload, because greater contractility in the presence of fixed peripheral (systemic) vascular resistance increases the blood pressure and the afterload.

The *ejection fraction* of the left ventricle, measured by radionuclide studies or indirectly by echocardiographic techniques, is frequently used but is not a sensitive parameter. The ejection fraction is the stroke volume expressed as a fraction of end-diastolic volume and is, therefore, an index of the extent of LV fiber shortening. Nonetheless, this index is easy to obtain and particularly useful in evaluating the course of chronic heart disease. Because the ejection fraction measures the contractile behavior of the heart during systole, it is, by definition, afterload sensitive. Another defect is that the ejection fraction relates systolic emptying to diastolic volume without measuring that volume, and the LV could, theoretically, be markedly enlarged yet have reasonable systolic function by this measure. Thus, the correlation between the degree of clinical heart failure and the decrease in the ejection fraction is often imperfect.

## Echocardiographic Indices of Contractile State

Echocardiographic indices are widely available and easy to measure. The *fractional shortening* uses the percentage of change of the minor axis (defined in the next paragraph) of the LV chamber during systole. An approximation clinicians often use but which requires that they make several assumptions, is to estimate the ejection fraction from fractional shortening. Despite such obvious defects, this easily defined index is useful in the management of heart failure. More accurate ejection fraction changes can be determined from volume measurements.

The *end-systolic volume* reflects contractile state, because the normal left ventricle ejects most of the blood present at the end of diastole (ejection fraction exceeds 55%). Impaired contractility, manifested as abnormally increased end-systolic volume, is a powerful predictor of adverse prognosis after myocardial infarction.[17] The *end-diastolic volume* is a less powerful predictor but is essential for accurate measurement of the ejection fraction.

Much more sophisticated measurements of the pumping function of the heart can be obtained with echocardiography. In particular, the velocity at which the circumference of the heart in its minor axis changes during systole is a useful index of myocardial contractility. The *minor axis* of the heart is the distance from the left side of the septum to the posterior endocardial wall. The *major axis* lies in the direction of the septum, which introduces an additional factor, septal contraction, so that major-axis changes cannot be used to assess contractile activity of the LV free wall. The mean *velocity of circumferential fiber shortening* (mean $V_{cf}$) can be determined from echocardiographic measurements of the end-diastolic and end-systolic sizes and the rate of change. The difference between the calculated circumferences is divided by the duration of shortening, which is the ejection time. The mean $V_{cf}$ compares favorably with more sophisticated invasive measurements of the contractile state.

## Contractility Indices Based on Pressure-Volume Loops

The pressure-volume loop discloses two fundamental aspects of the Frank-Starling relationship. First, as preload increases, volume increases. The loop is also

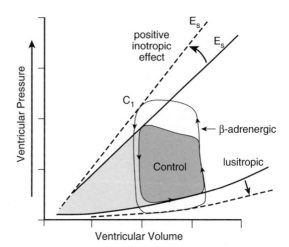

**Figure 3–9** ■ Pressure-volume loops: β-adrenergic stimulation, with both positive inotropic and increased lusitropic (relaxant) effects. Compare position of $C_1$ with C in Figure 3–2, and note increased slope of the index of contractility, $E_s$ (as defined in that figure).

an indirect measure of the Starling relationship between muscle length (measured indirectly by volume) and force (measured by the pressure). On the other hand, for any given preload (initial volume of contraction), a positive inotropic agent increases the amount of blood ejected, and, for the same final end-systolic pressure, there is a smaller end-systolic volume. Thus, a positive inotrope increases the slope of the end-systolic pressure-volume relationship ($E_s$; Fig. 3–9). It follows that the loop assesses both the Starling mechanism and the contractility of the left ventricle. Patients whose conditions are associated with higher contractile activity (increased inotropic state) have higher end-systolic pressures for a given end-systolic volume (with a steeper slope $E_s$) and have correspondingly higher oxygen uptake. Furthermore, pressure-volume loops, by assessing the sum of the internal and external work (see Fig. 3–2), indirectly measure work as another determinant of the myocardial oxygen demand.

Are invasive measurements necessary? The arterial systolic pressure and the end-systolic echocardiographic dimension give one fixed point, namely the end-systolic pressure-volume relation. But for the full loop, invasive measurements of the LV pressure are required. Although the loop is useful, like all systolic phase indices, it is not fully independent of the afterload.

## ■ DIASTOLE AND DIASTOLIC FUNCTION*

Among the many complex cellular factors that influence ventricular relaxation, four are of greater interest. First, the cytosolic calcium level must fall to cause the relaxation phase, a process that requires ATP and phosphorylation of phospholamban for uptake of calcium into the sarcoplasmic reticulum. Second, the inherent viscoelastic properties of the myocardium are important: in a hypertrophic heart, relaxation occurs more slowly. Third, increased phosphorylation of troponin 1 accelerates the rate of relaxation. Fourth, relaxation is influenced by the systolic load. The history of contraction affects crossbridge relaxation. Within limits, the greater the systolic load is, the faster the rate of relaxation. This complex relationship has been explored in detail by Brutsaert[2] but could, perhaps, be simplified as follows:

---

*Section modified from Opie LH: The Heart. Physiology, from Cell to Circulation, 3rd ed. Philadelphia: Lippincott-Raven, 1998: 374–378.

When the workload is high, peak cytosolic calcium is also thought to be high. A high end-systolic cytosolic calcium level means that the rate of fall of calcium also can be faster, provided that uptake mechanisms are functioning effectively. In this way a systolic pressure load and the rate of diastolic relaxation can be related. Furthermore, greater muscle length (when the workload is high) at the end of systole should produce more rapid relaxation by the opposite of length-dependent sensitization, so, the in early diastole, response to the rate of decline of calcium is more marked. Yet, when the systolic load exceeds a certain limit, the rate of relaxation is retarded, perhaps because of too much mechanical stress on the individual crossbridges. Thus, in congestive heart failure caused by an excessive systolic load, relaxation becomes increasingly afterload dependent, so therapeutic reduction of the systolic load should improve LV relaxation.

The *isovolumic relaxation* phase of the cardiac cycle is energy dependent, requiring ATP for uptake of calcium ions by the SR, which is an active, not a passive, process. Impaired relaxation is an early event in angina pectoris. A proposed metabolic explanation is that generation of energy is impaired, which effect diminishes the supply of ATP required for early diastolic uptake of calcium by the SR. The result is that the return to normal of the cytosolic calcium level (at a peak in systole) is delayed in the early diastolic period. In other conditions, too, there is a relationship between the rate of diastolic decay of the calcium transient and diastolic relaxation. In hypothyroidism the rate of return of the elevated cytosolic calcium during systole is delayed in early diastole, slowing the rate of relaxation; the opposite occurs in hyperthyroidism. In congestive heart failure, diastolic relaxation also is delayed and irregular, as is the rate of decay of the cytosolic calcium elevation. Most patients with coronary artery disease have a variety of abnormalities of diastolic filling that are probably related to those also associated with angina pectoris. Theoretically, such abnormalities of relaxation are potentially reversible, because they depend on changes in patterns of calcium ion movement.

## ■ PHASES OF DIASTOLE

Diastole can be divided into four hemodynamic phases, using the clinical definitions according to which diastole extends from aortic valve closure to the start of the first heart sound. The first phase of diastole (see preceding section) is the isovolumic phase, which, by definition, does not contribute to ventricular filling (Fig. 3–10). The second phase of early (rapid) filling provides most of the ventricular filling. At this stage, active ventricular relaxation may occur, which would explain ventricular suction. The third phase, slow filling or diastasis, accounts for only 5% of the total filling. The final atrial booster phase accounts for the remaining 15%.

### Atrial Function

The left atrium, well-known for its function as a blood-receiving chamber, also acts as follows: First, by presystolic contraction and its booster function, it helps to complete LV filling.[18] Second, it is the volume sensor of the heart, releasing atrial natriuretic peptide in response to intermittent stretch. Third, the atrium contains receptors for the afferent arms of various reflexes, including mechanoreceptors that increase sinus discharge rate, thus contributing to the tachycardia of exercise as the venous return increases (Bainbridge reflex).

The atria are different in structure and function from the ventricles in a number of respects, having smaller myocytes with shorter-lived action potential as well as a "more fetal type" of myosin (in both heavy and light chains). Furthermore, the atria are more reliant on the phosphatidylinositol signal transduction pathway, which may explain the relatively greater positive inotropic effect in the atria than

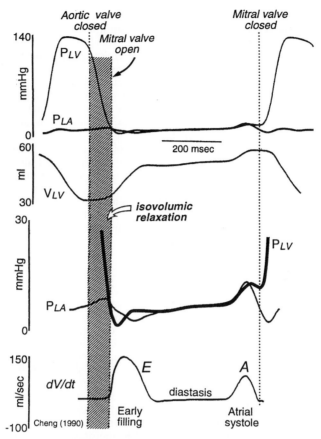

**Figure 3–10** ■ Diastolic filling phases. *Top panel,* Left ventricular pressure (P_LV), left atrial pressure (P_LA), and left ventricular volume (V_LV). *Middle panel,* Magnified scale of changes in P_LV and P_LA. *Lower panel,* Rate of change of left ventricular volume (dV/dt), an indication of the rate of left ventricular filling. Left ventricular filling, shown by an increased dV/dt, occurs early in diastole and during atrial systole in response to a pressure gradient from the left atrium to the left ventricle. In between is the phase of slow filling or diastasis. The early diastolic pressure gradient is generated as left ventricular pressure falls below left atrial pressure. The late diastolic gradient is generated as atrial contraction increases left atrial pressure above left ventricular pressure. (Data from Cheng CP, Freeman GL, Santamore WP, et al: Effect of loading conditions, contractile state and heart rate on early diastolic left ventricular filling in conscious dogs. Circ Res 1990;66:814. Copyright 1990 American Heart Association.)

in the ventricles in response to angiotensin II. The more rapid atrial repolarization is attributed to increased outward potassium currents, such as $I_{to}$ and $I_{kACh}$. In addition, some atrial cells have the capacity for spontaneous depolarization. In general, these histologic and physiologic changes can be related to the decreased need for the atria to generate high intrachamber pressures, rather being sensitive to volume changes, while retaining enough contractile action to help with LV filling and to respond to inotropic stimuli.

## Diastolic Dysfunction in Hypertrophy and Failure

In hypertrophic hearts like those affected by chronic hypertension or severe aortic stenosis, abnormalities of diastole are common and may antedate systolic failure. Diastolic dysfunction is marked by a number of important differences from systolic failure. The mechanism is not clear, though it is thought to be related to the extent of ventricular hypertrophy or, indirectly, to a stiff left atrium. Conceptually, impaired relaxation must be distinguished from prolonged systolic contraction with delayed onset of normal relaxation. Experimentally, several defects have been identified in early hypertensive hypertrophy, including decreased rates of contraction and relaxation and decreased peak force development. Loss of the load-sensitive component of relaxation may be due to impaired activity of the SR. Impaired relaxation is associated with a decrease in early filling and an apparent increase of the late (atrial) filling phase, so that E/A ratio, as derived from the mitral Doppler pattern, declines. In time, with both increased hypertrophy and the development of fibrosis, LV chamber compliance decreases and the E wave again becomes more prominent. Thus, it may be difficult to separate truly normal from *pseudonormal patterns of mitral inflow.*

In *myocardial failure*, many abnormalities can also be detected in the transmitral flow pattern, including an early change in the E/A ratio. It must be stressed that the E/A ratio changes considerably as LV failure becomes progressively more severe with late-phase "pseudonormalization."

## ■ COMPLIANCE

The diastolic volume of the heart is influenced not only by the loading conditions but also by the elastic properties of the myocardium. *Elasticity* enables the myocardium to recover its normal shape after removal of the systolic stress. *Compliance* is strictly defined as the relation between the change in stress and the resultant *strain* (percentage change in dimension or size). In clinical practice, compliance is taken as the ratio of dP to dV; that is, the rate of pressure change divided by the rate of volume change. The relation is curvilinear, as shown by the line *e-d-a* in Figure 3–2, and the initial slope of the change is gentle. As the pressure increases, the volume increases less and less, so that there is a considerable increase of pressure for only a small increase in volume. The term *diastolic distensibility* is often used interchangeably with *diastolic compliance*. Strictly, distensibility refers not to the slope of the pressure-volume relation but to the diastolic pressure required to fill the ventricle to a given volume. When compliance decreases, distensibility is reduced, as it is in a failing human heart. Resting *stiffness* may in part be attributed to the unique myocardial collagen network, which is thought to counteract the high systolic pressure normally developed in the ventricles. Pathologic loss of compliance is usually due to abnormalities of the myocardium. True loss of muscular compliance can have a variety of causes—acute ischemia, as in angina; fibrosis, as after myocardial infarction; or infiltrations that cause restrictive cardiomyopathy. In angina, the increased temporary stiffness may be caused by a combination of a rise in intracellular calcium and alterations in myocardial properties. With myocardial infarction, the connective tissue undergoes changes soon after occlusion. Eventually, healing and fibrosis permanently increase stiffness. When muscle stiffness increases, so does *chamber stiffness* (the chamber in this case being the ventricle).

The compliance of the heart affects the Starling curve, the pressure-volume loop, and the early diastolic filling rate of the heart. A stiffer heart will be on a lower Starling curve; the baseline of the pressure-volume loop will rise more abruptly, and higher left atrial pressure will be required for early diastolic filling. For these reasons, compliance fundamentally determines the mechanical properties of the heart.

## ■ CONTRACTILE PROPERTIES IN HUMAN HEART DISEASE

The failing human myocardium has impaired contractile properties, so that, even when the venous filling pressure is adequate, the stroke volume is less than it would normally be and the blood pressure tends to fall. An increase in heart rate compensates somewhat to help maintain cardiac output (and, in turn, blood pressure). Nonetheless, the treppe effect is lost and internal work is increased relative to external work. Homeostatic mechanisms that come into play sustain the blood pressure, but the severely failing myocardium does this at the cost of decreased efficiency of work. Other defects include an impaired response to increased preload, defective generation of cyclic AMP in response to β-adrenergic stimulation, and numerous defects of the patterns of handling of intracellular calcium. In response to increased afterload, the intracellular calcium transient of trabecular myocardium from the severely failing human heart shows an abnormally prolonged and exaggerated pattern of rise, despite poor generation of force. Whether the Frank-Starling response is truly defective or whether apparent defects can be explained by the decreased distensibility is a subject of debate.

In aortic valve disease, the increased volume load of aortic regurgitation contrasts with the pressure load of aortic stenosis. In aortic stenosis, kinetic work increases sharply as the cross-sectional area narrows, and pressure work increases as the gradient across the aortic valve rises. Therefore, both types of work increase myocardial oxygen demand. In aortic regurgitation, heart work and oxygen demand are increased by the increased wall stress that results from the greater ventricular volume and by increased afterload. The latter results both from the associated systolic hypertension and from the increased wall stress caused by the greater volume load.

# ■ REFERENCES

1. Katz AM: Physiology of the Heart, 2nd ed. New York: Raven, 1992:453.
2. Brutsaert DL, Sys SU, Gilbert TC: Diastolic failure: Pathophysiology and therapeutic implications. J Am Coll Cardiol 1993;22:318–325.
3. Frank O: Zur dynamik des Herzmuskels. Z Biol 1895;32:370–447.
4. Starling EH: The Linacre Lecture on the Law of the Heart. London: Longmans, 1918.
5. Fuchs F: Mechanical modulation of the $Ca^{2+}$ regulatory protein complex in cardiac muscle. NIPS 1995;10:6–12.
6. Solaro RJ, Rarick HM: Troponin and tropomysin: Proteins that switch on and tune in the activity of cardiac myofilaments. Circ Res 1998;83:471–480.
7. Fitzsimons DP, Moss RL: Strong binding of myosin modulates length-dependent $Ca^{2+}$ activation or rat ventricular myocytes. Circ Res 1998;83:602–607.
8. Luo W, Grupp IL, Harrer J, et al: Targeted ablation of the phospholamban gene is associated with markedly enhanced myocardial contractility and loss of beta-agonist stimulation. Circ Res 1994;75:401–409.
9. Mulieri LA, Leavitt BJ, Martin BJ: Myocardial force-frequency defect in mitral regurgitation heart failure is reversed by forskolin. Circulation 1993;88:2700–2704.
10. Fenelon G, Wijns W, Andries E, Brugada P: Tachycardiomyopathy: Mechanisms and clinical implications. PACE 1996;19:95–105.
11. Flamm SD, Taki J, Moore R, et al: Redistribution of regional and organ blood volume and effect on cardiac function in relation to upright exercise intensity in healthy human subjects. Circulation 1990;81:1550–1559.
12. Poliner LR, Dehmer GJ, Lewis SE, et al: Left ventricular performance in normal subjects: A comparison of the responses to exercise in the upright and supine positions. Circulation 1980;62:528–534.
13. Iskandrian AS, Hakki AH, DePace NL, et al: Evaluation of left ventricular function by radionuclide angiography during exercise in normal subjects and in patients with chronic coronary heart disease. J Am Coll Cardiol 1983;1:1518–1529.
14. Upton M, Rerych SK, Roeback JR Jr, et al: Effect of brief and prolonged exercise on left ventricular function. Am J Cardiol 1980;45:1154–1160.
15. Bar-Shlomo B-Z, Druck MN, Morch JE, et al: Left ventricular function in trained and untrained healthy subjects. Circulation 1982;65:484–488.
16. Vahl CF, Bonz A, Timek T, Hagl S: Intracellular calcium transient of working human myocardium of seven patients transplanted for congestive heart failure. Circ Res 1994;74:952–958.
17. Schiller NB, Foster E: Analysis of left ventricular systolic function. Heart 1996;(Suppl 2)75:17–26.
18. Hoit BD, Shao Y, Gabel M, Walsh RA: In vivo assessment of left atrial contractile performance in normal and pathological conditions using a time-varying elastance model. Circulation 1994;89:1829–1838.

19. Wiggers CJ: Modern Aspects of Circulation in Health and Disease. Philadelphia: Lea & Febiger, 1915.
20. Lind AR, McNicol GW: Muscular factors which determine the cardiovascular responses to sustained and rhythmic exercise. Can Med Assn J 1967;96:703–713.
21. Waldrop TG, Eldridge FL, Iwamoto GA, Mitchell JH: Central neural control of respiration and circulation during exercise. *In* Rowell LB, Shepherd JT (eds): Handbook of Physiology, Section 12. New York: Oxford University Press, 1996:333–380.

## ■ RECOMMENDED READING

Katz AM: Physiology of the Heart, 2nd ed. Chapters 13–17. New York: Raven, 1992.
Opie LH: The Heart. Physiology, from Cell to Circulation. Chapters 12–15. Philadelphia: Lippincott-Raven, 1998.
Opie LH: Mechanisms of cardiac contraction and relaxation. *In* Braunwald E (ed): Heart Disease, 5th ed. Philadelphia: WB Saunders, 1997:360–393.
Schlant R, Sonnenblick EH, Katz AM: Normal physiology of the cardiovascular system. *In* Alexander RW, Schlant RC, Fuster V (eds): The Heart, Arteries and Veins, 9th ed. New York: McGraw-Hill, 1998:81–124.

*Chapter* **4**

# Vascular Function

*Clive Rosendorff*

All blood vessels have an outer adventitia, a medial layer of smooth muscle cells, and an intima lined by endothelial cells. Contraction of the vascular smooth muscle causes changes in the diameter and the wall tension of blood vessels. In the aorta and large arteries, vascular smooth muscle contraction affects mainly the compliance (the reciprocal of stiffness) of the vessel. At the precapillary level, contraction of vascular smooth muscle regulates blood flow to different organs and contributes to the peripheral resistance. Compliance of large vessels and resistance of arterioles contribute most of the impedance of the vascular circuit, and, therefore, the afterload of the heart. The capacity of the circulation is determined by the degree of contraction of the veins ("capacitance vessels"), especially in the splanchnic area; this affects the venous filling pressure, or preload, of the heart.

## ■ TRANSMEMBRANE ION CONCENTRATIONS AND POTENTIALS

### Potassium[1]

The resting membrane potential ($E_m$) of excitable cells, including vascular smooth muscle cells (VSMC), depends on the concentration gradients between the extracellular fluid (o) and the cytoplasm (i), and relative permeabilities (P), of $Na^+$, $K^+$, and $Cl^-$ across the cell membrane, given by the Goldman constant field equation:

$$E_m = 61 \log \frac{P_{Na}[Na^+]_o + P_K[K^+]_o + P_{Cl}[Cl^-]_i}{P_{Na}[Na^+]_i + P_K[K^+]_i + P_{Cl}[Cl^-]_o}$$

In resting cells, $E_m$ is determined mainly by the $K^+$ permeability and gradient, because $P_K$ is very much greater than $P_{Na}$ or $P_{Cl}$. At rest, $P_K$ is directly related to the whole cell $K^+$ current $I_K = N\ i\ Pro$, where $N$ is the total number of membrane $K^+$ channels, $i$ is the single-channel current, and $Pro$ is the open state probability of a $K^+$ channel. Thus, when $K^+$ channels close, $Pro$, $I_K$, and $P_K$ decrease, and cell membranes depolarize toward their threshold for firing (i.e., become more excitable). Conversely, anything that opens $K^+$ channels hyperpolarizes the membranes and makes them less excitable.

In vascular smooth muscle cells (VSMC), this effect is amplified by the effect of the resting membrane potential on voltage-gated $Ca^{2+}$ channels. When closure or inactivation of $K^+$ channels lowers $E_m$, voltage-gated $Ca^{2+}$ channels open, producing vasoconstriction. Defective or attenuated $K^+$ channels have been described in some types of essential hypertension, primary pulmonary hypertension, and hypoxia- or fenfluramine-induced pulmonary hypertension. The opposite is also true. Agents that open $K^+$ channels hyperpolarize cells and render them less excitable. In VSMC, this translates to vasodilatation. Such agents include β-adrenergic agonists, muscarinic agonists, nitroglycerin, nitric oxide, prostacyclin, and "potassium-channel openers" such as cromakalim, now being developed as antihypertensive drugs.

## Sodium[2]

The major active transport pathway for $Na^+$ in mammalian cells is the $Na^+$ pump, or $Na^+$-$K^+$-adenosine triphosphatase ($Na^+$-$K^+$-ATPase)-dependent $Na^+$-$K^+$ exchanger ("$Na^+$ pump"; Fig. 4–1). This results in large concentration gradients for $Na^+$ (outside greater than inside) and $K^+$ (inside greater than outside), which keep the membrane polarized and result in a number of "passive" $Na^+$ transporters that allow movement of $Na^+$ from outside the cell to the interior along a concentration gradient.

All of these $Na^+$ fluxes have been studied intensively, mainly in red blood cells, in the context of human hypertension. In theory, any abnormality that reduces the electrochemical gradient for $Na^+$ across the vascular smooth muscle membrane (i.e., increases intracellular $Na^+$) lowers the threshold for those cells to contract. In the renal tubule cells, any increase in $Na^+$ influx (via passive $Na^+$ transport) on the luminal side of the cell or of $Na^+$ efflux (via the $Na^+$ pump) on the abluminal side causes $Na^+$ retention. Both vascular smooth muscle hypertonicity and renal $Na^+$ retention are important mechanisms of hypertension.

### Disorders of Active Sodium Transport

Many studies have shown increased $Na^+$ content of red blood cells in patients with hypertension, a finding ascribed to a deficiency of the $Na^+$-$K^+$-ATPase pump. It has been suggested that this may be due to a circulating endogenous ouabain-like hormone. In vascular smooth muscle, the increased intracellular $Na^+$ concentration

## Cellular Sodium Transport Pathways

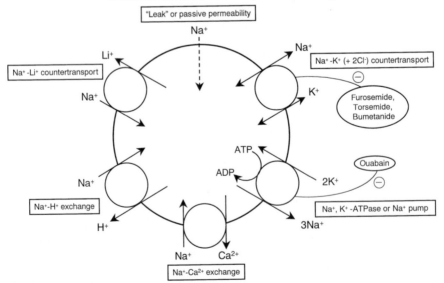

**Figure 4–1** ▪ Major cation transport pathways across cell membranes. For details, see text. ADP, adenosine diphosphate; ATP, adenosine triphosphate.

would reduce the resting membrane potential to lower the threshold of activation. Also, the increased cytosolic $Na^+$ would slow $Na^+$-$Ca^{2+}$ exchange, increasing intracellular free $Ca^{2+}$ levels. The result would be an increase in both cardiac and vascular smooth muscle contractility, and hypertension.

## Disorders of Passive Sodium Transport

**$Na^+$-$H^+$ Exchange.** The $Na^+$-$H^+$ antiporter is activated by several growth factors, including angiotensin II(A II), and the resulting change in intracellular pH is thought to be an important step in the sequence of events that leads to vascular smooth muscle hypertrophy/hyperplasia.

**$Na^+$-$K^+$ (+ $2Cl^-$) Cotransport.** This is inhibited by loop diuretics such as furosemide, torsemide, and bumetanide, and some hypertensive patients have been shown to have abnormal cotransport activity.

**$Na^+$-$Li^+$ Countertransport.** Some studies have shown abnormalities of this quantitatively minor transport pathway in red blood cells—and, by inference, in VSMC. Since $Na^+$-$Li^+$ countertransport seems to be controlled by a single gene, this has given rise to much work on $Na^+$-$Li^+$ countertransport as a potential genetic marker for hypertension, marred by the finding of considerable overlap between hypertensive and normotensive persons.

**Passive $Na^+$ Transport.** In some, but by no means all, patients with hypertension, there is increased passive inward flux (or "leak") of $Na^+$.

## ■ VASCULAR SMOOTH MUSCLE CONTRACTION AND RELAXATION[3]

The contractile activity of VSMC depends largely on changes in cytoplasmic calcium concentration, which in turn depends on calcium influx from the extracellular fluid or on release of calcium from intracellular stores, mainly in the endoplasmic reticulum. At rest, the plasma membrane of VSMC is relatively impermeable to $Ca^{2+}$. On activation, calcium channels open, allowing influx of $Ca^{2+}$ along a concentration gradient (Fig. 4–2). There are three types of calcium channels. The voltage-operated (or potential-operated) calcium channels are regulated by changes in membrane potential, and receptor-operated channels by transmitter-receptor or drug-receptor reactions. The third, much smaller, component is a passive leak pathway.

Release of $Ca^{2+}$ from the sarcoplasmic reticulum (SR) is activated by two mechanisms. First, influx of $Ca^{2+}$ through transmembrane $Ca^{2+}$ channels causes an increase in cytosolic calcium, a phenomenon called *$Ca^{2+}$-induced $Ca^{2+}$ release*, which amplifies the increase in cytosolic $Ca^{2+}$ produced by $Ca^{2+}$ flux across the membrane. Second, $Ca^{2+}$ release from the SR is controlled by a receptor on the SR, the inositol trisphosphate ($IP_3$) receptor discussed later.

The $Ca^{2+}$ released into the cytoplasm forms a complex with calmodulin, and this complex binds to and activates the catalytic subunit of myosin light chain kinase, which, in turn, phosphorylates myosin light chain, permitting ATPase activation of myosin crossbridges by actin.

Relaxation of vascular smooth muscle may occur by any combination of the following mechanisms: (1) hyperpolarization of the vascular smooth muscle membrane; (2) inhibition of $Ca^{2+}$ entry; (3) increase in the cytoplasmic concentration of cyclic 3',5'-adenosine monophosphate (cAMP); and (4) increased formation of cyclic 3',5'-guanosine monophosphate (cGMP).

## Hyperpolarization

The resting membrane potential in VSMC, as in all cells, depends on the transmembrane gradient of diffusible ions, particularly $Na^+$ and $K^+$. Changes in

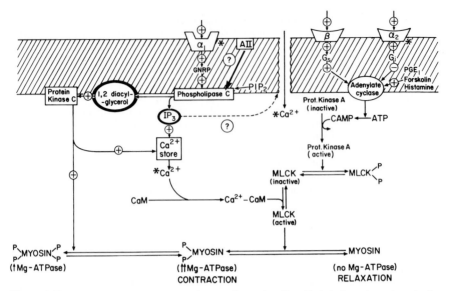

**Figure 4–2** ■ Adrenergic receptors on vascular smooth muscle cells, with their downstream transduction mechanisms. $\alpha_1$-Receptors, which mediate vasoconstriction, act via a guanine nucleotide regulatory protein (GNRP or G protein) to activate phospholipase C, the enzyme that converts phosphatidylinositol bisphosphate ($PIP_2$) to 1,2-diacylglycerol and inositol 1,4,5-trisphosphate ($IP_3$). $IP_3$ releases $Ca^{2+}$ from the endoplasmic reticulum, and may also open receptor-operated $Ca^{2+}$ channels. $Ca^{2+}$ forms complexes with calmodulin (CaM), and the complex activates myosin light-chain kinase (MLCK), which in turn phosphorylates myosin to facilitate contraction. $\beta$-Receptors, mainly $\beta_2$, act via a stimulatory G protein ($G_s$) to activate adenylate cyclase, increase cyclic AMP (cAMP), and thus activate protein kinase A. Protein kinase A phosphorylates and thus inactivates MLCK, causing relaxation of the smooth muscle cell. $\alpha_2$-Receptors, via an inhibitory G protein ($G_i$), inhibit adenylate cyclase and are, therefore, vasoconstrictors.

the resting membrane potential may affect the gating of calcium channels in the plasma membrane or may modify $Na^+$-$Ca^{2+}$ exchange. Hyperpolarization can be produced by activating the $Na^+$-$K^+$-ATPase system, whereby three $Na^+$ ions are extruded from the cell in exchange for two $K^+$ ions pumped in. This reduces calcium influx via voltage-operated calcium channels and stimulates $Na^+$-$Ca^{2+}$ countertransport to promote $Ca^{2+}$ efflux. This may be the mechanism of the relaxation induced by the endothelium-derived hyperpolarizing factor (EDHF). Another mechanism for hyperpolarization involves increased membrane permeability to $K^+$, which allows greater efflux of $K^+$ along its concentration gradient producing a greater (i.e., more negative) resting membrane potential. This action is the basis for the development of a new class of antihypertensive and vasodilator drugs such as cromakalim, pinacidil, and nicorandil, agents known as *K+-channel openers.*

## Inhibition of Calcium Entry

Calcium channel blockers, or calcium antagonists, block receptor-activated or voltage-activated $Ca^{2+}$ influx. They do not inhibit intracellular release of $Ca^{2+}$, reduce passive $Ca^{2+}$ entry ($Ca^{2+}$ leak), or stimulate $Ca^{2+}$ extrusion ($Ca^{2+}$-ATPase and $Na^+$-$Ca^{2+}$ countertransport).

## Increase in Cyclic Adenosine Monophosphate

Beta-adrenergic receptors on the plasma membrane promote conversion of ATP to cAMP via the enzyme adenylate cyclase. Adenylate cyclase is coupled to the receptor by a guanine nucleotide–binding protein (G protein). In the cell, cAMP binds to and activates cAMP-dependent protein kinase, which in turn phosphorylates myosin light chain kinase, blocking contraction and therefore reducing vasomotor tone (see Fig. 5–2).

## ■ ADRENERGIC NEUROTRANSMITTERS[4, 5]

Figure 4–3 shows the biosynthetic pathway of the synthesis of the catecholamines dopamine, norepinephrine (NE), and epinephrine (E), all of which play very important roles in cardiovascular functions. This biosynthesis occurs in adrenergic nerves (up to the NE stage) and in the adrenal medulla.

Catecholamines are stored in adrenergic nerve terminals and in adrenal chromaffin cells in storage vesicles together with ATP and storage proteins called *chromogranins*. Catecholamine concentrations in vesicles are continually being replenished by de novo synthesis from precursors (dopamine β-hydroxylase is localized in the vesicles) and by neuronal reuptake of released NE (called *uptake 1*). NE release and reuptake is described in Figure 4–4 and the metabolism of NE in Figure 4–5. Of the three enzymes principally responsible for the metabolism of NE, two have inhibitors that are used clinically. Monoamine oxidase (MAO) inhibitors work to treat depression by blocking NE metabolism in the central nervous system, and the MAO inhibitor selegiline is used as an adjunct to L-dopa to treat Parkinson's disease. For patients taking an MAO inhibitor, however, ingesting tyramine (for instance in cheese) can cause a life-threatening hypertensive crisis. Catechol-*o*-

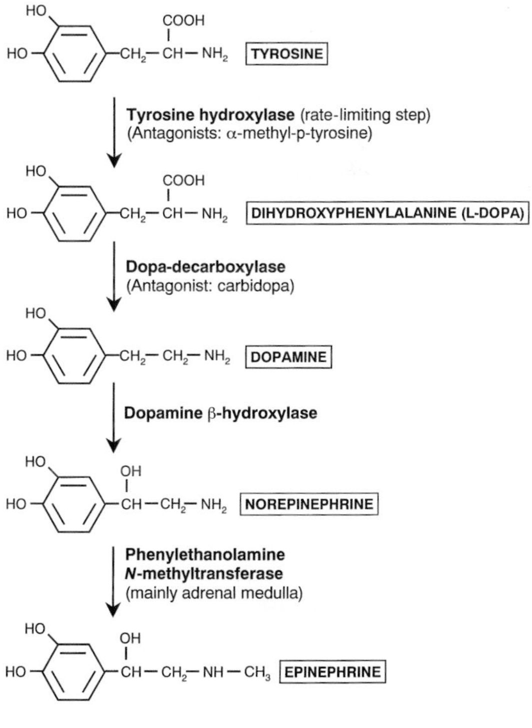

**Figure 4–3** ■ Biosynthesis of catecholamines.

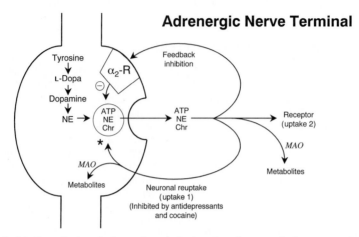

**Figure 4–4** ■ Biosynthesis and release of catecholamines from the sympathetic nerve terminal. Norepinephrine (NE) is stored in vesicles and co-released with ATP and chromogranins (Chr). After release, the NE may activate an adrenergic receptor (uptake 2), may be taken up by the neurone (uptake 1), may inhibit (via prejunctional $\alpha_2$-receptors) the further release of NE, or may be metabolized extraneuronally or intraneuronally. ★, Vesicular uptake of NE (blocked by reserpine).

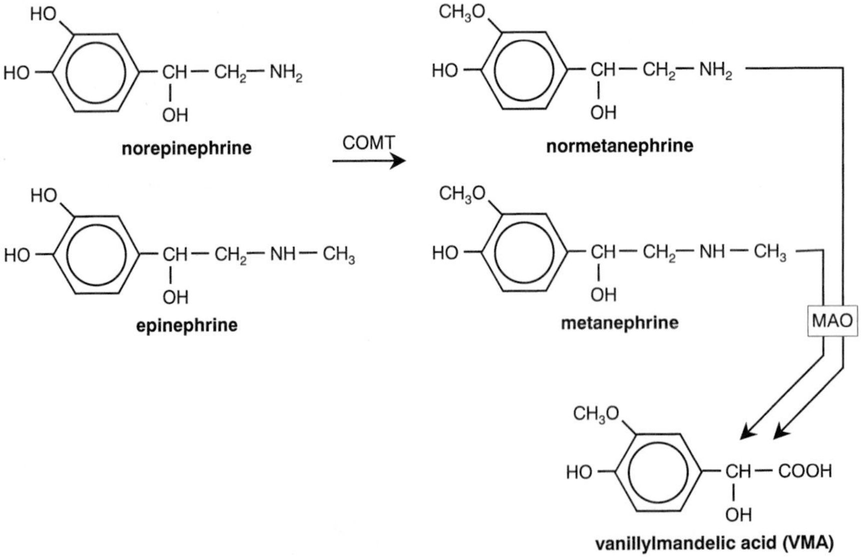

**Figure 4–5** ■ Metabolism of norepinephrine and epinephrine.

methyl transferase inhibitors are used with L-dopa for Parkinson's disease. Measurement of catecholamine metabolites such as vanillylmandelic acid, metanephrine, and normetanephrine in blood or urine is an essential part of the diagnosis of pheochromocytoma (see Chapter 31).

## Adrenergic Receptors

The main adrenergic receptors, $\alpha$ and $\beta$, are subdivided into $\alpha_1$-, $\alpha_2$-, $\beta_1$-, and $\beta_2$-adrenergic receptors. Currently, nine subtypes are known, $\alpha_{1A,B,C}$, $\alpha_{2A,B,C}$, and $\beta_{1,2,3}$. In VSMC, there are $\alpha_1$, $\alpha_2$, and $\beta_2$ receptors. In all three types, the actions on the VSMC are mediated by G proteins (Fig. 4–2).

Receptors designated $\alpha_1$ are more sensitive to NE than to E and are vasoconstrictors. Their action is mediated by a $G_q$ protein with activation of phospholipase C but also by direct activation of $Ca^{2+}$ channels, activation of $Na^+$-$H^+$ and $Na^+$-$Ca^{2+}$ exchange, and inhibition of $K^+$ channels. Phospholipase C catalyzes the conversion of phosphatidyl inositol bisphosphate (PIP$_2$) to inositol trisphosphate (IP$_3$) and 1,2,-diacylglycerol (DAG). IP$_3$ acts on an IP$_3$ receptor on the sarcoplasmic membrane to release $Ca^{2+}$ into the cytoplasm, which binds with calmodulin (CaM) to form a $Ca^{2+}$-CaM complex. This complex activates myosin light chain kinase (MLCK) to effect phosphorylation of myosin, and thus contraction. DAC activates protein kinase C (PKC). In addition to initiating VSMC contraction, sustained stimulation of $\alpha_1$ receptors also switches on cell processes that lead to hypertrophy or hyperplasia, via the released $Ca^{2+}$ and the PKC, both of which stimulate growth and proliferation through a variety of mechanisms, including the MAP-kinase system (see the Renin-Angiotensin System later).

Vascular $\beta$ receptors, mainly $\beta_2$, are linked to a $G_s$ (stimulatory) protein, and the $G_s$ protein activates adenylate cyclase, which converts ATP to cAMP. cAMP activates protein kinase A (PKA), which phosphorylates, and, therefore inactivates, MLCK. Stimulation of $\beta$ receptors thus causes vasodilation. Beta-adrenergic-blocking drugs are therefore directly vasoconstricting (and, so, are contraindicated in persons with peripheral vascular disease); their antihypertensive action is due to their actions on the heart to reduce cardiac output and on the kidneys to block renin release.

Alpha$_2$ receptors have a potency order E > NE and, like $\alpha_1$ receptors, are also vasoconstricting, but via a different mechanism. Alpha$_2$ receptors couple with inhibitory G proteins (G$_i$) to inhibit membrane-related adenylate cyclase, and, therefore, they have inhibitory actions on the formation of cAMP, activated PKA, and phosphorylated MLCK, all effects that cause vasoconstriction. There are also $\alpha_2$ adrenergic receptors (ARs) as autoreceptors on postganglionic sympathetic nerve terminals, which synthesize and release NE. These prejunctional $\alpha_2$-ARs respond to released (or circulating) catecholamines by inhibiting further release of NE. Also, activation of brain $\alpha_2$ ARs reduces sympathetic outflow, and stimulation of these receptors with clonidine and similar $\alpha_2$ agonists lowers blood pressure.

## Dopamine[7]

Dopamine is not only a precursor of NE and E; it is a neurotransmitter in its own right. VSMC contain both D$_1$ and D$_2$ receptors. D$_1$ receptors are located in the heart (myocardial cells and coronary vessels), VSMC, adrenal cortex (zona glomerulosa cells), and kidney tubule cells. Stimulation of D$_1$ receptors, as by dopamine, dobutamine, or fenoldopam, causes vasodilation by increasing adenylate cyclase and cAMP-dependent PKA, resembling in this respect the $\beta_2$ receptor. It also causes natriuresis and diuresis by affecting $Na^+$-$K^+$ antiport activity to decrease $Na^+$ reabsortion.

$D_2$ receptors are found in the endothelial and adventitial layers of blood vessels, where their function is unknown; on pituitary cells, where they inhibit prolactin secretion and where bromocriptine, a $D_2$ agonist, acts to reduce hyperprolactinemia; and in the zona glomerulosa of the adrenal gland, where they inhibit aldosterone secretion. There are also $D_2$ receptors on the sympathetic nerve terminal that inhibit NE release.

## ■ THE RENIN-ANGIOTENSIN SYSTEM[7-9]

The major components of the renin-angiotensin system are angiotensinogen, renin, angiotensin I (AI), angiotensin-converting enzyme (ACE), and A II. Angiotensinogen, a large, globular protein, is synthesized in the liver. The enzyme renin cleaves a leucine-valine bond in the N-terminal region of human angiotensinogen to produce the decapeptide A I. The major source of renin is the juxtaglomerular cells of the afferent arterioles of the kidneys. Translation of renin mRNA in these cells produces preprorenin, which in turn is converted to prorenin. Juxtaglomerular cells convert some prorenin to renin, and both are secreted. Prorenin is the more abundant circulating form of renin, however; the principal site of conversion of prorenin to renin is not known. Prorenin mRNA is expressed in very small amounts or is absent in blood vessels, but vascular tissue avidly takes up prorenin, which suggests that blood vessels may be the principal site of formation of renin from circulating prorenin. Some controversy surrounds whether renin is synthesized to any significant extent in cardiovascular tissue or is derived entirely from plasma uptake.

ACE converts A I to the octopeptide angiotensin II (A II) and inactivates bradykinin. Bradykinin stimulates the release of vasodilating prostaglandins and nitric oxide and may be responsible for ACE inhibitor–induced cough.

Some enzymatic pathways independent of ACE (tissue-type plasminogen activator [tPA], cathepsin, tonin, and elastase) allow for the formation of A II directly from angiotensinogen. Enzymes other than ACE (tPA, tonin, cathepsin G, chymase, and a chymostatin-sensitive A II-generating enzyme [CAGE]) catalyze the formation of A II from A I. The importance of these pathways is obscure; in particular, it is not known whether these non-ACE pathways are present in vivo or whether they are activated only when the conventional ACE pathway is blocked. Also, there is little if any experimental evidence that ACE-independent pathways contribute substantially to A II biosynthesis or to vascular hypertrophy.

### Angiotensin II Receptors

Two major A II receptor types exist, $AT_1$ and $AT_2$. The $AT_1$ receptors are found in vascular tissues and many others and are almost certainly the receptors that transduce A II–mediated cardiovascular actions, as discussed in the next section.

Less is known about $AT_2$ receptors. The fact that the $AT_2$-binding sites are much more abundant in fetal and neonatal tissue than in adult tissue, suggests that $AT_2$ has a role in development. Localization is mainly in the brain. It is probable, therefore, that $AT_2$ receptors have little to do with the acute cardiovascular actions of A II. Also, as described later, most of the growth-promoting effects of A II on arteries seem to be mediated by $AT_1$ receptors. Some recent evidence, however, indicates that $AT_2$ receptor expression is related to the suppression of VSMC growth, in contrast to the growth-promoting effect of stimulating $AT_1$ receptors.[10]

## Angiotensin II Signal Transduction Pathways for Mitogenesis and Growth

The $AT_1$ receptors are present in vascular tissues and many others and seem to mediate the vasoconstricting and growth-stimulating effects of A II in vascular smooth muscle. Like the $\alpha_1$ receptor, the $AT_1$ receptor is coupled to a G protein that activates phosphatidyl inositol bisphosphate ($PIP_2$) to inositol 1,4,5-trisphosphate ($IP_3$) and DAG; (Fig. 4–6). $IP_3$, acting through the $IP_3$ receptor ($IP_3R$) on the endoplasmic reticulum, stimulates the mobilization of $Ca^{2+}$ from intracellular stores, a process accelerated also by the influx of $Ca^{2+}$ through voltage-dependent $Ca^{2+}$ channels during activation. The increase the cytosolic $Ca^{2+}$ concentration is an essential component of both the activation of the contractile proteins of vascular smooth muscle and the mediation of growth-promoting actions of A II and other growth factors, at least partly through protein kinase C (PKC) activation.

An alternative pathway for the formation of DAG is the hydrolysis of phosphatidylcholine (PC) phospholipase C (PLC) or D (PLD). Both DAG and $Ca^{2+}$ activate a PKC that has many actions. PKC affects transmembrane $Na^+$-$K^+$ exchange to alkalinize the cytoplasm, which is important in mitogenesis. PKC activates a serum response element found on the promoter region of c-*fos*, an early-response proto-oncogene activated by A II that is thought to be a major factor in initiating the nuclear events that result in cell proliferation and growth.

There are alternative signal transduction pathways for A II. One of these is the mitogen-activate protein (MAP) kinase cascade. Although many components of this pathway have been identified, it is not known how A II (which binds to a G protein–coupled receptor that lacks intrinsic tyrosine kinase activity) feeds into the MAP kinase phosphorylation cascade. One possibility is PKC regulation of Raf-1 kinase. Convincing evidence, nevertheless, shows that the MAP kinase pathway mediates some of the vascular growth–promoting actions of A II. This pathway and related ones are shown in Figure 4–6.

We still do not know to what extent these signal transduction pathways are shared by receptors that mediate vasoconstriction, and possibly vascular hypertrophy, for example $AT_1$, $\alpha_1$-adrenergic receptors, and endothelin receptors. We also do not know much about the physiologic specificity of these pathways, such as which ones are essential for cell hypertrophy or hyperplasia, which activate c-*fos*, c-*jun*, or c-*myc* selectively, and which of the myriad intracellular events activated by A II depend on which pathway. It is obvious, however, that this is an area of research where there is enormous potential for the development of new and very precise gene and drug therapies for many clinical problems.

## Atherogenic Effects of Angiotensin II

Depending on what model is studied, A II can produce VSMC hypertrophy alone, hypertrophy and DNA synthesis without cell division (polyploidy), or DNA synthesis with cell division (hyperplasia). These different effects of A II on different cell and animal models of hypertension are difficult to explain. Several lines of evidence suggest, however, that A II stimulates both proliferative and antiproliferative cell processes. The proliferative actions include the stimulation via $AT_1$ receptors of the growth factors platelet-derived growth factor A chain (PDGF-A) and basic fibroblast growth factor (bFGF). The antiproliferative processes include transforming growth factor $\beta_1$ (TGF-$\beta1$). Another antiproliferative mechanism is the ability of the $AT_2$ receptor to mediate programmed cell death (apoptosis) by dephosphorylation of MAP kinase or to inhibit guanylate cyclase.

A II also has a profound effect on the composition of the extracellular matrix

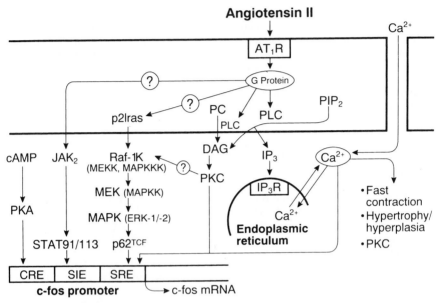

**Figure 4–6** ■ Signal transduction pathways for the angiotensin II receptor (subtype $AT_1$). The receptor is coupled to a guanine nucleotide–binding regulatory protein (G protein), which activates phospholipase C (PLC). PLC catalyzes the hydrolysis of phosphatidylinositol bisphosphate ($PIP_2$) to inositol 1,4,5-trisphosphate ($IP_3$) and 1,2-diacylglycerol (DAG). Inositol 1,4,5-trisphosphate, acting through the $IP_3$ receptor ($IP_3R$) on the endoplasmic reticulum, stimulates the mobilization of $Ca^{2+}$ from intracellular stores, a process also accelerated by the influx of $Ca^{2+}$ through voltage-dependent $Ca^{2+}$ channels during activation ($Ca^{2+}$-dependent $Ca^{2+}$ release). Free cytosolic $Ca^{2+}$ has many actions relating to contractility and cell hypertrophy or hyperplasia, including the activation of protein kinase C (PKC). An alternative pathway for the formation of DAG is hydrolysis of phosphatidylcholine (PC) by PLC. DAG activates PKC, which in turn may induce hypertrophy or hyperplasia through several mechanisms, one of which is the activation of a serum response element (SRE) on the c-*fos* promoter. The SRE also interacts with products of the mitogen-activated protein (MAP) kinase phosphorylation cascade. Both PKC and a small–molecular weight guanine nucleotide–binding protein, p21*ras*, regulate the serine/threonine kinase Raf kinase (Raf-1K), which acts as an MEK kinase (or MAP kinase kinase kinase). MEK (*MAP/ERK* kinase) is a MAP kinase kinase, and the MAP kinase has two active isoforms, *e*xtracellular signal-regulated *k*inases, ERK-1 and ERK-2. Activated MAP kinase substrates include the transcription factor p62[TCF], which forms a complex on the c-*fos* promoter SRE. Angiotensin II also stimulates the phosphorylation and activity of STAT 91 and STAT 113 through the action of *J*anus *k*inase 2 (JAK_2); this interacts with a *sis*-inducing element (SIE) on the c-*fos* promoter. Another c-*fos* promoter element is a cAMP response element (CRE) that is sensitive to protein kinase A (PKA). The significance of this pathway in angiotensin II cell signaling is not known. (Rosendorff C: Vascular hypertrophy in hypertension. Role of the renin-angiotensin system. Mt Sinai J Med 1998;65:108–117.)

of VSMC, including the synthesis and secretion of thrombospondin, fibronectin, and tenascin. Other processes of atherogenesis are stimulated by A II, such as migration of VSMC, the activation and release of tumor necrosis factor α (TNF-α), adhesion to endothelial cells by human peripheral blood monocytes, and thrombosis. A II increases plasminogen activator inhibitor type 1. All of these actions increase the probability that A II is atherogenic and prothrombotic and that ACE inhibitors or A II antagonists may exert some protective effect through these mechanisms.

## Effect of Angiotensin-Converting Enzyme Inhibitors on the Structure of Arteries

Hypertension produces consistent and major changes in the structural and functional properties of arteries and arterioles that increase arterial resistance and stiffness. The changes include these:

- Reductions in the external and internal diameters of the vessel wall without any increase in its cross-sectional area, a process known as *remodeling*
- Altered wall thickness, with medial hypertrophy, myointimal proliferation, and an increase in collagen content
- Increased passive stiffness of the vessel wall, probably caused by the increase in collagen and smooth muscle mass
- Increased active vascular muscle tone caused by a variety of local and extrinsic metabolic and neurohormonal factors.

Many studies show that ACE inhibitors counteract all these mechanisms. Is the prevention of vascular hypertrophy by ACE inhibitors in these animal models of hypertension unique to this class of antihypertensive agents, or is it a nonspecific consequence of blood pressure reduction? Pure vasodilators, such as hydralazine, which increase the plasma level of A II, do not prevent vessel wall thickening, despite the normalization of blood pressure, and ACE inhibitors have been shown to be more effective than other antihypertensive agents (α-blockers, vasodilators) in decreasing vascular hypertrophy, despite similar decreases in blood pressure.

## Angiotensin II Receptor Antagonists

A major advance in antihypertensive drug therapy has been the development of nonpeptide A II receptor antagonists (losartan, irbesartan, candesartan, valsartan) selective for the $AT_1$ receptor subtype, which mediates the vasoconstrictor actions of A II. A critical question is whether the hypertrophic action of A II can also be inhibited by selective $AT_1$ receptor antagonists. These drugs block A II–induced DNA and protein synthesis and intracellular $Ca^{2+}$ mobilization in cultured rat aortic smooth muscle cells, whereas $AT_2$ receptor antagonists have no effect. In intact animals, results have been consistent with those from cell culture; there is a reduction of medial thickness in the aorta and arteries of hypertensive rats after treatment with these agents.

Many questions remain. Is the improved compliance a measure of the regression of vascular smooth muscle hypertrophy or of a decrease in the elastin-collagen matrix, or both? Are the wall thickness changes caused by regression of early atherosclerotic lesions, remodeling of the hypertrophic media, a decrease in the number of individual smooth muscle cells, or a combination of these? To what extent do these changes described in larger arteries reflect those in small-resistance arteries and arterioles?

What do these data, obtained mainly from brachial and common carotid arteries, tell us about the coronary, intracerebral, and intrarenal arteries? Are these improvements in functional and morphologic properties of large arteries markers for improved clinical outcomes?

## ■ ENDOTHELIN[11, 12]

Endothelin is a 21–amino acid peptide (Fig. 4–7) with three isoforms—endothelin 1 (ET-1), endothelin 2 (ET-2), and endothelin 3 (ET-3). First discovered as products of endothelial cells, these peptides have since been shown also to be produced by other cells, including cardiac, renal tubule, and vascular smooth muscle cells. Endothelin is formed from proendothelin (39 aa) by the action of the endothelin-converting enzyme (ECE). Many factors stimulate endothelin release, including hormones (A II, vasopressin, cortisol, catecholamines, insulin), growth factors (transforming growth factor β, insulin-like growth factors), metabolic factors (glucose, low-density lipoprotein cholesterol), hypoxia, and changes in shear stress on the vascular wall (Fig. 4–8).

There are two endothelin receptors, $ET_A$ and $ET_B$. $ET_A$ receptors respond mainly to ET1, are found mainly on VSMC, and mediate vasoconstriction, proliferation, and cell hypertrophy. $ET_B$ receptors have two subtypes, an endothelial receptor activating the release of NO and a vascular smooth muscle receptor mediating vasoconstriction. The $ET_A$ receptor is the predominant type in adult cardiomyocytes, and ETs have both chronotropic and inotropic effects on cardiac muscle and stimulate cardiomyocyte expression of fetal genes, protein synthesis, and growth.

The downstream events initiated by the binding of endothelin to the $ET_A$ receptor (Fig. 4–8) involve activation of phospholipase C to hydrolyze phosphatidylinositol bisphosphate to form $IP_3$ and DAG. $IP_3$ promotes the release of $Ca^{2+}$ from endoplasmic reticulum stores, and $IP_3$ and G proteins may also open voltage-dependent calcium channels in the cell membrane, resulting in an increase in the cytosolic $Ca^{2+}$ concentration, which is essential both for the activation of the contractile proteins in the cell and for cell growth and proliferation. These signal transduction mechanisms of endothelin receptors are shared with $\alpha_1$-receptors and $AT_1$ receptors in the vasculature.

In addition to the pivotal role of cytosolic $Ca^{2+}$ in cell proliferation, the

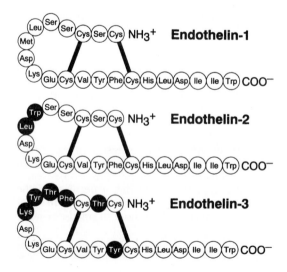

**Figure 4–7** ■ Molecular structure of endothelins 1, 2, and 3. (Rosendorff C: Endothelin, vascular hypertrophy and hypertension. Cardiovasc Drugs Ther 1996;10:795–802.)

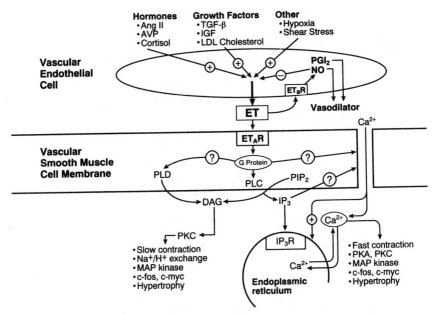

**Figure 4–8** ▪ Stimuli to endothelin (ET) release and ET signal transduction pathways. Hormones, such as angiotensin II (A II), arginine vasopressin (AVP), and cortisol; the growth factors, transforming growth factor beta (TGF-β), insulin-like growth factor (ILGF), and low-density lipoprotein (LDL) cholesterol; and other factors such as hypoxia and shear stress all stimulate ET production and release by vascular endothelial cells. The endothelial cell has $ET_B$ receptors ($ET_B R$), which may mediate vasodilatation by the release of nitric oxide (NO) and prostacyclin ($PGI_2$). NO also inhibits endothelial ET release. The predominant endothelin receptor in the vascular smooth muscle cell membrane is the $ET_A$ type, which is coupled to a guanine nucleotide-binding regulatory protein (G protein) that activates phospholipase C (PLC). PLC catalyzes the hydrolysis of phosphatidylinositol bisphosphate ($PIP_2$) to inositol 1,4,5-trisphosphate ($IP_3$) and 1,2-diacylglycerol (DAG). $IP_3$, acting via the $IP_3$ receptor ($IP_3 R$) on the endoplasmic reticulum membrane, stimulates the release of $Ca^{2+}$ into the cytosol, a process also accelerated by the influx of $Ca^{2+}$ through L-type voltage-dependent $Ca^{2+}$ channels during activation ($Ca^{2+}$-dependent $Ca^{2+}$ release). Free cytosolic $Ca^{2+}$ has a number of actions that relate to contractility and cell hypertrophy, possibly related to protein kinases A and C (PKA, PKC), mitogen-activated protein kinase (MAP kinase), and protooncogenes, such as *c*-fos and *c*-myc. DAG may be formed by the action of PLC or PLD, and it alkalinizes the cytoplasm ($Na^+$-$H^+$ exchange) and activates MAP kinase and protooncogenes, and thus contributes to hypertrophy. (Rosendorff C: Endothelin, vascular hypertrophy and hypertension. Cardiovasc Drugs Ther 1996;10:795–802.)

activation of PKC by DAG may also result in upregulation of the genes concerned with cell growth in both VSMC and cardiac myocytes. This effect may be mediated through a rise in intracellular pH and/or the activation of MAP kinases. MAP kinases are known to induce the phosphorylation of nuclear proteins; thus, the PKC-MAP kinase pathway could be a signaling system that links A II and endothelin activation of cell surface receptors with changes in nuclear activity.

## Endothelin in Hypertension

Convincing evidence for the role of endothelin in hypertension should include demonstration of increased levels of the peptide in plasma or in vascular tissue; potentiation of vasoconstrictor responses because of increased responsiveness of vascular smooth muscle or of a vascular proliferative effect; sustained increase in blood pressure during chronic intravenous infusion; or normalization of elevated blood pressure by endothelin receptor antagonists.

Plasma immunoreactive ET-1 concentration is very slightly increased or normal in most models of hypertension in rats. In hypertensive humans, plasma endothelin levels have been reported as normal or slightly raised or definitely elevated. This does not preclude an important role for endothelin in the pathogenesis of hypertension, because it has been suggested that endothelin release is mainly abluminal; that is, the paracrine release is *from* the endothelial cell *toward* the vascular media, and little if any spills over into the circulation.

Increased plasma endothelin levels (and sympathetic activity and plasma norepinephrine levels) in the offspring of hypertensive parents, but not in the offspring of normotensive parents, are suggestive of genetically determined dysregulation of endothelin release and of the sympathetic nervous system in response to certain stressful stimuli in the former group. The data on vascular responsiveness to endothelin in hypertension are not straightforward. In some animal models of hypertension, responsiveness to endothelin is enhanced, but in sodium and fluid overload models of hypertension in rats and in human hypertension, the ET-1 responses are attenuated. This may be due to downregulation of endothelin receptors in response to the increased production of endothelin.

Chronic intravenous infusion of ET-1 causes sustained hypertension in conscious rats, and endothelin receptor antagonists block the rise of blood pressure in some, but not all, rat models of hypertension. Nonpeptide receptor–selective antagonists are now available, and these will help to establish the importance of endothelin in human hypertension and may lead to the development of an important new class of antihypertensive drugs. Early clinical studies are already under way.

## Cardiac Hypertrophy and Heart Failure

In addition to causing coronary vasoconstriction and myocardial ischemia in persons with hypertension, ET-1, like A II, is a growth factor for cardiac myocytes and may be involved in myocardial hypertrophy. In heart failure, the neurohormonal activation includes the ET system. ET receptor antagonists improve cardiac function and hemodynamics in experimental animals and humans, but this may be due simply to blockade of endothelin-dependent systemic vasoconstriction with reduction of left ventricular afterload.

## Atherosclerosis

All of the main cell components of atherosclerotic lesions—endothelial cells, smooth muscle cells, and macrophages—can express ET-1. In atherosclerosis, ET-1 mRNA expression is increased, and ET-1 accumulates and acts as a chemoattractant for monocytes and macrophages. In animals, selective $ET_A$ receptor blockade decreases the number and size of macrophages and foam cells and reduces neointima formation.

## Coronary Artery Disease

Coronary atherosclerotic tissue has increased tissue endothelin-like immunoreactivity in smooth muscle cells, macrophages, and endothelial cells. Local ET-1 is also increased after coronary angioplasty, particularly in the neointima. $ET_A$ receptors predominate, although the population of $ET_B$ receptors is also increased, and there is some evidence that both are involved in neointima formation.

## Pulmonary Hypertension

Both ET-1 mRNA expression and ET-1 immunoreactivity have been documented in the lungs of patients with both primary and secondary pulmonary hypertension, and $ET_A$ receptor antagonists prevent and reverse chronic hypoxia-induced pulmonary hypertension in rats.

## Conclusion

ET-1 is generated by the endothelin-converting enzyme (ECE) in endothelial cells, VSMC, and cardiac myocytes. In the vasculature, ET-1 is vasoconstricting, activating the PLC-DAG-$Ca^{2+}$ axis with significant "crosstalk" with the tyrosine kinase–dependent pathways. ET promotes proliferation of VSMC, in hypertension and atherosclerosis and promotes smooth muscle cell migration, intimal hyperplasia, and macrophage recruitment. These atherogenic effects could, theoretically, be blocked by endothelin receptor antagonists or ECE inhibitors, but we do not yet know whether these drugs are effective.

## ■ NITRIC OXIDE[13–15]

In 1980, Furchgott and Zawadzki showed that simple mechanical disruption of the vascular endothelium (as by rubbing the endothelial surface with a cotton swab) abolished the vasodilator effect of acetylcholine, and they proposed that the normal response to acetylcholine involved release of an endothelium-derived relaxing factor (EDRF). Moncada and colleagues showed later that the EDRF is NO. In 1998, both Furchgott and Moncada received the Nobel Prize.

The enzyme nitric oxide synthase (NOS) catalyzes the conversion of l-arginine to l-citrulline and NO in endothelial and vascular smooth muscle cells and in neurons (Fig. 4–9). Three NOS isoforms have been identified. Endothelial cells contain a constitutive NOS, eNOS (NOS-III), and nNOS (NOS-I) is found in neurons; both require calcium and calmodulin for activity. Inducible NOS (iNOS or NOS-II) isoforms, mainly in VSMC and macrophages, are calcium independent and can produce high, sustained levels of NO.

Both endothelial cell and VSMC NO activate VSMC soluble guanylate cyclase, stimulating the conversion of guanosine triphosphate to cGMP. Increased cGMP levels cause smooth muscle relaxation, and thus vasodilatation, by activating c-GMP-dependent protein kinases, which do several things, including extruding intracellular $Ca^{2+}$ via a membrane-associated $Ca^{2+}$-$Mg^{2+}$-ATPase pump.

There is some evidence that underproduction of NO can cause hypertension in animals and in humans. Overproduction of NO by iNOS in macrophages and VSMC exposed to cytokines or lipopolysaccharide contribute to the vasodilatation and hypotension of septicemia.

There is also some evidence that NO is antiatherogenic. In animals, inhibitors of NOS such as N-nitro-l-arginine methyl ester (l-NAME) accelerate the development of atherosclerotic lesions and l-arginine slows it. In patients with atherosclerosis, endothelial NO production is deficient. In all arteries (including the coronary arteries), this is manifested by a constrictor response to acetylcholine (rather than the normal dilator response) that is due to release of little or no NO from damaged

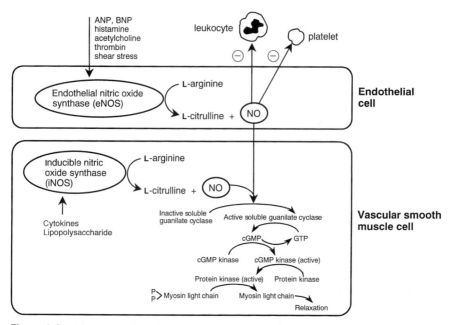

**Figure 4–9** ■ The nitric oxide and cyclic guanosine monophosphate (cGMP) signal transduction mechanism. Constitutive endothelial nitric oxide synthase (eNOS) synthesizes nitric oxide (NO) from ʟ-arginine. eNOS activity is stimulated by many factors (shown on the Figure). NO inhibits leukocyte and platelet activation and adhesion. NO diffuses to the subjacent vascular smooth muscle cell, where it activates a cascade of events, including cyclic guanosine monophosphate (cGMP) and an activated cGMP-dependent protein kinase, to cause vasodilatation. NO may also be synthesized by inducible nitric oxide synthase (iNOS) in vascular smooth muscle cells exposed to cytokines and/or lipopolysaccharides. ANP, atrial natriuretic peptide; BNP, brain natriuretic peptide. (Modified from Lloyd-Jones DM, Bloch KD: The vascular biology of nitric oxide and its role in atherogenesis. Annu Rev Med 1996;47:365–375.)

endothelial cells. Vasodilator responses to nitroglycerin are normal, since nitroglycerin acts directly on vascular smooth muscle.

What are the mechanisms of atherogenesis? First, NO inhibits oxidation of low-density lipoprotein (LDL) in vitro. This is true of the continuous generation of NO by the constitutive eNOS; however, when NO is present with superoxide or at low pH, as it is in active atherosclerotic lesions, both NO and its oxidized metabolite peroxynitrite (ONOO⁻) oxidize LDL, which is atherogenic. The second proposed mechanism is inhibition by NO of platelet activation and adhesion. NO also negatively regulates leukocyte adhesion and chemotaxis, limiting monocyte migration to the intima and macrophage and foam cell formation. NO also inhibits VSMC proliferation.

The mechanism of restenosis after percutaneous angioplasty may be denudation of the endothelium with poor NO production; leukocytes and platelets adhere to the damaged surface and release growth factors which lead to VSMC proliferation and migration into the intima. Several studies have shown slowing of neointima formation by NO donors (such as ʟ-arginine) or by transfer in vivo of the eNOS gene. Vascular injury also stimulates the expression of iNOS, which is a damage-limiting response.

All of these data suggest a promising therapeutic approach to a number of cardiovascular problems, particularly hypertension, atherosclerotic disease, coronary spasm, and post-angioplasty restenosis, that involves increasing vascular NO production. This could be achieved (1) by supplementing the NOS substrate l-arginine or cofactors such as tetrahydrobiopterin, (2) by using NO donor compounds (of which the most commonly used are nitrates) or inhibiting the conversion of NO to superoxide by superoxide dismutase, or (3) by stimulating overexpression of the NOS gene using intravascular gene therapy techniques. None of these approaches, however, has yet been shown to successfully slow or reverse atherosclerosis in humans. More successful has been treatment of endothelial dysfunction with cholesterol-lowering agents, particularly statins, or antioxidant therapy, or a combination of both.

## ■ THE ENDOTHELIUM AND ARTERIOSCLEROSIS

It is clear, then, that the endothelium plays a critical role in maintaining vascular health by secreting vasodilators, inhibitors of smooth muscle growth, and thrombolytic factors (Table 4–1).

It is also well-known that conditions such as hypertension, diabetes, dyslipidemia, and smoking cause the physiologic and structural changes in the vessel that lead to vascular disease. It has been suggested that one of the earliest changes to occur in each of these conditions is alteration of the oxidative metabolism of the endothelium, with increased oxidative stress. This causes endothelial dysfunction manifested as a decrease in vasodilators, inhibitors of growth, and thrombolytic factors and an increase in the synthesis and release of vasoconstrictor substances (which promote smooth muscle growth), adhesion molecules, and prothrombotic factors.

Table 4–1

### Factors Released by the Endothelium

| Vasodilators | Vasoconstrictors |
|---|---|
| Nitric oxide | Angiotensin II |
| Bradykinin | Endothelin |
| Prostacyclin | Thromboxane $A_2$, serotonin,* arachidonic |
| Endothelium-derived hyperpolarizing factor | acid, prostaglandin $H_2$, thrombin |
| Serotonin,* histamine, substance P | |
| C-type natriuretic peptide | |
| **Inhibitors of Smooth Muscle Cell Growth** | **Promoters of Smooth Muscle Cell Growth** |
| Nitric oxide, prostacyclin, bradykinin | Platelet-derived growth factor |
| Heparan sulfate | Basic fibroblast growth factor |
| Transforming growth factor β | Insulin-like growth factor I |
| C-type natriuretic peptide | Endothelin, angiotensin II |
| **Inhibitors of Inflammation or Adhesion** | **Promoters of Inflammation or Adhesion** |
| Nitric oxide | Superoxide radicals |
| | Tumor necrosis factor α |
| | Endothelial leukocyte adhesion molecule |
| | Intercellular adhesion molecule (ICAM) |
| | Vascular cell adhesion molecule (VCAM) |
| **Thrombolytic Factors** | **Thrombotic Factors** |
| Tissue-type plasminogen activator | Plasminogen activator inhibitor 1 |

*Serotonin functions mostly as a vasodilator in normal blood vessels, but it produces paradoxical vasoconstriction when the endothelium is damaged by hypertension, hypercholesterolemia, or another condition that is a risk factor for cardiovascular disease.

Modified and reprinted from Am J Cardiol 82; Drexler H: Factors involved in the maintenance of endothelial function, 3S-4S, 1998, with permission from Excerpta Medica.

In particular, there is a decrease in NO formation and activation of vascular ACE and endothelin. The result is vasoconstriction, vascular hypertrophy and/or hyperplasia (vascular remodeling) due to A II, endothelin, and other growth factors, and also inflammatory changes including monocyte adhesion and infiltration, due to adhesion molecules and cytokines. Eventually, if the patient is unlucky, the plaque ruptures due to proteolysis, and thrombosis is caused by tissue factor release from the atherosclerotic plaque, and excess plasminogen activator inhibitor 1 (PAI-1).

## ■ ACETYLCHOLINE[16]

Acetylcholine (ACh) is the neurotransmitter for postganglionic parasympathetic neurons (acting on muscarinic receptors), both sympathetic and parasympathetic preganglionic neurons (acting on nicotinic receptors), preganglionic autonomic neurons innervating the adrenal medulla, motor end plates in skeletal muscle, and some neurons in the central nervous system. ACh is synthesized by acetylation of choline, stored in vesicles, and released from cholinergic nerves when they are depolarized. After acting on the ACh receptor, ACh is rapidly degraded by acetylcholinesterase.

### Muscarinic Receptors

At least five subtypes of muscarinic receptors are known, $M_1$ to $M_5$. Although several vascular effects of ACh have been described—notably release of NO from endothelial cells to produce vasodilatation—the administration of atropine, a muscarinic antagonist, has no significant effect on vascular resistance. It is, therefore, unlikely that ACh has a major role in vascular homeostasis. However, the intense negative cardiac inotropic and chronotropic effects of parasympathetic (vagal) stimulation, opposed by atropine, are well-known.

### Nicotinic Receptors

All autonomic ganglionic neurotransmission is mediated by nicotinic cholinergic receptors. Ganglion-blocking drugs such as trimethophan and mecamylamine were once among the few agents available for the treatment of hypertension. They caused blood pressure to drop, but what is effectively blockade of the efferent pathway of the baroreceptor reflex frequently caused profound postural hypotension, dizziness, and syncope. These drugs are no longer used.

## ■ SEROTONIN[17]

Serotonin, or 5-hydroxytryptamine (5-HT), is found in the central and the peripheral nervous system, in the enterochromaffin cells of the gastrointestinal tract, and in platelets. It is synthesized by hydroxylation of tryptophan to 5-hydroxytryptophan and then by decarboxylation to 5-HT. The cardiovascular actions of 5-HT are complex. At least 14 different 5-HT receptors are known. Activation of central nervous system $5\text{-HT}_{1A}$ receptors causes hypotension; $5\text{-HT}_{1B}$ receptors decreased ACh and NE release from nerve terminals, and $5\text{-HT}_{1C}$ receptors mediate endothelium-dependent vasodilatation. Receptors for $5\text{-HT}_2$ are involved with direct arterial and venous constriction, and $5\text{-HT}_3$ receptor activation causes bradycardia and hypotension. Intravenous dosing with 5-HT causes a brief depressor phase mediated by $5\text{-HT}_3$ receptors, which is followed by a brief pressor effect due to $5-HT_2$ receptors in the renal, splanchnic, and cerebral circulation. Next is a more prolonged fall in blood pressure that is due to vasodilatation in skeletal muscle, probably mediated by $5-HT_{1C}$ receptors. Ketanserin is a $5-HT_2$ (and $\alpha_1$-adrenergic) receptor antagonist, which is used as an antihypertensive agent.

## ■ ADENOSINE[18]

Adenosine, made up from adenine and d-ribose, is distributed throughout all body tissues and (aside from its importance in AMP, ADP, and ATP) is a potent vasodilator with a short half-life (not more than 6 seconds). It also has negative inotropic and chronotropic effects on the heart and is used to treat supraventricular tachycardias. There are four adenosine receptors: $A_1$, $A_{2a}$, $A_{2b}$, and $A_3$. $A_1$ and $A_3$ receptors in the heart inhibit adenylate cyclase and activate $K^+$ channels to decrease inotropy and to suppress sinus mode automaticity and atrioventricular node conduction. The vasodilatation is mediated via $A_{2a}$ and $A_{2b}$ receptors, which activate adenylate cyclase via a $G_s$ protein.

## ■ γ-AMINOBUTYRIC ACID[19]

Gamma-aminobutyric acid (GABA) is an inhibitory amino acid found throughout the central nervous system. GABA-ergic neurons in the posterior hypothalamus and ventral medulla exert a tonic inhibitory effect on blood pressure, and GABA antagonists raise blood pressure.

## ■ ENDOGENOUS OUABAIN[20]

The plant glycoside ouabain has digitalis-like actions, particularly inotropic effects. Recently, an endogenous ouabain-like (EO) steroid hormone was discovered that is a high-affinity, selective inhibitor of $Na^+-K^+$-ATPase, is positively inotropic, and is vasopressor. All of these actions would be expected to cause hypertension, and this has been shown with sustained infusions of EO in rats. Elevated EO levels have been described in 30% to 45% of humans with hypertension. The primary site of EO production seems to be the adrenal zona glomerulosa, and EO release can be stimulated by adrenocorticotropin (ACTH) and A II via $AT_2$ receptors.

## ■ EICOSANOIDS[21, 22]

Prostacyclin ($PGI_2$) is an eicosanoid prostaglandin (Fig. 4–10) that is rapidly released from endothelial cells in response to a variety of humoral and mechanical stimuli. $PGI_2$ is the major product of arachidonic acid metabolism through the cyclooxygenase pathway in blood vessels. It is a vasodilator, but it also retards platelet aggregation and adhesion. This action is the opposite of that of the major metabolite of arachidonic acid in platelets, thromboxane $A_2$, which is vasoconstricting and stimulates platelet aggregation. Although the $PGI_2$ receptor is present in the arterial vascular wall, $PGI_2$ is not constitutively expressed and therefore is not involved in the regulation of systemic vascular tone. Rather, it is released in response to short-term perturbations of tone. Recently, however, an enzyme, prostaglandin H synthase II (PHS-II), has been identified. This is an inducible form of a key enzyme in $PGI_2$ synthesis, which provides a mechanism for the sustained production of $PGI_2$ in chronic inflammation and vascular injury.

Other physiologically important eicosanoids are synthesized from arachidonic acid by cytochrome $P_{450}$ oxygenases. These are (1) 5,6-epoxy-eicosatrienoic acid

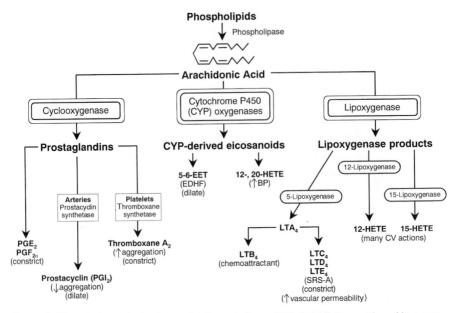

**Figure 4–10** ■ The biosynthesis of prostaglandins, cytochrome P450–derived eicosanoids, and lipoxygenase products from arachidonic acid. PG, prostaglandin. For other abbreviations, see text.

(5,6-EET), the endothelium-derived hyperpolarizing factor, which, like $PGI_2$, is vasodilator; (2) 12(R)-hydroxyeicosatetraenoic acid (12R-HETE), which inhibits $Na^+$-$K^+$-ATPase; and (3) 20-HETE, which elevates blood pressure via several different mechanisms, both directly and via the kidneys. The third enzyme pathway for the production of vasoactive arachidonic acid products is lipoxygenases, of which there are three, designated 5-, 12-, and 15-lipoxygenase. The 5-lipoxygenase pathway produces leukotriene $A_4$ ($LTA_4$), which is then converted to $LTB_4$, a potent chemoattractant substance that causes polymorphonuclear cells to bind to vessel walls and may therefore be important in atherogenesis. $LTA_4$ can also be converted to $LTC_4$, $LTD_4$, or $LTE_4$, formerly known collectively as "slow-reacting substance of anaphylaxis," which are made by mast cells, neutrophils, eosinophils, and macrophages, and are potent vasoconstrictors and increase microvascular permeability. The 12- and 15-lipoxygenase pathways produce 12-HETE and 15-HETE, respectively, in VSMC and endothelial cells. Also, platelets, adrenal glomerulosa cells, and renal mesangial and glomerular cells can make 12-HETE, and monocytes can make 15-HETE. These two lipoxygenase products have several possible roles in vascular disease. The substance 12-HETE may activate mitogen-activated protein kinase, suggesting a role in cell proliferation and atherogenesis. Both 12- and 15-HETE inhibit prostacyclin synthesis and vasoconstrict certain vascular beds. They are growth promoting on VSMC, may increase monocyte adhesion to endothelial cells, and may be involved in the oxidation of LDL.

## ■ KININS[23]

Kinins are vasodilator peptides that are released from substrates known as *kininogens* by serine protease enzymes known as *kininogenases*. There are two main kininogenases, plasma kallikrein and tissue kallikrein, and these produce bradykinin and lys-bradykinin from the high– or low–molecular weight kininogens made in the liver that circulate in the plasma (Fig. 4–11). Kinins are broken down by enzymes known as *kininases,* one of which is kininase II, also known as ACE. Others include neutral endopeptidases (NEP) 24.11 and 24.15. Most kininases are found in the endothelial cells of lung capillaries.

Kinins activate $B_1$ and $B_2$ receptors. $B_1$ receptors are involved with inflammatory responses to bacterial endotoxins. $B_2$ receptors mediate vasodilator responses, particularly in salivary glands, gastrointestinal tract, and kidneys. In the kidney, kinins are vasodilator, natriuretic, and diuretic, actions which are possibly mediated by the kinin-induced release of prostaglandin $E_2$ and NO.

In children low urinary kallikrein excretion is an important genetic marker for primary hypertension, so kinins may play some role in hypertension. At least some of the antihypertensive activity of both ACE inhibitors and NEP inhibitors may be potentiation of the effects of kinins.

Tissue kallikrein is present in heart, arteries, and veins. Kinin production is increased in myocardial ischemia. It may be an important mediator of myocardial preconditioning (protection from damage during subsequent ischemic episodes) and may contribute to the beneficial effect of ACE inhibitors in reversing ventricular remodeling and improving cardiac function. Kinins also have several important functions in hemostasis. Plasma kallikrein and high–molecular weight kininogen are involved with the intrinsic pathway of blood coagulation. Kinins also promote NO and prostaglandin 2 ($PGI_2$) formation, both of which inhibit platelet aggregation and adhesion, and kinins stimulate release of tissue plasminogen activator to promote fibrinolysis. All of these effects are enhanced by inhibitors of kininases, such as ACE inhibitors and NEP inhibitors.

## ▪ ENDOGENOUS NATRIURETIC PEPTIDES[24]

There are three structurally and functionally similar natriuretic peptides, atrial natriuretic peptide (ANP), brain natriuretic peptide (BNP), and C-type natriuretic

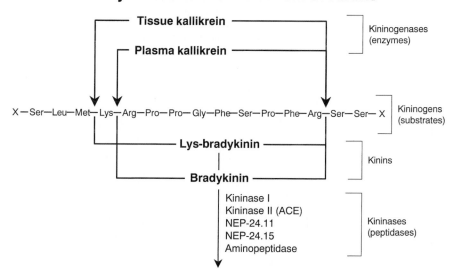

**Biosynthesis and Metabolism of Kinins**

**Figure 4–11** ▪ Biosynthesis and metabolism of kinins. For description, see text.

peptide (CNP), which all induce natriuresis and are vasodilators. ANP is released from atrial and ventricular myocytes in response to stretch (making the heart a true endocrine organ). The ANP prohormone contains 126 amino acids and is cleaved in cardiac myocytes to two fragments. The C-terminal, 28–amino acid peptide is the active hormone. BNP, structurally similar to ANP, is synthesized and stored in the brain and in cardiac myocytes and is also released in response to atrial and ventricular stretch, although in lower concentrations than is ANP. The third member of the group, CNP, is made not in the heart but in the endothelium of blood vessels, and it probably acts not as a circulating hormone but in a paracrine manner, acting on adjacent VSMC.

ANP and BNP bind to ANPR-A receptors, which are located on vascular endothelial and renal epithelial cells. CNP binds to the ANPR-B receptor found on VSMC. Both ANPR-A and ANPR-B receptors activate guanilyl cyclase and GMP to cause natriuresis, diuresis, and vasodilation. They inhibit the renin-angiotensin system, endothelin, and sympathetic function and are antimitogenic in VSMC.

ANP and BNP levels are elevated in congestive heart failure, but they seem disproportionately low for the degree of cardiomegaly. New agents are in development that will enhance ANP and BNP activity, among them drugs that inhibit the enzyme that degrades the peptides, neutral endopeptidase, including some drugs that combine ACE-inhibition and NEP-inhibition, for the treatment of hypertension and congestive heart failure.

## ■ VASOPRESSIN[25]

Arginine vasopressin (AVP), also known as antidiuretic hormone (ADH), is released from the posterior pituitary in response to increased plasma osmolality via osmoreceptors in the hypothalamus, reduced blood volume sensed by atrial stretch receptors, and decreased blood pressure via aortic and carotid baroreceptors. In addition to promoting water reabsorption in renal collecting ducts (via $V_2$ receptors), AVP activates blood vessel $V_{1a}$ receptors to cause vasoconstriction, but it also stimulates hepatic glycogenolysis and renal tubular $PGE_2$ generation. The $V_{1a}$ receptors are coupled to membrane G proteins, phosphatidylinositol phosphate (PIP), phospholipase C (PLC), and increased free cytosolic $Ca^{2+}$ release from the endoplasmic reticulum. The $V_2$ receptors, which mediate water permeability of the collecting ducts and vasodilatation in skeletal muscle, are coupled to adenylate cyclase and cAMP.

The normal concentration of AVP is 1 to 3 pg/ml (10 to 12 mol/L), and concentrations within the physiologic range (10 to 20 pg/ml) can produce significant vasoconstriction in skin, splanchinic, renal, and coronary beds and some $V_2$ receptor–mediated skeletal muscle vasodilatation, with variable effects on arterial blood pressure. AVP also enhances sympathoinhibitory responses to baroreceptor stimulation, so that quite high plasma AVP concentrations are not accompanied by hypertension, which allows the antidiuretic action of AVP to proceed unopposed by any pressure-induced diuresis. The role of AVP in human hypertension is not clear. In a small percentage of patients with primary hypertension (30% of males, 7% of females) there is significant elevation (5 to 20 pg/ml) of plasma AVP, but it is not known whether these changes in AVP concentrations are primary or secondary. These concentrations are lower than those required to increase blood pressure in normal humans but may contribute to the fluid retention and volume expansion seen in many hypertensive patients. There is, however, the phenomenon of "vasopressin escape": the AVP-induced pressure diuresis overcomes the fluid-retaining effects of AVP, so that, after a few weeks, extracellular fluid volume returns to normal.

# ■ NEUROPEPTIDE Y[26]

Neuropeptide Y (NPY) is a 36–amino acid vasoconstrictor peptide that is coreleased with norepinephrine and ATP from sympathetic nerve terminals innervating small arteries, heart, and kidneys. It is also abundant in the brain (hypothalamus, ventrolateral medulla, and locus coeruleus) and in sympathetic ganglia. $Y_1$ receptors in blood vessels inhibit adenylate cyclase and increase intracellular free $Ca^{2+}$ to cause vasoconstriction. The $Y_2$ receptors are on the sympathetic nerve terminal and mediate feedback inhibition of neurotransmitter release.

In the central nervous system, NPY probably acts to lower blood pressure and heart rate. Unlike most other vasoconstrictor agents, NPY is diuretic and natriuretic. Plasma concentrations of NPY are elevated in some patients with hypertension, but the significance of this finding is unknown.

# ■ REFERENCES

1. Nelson MT, Quayle JM: Physiological roles and properties of potassium channels in arterial smooth muscle. Am J Physiol 1995;268:C799–C822.
2. Lijnen P: Alterations in sodium metabolism as an etiological model for hypertension. Cardiovasc Drugs Ther 1995;9:377–399.
3. Stamler JS, Dzau VJ, Loscalzo J: The vascular smooth muscle cell. In Loscalzo J, Creager MA, Dzau VJ (ed): Vascular Medicine: A Textbook of Vascular Biology and Diseases. Boston: Little Brown, 1992.
4. Insel PA: Adrenergic receptors: Evolving concepts and clinical applications. N Engl J Med 1996;334:580–585.
5. Day MD: Autonomic Pharmacology, Experimental and Clinical Aspects. Edinburgh: Churchill Livingstone, 1979.
6. Alexander SPH, Peters JA: Receptor and Ion Channel Nomenclature. Trends in Pharmacologic Sciences, Supplement, 1997, pp 9–13.
7. Rosendorff C: The renin-angiotensin system and vascular hypertrophy. J Am Coll Cardiol 1996;28:803–812.
8. Rosendorff C: Vascular hypertrophy in hypertension. Role of the renin-angiotensin system. Mt Sinai J Med 1998;65:108–117.
9. Atlas SA, Rosendorff C: The renin-angiotensin system—from Tigerstedt to Goldblatt to ACE inhibition and beyond. Mt Sinai J Med 1998;65:81–86.
10. Horiuchi M, Akashita M, Dzau VJ: Recent progress in angiotensin II type 2 receptor research in the cardiovascular system. Hypertension 1999;33:613–621.
11. Rosendorff C: Endothelin, vascular hypertrophy and hypertension. Cardiovasc Drugs Ther 1996;10:795–802.
12. Schiffrin EL, Touyz RM: Vascular biology of endothelin. J Cardiovasc Pharmacol 1998;32(Suppl 3):S2–S13.
13. Lloyd-Jones DM, Bloch KD: The vascular biology of nitric oxide and its role in atherogenesis. Annu Rev Med 1996;47:365–375.
14. Radomski MW, Moncada S: The biological and pharmacological role of nitric oxide in platelet function. In Authi KS (ed): Mechanisms of Platelet Activation and Control. New York: Plenum, 1993:251–264.
15. Scott-Burden T, Vanhoutte PM: The endothelium as a regulator of vascular smooth muscle proliferation. Circulation 1993;87(Suppl V):V51–V55.
16. Lefkowitz RJ, Hoffman BB, Taylor P: Neurohumoral transmission: The autonomic and somatic motor nervous systems. In Gilman AG, Rall TW, Nies AS, Taylor P (eds): The Pharmacologic Basis of Therapeutics, 8th ed. New York: Pergamon Press, 1992, 84–121.
17. Hollenberg N: Serotonin and vascular responses. Ann Rev Pharmacol Toxicol 1988;28:41–59.
18. Olah ME, Stiles GL: Adenosine receptor subtypes: Characterization and receptor regulation. Annu Rev Pharmacol Toxicol 1995;35:581–606.
19. Peng YJ, Gong QL, Li P: GABA (A) receptors in the rostral ventrolateral medulla mediate the depressor response induced by stimulation of the greater splanchnic nerve afferent fibres in rats. Neurosci Lett 1998;249:95–98.
20. Hamlyn JM, Lu ZR, Manunta P: Observations on the nature, biosynthesis, secretion and significance of endogenous ouabain. Clin Exp Hypertens 1998;20(5-6):523–533.
21. Nasjletti A: The role of eicosanoids in angiotensin-dependent hypertension. Hypertension 1997;31:194–200.
22. Lewis RA, Austen KF, Soberman RJ: Leukotrienes and other products of the 5-lipoxygenase pathway: Biochemistry and relation to pathobiology of human diseases. N Engl J Med 1990;323:645–655.
23. Margolius HS: Kallikreins and kinins. Some unanswered questions about system characteristics and roles in human disease. Hypertension 1995;26(2):221–229.

24. Wilkins MR, Redondo J, Brown LA: The natriuretic-peptide family. Lancet 1997;349:1307–1310.
25. Cowley AW Jr: Vasopressin and neuropeptide Y. *In* Izzo JL, Black HR (eds): Hypertension Primer, 2nd ed. Baltimore: Williams & Wilkins, 1999:38–39.
26. Michel MC, Rascher W: Neuropeptide Y: A possible role in hypertension. J Hypertens 1995;13:385–395.

# ■ RECOMMENDED READING

Cines DB, Pollak ES, Buck CA, Loscalzo J, et al: Endothelial cells in physiology and in the pathophysiology of vascular disorders. Blood 1998;91:3527–3561.
O'Rourke ST, Vanhoutte PM: Vascular pharmacology. *In* Loscalzo J, Creager MA, Dzau VJ (eds): Vascular Medicine: A Textbook of Vascular Biology and Diseases. Boston: Little, Brown, 1992.
Stamler JS, Dzau VJ, Loscalzo J: The vascular smooth muscle cell. *In* Loscalzo J, Creager MA, Dzau VJ (eds): Vascular Medicine: A Textbook of Vascular Biology and Diseases. Boston: Little, Brown, 1992.
A Symposium: Endothelial function and cardiovascular disease: Potential mechanisms and interventions. Am J Cardiol 1998;82(10A):1S–64S.

*Chapter 5*

# Thrombosis

*Yale Nemerson* ▪ *Mark B. Taubman*

Thrombosis and hemostasis are similar processes, the former being pathologic and involving intravascular formation of aggregates of platelets and fibrin and the latter resulting in the cessation of bleeding after external injury to the vasculature. While it is not clear that these processes involve precisely the same biochemical and biophysical events, they appear to be sufficiently similar to be considered as a single process that results in quite different structures owing to the local environment, either within a vessel or at the site of bleeding.

The initial event in both instances is the exposure of tissue factor (TF) at the site of injury.[1, 2] In arterial thrombosis, the most frequent initiating event appears to be rupture or fissuring of an atheromatous plaque, which exposes TF,[3] an event that enables the circulating blood to contact TF, thus activating the coagulation cascade.

## ▪ A BRIEF VIEW OF THE MECHANISM OF BLOOD COAGULATION

Although for many years it was thought that coagulation was initiated via the so-called intrinsic system (so named because it was believed that all the components required for coagulation were "intrinsic" to the blood), it is generally recognized that this system was an artifact of glass activation.[1] The prevailing view is that coagulation via the TF pathway is the principal means of thrombin production. Some patients are, however, deficient in factor XI and have some hemorrhage symptoms. Until recently, it was thought that factor XI was activated mainly when the blood contacted glass or a similar surface by a mechanism independent of TF. Two findings, however, offer alternative schemes, each consistent with TF's being the only physiologic activator of the coagulation system. First, it was shown that factor XI could be activated on platelets via a mechanism independent of factor XII or glass. Interestingly, platelet factor XI is an alternatively spliced form of plasma factor XI,[4] and its synthesis is independent.[5] Alternatively, the major catalyst of factor XI activation may be thrombin, which activates this zymogen via limited proteolysis.[6]

Formation of a thrombus involves many circulating proteins, blood platelets, and damage to the arterial wall with consequent exposure of TF. Because of this complexity, it is difficult to describe the entire process precisely. The clinical efficacy of anticoagulant and antiplatelet agents indicates that perhaps all of these components are necessary but that none alone is sufficient.

TF forms a complex with activated factor VII (VIIa), thereby forming a holoenzyme that initiates the coagulation cascade by activating factors IX and X (Fig. 5–1). The TF:VIIa complex has a regulatory subunit, TF, and a catalytic subunit, VIIa. The latter is a serine protease that has essentially no procoagulant activity unless it is in complex with TF. This theme—the assembly of holoenzymes from regulatory and enzymatic species—is central to the understanding of coagulation, because it occurs three times in the coagulation scheme.

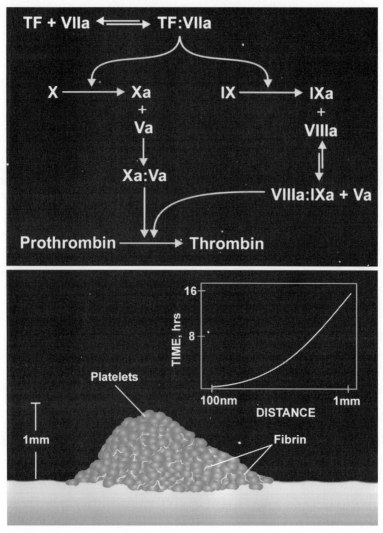

**Figure 5–1** ■ *Upper panel,* Schematic view of blood coagulation with tissue factor (TF) as the initiating species. Note that TF is shown as a complex with activated factor VII (VIIa) and that small amounts of this enzyme are present in normal blood. *Lower panel,* Schematic view of a thrombus. Note that the inset indicates the relationship between the time it takes a diffusing molecule to traverse a given distance. This relationship is such that, as the distance doubles, the time to capture is squared.

The vast majority of circulating factor VII is in the zymogen, or unactivated, form, but small amounts of VIIa also circulate,[7, 8] and it is probably responsible for the initial activity of the TF complex. When factor VII is bound to TF, it has little or no enzymatic activity; however, in this bound state (whose crystal structure has been described[9]), zymogen factor VII is in a conformation that renders it liable to limited proteolysis that results in its conversion to its active enzymatic form, VIIa.[10, 11] The complex of TF:VIIa has two substrates, factors IX and X. Their activated forms, IXa and Xa, respectively, form complexes with two circulating regulatory proteins; IXa with the antihemophilic factor, factor VIII, and Xa with factor V, forming the so-called prothrombinase complex. These complexes are similar to the TF:VIIa complex inasmuch as each contains a serine protease (factors IXa and Xa, respectively) and a regulatory protein (factors VIIIa and Va) respectively. Both factors VIII and V circulate as "pro-cofactors" and must be activated via limited proteolysis to function in these complexes. Thrombin is likely the enzyme that is mainly responsible for activating these cofactors; thus, strong positive feedback results in explosive formation of thrombin. The last event in this cascade is the crosslinking of fibrin via the action of factor XIII, which, after being activated by thrombin, crosslinks the fibrin monomers. Once crosslinked, fibrin becomes resistant to lysis by plasmin, which is one explanation for lytic therapy losing efficacy over time.

This concert of events, during which the platelets become activated, enables them to support coagulation and to form a nidus for thrombus formation via the action of the IIb/IIIa receptor that facilitates the formation of platelet masses by interacting with fibrin. The IIb/IIIa receptor is the target of the clinically effective antithrombotic monoclonal antibody Rheopro.

Leukocytes are also involved in thrombus formation. It is noteworthy that a blocking antibody to P selectin inhibited fibrin formation in an arteriovenous shunt model in vitro.[12] P selectin is a protein stored in platelet granules that translocates to the plasma membrane upon platelet activation. When on the platelet surface, P selectin interacts with its cognate ligand, CD-15, on the surface of leukocytes. This observation raises the issue of the role of leukocytes in thrombus formation, which is addressed later.

## ■ THE NATURAL ANTICOAGULANT SYSTEMS

Natural anticoagulant systems can conveniently be divided into two classes, one that circulates as inhibitory species and those that are activated during coagulation. Of those that require activation, that best studied is protein C, which, like factors VII, IX, and X, is a vitamin K–dependent zymogen that must be activated by limited proteolysis (for a recent review see reference 13). The activation of protein C is accomplished by thrombin that is complexed with an endothelial surface protein, thrombomodulin. When thrombin is in this complex, the substrate specificity of thrombin is altered so that it activates protein C and thrombin-activatable fibrinolysis inhibitor (TAFI)[14] but does not clot fibrinogen. Activated protein C is a serine protease that attacks activated factors V and VIII, thus shutting down the coagulation cascade. Factor V Leiden is a genetic variant of factor V that is resistant to proteolysis by activated protein C. Those with this mutation exhibit increased thrombosis, mostly venous, although serious arterial thrombosis is also increased.[15–17] This is a reasonably common mutation: some 5% to 6% of whites possess it.[18] Deficiencies of protein C are associated mainly with venous thromboembolic disease, although instances of arterial thrombosis have been reported.[19]

TAFI is a recently described fibrinolysis inhibitor that is a form of procarboxidase B. When activated by thrombin or (>1000-fold faster) by thrombomodulin-thrombin complex, the resultant enzyme attacks the carboxy-terminal residues of proteins, resulting, in this case, in reduced plasmin/plasminogen and tissue plasminogen activator (tPA) binding to fibrin.[20] Thus, the formation of the thrombin-thrombomodulin complex results in the generation of an anticoagulant, activated protein C, and the antifibrinolytic (prothrombotic) species TAFI. Clearly, sorting out these phenomena with respect to thrombogenesis will be most difficult.

The blood also contains an inhibitory protein, tissue factor pathway inhibitor (TFPI), whose functioning is complex: TFPI has modest affinity for TF and thus it is not directly inhibitory. TFPI is in its most effective form when it is bound to Xa; this binary complex then attacks TF:VIIa, with which it forms an inactive quaternary complex, thus damping TF initiated coagulation.[21, 22] No clinical deficiency states of TFPI have yet been reported, so it is difficult to assess its role in preventing thrombosis. It is noteworthy, however, that mice whose gene for TFPI has been knocked out die in utero.[23]

The other major circulating anticoagulant is antithrombin III, which forms a stable complex with several of the coagulation enzymes, most prominently thrombin and activated factor X. This reaction is markedly accelerated by heparin and similar compounds and is the mechanism by which heparin exerts its anticoagulant activity.[24] Like deficiencies of protein C, antithrombin III deficiencies are associated mainly with venous thrombosis, although recent data indicate that low levels of this protein are predictive of future cardiac events.[25]

## ■ FIBRINOLYSIS

Just as coagulation involves multiple enzymatic and regulatory proteins, fibrinolysis, the process by which fibrin is lysed to reestablish blood flow, involves multiple proteins and reactions, the details of which are beyond the scope of this chapter. Plasminogen is the circulating zymogen of plasmin, a serine protease that has high specificity for fibrin. It is activated in vivo by plasminogen activators that are released from tissue stores by ischemia. The activators generate plasmin, the active fibrinolytic enzyme, from the zymogen plasminogen. Plasminogen activation inhibitors 1 and 2 oppose the activation of plasmin and thus are prothrombotic.[26–28] These inhibitors appear to be the major components of the fibrinolytic system that are associated with thrombotic risk.

## ■ TISSUE FACTOR AND THE ATHEROSCLEROTIC PLAQUE

As noted above, occlusive thrombi of the coronary arteries are thought to be a consequence of plaque rupture[3] and are the leading cause of death in the western world; because of this and because TF in plaques is felt to be necessary for thrombosis, many studies have focused on the presence of this protein in plaques. As early as 1972, TF was detected in plaque by immunostaining, although the antibody was undoubtedly polyspecific.[29] Subsequent experiments with antibodies raised against pure TF confirmed these findings,[30] as did results obtained with monoclonal antibodies and the use of haptene-labeled factor VIIa, a specific probe for TF.[31] Because these experiments reflect only localization of antigen, in the case of the immunostaining, and binding of VIIa to TF, in the latter instance, neither of these techniques demonstrates TF *activity* in plaque. Direct enzymatic assay of TF harvested from plaque has been reported, and the majority of samples demonstrated activity.[32, 33] The activity, however, was low, and it is not certain that the specimens contained only plaque; thus, the meaning of these findings is somewhat questionable. What clearly is required to demonstrate unambiguously active TF in plaque is an enzyme histochemical assay for TF, which, however, has not been reported.

### Circulating Tissue Factor: A Thrombogenic Species

Recent experiments have demonstrated that native, normal human blood forms TF-dependent thrombi on collagen-coated glass slides in a laminar flow chamber. The fact that these thrombi contain fibrin indicates that the deposited TF is biochemically active; furthermore, inclusion of active site inhibited VIIa (a potent TF inhibitor) essentially abolished both fibrin and thrombus formation in the perfusions.[34] This finding contradicts many statements in the literature, including our own, that circulating TF is of no consequence. Further, these experiments suggest that exposure of collagen on blood vessels may be sufficient to initiate thrombus formation, although it seems likely that vessel wall TF initiates thrombus formation whereas circulating TF may be responsible for its propagation. The apparent mechanism by which bloodborne TF can initiate thrombosis ex vivo works as follows: the first event appears to be binding of platelets to collagen; thereafter, neutrophils and monocytes bind to the platelets (probably via P selectin and other molecules as yet to be identified). The leukocytes, which contain TF, apparently deposit TF-containing membranous structures on the platelets, thus rendering them highly thrombogenic. These experiments were designed to mimic thrombosis in vivo in the sense that they involved laminar flow at arteriolar shear rates (1000 to 2000 per second). We imagine that the shear field, which is also encountered in mildly stenosed coronary arteries, favors (1) delivery of leukocytes to the nascent thrombus and (2) their fragmentation in situ. Thus, as the thrombus grows, the platelets become surrounded with TF-containing vesicles and membranous structures that are competent to initiate coagulation and thrombus propagation.

## Encryption of Cell Surface Tissue Factor: What Is the Biologically Active Species?

The fact that bloodborne TF is active in experimental thrombogenesis suggests that there is a mechanism for controlling its activity in blood cells. One possibility is that cell surface TF in vivo is entirely encrypted, by which we mean that, while it is capable of binding VIIa and specific antibodies, cell surface TF is catalytically inactive. The phenomenon of encryption or dormancy on the cell surface was suggested many years ago[35] and was subsequently explored and documented using contemporary techniques.[36-38] It has been suggested that on the surface TF exists as inactive dimers and that it must be monomerized to exhibit procoagulant activity.[39] Quantitative studies using cultured cells have shown that the majority of surface TF is encrypted. One possibility that is difficult to explore is that, in vivo, cell surface TF is inactive; if so, that fact raises the question of the state of the active species. Extracellular TF has been noted in arterial adventitia and in the plaque, which raises the possibility that it is the active pool.[31] It is well documented that, for optimal activity, TF requires acidic phosphatides to be exposed. Normally, it is presumed that these molecules are on the inner leaflets of plasma membranes and render these membranes more or less inactive. Extracellular TF, however, is present on membrane fragments and vesicles, which lack the energy necessary to maintain phospholipid asymmetry; therefore, one expects acidic phosphatides to be randomly distributed, the net result being that extracellular TF quite likely is procoagulant.

## Tissue Factor in Arterial Injury

In addition to its association with acute coronary syndromes such as myocardial infarction and unstable angina, thrombosis is also a concomitant of acute arterial injury, such as that produced by coronary angioplasty, directional atherectomy, and coronary artery stenting.[40-42] TF antigen is induced in the smooth muscle cells near the luminal border in rat,[43] rabbit,[44-46] and porcine[47] models of arterial injury. The significance of this induction is subject to the same concerns raised earlier in the discussion of the atherosclerotic plaque. It has been demonstrated that TF activity in the injured rat aortic media increased coordinately with TF mRNA and antigen[43]; however, activity was measured in homogenized aortic sections and therefore could have come from encrypted or intracellular stores not capable of initiating coagulation in vivo.

The relevance of TF induction after balloon injury can be questioned on the grounds that injury to normal rat and rabbit arteries does not result in deposition of fibrin, the end product of TF activation, even when medial smooth muscle is injured.[48–50] However, fibrin deposition occurs rapidly when previously injured rabbit arteries are subjected to a second injury 1 to 2 weeks later.[48, 49, 51] Fibrin deposition and microthrombi were not seen at any time after single injuries to normal rat aortas but were present on the luminal surface within 30 minutes of a second injury. TF antigen was not detectable in the endothelium or media during the first 4 hours after injury. TF antigen was abundant in the media by 24 hours and then returned to baseline amount over the next 2 days. TF antigen subsequently accumulated in the developing intima and was abundant throughout the intima after 2 weeks, at the time of the second injury. Whole-mount preparations showed minimal TF antigen on the surface of uninjured or once injured vessels, but the second injury rapidly exposed surface TF antigen. Rapid exposure of intimal TF to the circulation may be necessary to generate fibrin and produce thrombosis.

Other studies have suggested that the induction of TF by arterial injury is functionally important. Antibodies to TF inhibited the variations in cyclic flow in rabbits subjected to arterial injury and mechanical stenosis[44] and inhibited thrombus formation in a rabbit femoral artery eversion graft preparation.[52] TFPI has also been shown to inhibit angiographic restenosis and intimal hyperplasia in balloon-injured atherosclerotic rabbits[53] and to attenuate stenosis in balloon-injured hyperlipidemic pigs.[54] Once again, the precise location of the functionally important TF remains to be determined and awaits the development of an in situ activity assay.

## ■ REFERENCES

1. Nemerson Y: Tissue factor and hemostasis [published erratum appears in Blood 1988;71(4):1178]. Blood 1988;71:1.
2. Edgington TS, Ruf W, Rehemtulla A, et al: The molecular biology of initiation of coagulation by tissue factor. Curr Stud Hematol Blood Transfus 1991;58:15.
3. Fuster V, Fallon JT, Nemerson Y: Coronary thrombosis. Lancet 1996;348(Suppl 1):s7.
4. Hsu TC, Shore SK, Seshsmma T, et al: Molecular cloning of platelet factor XI, an alternative splicing product of the plasma factor XI gene. J Biol Chem 1998;273:13787.
5. Hu CJ, Baglia FA, Mills DC, et al: Tissue-specific expression of functional platelet factor XI is independent of plasma factor XI expression. Blood 1998;91:3800.
6. Gailani D, Broze GJ Jr: Factor XI activation in a revised model of blood coagulation. Science 1991;253:909.
7. Wildgoose P, Nemerson Y, Hansen LL, et al: Measurement of basal levels of factor VIIa in hemophilia A and B patients [see Comments]. Blood 1992;80:25.
8. Morrissey JH: Plasma factor VIIa: Measurement and potential clinical significance. Haemostasis 1996;26:66.
9. Banner DW: The factor VIIa/tissue factor complex. Thromb Haemost 1997;78:512.
10. Nemerson Y, Repke D: Tissue factor accelerates the activation of coagulation factor VII: The role of a bifunctional coagulation cofactor. Thromb Res 1985;40:351.
11. Rao LV, Rapaport SI: Activation of factor VII bound to tissue factor: A key early step in the tissue factor pathway of blood coagulation. Proc Natl Acad Sci USA 1988;85:6687.
12. Palabrica T, Lobb R, Furie BC, et al: Leukocyte accumulation promoting fibrin deposition is mediated in vivo by P-selectin on adherent platelets. Nature 1992;359:848.
13. Esmon CT, Gu JM, Xu J, et al: Regulation and functions of the protein C anticoagulant pathway. Haematologica 1999;84:363.
14. Bajzar L, Morser J, Nesheim M: TAFI, or plasma procarboxypeptidase B, couples the coagulation and fibrinolytic cascades through the thrombin-thrombomodulin complex. J Biol Chem 1996;271:16603.
15. Heresbach D, Pagenault M, Gueret P, et al: Leiden factor V mutation in four patients with small bowel infarctions. Gastroenterology 1997;113:322.

16. Rosendaal FR: Thrombosis in the young: Epidemiology and risk factors. A focus on venous thrombosis. Thromb Haemost 1997;78:1.
17. Eskandari MK, Bontempo FA, Hassett AC, et al: Arterial thromboembolic events in patients with the factor V Leiden mutation. Am J Surg 1998;176:122.
18. Heijmans BT, Westendorp RG, Knook DL, et al: The risk of mortality and the factor V Leiden mutation in a population-based cohort. Thromb Haemost 1998;80:607.
19. Coller BS, Owen J, Jesty J, et al: Deficiency of plasma protein S, protein C, or antithrombin III arterial thrombosis. Arteriosclerosis 1987;7:456.
20. Bajzar L, Nesheim M, Morser J, et al: Both cellular and soluble forms of thrombomodulin inhibit fibrinolysis by potentiating the activation of thrombin-activable fibrinolysis inhibitor. J Biol Chem 1998;273:2792.
21. Broze GJJ, Miletich JP: Characterization of the inhibition of tissue factor in serum. Blood 1987;69:150.
22. Rapaport SI: The extrinsic pathway inhibitor: A regulator of tissue factor-dependent blood coagulation. Thromb Haemost 1991;66:6.
23. Huang ZF, Higuchi D, Lasky N, et al: Tissue factor pathway inhibitor gene disruption produces intrauterine lethality in mice. Blood 1997;90:944.
24. Rosenberg RD: Biochemistry of heparin antithrombin interactions, and the physiologic role of this natural anticoagulant mechanism. Am J Med 1989;87:2S.
25. Thompson SG, Fechtrup C, Squire E, et al: Antithrombin III and fibrinogen as predictors of cardiac events in patients with angina pectoris. Arterioscler Thromb Vasc Biol 1996;16:357.
26. Geppert A, Graf S, Beckmann R, et al: Concentration of endogenous tPA antigen in coronary artery disease: Relation to thrombotic events, aspirin treatment, hyperlipidemia, and multivessel disease. Arterioscler Thromb Vasc Biol 1998;18:1634.
27. Zhu Y, Carmeliet P, Fay WP: Plasminogen activator inhibitor-1 is a major determinant of arterial thrombolysis resistance. Circulation 1999;99:3050.
28. Cushman M, Lemaitre RN, Kuller LH, et al: Fibrinolytic activation markers predict myocardial infarction in the elderly. The Cardiovascular Health Study. Arterioscler Thromb Vasc Biol 1999;19:493.
29. Zeldis SM, Nemerson Y, Pitlick FA, et al: Tissue factor (thromboplastin): Localization to plasma membranes by peroxidase-conjugated antibodies. Science 1972;175:766.
30. Wilcox JN, Smith KM, Schwartz SM, et al: Localization of tissue factor in the normal vessel wall and in the atherosclerotic plaque. Proc Natl Acad Sci USA 1989;86:2839.
31. Thiruvikraman SV, Guha A, Roboz J, et al: In situ localization of tissue factor in human atherosclerotic plaques by binding of digoxigenin-labeled factors VIIa and X [published erratum appears in Lab Invest 1997;76(2):297]. Lab Invest 1996;75:451.
32. Annex BH, Denning SM, Channon KM, et al: Differential expression of tissue factor protein in directional atherectomy specimens from patients with stable and unstable coronary syndromes. Circulation 1995;91:619.
33. Marmur JD, Thiruvikraman SV, Fyfe BS, et al: Identification of active tissue factor in human coronary atheroma. Circulation 1996;94:1226.
34. Giesen PL, Rauch U, Bohrmann B, et al: Blood-borne tissue factor: Another view of thrombosis. Proc Natl Acad Sci USA 1999;96:2311.
35. Maynard JR, Heckman CA, Pitlick FA, et al: Association of tissue factor activity with the surface of cultured cells. J Clin Invest 1975;55:814.
36. Bach R, Rifkin DB: Expression of tissue factor procoagulant activity: Regulation by cytosolic calcium. Proc Natl Acad Sci USA 1990;87:6995.
37. Le DT, Rapaport SI, Rao LV: Relations between factor VIIa binding and expression of factor VIIa/tissue factor catalytic activity on cell surfaces. J Biol Chem 1992;267:15447.
38. Schecter AD, Giesen PL, Taby O, et al: Tissue factor expression in human arterial smooth muscle cells. TF is present in three cellular pools after growth factor stimulation. J Clin Invest 1997;100:2276.
39. Bach RR, Moldow CF: Mechanism of tissue factor activation on HL-60 cells. Blood 1997;89:3270.
40. Carrozza JP Jr, Baim DS: Complications of directional coronary atherectomy: incidence, causes, and management. Am J Cardiol 1993;72:47E.
41. Losordo DW, Rosenfield K, Pieczek A, et al: How does angioplasty work? Serial analysis of human iliac arteries using intravascular ultrasound. Circulation 1992;86:1845.
42. Nath FC, Muller DW, Ellis SG, et al: Thrombosis of a flexible coil coronary stent: Frequency, predictors and clinical outcome. J Am Coll Cardiol 1993;21:622.
43. Marmur JD, Rossikhina M, Guha A, et al: Tissue factor is rapidly induced in arterial smooth muscle after balloon injury. J Clin Invest 1993;91:2253.
44. Pawashe AB, Golino P, Ambrosio G, et al: A monoclonal antibody against rabbit tissue factor inhibits thrombus formation in stenotic injured rabbit carotid arteries. Circ Res 1994;74:56.
45. Speidel CM, Eisenberg PR, Ruf W, et al: Tissue factor mediates prolonged procoagulant activity on the luminal surface of balloon-injured aortas in rabbits. Circulation 1995;92:3323.
46. Speidel CM, Thornton JD, Meng YY, et al: Procoagulant activity on injured arteries and associated thrombi is mediated primarily by the complex of tissue factor and factor VIIa. Coron Artery Dis 1996;7:57.
47. Gallo R, Fallon JT, Gertz SD, et al: Bi-phasic increase of tissue factor activity after angioplasty in porcine coronary arteries. Circulation 1995;92:I.

48. Stemerman MB: Thrombogenesis of the rabbit arterial plaque. An electron microscopic study. Am J Pathol 1973;73:7.
49. Richardson M, Kinlough-Rathbone RL, Groves HM, et al: Ultrastructural changes in re-endothelialized and non-endothelialized rabbit aortic neo-intima following re-injury with a balloon catheter. Br J Exp Pathol 1984;65:597.
50. Clowes AW, Reidy MA, Clowes MM: Kinetics of cellular proliferation after arterial injury. I. Smooth muscle growth in the absence of endothelium. Lab Invest 1983;49:327.
51. Groves HM, Kinlough-Rathbone RL, Richardson M, et al: Thrombin generation and fibrin formation following injury to rabbit neointima. Studies of vessel wall reactivity and platelet survival. Lab Invest 1982;46:605.
52. Jang IK, Gold HK, Leinbach RC, et al: Antithrombotic effect of a monoclonal antibody against tissue factor in a rabbit model of platelet-mediated arterial thrombosis. Arterioscler Thromb 1992;12:948.
53. Jang Y, Guzman LA, Lincoff AM, et al: Influence of blockade at specific levels of the coagulation cascade on restenosis in a rabbit atherosclerotic femoral artery injury model. Circulation 1995;92:3041.
54. Oltrana L, Speidel CM, Recchia D, Abendschein DR: Inhibition of tissue factor-mediated thrombosis markedly attenuates stenosis after balloon-induced arterial injury in hyperlipidemic minipigs. Circulation 1994;90:I.
55. Giesen PL, Rauch U, Bohrmann B, et al: Blood-borne tissue factor: Another view of thrombosis. Proc Natl Acad Sci USA 1999;96:2311.
56. Taubman MB, Fallon JT, Schecter AD, et al: Tissue factor in the pathogenesis of atherosclerosis. Thromb Haemost 1997;78:200.
57. Dahlback B: Activated protein C resistance and thrombosis: Molecular mechanisms of hypercoagulable state due to FVR506Q mutation. Semin Thromb Hemost 1999;25:273.

## ■ RECOMMENDED READING

Dahlback B: Activated protein C resistance and thrombosis: Molecular mechanisms of hypercoagulable state due to FVR506Q mutation. Semin Thromb Hemost 1999;25:273.
Esmon CT, Gu JM, Xu J, et al: Regulation and functions of the protein C anticoagulant pathway. Haematologica 1999;84:363.
Fuster V, Fallon JT, Nemerson Y: Coronary thrombosis. Lancet 1996;348(Suppl 1):s7.
Giesen PL, Rauch U, Bohrmann B, et al: Blood-borne tissue factor: Another view of thrombosis. Proc Natl Acad Sci USA 1999;96:2311.
Taubman MB, Fallon JT, Schecter AD, et al: Tissue factor in the pathogenesis of atherosclerosis. Thromb Haemost 1997;78:200.

*Chapter 6*

# The Medical History and Symptoms of Heart Disease

*H. J. C. Swan*

It is accepted as a truism that the medical history and physical examination provide the most fundamental information on personal health and the need for specific medical care. Although it may appear trite, unnecessary, and perhaps presumptuous, it is the purpose of this chapter, first, to restate and underscore the objective of the taking of a medical history in general, and, then, to a lesser extent, to consider the nature of complaints that may be associated with cardiovascular disease in adults. The specific symptom profiles and presentations are best discussed in association with specific clinical entities, including the chapters concerning ischemic heart disease, acute myocardial infarction, and congestive heart failure. Symptoms related to congenital malformations with associated cardiac lesions, including failure to thrive, cyanosis, and heart failure in the neonate are not considered here. The principal symptoms are summarized in tabular form, followed by a short comment on general issues. The onset and severity of a principal complaint may dominate the initial history taking, and relief of distressing symptoms becomes the first priority; however, it is essential, next, to take complete and comprehensive medical and cardiac histories.

## ▪ HISTORY

### Relevance

The medical history directs the physician's assessment of the initial presentation. The purpose is to exclude the most unlikely diagnoses and further investigate the more likely ones, and in each case to achieve a level of confidence sufficient to allow an action—optimal management decisions, including reassurance, lifestyle modification, additional testing, medical treatment, or the need for interventional procedures. Each conceptual step takes the form of *"What if"* and *"If, then"* clinical reasoning. Specific tests of cardiac or vascular function include exercise electrocardiography (ECG), echocardiography (transthoracic, or, when indicated, transesophageal), arrhythmia monitoring, radioisotope and magnetic resonance imaging. More advanced testing strategies must follow, and not precede, a careful consideration of the initial history, the physical examination, ECG, chest radiography, and basic blood and urine tests and, ideally, should be structured to increase confidence in the probability that a particular diagnosis is correct or can be excluded.

## The Medical Interview[1]

This encounter initiates a process of interaction and confidence building between patient and physician. The goal of the interview is to establish, with a reasonable degree of certainty, the presence or absence of disorders of body structure or function that might cause the complaint, the significance of such diseases and disorders for the patient's well-being; the implications of these findings for management strategies; and how the proposed strategies might relieve symptoms and foster good health by increasing longevity and improving the quality of life. The process is to progressively exclude/include possible causes based on the information gathered as the physician proceeds from an initial introduction through a detailed history, physical examination, and routine testing to approaches specific to cardiovascular disease.

History taking is far more art than science.[2] It is an exercise in unstructured probabilistics and should be so regarded. In all of this, the opportunity to establish a sense of trust and confidence between physician and patient is paramount. After all, it is the patient who has "hired" the doctor. As Claude Bennett put it, "the good doctor" becomes a friend and resource for his patient with respect to family, suffering, aging, and dying.[3] In a recent commentary, "Humility and the Practice of Medicine," James Li[4] suggests that the overconfident physician who believes that medical science and technology are sufficient, subordinates the patient-physician relationship.[5] Competence, concern, compassion, and caring are the hallmark of medical practice, but there is a place for the honest "I don't know," tactfully stated.

## Initial Presentation

The history taking from a "first visit" patient is a vital part of the practice of medicine. Clearly, the history taking is different for initial elective conditions, follow-up, "consultation," and the emergent presentation of a patient. In a first visit, the physician assesses the general health of the patient and develops impressions of his educational and intellectual background, and thus the accuracy and credibility of "the story." The attitudinal, social, and emotional makeup of the patient is elucidated by nonverbal—as well as verbal—communication. At the same time, the prudent patient assesses, not only the physician's professional competence, but also his ability to communicate and to address appropriately his needs and concerns. While personalities and attitudes differ widely between patients and physicians, every patient must feel that the physician is "on her side." A physician who claims to be objective and takes an intellectual or strictly academic approach (the most recent clinical trial results for example), may not meet a fundamental emotional need of the patient. In "The Ballad of Reading Gaol," Irish poet Oscar Wilde wrote,[6] "Something was dead in each of us, and what was dead was *hope*," that never-to-be-forgotten or ever-to-be ignored yearning of each and every person. Many years ago, the famed surgeon William James Mayo, of Rochester, Minnesota, characterized his fellow doctors[7]: "One meets with many men who have been fine students, and have stood high in their classes, who have had great knowledge of medicine but very little wisdom in its application. They have mastered the science and have failed in their understanding of the human being."

## The Complaint

A *complaint* is defined as "an expression of discontent, regret, pain, censure, resentment, or grief."[8] Each of these elements enters into the complaint and thus into the analysis of symptoms, but the fundamental objective remains, to effect a reduction or increase in the probability/possibility of a specific organic or functional cause for the complaint and to establish as accurate and complete a diagnosis as possible. Just as the nature of man is best understood by the company he keeps, so it is with the medical history. The commitment of appropriate time for an initial history is essential. The patient expects to be listened to, and to have his concerns respected and understood. A careful and complete history is the shortcut to appropriate additional testing and the defense against waste of resources. Specific complaints must be considered in the context of patient's background and demography if their significance is to be analyzed effectively. The initial history for any patient must include, and record with accuracy, the elements of age, gender, racial origin, education, occupation, socioeconomic status, family status, satisfaction with occupation and family, and physical activities and hobbies.

The "noncardiovascular history" must be incorporated, since many complaints commonly associated with cardiovascular disease can be due to other disorders. For example, dyspnea is common in emphysema and bronchitis and ankle edema in patients with renal insufficiency, obesity, or venous varicosities. Detailed inquiry into past and current medications must be made. All medications taken by the patient must be listed. From time to time, patients referred for a "cardiology" consultation feel that medications for noncardiovascular complaints may not be relevant and may fail to report them. The family history requires careful exploration, since, in the United States, many patients are far removed from their place of origin. A spouse or another family member may provide unexpected information—for example, a history of premature heart disease or death in blood relatives. In patients who have cardiovascular disease, considering the chief complaint alone is likely to result in significant error. Nonverbal communication between spouses may be a useful clue to future compliance with recommended treatment. In all of these matters, a physician's behavior influences a patient's response. Patients who suspect or are suspected of having heart disease come with a sense of uncertainty, or even fear. Simple open-ended questions—Tell me how you feel, How can I help you?—are important, since they communicate the physician's concern and invite the patient to express himself in his own way. Then the physician can inquire further about the complaint. While every effort must be made not to "lead the patient," it is essential to understand the intrinsic limitations of the patient's understanding of medical questions and when specific direct inquiry is in order. A good example is a heart failure patient who no longer complains of shortness of breath because his activity level has now been reduced to a degree appropriate to his residual ventricular function. It is a useful exercise to "live through a day" with the patient by eliciting a brief verbal "diary" of his activities and attitudes. A knowledge of the issues that disturb or please the patient enhances the overall assessment. It also provides information on physical activity. In patients with existing disabilities, the impact of emotional, social, and functional limitations in matters large and small has become the continued living experience. Many may have been tested for heart disease, including exercise stress testing, angiography, cardiovascular intervention procedures, and vascular scanning to estimate the status of the carotid and systemic arteries. Tests for coronary calcification are now available (and increasingly common) and such findings may be the precipitating reason for a patient's visit. Each test should be documented with care and entered into the medical record. Whenever possible, original copies of such reports must be obtained.

## Follow-up, Emergent, and Consulting Visits

While the initial visit provides the bedrock of understanding, the circumstances of presentation determine the nature and purpose of the later medical history.

Follow-up visits are usually structured to document responses to treatment, since, an effective practitioner should have an accurate profile that should be available for comparison. The time commitment of an initial visit may not be necessary. A careful record of current medications and laboratory and other test results is made by a specialty nurse and, when appropriate, reported to the patient. Such a visit is always worth a "How are you doing?" from the physician, with specific inquiry about changes in a principal complaint, a new event, new test results, or response to medication. Emergent visits assume the availability of at least a minimum of prior information; usually the issues at hand are specific. When a patient's survival is in question, obtaining complete historical details will, of necessity, be deferred. In contrast, a formal consultation requires a clear definition of purpose—diagnosis, management, procedure, reassurance. Here, the interview establishes, in great detail and with precision, the nature and significance of complaints and the relation of physical examination data and other relevant findings to developing an optimal strategy.

## Questionnaires, Nurse Practitioners, and Physician Extenders

History taking may be facilitated by a questionnaire, which is best sent to a patient several days before a first visit. A questionnaire raises important general issues in a patient's mind and provides an opportunity for unhurried thought and discussion with a family member. It also promotes careful completion of essential demographic questions, inclusion of secondary complaints, and a considered review by patient and spouse of family and patient histories and medications. A trained physician's assistant may review the responses and obtain clarification when necessary. The interview must be unhurried: the patient must be given sufficient time to express himself and to clarify questions in his mind. Since accurate and specific information is required and patients may be unfamiliar with symptoms and their significance, direct inquiry is usually necessary. Patients feel (properly) dissatisfied if the initial consultation is so brief that many of their concerns go unaddressed and unanswered. There may be important advantages if a spouse or family member is involved in an initial interview or at least is present for the physician's summation and recommendations. When a physician interviews a patient absent a spouse, symptoms and other important information may go unreported. On the other hand, the interview with the patient may be more open. Elements of family history may be denied or forgotten by the patient. Interspousal and personal dynamics that may be relevant to future management and compliance also become evident. A younger person sometimes provides better reporting of an elderly patient's complaints. A third person is even more essential for patients whose first language is not the physician's. While an interpreter may translate, the connotations of the words can be lost. An experienced physician's assistant can contribute to the process, but an initial interview is best concluded personally by the physician—and always when that person is a consulting subspecialist. The needs of the poor and underserved pose a major challenge to providers and require innovative approaches. The important and expanding role of nurse practitioners in primary care, follow-up, and extended care giving is predicated on the confidence of the patient in a team approach supported by prompt physician participation.

## ■ THE MEDICAL RECORD

Clinical information is subject to variations in accuracy, precision, variability, sensitivity, and specificity.[9] In this respect, the veracity of the medical record is paramount. To *record*[8] is "to set down in writing or the like, as to the purpose of presenting evidence." This definition implies that the facts be described accurately and be complete, inclusive, and, when proper, available and understandable to persons of like background to the originator of the record. Also, it should be readily available. Current medical records seldom fulfill these criteria: they are usually incomplete, not easily available, frequently handwritten, and many times only partially legible. This is a particular problem with emergency room reports, which may contain critical information for later admission or call for a cardiac consultation. In legal disputes, a physician may be required to read his notes into the court record to allow reasonable interpretation, even by other physicians. *It is essential that this serious deficiency of record completeness and legibility be corrected*, since an accurate record is vital to the provision of immediate *and* long-term medical care. Desktop and hand-held automated devices are now available for effective collection of diagnostic information of all sorts, including a detailed medical history. Thus, reliable, systematic, comprehensive, and legible record systems are now available. They are easy to learn and should become a standard of care, as younger, computer-literate physicians enter practice. Useful diagnostic logic and medication data can also be programmed to assess common complaints and drug side effects.

## ■ CORONARY RISK

Because of the overall primacy of atherosclerotic disease[10] as a cause of heart disease, specific inquiries must be made to include risk evaluation for coronary artery disease and atherosclerosis.[11] It is now clear that coronary risk can be modified, but it is essential to recognize that the intensity of treatment must be tailored to the hazard for coronary disease events.[12] On the basis of available knowledge and current costs of effective medications, it is neither desirable nor possible to treat all patients, including those at low risk for coronary disease events. Thus, selection must be based on risk. The factors currently deemed most important are listed in Table 6–1, but it is the presence of multiple risk factors in a single patient that confers the highest risk, and for such patients rigorous and directed inquiry is in order.

## ■ AFTER THE HISTORY

An effective history includes other factual observations, including the findings on physical examination, the standard 12-lead ECG, the chest film, and basic laboratory data, including a blood lipid panel and blood glucose. Each of these

Table 6–1

**Atherosclerosis Risk Factors**

Increasing age and male gender

Past cardiovascular events: stable angina pectoris, unstable angina, acute myocardial infarction, revascularization procedures, prior positive testing for ischemia, emergency room visit for chest pain (rule out acute myocardial infarction), family history of premature events

Current symptoms and medications: chest discomfort or pain requiring antiangina medication, hypertension requiring medication, familial hyperlipidemia

Conventional metabolic and endocrine factors: blood lipids, elevated low-density lipoprotein, low high-density lipoprotein, elevated triglycerides, elevated blood glucose, glucose intolerance, hyper- and hypothyroidism, menopausal status, obesity

Personal habits: cigarette smoking history, diet, activity level, alcohol use

Type A personality

Psychosocial, familial, or occupational stress

Table 6–2

**Symptoms Associated with Cardiovascular Disease**

| | |
|---|---|
| Pain (in the chest and elsewhere) | Embolic manifestations |
| Dyspnea of effort, orthopnea, paroxysmal nocturnal dyspnea | Symptoms related to systemic disorders that may have a cardiovascular cause or relationship |
| Fatigue on exertion or at rest | |

contributes to the ongoing process of qualitative, unstructured probabilistics relative to a specific anatomic or functional diagnosis. Physicians must recognize the intrinsic reality of such a process and apply scientific reasoning whenever possible. This will allow conclusions as to appropriate areas for further investigation, so as to improve or cast doubt on the direction of diagnostic inquiry. In particular, such an analytic approach usually allows a physician to exclude the least probable causes and to logically proceed to a correct diagnosis.

## ■ CARDIAC SYMPTOMS

The principal symptoms associated with cardiovascular disorders are listed in Table 6–2. Each is considered briefly for what it may suggest about a cause. Also, it is essential to distinguish between the far more frequent noncardiac causes and the far more serious cardiac ones. Symptoms associated with heart disease are frequently activity related, like those of angina pectoris and heart failure and certain dysrhythmias, but a particular symptom, or its absence, may favor certain possibilities over others.

### Chest Pain

The principal causes of chest pain or discomfort are listed in Table 6–3 and specific directions of inquiry in Table 6–4. Chest pain is one of the symptoms that most often precipitate a visit to a physician or cardiologist. It is a common, and

Table 6–3

**Causes of Discomfort in the Chest**

| | |
|---|---|
| **Chest Wall** | Pericardial |
| |   Acute subacute pericarditis |
|   Cervicodorsal osteoarthritis |   Malignancy |
|   Intervertebral disc disease | Other |
|   Intercostal neuritis |   Mitral valve prolapse |
|   Rib fracture |   Hypertrophic cardiomyopathy |
|   Costochondritis | |
|   Herpes zoster | **Intrathoracic Pulmonary** |
| **Intrathoracic Cardiovascular** |   Acute pneumothorax |
| |   Pleurisy and pleural effusion |
|   Vascular |   Pneumonia |
|     Aortic dissection |   Pulmonary embolism |
|     Pulmonary hypertension | |
|   Myocardial | **Referred from Other Organs** |
|     Stable angina pectoris |   Gastric reflux |
|     Unstable angina |   Esophagitis and esophageal spasm |
|     Prolonged myocardial |   Peptic ulcer disease |
|       ischemia |   Pancreatitis |
|     Acute myocardial infarction |   Gallbladder disease |

Table 6–4

**Variables Associated with Discomfort in the Chest**

Intensity: Severity, temporal features (continuous sporadic) easing, worsening
Quality: Visceral, superficial, pressure, crushing, stabbing, burning, tearing
Location: Retrosternal, suprasternal, epigastric
Sites of referred pain: chest wall, back, right shoulder, right arm, both arms, jaw, occiput, head,
  epigastrium, right or left subcostal area, abdomen
Onset: Sudden, gradual
Precipitating cause (if any)
Aggravating factors: Activity, breathing, posture
Associated finding: Anxiety, coughing, dyspnea, nausea, vomiting, diarrhea, sweating, pallor, cold
  extremities, rapid or slow heart rate

possibly the most important, symptom associated with heart disease, yet it is neither very sensitive nor very specific for any diagnosis. Chest pain may range from brief, transient, mild discomfort to continuous, excruciating pain. In general, the more severe the pain, the greater is the likelihood of important underlying disease.

## Cardiac Ischemia

Although many forms of heart disease are associated with discomfort in the chest, the most important by far is that associated with vascular narrowing due to coronary atherosclerosis. Ischemic pain is the sensation caused by an imbalance between available oxygen supply and the metabolic demand of working myocardium. The afferent pathway is complex, and the resulting symptoms are complex and variable in intensity, location, and radiation. Is the pain continuous or intermittent? The onset characteristics may be defining. Transient substernal chest discomfort on activity or stair climbing, in response to excitement, anxiety, or cold, or postprandial discomfort favors angina pectoris. The association of new onset or more severe angina with fever, tachycardia, or anemia is also common. In general, the pain of angina pectoris appears at some level of activity or emotional stress, rapidly regresses when the activity ceases, and is reproducible under comparable circumstances. Effort-related angina is usually short-lived and self-limited and is described as pressure, constriction, squeezing, and unlike anything the patient has experienced before. Severe, unrelenting pain is suggestive of ongoing severe myocardial ischemia and acute myocardial infarction. Intermittent recurrent pain may be associated with angina pectoris or unstable angina.

Other descriptors of angina pectoris include *new, accelerated, progressive, unstable, preinfarction,* and *nocturnal.* "Angina equivalent" refers to dyspnea as an alternative symptom that develops under circumstances similar to those that precipitate common angina pectoris. "Unstable angina" refers to angina of new onset (less than 1 month), with symptoms that increase in severity, frequency, and intensity and a changing pattern of radiation, in the absence of enzymatic evidence infarction. It is due to partial and transient thrombotic occlusion of a diseased vessel and may progress to a completed infarction.

## Location and Radiation

Ischemic chest pain is usually substernal with variable radiation patterns, commonest being into the left shoulder and the ulnar aspect of the left arm. It is usually perceived as pressing, constricting, and heavy, frequently associated v

activity but not necessarily so. Although centrally located pain is characteristic of ischemia, pain may be limited to the neck and jaw, the xyphoid region, or the left shoulder and arm, and it may or may not radiate. Atypical distribution patterns are not rare and include the right chest alone and the epigastrium without radiation to the neck or arms. In "demographically appropriate" persons (e.g., a man 60 years of age), the presence of any chest pain raises the possibility of underlying coronary disease. Other causes of chest pain, the acute tearing pain of aortic dissection or aneurysm, and pain associated with respiration, like that of pneumothorax, pleurisy, pneumonia, pericarditis, or pulmonary embolus, may be identified by their specific characteristics. The initial pain of aortic dissection may be described as the worst possible and may be localized or radiate to the back. Pleuritic chest pain is worse on inspiration or with coughing. The severity and duration of pain help to clarify cause. Rapid relief suggests angina pectoris. More prolonged pain, yet with relief, is seen in unstable or progressive angina, and severe, persistent, prolonged pain in myocardial infarction. The association of nausea, vomiting, sweating, and anxiety with chest pain is suggestive of evolving myocardial infarction. Angina at rest is usually caused by severe, prolonged myocardial ischemia, may be spontaneous, and often occurs at night, waking the patient from sleep. Chest pain associated with nausea, vomiting, palpitations, and feelings of weakness and fear is common in acute infarction.

## Noncardiac Chest Pain

Chest pain secondary to peptic ulcer, gallbladder disease, gastric reflux or esophagitis, or spinal disease or costochondritis is more common than cardiac chest pain. In these conditions pain may be spontaneous, due to hunger, associated with recumbency (reflux), and relieved by antacids or by eating. The pain and discomfort of esophageal spasm may be relieved by nitroglycerin. Chest pain associated with ingestion of food, swallowing, coughing, or position changes is less likely to be of cardiac origin. Musculoskeletal pain is variable in site and severity and is exacerbated by respiration, other movements, and localized pressure. Attention to simple demographics (age, gender, history) is helpful in most cases but, uncommonly, may mislead. While, for example, acute infarction is uncommon in younger women, failure to entertain the possibility has resulted in tragic outcomes. Ischemia must always be considered when an older patient reports new-onset chest pain. The key is awareness of such possibilities, but in many cases the cause can be established with confidence from the history alone. Anxiety (which frequently is justified) can affect the symptoms. Pain due to pneumothorax, pleurisy, pneumonia, or pulmonary embolism is worse on inspiration, and patients minimize the effort of breathing with unilateral chest splinting. Pain of pulmonary origin generally does not radiate, is localized to one side or the other, and is seldom substernal. The discomfort associated with other forms of heart disease—mitral valve prolapse, pulmonary hypertension, and hypertrophic cardiomyopathy—is usually not sufficient to cause severe distress. Functional chest pain associated with fear of heart disease or with anxiety is usually acute, sharp, and stabbing, and frequently is localized to the cardiac apex. At times, it is associated with hyperventilation, but it is not usually exercise related, although it may subside relatively rapidly. Anxiety and hyperventilation are more common in younger females, and, rarely, chest pain may be factitious or a component of an abnormal psychological state. Factors associated with relief of pain are all important. Relief on cessation of activity and nitroglycerin suggests angina pectoris. Increasing or persistent pain under those circumstances is consistent with unstable angina, myocardial infarction, or aortic dissection. Acute pericarditis may be relieved by leaning forward. In brief, any patient whose complaint includes chest pain deserves careful interrogation and evaluation.

## Dyspnea

Dyspnea is an uncomfortable awareness of the necessity of breaking. It is a common symptom of both cardiac and pulmonary disorders and a response to anxiety. It is frequently associated with increased pulmonary venous pressure. The principal causes are listed in Table 6–5.

Dyspnea, by itself, is not abnormal, since it is inevitable with vigorous exercise, including treadmill testing, even in trained athletes. At rest, however, awareness of an abnormal need for breathing under conditions of mild or moderate exertion becomes significant. Acute-onset dyspnea usually has a pulmonary cause—for example, acute pneumothorax, pleurisy, pneumonia, or pulmonary embolus—but it may also be a major, early feature of an extensive myocardial infarction. The dyspnea of congestive heart failure is experienced at decreasing levels of external work and, finally, at rest. Dyspnea may be associated with chest pain of cardiac causes. A history of smoking is associated with recurrent chest infections and emphysema. Mild dyspnea results from early congestive heart failure. Each may be worsened by new onset myocardial ischemia. Again, relief of dyspnea should occur when the precipitating symptom is removed or alleviated. Several factors contribute to dyspnea, including deconditioning and obesity, fever, tachycardia, and anemia. Anxiety-induced hyperventilation is often mistaken for dyspnea. Orthopnea is severe dyspnea that renders patients unable to lie flat and forces them to recline in a semiupright position. Paroxysmal nocturnal dyspnea is usually associated with chronic heart failure. It begins shortly after the patient lies down to sleep and is relieved by assuming an upright position. In addition, a fast-acting diuretic may be necessary. The common mechanism is increased pulmonary venous pressure due to mitral valve disease or left ventricular dysfunction. Acute pulmonary edema is an expression of pulmonary venous hypertension with transudation of large quantities of fluid into the alveoli that precipitates severe coughing with expectoration of frothy fluid (which may be blood stained) and extreme anxiety. "Functional" dyspnea often occurs at rest and is associated with apical stabbing or prolonged chest wall pains.

### Table 6–5

#### Causes of Dyspnea

| Pulmonary Disease | Cardiac Disease |
|---|---|
| Acute | Acute |
| Spontaneous pneumothorax | Pulmonary edema |
| Pulmonary embolus | Aortic/mitral valve insufficiency |
| Pneumonia | Prosthetic valve dysfunction |
| Airway obstruction | Left atrial thrombosis |
| Subacute | Left atrial myxoma |
| Airway obstruction | Subacute |
| Chronic obstructive lung disease | Left ventricular failure |
| Emphysema | Myocardial infarction |
| Pulmonary fibrosis | Pericardial effusion |
| Chronic bronchitis | Constrictive pericarditis |
| Bronchiectasis | |
| | **Other Causes** |
| | Intrathoracic malignancy |
| | Rib fracture, chest trauma |
| | Anxiety |
| | Hyperventilation |

## Fatigue

Fatigue, transient weariness during exertion, is due to an imbalance between the metabolic demands of working skeletal muscle and the available blood flow to deliver oxygen and remove products of muscle metabolism. The symptom may be due to deconditioning, as with prolonged bed rest, and it is the presenting symptom of anemia of any cause. Circulatory dynamics favor coronary and cerebral blood flow. When cardiac output is reduced from any cause and cannot increase, the skeletal muscle metabolic demand during activity cannot be met. Obstructive vascular disease also limits the availability of blood flow and is a common cause of limb fatigue and of intermittent claudication.

## Palpitations

Palpitations, perceived unusual or prominent heartbeats, are commonplace and may be benign or a sign of important heart disease. In general, the term refers to an awareness of an irregular heartbeat. The patient is also aware of either severe tachycardia or bradycardia and associated lightheadedness, or even syncope. As with the other symptoms of heart disease, the nature of the occurrence, the precipitating and resolving factors, and the medical history are vital. The underlying causes of palpitations include ectopic beats, transient atrial fibrillation, and heart block. Sudden onset and cessation favors paroxysmal atrial tachycardia or atrial flutter or fibrillation. Flip-flops favor premature ventricular contractions. A moderate unexplained increase in heart rate may favor an anxiety state. Again, the influence of other factors, including fever, anemia and hyperthyroidism, must be considered.

## Syncope

Syncope is defined as loss of consciousness secondary to underperfusion of the brain. It may be due to a Stokes-Adams attack associated with heart block or in response to ventricular flutter or fibrillation. Syncope after effort is associated with aortic stenosis and with hypertrophic cardiomypathy and pulmonary hypertension. The differential diagnosis includes the common faint (vasovagal attack) and seizure disorders.

Other "remote" manifestations of heart and vascular diseases are listed in Table 6–6. Embolic stroke always requires a search for an intracardiac cause, particularly in patients who have atrial fibrillation and infective endocarditis, but also in those with carotid artery disease or after myocardial infarction. The left atrium, left ventricle, mitral and aortic valves, and the aorta and carotid arteries are sources of calcific embol. Paradoxical embolism occurs by way of a patent foramen ovale. Systemic findings of fever, chills, and tachycardia associated with a new or changing murmur suggest infective endocarditis, but they also characterize rheumatic fever and atrial myxoma. Cardiac involvement may occur in a number of systemic disorders, including rheumatoid arthritis, systemic lupus erythematosus, and scleroderma.

## Hematologic Disorders

Blood disorders include polycythemia vera, sickle cell anemia, and thalassemia. Cardiac involvement is common in cancer patients overall. Acute leukemia, malignant melanoma, and Hodgkin's disease are frequent causes, as are intrathoracic

Table 6–6

**Other Conditions and Symptoms Associated with Heart Disease**

| General Symptoms of Infection | Embolic Disorders |
|---|---|
| Fever | Cerebral |
| Sweating | Hemiparesis |
| Malaise | Transient or persistent visual |
| Rheumatic fever | disorders |
| Infective endocarditis | **Manifestations of Septic Emboli** |
| Atrial myxoma | |
| **General Manifestations of Rheumatic Diseases** | Skin |
| | Digits, nailbeds |
| Systemic lupus erythematosus | Spleen |
| Scleroderma | Kidneys |
| Polymyositis | Limbs |
| Polyarteritis nodosa | |
| Muscular dystrophies—progressive, myotonic, | |
| Friedrich's ataxia | |

malignancies, in particular broncogenic carcinoma and metastatic breast disease. Infiltrative disorders of the myocardium include amyloidosis and hemochromatosis.

## Conclusion

The evaluation of the complaints of any patient reduces to detection—a "Whodunit." An astute clinician considers the medical history the primary evidence and then seeks new clues from forensic tests and the like. Sometimes he revisits "the scene of the crime" with a second interview—"I didn't understand how your father died. Please tell me again." We all rely on likelihoods structured or unstructured, intuitive, instinctive, or scientifically derived. Nevertheless, the taking of a medical history remains an art that must be learned. It is application of a true "uncertainty principle," inexactitudes in action. Yet, from the patient's perspective, "the verdict"—a solution to a specific complaint, is the goal. This also is basic to our purposes and to whether or not our derived conclusions are correct and our recommended treatments effective. But diagnosis and treatment are not the only outcomes to be fostered by the medical history. It should also be the basis for a continuing interaction between doctor and patient aimed at achieving a net gain in individual personal health, which is the fundamental purpose of medical practice.

## ■ REFERENCES

1. Swartz MH: The art of interviewing. pages 1-81 *In* Swartz MH (Ed): Textbook of Physical Diagnosis, History and Examination, 3rd ed. Philadelphia: WB Saunders, 1998:1–81.
2. Smith LH Jr: Medicine as an art. *In* Wyngaarden JB, Smith LH Jr, Bennett CJ (Eds): Cecil Textbook of Medicine, 19th Ed. Philadelphia: WB Saunders, 1992:6–9.
3. Bennett JC: The social responsibilities and humanistic qualities of "the good doctor." *In* Wyngaarden JB, Smith LH Jr, Bennett CJ (Eds): Cecil Textbook of Medicine, 19th ed. Philadelphia: WB Saunders, (1992):2–6.
4. Li JTC: Humility and the practice of medicine. Mayo Clin Proc 1999;74:529–530.
5. Merkle WT, BB Margolis, RC Smith: Teaching humanistic and psychosocial aspects of care. J Gen Intern Med 1990;5:34–50.
6. Wilde O: The Ballad of Reading Gaol. *In* The Works of Oscar Wilde. Ware: The Wordsworth Poetry Library, 1994:136–152.
7. Willius FW (Ed): Aphorisms, 2nd Ed. Rochester: Mayo Foundation 1990:67.
8. Webster's College Dictionary. New York: Random House, 1992.
9. Bland M: Introduction to Medical Statistics, 2nd ed. Oxford: Oxford University Press, 1995.

10. Prevention of coronary heart disease in clinical practice. Recommendations of the Second Joint Task Force of European and Other Societies on Coronary Prevention. Eur Heart J 1998;19:1434–1503.
11. Wilson PWF, D'Agostino RB, Levy D, et al: Prediction of coronary heart disease using risk factor categories. Circulation 1998;97:1837–1847.
12. Pearson TA, Fuster V: American College of Cardiology 27th Bethesda Conference: Matching the intensity of risk factor management with the hazard for coronary disease events. Executive summary. J Am Coll Cardiol 1996;27:958–1047.

## ■ RECOMMENDED READING

Bickley LS, Hokelman RA: Interview and the health history. *In* Bickley LS, Hoekleman RA (Eds). Physical Examination and History Taking. Philadelphia: JB Lippincott, 1999: 1–40.
Fletcher RH, Fletcher SW, Wagner EH: Clinical Epidemiology. The Essentials, 3rd ed. Baltimore: Williams & Wilkins, 1996.
Gross RA: Making Medical Decisions. An Approach to Clinical Decision Making. Philadelphia: American College of Physicians-American Society of Internal Medicine, 1999.
Meador CK: A Little Book of Doctors' Rules. Philadelphia: Hanley and Belfus, 1992.
Seidel HM, Ball JW, Daims JE, Benedict GW (Eds): Mosby's Guide to Physical Examination. St. Louis: Mosby–Year Book, 1999.

*Chapter 7*

# Physical Examination of the Heart and Circulation

*Jonathan Abrams*

## ▪ GENERAL COMMENTS

The examination of the heart and circulation has a long and rich tradition in clinical medicine. Most of the cardinal signs of cardiovascular disease detectable on the physical examination were described and documented by master physicians during the 19th and early 20th centuries. Subsequently, echocardiography and cardiac catheterization studies have demonstrated that the presumed pathogenesis of many or most cardiovascular abnormalities detected on the physical examination were accurately and presciently described before these modern techniques became available. In the past, generations of internists and cardiologists were well-trained in the skills of cardiac examination; there was no ultrasound technology, so there was an emphasis on expertise in cardiac physical diagnosis. Unfortunately, clinical skills in this area are no longer emphasized in medical education, in part owing to the burgeoning of other aspects of medical science that must be taught in the medical student curriculum. The ready availability of two-dimensional echocardiography has clearly contributed to the demise of cardiac physical diagnosis skills among physicians, a phenomenon well-documented in recent published studies.

In this chapter I will highlight the core components of the cardiac physical examination and will focus on a practical assessment of the heart and circulation in health and disease. *My assumption is that readers already possess a basic knowledge of the cardiac examination and of structural heart disease.* It is hoped that physicians will redouble their efforts in applying the well-known components of the cardiac examination to their patients. The rewards are many, in particular, a feeling of real satisfaction in making a diagnosis of organic heart disease with one's own hands and ears.

### Limitations of the Cardiac Physical Examination

Echocardiography has clearly demonstrated that much cardiovascular disease is not detectable or accurately quantifiable, even to the expert, on physical examination. For instance, mitral and aortic regurgitation are often missed; left ventricular function may be significantly depressed without producing a detectable abnormality on examination. *Thus, it is best to consider the physical examination and the echocardiogram as complementary.* For the experienced clinician, the findings on the cardiac examination often predict what will be noted on the ultrasound study. Nevertheless, if significant heart disease is suspected, a complete two-dimensional Doppler echocardiographic examination is often indicated. Conversely, with a negative cardiac physical examination in the setting of a normal electrocardiogram, an echocardiogram can be avoided in many instances.

Table 7–1

**The Cardiac Physical Examination**

- Overall assessment of the patient
  —General features (e.g., dyspnea, cyanosis, edema)
  —Special features (e.g., unusual facies, lipid deposits)
- Blood pressure
  —Supine, upright
  —Leg pressure (if coarctation is suspected)
- Arterial pulses
  —Contour, volume
- Precordial motion
  —LV apex impulse (PMI)
  —RV activity
  —Ectopic impulses
  —Thrills (loud murmur)
- Heart sounds
  —Characteristics of $S_1$, $S_2$
  —Is an $S_3$ or $S_4$ present?
  —Ejection or nonejection clicks
  —Opening snap
- Heart murmurs
  —Systolic
  —Diastolic
  —Continuous
  —Timing in cardiac cycle
  —Quality
  —Length
  —Radiation
  —Effect of inspiration

## The Cardiac Examination

The components of the cardiac physical examination are standard (Table 7–1). Physicians are urged to conduct the cardiac examination in a systematic and sequential fashion. After a general assessment of the patient, the arterial pulses, blood pressure, and venous pulsations are evaluated, followed by careful inspection and palpation of the precordium. Auscultation is the last, but most important, component of the cardiac examination.

## ■ EVALUATION OF THE ARTERIAL PULSE

An accurate determination of arterial pressure is part of the cardiac physical examination. Careful attention to the details of the technique of taking the blood pressure is important (see Chapter 31). Abnormalities of blood pressure are a feature of several types of structural heart disease (Table 7–2). Assessment of the severity of aortic regurgitation or detection of pulsus paradoxus are two situations where the blood pressure can provide important information.

## The Examination

The physician must become familiar with the normal volume and rate of rise of the arterial pulse. In general, the carotid artery is the only artery that should be utilized for detection of cardiovascular abnormalities. Because of delay of transmission of the pulse wave in the periphery and the distal decrease in arterial diameter,

Table 7–2

**Blood Pressure and Peripheral Arterial Examination: Clues to Cardiovascular Disease**

| Disease | Findings |
| --- | --- |
| Coarctation of the aorta | Hypertension in upper extremities; brachial–femoral delay |
| Aortic regurgitation | Wide pulse pressure with increased systolic and decreased diastolic pressure |
| | Increased volume, rate of rise of arterial pulses with exaggerated collapse |
| Pulsus or mechanical alternans | Beat-to-to beat alternation in peak pressure and pulse volume (detected by palpation, not cuff) |
| Pulsus paradoxus | Exaggerated inspiratory decline (>10 mm Hg) in peak systolic pressure measured carefully by cuff; palpation alone may detect severe cases |
| Hypertension | Elevated systolic and diastolic pressures. Increased systolic pressure with normal diastolic pressure (isolated systolic hypertension of the elderly) |

the assessment of the radial or brachial arterial pulses usually is of little value (except in the assessment of pulsus alternans, pulsus paradoxus, or cardiogenic shock). In hypertensive patients, simultaneous assessment of the brachial and femoral arterial pulses is useful to rule out significant coarctation of the aorta. *In such cases, the femoral pulse wave peak will* clearly follow *the palpable brachial artery impulse; a delay indicates probable obstruction in the aorta.*

The contour of the aortic pulse is important in the assessment of aortic valve disease. *Aortic stenosis characteristically produces a small volume, late peaking or delayed carotid upstroke, often with a palpable shudder or thrill* (Fig. 7–1). Remember that in healthy older subjects, decreased compliance and increased arterial stiffness typically result in an increase in arterial pulse amplitude and pulse pressure. This can readily mask the typical abnormalities of aortic stenosis. Aortic regurgitation, when significant, typically results in an arterial pulse with increased amplitude and rate of rise and a collapsing quality. *In severe aortic regurgitation, the aortic pulsations may be abnormal throughout the arterial system (Table 7–3). A prominent (often visible), high-amplitude, full-volume carotid arterial pulse, coupled with a wide pulse pressure (diastolic blood pressure 60 mmHg or less) is very suggestive of severe aortic regurgitation. A double-peaking (or bisferiens) pulse is common in advanced aortic regurgitation (Fig. 7–2).*

## Pulsus Paradoxus

A greater than normal difference in systolic blood pressure between inspiration and expiration is known as *pulsus paradoxus.* This is common whenever there are

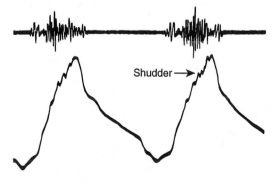

**Figure 7–1** ▪ The arterial pulse in aortic stenosis. Note the delayed upstroke and the jagged contour representing a palpable shudder or transmitted thrill. The pulse volume is usually decreased as well.

Shudder ⟶

Table 7–3

**Peripheral or Nonauscultatory Signs of Severe Aortic Regurgitation: A Glossary**

| | |
|---|---|
| Bisferiens pulse | A double or bifid systolic impulse felt in the carotid arterial pulse |
| Corrigan's sign | Visible pulsations of the supraclavicular and carotid arteries |
| Pistol shot of Traube | A loud systolic sound heard with the stethoscope lightly placed over a femoral artery |
| Palmar click | A palpable, abrupt flushing of the palms in systole |
| Quincke's pulse | Exaggerated sequential reddening and blanching of the fingernail beds when light pressure is applied to the tip of the fingernail. A similar effect can be induced by pressing a glass slide to the lips |
| Duroziez's sign | A to-and-fro bruit heard over the femoral artery when light pressure is applied to the artery by the edge of the stethoscope head. This bruit is caused by the exaggerated reversal of flow in diastole. |
| De Musset's sign | Visible oscillation or bobbing of the head with each heartbeat |
| Hill's sign | Abnormal accentuation of leg systolic blood pressure, with popliteal pressure 40 mm Hg or higher than brachial artery pressure |
| Water-hammer pulse | The high-amplitude, abruptly collapsing pulse of aortic regurgitation. This term refers to a popular Victorian toy comprised of a glass vessel partially filled with water, which produced a slapping impact on being turned over. |
| Müller's sign | Visible pulsations of the uvula |

major fluctuations of intrathoracic pressure or in pericardial tamponade. *Careful auscultation is mandatory to detect significant pulsus paradoxus (>10 mm Hg). Palpation is less sensitive but may be useful when the respiratory differences in peak systolic pressures are large.* Normally, there is a slight physiologic respiratory difference between inspiration and expiration, typically 6 to 8 mm Hg or less during quiet respiration. Pulsus paradoxus may be associated with severe congestive heart failure, decompensated chronic obstructive lung disease, asthma, and occasionally, extreme obesity. Paradoxus must always be sought when a pericardial effusion is known or suspected.

### Pulsus Alternans

In a setting of severe left ventricular systolic dysfunction, beat-to-beat alteration in the peak amplitude of the arterial pulse may be noted (Fig. 7–3). It can be palpated in the brachial or radial arteries but usually goes undetected. It is most likely to be associated with a left ventricular heave and a third heart sound. Careful palpation of the radial artery is recommended.

Determination of pulsus paradoxus or mechanical pulsus alternans are two exceptions to the rule of always using the carotid arteries for arterial pulse analysis. Table 7–2 lists conditions when arterial pulse wave analysis is particularly valuable.

### ■ EVALUATION OF THE VENOUS PULSE

Most physicians do a poor job of the venous examination, and many are intimidated by the presumed difficulty of assessing the jugular venous pulse (JVP). The following key points should help to make the JVP examination straightforward:

1. The A wave (produced by right atrial contraction) is normally larger or taller than the V wave in normal subjects. *The examiner should expect to visualize a dominant A wave in most instances (Fig. 7–4).*
2. Conditions of decreased right ventricular compliance, such as right ventricu-

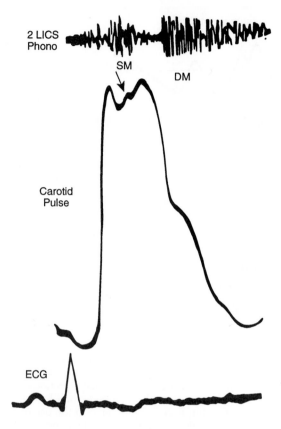

**Figure 7–2** ■ Bisferiens pulse of aortic regurgitation. Note the bifid systolic pulse wave, which is best detected using light finger pressure over the carotid arteries. This contour is usually associated with increased pulse volume. The bisferiens pulse must be differentiated from a transmitted systolic murmur or palpable thrill. Note the soft $S_1$ and $S_2$. SM, systolic murmur; DM, diastolic murmur; 2 LICS, second left intercostal space; Phono, phonocardiogram.

lar hypertrophy or pulmonary disease, may augment the A wave amplitude and prominence, particularly in the setting of pulmonary hypertension.

3. *Detection of the A wave is easy if the examiner remembers that it immediately precedes the palpable carotid arterial pulse (one must use simultaneous inspection and palpation of the carotid upstroke). Conversely, the V wave of the jugular venous pulse is simultaneous with the carotid upstroke (systolic in timing).*

4. *When the V wave is the predominant waveform* and is greater than the A wave (in the absence of atrial fibrillation), it is likely that significant tricuspid regurgitation is present, even in the absence of a typical murmur of tricuspid regurgitation (see Fig. 7–13).

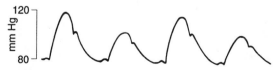

**Figure 7–3** ■ Pulsus alternans. Note that every other beat has a lower systolic pressure. The rate of rise of the second pulse wave is slower, relating to decreased contractile force in alternate beats. Pulsus alternans is an important sign of severe left ventricular dysfunction. It is best detected in a peripheral vessel such as the radial artery. Heart sounds and murmurs may also alternate in intensity.

Jugular Venous Pulse

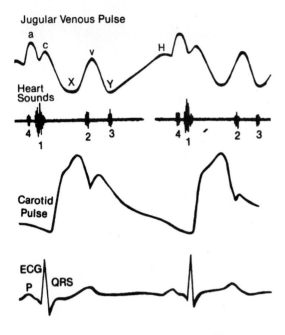

**Figure 7–4** ■ Normal jugular venous pulse. Note the biphasic venous waveform with a large A wave immediately preceding the carotid arterial upstroke and roughly coinciding with $S_1$, and a smaller V wave that peaks almost coincident with $S_2$. The jugular X descent occurs during systole and in some individuals may be quite prominent. The Y descent occurs during early diastole; the nadir of the Y descent times with $S_3$. The C wave and H wave are not visible to the eye but are often recordable in venous pulse tracings.

5. Mean jugular pressure is relatively easy to measure (Fig. 7–5). *It is most important to determine if the mean venous pressure is normal or elevated*; quantification of the precise degree of venous pressure elevation is less important, although often this can be accomplished.

Dr. Gordon Ewy has emphasized the use of abdominal or hepatic compression to bring out latent or borderline elevation of the jugular venous pressure, which may be important to assess if a volume overload state or heart failure is suspected.

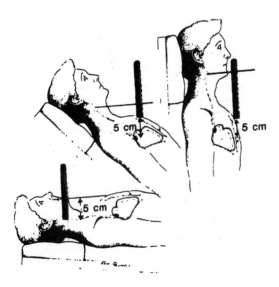

**Figure 7–5** ■ Estimation of mean venous pressure. The right atrium is approximately 5 cm below the sternal angle of Louis with the subject in any position. Thus, with a patient supine or erect, the height of the venous pulsations from the sternal angle can be measured; by adding 5 cm to this value, one can estimate the actual venous pressure. The thorax and neck should be positioned until the peak of the venous column is readily identified. In subjects with normal venous pressure, only the peaks of the A and V waves may be seen when the patient is sitting up at 45 degrees or greater. When the venous pressure is abnormally high, the thorax and head must be elevated to accurately identify the true peak of the venous column.

The technique is simple: steady pressure is applied with the hand over the upper abdomen for 60 seconds while carefully observing the jugular venous pulsations. The normal response is a brief rise and a decline in the mean jugular venous pressure. An abnormal result consists of a progressive and sustained rise in the mean venous pressure for as long as 1 minute.

*Abnormalities of the venous contour or pressure reflect right heart events. While it is true that left heart disease, particular left ventricular failure, is the most common cause of right ventricular failure, increased venous pressure does not necessarily imply left ventricular systolic failure.* Fluid or volume overload in the setting of normal cardiac function, left ventricular diastolic dysfunction, primary or significant secondary pulmonary hypertension, severe tricuspid regurgitation, or isolated right heart failure due to the pulmonary hypertension of pulmonary disease (cor pulmonale) can all increase jugular venous pressure in the absence of left ventricular disease. Nevertheless, increased jugular venous pressure is one of the hallmarks of congestive heart failure, often a left heart problem in adults.

## ■ PRECORDIAL MOTION

### The Left Ventricle

By far the most important aspect of inspection and palpation of the heart is determining whether the left ventricle is grossly normal or abnormal. Left ventricular hypertrophy and dilatation are the commonest causes of an abnormal PMI (*point of maximal impulse*, an old-fashioned term that nevertheless is still useful), also known as the *left ventricular apical impulse.* The normal left ventricle is felt over a small area, (<3 cm), is not displaced beyond the midclavicular line, is not sustained into late systole, and is not hyperdynamic (Table 7–4, Fig. 7–6). *Often, the left ventricle is not palpable with the patient in the supine position; the examiner must then ask the patient to turn onto the left side with the left arm elevated for optimal assessment of the precordium (Fig. 7–7). Usually, but not always, the left ventricular impulse then becomes apparent in this position.* Subjects older than 50 years, and those with large chests, prominent musculature, or obesity, or large breasts, all have a decreased likelihood of a detectable the PMI.

Abnormalities of the apical impulse are listed in Table 7–5. *Third and fourth heart sounds are more often palpable than physicians realize,* particularly in the left lateral position, and represent important findings suggesting abnormal left ventricular size, function, or compliance. Leftward *displacement* of the apical or LV impulse (1 to 2 cm beyond the midclavicular line) reflects cardiac (left ventricular) enlargement or dilatation. *Increased forcefulness* of the apical impulse is usually a sign of left ventricular hypertrophy. In coronary artery disease, an ectopic or bifid (double) left ventricular impulse is related to dyskinesis or akinesis caused by a prior

Table 7–4

**The Normal Supine Apical Impulse**

A gentle, nonsustained tap
Early systolic anterior motion that ends before the last third of systole
Located within 10 cm of the midsternal line in the fourth or fifth left intercostal space
A palpable area <2 to 2.5 cm² and detectable in only one intercostal space
Right ventricular motion normally not palpable
Diastolic events normally not palpable
May be completely absent in older persons

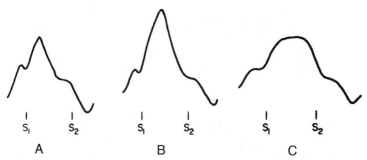

**Figure 7-6** ■ Major variants of left ventricular precordial motion: *A*, normal; *B*, hyperdynamic; *C*, sustained. With the patient in the supine position, sustained left ventricular activity detectable in the latter half of systole is distinctly abnormal. Some experts believe that palpation of a sustained impulse when patients are in the left lateral decubitus position may have less specificity for underlying left ventricular enlargement. (From Abrams J: Precordial palpation. *In* Horwitz LD, Groves BM [eds]: Signs and Symptoms in Cardiology. Philadelphia: JB Lippincott, 1985.)

myocardial infarction. A palpable $S_4$ is an important observation in aortic valve disease (suggesting severe aortic stenosis or regurgitation) and in coronary artery disease (suggesting decreased left ventricular compliance).

A meticulous search for the apical impulse can be quite rewarding and may suggest left ventricular enlargement or hypertrophy with high specificity. Absence of an abnormal left ventricular impulse in a thin person is useful in *ruling out* significant aortic stenosis, hypertrophic cardiomyopathy, or severe mitral regurgitation in a patient with a prominent systolic murmur.

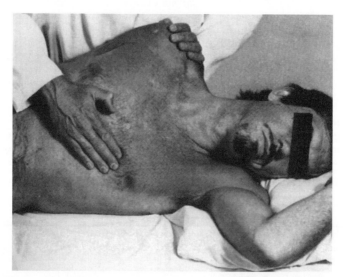

**Figure 7-7** ■ Palpation of the apex impulse, left lateral decubitus position. This maneuver should be used whenever left ventricular disease is suspected. The patient should be turned 45 to 60 degrees onto the left side with the left arm extended above the head. (From Abrams J: Precordial palpation. *In* Horwitz LD, Groves BM [eds]: Signs and Symptoms in Cardiology. Philadelphia, JB Lippincott Co, 1985.)

Table 7–5

**Causes of Palpable Precordial Abnormalities**

Left ventricular hypertrophy and / or dilatation
Left ventricular wall motion abnormalities (fixed or transient)
Increased force of left atrial contraction (palpable $S_4$)
Accentuated diastolic rapid filling (palpable $S_3$)
Anterior thrust of the heart from severe mitral regurgitation
Right ventricular hypertrophy and / or dilatation
Loud murmurs (thrills)
Loud heart sounds (normal and abnormal)
Dilated or hyperkinetic pulmonary artery
Dilated aorta

## The Right Ventricle

Right ventricular activity is not usually detectable in normal subjects, except in young or thin people, when a gentle parasternal impulse may be found. Technique is important in the detection of a right ventricular impulse; firm pressure over the lower parasternal region is the key while the patient's breath is held in end expiration (Fig. 7–8). The examining hand should be observed for upward or anterior motion, which can be quite subtle. Subxiphoid palpation with two or three fingers may be used in patients who have a large chest or chronic obstructive pulmonary disease.

*Detection of right ventricular hypertrophy generally implies pulmonary hypertension in an adult.* Severe mitral regurgitation can occasionally result in a recoil phenomenon related to left atrial expansion as the regurgitant jet of blood "pushes" the heart forward.

## Palpable Heart Sounds

The experienced examiner is familiar with palpable heart sounds that can be felt with the hand or fingers as discrete deflections. Thus, a loud $S_1$, $S_2$, or opening

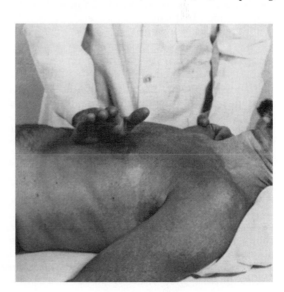

**Figure 7–8** ■ Precordial palpation for detection of parasternal or right ventricular activity. Use firm downward pressure with the heel of the hand while the patient's breath is held in end expiration. (From Abrams J: Examination of the precordium. Prim Cardiol 1982;8:156–168.)

snap is often palpable. An $S_3$ or $S_4$ may be detectable in the left lateral position. Mitral stenosis can be strongly suspected solely on the basis of a palpable $S_1$ or opening snap, diastolic apical thrill, and a right ventricular lift.

# ■ HEART SOUNDS

## Normal and Abnormal

Abrupt intracardiac pressure changes and the subsequent valve motion related to alterations in hemodynamics are responsible for most normal and abnormal heart sounds. Thus, closure of the atrioventricular and semilunar valves ($S_1$, $S_2$) and the opening motion of thickened and noncompliant aortic and mitral valve leaflets (aortic ejection click, mitral opening snap) produce commonly heard sounds.

$S_1$ is often heard as a "split" sound of two high-frequency components close together. The first of these sound transients reflects mitral valve closure and the second is produced by tricuspid closure. In general, assessment of $S_1$ splitting characteristics is unrewarding. The two components of $S_2$ are far more valuable for the physician to evaluate carefully. The first, $A_2$, coincides with abrupt closure of the aortic valve leaflets. The second, $P_2$, reflects closure of the semilunar pulmonic valve. The normal respiratory delay between $A_2$ and $P_2$ relates to increased right ventricular ejection time during inspiration (due to enhanced right ventricular filling) and, to a lesser degree, to decreased left ventricular filling during inspiration. Differences in compliance between the proximal aorta and pulmonary artery also affect the inspiratory splitting and fusion (single $S_2$) during expiration. The loudness or audibility of the two second heart sounds, as well as their behavior during the respiratory cycle, may be influenced by electrical conduction disturbances (e.g., left or right bundle branch block), ventricular ejection characteristics, and the vascular compliance of the two great vessels (see Table 7–6).

The $S_3$ and $S_4$ are due to left ventricular filling transients produced by left atrial contraction ($S_4$) and passive left ventricular inflow after mitral valve opening ($S_3$). These sounds are low-frequency and dull, and are best heard with the bell of the stethoscope (light pressure) with the patient in the left lateral position. Conversely, the first and second heart sounds, aortic and pulmonary ejection clicks, and opening snap are high-frequency sounds, and are best heard with the diaphragm of the stethoscope (firm pressure).

## First Heart Sound (S₁)

The $S_1$ is directly related to vibrations of the atrioventricular valves and myocardium produced by atrioventricular closure and in general has little diagnostic usefulness. A loud $S_1$ is common in mitral stenosis and in persons with a short PR interval, owing to increased excursion velocity of the mitral valve leaflets in late diastole. A soft $S_1$ is common when there is decreased left ventricular systolic function or first-degree atrioventricular block (the mitral leaflets are almost closed at the onset of left ventricular contraction).

## Second Heart Sound (S₂)

Although assessment of the respiratory movement and intensity of the two components of $S_2$ is a well-known aspect of auscultation, for practical purposes analysis of $S_2$ is helpful in relatively few conditions (see Table 7–6). *The physician should focus on the relative intensity of aortic and pulmonary components ($A_2$, $P_2$) and the possible presence of* reversed or paradoxical splitting, characterized by inspiratory

Table 7–6

**Assessment of the Second Heart Sound (S₂): A Practical Approach**

| Character* | Significance |
|---|---|
| Abnormalities of respiratory variation | |
| Wide splitting, inspiratory increase in $A_2$–$P_2$ interval | Right ventricular conduction delay (e.g., incomplete or total right bundle branch block—important clue) |
| | Idiopathic dilatation of the pulmonary artery |
| | Small atrial septal defect (unusual) |
| | Pulmonic stenosis |
| Wide splitting, fixed $A_2$–$P_2$ interval | Atrial septal defect (important clue) |
| Single $S_2$ | Often normal in older patients |
| | Aortic stenosis |
| | Mild left ventricular conduction delay |
| | Severe pulmonary hypertension ($A_2$ "masked") |
| Reversed or paradoxical splitting | Left bundle branch block (important clue) |
| | Left ventricular systolic dysfunction (important in acute ischemia) |
| Abnormalities of intensity | |
| Loud $A_2$ | Dilated aorta |
| | Hypertension |
| | Tetralogy of Fallot |
| Loud $P_2$ | Pulmonary hypertension (important clue) |
| | Atrial septal defect |
| | Dilated pulmonary artery |
| Soft $A_2$ | Aortic sclerosis or stenosis |
| | Hypotension |
| Soft $P_2$ | Pulmonic stenosis |

*The physician must differentiate between decreased intensity of *all* cardiac sounds vs. a *selective* decrease in the loudness of $A_2$ or $P_2$.

narrowing and expiratory widening of the two components of $S_2$. Paradoxical splitting is an important clue to an underlying left bundle branch block or significant aortic stenosis in a patient with a systolic ejection murmur. *A loud $P_2$, particularly when $P_2$ is louder than $A_2$ at the base and apex, suggests significant pulmonary hypertension.*

### Third Heart Sound (S₃)

The low-pitched early diastolic third heart sound can be a normal finding or a significant cardiovascular abnormality. With depression of left ventricular systolic function or overt heart failure, an $S_3$ is common and in general is a poor prognostic finding. An $S_3$ may be audible with severe mitral or aortic regurgitation, reflecting increased volume of diastolic blood flow to the left ventricle, but not necessarily left ventricular systolic dysfunction. In children and young adults, an $S_3$ is normal. The $S_3$ is most easily heard by turning the patient into the left lateral position, identifying the apex impulse with a finger, and carefully applying the bell of the stethoscope with light pressure (see Fig. 7–7).

### Fourth Heart Sound (S₄)

The atrial sound or $S_4$ is caused by augmentation of late LV diastolic filling resulting from left atrial contraction. Audibility is correlated with increased left

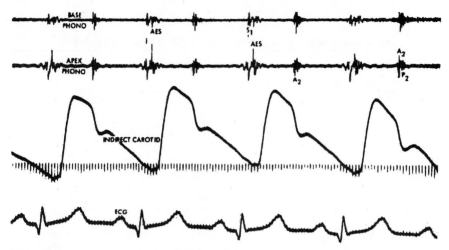

**Figure 7–9** ■ Aortic ejection sound. This phonocardiogram and carotid arterial pulse tracing demonstrates a prominent, discrete aortic ejection sound (AES) that is better heard and recorded at the apex than at the base. This is characteristic of aortic ejection sounds or clicks. Note the prominent separation of the ejection sound from $S_1$ by approximately 40 to 50 msec. (From Shaver JA, Griff FW, Leonard JJ: Ejection sounds of left-sided origin. *In* Leon DF, Shaver JA [eds]: Physiologic Principles of Heart Sounds and Murmurs. American Heart Association Monograph No.46, Dallas, TX, 1975.)

ventricular stiffness or decreased compliance; thus, $S_4$ is a useful finding in hypertension or in coronary artery disease, where it suggests increased left ventricular end-diastolic pressure or hypertrophy. The $S_4$ (and $S_3$) may be palpable. The $S_4$ is felt as a *presystolic* outward thrust just before the palpable left ventricular impulse and is noted as a double early systolic left ventricular impulse. It is important to use the left lateral position for optimal detection by palpation or auscultation of both the $S_3$ and $S_4$ (see Fig. 7–7).

## Ejection Sounds

These are high-frequency, discrete, audible sounds that occur immediately after $S_1$ (Fig. 7–9). They are usually caused by stiff or malformed semilunar leaflets, such as a bicuspid aortic valve or valvar pulmonic stenosis. Importantly, ejection sounds may be detected in the presence of a dilated great vessel (aorta or pulmonary artery), particularly if systolic pressure is elevated. An isolated ejection sound or click in a patient with or without a systolic ejection murmur suggests a congenitally deformed aortic valve, typically biscuspid.

## ■ HEART MURMURS

Physicians are usually more focused on heart murmurs than on any other aspect of the cardiac physical examination. Nevertheless, recent studies confirm that physicians' skills in cardiac auscultation are poor, probably worse than in earlier decades. The widespread availability and utilization of two-dimensional echocardiography is certainly a significant contributor to this decline in expertise. In addition, the teaching of the cardiac physical examination in medical schools takes up progressively less of the curriculum.

Murmurs are a result of turbulence of blood flow; thus, systolic murmurs are by far the most common and are related to ejection of blood across the aortic and pulmonic valves in a normal or structurally abnormal heart. Abnormal aortic or pulmonic valves frequently produce systolic ejection murmurs, which must be differentiated from functional or flow murmurs. Mitral insufficiency, with regurgitant flow into the left atrium throughout systole, is a common cause of systolic murmurs. *Thus, a systolic murmur may be normal or abnormal. On the other hand,* all *diastolic murmurs are abnormal,* as there is no physiologic explanation for normal flow of sufficient turbulence during diastole to produce a murmur.

## Classification of Murmurs (Fig. 7–10)

### Systolic Murmur

A systolic ejection murmur is characterized by a crescendo-decrescendo contour and a gap between the end of audible sound and $S_2$ (see Figs. 7–10 and 7–11). This sound-free period is the critical feature that distinguishes a systolic ejection murmur from a mitral or tricuspid regurgitant systolic murmur, where sound continues up to $S_2$ (holosystolic, pansystolic; see Fig. 7–10A). Distinguishing between the two is not

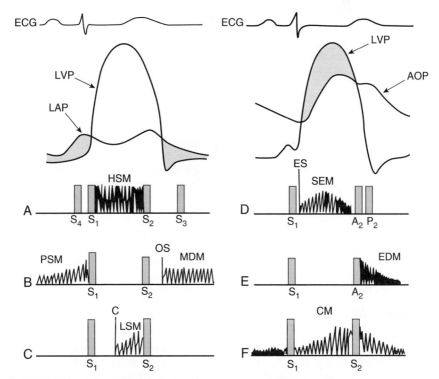

**Figure 7–10** ■ Intracardiac pressures and heart murmurs of the major cardiac valve abnormalities. See text for discussion of specific murmurs. LVP, left ventricular pressure; LAP, left atrial pressure; AOP, aortic pressure; HSM, holosystolic murmur; PSM, presystolic murmur; OS, opening snap; MDM, middiastolic murmur; C, midsystolic click; LSM, late systolic murmur; ES, ejection sound; SEM, systolic ejection murmur; EDM, early diastolic murmur; CM, continuous murmur. (From Crawford MH, O'Rourke RA: A systematic approach to the bedside differentiation of cardiac murmurs and abnormal sound. Curr Prob Cardiol 1979; 1:1.)

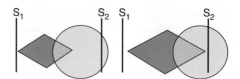

**Figure 7–11** ■ Importance of late systole in evaluation of systolic murmurs. It is essential to assess the last part of systole to determine whether a murmur is ejection in quality or is holosystolic, or, as in this figure, to distinguish between ejection murmurs that indicate lesions of different severity. On the left, an early-peaking murmur ends before the last third of systole. This is the rule in functional murmurs or with mild aortic or pulmonic valve stenosis. On the right, a long ejection murmur is shown, which peaks later in systole. Sound vibrations extend to $S_2$, suggesting severe obstruction to ventricular outflow. In severe aortic or pulmonic valve stenosis, the vibrations may extend beyond $S_2$. (From Abrams J: Auscultation of heart murmurs. Prim Cardiol 1981;7:21–43.)

always possible, even by an expert in cardiac physical diagnosis. Nevertheless, the large majority of systolic murmurs can be correctly identified with careful cardiac examination.

The *functional heart murmur*, also known as an *innocent or physiologic murmur*, is usually not very loud (grade 1 to 3 intensity), is best heard at or near the base of the heart and is not associated with other cardiac abnormalities. It is thought that functional murmurs are related to normal turbulent blood flow across semilunar valves. Thus, anxiety, fever, anemia, excitement, pregnancy, or exercise can create a functional murmur. Younger persons (children, teens, young adults) commonly have a functional or innocent murmur. The occasional individual with mitral valve prolapse (see Fig. 7–10C and Fig. 7–14) can be confusing. The systolic murmur of prolapse typically begins late in systole and extends up to $S_2$.

## Diastolic Murmurs

The most common audible diastolic murmur is the blowing or high-pitched decrescendo murmur of aortic regurgitation (see Figs. 7–2, 7–10D). This can be difficult to hear and should be sought out by the clinician in a quiet room with the subject sitting up, leaning forward, and holding the breath in end expiration to enhance detection of these murmurs, which can be quite soft and are typically of high frequency. Thus, an inexperienced or distracted physician often misses a grade 1 or 2 aortic regurgitation murmur. Furthermore, echocardiography confirms that mild to moderate aortic regurgitation is often silent to examination.

Mitral stenosis produces a diastolic murmur, which is different from the murmur of aortic regurgitation. The classic mitral stenosis rumble, a low-frequency sound, begins after the early diastolic opening snap and is often heard *only* at the cardiac apex in the left lateral position (see Figs. 7–10B, 7–12).

## Continuous Murmur

These unusual murmurs are caused by late systolic flow and persistent blood flow from one cardiac chamber or great vessel to another after ventricular ejection has been completed (Table 7–7). Thus, *a continuous murmur typically is heard in late systole and extends into diastole* (Fig. 7–10F). These murmurs are often phasic in intensity and may be audible at sites away from the classic valve areas. The murmur of patent ductus arteriosus is usually very loud and harsh and maximal at the upper left infraclavicular area and left scapular area. Aortic valve disease with both stenosis and regurgitation may simulate a continuous murmur, especially at fast heart rates.

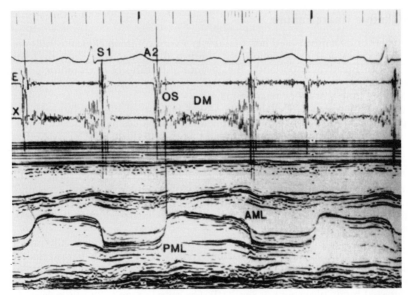

**Figure 7–12** ■ Echocardiographic correlates of the loud first sound and opening snap (OS) in mitral stenosis. $S_1$ is produced by mitral valve closure and is accentuated and delayed to elevation owing of left atrial pressure and the loss of valve compliance. A prominent presystolic diastolic murmur merges with $S_1$; this represents augmented transmitral flow with left atrial contraction. The opening snap times precisely with the maximum opening excursion of the anterior leaflet of the mitral valve (AML) and is produced by tensing of the valve cusps during early diastole. Left ventricular filling and the resultant early to mid-diastolic murmur (DM) follows the OS. $S_1$, first heart sound; $A_2$, aortic component of second heart sound; PML, posterior mitral leaflet. (From Reddy PS, Salerni R, Shaver JA: Normal and abnormal heart sounds in cardiac diagnosis. Part II. Diastolic sound. Curr Prog Cardiol 1985; 10:1.)

## ■ THE CARDIAC PHYSICAL EXAMINATION IN SPECIFIC CARDIOVASCULAR CONDITIONS

The cardinal physical findings in a variety of common cardiac syndromes and conditions are summarized below. *It is important to recognize that typical or classic features of structural heart disease are not always present on examination.* In many instances, atypical characteristics or absence of specific features (e.g., "silent" valve disease) can produce considerable diagnostic confusion or error.

Table 7–7

**Common Causes of a Continuous Murmur***

| |
|---|
| Patent ductus arteriosus |
| Arteriovenous fistula, congenital or acquired, systemic or pulmonary |
| Ruptured aneurysm of the sinus of Valsalva (communication usually into right atrium or right ventricle) |
| Venous hum (innocent finding in children) |
| Anomalous origin of the coronary artery from the pulmonary artery |
| Coronary arteriovenous fistula |
| "Mammary *souffle*" of pregnancy |
| Systemic arterial-pulmonary arterial collaterals or bronchial arterial collaterals in congenital defects |
| Coarctation of the aorta: coarctation site and/or collateral vessel flow |

*Pseudocontinuous murmur suggests aortic stenosis and regurgitation.

## Congestive Heart Failure

Overt or decompensated heart failure is a very common clinical condition, and the cardiac physical examination can confirm this diagnosis when the patient's history is suggestive. Importantly, the absence of features of heart failure on examination may suggest another cause for the patient's complaints, such as chronic obstructive lung disease or pneumonia.

*General Appearance.* The decompensated patient is often tachypneic and orthopneic and has lower extremity peripheral edema. Rales may be heard at the lung bases; percussion dullness and decreased breath sounds suggest pleural effusions.

*Jugular Venous Pulse.* Elevation of the mean venous pulse is the *sine qua non of* right heart failure. The A wave may be prominent, suggesting right atrial pressure elevation (see Fig. 7–4). Tricuspid regurgitation in subjects with heart failure is common and may produce a dominant systolic jugular V wave, typically seen simultaneously with the palpable carotid arterial upstroke (Fig. 7–13). A large systolic V wave is often present in persons with heart failure but is frequently missed by the examiner.

*Precordial Impulse.* The examiner should actively seek an abnormally prominent left ventricular impulse (left ventricular hypertrophy) and a parasternal heave (right ventricular hypertrophy) and should look for findings on the examination that confirm structural heart disease, such as murmurs or cardiac enlargement (manifested by displacement of the PMI). On occasion, an $S_3$ can be palpated with the patient in the left lateral position. In the presence of hypertensive heart disease or coronary artery disease, a hypertrophic or dilated left ventricle may result in prominent or displaced left ventricular thrust. Leftward displacement of the PMI indicates left ventricular enlargement (see section on Precordial Motion). Remember that heart failure can be due to diastolic dysfunction (a stiff left ventricle with normal systolic function).

*Heart Sounds.* An $S_3$ or $S_4$ is common: An $S_3$ has adverse prognostic implications. An $S_4$ (audible or palpable) indicates decreased left ventricular compliance and left ventricular hypertrophy. $S_1$ may be diminished with heart failure.

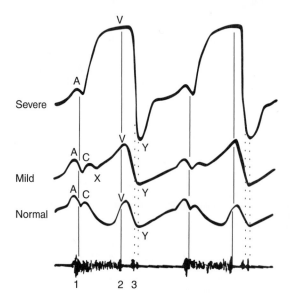

Severe

Mild

Normal

1  2 3

**Figure 7–13** ■ The large V wave of tricuspid regurgitation. As reflux across the tricuspid wave increases in severity, the systolic V wave becomes higher and broader. The X descent disappears, and the Y descent is progressively accentuated with increasing severity of tricuspid reurgitation. With severe tricuspid regurgitation, the systolic wave may be so dominant as to mimic the carotid arterial pulsations; the entire lower neck and earlobe will pulsate with each right ventricular systole. A, A wave; C, C wave (not usually visible).

*Murmurs.* Mitral and tricuspid regurgitation, perhaps due to stretching of the valve annulus, are common in the dilated failing heart, but often these regurgitant murmurs are nondescript or inaudible. If congestive heart failure is due to an underlying valve lesion, specific features of that structural abnormality may be prominent. In the setting of heart failure due to decreased left ventricular systolic function, the murmur of severe aortic regurgitation, aortic stenosis, or mitral regurgitation may be unimpressive or even inaudible in spite of a major hemodynamic burden due to the valve lesion.

## Coronary Artery Disease

Unless there is left ventricular damage from a previous infarction or earlier episodes of myocardial stunning or hibernation, the cardiac examination findings in patients with coronary disease are usually unremarkable. Signs of hypercholesterolemia should be sought, such as arcus senilis, xanthelasma, and tendon xanthomas. In patients with left ventricular dysfunction, an ectopic cardiac impulse or enlarged apical impulse may be noted. An $S_4$ is common, but this finding is not specific enough to be diagnostically helpful. A third heart sound may be heard, but only if severe left ventricular dysfunction is present. Mitral regurgitation is common in patients with depressed systolic function and left ventricular dilatation; a late systolic murmur of papillary muscle dysfunction should be sought. It is important to examine all persons with coronary heart disease in the left lateral position to "bring out" the left ventricular impulse and the third and fourth heart sounds (see Fig. 7–7).

## Mitral Stenosis

Mitral stenosis is easily identified by experienced examiners and usually is missed by inexperienced ones. The classic features include a very loud (often palpable), $S_1$ and an increased $P_2$ and an early diastolic sound, the opening snap. The typical murmur of mitral stenosis is a mid- to late diastolic, low-frequency "rumble," that is best (or only) heard at the left ventricular apex with the subject in the left lateral position (see Fig. 7–10B). A right ventricular lift is common; in pure mitral stenosis, the left ventricular impulse is not abnormal and may be indetectable. Coexisting mitral regurgitation may confuse the auscultatory findings, usually producing an apical murmur that typically is holosystolic. Many physicians have difficulty assessing the timing of the acoustic events in mitral stenosis, confusing systole with diastole.

## Mitral Regurgitation

This lesion is ubiquitous and occurs in many forms. In long-standing severe mitral regurgitation the left ventricle dilates. Thus, careful evaluation of the apical impulse is important: the examiner seeks a left ventricular heave, a palpable $S_3$, or an apical systolic thrill. A right ventricular lift is common with chronic severe mitral regurgitation. The murmur of mitral regurgitation is typically holosystolic at the apex (see Fig. 7–10A), but variants of the classic murmur can confuse the picture. Myxomatous mitral valve prolapse may produce a mid- to late-systolic murmur that can radiate to the aortic area if there is selective posterior leaflet prolapse. The mitral regurgitation murmur may vary in intensity, particularly in persons with left ventricular dysfunction; when mitral regurgitation is secondary to left ventricular dysfunction, the murmur is loudest during decompensated heart failure. Conversely, organic mitral regurgitation murmurs are usually loudest after heart failure has been effectively treated and left ventricular function has improved.

## Mitral Valve Prolapse

The cardinal features of mitral valve prolapse include a mid- to late systolic murmur and one or more mid- to late systolic clicks (see Figs. 7–10C, 7–14). The latter may or may not be present or can be variably audible from day to day. The clicks are often confusing to the uninitiated; they may be "close to the ear," quite high in frequency, sounding like extracardiac phenomena. Typically, the systolic murmur begins well after $S_1$ and may vary in length and intensity, especially in response to specific maneuvers that alter left ventricular volume or systemic resistance (e.g., going from supine to upright position, squatting, Valsalva maneuver, sustaining a hand grip).

## Aortic Stenosis

Classic features of valvar aortic stenosis include a small and slow rising carotid arterial upstroke (see Fig. 7–1); a left ventricular lift; a palpable $S_4$; a palpable basal systolic thrill; and a loud, often harsh, systolic murmur at the aortic area radiating into the neck (see Fig. 7–10D). The murmur of aortic stenosis is often more a high-

## LATE SYSTOLIC MURMUR OF MVP

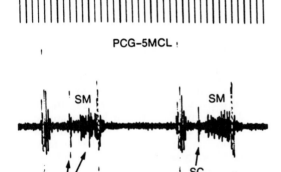

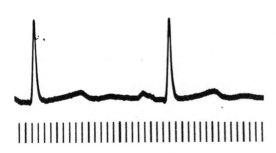

**Figure 7–14** ■ The classic late systolic murmur of mitral valve prolapse. Note the crescendo configuration of the murmur, which begins in midsystole following the first systolic click. The frequency of this murmur is usually relatively pure. SM, systolic murmur; SC, systolic click; PCG-5MCL, phonocardiogram, 5th interspace, midclavicular line. (From Delman AJ, Stein E: Dynamic cardiac auscultation and phonocardiography. Philadelphia: WB Saunders, 1979.)

frequency sound and pure in pitch at the apex (where it is often confused with mitral regurgitation). The length of the murmur is key; functional or aortic sclerosis murmurs are not very long and do not peak late; moderate to severe aortic stenosis murmurs typically take up much of systole, and their peak intensity is later than normal (see Fig. 7–11). These murmurs can be quite harsh and grunting above the right clavicle and usually radiate into the carotids.

## Hypertrophic Cardiomyopathy

These patients have an extremely prominent left ventricular heave, a very loud and usually palpable fourth heart sound, and a loud, long systolic murmur that is best heard at the left sternal region and apex. The murmur typically changes with body position, the Valsalva maneuver, or after premature ventricular contractions. *The murmur may have characteristics of both mitral regurgitation and aortic stenosis.* The ejection component (similar in contour to aortic stenosis) is due to increased velocity of blood flow in the left ventricular outflow tract. Mitral regurgitation is common in subjects who have an obstructive component. The carotid upstrokes are brisk and not delayed. Experienced examiners should be able to differentiate valvar aortic stenosis from hypertrophic cardiomyopathy.

## Aortic Regurgitation

The first clue to the recognition of significant aortic regurgitation is an abnormal carotid arterial pulse characterized by a full-volume, high-amplitude impulse, often with a double (or bisferiens) contour (see Fig. 7–2). Signs of left ventricular enlargement signify a major degree of regurgitation. A third heart sound is a poor prognostic finding. Fourth heart sounds are commonly heard. A high-frequency, blowing, decrescendo diastolic murmur beginning with $S_2$ is the typical finding of aortic regurgitation (see Fig. 7–10E). This murmur is usually soft.

Careful technique is necessary to hear the often soft murmur of aortic regurgitation. The optimal patient position for examination is sitting up, leaning forward, with the breath held in end expiration. An associated aortic systolic murmur is common.

## ■ RECOMMENDED READING

Abrams J: Essentials of Cardiac Physical Diagnosis. Philadelphia: Lea & Febiger, 1987.

Crawford MH, O'Rourke RA: A systematic approach to the bedside differentiation of cardiac murmurs and abnormal sounds. Curr Prob Cardiol 1977;1:1.

Lembo NJ, Dell'Italia LJ, Crawford MH, O'Rourke RA: Bedside diagnosis of systolic murmurs. N Engl J Med 1988;318:1572.

Leon DF, Shaver JA (eds): Physiologic Principles of Heart Sounds and Murmurs. American Heart Association Monograph No. 46. Dallas, TX, 1975.

Mangione S, Nieman LZ, Gracely E, et al: The teaching and practice of cardiac auscultation during internal medicine and cardiology training. Ann Intern Med 1993;119:1.

Perloff JK: Physical Examination of the Heart and Circulation. Philadelphia: WB Saunders, 1982.

Shaver JA, Salerni R, Reddy PS: Normal and abnormal heart sounds in cardiac diagnosis. Part I: Systolic sounds. Part II. Diastolic sounds. Curr Prob Cardiol 1985;10:1.

# Chapter 8

# Electrocardiography

*Alexander Ivanov* ▪ *James F. Burke* ▪ *Peter R. Kowey*

The electrocardiogram (ECG) records electric potential changes in the electrical field produced by the heart. Although it records only the *electrical* behavior of the heart, it can be used to identify numerous metabolic, hemodynamic, and anatomic changes. Electrocardiography is considered the "gold standard" for the diagnosis of arrhythmias (see Chapter 17). In this chapter, mostly "nonarrhythmic" ECG changes are reviewed. Abbreviations and acronyms used in this chapter can be found in Table 8–1.

## ▪ LEADS

The standard 12-lead ECG consists of tracings obtained from the bipolar recording leads (I, II, and III), the unipolar limb leads (aVR, aVL, and aVF), and, usually, six unipolar chest (precordial) leads ($V_1$ through $V_6$). The *bipolar limb leads* (I, II, III), respectively, register potential differences between the right arm and left arm, right arm and left leg, and left arm and left leg. The axis of a bipolar lead is an imaginary vector directed from the electrode assumed to be negative to the electrode assumed to be positive (Fig. 8–1). To record *unipolar limb leads*, these three extremities are connected to a central terminal used as the indifferent electrode. Then, the exploring electrode (called *positive*) can be placed on one of the three extremities to register the heart potentials transmitted to that particular limb. The letter *V* denotes a unipolar lead. The letters *R*, *L*, and *F* identify the right arm, left

Table 8–1

**Abbreviations and Acronyms Used in Electrocardiography**

| | | | |
|---|---|---|---|
| 1° | First-degree | LAD | Left axis deviation |
| 2° | Second-degree | LAFB | Left anterior fascicular block |
| > | More than | LBBB | Left bundle branch block |
| ≥ | More than or equal to | LPFB | Left posterior fascicular block |
| < | Less than | LV | Left ventricle |
| ≤ | Less than or equal to | LVH | Left ventricular hypertrophy |
| AV | Atrioventricular | MI | Myocardial infarction |
| CAD | Coronary artery disease | RA | Right atrium |
| cm | centimeter(s) | RAA | Right atrial abnormality |
| CNS | Central nervous system | RAD | Right axis deviation |
| COPD | Chronic obstructive pulmonary disease | RBBB | Right bundle branch block |
| ECG | Electrocardiogram | RV | Right ventricle |
| ICS | Intercostal space | RVH | Right ventricular hypertrophy |
| IVCD | Interventricular conduction disturbance | QTc | QT interval corrected for the patient's heart rate |
| $K^+$ | Potassium | sec | Second |
| LA | Left atrium | VT | Ventricular tachycardia |
| LAA | Left atrial abnormality | WPW | Wolff-Parkinson-White syndrome |

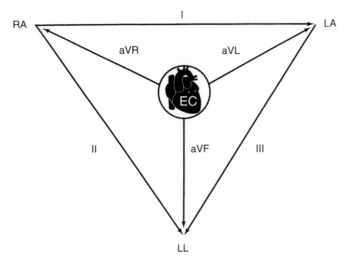

**Figure 8–1** ▪ Frontal lead axes. Leads I, II, and III are formed by connecting the right arm (RA) to the left arm (LA), the RA to the left leg (LL), and LA to LL, respectively. Arrows indicate the axes of these leads in relation to the theoretical electrical center (EC) of the heart. The indifferent electrode of the unipolar system is obtained by connecting RA, LA, and LL to a central terminal.

arm, and left leg (foot), respectively. The letter *a* means that the potential difference was electrically *a*ugmented.[1] The axis of a unipolar lead is an imaginary vector directed from the indifferent electrode to the exploring (positive) electrode.

When the exploring electrode is situated on the chest, it records potential from that particular site on the chest wall. Figure 8–2 demonstrates the precordial ECG lead axes, and Table 8–2 describes their placement. Typically, limb leads record

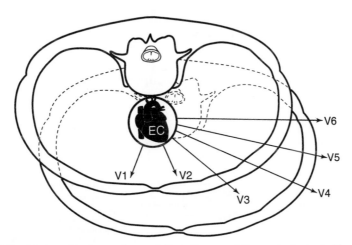

**Figure 8–2** ▪ Horizontal lead axes. Arrows indicate the axes of these unipolar leads. The indifferent electrode is obtained by connecting the precordial surface leads to a central terminal. Since the precordial electrodes are placed at different levels in relation to the electrical center (EC) of the heart, these leads also record some *frontal* vectors in addition to horizontal ones.

Table 8–2

**Precordial Lead Placement***

| Name | Leads | Location |
|---|---|---|
| Septal | $V_1-V_2$ | $V_1$ is in the fourth intercostal space (ICS) to the right of the sternum. $V_2$ is in the fourth ICS to the left of the sternum. |
| Anterior (transitional or midprecordial) | $V_3-V_4$ | $V_3$ is midway between $V_2$ and $V_4$. $V_4$ is in the fifth ICS at the midclavicular line. |
| Lateral | $V_5-V_6$ | $V_5$ is at the anterior axillary line at the same *horizontal level* at $V_4$ (but not necessarily in the same ICS). $V_6$ is at the midaxillary line at the level of $V_4$. |
| Right-sided | $V_2$, $V_1$, $V_3R$, $V_4R$, $V_5R$, $V_6R$ | The same as standard precordial but on the right side of the chest |

*See also Figure 8–2.

electrical forces of the anatomic frontal plane, and precordial leads reflect potentials of the horizontal plane. Inferior limb leads (II, III, and aVF) preferentially record the activity of the inferior wall of the heart because of their proximity to that wall.

## ■ GENERATION OF THE TRACING

Before attempting to understand the electrical activity of the whole heart, the reader should consider electrical activation of an isolated cardiac muscle strip (Fig. 8–3). A resting or polarized muscle strip is positively charged on the outside and negatively charged inside. Therefore, there is no potential difference *along* the uniformly charged surface of the resting muscle strip. Electrical activation at any given site of the strip produces depolarization that results in a negative charge

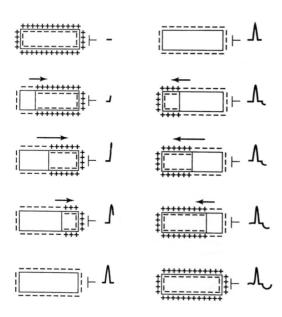

**Figure 8–3** ■ Potential generated during depolarization (*left vertical sequence*) and repolarization (*right vertical sequence*) recorded with an exploring electrode located at one end of the muscle strip. (Modified from Fisch C: Electrocardiography. *In* Braunwald E (ed): Heart Disease: A Textbook of Cardiovascular Medicine, 5th ed. Philadelphia: WB Saunders, 1997:109.)

*outside* the depolarized portion of the membrane. The membrane at this site of excitation is said to be *negatively charged*. During spread of the depolarization wave, a potential difference develops between already depolarized and still polarized (resting) portions of the membrane. An electric current flows from the negatively charged portions of the membrane to the positively charged ones. This current can be represented by a dipole or vector.

This vector moves along the muscle strip from the point of excitation and reflects constantly changing electrical activity of the strip.[1] A larger number of negative-positive ionic couples produces a larger vector. The magnitude and direction of these changes can be recorded as positive or negative deflections from the baseline of the ECG tracing. By convention, a positive deflection is recorded if the vector that is directed from the negative (depolarized) to the positive (resting) portion of the muscle strip points in the same direction as the axis of the recording lead. A negative deflection is recorded if the vector is directed opposite to that of the axis of the recording lead. No deflection is produced if the vector is perpendicular to the axis of the lead. At any given moment, the magnitude of the deflection depends on the strength of the electrical source, the distance from the source, and the cosine of the angle between the vector and the axis of the recording lead.[1]

Repolarization is a process of restitution of membrane positivity. Repolarization of the muscle strip is accompanied by a wave of positivity that proceeds in the same direction as the wave of negativity (depolarization) but has the opposite potential vector. This happens because positive potentials produced outside the membrane during repolarization spread from the site of *initial* depolarization toward the still depolarized portion of the membrane (Fig. 8–3). Thus, the net area of the tracing deflection caused by repolarization equals the area inscribed by depolarization. However, the deflections of depolarization and repolarization have the opposite directions.[1]

In the intact ventricles, the subendocardial action potential normally lasts longer than the subepicardial one. Therefore, the *process* of repolarization proceeds from subepicardium to subendocardium, in a direction approximately opposite to that of depolarization. Consequently, the *vector* of repolarization has a direction more or less similar to that of the depolarization vector. Thus, the ECG deflections of depolarization and repolarization (represented by the QRS complex and T wave) have the same polarity but unequal shapes and areas under the curve. Furthermore, since the intact heart contains more than one muscle strip, the net ECG tracing reflects contributions of all such portions of the myocardium.[1]

In the thin-walled atria, the durations of the action potentials of the subendocardium and subepicardium are equal. Thus, the ECG deflections of depolarization and repolarization have opposite polarities, as in the isolated muscle strip. The deflection of atrial *de*polarization is called the *P wave*. The wave of atrial *re*polarization is usually hidden within the large QRS complex of ventricular depolarization.

### ▪ AXIS DETERMINATION

The amplitude of an ECG deflection depends on the strength of the source and the angle between the axis of the electrical vector and the axis of the recording lead. Thus, the heart chamber with the most significant electrical contribution produces the largest deflection (especially if the recording lead is very close to that chamber). Also, the lead whose axis is most nearly parallel to the electrical vector of the heart will record the largest ECG deflection (Fig. 8–4). The approximate spatial orientation of the lead axes is known (see Fig. 8–4). Therefore, by comparing the amplitudes of a deflection in different leads, one can infer the direction and amplitude of the electrical vector at any given moment.

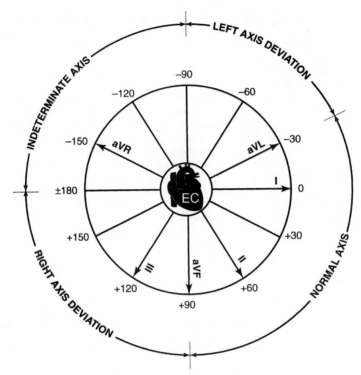

**Figure 8–4** ■ The frontal plane hexaxial reference system. It represents the limb leads where axes are drawn with intersection at the electrical center (EC) of the heart. (Modified from Fisch C: Electrocardiography. *In* Braunwald E (ed): Heart Disease: A Textbook of Cardiovascular Medicine, 5th ed. Philadelphia: WB Saunders, 1997:113.)

Summation of *instantaneous* vectors of atrial or ventricular depolarization or repolarization over time is reflected by typical ECG deflections such as the P waves, QRS complexes, and T waves (see section on Generation of the Tracing). The direction of the *mean* vector of any of these deflections is called the *axis* of that deflection. The mean vector (axis) of a wave is easy to calculate, so, it can be used in everyday practice to assess the relative electrical contributions of the atria or ventricles throughout depolarization or repolarization. Relative contribution of the chambers to the electrical events in the heart commonly changes in the presence of abnormalities of those chambers.

By convention, the axes of the P, QRS, and T waves are calculated using the *hexaxial system* of the frontal plane leads (see Fig. 8–4). The following two rules are frequently utilized to calculate an electrical axis (Fig. 8–4). First, the axis of an ECG deflection is perpendicular to the axis of the lead and the algebraic sum of deflections equals zero (*isoelectric* complexes). Second, the axis is parallel to and has the same direction as the axis of the lead with the largest positive deflection. Combining both methods improves accuracy of axis determination. For axis determination, the *area* of the deflection is more important than the *amplitude*. The normal QRS axis in the frontal plane is −30 to +90 degrees. When R wave equals S wave in all three *bipolar* limb leads, the QRS axis is considered indeterminate.

## ■ STANDARDIZATION OF THE ELECTROCARDIOGRAPHIC RECORDING

When potentials registered by the leads are recorded on paper, a 1 mm vertical deflection on the paper represents a 1 mV potential difference. Most often, millimeters are used to describe amplitude of ECG deflections.

## ■ HEART RATE MEASUREMENT

The heart rate can easily be determined utilizing two rules. The first one assumes that the distance between two thick lines on standard ECG paper is 0.5 cm. The standard paper speed is 2.5 cm/sec; so, if the distance between two consecutive R waves equals 0.5 cm (two thick lines), the heart rate is 300 bpm. If the distance is 1 cm, the heart rate is 150 bpm; 1.5 cm, 100; 2 cm, 75; 2.5 cm, 60; 3 cm, 50; 3.5 cm, 43; 5 cm, 30 bpm. This method is not accurate when the heart rate is irregular. To estimate the heart rate when the rhythm is *irregular*, the number of QRS complexes between the 3-second marks (7.5 cm apart) on the paper can be measured and multiplied by 20. This method is not accurate for slow heart rates. One can also use these two methods to determine the rate of P waves.

## ■ P WAVE

### Normal P Wave

Atrial depolarization begins within the SA node in the subendocardium and spreads to the right atrium (RA), then to the interatrial septum, and then to the left atrium (LA). Therefore, the mean vector of normal atrial depolarization is directed leftward and downward, producing a positive ECG deflection in the leads with the same axis (such as I and II). The vector of atrial repolarization, which is opposite to the vector of depolarization, produces an ECG deflection opposite to the deflection of depolarization (see section on Generation of the ECG Tracing). It may be seen occasionally after the P wave in long PR interval when the QRS complex does not obscure this small wave. Table 8–3 lists the criteria for the normal P wave.

### Right Atrial Abnormality or Enlargement

Right atrial abnormality (RAA) implies RA hypertrophy, dilatation, or primary intraatrial conduction abnormality (Table 8–4). Forces of the RA (which is located anteriorly, rightward, and inferiorly to the LA) dominate forces of the LA.

### Left Atrial Abnormality or Enlargement

Left atrial abnormality (LAA) implies LA hypertrophy, dilatation, or primary intraatrial conduction abnormality (Table 8–5). Forces of the LA (which is located

---

Table 8–3

**Criteria for Normal P Wave**

1. Duration 0.08–0.11 sec
2. Axis 0 to +75 degrees (always upright in I and II)
3. Early (right atrial) forces are positive in $V_1$. Later (left atrial) forces are negative in $V_1$. Entirely positive or negative P waves also may be seen in $V_1$.

Table 8–4

**Criteria for Right Atrial Abnormality**

1. Normal duration
2. P wave axis $> +75$ degrees (**rightward axis**)
3. Amplitude $>2.5$ mm in II, III, and aVF
4. Positive deflection in $V_1$ or $V_2$ $>1.5$ mm

posteriorly and leftward to the RA) dominate forces of the RA. If evidence of LAA and RAA appears simultaneously, **biatrial** enlargement can be suspected.

# ■ NORMAL PR INTERVAL

The normal PR interval is the time from the beginning of atrial activation to the beginning of ventricular activation. During this time, the impulse travels from the sinoatrial node through the atria, atrioventricular (AV) node, and His-Purkinje network toward the ventricular myocytes. Normal PR duration is 0.12 to 0.20 sec (but longer with slower heart rates and more advanced age).

# ■ QRS COMPLEX

## Normal QRS

The sequence of normal ventricular depolarization that produces waves Q, R, and S may be described as follows (Fig. 8–5): Ventricular excitation begins predominantly in the middle third of the left side of the interventricular septum. From there, the initial wave of depolarization spreads toward the right side of the septum. A small resultant vector, which is rightward, anterior, and superior or inferior, produces the initial QRS deflection of the ECG.

After that, the impulse spreads throughout the apical and free walls of both ventricles in the endocardial-to-epicardial direction. Because of the much larger mass of the left ventricle (LV), the resultant mean vector is leftward and inferior. It produces the major deflection of the QRS complex.

Finally, the wave of depolarization arrives at the posterobasal LV wall and posterobasal septum. A small resultant vector is directed posteriorly and superiorly, producing the latest QRS deflection.[2] The criteria of the normal QRS complex are listed in Table 8–6.

## Low Voltage

A low voltage ECG is defined as an amplitude of the whole QRS complex (R plus S) of less than 5 mm in all limb leads and less than 10 mm in all precordial

Table 8–5

**Criteria for Left Atrial Abnormality**

1. Notched P waves with duration $\geq 0.12$ sec in II, III, and aVF
2. Terminal force of the P wave in $V_1$ with a negative deflection
   $\geq 1$ mm deep *and* $\geq 0.04$ sec long

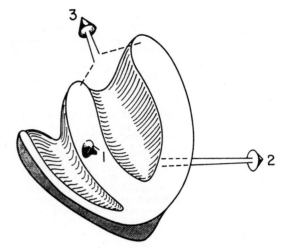

**Figure 8–5** ▪ Sequence and vectors of ventricular activation. Vector 1 represents the resultant force of the initial septal and paraseptal activation; vector 2, the activation of the free wall of the ventricles; vector 3, the basal portion of the ventricles. (Chou TC, Knilans TK: Electrocardiography in Clinical Practice: Adult and Pediatric, 4th ed. Philadelphia: WB Saunders, 1996:5.)

leads. Low ECG voltage is associated with chronic lung disease, myocardial loss due to multiple myocardial infarctions (MI), pericardial effusion, and myxedema.

## Axis Deviation

In patients with left axis deviation (LAD), the QRS axis is −30 to −90 degrees. Common causes of LAD include LV hypertrophy (LVH), left anterior fascicular block (LAFB), and inferior MI (when superior and leftward forces dominate). In patients with right axis deviation (RAD), the QRS axis is +90 to +180 degrees. Causes that are more common include RV hypertrophy (RVH), vertical heart, chronic obstructive pulmonary disease (COPD), and lateral MI.

## R Wave Progression

In early R wave progression, there is a shift of the transitional zone to the right of $V_2$ (counterclockwise rotation of the heart when looking up from the apex). R is bigger than S in $V_2$, and possibly in $V_1$. The differential diagnosis of early R wave progression includes lead malposition, normal variant, RVH, and posterior MI. In late or poor R wave progression, there is a shift of the transitional zone to the left of $V_4$ (clockwise rotation). Here, the diagnosis could be lead malposition, mild RVH (as in COPD), left bundle branch block (LBBB), LAFB, LVH, and anteroseptal MI.

Table 8–6

### Criteria for Normal QRS Complex

1. Duration 0.06–0.10 sec
2. Axis −30 to approximately +100°
3. Transitional zone between $V_2$ and $V_4$*

*__Transitional zone__ is the precordial lead having equal positive and negative deflections.

Table 8–7

### Criteria for Left Ventricular Hypertrophy

1. Amplitude of R wave in lead aVL >11 mm
2. Amplitude of R wave in lead I >13 mm
3. Amplitude of S wave in lead aVR >14 mm
4. Amplitude of R wave in lead aVF >20 mm
5. Sum of R wave in lead I and S wave in lead II >25 mm
6. Sum of R wave in $V_5$ or $V_6$ and S wave in $V_1$ >35 mm
7. Amplitude of R wave in $V_5$ >26 mm
8. Sum of maximum R wave and deepest S wave in the precordial leads >45 mm

*Supportive evidence:*

1. R wave in lead $V_6$ is taller than R wave in $V_5$ (both leads with dominant R waves)
2. Downsloping ST segment depression with upward *convexity* and/or asymmetric T wave inversion in leads I, aVL, and/or $V_4$ through $V_6$. This shape of ST-T changes is called the **strain pattern** or **secondary ST-T changes**. Reciprocal ST elevation and/or T positivity may be seen in the leads with the opposite axis (such as III, aVF, and/or $V_1$–$V_2$). T waves may even become tall in these leads (see Fig. 8–8D). In the patient with a vertical heart, typical ST depression and T inversion may be seen in leads II, III, and aVF.
3. Left atrial abnormality
4. Left axis deviation
5. Absent or decreased R wave amplitude in $V_1$ to $V_3$
6. Prolonged QRS duration, particularly initial portion

## Left Ventricular Hypertrophy

Leftward and posterior electrical forces increase owing to increased LV mass. Delay in completion of subendocardial-to-subepicardial *de*polarization may result in *re*polarization beginning in the subendocardium instead of the subepicardium. Reversal of repolarization forces ensues with consequent opposite direction of the QRS complex and the T wave. (See Table 8–7 for common LVH criteria.[3, 4]) In subjects younger than 30 years or when LVH is accompanied by LBBB or right bundle branch block (RBBB), the usual voltage criteria for LVH no longer apply.

## Right Ventricular Hypertrophy

In RVH, anterior and rightward forces increase owing to increased RV mass. Usually, they are masked by LV forces unless RVH is significant. Occasionally, posterior and rightward forces also increase owing to posterior tilt of the cardiac apex. Delay in completion of subendocardial-to-subepicardial depolarization may result in repolarization beginning in the subendocardium instead of the subepicardium. Reversal of repolarization forces ensues, with consequent opposite direction

Table 8–8

### Criteria for Right Ventricular Hypertrophy

1. RAD ≥ +110 degrees
2. R > S in $V_1$
3. R < S in $V_6$
4. qR in $V_1$ without prior anteroseptal myocardial infarction
5. Right atrial abnormality
6. Secondary ST-T changes; namely, downsloping ST depression with upward convexity and asymmetric T wave inversion in the right precordial and inferior leads
7. $S_I S_{II} S_{III}$ pattern (R ≤ S in I, II, and III)

Table 8–9

### Criteria for Right Bundle Branch Block*

1. Prolonged QRS ($\geq 0.12$ sec)
2. R′ (**secondary R wave**) taller than initial R wave in right precordial leads
3. Wide S wave in I, $V_5$, $V_6$
4. Axis of initial 0.06–0.08 sec of QRS should be normal
5. Secondary ST-T changes (downsloping ST depression with upward convexity and asymmetric T inversion) in inferior and posterior leads
6. In **incomplete RBBB**, QRS complex has typical RBBB morphology but QRS duration is only 0.09–0.11 sec

*See Figure 8–6.

of the QRS complex and the T wave. The diagnosis of RVH requires two or more of the criteria to be present (Table 8–8).[3, 4] In a patient with combined RVH and LVH, LV and RV forces try to cancel each other. The LV usually "wins."

## Right Bundle Branch Block

The right bundle of His does not contribute significantly to septal activation. Therefore, the *early* part of the QRS complex is unchanged in RBBB. LV activation proceeds normally. The RV, which is located anteriorly and to the right of the LV, is activated late and from left to right. Therefore, terminal forces are directed anteriorly and rightward. In addition, this late (terminal) depolarization of RV proceeds by slow muscle-to-muscle conduction without utilizing the right-sided His-Purkinje system. This gives wide and slurred terminal deflections of the QRS complex. *R*epolarization proceeds from the subendocardium to the subepicardium owing to alteration of the recovery process (see section on Generation of the Electrocardiogram Tracing for comparison with *normal* repolarization). Thus, the ST and T vectors are opposite to the terminal part of the QRS complex. Table 8–9 lists the RBBB criteria. The diagnosis requires all of the criteria to be present (see Fig. 8–6 for an example.[3, 4])

## RSR′ Pattern in $V_1$

RSR′ pattern in $V_1$ is a common ECG pattern, which may be seen as a normal variant or in association with abnormalities of the RV or the posterior wall of the LV.

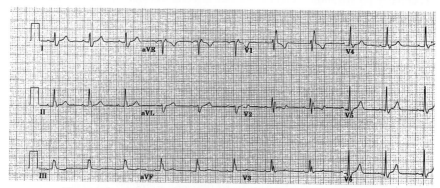

**Figure 8–6** ■ Complete right bundle branch block. (See text for description.)

Table 8–10

**Criteria for Left Anterior Fascicular Block**

1. Mean QRS axis of $-45$ to $-90$ degrees ($S_{II} < S_{III}$).
2. qR complex (or a pure R wave) in I and aVL; rS complex in leads II, III, and aVF
3. Normal to slightly prolonged QRS duration (0.08–0.12 sec)
4. Deep S waves may be seen in the left precordial leads (owing to occasional extreme superior direction of the mean QRS vector in the frontal plane).

## Left Anterior Fascicular Block

The left anterior fascicle travels toward the anterolateral papillary muscle (i.e., superiorly, anteriorly, and leftward). Thus, in LAFB, the *initial* depolarization is directed inferiorly, posteriorly, and rightward through the posterior division. *Delayed* depolarization of both anterior and lateral walls is directed leftward and superiorly. Therefore, leftward and superior terminal forces of the LV free wall are unopposed and prominent. The LAFB criteria are listed in Table 8–10.[3, 4]

## Left Posterior Fascicular Block

True left posterior fascicular block (LPFB) is rare. In differential diagnosis, one should consider asthenic persons, COPD, RVH, and extensive lateral MI. Table 8–11 lists the LPFB criteria. The transitional zone is often displaced leftward, so Q waves in the left precordial leads may disappear. This happens because the mean QRS vector is directed posteriorly in the horizontal plane (see Fig. 8–2).

## Left Bundle Branch Block

Normally, the left bundle *does* contribute to septal activation. Thus, in LBBB, septal activation develops late. Therefore, early forces manifested on ECG originate from the RV apex, which is located to the left, in front of and below the electrical center of the heart. Depolarization spreads from the subendocardium to the RV apex to the subepicardium. Consequently, the resultant vector of early forces is directed leftward, forward, and down. Leftward orientation of the electrical forces remains as depolarization progresses. *Terminal* depolarization proceeds by slow muscle-to-muscle conduction, resulting in slurring and widening of the terminal deflection. *Repolarization* proceeds from the subendocardium to the subepicardium owing to changes in the course of the recovery process (see section on Generation of the Tracing for comparison to *normal* repolarization). Thus, the ST and T vectors are opposite to the terminal part of the QRS (Fig. 8–7). Table 8–12 lists LBBB criteria. All the criteria should be present to diagnose LBBB.[3, 4] **Nonspecific intraventricular conduction disturbance** (IVCD) is characterized by QRS duration longer than 0.11 sec when the QRS morphology does not satisfy the criteria for either LBBB or RBBB.

Table 8–11

**Criteria for Left Posterior Fascicular Block**

1. Frontal plane QRS axis of $+100$ to $+180$ degrees
2. $S_I Q_{III}$ pattern (as opposed to left anterior fascicular block)
3. Normal or slightly prolonged QRS duration (0.08–0.12 sec)

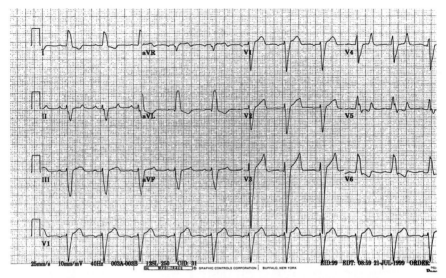

**Figure 8–7** ▪ Complete left bundle branch block. (See text for description.)

Common **causes** of various blocks below the AV node include coronary artery disease (CAD), hypertensive heart disease, aortic valve disease, cardiomyopathy, sclerosis of the conduction tissue or cardiac skeleton usually seen in elderly people, and surgical trauma.[3] **Heart rate–related RBBB** (and less commonly LBBB) and other conduction abnormalities are not rare in clinical practice.

## Abnormal/Pathological Q Wave

An electrically inert myocardium, like that affected by MI, fails to contribute to normal electrical forces. Thus, the vector of the opposite wall takes over. The Q wave is bigger. The R wave may become smaller. Bigger S waves are often obscured by ST changes. Table 8–13 lists the criteria for abnormal Q waves.

In a normally positioned heart, leads $V_3R$ and $V_4R$ are located over the mid-RV. $V_1$ is located over the high RV or septum and opposite the posterior LV wall. $V_2$ is placed over the septum and opposite the posterior wall. Leads $V_3$ and $V_4$ are over the middle anterior LV. $V_5$ and $V_6$ are situated over the *low* lateral LV, and I and aVL across the *high* lateral aspect. Leads II, III, and aVF are closest to the inferior LV. Therefore, the location of the infarction may be deduced from the location of abnormal Q waves (Table 8–14).

Table 8–12

**Criteria for Left Bundle Branch Block***

1. Prolonged QRS duration (>0.12 sec)
2. Broad monophasic R in leads I, $V_5$, or $V_6$ that is usually notched or slurred
3. Absence of any Q waves in I and $V_5$–$V_6$
4. Direction of the ST segment shift and the T wave is opposite to that of the QRS complex. T waves in "lateral" leads (i.e., I, aVL, $V_4$–$V_6$) may become tall (Fig. 8–8E).

*See Figure 8–7.

Table 8–13

**Criteria for Q Wave Abnormality**

1. Duration of Q wave ≥0.04 sec
2. Amplitude of the Q wave in the limb leads ≥4 mm or ≥25% of the R wave in that lead (even deeper required for leads III, aVF, and aVL)
3. Normally, QRS in $V_2$–$V_4$ begins with R wave. Thus, even small Q waves are abnormal if seen in $V_2$–$V_4$ (unless the transitional zone is markedly shifted owing to another cause).

Note that new myocardial infarction may mask a previous one.

In posterior MI, reciprocal changes of the ST segment (i.e., depression in the anteroseptal leads) are often seen with *acute* ischemia/injury. When diagnosing posterior MI, one should rule out juvenile ECG, early R wave progression, and RVH. RV infarction is characterized by ST elevation greater than 1 mm in the right precordial lead(s). $V_4R$ is considered more sensitive and specific than $V_1$ for this diagnosis.

## ■ ST SEGMENT AND T WAVE CHANGES

**The normal ST segment** reflects *steady* membrane polarization from the end of depolarization to the beginning of repolarization. Usually, the ST segment is almost absent, because the ascending limb of the T wave begins right at the J point (the junction of the end of the QRS and the beginning of the ST segment).

**Normal T wave** represents ventricular repolarization. Owing to a longer action potential duration in the ventricular subendocardium than in the subepicardium, repolarization proceeds in the direction opposite that of depolarization (i.e., it begins in the subepicardium and spreads toward the subendocardium; see section on Generation of the Tracing). Therefore, the vector of repolarization (T wave) has the same direction as the vector of depolarization (QRS). Usually, the T wave is asymmetric, the ascending limb being longer than the descending one. It is at least 0.5 mm tall in I, II, and the left precordial leads[3] but may be slightly inverted or biphasic in other leads.

**Juvenile T waves** are a normal variant that is characterized by persistence of negative T waves in $V_1$ to $V_3$ after approximately age 20 years. They are usually neither symmetric nor deep. The degree of the T wave inversion decreases progres-

Table 8–14

**Electrocardiographic Localization of Q Wave Myocardial Infarction**

| Site of Infarct | Signs of Electrically Inert Myocardium |
|---|---|
| Anteroseptal | Pathologic Q or QS in $V_1$–$V_3$, and sometimes $V_4$ |
| Anterior | Absence of Q in $V_1$, QS, or QR in $V_2$–$V_4$. Late R progression or reversal of R progression in precordial leads may also be present. |
| Anterolateral | Abnormal Q in $V_4$–$V_6$ |
| Lateral | Abnormal Q in $V_5$ and $V_6$ |
| Extensive anterior | Abnormal Q in $V_1$–$V_6$ |
| High lateral | Abnormal Q in I and aVL |
| Inferior | Pathologic Q in II, III, aVF (Q in III and aVF >25% of amplitude of R wave) |
| Inferolateral | Abnormal Q in II, III, aVF, $V_5$, and $V_6$ |
| Posterior | Initial R wave in $V_1$ and $V_2$ >0.04 sec with R larger than S |

sively from $V_1$ to $V_4$. In normal tracings, however, the T waves are always upright in I, II, and the left precordial leads.

**Peaked T waves** may also be a normal variant. In this case, the T wave is more than 6 mm in the limb leads or more than 10 mm in the precordial leads (Fig. 8–8A).[1] **Early repolarization** is due to dominant parasympathetic effect on the heart.[5] This normal variant (Fig. 8–9A) is characterized by (1) an elevated J point and ST segment, (2) a distinct notch or slur on the downstroke of the R wave; and (3) upward *concavity* of the ST segment. There are no reciprocal (i.e., in the leads with opposite axes) changes of the ST segment. **Increased vagal tone** is accompanied by tall, peaked T waves. Usually, it is associated with a characteristic ST segment elevation (when it is called *early repolarization*).

**Nonspecific ST segment and/or T wave abnormalities** may show any of the following features: (1) slight ST depression or elevation (<1 mm) or (2) flattening, decreased amplitude, or slight inversion of the T wave. On a normal ECG, the T wave should be at least 0.5 mm tall in I, II, and the left precordial leads. ST/T changes may be local or diffuse. Numerous physiologic and pathologic conditions can cause this entity.

### ST Segment and T Wave Changes in Ischemia or Injury

Any **ischemic area** exhibits prolonged repolarization (phase III of the action potential).[6] This prolongation results in a difference of potential between the ischemic and normal areas during this phase of action potential with resultant T wave changes and QT interval prolongation.

An **injured area** has reduced resting potential, which results in a difference in potentials between the injured and uninjured areas (producing a diastolic or resting current of injury). The ECG machine automatically adjusts for this baseline shift by shifting the tracing in the opposite direction. Therefore, the whole QRS-T complex is shifted to keep the baseline (TQ segment) at the same level. This causes the ST segment to look elevated or depressed depending on what layer of the myocardial wall is involved. Second, the injured area shows early completion of repolarization or diminished depolarization. Thus, phase II (plateau) is shortened. Systolic difference in potentials between the injured and uninjured areas ensues. The second mechanism (systolic current of injury) plays a lesser role.[1]

**T wave abnormalities suggesting myocardial ischemia** may include (1) abnormally tall upright T waves (see Fig. 8–8 for common types of tall T waves); (2) symmetrically or deeply inverted T waves, (3) "pseudonormalization" of inverted T waves (when previously inverted T waves become positive owing to ischemia-induced changes in repolarization), and (4) nonspecific T wave abnormalities. Hyperacute T waves may be seen occasionally in the earliest stage of coronary

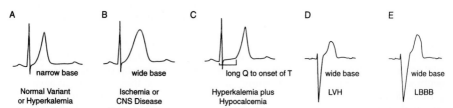

**Figure 8–8** ■ Some examples of tall T waves. CNS, central nervous system; LVH, left ventricular hypertrophy; LBBB, left bundle branch block.

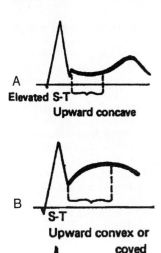

A
**Elevated S-T**
**Upward concave**

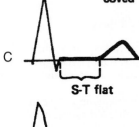

B
**S-T**
**Upward convex or**
**coved**

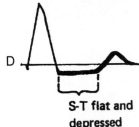

C
**S-T flat**

D
**S-T flat and**
**depressed**

**Figure 8–9** ■ Early repolarization and the ST segment changes in injury/ischemia. (See text for description.) (Modified from Constant J: Learning Electrocardiography: A Complete Course, 2nd ed. Boston: Little, Brown, 1981:242.)

occlusion. They are tall, symmetric or asymmetric, and peaked or blunted.[1,3] More often, however, T waves on the initial ECG are isoelectric, biphasic, or inverted. T wave changes of angina may be transitory or persistent. **ST segment abnormalities suggesting myocardial injury** include acute ST segment elevation with upward convexity in the leads facing the area of transmural or subepicardial injury (see Fig. 8–9B). There may be reciprocal ST depression. Posterior wall transmural or subepicardial injury may cause ST segment *depression* in $V_1$–$V_3$. It is important to realize that, in real life (as opposed to experimental coronary occlusion), any ST or T changes may reflect CAD. The ECG may also be completely normal. Subendocardial injury, ischemia, and necrosis commonly cause horizontal or down-sloping ST segment depression and/or flattening, with or without the T wave changes described above (see Figs. 8–9B–D for some examples). Usually, the depressed ST segment is flat or sagging, in contrast to the upward convexity of the "strain pattern." To diagnose CAD, ECG changes should be present in at least two contiguous leads.

## ■ QT INTERVAL

The QT interval represents the duration of the whole of electrical systole of the ventricle (depolarization plus repolarization). The normal QT interval corrected for the heart rate is less than 0.44 sec. Usually, the normal QT interval is less than half of the RR interval. A **prolonged QT interval** may be caused by asynchrony or prolongation of ventricular repolarization. The corrected QT interval, which is significantly longer than normal (<0.48 to 0.50 sec), is associated with numerous pathologic conditions, such as ischemia, infarction (the most common causes), and central nervous system (CNS) disorders. In hypokalemia, prominent U waves merge with T waves and result in *pseudo*–QT prolongation. In this case, "bifid T waves" may be present. A **shortened QT interval** is most often caused by digitalis or hypercalcemia.

## ■ U WAVE

The **normal U wave** represents afterpotentials of the ventricular myocardium or delayed repolarization of the Purkinje fibers. Normally, it should be upright in all leads except aVR. **Prominent U waves** often have amplitude larger than 25% of the T wave in the same lead or larger than 1.5 mm. Common causes include bradycardia, hypokalemia, and LVH. **U wave inversion** is very specific for organic heart disease.

## ■ NORMAL ECG

**Normal variants** of ECG include early repolarization, juvenile T waves, occasionally $S_I$, $S_{II}$, $S_{III}$ pattern, rSr′ in $V_1$, and the "athlete's heart." The mechanism of ECG changes in the **athlete's heart** reflects increased vagal tone, RVH or LVH, and asymmetry of ventricular repolarization. In this condition one may see sinus bradycardia with junctional escape rhythm, first-degree AV block or second-degree type I AV block, and increased P wave and QRS amplitude. Early repolarization is more common in athletes. T waves in the precordial leads may be tall, inverted, or biphasic.

**Incorrect electrode placement** in a normal healthy person may produce characteristic ECG changes. The most common mistake is reversal of the right and left arm leads with resultant P, QRS, and T inversion in leads I and aVL. **Parkinson's tremor** can simulate atrial flutter or ventricular tachycardia (VT) with a rate of 330 bpm.

## ■ MYOCARDIAL INFARCTION

The distinction between **Q wave** and **non–Q wave MI** may be less relevant clinically than investigators once thought. Subendocardial or nontransmural MI often shows abnormal Q waves, whereas transmural MI may not.

The typical **evolution of the ECG in acute Q wave MI** includes these stages:

1. **Tall T waves** (see Fig. 8–8B) may appear within the first minutes or hours, but, more often, isoelectric, negative, or biphasic T waves are seen on the ECG at the presentation.
2. **ST segment elevation** (see Fig. 8–9B) appears within hours after coronary occlusion and lasts approximately 2 weeks. If it lasts longer than 2 weeks, ventricular aneurysm, pericarditis, or concomitant early repolarization

should be considered. If reciprocal ST segment depression is also seen, the infarction is probably extensive.

3. **Abnormal Q waves** appear within hours or days after MI and, typically, persist indefinitely.
4. **Decline in the ST segment elevation** occurs at the same time or after the start of the T wave inversion. In acute pericarditis, in contrast, the ST segment becomes isoelectric *before* the T wave becomes inverted.
5. **Isoelectric ST segment with symmetric T wave inversion** that may last months to years or persist indefinitely.

The ECG interpretation can be complicated by the fact that the QRS wave, ST segment, and T wave may normalize transiently in the course of MI evolution. If the ST segment is elevated, the infarction is probably **recent or acute** (within approximately two weeks) (Fig. 8–10). If there is no ST segment elevation on the ECG, the infarction is probably **old or of indeterminate age**. Another caveat is that traditional teaching holds that T wave changes reflect ischemia, ST segment changes reflect injury, and abnormal Q waves reflect necrosis. This is an overly simplistic and artificial approach, however. For example, both T wave and ST segment changes may be due to ischemia, injury, or necrosis. The Q wave may reflect temporary electrical silence and not necessarily necrosis.

## Differential Diagnosis

**LVH** can be indicated by a QS pattern in the right precordial leads or by late R wave progression. In LVH, however, this pseudoinfarction pattern is not present in the chest leads recorded one interspace lower than usual. Also, the "strain" pattern of LVH may mimic or mask ischemia or injury. Ischemia or subendocardial injury is favored over hypertrophy with the "strain" pattern when (1) the ST segment changes are disproportional to the R wave amplitude in the same lead, (2) ST segment depression is present without T wave inversion, and (3) T wave inversion is *symmetric*.

In **RVH**, T wave inversion in the right precordial or inferior leads may imitate CAD; however, in RVH other ECG changes often suggest this diagnosis. In patients with **pulmonary disease**, late R wave progression in the precordial leads may be mistaken for an anterior MI, although in COPD and cor pulmonale this "abnormal-

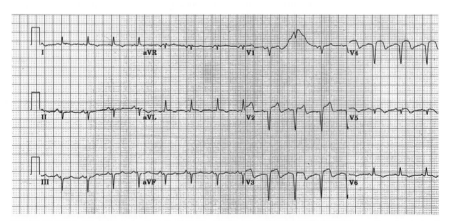

**Figure 8–10** ■ Acute extensive anterior MI. Note upward convexity of the ST segment elevation in leads V₄ and V₅, which is typical for myocardial injury. Also, note that upward convexity is obscured by tall acute T waves in lead V₂. Motion artifact is apparent in lead V₁.

ity" disappears when the leads are placed one interspace lower than usual. Also, with pulmonary diseases there may be other signs of RV involvement. Sometimes, in patients with pulmonary diseases abnormal Q waves in the inferior leads may mimic inferior infarction; however, in pulmonary disease, abnormal Q waves are rarely seen in lead II. Abnormal Q waves and ST/T changes may appear in **myocardial diseases** secondary to localized fibrosis and repolarization abnormalities.

In **Wolff-Parkinson-White** (WPW) syndrome, preexcitation of a ventricle significantly changes the initial QRS forces. The resultant delta wave can mimic an abnormal Q wave if the delta wave is a negative deflection. An upward delta wave may mask abnormal Q waves. The degree of preexcitation (and ST/T changes) may vary in any given person, a finding that mimics evolutionary changes of an acute ischemic event. In WPW, however, the PR interval is usually short and the QRS complex is wide with initial slurring. Also, marked ST segment elevation in the leads with an upright QRS complex or ST depression in the leads with a downward QRS complex is very unlikely in WPW syndrome.

Among **CNS disorders**, ECG changes are most often present in subarachnoid or intracranial hemorrhage. One can observe ST segment elevation or depression, large, wide, inverted, or upright T waves (see Figure 8B for an example), long QT, and occasionally, abnormal Q waves. Often, only the clinical picture helps to make a definitive diagnosis.

In **hyperkalemia**, the T wave is tall, and the ST segment may be elevated or depressed. In contrast to ischemia, however, the QT interval is normal or shortened (if there is no QRS complex prolongation or other reasons for QT lengthening). In addition, the T wave is narrow-based (see Fig. 8–8A). ST segment depression is upsloping, not horizontal or downsloping as it is in ischemia. Presence of the U waves tends to rule out hyperkalemia.

Patients with **acute pericarditis** very often have ST segment elevation that mimics acute injury. In pericarditis, however, ST segment elevation is usually present in almost all leads on the ECG and there is no reciprocal ST segment depression. Also, in contrast to MI, the ST segment elevation in pericarditis has an upward *concavity* and is usually less than 4 to 5 mm from the baseline. T wave inversion tends to be less pronounced but more diffuse in pericarditis than in ischemia.

**Digitalis effect or toxicity** may cause horizontal or downsloping ST segment depression that looks similar to MI; however, digitalis-induced ST segment depression often has a sagging and upwardly concave shape. In addition, the QT interval is often shortened. In **RBBB**, the initial forces are not altered. In MI, they are abnormal. Therefore, RBBB usually does not interfere with signs of MI. In **LAFB and LPFB**, the initial forces may occasionally be altered. Thus, both LAFB and LPFB can imitate or mask MI. Abnormal Q waves may be prominent if the precordial leads are accidentally recorded one interspace higher than usual.

Both **LBBB and pacing** cause significant alterations of both initial and late QRS complex forces. Therefore, both LBBB and pacing may imitate or mask MI. In the presence of these conditions, correct diagnosis of MI from the ECG alone is usually impossible. Occasionally, MI can be diagnosed in the presence of LBBB or pacing by the presence of (1) pathologic Q waves, (2) ST-T deflections that have the same direction as the QRS complex, (3) ST segment elevation disproportionate to the amplitude of the QRS complex (greater elevation is required for leads $V_{1-2}$), or (4) notched upstroke of the S wave in two precordial leads.

## ■ DRUG EFFECTS

**Digitalis** increases vagal tone and the amount of calcium in myocytes. It may also improve bypass tract conduction. In the case of digitalis toxicity, automaticity of the myocytes is increased or conduction in the His-Purkinje system impaired, or both. Digitalis **effect** may be accompanied by QT interval shortening, PR interval lengthening, and increased U wave amplitude. Another characteristic finding is a sagging ST segment depression with upward concavity, a finding that may also be seen in CAD. Almost all types of cardiac arrhythmias except atrial flutter and bundle branch block may be present in digitalis **toxicity**. Ventricular premature depolarizations are common. Tachyarrhythmias with different degrees of AV block are considered diagnostic.

## ■ METABOLIC ABNORMALITIES

In **hyperkalemia**, the main electrophysiologic abnormality is shortening of phase III of the action potential, the phase when the T waves of the ECG are generated. Therefore, the earliest and most prominent ECG findings involve the T waves. The ECG criteria for hyperkalemia are listed in Table 8–15.[4] In **hypokalemia**, phase III of the action potential is prolonged. Therefore, many of the ECG changes are opposite to those of hyperkalemia. Prominent U waves with decreased T wave amplitude are typical. In **hypercalcemia**, the main electrophysiologic finding is shortening of phase II of the action potential. This "plateau" phase is not usually accompanied by significant deflections of the ECG tracing. The ST segment is shortened or nearly absent and the whole QT interval consequently shortened. There will be little effect on the QRS complex or the P or T waves. **Hypocalcemia** is usually accompanied by the opposite ECG changes (i.e., a prolonged QT interval due to a long ST segment). The combination of hyperkalemia and hypercalcemia (often seen in renal disease) causes QT prolongation combined with peaked T waves, which occasionally may be tall (see Fig. 8–8C).

## ■ PULMONARY DISEASES

### Chronic Lung Disease

In patients with lung diseases, ECG changes may be caused by a possible vertical heart position (due to hyperinflation of the lungs), RVH or RAA. The ECG criteria for pulmonary disease are listed in Table 8–16.

### Table 8–15

#### Criteria for Hyperkalemia

| Serum Potassium (mEq/L) | ECG Findings |
| --- | --- |
| 5.5–7.5 | 1. Tall, peaked, narrow-based, and symmetric T waves (Fig. 8–9A). Usually most prominent in the precordial leads. Normal QTc (unless QRS is prolonged or there is another reason for QT prolongation; see Fig. 8–8A). No prominent U waves.<br>2. Left anterior or posterior fascicular block |
| 7.5–10.0 | 1. First-degree AV block<br>2. Flattening and widening of the P wave (with worsening of hypercalcemia, P wave disappears)<br>3. Upsloping ST segment depression. |
| >10.0 | 1. Left or right bundle branch block, markedly widened QRS, and diffuse interventricular conduction disturbance<br>2. Ventricular tachycardia, ventricular fibrillation, or idioventricular rhythm |

Table 8–16

### Criteria for Chronic Obstructive Pulmonary Disease

1. P wave axis is farther right than +75 degrees
2. Any right ventricular hypertrophy criteria. *Increased R/S ratio in $V_1$* is the least common right ventricular hypertrophy pattern in COPD
3. Late R wave progression in precordial lead
4. Low voltage
5. Abnormal Q waves in inferior or anterior leads
6. Supraventricular arrhythmias, especially atrial tachycardia, multifocal atrial tachycardia, or atrial fibrillation

## Acute Cor Pulmonale, Including Pulmonary Embolism

Mechanisms of ECG changes in acute cor pulmonale involve RV dilatation with clockwise rotation, a vertical heart position, and RV conduction abnormality. ECG abnormalities in these patients are frequently transitory. See Table 8–17 for the diagnostic criteria.[4]

## ■ ACUTE PERICARDITIS

ECG changes in pericarditis reflect subepicardial myocarditis with subepicardial injury. Typically, the ECG in acute pericarditis has the following evolution:

**Stage 1:** The ST segment becomes elevated (upwardly concave) in almost all leads except aVR. Reciprocal changes are absent.

**Stage 2:** The ST segment returns to the baseline, and the T wave amplitude begins to decrease. At this point, the ECG may look completely normal.

**Stage 3:** The T wave inverts.

**Stage 4:** Electrocardiographic resolution may occur (but does not necessarily). Other clues may also help in the diagnosis. In the early stages, PR segment depression reflects atrial injury (as ST elevation reflects ventricular injury). Low-voltage QRS complexes and electrical alternans of ECG waves may occur in pericardial effusion. Sinus tachycardia and atrial arrhythmias are very common.[4]

The differential diagnosis of acute pericarditis should include early repolarization. The absence of serial ST/T changes, the presence of tall T waves, and a characteristic notching of the terminal QRS favor early repolarization. PR segment depression in *both* limb *and* precordial leads (as opposed to *either* limb *or* precordial leads) favors pericarditis. In addition, ST segment depression in lead $V_1$, occasionally present in pericarditis, is not present in early repolarization.

Table 8–17

### Criteria for Acute Cor Pulmonale

1. Sinus tachycardia (most common ECG sign)
2. Transient right bundle branch block (incomplete or complete)
3. Inverted T waves in $V_1$–$V_3$
4. The $S_IQ_{III}$ or $S_IQ_{III}T_{III}$ pattern with pseudoinfarction in the inferior leads
5. Right axis deviation
6. Right atrial abnormality with various supraventricular tachyarrhythmias
7. (Occasionally) late R wave progression, left axis deviation, signs of right ventricular hypertrophy, and ST elevation or depression in right or left precordial leads

Table 8–18

**Criteria for Wolff-Parkinson-White Syndrome**

1. Normal P wave with PR interval generally <0.12 sec
2. Initial slurring of the QRS (delta wave)
3. Wide QRS interval >0.10 sec (unless septal insertion of the bypass tract)
4. Secondary ST/T changes (similar to the "strain pattern")
5. Atrioventricular reentrant tachycardias (most common arrhythmias)
6. Atrial fibrillation or flutter with a wide QRS complex and a rate >200 bpm is suggestive.

# ■ CENTRAL NERVOUS SYSTEM DISORDERS

The most common CNS disorders associated with ECG abnormalities are subarachnoid and intracranial hemorrhage. The mechanism of ECG changes in these patients includes altered autonomic tone and resultant changes in repolarization. The most common ECG findings are deeply inverted T waves and a markedly prolonged QT interval. Sometimes the T waves may be upright and tall (see Fig. 8–8B).

# ■ PREEXCITATION (WOLFF-PARKINSON-WHITE) SYNDROME

In WPW syndrome, one or more accessory AV pathways allow the atrial impulse to bypass the AV node and activate the ventricles prematurely. AV delay is shortened. Ventricular activation may follow the usual course through the normal conduction system; or it may begin from the site of attachment of the bypass tract within one of the ventricles. Commonly, both pathways contribute to the QRS complex (see Table 8–18).

# ■ REFERENCES

1. Fisch C: Electrocardiography. *In* Braunwald E (ed): Heart Disease: A Textbook of Cardiovascular Medicine, 5th ed. Philadelphia: WB Saunders, 1997:108.
2. Durrer D, et al: Total excitation of the isolated human heart. Circulation 1970;41:899.
3. Chou TC, Knilans TK: Electrocardiography in Clinical Practice: Adult and Pediatric, 4th ed. Philadelphia: WB Saunders, 1996.
4. O'Keefe Jr, James H, et al: ECG Board Review and Study Guide: Scoring Criteria and Definitions. Armonk, NY: Futura, 1994.
5. Mason JW, et al: Electrocardiography Self-Assessment Program. Bethesda, MD: Copyright 1995 American College of Cardiology.
6. Antzelevitch C, Sicouri S, Lukas A, et al: Clinical implications of electrical heterogeneity in the heart: The electrophysiology and pharmacology of epicardial, M, and endocardial cells. *In* Podrid PJ, Kowey PR (eds): Cardiac Arrhythmia: Mechanisms, Diagnosis, and Management. Baltimore: Williams & Wilkins, 1995:88–107.

*Chapter* 9

# Echocardiography

*Daniel G. Blanchard* ◾ *Anthony N. DeMaria*

Echocardiography is the evaluation of cardiac structures and function utilizing images produced by ultrasound (US) energy. Echocardiography started as a crude one-dimensional technique but has evolved into one that images in two and three dimensions (2D, 3D) and that can be performed from the chest wall, from the esophagus, and from within vascular structures. Clinically useful M-mode recordings became available in the late 1960s and early 1970s. In the mid-1970s, linear-array scanners that could produce 2D images of the beating heart were developed. Eventually, these evolved into the phased-array instruments currently in use. In addition to 2D imaging, the Doppler examination has become an essential component of the complete echocardiographic evaluation. Doppler US technology blossomed in the early 1980s with the development of pulsed-wave (PW), continuous-wave (CW), and 2D color-flow imaging. The field of cardiac US continues to grow rapidly: new techniques under active investigation include 3D imaging, contrast echocardiography, and harmonic imaging.

## ◾ PHYSICS AND PRINCIPLES

US is sonic energy with a frequency higher than the audible range (greater than 20,000 Hz). US is created by a transducer that consists of electrodes and a piezoelectric crystal that deforms when exposed to an electric current. This crystal creates US energy and then generates an electrical signal when struck by reflected US waves. US is useful for diagnostic imaging because, like light, it can be focused into a beam that obeys the laws of reflection and refraction. A US beam travels in a straight line through a medium of homogeneous density, but if the beam meets an interface of different acoustic impedance, part of the energy is reflected. This reflected energy can then be evaluated and used to construct an image of the heart.[1]

Because the velocity of sound in soft tissue is relatively constant (approximately 1540 m/sec), the distance from the transducer to an object that reflects US can be calculated using the time a sound wave takes to make the "round trip" from the transducer to the reflector and back again. Sophisticated computers can examine reflections from multiple structures simultaneously and display them on a screen as one-dimensional images. If the US beam is then electronically swept very rapidly across a sector, a 2D image can be generated.

Several characteristics of US are important in obtaining high-quality images. High-frequency US energy yields excellent resolution, and such beams tend to diverge less over distance than low-frequency signals. High-frequency beams, however, tend to reflect and scatter more as they pass through tissue and are thus subject to greater attenuation than low-frequency signals. Therefore, echocardiographic examinations should utilize the highest frequency that is capable of obtaining signals from the targets in the US field of interest.[1]

## ■ TWO-DIMENSIONAL ECHOCARDIOGRAPHY: THE STANDARD EXAMINATION

A US beam can image the heart from multiple areas on the chest wall. Several years ago, M-mode imaging (which detects motion along a single beam of US) was the primary tool of clinical echocardiography. M-mode has been largely supplanted by 2D imaging. To help standardize the 2D examination, the American Society of Echocardiography recognizes three orthogonal imaging planes: the long-axis, the short-axis, and the four-chamber planes (Fig. 9–1).[2] *It is important to remember that the long and short axes are those of the heart, not of the entire body.* These three planes can be imaged in four basic transducer positions: parasternal, apical, subcostal, and suprasternal (Fig. 9–2). From these standard positions, the transducer angle can be modified to obtain views through the base of the heart and through the tricuspid valve and to modulate the four-chamber view (the so-called two-chamber and three-chamber views; Fig. 9–3). The transducer can also be placed in the suprasternal position to image the thoracic aorta and great vessels.

A complete examination utilizing these imaging planes and transducer positions visualizes the cardiac valves, chamber sizes, and ventricular function in the great majority of cases. Echocardiography has become an accepted method for evaluating cardiac systolic function, and assessments of ejection fraction and regional ventricular dysfunction correlate well with those made with angiographic and radionuclide methods. In occasional patients, however, examination is limited owing to US artifacts, marked obesity, severe lung disease (with lung tissue interposed between chest wall and heart), or chest wall deformities.

A recent advance that has improved imaging quality is termed *harmonic imaging*. In usual practice, the US transducer transmits and receives at the same frequency. In harmonic imaging, the transducer transmits at a given frequency but receives at a harmonic frequency (for example, transmission at a frequency of

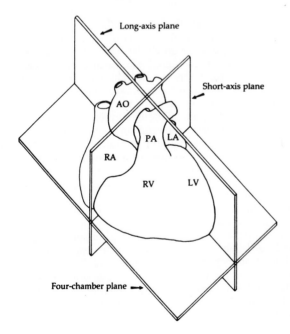

**Figure 9–1** ■ The three basic tomographic imaging planes used in echocardiography: long-axis, short-axis, and four-chamber. LV, left ventricle; LA, left atrium; RV, right ventricle; RA, right atrium; PA, pulmonary artery; AO, aorta. (From DeMaria AN, Blanchard DG: The echocardiogram. *In* Schlant RC, Alexander RW, Fuster V [eds]: Hurst's The Heart, 9th ed. New York: McGraw-Hill, 1998:415–517, with permission.)

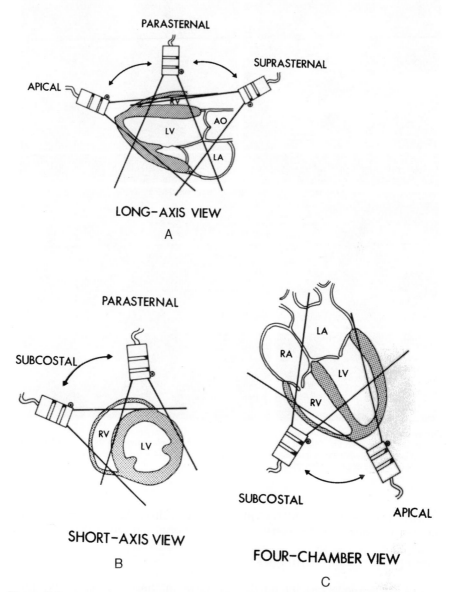

**Figure 9–2** ▪ Visualization of the heart's basic tomographic imaging planes by various transducer positions. The long-axis plane *(A)* can be imaged in the parasternal, suprasternal, and apical positions; the short-axis plane *(B)* in the parasternal and subcostal positions; and the four-chamber plane *(C)* in the apical and subcostal positions.

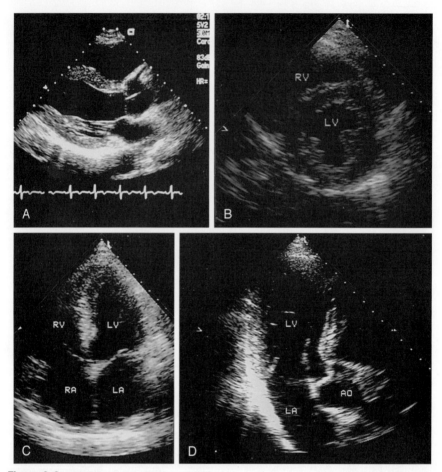

**Figure 9–3** ■ *(A)* Two-dimensional image of the heart in the parasternal long-axis view. The cardiac chambers correlate with the diagram in Figure 9–2A. *(B)* Short-axis plane through the heart at the level of the papillary muscle. *(C)* Two-dimensional image of the apical four-chamber plane. *(D)* Two-dimensional image of the apical three-chamber plane.

2.5 MHz and reception at 5 MHz). This technology helps to limit artifacts and often improves visualization of regional ventricular function and cardiac anatomy.[3]

## ■ DOPPLER ECHOCARDIOGRAPHY

Two-dimensional imaging provides abundant information about cardiac structure but no direct data on blood flow. This important area of cardiac imaging is addressed by Doppler echocardiography. When a sound signal strikes a moving object, the frequency of the reflected signal is altered in a way that is proportional to the velocity at which the object is moving and its direction. The velocity of the moving object can be calculated by the Doppler equation:

$$v = f_d.c/2f_o \text{ (cos } \theta),$$

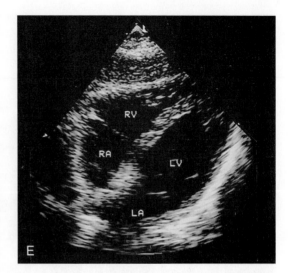

**Figure 9–3** *Continued* ■ *(E)* Two-dimensional image of the subcostal four-chamber plane. RA, right atrium; RV, right ventricle; LV, left ventricle; LA, left atrium; AO, aorta. (From DeMaria AN, Blanchard DG: The echocardiogram. *In* Schlant RC, Alexander RW; Fuster V [eds]: Hurst's The Heart, 9th ed. New York: McGraw-Hill, 1998: 515–517, with permission.)

where $v$ is the velocity of red blood cells under examination, $f_d$ is the Doppler frequency shift recorded, $f_o$ the transmitted frequency, and c the velocity of sound.[4] The angle $\theta$ is the angle between the US beam and the direction of red blood cell flow (i.e., if the US beam is directed parallel to blood flow, the angle is 0 degrees). The importance of this angle cannot be overstated, as echocardiography computer systems assume it to be zero degrees. If the angle $\theta$ is greater than 20 degrees, significant errors in velocity calculation occur.[5]

Thus, the echocardiography system evaluates the change in frequency (the Doppler shift) of US reflected by red blood cells and translates this into velocity of blood flow. By convention, spectral Doppler tracings (1) plot velocity with respect to time and (2) display blood flow toward the transducer above an arbitrary "zero" line and flow away from the transducer below this line. As an example, Figure 9–4 shows a normal Doppler tracing of blood flow through the mitral valve and the typical early filling (E) and late filling from atrial contraction (A). In this example, the transducer is in the apical position.

There are three main forms of Doppler imaging: PW, CW, and color-flow Doppler. Through a technique called *range gating*, PW Doppler can examine flow in discrete, specific areas in the heart and vasculature. This capability is extremely useful in assessing local flow disturbances, but, because of the phenomenon of "aliasing," high velocities cannot be accurately recorded (for a more complete discussion of this phenomenon, the reader is referred to references 5 and 6). The normal velocity of flow through the tricuspid valve is 0.3 to 0.7 m/sec and through the pulmonary artery 0.6 to 0.9 m/sec. Normal flow velocity through the mitral valve is 0.6 to 1.3 m/sec and 1.0 to 1.7 m/sec through the LV outflow tract.

Unlike PW Doppler, CW records all blood flow velocities encountered along the Doppler US beam. Therefore, there is ambiguity of flow location, but CW Doppler is free from "aliasing" and can successfully record very high flow velocities. Color-flow imaging, a major advance in echocardiography, is an extension of PW Doppler. This technique assesses the velocity of flow in multiple sample volumes along multiple beam paths and then assigns a color to each velocity. This color "map" is then superimposed on the 2D image to obtain a real-time, moving description of blood flow.[7] By convention, flow moving toward the transducer is

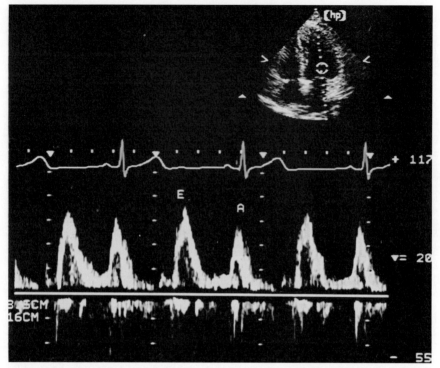

**Figure 9–4** ■ Normal pulsed-wave Doppler tracing from the left ventricular inflow tract displays the early rapid filling (E) and atrial contraction (A) phases of diastolic flow. The transducer is in the apical position, and the sample volume is at the mitral leaflet tips. (From DeMaria AN, Blanchard DG: The echocardiogram. *In* Schlant RC, Alexander RW, Fuster V [eds]: Hurst's The Heart, 9th ed. New York: McGraw-Hill, 1998:415–517, with permission.)

color coded in shades of red, flow moving away from the transducer in blue (Fig. 9–5). Very high-velocity flow is assigned a speckled or green color. Color-flow Doppler has become an essential part of the complete echocardiographic examination and is an excellent tool for both screening and semiquantitation of valvular regurgitation and stenosis.

Recently, there has been much interest in using mitral inflow velocity patterns to evaluate left ventricular (LV) diastolic function.[8] Normally, the E wave is larger than the A wave (see Fig. 8–4). In cases of LV relaxation impairment, the early diastolic transmitral pressure gradient is blunted, causing a decrease in the peak E wave velocity and the rate of flow deceleration. Accompanying this, the peak A wave velocity increases (Fig. 9–6A). In patients with advanced diastolic dysfunction and markedly increased left atrial pressure and LV stiffness, the E-A ratio becomes abnormally high and the E wave develops a very rapid deceleration of flow velocity (i.e., a short deceleration time). This is the so-called "restrictive" filling pattern (Fig. 9–6B). In general, the former "relaxation" abnormality (small E, large A) represents mild diastolic dysfunction whereas the "restrictive" pattern indicates a noncompliant LV and significantly elevated left atrial pressure. It can occur in cases of restrictive cardiomyopathy, advanced LV systolic dysfunction, pericardial disease, and severe valvular disease (e.g., severe mitral or aortic regurgitation). The restric-

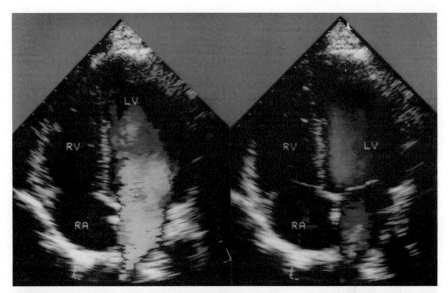

**Figure 9–5** ■ Apical four-chamber images with color-flow Doppler during diastole and systole. Red flow indicates movement toward the transducer (diastolic filling); blue flow indicates movement away from the transducer (systolic ejection). RA, right atrium; RV, right ventricle; LV, left ventricle. (See Color Figure 9–5.) (From DeMaria AN, Blanchard DG: The echocardiogram. *In* Schlant RC, Alexander RW, Fuster V [eds]: Hurst's The Heart, 9th ed. New York: McGraw-Hill, 1998:415–517, with permission.)

tive pattern also has been associated with increased risk of death in patients with advanced heart failure.

Despite the utility of transmitral flow patterns in assessing diastolic properties, these should not be interpreted as pathognomonic findings of diastolic dysfunction but rather as a component of a complete clinical and echocardiographic evaluation. In this regard, pulmonary vein flow patterns are also quite useful and may help detect elevated left atrial pressure when mitral inflow patterns are equivocal or (falsely) appear normal.[8]

## The Bernoulli and Continuity Equations

The *modified Bernoulli equation* states that the gradient across a discrete stenosis in the heart or vasculature can be estimated thus:

$$\text{Pressure gradient} = 4 \; ([\text{Stenotic orifice velocity}]^2 - [\text{Proximal velocity}]^2).$$

If the blood velocity proximal to the stenosis is less than 1.5 m/sec, this proximal velocity term can be ignored. The resulting equation states that the pressure gradient across a discrete stenosis is four times the square of the peak velocity through the orifice. This equation can be used to calculate pressure gradients across any flow-limiting orifice.[9] In addition, if valvular regurgitation is present, the Bernoulli equation can be used to calculate pressure gradients across the tricuspid and mitral valves. This is quite helpful in measuring pulmonary artery pressure, as the peak right ventricular (RV) and pulmonary artery pressures equal 4 (peak TR)$^2$ plus the right atrial pressure (which can be estimated on physical examination).

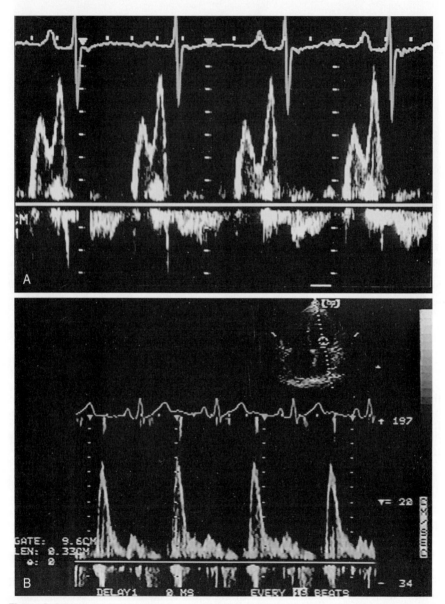

**Figure 9–6** ▪ (A) Pulsed-wave Doppler tracing of diastolic relaxation abnormality. The transducer is in the apical position with the sample volume at the mitral leaflet tips. (B) Pulsed-wave Doppler tracing of diastolic restrictive abnormality. (From DeMaria AN, Blanchard DG: The echocardiogram. In Schlant RC, Alexander RW, Fuster V [eds]: Hurst's The Heart, 9th ed. New York: McGraw-Hill, 1998:415–517, with permission.)

The *continuity equation* states that the product of cross-sectional area and velocity is constant in a closed system of flow:

$$A_1 \, V_1 = A_2 \, V_2$$

The most common use of the continuity equation is calculating aortic valve area, where the product of the cross-sectional area and flow velocity of the LV outflow tract (LVOT) equals the product of the cross-sectional area and velocity of the aortic valve orifice.[10] LVOT area is defined as $\pi(d/2)^2$. This area is multiplied by the LVOT peak systolic velocity (measured by PW Doppler) and then divided by the peak velocity through the stenotic orifice (measured by CW Doppler) to obtain the aortic valve area.

## ■ TRANSESOPHAGEAL ECHOCARDIOGRAPHY

Occasionally transthoracic echocardiography (TTE) does not provide adequately detailed information regarding cardiac anatomy. This is most often true in the evaluation of posterior cardiac structures (e.g., the left atrium and mitral valve), prosthetic cardiac valves, small vegetations or thrombi, and the thoracic aorta. Transesophageal echocardiography (TEE) is well-suited for these situations, as the esophagus is for much of its course immediately adjacent to the left atrium and the thoracic aorta.[11]

TEE images can be recorded from a variety of positions, but most authorities recommend three basic positions: (1) posterior to the base of the heart, (2) posterior to the left atrium, and (3) inferior to the heart (Fig. 9–7B). There are several specific instances where TEE is recommended. These include assessment and evaluation of: (1) cardiac anatomy when TTE is inadequate, (2) valvular vegetations and infective intracardiac abscesses (Fig. 9–8A), (3) prosthetic valve function, (4) cardiac embolic sources, including atrial appendage thrombi (Fig. 9–8B), patent foramen ovale, and interatrial septal aneurysm, and (5) aortic dissection and atherosclerosis (Fig. 9–8C).[12]

## ■ CONTRAST ECHOCARDIOGRAPHY

Contrast echocardiography has grown explosively in the last few years. Until recently, the main agent used for echocardiographic "contrast" injection was agitated saline, which contains numerous air microbubbles that are strong reflectors of US energy. When injected intravenously, agitated saline produces dense opacification of the right heart structures and is an excellent method for detecting intracardiac shunts. As the air microbubbles dissolve rapidly into the bloodstream, they do not pass through the pulmonary circulation. Therefore, any air microbubbles entering the left side of the heart must arrive there through a shunt (Fig. 9–9).

Direct injection of agitated saline into the aorta or left ventricle produces US opacification of the myocardium and LV cavity, respectively.[13] LV opacification markedly enhances US images and endocardial border definition, but intraarterial contrast injection is clearly impractical for routine use. Thus, extensive research has focused on creating echocardiographic contrast agents that reach the left side of the heart after intravenous injection. The first commercially available agent, Albunex, consisted of air microbubbles in albumin shells. These stabilized microbubbles survived transit through the pulmonary circulation and reached the left ventricle, but dense opacification was often not achieved. The newer generation of agents, such as Optison, use various perfluorocarbon gases instead of air. The fact that these gases are dense and much less soluble in blood than in air enables them to

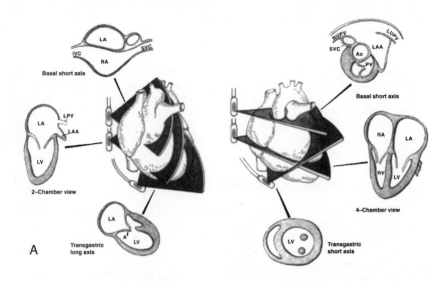

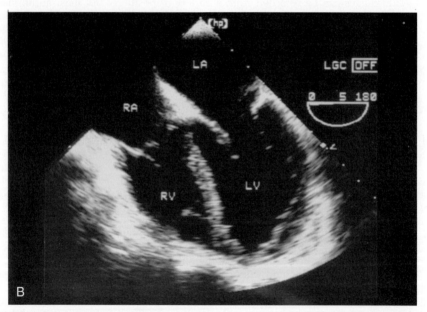

**Figure 9–7** ■ *(A)* Standard TEE imaging planes in transverse and longitudinal axes. *(B)* Transverse four-chamber TEE plane; SVC, IVC, superior and inferior vena cava; LAA, left atrial appendage; RUPV, LUPV, right and left upper pulmonary vein; LA, left atrium; LV, left ventricle; RA, right atrium; RV, right ventricle. *(A,* Fisher EA, Stahl JA, Budd JH, Goldman ME: Transesophageal echocardiography: Procedures and clinical applications. J Am Coll Cardiol, 1991;18:1333–1348; *B,* DeMaria AN, Blanchard DG: The echocardiogram. *In* Schlant RC, Alexander RW, Fuster V [eds]: Hurst's The Heart, 9th ed. New York: McGraw-Hill, 1998:415–517, with permission.)

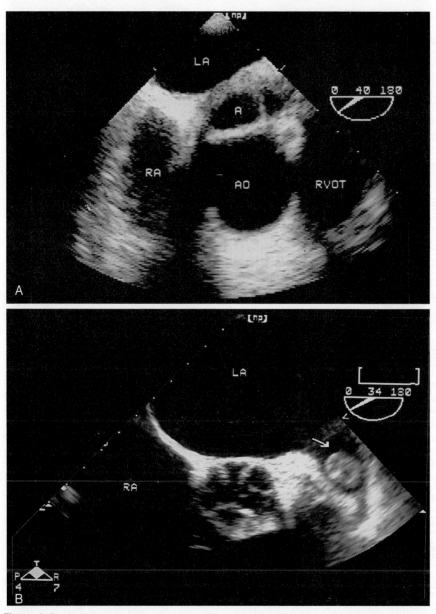

**Figure 9–8** ▪ *(A)* Short-axis TEE image through the cardiac base. A large septated abscess cavity *(A)* is present between the aortic root (AO) and the left atrium (LA). *(B)* TEE image of a thrombus in the left atrial appendage *(arrow).* RVOT, right ventricular outflow tract. (From DeMaria AN, Blanchard DG: The echocardiogram. *In* Schlant RC, Alexander RW, Fuster V [eds]: Hurst's The Heart, 9th ed. New York: McGraw-Hill, 1998:415–517, with permission.)

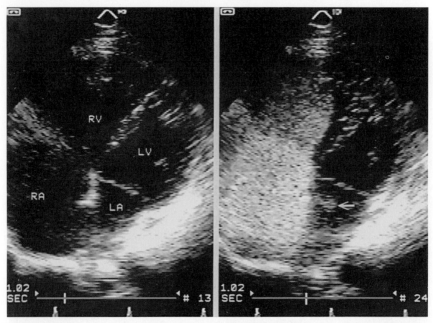

**Figure 9–9** ▪ Contrast microbubble injection demonstrating a shunt *(arrow)* from the right atrium (RA) to the left atrium (LA). RV, right ventricle; LV, left ventricle. (From DeMaria AN, Blanchard DG: The echocardiogram. *In* Schlant RC, Alexander RW, Fuster V [eds]: Hurst's The Heart, 9th ed. New York: McGraw-Hill, 1998:415–517, with permission.)

persist in the circulation, producing consistent and dense opacification of the LV cavity. In addition, harmonic imaging enhances the US backscatter from contrast microbubbles (which resonate in a US field) while it decreases the signal returning from the myocardium (which does not resonate).[14] Echocontrast agents are especially useful in stress echocardiography, as the enhanced LV endocardial border definition improves detection of regional dysfunction. In the near future, direct assessment of myocardial perfusion via contrast echo will likely become available.

## ▪ VALVULAR HEART DISEASE

### Aortic Valve

#### Aortic Stenosis

The thin leaflets of the aortic valve are usually well-visualized by echocardiography. Aortic valve disease is often best imaged from the parasternal views. In cases of acquired (calcific) aortic stenosis (AS), the valve leaflets are markedly thickened and calcified, and their motion severely restricted (Fig. 9–10). In congenital AS, systolic "doming" of the leaflets is seen, often along with congenital anomalies of the valve leaflets (e.g., bicuspid, unicuspid). Attempts at valve area planimetry by transthoracic echocardiography (TTE) have generally been unsuccessful, although planimetry with TEE has yielded better results. Thus, standard 2D imaging accurately detects AS, but not its severity.

The cornerstone of quantification is the Doppler examination. CW Doppler can

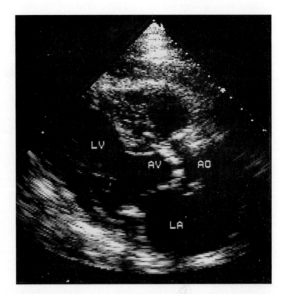

**Figure 9–10** ■ Parasternal long-axis view demonstrates a thickened, stenotic aortic valve (AV). AO, aorta; LV, left ventricle; LA, left atrium. (From DeMaria AN, Blanchard DG: The echocardiogram. *In* Schlant RC, Alexander RW, Fuster V [eds]: Hurst's The Heart, 9th ed. New York: McGraw-Hill, 1998:415–517, with permission.)

record the peak velocity of blood flow through the aortic valve, which with the modified Bernoulli equation then can be used to calculate the peak instantaneous systolic gradient. The aortic valve orifice area is then calculated via the continuity equation in the following manner:

First, the area of the LVOT just proximal to the aortic valve is calculated using this equation: $\pi r^2$ (where $r$ is half of the diameter of the LVOT measured in the parasternal long axis view); next, the velocity of flow in the LVOT is measured using PW Doppler; finally, the area of the valve orifice is calculated by multiplying the LVOT area by the LVOT velocity and dividing the result by the peak flow velocity through the stenotic orifice.[9, 10] These calculations correlate quite well with catheterization-derived values and are valid as long as the LVOT flow velocity is less than 1.5 m/sec.

## Aortic Insufficiency

Two-dimensional imaging may show a normal aortic valve in cases of aortic insufficiency (AI), but it can also demonstrate leaflet abnormalities, aortic root enlargement, LV dilatation, and diastolic "flutter" of the anterior mitral valve leaflet. In acute severe AI, M-mode imaging can reveal early diastolic closure of the mitral valve (an uncommon but extremely important finding). Although 2D imaging provides clues to the presence of AI, the Doppler examination is much more useful and easily detects the abnormal flow. Indeed, color-flow Doppler is a very rapid screening tool that detects AI with nearly 100% sensitivity. Quantitation of AI, however, is considerably more difficult.

There are several approaches for semiquantitation of AI by echocardiography. The first utilizes color-flow imaging. In the parasternal views, severity can be estimated by the diameter (or cross-sectional area) of the color jet in the LVOT. Mild AI generally has a jet diameter smaller than 25% of the outflow tract diameter (Fig. 9–11A), whereas a severe AI color jet often occupies more than 75% of the outflow tract during diastole. Findings with moderate AI fall between these.

A second method uses CW Doppler to calculate the AI "pressure half-time" (see Mitral Stenosis below). This parameter is a function of the gradient between

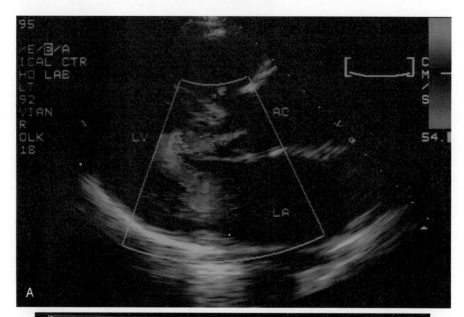

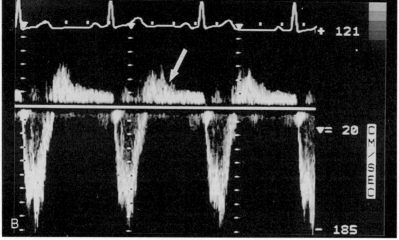

**Figure 9–11** ■ *(A)* Parasternal long-axis image showing a multicolored jet (indicating turbulent flow) of aortic regurgitation in the left ventricular outflow tract. The jet is narrow in width, suggesting mild regurgitation. *(B)* Pulsed-wave Doppler tracing (from the suprasternal transducer position) in a case of severe aortic regurgitation. The sample volume is in the descending thoracic aorta, and holodiastolic flow reversal *(arrow)* is present. AO, aorta; LA, left atrium; LV, left ventricle. (See Color Figure 9–11.) (From DeMaria AN, Blanchard DG: The echocardiogram. *In* Schlant RC, Alexander RW, Fuster V [eds]: Hurst's The Heart, 9th ed. New York: McGraw-Hill, 1998:415–517, with permission.)

the aorta and left ventricle during diastole. In severe AI, this gradient decreases very quickly (producing a short pressure half-time) but with mild AI decreases much more slowly (producing a long pressure half-time). In general, a pressure half-time of 200 to 250 msec or less strongly suggests severe aortic insufficiency.

In the third method, PW Doppler is utilized to detect diastolic reversal of flow in the descending aorta. Holodiastolic flow reversal suggests severe AI (Fig. 9–11B). Several other techniques for evaluating severity of AI (e.g., calculation of regurgitant flow volume and orifice area using flow convergence measurements) are beyond the scope of this chapter.[1]

Although echocardiographic assessment of aortic stenosis is quantitative and generally accurate, assessment of AI is semiquantitative at best. Clinical examination and correlation are, therefore, essential. Despite this, echocardiography is quite useful with aortic valve disease and can help to determine proper timing of valve surgery.

## Mitral Valve

### Mitral Stenosis

Detection of mitral stenosis (MS) was one of the earliest clinical applications of cardiac US. Rheumatic MS is characterized by tethering and fibrosis of the mitral leaflets, principally at the distal tips. The leaflets are sometimes calcified and usually thickened and display characteristic "doming" during diastole (Fig. 9–12A). The posterior leaflet of the valve may be pulled anteriorly during diastole secondary to commissural fusion with the longer anterior leaflet. The left atrium is almost always enlarged. In the parasternal short-axis view, the commissural fusion is apparent and produces a "fish-mouth" appearance of the orifice (Fig. 9–12B).[15] Doppler examination reveals abnormally high diastolic flow velocity through the mitral valve and often detects coexistent mitral regurgitation.

Echocardiographic quantitation of MS severity is done in two ways. First, the mitral orifice area can be measured directly via planimetry in the parasternal short-axis view. Gain artifacts must be avoided, and care must be taken to find the smallest orifice area at the distal end of the leaflets. Properly done, this technique is accurate and correlates well with catheterization data. The second commonly used technique is the "pressure half-time" method. The pressure half-time is the interval required for transmitral flow velocity to decrease from its maximum to the velocity that represents half of the pressure equivalent. As the severity of MS increases, the rate of flow deceleration decreases (i.e., the pressure gradient between left atrium and LV remains high during diastole), prolonging the pressure half-time. The pressure half-time method also correlates with planimetry measurements, but it is not accurate immediately after mitral valvuloplasty.

In addition to valve area quantitation, echocardiography is useful in predicting success of percutaneous mitral valvuloplasty. A score based on four variables (mitral valvular thickening, calcification, mobility, and subvalvular involvement) has been devised and tested. Each variable is rated on a scale of 1 to 4 (where 4 is most severe) and the individual components are summed. A score of 8 to 12 or greater predicts a poor response to valvuloplasty and an increased risk of complications.

### Mitral Regurgitation

As it is for AI, echocardiography is extremely accurate for detecting mitral regurgitation (MR), but quantitation is more difficult. Two-dimensional imaging in MR may reveal thickened, abnormal mitral valve leaflets (for example, in cases of

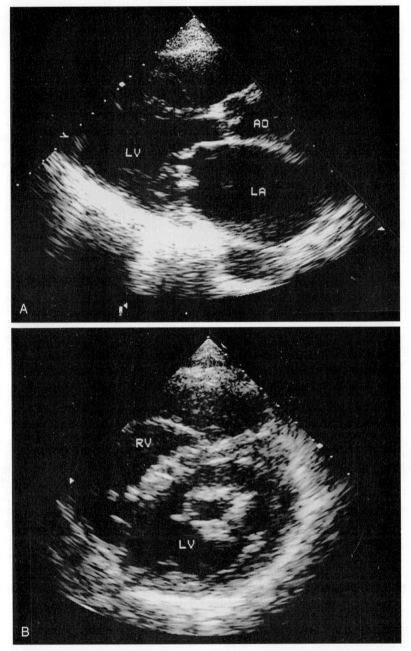

**Figure 9–12** ▪ *(A)* Parasternal long-axis view of mitral stenosis. The left atrium (LA) is enlarged, mitral opening is limited, and "doming" of the anterior mitral leaflet is present. *(B)* Parasternal short-axis plane in mitral stenosis. RV, right ventricle; LV, left ventricle; AO, aorta. (From DeMaria AN, Blanchard DG: The Echocardiogram. *In* Schlant RC, Alexander RW, Fuster V [eds]: Hurst's The Heart, 9th ed. New York: McGraw-Hill, 1998:415–517, with permission.)

rheumatic disease, myxomatous degeneration, mitral valve prolapse, or ruptured mitral chordae tendineae). With severe MR, the left atrium and ventricle are often enlarged. Doppler echocardiography is the primary method of semiquantitation of MR. Color-flow imaging shows a jet of aliased flow in the left atrium during systole, and the size of this color jet correlates roughly with angiographic MR severity (Fig. 9–13).[17] Eccentrically directed MR, however, may produce a color jet of misleadingly small cross-sectional area on US imaging, even when left ventriculography demonstrates severe MR.

Volumetric analysis with PW Doppler can be used to calculate regurgitant volumes, but its accuracy is limited. PW Doppler interrogation of the pulmonary veins (by TTE or TEE) is helpful in quantifying MR, as systolic flow reversal within the vein is quite specific for severe regurgitation. Recent work has shown that flow convergence is a useful marker in cases of valvular regurgitation.[18] With significant MR, there is often a large zone of high-velocity (aliased) color flow proximal to the mitral valve leaflets. This finding (even with a relatively small color jet in the left atrium) often indicates MR of at least moderate severity.

## Mitral Valve Prolapse

Echocardiography is the diagnostic procedure of choice for mitral valve prolapse.[19] This condition is defined by the bulging back of the mitral valve leaflets into the left atrium, with a portion of the leaflets passing the level of the mitral valve annulus on the parasternal long-axis view (Fig. 9–14). M-mode imaging also can detect mitral valve prolapse, but it is less sensitive than 2D imaging.

Rupture of a chordae tendineae is well-visualized by US. Imaging usually reveals the involved chord and leaflet as well as the severity of MR. TEE is especially beneficial for assessing the feasibility of mitral valve repair.

## Prosthetic Cardiac Valves

Echocardiography can assess the anatomy and function of bioprosthetic and mechanical heart valves. In general, however, evaluation is considerably more

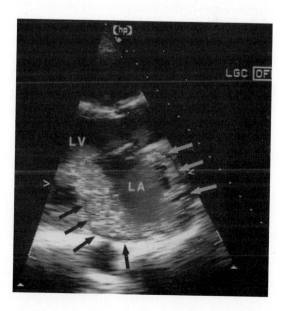

**Figure 9–13** ■ Parasternal long-axis view in a case of severe mitral regurgitation. The color Doppler jet is directed posteriorly and is eccentric (*black arrows*). The jet "hugs" the wall of the left atrium (LA) and wraps around all the way to the aortic root (*white arrows*). LV, left ventricle. (See Color Figure 9–13.) (From DeMaria AN, Blanchard DG: The echocardiogram. *In* Schlant RC, Alexander RW, Fuster V [eds]: Hurst's The Heart, 9th ed. New York: McGraw-Hill, 1998: 415–517, with permission.)

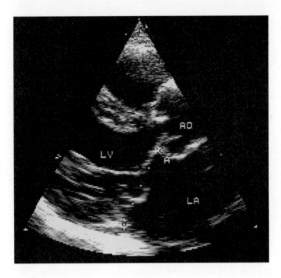

**Figure 9–14** ■ Parasternal long-axis image through the mitral valve in late systole. The plane of the annulus (A) is drawn in a dotted line. The posterior leaflet prolapses past the level of the annulus. LA, left atrium; AO, aorta; LV, left ventricle. (From DeMaria AN, Blanchard DG: The echocardiogram. *In* Schlant RC, Alexander RW, Fuster V [eds]: Hurst's The Heart, 9th ed. New York: McGraw-Hill, 1998:415–517, with permission.)

limited than it is for native valves. Because of acoustic shadowing, the areas distal to prosthetic (especially mechanical) valves are obscured, limiting detection of valvular regurgitation, thrombi, and vegetations. Because of this, TEE has become indispensable in the evaluation of prosthetic valve dysfunction and associated abnormalities.

### Right-Sided Valvular Disease and Pulmonary Hypertension

Echocardiography can detect rheumatic involvement of the tricuspid and pulmonic valves and congenital pulmonic stenosis. Color-flow imaging detects and helps to semiquantify tricuspid and pulmonic regurgitation, similar to insufficiency of the mitral and aortic valves. Measurement of the peak tricuspid regurgitation velocity by CW Doppler is helpful for estimating peak systolic pulmonary artery and right ventricular pressures (via the modified Bernoulli equation).[9]

The 2D findings associated with right ventricular overload and pulmonary hypertension include enlargement of the right ventricle and right atrium, dilatation of the pulmonary artery and inferior vena cava, flattening of the interventricular septum (with loss of the normal curvature toward the right), and hypertrophy of the right ventricular free wall. Doppler examination often shows moderate or severe tricuspid regurgitation in these cases.

### ■ DISEASES OF THE AORTA

#### Aortic Dissection

In the last several years, echocardiography has fundamentally changed the diagnostic approach to suspected aortic dissection. TTE is a reasonably accurate screening tool for ascending aortic dissection (type A) but is not sensitive for detecting descending dissection (type B). Diagnostic findings include a dilated aorta with a thin, linear mobile signal in the lumen representing the dissected intimal flap. Color Doppler imaging may reveal normal or high-velocity flow in the true lumen and slow (stagnant) flow in the false channel. Occasionally, the entrance into the false channel is defined. Although TTE is sometimes helpful, TEE has become a diagnostic procedure of choice for aortic dissection.[12] Its sensitivity and specificity rival those of magnetic resonance imaging, and TEE has the advantage of being portable and rapid. In addition, LV and valvular function can be defined during the examination. TEE can also help detect thrombosis of the false lumen, traumatic transection of the aorta, and intramural aortic hemorrhage (an increasingly recognized disorder whose prognosis is similar to that of dissection).

## Aortic Aneurysm and Atherosclerosis

Aneurysms of the aorta may appear saccular or fusiform, and on echocardiography are seen as focal or diffuse areas of aortic enlargement. TTE is useful for detecting ascending aortic dilatation and can sometimes visualize descending thoracic and abdominal aortic aneurysms (Fig. 9–15). Sinus of Valsalva aneurysms (asymmetric dilatations of the aortic root) are also well-visualized, and the aortic insufficiency or shunts often associated with these aneurysms are well-defined. Echocardiography has been used extensively to aid decision making on the timing of aortic valve and root replacement in patients with Marfan's syndrome.[12]

TEE has played a major role in the detection of aortic atherosclerosis. This disease has been underappreciated in the past but appears to be a powerful risk factor for stroke and peripheral emboli. TEE is currently the procedure of choice for detecting aortic atheromas, which characteristically appear as asymmetric, calcified plaques that protrude into the aortic lumen.[12]

## ▪ INFECTIVE ENDOCARDITIS

Echocardiography is an integral part of the diagnosis and management of infective endocarditis. Clearly, the diagnosis remains a clinical one, but echocardiographic detection of vegetations is now included in most modern diagnostic algorithms and strategies. The hallmark of endocarditis is an infective valvular vegetation (Fig. 9–16), and TTE detects these with reasonable sensitivity (although as

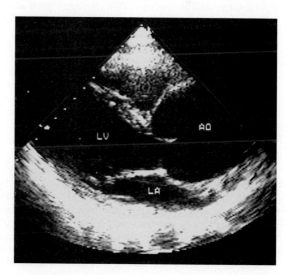

**Figure 9–15** ▪ Parasternal long-axis image demonstrates severe aortic root (AO) enlargement. LA, left atrium; LV, left ventricle. (From DeMaria AN, Blanchard DG: The echocardiogram. *In* Schlant RC, Alexander RW, Fuster V [eds]: Hurst's The Heart, 9th ed. New York: McGraw-Hill, 1998:415–517, with permission.)

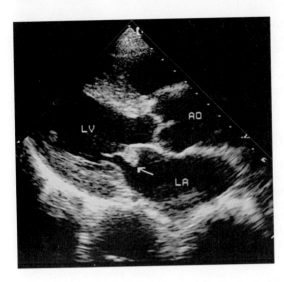

**Figure 9–16** ■ Parasternal long-axis view demonstrates a vegetation (*arrow*) on the anterior mitral valve leaflet. AO, aorta; LV, left ventricle; LA, left atrium. (From DeMaria AN, Blanchard DG: The echocardiogram. *In* Schlant RC, Alexander RW, Fuster V [eds]: Hurst's The Heart, 9th ed. New York: McGraw-Hill, 1998:415–517, with permission.)

many as 20% of patients with proven native valve endocarditis may have unremarkable TTE findings).

TEE is considerably more accurate than TTE for visualizing vegetations and is significantly better in detecting valvular abscesses and prosthetic valve endocarditis (see Fig. 9–8A).[20] Echocardiography also helps to visualize associated abnormalities such as valvular regurgitation, purulent pericarditis, and intracardiac fistulas. Accurate visualization of these abnormalities helps to guide management and is useful in assessing the need for cardiac surgery. A common clinical dilemma concerns the appropriate use of TEE in persons with endocarditis. It seems reasonable to use TTE as the first screening test for most patients with suspected endocarditis. If the study is technically limited or findings are equivocal or diagnostic of vegetations in patients at high risk for perivalvular complications, TEE should be performed. If TTE findings are unremarkable or vegetations are detected in patients at low risk for complications, TEE is probably unnecessary. Patients at high risk (e.g., those with prosthetic cardiac valves, congenital heart disease, or infection with virulent organisms) should undergo TEE if endocarditis is strongly suspected, even if TTE results are unremarkable.[20]

Despite all technologic advances, infective endocarditis remains a clinical diagnosis, and the utility of echocardiography should not be overestimated. Myxomatous valvular degeneration can masquerade as vegetations, and an old, healed vegetation can be mistaken for an active lesion. Therefore, echocardiographic results should be integrated with all available clinical data.

## ■ ISCHEMIC HEART DISEASE

In the last several years, echocardiography has become an important technique for detecting and measuring myocardial ischemia and infarction (MI). LV ischemia quickly produces dysfunction and hypokinesis of the involved ventricular segment. If coronary flow is not restored, permanent damage occurs with resulting akinesis and thinning of the affected myocardial segment. If the region of dysfunctional myocardium is identified, the infarct-related coronary artery often can be inferred.[21] Echocardiography detects these abnormalities and the LV dilatation and depression of ejection fraction that accompany severe ischemic heart disease. The LV myocardium can be divided into 16 wall segments according to a format adopted by the American Society of Echocardiography (Fig. 9–17).[21] By grading the contraction of each of these segments, a semiquantitative wall motion score can be calculated. This parameter has been used to assess prognosis for both acute MI and chronic ischemic heart disease.

Although echocardiography can help to estimate the extent of damage in acute MI, the technique is also valuable for detecting post-MI complications. Easily visualized findings include pericardial effusion (from pericarditis or LV free wall rupture), ventricular septal rupture, mitral regurgitation (from LV enlargement or papillary ischemia), LV pseudoaneurysm, and RV dysfunction associated with inferior wall MI. Long-term LV remodeling and aneurysm formation can also be assessed (Fig. 9–18).[22]

## Stress Echocardiography

Recently, echocardiography has been combined with stress testing to increase the accuracy of ischemia detection.[23] In this technique, side-by-side cine loops of 2D images made before and after (or during) stress are displayed on a video monitor. Normally, the LV myocardium becomes hypercontractile with exercise and end-diastolic LV cavity size decreases. Stress-induced segmental hypokinesis is abnormal, and the affected coronary artery can be predicted from which particular area(s) exhibit inducible ventricular dysfunction. Multiple wall segment abnormalities and LV dilatation with stress are ominous findings that suggest severe stenoses

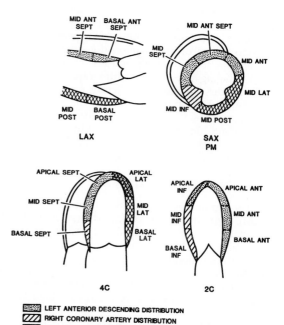

**Figure 9–17** ■ Sixteen-segment format for identification of left ventricular wall segments. Coronary arterial territories are also included. LAX, parasternal long-axis; SAX PM, short-axis at papillary muscle level; 4C, apical four-chamber; 2C, apical two-chamber; ANT, anterior; SEPT, septal; POST, posterior; LAT, lateral; INF, inferior. (From Segar D, Brown S, Sawada S, et al: Dobutamine stress echocardiography: Correlation with coronary lesion severity as determined by quantitative angiography. J Am Coll Cardiol 1992;19:1197.)

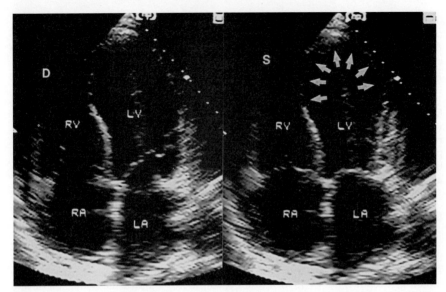

**Figure 9–18** ■ Apical four-chamber images of a large apical infarction with aneurysm. Diastole (D) is displayed on the left, systole (S) on the right. During systole, the base on the ventricle contracts but the apex is dyskinetic *(arrows)*. RA, right atrium; RV, right ventricle; LV, left ventricle; LA, left atrium. (From DeMaria AN, Blanchard DG: The echocardiogram. *In* Schlant RC, Alexander RW, Fuster V [eds]: Hurst's The Heart, 9th ed. New York: McGraw-Hill, 1998:415–517, with permission.)

in multiple coronary arteries and widespread ischemia.[23] An example of inducible apical hypokinesis is seen in Figure 9–20.

Stress echocardiography can be performed with either exercise or a graded infusion of a drug (most often dobutamine). In general, both types of stress are safe and are tolerated well, and accuracy rates compare well with those of nuclear stress imaging. Stress echocardiography tends to be slightly less sensitive than nuclear stress imaging but slightly more specific. Dobutamine echocardiography has assumed an important role in the detection of myocardial viability and the phenomenon of "hibernation."[24] Recent technical innovations such as harmonic imaging and contrast echocardiography have increased the accuracy and applicability of stress echocardiography. In addition, US contrast agents may facilitate direct quantitation of myocardial perfusion during stress.

## ■ THE CARDIOMYOPATHIES

The cardiomyopathies are generally separated into three categories: dilated (DCM), hypertrophic (HCM), and restrictive (RCM). Echocardiography plays an important role in the clinical evaluation, providing information on cavity size, ventricular wall thickness, valvular lesions, and systolic function. In cases of classic HCM, echocardiography alone may be diagnostic. In cases of dilated, restrictive, and non-classic HCM, however, additional clinical information may be needed to arrive at a firm diagnosis. These diseases are discussed in further detail in Chapter 33. In this section, we focus primarily on their US features.

### Hypertrophic Cardiomyopathy

HCM is a primary abnormality of the myocardium that exhibits unprovoked hypertrophy and often affects the septum disproportionately. The first and fundamental echocardiographic abnormality is LV hypertrophy, which is often severe. Classically, the septum is involved more extensively than other areas (Fig. 9–19A), but the hypertrophy may also be concentric or apical. Asymmetric septal hypertrophy leads to the second classic US feature of HCM: dynamic LVOT obstruction. This is associated with systolic anterior motion (SAM) of the mitral valve (see *arrow*, Fig. 9–19A). Systolic encroachment of the abnormally thickened septum into the LVOT creates a pressure drop by the Venturi effect, which then draws the mitral leaflets toward the septum, causing dynamic obstruction. Like severe LVH, SAM is not pathognomonic for HCM and can occur in other conditions such as hypovolemia and hyperdynamic states.[1]

The third manifestation of classic HCM is midsystolic closure of the aortic valve. This appears to occur only in obstructive HCM cases and is probably a manifestation of the sudden late systole pressure drop caused by SAM. Therefore, when this sign is present, significant LVOT obstruction is likely.[25] The fourth sign of HCM is seen on CW Doppler imaging through the LVOT. Normally, flow velocity in this area peaks early during systole and has a maximum of 1.7 m/sec. In HCM with outflow tract obstruction, the peak systolic flow velocity is abnormally high. As opposed to valvular aortic stenosis, however, the CW spectral tracing of obstructive HCM peaks late in systole, creating a characteristic "sabertooth" pattern (Fig. 9–21B). Catheterization data would predict this type of tracing, as the outflow tract gradient is not severely elevated in early systole but rises in mid- and late systole because of dynamic obstruction. The peak CW velocity can be used to calculate the systolic gradient via the modified Bernoulli equation, although recent studies have suggested that this calculation may not be consistently accurate in HCM.

## Dilated Cardiomyopathy

Echocardiographic findings in DCM include four-chamber cardiac dilatation and marked LV enlargement. Systolic function is depressed, often severely. In addition, the LV walls are often thin, with concomitant left atrial enlargement, limited mitral and aortic valve opening (due to low stroke volume), and mitral annular dilatation (with secondary mitral regurgitation).[26] Unfortunately, these findings are not specific for DCM and can be caused by severe ischemic heart disease, viral myocarditis, cardiac toxins, and nutritional deficiencies. Ischemic heart disease can often be predicted by the presence of regional LV dysfunction, but, again, this finding is not always reliable. Diastolic dysfunction is common in DCM, and Doppler interrogation of mitral inflow may show an abnormal relaxation, restrictive, or "pseudonormal" pattern, depending on left atrial pressure and loading conditions. A restrictive pattern of inflow is associated with poor prognosis for DCM.

## Restrictive Cardiomyopathy

RCM is a fairly rare condition that is characterized on US by (1) a diffuse increase in LV wall thickness in the absence of severe cavity dilatation and (2) marked biatrial enlargement.[27] Systolic function may be normal or modestly decreased. Doppler examination may show a mitral inflow relaxation abnormality early in the course of RCM, but this tends to evolve into a restrictive pattern as the disease progresses. RCM may be idiopathic or secondary to infiltrative diseases such as hemochromatosis and hypereosinophilic endocardial disease. The most common cause of RCM, however, is amyloidosis, which causes biventricular hypertrophy and diffuse thickening of the interatrial septum and cardiac valves (Fig.

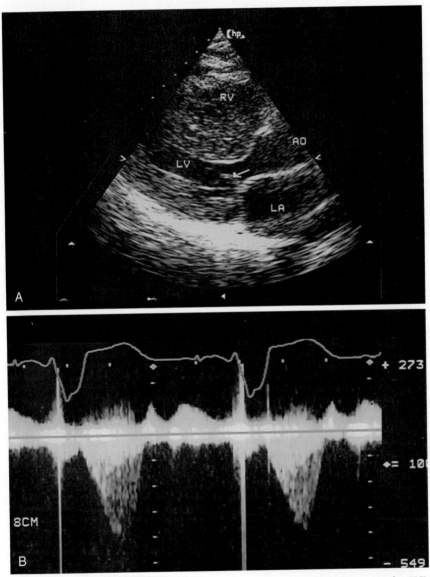

**Figure 9–19** ■ *(A)* Parasternal long-axis view (during systole) of hypertrophic cardiomyopathy (HCM). Asymmetric septal hypertrophy is present, as well as systolic anterior motion of the anterior mitral leaflet *(arrow)*. *(B)* Continuous-wave Doppler tracing through the left ventricular outflow tract (from the apical transducer position) in hypertrophic obstructive cardiomyopathy. In comparison to valvular aortic stenosis, the rise in velocity is delayed (reflecting dynamic rather than fixed outflow obstruction). LV, left ventricle; LA, left atrium; RV, right ventricle; AO, aorta. (From DeMaria AN, Blanchard DG: The echocardiogram. *In* Schlant RC, Alexander RW, Fuster V [eds]: Hurst's The Heart, 9th ed. New York, McGraw-Hill, 1998:415–517, with permission.)

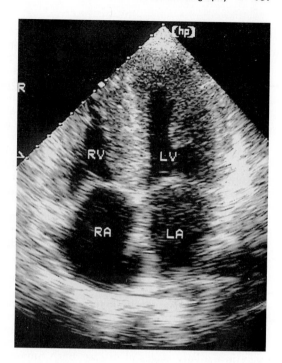

**Figure 9–20** ■ Apical four-chamber view of cardiac amyloid. RV, right ventricle; RA, right atrium; LA, left atrium; LV, left ventricle. (From De-Maria AN, Blanchard DG: The echocardiogram. *In* Schlant RC, Alexander RW, Fuster V [eds]: Hurst's The Heart, 9th ed. New York: McGraw-Hill, 1998: 415–517, with permission.)

9–20). A "ground-glass" or speckled appearance of the myocardium has been described with amyloid, but this sign has minimal clinical usefulness. As with the other cardiomyopathies, the echocardiographic findings in RCM are often helpful but ultimately nonspecific.

## ■ CARDIAC MASSES

Echocardiography has become the procedure of choice for the detection of intracardiac thrombi, vegetations, and tumors. It also visualizes a number of "pseudomasses" or benign anatomic variants (e.g., prominent eustachian valve, Chiari network, prominent right ventricular moderator band, and LV false chordae tendineae). US can also detect intracardiac foreign bodies, including pacemaker leads, intracardiac catheters, and endomyocardial bioptomes.

### Intracardiac Thrombi

Thrombi can develop in any chamber of the heart and may cause embolic events.[28] The major predisposing factors for intracardiac thrombi formation include low cardiac output, localized stasis of flow, and myocardial injury. The echocardiographic appearance of thrombi is quite variable: thrombi can be freely mobile or attached to the endocardium, and they may be laminar and homogeneous in density or heterogeneous with areas of central liquefaction or calcification. Thrombi typically have identifiable borders on US and should be visible in multiple imaging planes.[28]

Thrombi within the right heart are often laminar but can be quite mobile (especially venous thromboemboli that have migrated to the right side of the heart), and they increase the risk of pulmonary embolism. Left atrial thrombi occur most often in the setting of LV systolic dysfunction, mitral stenosis, atrial fibrillation, and severe left atrial enlargement. TEE is clearly superior to TTE for detecting these thrombi, especially those within the left atrial appendage (see Fig. 9–8B). Because approximately 50% of left atrial thrombi are limited to the appendage, TEE is the procedure of choice for detecting them. Left atrial thrombi are often accompanied by spontaneous US contrast (or "smoke") in the left atrium, which indicates stagnant flow and increased likelihood of embolic events.

LV thrombi usually occur in settings of systolic dysfunction,[28] including DCM, acute MI, and chronic LV aneurysm. Most LV thrombi are located in the apex and thus are best visualized in the apical views. LV thrombi may be laminar and fixed, protruding or mobile, and homogeneous or heterogeneous in US density. Artifacts can sometime mimic apical thrombi. A true LV thrombus has a density that is distinct from that of the myocardium, moves concordantly with the underlying tissue, and is visible in multiple imaging planes. Finally, an LV thrombus rarely occurs in areas of normally functioning myocardium.

## Cardiac Tumors

Cardiac tumors can be benign or malignant, and the malignancies may be primary, metastatic, or the result of direct extension from adjacent tumors. Although primary cardiac malignancies are exceedingly rare, metastatic spread to the heart from lung cancer, breast cancer, lymphoma, or melanoma is fairly common, especially in the later stages of disease. Such tumors may be seen within the cardiac chambers, but pericardial or epicardial involvement is more common.

Myxomas are by far the most common primary cardiac tumors, and about 75% are found in the left atrium.[29] On 2D imaging, these tumors generally appear gelatinous, speckled, and sometimes globular. Tissue heterogeneity is frequently seen, but calcifications are rare. Although they can originate from any portion of the atrial wall, myxomas are usually attached by a pedicle to the interatrial septum. Large myxomas are almost always mobile and may move back and forth into the mitral annulus. Doppler examination may demonstrate valvular regurgitation, obstruction, or both. TTE accurately detects most large myxomas (see Fig. 9–21), but TEE is superior for delineating small tumors.[29] Less common benign primary cardiac tumors include rhabdomyomas (associated with tuberous sclerosis), fibromas (which tend to grow within the LV myocardial wall), and papillary fibroelastomas (which grow on valves and tend to embolize systemically).

## ▪ CONGENITAL HEART DISEASE*

In this section we focus primarily on the echocardiographic recognition of the more common congenital lesions seen in adults.

## Atrial Septal Defect

Most ostium secundum and ostium primum atrial septal defects (ASD) are easily seen with TTE.[30] Sinus venosus defects, however, can be difficult to detect without TEE. As the normal interatrial septum is thin and parallel to the US beam from the apical position, artifactual "dropout" in the area of the fossa ovalis can be

---

*For a more complete discussion of congenital heart disease, the reader should see Chapter 21.

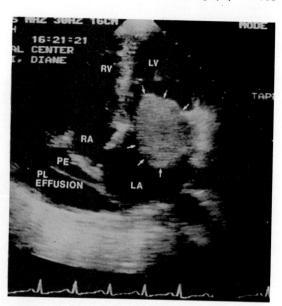

**Figure 9–21** ▪ Apical four-chamber view of a large left atrial myxoma *(arrows)* that is attached to the lateral wall of the left atrium (LA). RA, right atrium; RV, right ventricle; LV, left ventricle; PE, pericardial effusion; PL, pleural. (From DeMaria AN, Blanchard DG: The echocardiogram. *In* Schlant RC, Alexander RW, Fuster V [eds]: Hurst's The Heart, 9th ed. New York: McGraw-Hill, 1998:415–517, with permission.)

mistaken for ASD. Therefore, subcostal imaging is usually superior. Ostium secundum defects (the most common form of ASD) are distinguished by localized absence of tissue in the middle portion of the interatrial septum (Fig. 9–22A). The absence of any septal tissue interposed between the defect and the base of the interventricular septum suggests an ostium primum defect, which is frequently associated with a cleft anterior mitral valve leaflet, mitral regurgitation, and sometimes an inlet ventricular septal defect (VSD). Sinus venosus ASDs are seen in the superior and posterior portions of the interatrial septum and are usually associated with anomalous drainage of one or more pulmonary veins into the right atrium.[1]

Additional 2D findings seen in ASD include right atrial and RV enlargement, flattening of the interventricular septum, and paradoxical septal motion. Doppler interrogation often demonstrates blood flow through the defect, but inflow from the vena cava and pulmonary veins sometimes mimics ASD. To prevent misdiagnosis of ASD, intravenous injection of agitated saline is recommended (see section on Contrast Echocardiography). Finally, Doppler and 2D imaging can be used to estimate roughly the pulmonary-to-systemic blood flow ratio in patients with ASD or other intracardiac shunts.

## Ventricular Septal Defect

The majority of VSDs in adults are perimembranous. Inlet (AV canal), trabecular, and outlet (supracristal) defects are much rarer. Although large VSDs are often visible on 2D imaging alone (Fig. 9–22B), color-flow imaging is essential for detection of small defects.[31] CW Doppler measurement of peak systolic flow velocity through a VSD can be used to estimate the pressure gradient between the two ventricles via the modified Bernoulli equation (the estimated RV systolic pressure is the systolic arterial pressure minus the calculated Bernoulli gradient).[9] Associated 2D and Doppler findings include cardiac enlargement (possibly with RV pressure overload), mitral and tricuspid valvular abnormalities and regurgitation, coexistent ASD (most often with inlet VSD), ventricular septal aneurysms, and aortic insuffi-

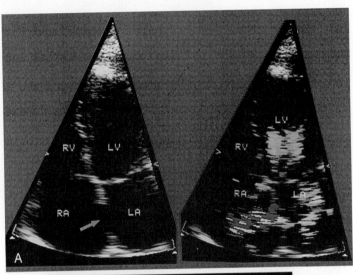

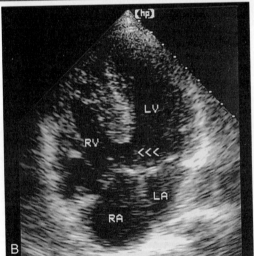

**Figure 9–22** ■ *(A)* Apical four-chamber view of an ostium secundum atrial septal defect. On the left, a defect in the mid-atrial septum is present *(arrow)*. On the right, there is color flow through the shunt. RA, right atrium; RV, right ventricle; LA, left atrium; LV, left ventricle. *(B)* Apical four-chamber image of an inlet ventricular septal defect. RV, right ventricle; RA, right atrium; LA, left atrium; LV, left ventricle. (See Color Figure 9–22.) (From DeMaria AN, Blanchard DG; The echocardiogram. *In* Schlant RC, Alexander RW, Fuster V [eds]: Hurst's The Heart, 9th ed. New York: McGraw-Hill, 1998:415–517, with permission.)

ciency (especially with supracristal VSD). During intravenous injection of agitated saline, "negative" contrast jets are sometimes seen at the mouth of the VSD.

## Patent Ductus Arteriosus

Patent ductus arteriosus (PDA) is a connection between the distal portion of the aortic arch and the pulmonary artery (usually just to the left of its bifurcation). Two-dimensional imaging occasionally detects a PDA, but color Doppler interrogation is considerably more likely to demonstrate the characteristic high-velocity diastolic flow in the proximal pulmonary artery.[32] Additional 2D findings include LV enlargement and volume overload. If "Eisenmenger physiology" supervenes, the right side of the heart enlarges and LV dilatation may reverse to some degree. Therefore, absence of LV or RV enlargement suggests a small shunt.

## Conotruncal and Aortic Abnormalities

The most common congenital cardiac anomaly in adults is a bicuspid aortic valve (prevalence of 1% to 2% in men and somewhat less in women). This anomaly is often associated with aortic insufficiency or stenosis, as well as coarctation of the aorta. Tetralogy of Fallot is one of the more frequent conotruncal abnormalities. The classic echo features include a large perimembranous VSD, pulmonic stenosis, RV enlargement and hypertrophy, and anterior displacement of the aortic valve. Coarctation of the aorta, which is often associated with a bicuspid aortic valve, is best visualized from the supersternal position. Two-dimensional imaging sometimes detects the coarctation, but acoustic shadowing and dropout may limit evaluation of the descending aorta. Doppler examination is more reliable and shows abnormally high flow velocity in the descending aorta. A classic finding in coarctation is holodiastolic antegrade flow in the descending aorta, indicating a pressure gradient throughout diastole and, therefore, severe stenosis. Another congenital abnormality seen occasionally in adult patients is Ebstein's anomaly. Two-dimensional imaging in classic cases reveals a deformed tricuspid valve, including an elongated anterior leaflet and an apically displaced septal leaflet. Associated findings include enlargement of the right side of the heart and tricuspid regurgitation. ASDs are present in a significant minority of cases.

## ■ PERICARDIAL DISEASE

Echocardiography is an accurate, reliable tool for the detection of pericardial effusion, intrapericardial masses, and cardiac tamponade. Pericardial fluid is identified as a "dark" or echo-free space immediately adjacent to the epicardium (Fig. 9–23). Pericardial effusions may be concentric or loculated and vary much in size. Large, nonloculated effusions generally contain at least 400 ml of fluid and often allow free motion of the heart within the pericardial space. Multiple fibrinous strands in the pericardial effusion raise the possibility of infection, hemorrhage, or malignancy.

There are several echocardiographic clues to the presence of tamponade. Collapse of the right atrial wall (especially with associated tachycardia) is a sensitive, although not specific, sign of increased pericardial pressure. A more specific sign of tamponade is RV free wall diastolic collapse or compression, which indicates marked elevation of intrapericardial pressure. Finally, PW Doppler interrogation of mitral inflow in cardiac tamponade demonstrates an abnormal respiratory variation of peak velocity.[33] A respiratory variation in peak E velocity greater than 20%

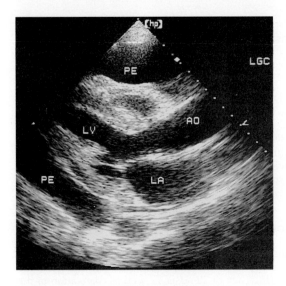

**Figure 9–23** ■ Parasternal long-axis image of a large pericardial effusion (PE). LV, left ventricle; LA, left atrium; AO, aorta. (From DeMaria AN, Blanchard DG: The echocardiogram. *In* Schlant RC, Alexander RW, Fuster V [eds]: Hurst's The Heart, 9th ed. New York: McGraw-Hill, 1998:415–517, with permission.)

suggests cardiac tamponade when an effusion is present (and pericardial constriction when an effusion is absent or minimal). This Doppler finding is useful for differentiating constrictive pericarditis from restrictive cardiomyopathy, as exaggerated respiratory variation of mitral inflow velocity is not seen in the latter.[34]

## ■ REFERENCES

1. DeMaria AN, Blanchard DG: The echocardiogram. *In* Schlant RC, Alexander RW, Fuster V (eds): Hurst's The Heart, 9th ed. New York: McGraw-Hill, 1998:415–517.
2. Henry WL, DeMaria A, Gramiak R, et al: Report of the American Society of Echocardiography: Nomenclature and standards in two-dimensional echocardiography. Circulation 1980;62:212.
3. Thomas JD, Rubin DN: Tissue harmonic imaging: Why does it work? J Am Soc Echocardiogr 1998;11:803–808.
4. Burns PM: The physical principles of Doppler and spectral analysis. J Clin Ultrasound 1987;15:567–590.
5. Nishimura RA, Miller FA Jr, Callahan MJ, et al: Doppler echocardiography: Theory, instrumentation, technique, and application. Mayo Clin Proc 1985;60:321–343.
6. Bom K, deBoo J, Rijsterborgh H: On the aliasing problem in pulsed Doppler cardiac studies. J Clin Ultrasound 1984;12:559–567.
7. Omoto R, Kasai C: Physics and instrumentation of Doppler color flow mapping. Echocardiography 1987;4:467.
8. Rakowski H, Appleton C, Chan K-L, et al: Canadian consensus recommendations for the measurement and reporting of diastolic dysfunction by echocardiography. J Am Soc Echocardiogr 1996;9:736–760.
9. Hegrenaes L, Hatle L: Aortic stenosis in adults. Non-invasive estimation of pressure differences by continuous wave Doppler echocardiography. Br Heart J 1985;54:396–404.
10. Richards KL, Cannon SR, Miller JF, Crawford MH: Calculation of aortic valve area by Doppler echocardiography: A direct application of the continuity equation. Circulation 1986;73:964–969.
11. Daniel WG, Mügge A: Transesophageal echocardiography. N Engl J Med 1995;332;1268–1279.
12. Blanchard DG, Kimura BJ, Dittrich HC, DeMaria AN: Transesophageal echocardiography of the aorta. JAMA 1994;272:546–551.
13. Gramiak R, Shah PM: Echocardiography of the aortic root. Invest Radiol 1968;3:356–366.
14. Mulvagh SL, Foley DA, Aeschbacher BC, et al: Second harmonic imaging of intravenously administered echocardiographic contrast agent: Visualization of coronary arteries and measurement of coronary blood flow. J Am Coll Cardiol 1996;27:1519–1525.
15. Glover MU, Warren SE, Vieweg WVR, et al: M-mode and two-dimensional echocardiographic correlation with findings at catheterization and surgery in patients with mitral stenosis. Am Heart J 1983;105:98–102.
16. Hatle L, Angelsen B, Tromsdal A: Noninvasive assessment of atrioventricular pressure half-time by Doppler ultrasound. Circulation 1979;60:1096–1104.

17. Spain MG, et al: Quantitative assessment of mitral regurgitation by Doppler color flow imaging: Angiographic and hemodynamic correlations. J Am Coll Cardiol 1989;13:585.
18. Bargiggia GS, Tronconi L, Sahn DJ, et al: A new method for quantitation of mitral regurgitation based on color flow Doppler imaging of flow convergence proximal to regurgitant orifice. Circulation 1991;84:1481–1489.
19. Devereux RB, Kramer-Fox R, Kligfield P: Mitral valve prolapse: Causes, clinical manifestations, and management. Ann Intern Med 1989;111:305–317.
20. Yvorchuk KJ, Chan K-L: Application of transthoracic and transesophageal echocardiography in the diagnosis and management of infective endocarditis. J Am Soc Echocardiogr 1994;14:294–308.
21. Segar DS, Brown SC, Sawada SG, et al: Dobutamine stress echocardiography: Correlation with coronary lesion severity as determined by quantitative angiography. J Am Coll Cardiol 1992;19:1197–1202.
22. Matsumoto M, Watanabe F, Gotto A, et al: Left ventricular aneurysm and the prediction of left ventricular enlargement studied by two-dimensional echocardiography; Quantitative assessment of aneurysm size in relation to clinical course. Circulation 1985;72:280–286.
23. Quinones MA, Verani MS, Haichin RM, et al: Exercise echocardiography versus T1-201 single photon emission computerized tomography in evaluation of coronary artery disease. Analysis of 292 patients. Circulation 1992;85:1026–1031.
24. Bax JJ, Cornel JH, Visser FC, et al: Prediction of recovery of myocardial dysfunction after revascularization: Comparison of fluorine-18 fluorodeoxyglucose/thallium-201 SPECT, thallium-201 stress-reinjection SPECT and dobutamine echocardiography. J Am Coll Cardiol 1996;28:558–564.
25. Maron BJ, Epstein SE: Hypertrophic cardiomyopathy: Recent observations regarding the specificity of three hallmarks of the disease: Asymmetric septal hypertrophy, septal disorganization and systolic anterior motion of the anterior mitral leaflet. Am J Cardiol 1980;45:141.
26. Shah PM: Echocardiography in congestive or dilated cardiomyopathy. J Am Soc Echocardiogr 1988;1:20–27.
27. Picano E, Pinamonti B, Ferdeghini EM, et al: Two-dimensional echocardiography in myocardial amyloidosis. Echocardiography 1991;8:253–262.
28. Haugland JM, Asinger RW, Mikell FL, et al: Embolic potential of left ventricular thrombi: detection by two-dimensional echocardiography. Circulation 1984;70:588–598.
29. Reynen K: Cardiac myxomas. N Engl J Med 1995;1610–1617.
30. Shub C, Dimopoulos IN, Seward JB, et al: Sensitivity of two-dimensional echocardiography in the direct visualization of atrial septal defect utilizing the subcostal approach: Experience with 154 patients. J Am Coll Cardiol 1983;2:127–135.
31. Linker DT, Rossvoll O, Chapman JV, Angelsen B: Sensitivity and speed of color Doppler flow mapping compared with continuous wave Doppler for the detection of ventricular septal defects. Br Heart J 1991;65:201–203.
32. Liao P-K, Su W-J, Hung J-S: Doppler echocardiographic flow characteristics of isolated patent ductus arteriosus: Better delineation by Doppler color flow mapping. J Am Coll Cardiol 1988;12:1285–1291.
33. Appleton CP, Hatle LK, Popp RL: Cardiac tamponade and pericardial effusion: Respiratory variation in transvalvular flow velocities studied by Doppler echocardiography. J Am Coll Cardiol 1988;11:1020–1030.
34. Oh JK, Hatle LK, Seward JB, et al: Diagnostic role of Doppler echocardiography in constrictive pericarditis. J Am Coll Cardiol 1994;23:154–162.

# ■ RECOMMENDED READING

Blanchard DG, DeMaria AN: Cardiac and extracardiac masses: Echocardiographic evaluation. In Skorton DJ, Schelbert HR, Wolf GL, Brundage BH (eds): Marcus' Cardiac Imaging, 2nd ed. Philadelphia: WB Saunders, 1996:452–480.
DeMaria AN, Blanchard DG: The echocardiogram. In Schlant RC, Alexander RW, Fuster V (eds): Hurst's The Heart, 9th ed. New York: McGraw-Hill, 1998:415–517.
Nishimura RA, Miller FA Jr, Callahan MJ, et al: Doppler echocardiography: Theory, instrumentation, technique, and application. Mayo Clin Proc 1985;60:321–343.
Oh JK, Seward JB, Tajik AJ: The Echo Manual. Boston: Little, Brown, 1994.

# Chapter 10

# Exercise Testing

*Victor Froelicher*

Exercise can be considered the true test of the heart because it is the most common everyday stress that humans undertake. The exercise test is the most practical and useful procedure in the clinical evaluation of cardiovascular status.

Despite the many recent advances in technology related to the diagnosis and treatment of cardiovascular disease, the exercise test remains an important diagnostic modality. Its many applications, widespread availability, and high yield of clinically useful information continue to make it an important "gatekeeper" to more expensive and invasive procedures. The numerous approaches to the exercise test, however, have been a drawback to its proper application. Excellent up-to-date guidelines based on a multitude of research studies over the last 20 years have led to greater uniformity among methods.

## ■ ADVANTAGES AND DISADVANTAGES

The standard exercise test, surprisingly, has characteristics that are not dissimilar from those of newer more expensive tests. Table 10–1 lists its disadvantages and advantages.

## ■ INDICATIONS

The common clinical applications of exercise testing that are discussed in this chapter are diagnosis and prognosis. The other applications (listed in Table 10–2) are discussed elsewhere.[1] The ACC/AHA Guidelines will be followed in regard to diagnosis and prognosis.

## ■ METHODS

### Safety Precautions and Risks

The safety precautions outlined by the American Heart Association (AHA) are very explicit with respect to the requirements for exercise testing. Everything

Table 10–1

**Advantages and Disadvantages of the Standard Exercise Test**

| Advantages | Disadvantages |
|---|---|
| Low cost | Relatively limited sensitivity and specificity |
| Ready availability of trained personnel | No localization of ischemia or coronary lesions |
| Exercise capacity determined | No estimate of left ventricular function |
| Patient acceptability | Not suitable for certain groups |
| Takes less than an hour | Requires patient cooperation and the ability to walk long |
| Convenience | enough to produce strenuous exercise |
| Availability | |

Table 10–2

**Additional Applications of the Exercise Test**

| | |
|---|---|
| Treatment evaluation | Exercise prescription |
| Exercise capacity determination | Arrhythmia evaluation |
| After myocardial infarction | Intermittent claudication |
| Screening | Preoperative evaluation |
| Cardiac rehabilitation | |

necessary for cardiopulmonary resuscitation must be available, and regular drills should be performed to ensure that both personnel and equipment are ready to handle a cardiac emergency. The classic survey of clinical exercise facilities by Rochmis and Blackburn[2] showed exercise testing to be a safe procedure: for every 10,000 tests one death and five nonfatal complications are reported. Perhaps because of expanded knowledge about indications, contraindications, and end points, maximal exercise testing appears safer today than it was 20 years ago. Gibbons and coworkers reported the safety of exercise testing in 71,914 tests conducted over a 16-year period.[3] The complication rate was 0.8 per 10,000 tests. Cobb and Weaver[4] estimated the risk of a cardiac event to be over 100 times and point out the dangers of the recovery period. The risk of exercise testing in coronary artery disease patients cannot be disregarded, even with its excellent safety record.

Most problems can be avoided by having an experienced physician, nurse, or exercise physiologist standing next to the patient, measuring blood pressure, and assessing the patient's appearance during the test. The exercise technician should operate the recorder and treadmill, take the appropriate tracings, enter data on a form, and alert the physician to any abnormalities that may appear on the monitor scope. If the patient's appearance is worrisome, if systolic blood pressure drops or plateaus, if there are alarming electrocardiographic (ECG) abnormalities, if chest pain occurs and becomes worse than the patient's usual pain, or if the patient wants to stop the test for any reason, it should be stopped, even at a submaximal level. In most instances, a symptom-limited maximal test is preferred, but it is usually advisable to stop if 0.2 mV of additional ST-segment elevation occurs or 0.2 mv of flat or downsloping ST depression. In some patients, estimated to be at high risk because of their clinical history, it may be appropriate to stop at a submaximal level, since it is not unusual for severe ST-segment depression, dysrhythmias, or both to occur only after exercise. If measurement of maximal exercise capacity or other information is necessary, it is better to repeat the test later, once the patient has demonstrated safe performance of a submaximal workload.

Exercise testing should be an extension of the history and physical examination. A physician obtains the most information by being present to talk with, observe, and examine the patient in conjunction with the test. A physical examination should always be performed to rule out significant obstructive aortic valve disease. In this way, patient safety and an optimal yield of information are ensured. In some instances, as when asymptomatic, apparently healthy subjects are being screened or during a repeat treadmill test on a patient whose condition is stable, a physician need not be present but should be nearby and prepared to respond promptly. The physician's reaction to signs or symptoms should be tempered by the information the patient gives about his usual activities. If abnormal findings occur at accustomed levels of exercise, it may not be necessary to stop the test for them. Also, the patient's activity history should help to determine appropriate work rates for testing.

## Contraindications

Table 10–3 lists the absolute and relative contraindications to performing an exercise test and what factors to consider when assessing the degree of exercise. Good clinical judgment should be foremost in deciding the indications and contraindications for exercise testing. In selected cases with relative contraindications, testing can provide valuable information even if performed submaximally.

## Patient Preparation

1. The patient should be instructed not to eat or smoke at least 2 to 3 hours before the test and to come dressed for exercise.
2. A history and physical examination (particularly for systolic murmurs) should be accomplished to rule out any contraindications to testing
3. Specific questioning should determine which drugs are being taken, and potential electrolyte abnormalities should be considered. The labeled medication bottles should be brought along so that they can be identified and recorded. Because of the life-threatening rebound phenomena associated with beta-blockers, they should not be stopped in anticipation of testing. If testing is performed for diagnostic purposes, however, they can be stopped gradually if a physician or nurse carefully supervises the tapering.
4. If the reason for the exercise test is not apparent, the referring physician should be contacted.
5. A 12-lead ECG should be obtained with the patient (1) supine and (2) standing. The latter is an important rule, particularly in patients with known heart disease, since an abnormality may prohibit testing. On occasion, a patient referred for an exercise test is instead admitted to the coronary care unit.
6. There should be careful explanations of why the test is being performed, of the testing procedure (including risks and possible complications), and of how to perform it. This should include a demonstration of getting on and

Table 10–3

**Contraindications to Exercise Testing**

**Absolute**
  Acute myocardial infarction (within 2 days)
  Unstable angina not stabilized by medical therapy
  Uncontrolled cardiac arrhythmias that cause symptoms or hemodynamic compromise
  Symptomatic severe aortic stenosis
  Uncontrolled symptomatic heart failure
  Acute pulmonary embolus or pulmonary infarction
  Acute myocarditis or pericarditis
**Relative**
  Left main coronary stenosis or its equivalent
  Moderate stenotic valvular heart disease
  Electrolyte abnormalities
  Severe arterial hypertension†
  Tachyarrhythmias or bradyarrhythmias
  Hypertrophic cardiomyopathy and other forms of outflow tract obstruction
  Mental or physical impairment leading to inability to exercise adequately
  High-degree atrioventricular block

*Relative contraindications can be superseded if benefits outweigh risks of exercise.
†In the absence of definitive evidence, a systolic blood pressure of 200 mm Hg and a diastolic blood pressure of 110 mm Hg seem reasonable criteria.

off the treadmill and walking on it. The patient should be told that he or she can hold on to the rails initially but later should use them only for balance.

## Protocols

The many different exercise protocols in use have led to some confusion over how physicians compare results between patients and from serial tests of one patient. The most common protocols, their stages, and the predicted oxygen cost of each stage are illustrated in Figure 10–1. When treadmill and cycle ergometer testing were first introduced into clinical practice, practitioners adopted protocols used by major researchers (i.e., Balke,[5] Astrand,[6] Bruce,[7] and Ellestad[8] and their coworkers). In 1980, Stuart and Ellestad[9] surveyed 1375 exercise laboratories in North America and reported that, of those performing treadmill testing, 65.5% use the Bruce protocol for routine clinical testing. This protocol uses relatively large and unequal 2- to 3-MET (metabolic equivalent) increments in work every 3 minutes. Large and uneven work increments like these have been shown to result in a tendency to overestimate exercise capacity.[10] Investigators have since recommended protocols with smaller and more equal increments.[11, 12]

## Ramp Testing

An approach to exercise testing that has gained interest is the ramp protocol, in which work increases constantly and continuously (Fig. 10–2). The recent call for "optimizing" exercise testing would appear to be facilitated by the ramp approach, since work increments are small. Also, since it allows increases in work to be individualized, a given test duration can be targeted.

To investigate this, our laboratory compared ramp treadmill and bicycle tests

| FUNCTIONAL CLASS | CLINICAL STATUS | O2 COST ml/kg/min | METS | BICYCLE ERGOMETER | BRUCE 3 MIN STAGES MPH %GR | BALKE-WARE % GRADE AT 3.3 MPH 1 MIN STAGES | USAFSAM MPH %GR | "SLOW" USAFSAM MPH %GR | McHENRY MPH %GR | STANFORD % GRADE AT 3 MPH / AT 2 MPH | ACIP MPH %GR | CHF MPH %GR | METS |
|---|---|---|---|---|---|---|---|---|---|---|---|---|---|
| NORMAL AND I | HEALTHY, DEPENDENT ON AGE ACTIVITY | 56.0 | 16 | | 5.5 20 | 26 | | | | | | | 16 |
| | | 52.5 | 15 | | 5.0 18 | 25 | 3.3 25 | | | | 3.4 24.0 | | 15 |
| | | 49.0 | 14 | 1500 | | 24 | | | 3.3 21 | | 3.1 24.0 | | 14 |
| | | 45.5 | 13 | | 4.2 16 | 23 22 21 | | | | | | | 13 |
| | | 42.0 | 12 | 1350 | | 20 | 3.3 20 | | 3.3 18 | 22.5 | 3.0 21.0 | | 12 |
| | SEDENTARY HEALTHY | 38.5 | 11 | 1200 | | 19 18 17 16 | | | | 20.0 | | | 11 |
| | | 35.0 | 10 | 1050 | 3.4 14 | 15 14 | 3.3 15 | 2 25 | 3.3 15 | 17.5 | 3.0 17.5 | 3.4 14.0 | 10 |
| | | 31.5 | 9 | 900 | | 13 12 | | | 3.3 12 | 15.0 | 3.0 14.0 | 3.0 15.0 | 9 |
| | | 28.0 | 8 | 750 | | 11 | 3.3 10 | 2 20 | | 12.5 | | 3.0 12.5 | 8 |
| | | 24.5 | 7 | 600 | 2.5 12 | 10 9 | | | 3.3 9 | 10.0 / 17.5 | 3.0 10.5 | 3.0 10.0 | 7 |
| II | LIMITED | 21.0 | 6 | | | 8 7 | 3.3 5 | 2 15 | 3.3 6 | 7.5 / 14.0 | 3.0 7.0 | 3.0 7.5 | 6 |
| | | 17.5 | 5 | 450 | 1.7 10 | 6 5 | | 2 10 | | 5.0 / 10.5 | 3.0 / | 2.0 10.5 | 5 |
| III | SYMPTOMATIC | 14.0 | 4 | 300 | 1.7 5 | 4 3 | | 2 5 | | 2.5 / 7.0 | 2.5 2.0 | 2.0 7.0 | 4 |
| | | 10.5 | 3 | 150 | 1.7 0 | 2 | 3.3 0 | 2 0 | 2.0 3 | 0 / 3.5 | 2.0 0.0 | 2.0 3.5 | 3 |
| | | 7.0 | 2 | | | 1 | 2.0 0 | | | | | 1.5 0.0 | 2 |
| IV | | 3.5 | 1 | | | | | | | | | 1.0 0.0 | 1 |

USAFSAM = United States Air Force School of Aerospace Medicine
ACIP = Asymptomatic Cardiac Ischemia Pilot
CHF = Congestive Heart Failure (Modified Naughton)
Kpm/min = Kilopond meters/minute
%GR = percent grade
MPH = miles per hour

**Figure 10–1** ■ The most common protocols, their stages, and the predicted oxygen cost of each stage.

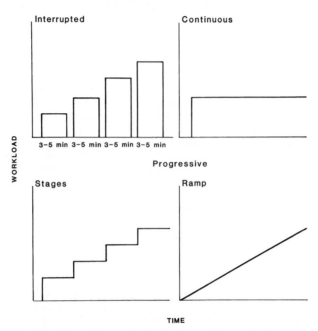

**Figure 10–2** ■ An approach to exercise testing that has attracted interest is the ramp protocol, in which work increases at a constant rate.

to more commonly used clinical protocols. Ten patients with chronic heart failure, 10 with coronary artery disease who were limited by angina during exercise, 10 with coronary artery disease who were asymptomatic during exercise, and 10 age-matched normal subjects performed three bicycle tests (25 W per 2-minute stage, 50 W per 2-minute stage, and ramp) and three treadmill tests (Bruce, Balke, and ramp) in random order on different days. For the ramp tests, ramp rates on the bicycle and treadmill were individualized to yield a test duration of approximately 10 minutes for each subject. Maximal oxygen uptake was significantly higher (18%) on the treadmill protocols than on the bicycle protocols collectively, a finding that confirmed previous observations. Only minor differences in maximal oxygen uptake, however, were observed between the treadmill protocols themselves or between the cycle ergometer protocols themselves.

Because this approach appears to offer several advantages, we presently perform all our clinical and research testing on the ramp. This approach is empirical, however, and more data from other laboratories are necessary to confirm its utility. A number of equipment manufacturers have developed or are in the process of developing treadmills that can perform ramping. The ramp appears to offer a better way of testing patients than traditional, single-protocol approaches.

## Hemodynamic Responses

Age-predicted maximal heart rate targets are relatively useless for clinical purposes, and it is surprising how much steeper the age-related decline in maximal heart rate (HR) is in referred populations as compared with age-matched normal persons or volunteers. A consistent finding in population studies has been a relatively poor relationship of maximal HR to age. Correlation coefficients of -.4 are usually found with a standard error of the estimate of 10 to 25 bpm.

Exertional hypotension, best defined as a drop in systolic blood pressure below standing rest or a drop of 20 mm Hg after a rise, is very predictive of severe angiographic CAD and a poor prognosis. Failure of systolic blood pressure to rise is particularly worrisome after a myocardial infarction (MI). Until automated devices are adequately validated, we strongly recommend that blood pressure be taken manually with a cuff and stethoscope.

Reporting exercise capacity as a percentage, with 100% as normal for age, is highly recommended. A nomogram is available in the guidelines.

## ST Analysis

ST-segment depression is a representation of global subendocardial ischemia, with an ST vector direction determined largely by the placement of the heart in the chest. ST depression does not localize coronary artery lesions. The lead V5 predominates in significant ST depression. Depression isolated to other leads is usually due to Q-wave distortion on the resting ECG. ST depression in the inferior leads (II, AVF) is most often due to the atrial repolarization wave, which begins in the PR segment and can extend to the beginning of the ST segment. When ST depression is isolated to these leads and there are no diagnostic Q waves, it is usually a false positive, whereas ST segment depression limited to the recovery period does not generally represent a false-positive response. Inclusion of analysis during this period increases the diagnostic yield of the exercise test.

When the resting ECG shows Q waves of an old MI, ST elevation is due to wall motion abnormalities, whereas accompanying ST depression can be due to a second area of ischemia or reciprocal changes. When the resting ECG is normal, ST elevation is due to severe ischemia (spasm or a critical lesion), though accompanying ST depression is reciprocal. Such ST elevation is uncommon, very arrhythmogenic, and it localizes the involved coronary artery. Exercise-induced ST elevation (not over diagnostic Q waves) and ST depression both represent ischemia, but they are quite distinctive: *Elevation* is due to transmural ischemia, is arrythmogenic, has a 0.1% prevalence, and localizes the artery where there is spasm or a tight lesion. *Depression* is due to subendocardial ischemia, is not arrythmogenic, has 5% to 50% prevalence, is rarely due to spasm, and does not localize. Figure 10–3 illustrates the various patterns. The standard criterion for abnormal is 1 mm of horizontal or downsloping ST depression below the PR isoelectric line or 1 mm further depression if there is baseline depression. Most information is available in lead V5, maximal exercise and 3 minutes recovery being the most important times to look for ST depression.[13] ECG recordings should continue for 5 minutes in recovery or until any new changes from baseline stabilize.

Unsustained ventricular tachycardia is uncommon during routine clinical treadmill testing (prevalence less than 2%), is tolerated well, and its prognosis is determined by the accompanying ischemia and left ventricular (LV) damage.[14]

## ■ DIAGNOSTIC EXERCISE TESTING

### The ACC/AHA Guidelines for Diagnostic Use of the Standard Exercise Test

The task force to establish guidelines for the use of exercise testing produced guidelines in 1986 and 1997.[15] The most recent publication had some dramatic

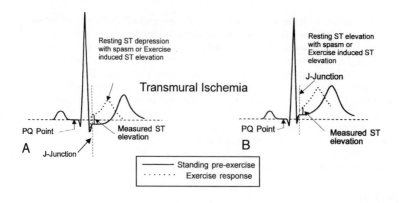

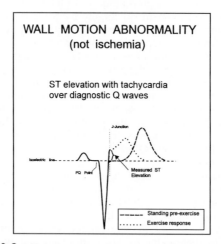

**Figure 10–3** ▪ Various patterns of exercise ST shifts possible with ischemia.

changes from the first, including the recommendation that the standard exercise test—not imaging studies—be the first diagnostic procedure for women and for most patients with resting ECG abnormalities. The following is a synopsis of these evidence-based guidelines.

**Class I (Definitely Appropriate).** Conditions for which there is evidence and/ or general agreement that the standard exercise test is useful and helpful for the diagnosis of coronary artery disease.

Adult male or female patients (including those with complete right bundle branch block or with less than 1 mm of resting ST depression) with an *intermediate pretest probability* of coronary artery disease based on gender, age, and symptoms* (specific exceptions are noted under Class II and III below).

**Class IIa (Probably Appropriate).** Conditions for which there is conflicting evidence or a divergence of opinion that the standard exercise test is useful and

---

* Pretest probability was determined from the Diamond-Forrester estimates tabulated in the guidelines (Table 10–4).

Table 10–4

**Pretest Probability of Coronary Disease by Symptoms, Gender, and Age\*†**

| Age (yr) | Gender | Typical/Definite Angina Pectoris | Atypical/Probable Angina Pectoris | Nonanginal Chest Pain | No Symptoms |
|---|---|---|---|---|---|
| 30–39 | Male | Intermediate | Intermediate | Low (<10%) | Very low (<5%) |
| | Female | Intermediate | Very low | Very low | Very low |
| 40–49 | Male | High | Intermediate | Intermediate | Low |
| | Female | Intermediate | Low | Very low | Very low |
| 50–59 | Male | High | Intermediate | Intermediate | Low |
| | Female | Intermediate | Intermediate | Low | Very low |
| 60–69 | Male | High | Intermediate | Intermediate | Low |
| | Female | High | Intermediate | Intermediate | Low |

\*High, >90%; intermediate, 10–90%; low, <10%; very low, <5%.
†There are no data for patients younger than 30 or older than 69, but it can be assumed that coronary artery disease prevalence increases with age.

helpful for diagnosis but the weight of evidence for usefulness or efficacy favors the exercise test.

Patients with vasospastic angina.

**Class IIb (May be Appropriate).** Conditions for which there is conflicting evidence or a divergence of opinion that the standard exercise test is useful and helpful for the diagnosis of coronary artery disease but the usefulness/efficacy is less well-established.

1. Patients taking digoxin with less than 1 mm of baseline ST depression.
2. Patients with ECG criteria for left ventricular hypertrophy and less than 1 mm of baseline ST depression.
3. Patients with high pretest probability of coronary artery disease relative to age, symptoms, and gender.
4. Patients with a low pretest probability of coronary artery disease relative to age, symptoms, and gender.

**Class III (Not Appropriate).** Conditions for which there is evidence or general agreement that the standard exercise test is not useful and helpful for the diagnosis of coronary artery disease and in some cases may be harmful.

1. To use the ST-segment response in the diagnosis of coronary artery disease in patients who demonstrate the following baseline ECG abnormalities:
   Preexcitation (Wolff-Parkinson-White) syndrome
   Electronically paced ventricular rhythm
   More than 1 mm of resting ST depression
   Complete left bundle branch block
2. To use the ST-segment response for the diagnosis of coronary artery disease in patients who have had a well-documented myocardial infarction. (Though the diagnosis of coronary artery disease is established by the MI, ischemia and risk can be determined by testing.)

## Test Performance Definitions

Sensitivity and specificity are the terms used to define how reliably a test identifies disease. They are parameters of the accuracy of a diagnostic test. Sensitivity is the percentage of times that a test gives an abnormal ("positive") result when persons who have the disease are tested (i.e., a true-positive result). Specificity is the percentage of times that a test gives a "normal" (negative) result when those

Table 10–5

**Definitions and Calculation of the Terms Used to Quantify Test Diagnostic Accuracy**

True positive (TP) = Number of patients with the disease and a positive result
False negative (FN) = Number of patients with the disease and a negative result
True negative (TN) = Number of patients without the disease and a negative result
False positive (FP) = Number of patients without the disease and a positive result
TP + FN + TN + FP = Total population
Sensitivity = The percentage of those with the disease who test positive: TP/(TP + FN) × 100
Specificity = The percentage of those without the disease who test negative: TN/(FP + TN) × 100
Positive predictive value (PV+) = The percentage of those with a positive result who have the disease: TP/(TP + FP) × 100
Negative predictive value (PV−) = The percentage of those with a negative result who do not have the disease: TN/(TN + FN) × 100
Predictive accuracy (PA) = The percentage of correct classifications, both positive and negative: (TP + TN)/Total population × 100
Risk ratio (RR) = The ratio of disease rate in those with a positive result compared to those with a negative result: TP/(TP + FP)/FN/(FN + TN) = PV +/FN/(FN + TN)
Range of characteristics (ROC) = A plot of sensitivity versus specificity for the range of measurement cutpoints

without the disease are tested (i.e., a true-negative result). This is quite different from the colloquial use of the word *specific*.

The method of calculating these terms is shown in Table 10–5. Tables 10–6 and 10–7 show the effect of prevalence on predictive value.

## Feinstein's Methodologic Standards for Studies of Diagnostic Test Performance

Of these seven methodologic standards for research design, only the requirement for an adequate variety of anatomic lesions was followed by most investigators. Only one study met as many as five of the seven standards. Reid, Feinstein, and colleagues updated these criteria for "methodologic standards" for diagnostic tests in 1995.[16] Their purpose in refining these standards was to improve patient

Table 10–6

**The Predictive Value of a Positive Test Result Varies Directly with the Prevalence of Disease in a Population**

| Population | Disease | Test Result | |
|---|---|---|---|
| *Assuming a CAD prevalence of 5%, sensitivity of 50%, and specificity of 90%* | | | |
| 10,000 patients | 500 with CAD | 250+ | (TP) |
| | | 250− | (FN) |
| | 9500 without CAD | 950+ | (FP) |
| | | 8550− | (TN) |
| Predictive Value of a Positive Result = [250/(250 + 950)] × 100 = 21% | | | |
| *Assuming a CAD prevalence of 50%, sensitivity of 50%, and specificity of 90%* | | | |
| 10,000 patients | 5000 with CAD | 2500+ | TP |
| | | 2500− | FN |
| | 5000 without CAD | 500+ | FP |
| | | 4500− | TN |
| Predictive value of a positive result = 2,500/(2,500 + 500) × 100 = 83% | | | |

Table 10–7

**The Effect of Disease Prevalence on the Predictive Value of a Test***

| Disease Prevalence Sensitivity (%)/Specificity (%) | Predictive Value of (%) | an Abnormal Test (%) | Risk (%) | Ratio (%) |
|---|---|---|---|---|
| | 5 | 50 | 5 | 50 |
| 70/90 | 27 | 88 | 27x | 3x |
| 90/70 | 14 | 75 | 14x | 5x |
| 90/90 | 32 | 90 | 64x | 9x |
| 66/84 | 18 | 80 | 9x | 3x |

*Calculation of the predictive value of an abnormal test (positive predictive value) using a test with a sensitivity of 50% and a specificity of 90% in two populations of 10,000 patients: one with a coronary artery disease prevalence of 5% and the other with a 50% prevalence. This demonstrates the important influence that prevalence has on the positive predictive value. The sensitivity and specificity values were obtained from various metaanalyses and published results of commonly used diagnostic tests. The last set were specifically from the metaanalysis of the standard exercise test.

care, reduce health care costs, improve the quality of diagnostic test information, and eliminate useless tests or testing methods.

## Conclusions Regarding Standards Criteria

Most of the diagnostic test standards, such as blinding to test interpretation, exclusion of patients with prior MIs, and chest pain classification, are very logical and easy to appreciate. The two subtle standards that are least understood but affect test performance drastically and most often are not fulfilled are *limited challenge and workup bias*. Limited challenge actually could be justified as the first step in looking at a new measurement or test. An investigator may choose healthy persons and sick ones, test them with the new measurement, and see if results are different. If no difference is noted then further investigation is not indicated. Such a subject choice favors the measurement, but its true test is applying it to consecutive patients who present for evaluation. A measurement or test may function well to separate those at the extremes and still fail in clinical use. Workup bias means simply that who goes to catheterization is a decision made by the physician using the test and her clinical acumen. Thus, the patients in the study are different from those who present for evaluation before this selection process occurs. This can only be avoided by having patients agree to both procedures before any testing is performed.

*Populations chosen for test evaluation that fail to avoid limited challenge will result in predictive accuracies and ROC curves greater than those actually associated with the test measurement. While this is not the case for populations with workup bias, calibration of the measurement cutpoints can be affected. That is, a score or ST measurement can have different sensitivity and specificity for a particular cutpoint when workup bias is present.*

The two studies that have removed workup bias by protocol have included 2000 patients and have considerably different test characteristics.[17]

## Further Clinical Metaanalysis of Exercise Testing Studies

Following Feinstein's approach but considering more of the clinical and test methodologic issues, Gianrossi and coworkers investigated the variability of the reported diagnostic accuracy of the exercise ECG by applying metaanalysis.[18] One hundred forty-seven consecutively published reports involving 24,074 patients who underwent both coronary angiography and exercise testing were summarized and the results entered into a computer spreadsheet. Details about population characteristics and methods were entered, including publication year, number of ECG leads, exercise protocol, preexercise hyperventilation, definition of an abnormal ST response, exclusion of certain subgroups, and blinding of test interpretation. Wide variations in sensitivity and specificity were found (mean sensitivity 68%, range 23% to 100%, standard deviation 16%; mean specificity 77%, range 17% to 100%, standard deviation 17%). Though such data were not provided, the median predictive accuracy (percentage of total true calls) is approximately 73%.

To more accurately portray the performance of the exercise test, only the results of 41 studies out of the original 147 were considered. These 41 studies removed patients who had a prior MI from this metaanalysis (fulfilling one of the criteria for evaluating a diagnostic test) and provided all of the numbers for calculating test performance. These 41 studies, including nearly 10,000 patients, demonstrated **lower mean sensitivity (68%) and lower mean specificity (74%); this means that predictive accuracy is also lower (71%).** In several studies where workup bias has been lessened (fulfilling the other major criterion), **sensitivity is approximately 50% and specificity 90% while predictive accuracy stays at 70%.**[19] *This demonstrates that the key feature of the standard exercise test for clinical utility is its high specificity and that its low sensitivity is a problem.*

## Effects of Digoxin, Left Ventricular Hypertrophy, and Resting ST Depression

For resolving the issues of left ventricular hypertrophy (LVH), resting ST depression, and digoxin, the results from the metaanalysis were considered. Of the appropriate studies, only those that provided sensitivity, specificity, and total patient numbers and that included more than 100 patients were considered. The conclusion from this analysis was that only digoxin and more than 1 mm of resting ST depression had a major effect on test performance.

## Gender

There has been controversy over the use of the standard exercise ECG test in women. In fact, some experts have recommended that only imaging techniques be used to test women because of the impression that the standard exercise ECG did not perform as well in them as it did in men. The recent ACC/AHA guidelines reviewed this subject in detail and came to another conclusion. This position was based on evidence and used information from metaanalysis, as well as fifteen studies that considered only women. The recent guidelines have definitely stated that exercise testing for the diagnosis of significant obstructive coronary disease in adult patients, including women, with symptoms or other clinical findings suggestive of coronary artery disease is a Class I indication (i.e., definitely indicated). Women in the intermediate class are those aged 30 to 59 years with typical or definite angina pectoris, those aged 30 to 69 with atypical or probable pectoris, and those aged 60 to 68 with nonanginal chest pain (see Table 10–4).

## Comparison with Other Diagnostic Tests

### Nuclear Perfusion and Echocardiography

Investigators from the University of California San Francisco reviewed the contemporary literature to compare the diagnostic performance of exercise echocardiography (ECHO) and exercise nuclear perfusion scanning (NUC) in the diagnosis of coronary artery disease.[20] Studies published between January 1990 and October 1997 were identified from MEDLINE search; bibliographies of reviews and original articles; and suggestions from experts in each area. Articles were included if they discussed exercise ECHO or exercise NUC imaging with thallium or sestamibi for detection or evaluation of coronary artery disease, if data on coronary angiography were presented as the reference test, and if the absolute numbers of true-positive, false-negative, true-negative, and false-positive observations were available or derivable from the published data. Studies performed exclusively in patients who had had a myocardial infarction, had undergone percutaneous transluminal coronary angioplasty or coronary artery bypass grafting, or recently had an unstable coronary syndrome were excluded. The results are presented in Table 10–8. In models comparing the discriminatory abilities of exercise ECHO and exercise NUC with exercise testing without imaging, both ECHO and NUC performed significantly better than the exercise ECG. While the nonexercise stress tests are very useful, the results presented are probably better than their actual performance because of patient selection.

## Exercise Test Scores

The exercise testing studies that have considered other information in addition to the ST response have been reviewed and demonstrate the improved test characteristics obtained using this approach.[21] Recent publications have extended the Duke prognostic score to diagnosis,[22] and a consensus approach that uses a number of equations appears to make the scores more portable to other populations.[23]

## Summary of the Diagnostic Utilization of Exercise Testing

It is appropriate to compare the newer diagnostic modalities with the standard exercise test, since it is a mature, established technology. Equipment and personnel

Table 10–8

**Comparison of Exercise Testing Subgroups and Different Test Modalities**

| Grouping | Studies (No.) | Patients (No.) | Sensitivity (%) | Specificity (%) | Predictive Accuracy (%) |
|---|---|---|---|---|---|
| Metaanalysis of standard ET | 147 | 24,047 | 68 | 77 | 73 |
| • Metaanalysis w/o MI | 58 | 11,691 | 67 | 72 | 69 |
| ⇒ Metaanalysis w/o workup bias | 3 | >1000 | 50 | 90 | 69 |
| ⇒ Metaanalysis w/ST depression | 22 | 9153 | 69 | 70 | 69 |
| ⇒ Metaanalysis w/o ST depression | 3 | 840 | 67 | 84 | 75 |
| ⇒ Metaanalysis w/Digoxin | 15 | 6338 | 68 | 74 | 71 |
| ⇒ Metaanalysis w/o Digoxin | 9 | 3548 | 72 | 69 | 70 |
| ⇒ Metaanalysis w/LVH | 15 | 8016 | 68 | 69 | 68 |
| ⇒ Metaanalysis w/o LVH | 10 | 1977 | 72 | 77 | 74 |
| Metaanalysis of treadmill scores | 24 | 11,788 | | | 80 |
| Consensus | 1 | 2000 | 85 | 92 | 88 |
| Electron beam computed tomography | 4 | 1631 | 90 | 45 | 68 |
| Thallium scintigraphy | 59 | 6038 | 85 | 85 | 85 |
| SPECT w/o MI | 27 | 2136 | 86 | 62 | 74 |
| Persantine thallium | 11 | | 85 | 91 | 87 |
| Exercise echocardiography | 58 | 5000 | 84 | 75 | 80 |
| Exercise echocardiography w/o MI | 24 | 2109 | 87 | 84 | 85 |
| Dobutamine echocardiography | 5 | | 88 | 84 | 86 |

ET, Exercise test; MI, myocardial infarction; LVH, left ventricular hypertrophy; w, with; w/o, without; SPECT, single photon emission computed tomography.

are readily available. Exercise testing equipment is relatively inexpensive, so replacement or updating is not a major limitation. The test can be performed in the doctor's office and does not require injections or exposure to radiation. It can be an extension of the medical history and physical examination that provides more than simple diagnostic information. Furthermore, it can determine the degree of disability and impairment in quality of life.

With patients subgrouped according to β-blocker administration as instituted by their referring physician, no differences in test performance were found in a consecutive group of males being evaluated for possible coronary artery disease. Though stopping β-blockers before testing might be optimal, for routine exercise testing it appears unnecessary for physicians to accept the risk when a patient is exhibiting symptoms that might reflect ischemia.

Studies considering non-ECG data consistently demonstrate that the multivariable equations outperform simple ST diagnostic criteria. Generally, these equations have predictive accuracy of 80%. A limitation of the equations is their complexity; however, a computer program can simplify the use of the equations.

To obtain the best diagnostic characteristics with the exercise test, clinical and non-ECG test responses should be considered. Computerized ECG measurements and ECG scores are not superior to visual analysis but can duplicate the results of expert readers. Multivariate scores using computers to make the calculations from logistic regression equations appear to improve significantly on test characteristics. Early experience with consensus of three equations appears to diagnose disease well and provide a logical plan for going on to further testing.

The summary from the guidelines is clearly stated regarding testing women: concern about false-positive ST responses may be addressed by careful assessment of posttest probability and selective use of stress imaging before proceeding to angiography. Although the optimal strategy for circumventing false-positive test results for the diagnosis of coronary disease in women has yet to be defined, data are currently insufficient to justify routine stress imaging test as the initial test for coronary disease in women.

## ■ PROGNOSTIC USE OF THE EXERCISE TEST

### The ACC/AHA Guidelines

Indications for exercise testing to assess risk and prognosis in patients with symptoms or a history of coronary artery disease:

**Class I (Definitely Appropriate).** Conditions for which there is evidence or general agreement that the standard exercise test is useful and helpful for assessing risk and prognosis in patients with symptoms or a history of coronary artery disease

- Patients undergoing initial evaluation for suspected or known coronary artery disease. Specific exceptions are noted below in Class IIb.
- Patients with suspected or known CAD previously evaluated with significant change in clinical status.

**Class IIb (May be Appropriate).** Conditions for which there is conflicting evidence or a divergence of opinion about whether the standard exercise test is useful and helpful for assessing risk and prognosis for patients with symptoms or history of coronary artery disease but whose usefulness/efficacy is less well-established.

- Patients who demonstrate the following ECG abnormalities:
    - Preexcitation (Wolff-Parkinson White) syndrome
    - Electronically paced ventricular rhythm
    - More than 1 mm of resting ST depression

- Complete left bundle branch block
- Patients with a stable clinical course who undergo periodic monitoring to guide management

**Class III (Not Appropriate).** Conditions for which there is evidence or general agreement that the standard exercise test is not useful or helpful for assessing risk and prognosis in patients with symptoms or a history of coronary artery disease and in some cases may be harmful.

- Patients with severe comorbidity likely to limit life expectancy or candidacy for revascularization.

## The Duke Treadmill Score and Nomogram

Mark and coworkers studied 2842 consecutive patients who underwent cardiac catheterization and exercise testing and whose data were entered into the Duke computerized medical information system.[24] Median follow-up for the study population was 5 years, and it was 98% complete. All patients underwent a Bruce protocol exercise test and had standard ECG measurements recorded. A treadmill angina index was assigned a value of 0 if angina was absent, 1 if typical angina occurred during exercise, and 2 if angina was the reason the patient stopped exercising. Before the test, 54% of the patients had taken propranolol and 11% had taken digoxin. ST measurements considered were sum of the largest net ST depression and elevation, sum of the ST displacements in all 12 leads, the number of leads showing ST displacement of 0.1 mV or more, and the product of the number of leads showing ST displacement and the largest single ST displacement in any lead. This nomogram and an example are shown in Figure 10–4.

On the basis of clinical and exercise test data, patients with signs and symptoms of coronary heart disease can be assigned to low- and high-risk categories. Those at high risk clearly should be considered for cardiac catheterization; the others should not, unless their symptoms dictate otherwise. The problem lies

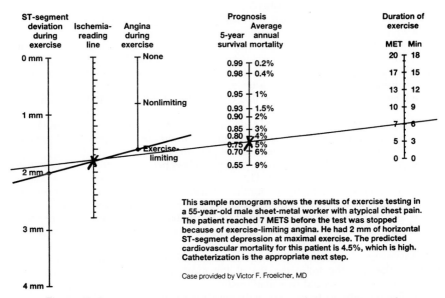

**Figure 10–4** ■ The Duke treadmill prognostic nomogram and a patient-case example.

in justifying intervention to improve survival for patients whose symptoms are satisfactorily managed medically. Our study demonstrates that simple clinical indicators can stratify these patients with stable coronary artery disease into high- and low-risk groups. Cardiac catheterization is not needed to do so in the majority of such patients. In our Veterans Administration population, we consider a history of congestive heart failure or digoxin administration and three exercise tests responses as the most important predictors of cardiovascular death.[25] Clinical judgment must be applied to decide whether intervention is likely to improve survival for our high-risk patients. The Duke and Veterans Administration predictive equations appear to be the best and represent the "state of the art" in prognostication. Recent work suggests that measured METS (ventilatory oxygen consumption) is more predictive of cardiac events than estimated METS from treadmill speed and grade.[26]

## Summary

It appears that 50% of internists and family practitioners are performing exercise tests, and it is important to see that they are properly trained to do so. They have to learn so much these days that it is difficult for them to set aside enough time to become comfortable with doing the test. In fact, they are most comfortable testing low-risk patients who probably least need the test. Many physicians have learned from experience, however, that the exercise test complements the medical history and the physical examination as no other test can, so it remains the second most-performed cardiac investigation next to routine ECG. The renewed efforts to control costs will undoubtedly win over more to this group of enlightened physicians, as will the convincing evidence that treadmill scores enhance the diagnostic and prognostic power of the exercise test. There is also evidence that measurement of expired gases improves the prognostic power of the test in certain patients.

The following rules are important for getting the most value out of the standard exercise test:

- The treadmill protocol should be adjusted to the patient, and one protocol is not appropriate for all patients.
- Exercise capacity is reported in METS, not minutes of exercise.
- Hyperventilation before testing is not indicated.
- ST measurements should be made at ST0 (J junction), and ST depression should be considered abnormal only when horizontal or downsloping.
- For the test to have the greatest diagnostic value, patients should be placed supine as soon as possible after exercising, without a cool-down walk.
- The 3-minute recovery period is critical information to include in analysis of the ST response.
- Measurement of systolic blood pressure during exercise is extremely important, and exertional hypotension is ominous. At this point, only manual blood pressure measurement techniques are valid.
- Age-predicted HR targets are largely useless because of the wide scatter for any age. A relatively slow HR can be maximal for one patient of a given age and submaximal for another. Thus, a test should not be considered nondiagnostic if 85% of age-predicted maximal HR is not reached.
- The Duke treadmill score should be calculated automatically for every test.
- Other predictive equations should be considered as part of the treadmill report.

To ensure the safety of exercise testing and reassure noncardiologists who perform the test, the following list of the most dangerous circumstances in the exercise testing lab should be considered:

- Testing patients with aortic valvular disease should be done with great care, because they can have cardiovascular collapse and it is extremely hard to resuscitate them owing to the outflow obstruction. Because of this, physical examination, including assessment of systolic murmurs, should be done before every exercise test. If a significant murmur is heard, echocardiography should be considered.

■ When patients exhibit ST-segment elevation without diagnostic Q waves (which is due to transmural ischemia), this can be associated with dangerous arrhythmias and infarction. It occurs in about one in 1000 clinical tests.

■ When a patient with an ischemic cardiomyopathy exhibits severe chest pain due to ischemia (angina pectoris), a cool-down walk is advisable, since the ischemia can worsen during recovery.

■ When a patient develops exertional hypotension accompanied by ischemia (angina or ST depression) or when it occurs in a patient with a history of congestive heart failure, cardiomyopathy, or recent MI.

■ When a patient with a history of sudden death or collapse during exercise develops premature ventricular contractions that become frequent, a cool-down walk is advisable since the PVCs can increase during recovery, particularly after abrupt cessation of exercise.

Appreciation of these circumstances can help to avoid any complications in the exercise lab.

# ■ REFERENCES

1. Froelicher VF, Myers J: Exercise and the Heart, 4th ed. Philadelphia: Saunders/Mosby–Year Book, 1999.
2. Rochmis P, Blackburn H: Exercise tests: A survey of procedures, safety, and litigation experience in approximately 170,000 tests. JAMA 1971;217:1061–1066.
3. Gibbons L, Blair SN, Kohl HW, Cooper K: The safety of maximal exercise testing. Circulation 1989;80:846–852.
4. Cobb LA, Weaver WD: Exercise: A risk for sudden death in patients with coronary heart disease. J Am Coll Cardiol 1986;7:215–219.
5. Balke B, Ware R: An experimental study of physical fitness of air force personnel. US Armed Forces Med J 1959;10:675–688.
6. Astrand PO, Rodahl K: Textbook of Work Physiology. New York: McGraw-Hill, 1986:331–365.
7. Bruce RA: Exercise testing of patients with coronary heart disease. Ann Clin Res 1971;3:323–330.
8. Ellestad MH, Allen W, Wan MCK, Kemp G: Maximal treadmill stress testing for cardiovascular evaluation. Circulation 1969;39:517–522.
9. Stuart RJ, Ellestad MH: National survey of exercise stress testing facilities. Chest 1980;77:94–97.
10. Sullivan M, McKirnan MD: Errors in predicting functional capacity for postmyocardial infarction patients using a modified Bruce protocol. Am Heart J 1984;107:486–491.
11. Webster MWI, Sharpe DN: Exercise testing in angina pectoris: The importance of protocol design in clinical trials. Am Heart J 1989;117:505–508.
12. Panza JA, Quyyumi AA, Diodati JG, et al: Prediction of the frequency and duration of ambulatory myocardial ischemia in patients with stable coronary artery disease by determination of the ischemic threshold from exercise testing: Importance of the exercise protocol. J Am Coll Cardiol 1991;17:657–663.
13. Lachterman B, Lehmann KG, Abrahamson D, Froelicher VF: "Recovery only" ST-segment depression and the predictive accuracy of the exercise test. Ann Intern Med 1990;112(1):11–16.
14. Yang JC, Wesley RC, Froelicher VF: Ventricular tachycardia during routine treadmill testing. Risk and prognosis. Arch Intern Med 1991;151:349–353.
15. Gibbons RJ, Balady GJ, Beasley JW, et al: ACC/AHA Guidelines for Exercise Testing. A report of the American College of Cardiology/American Heart Association Task Force on Practice Guidelines (Committee on Exercise Testing). J Am Coll Cardiol 1997;30(1):260–311.
16. Reid M, Lachs M, Feinstein A: Use of methodological standards in diagnostic test research. JAMA 1995;274:645–651.
17. Froelicher VF, Lehmann KG, Thomas R, et al: The electrocardiographic exercise test in a population with reduced workup bias: Diagnostic performance, computerized interpretation, and multivariable prediction. Veterans Affairs Cooperative Study in Health Services #016 (QUEXTA) Study Group. Quantitative Exercise Testing and Angiography. Ann Intern Med 1998;128(12 Pt 1):965–974.
18. Gianrossi R, Detrano R, Mulvihill D, et al: Exercise-induced ST depression in the diagnosis of coronary artery disease: A meta-analysis. Circulation 1989;80:87–98.
19. Morise A, Diamond GA: Comparison of the sensitivity and specificity of exercise electrocardiography in biased and unbiased populations of men and women. Am Heart J 1995;130(4):741–747.

20. Fleischmann KE, Hunink MG, Kuntz KM, Douglas PS: Exercise echocardiography or exercise SPECT imaging? A meta-analysis of diagnostic test performance. JAMA 1998;280(10):913–920.
21. Yamada H, Do D, Morise A, Froelicher V: Review of studies utilizing multi-variable analysis of clinical and exercise test data to predict angiographic coronary artery disease. Progr Cardiovasc Dis 1997;39:457–481.
22. Shaw LJ, Peterson ED, Shaw LK, et al: Use of a prognostic treadmill score in identifying diagnostic coronary disease subgroups. Circulation 1998;98(16):1622–1630.
23. Do D, West JA, Morise A, Froelicher V: A consensus approach to diagnosing coronary artery disease based on clinical and exercise test data. Chest 1997;111(6):1742–1749.
24. Mark DB, Hlatky MA, Harrell FE, et al: Exercise treadmill score for predicting prognosis in coronary artery disease. Ann Intern Med 1987;106:793–800.
25. Morrow K, Morris CK, Froelicher VF, Hideg A: Prediction of cardiovascular death in men undergoing noninvasive evaluation for CAD. Ann Intern Med 1993;118(9):689–695.
26. Myers J, Gullestad L, Vagelos R, et al: Clinical, hemodynamic, and cardiopulmonary exercise test determinants of survival in patients referred for evaluation of heart failure. Ann Intern Med 1998;129(4):286–293.

# ■ RECOMMENDED READING

Atwood JE, Do D, Froelicher V, et al: Can computerization of the exercise test replace the cardiologist? Am Heart J 1998;136(3):543–552.
Dat Do BS, Rachel Marcus R, Froelicher V, et al: Predicting severe angiographic coronary artery disease using computerization of clinical and exercise test data. Chest 1998;114(5):1437–1445.
Do D, West JA, Morise A, Froelicher VF: A consensus approach to diagnosing coronary artery disease based on clinical and exercise test data. Chest 1997;111(6):1742–1749.
Fletcher GF, Froelicher VF, Hartley LH, et al: Exercise Standards. A statement for health professionals from the American Heart Association. Circulation 1990;82:2286–2321. Revised Circulation 1995,91:580–632.
Froelicher VF: Manual of Exercise Testing, 2nd ed. St. Louis:Mosby–Year Book, 1995.
Froelicher VF, Quaglietti S: Handbook of Exercise Testing. Boston: Little, Brown, 1995.
Froelicher VF, Myers J: Research as part of clinical practice: Use of Windows-based relational data bases. Veterans Health System Journal 1998;March:53–57.
Marcus R, Lowe R, Froelicher VF, Do Dat: The exercise test as gatekeeper. Limiting access or appropriately directing resources? Chest 1995;107(5):1442–1446.
Miranda CP, Lehmann KG, Froelicher VF: The effect of resting ST-depression, digitalis, and left ventricular hypertrophy on the standard exercise test. Am Heart J 1991;122:1617–1628.
Morris CK, Ueshima K, Kawaguchi T, et al: The prognostic value of METs: A review. Am Heart J 1991;122:1423–1431.
Morrow K, Morris CK, Froelicher VF, Hideg A: Prediction of cardiovascular death in men undergoing noninvasive evaluation for CAD. Ann Intern Med 1993;118(9):689–695.
Myers J, Buchanan N, Walsh D, et al: A comparison of the ramp versus standard exercise protocols. J Am Coll Cardiol 1991;17:1334–1342.

*Chapter* 11

# Radiology of the Heart

*Gautham P. Reddy* ▪ *Robert M. Steiner*

Imaging plays a critical role in the diagnosis of heart disease. In the past 20 to 30 years, advanced imaging modalities such as digital angiography, echocardiography, magnetic resonance imaging (MRI), computed tomography (CT), and nuclear cardiology have become important in the evaluation of the heart. The conventional radiographic examination remains the mainstay of cardiac imaging, however. In this chapter we discuss the role of the chest radiograph in the diagnosis of cardiac disease in adults, with emphasis on both normal and pathologic cardiovascular anatomy in a variety of diseases. Correlation will be made with cross-sectional imaging to illustrate important anatomic points.

## ▪ NORMAL ANATOMY

The standard radiographic examination of the chest consists of upright frontal (posteroanterior) and lateral projections (Fig. 11–1). If a patient is acutely ill or is unable to stand upright, an anteroposterior frontal radiograph may be obtained with the patient in the supine position, and the lateral radiograph is usually omitted. It is important to ensure that the patient is properly positioned for both the frontal and the lateral views so that cardiac structures can be evaluated accurately. In the past, left and right anterior oblique projections were obtained routinely, often with contrast medium in the esophagus. With the advent of echocardiography, however, the current role of oblique radiographs is limited.

In the normal chest radiograph, there is excellent inherent contrast between the air-filled lungs, pulmonary vessels, and mediastinum. The chest film, therefore, is the primary imaging study for the lung parenchyma and vessels; however, structures in the mediastinum, including the heart, the blood, and the fat, have similar radiographic densities and cannot easily be distinguished on chest radiographs. Nevertheless, the margins of the heart and mediastinal vessels are clearly demarcated, and variation from the normal appearance suggests disease.

### Left Subclavian Artery

On the frontal chest radiograph, the left subclavian artery forms the superior portion of the left mediastinal border above the aortic arch (see Fig. 11–1A). This artery usually forms a concave border with the lung, although a convex border may be seen if blood flow is increased (as in coarctation of the aorta) or if the vessel is tortuous because of atherosclerosis or hypertension. A persistent left superior vena cava is suggested by a straight or convex left supraaortic border.

### Aorta

On the frontal view, the ascending aorta forms a convex margin above the right heart border (see Fig. 11–1A). When the ascending aorta is enlarged, it projects

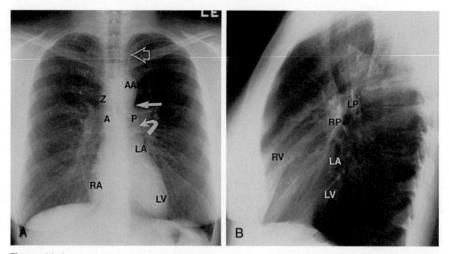

**Figure 11–1** ■ Normal chest radiograph of a 36-year-old woman. *(A)* Posteroanterior frontal projection; *(B)* lateral projection. A, ascending aorta; AA, aortic arch; LA, left atrium; LP, left pulmonary artery; LV, left ventricle; P, main pulmonary artery; RA, right atrium; RP, right pulmonary artery; RV, right ventricle; Z, azygos vein. *Open arrow,* left subclavian artery; *straight arrow,* aorticopulmonary window; *curved arrow,* left mainstem bronchus.

farther to the right. On the lateral view, the anterior margin of the ascending aorta lies above the right ventricle but is not seen in normal persons owing to the abundant mediastinal fat.

The aortic arch, or "knob," forms a convex border just below the left subclavian artery on the frontal radiograph. The aortic arch displaces the trachea slightly to the right. In a patient with a right aortic arch, the trachea deviates slightly to the left.[1] The arch is usually small in young, healthy persons. An enlarged arch is higher and wider than the normal aorta.

The ascending aorta or arch may be enlarged on the frontal view in association with aortic aneurysm, aortic regurgitation, systemic hypertension, or atherosclerosis. Immediately below the aortic arch along the left mediastinal border is an indentation known as the *aorticopulmonary window,* which is bordered by the lower margin of the aortic arch and by the superior margin of the left pulmonary artery. Convex bulging of the aorticopulmonary window may reflect a ductus diverticulum, lymphadenopathy, or another mass.[2]

## Pulmonary Vasculature

The main pulmonary artery forms a slightly convex border along the left side of the mediastinum between the aortic knob and the left atrial appendage (see Fig. 11–1A). A prominent convex bulge in this location indicates enlargement of the main pulmonary artery. A large main pulmonary artery may be related to pulmonary arterial hypertension; increased blood flow, as in anemia or a left-to-right shunt; or turbulent flow, as with pulmonary valvular stenosis. On the other hand, the main pulmonary artery border may be flat or convex in patients with transposition of the great vessels, truncus arteriosus, tetralogy of Fallot, or pulmonary atresia. On the lateral projection, the anterior border of the main pulmonary artery, located above the right ventricle, is obscured by mediastinal fat.

The left pulmonary artery is visualized as a smooth arc just inferior to the aorticopulmonary window. The left pulmonary artery arches over the left mainstem bronchus, as seen on the lateral projection (see Fig. 11–1B). The right pulmonary artery is a round or oval opacity anterior to the right mainstem bronchus on the lateral view.

The intrapulmonary branch arteries run parallel to the airways and gradually decrease in size toward the lung periphery. Because the arteries and bronchi are approximately the same size at any given level, comparison of arterial and bronchial diameters is useful when assessing increases in or redistribution of blood flow. When a patient is upright, lower lobe vessels are larger than upper lobe vessels owing to differences in blood flow that are partly due to the effects of gravity.[3]

## Heart

On the posteroanterior frontal radiograph, the normal heart usually occupies no more than 50% of the transverse diameter of the thorax.[4] The respective widths of the heart and the chest can be measured to determine the cardiothoracic ratio: the maximum transverse diameter of the heart is divided by the maximum width of the thorax.[4] In practice, the size of the heart is usually assessed subjectively. Low lung volumes, lordotic projection of the radiograph, or pectus excavatum deformity can cause the heart to appear larger than it really is. A large heart may appear to be of normal size if the lungs are hyperinflated, as in patients with emphysema, or if the cardiac apex is displaced inferiorly. Anyone evaluating the size of the heart should keep in mind that anteroposterior frontal projections magnify the cardiac silhouette by 10% to 13%.[5]

## Left Atrium

The left atrial appendage is identified as a smooth, slightly concave segment of the left heart border immediately inferior to the left mainstem bronchus in the frontal view (see Fig. 11–1A). When the left atrial border is straightened or convex, atrial enlargement is suggested. It is important to recognize that noncardiac disease such as a pericardial cyst or lymphadenopathy on the frontal radiograph may mimic enlargement of the left atrial appendage. The right-side margin of the normal left atrium is visualized deep to the right atrial border as a convex "double" density. If the left atrium is severely dilated, the left atrial border may project lateral to the margin of the right atrium.[6] Elevation of the left mainstem bronchus is another sign of left atrial enlargement.[7] On the lateral projection, the normal left atrium forms a slight bulge at the upper posterior cardiac border (see Fig. 11–1B). Enlargement of the left atrium results in posterior displacement of the esophagus, which is most easily seen when the esophagus is filled with contrast medium.

### Left Ventricle

The borders of the left ventricle blend with the left atrial margins on both the frontal and lateral radiographs (see Fig. 11–1). On both projections, the slightly convex left ventricular border extends to the diaphragm. The cardiac apex can be displaced inferiorly and laterally when the left ventricle is dilated owing to aortic or mitral regurgitation. When the ventricle is hypertrophic because of aortic stenosis or hypertrophic cardiomyopathy, it may be rounded and the apex may be elevated.

### Right Atrium

The right atrium forms a slightly convex border with the right lung (see Fig. 11–1A). The margins of the right atrium blend with the inferior and superior venae cavae. The border of the inferior vena cava below the right atrium is usually straight.[8] On the lateral view, the right atrium is not seen directly because it does not form the cardiac border.

## Right Ventricle

The right ventricle cannot be visualized directly on the frontal projection because it is not border forming in the frontal projection. A large right ventricle can displace the left ventricle posteriorly and to the left causing widening of the cardiac silhouette on the frontal view. On the lateral view, the right ventricle comprises the anterior margin of the heart in the subxyphoid area, occupying the inferior third of the thorax (see Fig. 11–1B). A dilated right ventricle extends farther up into the retrosternal space.[9]

### Azygos Vein

The azygos vein is an oval structure seen in the frontal radiograph at the right tracheobronchial angle (see Fig. 11–1A). Its size is a good marker of cardiovascular dynamics. It enlarges in left or right heart failure, obstruction of the superior vena cava, or absence of the intrahepatic segment of the inferior vena cava.[10] A change in the size of the azygos vein parallels changes in pulmonary venous pressure, making it a useful radiographic indicator of congestive heart failure.

## ■ SPECIFIC ABNORMALITIES

### Abnormal Pulmonary Blood Flow and Pulmonary Edema

Pulmonary blood flow reflects the hemodynamics of the heart itself. Increased, decreased, or asymmetric pulmonary blood flow can be recognized on chest radiographs and correlated with other signs of disease. The size of the pulmonary arteries is related to both blood flow and blood pressure or to pressure alone.[4] Enlarged pulmonary arteries are present in a variety of conditions, including left-to-right shunt, increased cardiac output due to chronic anemia or pregnancy, and pulmonary arterial hypertension, which may be primary or secondary to conditions such as chronic interstitial lung disease, emphysema, Eisenmenger's syndrome, or chronic thromboembolism (Fig. 11–2). Central pulmonary artery calcification indicates chronic, severe pulmonary arterial hypertension.[11]

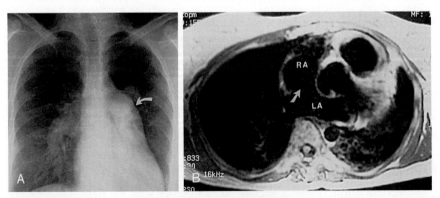

**Figure 11–2** ■ Pulmonary arterial hypertension secondary to Eisenmenger's syndrome in a 32-year-old woman with atrial septal defect. *(A)* Frontal chest radiograph. The main *(arrow)*, left, and right pulmonary arteries are enlarged. *(B)* Transverse electrocardiographically gated spin echo MRI image shows a large defect *(arrow)* of the atrial septum. LA, left atrium; RA, right atrium.

Elevation of pulmonary venous pressure can be due to left ventricular failure, mitral stenosis, or another cause of vascular obstruction distal to the pulmonary arterial bed. When pressure rises to 12 to 18 mm Hg, there is a redistribution of pulmonary blood flow to the upper lobes, which is manifested radiographically as enlargement of the upper lobe vessels ("cephalization").[12] As pulmonary venous pressure rises above 18 mm Hg, pulmonary interstitial edema develops. Radiographically, thin horizontal interlobular septal lines, called *Kerley B lines*, are visible at the lung bases (Fig. 11–3).[13] With elevation of pulmonary venous pressure above 25 mm Hg, alveolar edema ensues. In persons with alveolar edema, chest radiographs demonstrate opacities that typically involve the central portions of the lungs, sometimes producing a "bat-wing" appearance. If the pulmonary edema is related to heart failure, the heart may be enlarged (see Fig. 11–3).

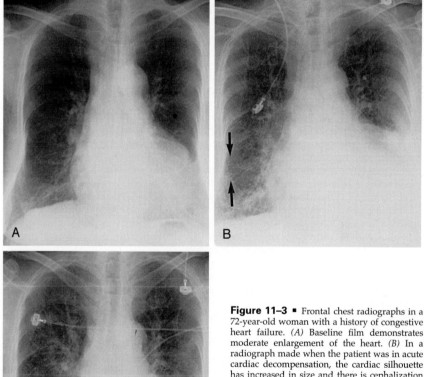

**Figure 11–3** ■ Frontal chest radiographs in a 72-year-old woman with a history of congestive heart failure. (A) Baseline film demonstrates moderate enlargement of the heart. (B) In a radiograph made when the patient was in acute cardiac decompensation, the cardiac silhouette has increased in size and there is cephalization of the pulmonary vasculature. Kerley B lines *(between arrows)* are identified in the right lower lobe, indicating pulmonary interstitial edema. (C) Film obtained the next day shows progression of pulmonary edema with alveolar opacities.

## Valvular Heart Disease

Stenosis of the aortic valve is most frequently related to a congenital bicuspid valve. Less commonly, a tricuspid aortic valve can degenerate, sometimes because of rheumatic valvulitis. Mild to moderate aortic stenosis causes left ventricular hypertrophy. Radiographically, the valve may be calcified, and typically the right side of the ascending aorta bulges owing to poststenotic dilatation. The left ventricular border may be rounded or the cardiac apex elevated secondary to concentric hypertrophy of the left ventricle.[14] More severe narrowing of the valve can lead to enlargement of the left ventricle and atrium that is proportionate to the degree of stenosis and the severity of associated mitral regurgitation.[15] Pulmonary venous hypertension and pulmonary edema also can develop in patients with severe aortic stenosis.

Aortic regurgitation can develop in a stenotic bicuspid valve, or it can be due to rheumatic valvulitis, infective endocarditis, or annular dilatation resulting from enlargement of the ascending aorta in conditions such as annuloaortic ectasia. Aortic dissection also can cause aortic insufficiency. With mild aortic regurgitation, the heart size usually remains normal and the ascending aorta is normal or slightly dilated. Enlargement of the left atrium suggests intercurrent mitral regurgitation. In moderate or severe cases, the left ventricle and the aorta are enlarged. In contrast to aortic stenosis, diffuse dilatation of the aorta can occur with aortic regurgitation. In patients with annuloaortic ectasia, the aortic root is disproportionately enlarged. Valve calcification often occurs in patients with aortic insufficiency that is due to a congenital bicuspid valve or to rheumatic valve disease. With chronic aortic regurgitation, the left ventricle enlarges but the lungs appear essentially normal.[16] When aortic regurgitation is acute, as with trauma or dissection, chest radiographs demonstrate pulmonary venous hypertension and pulmonary edema without left ventricular enlargement.

Mitral stenosis is most frequently secondary to rheumatic heart disease. Mild enlargement of the left atrium is one of the initial radiographic manifestations of mitral stenosis. When the stenosis is more severe, the left atrium dilates further and the left atrial appendage can enlarge disproportionately.[17] Pulmonary venous hypertension and cephalization can develop, and the central pulmonary arteries can enlarge. The mitral valve is frequently calcified. The left ventricle appears normal in most patients with mitral stenosis.

Chronic mitral regurgitation can be due to a variety of causes, including ischemic cardiomyopathy, rheumatic heart disease, valve prolapse secondary to myxomatous degeneration, and calcification of the mitral annulus. Chest radiographs exhibit enlargement of both the left atrium and the left ventricle (Fig. 11–4). Because of volume overload and elevated pressure, chamber enlargement can be severe. Acute mitral regurgitation can be caused by rupture of the chordae tendineae or papillary muscles, ischemic dysfunction, and bacterial endocarditis. Although the heart may be normal in size, these patients have left heart failure that causes severe pulmonary alveolar edema. Occasionally, asymmetric pulmonary edema, more severe in the right upper lobe, can result from selective retrograde flow from the mitral valve into the right upper lobe pulmonary veins.[18] The valve can be evaluated and the regurgitant flow quantified with either echocardiography or MRI.

Tricuspid valve regurgitation (see Fig. 11–4) can be due to ischemic cardiomyopathy, rheumatic heart disease, Ebstein's anomaly, or another cause. Typically, the right-sided chambers enlarge, and the right atrium can be disproportionately dilated.[19] Patients with tricuspid regurgitation can have massive cardiac enlargement, a finding known as *wall-to-wall heart*.

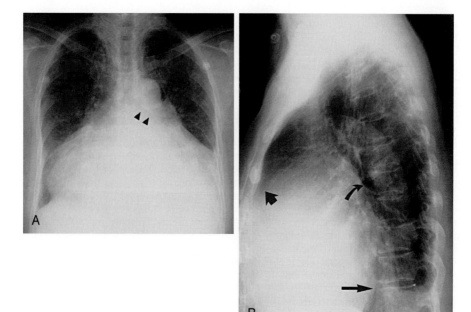

**Figure 11–4** ■ Severe tricuspid and mitral regurgitation. *(A)* Frontal projection reveals a markedly enlarged cardiac silhouette with global cardiomegaly. The prominent right heart border indicates severe right atrial dilatation. The elevation of the left mainstem bronchus *(arrowheads)* suggests left atrial enlargement. *(B)* Lateral view demonstrates enlargement of the right ventricle *(short, wide arrow)*, left ventricle *(long, straight arrow)*, and left atrium *(curved arrow)*.

## Ischemic Heart Disease

Several imaging techniques can be used to evaluate patients with ischemic heart disease, including coronary angiography, radionuclide scintigraphy, echocardiography, electron-beam CT, and MRI. Chest films can be completely normal in patients with ischemic cardiomyopathy, even those who have severe disease; however, many of these patients have cardiomegaly, especially left ventricular enlargement. They may also have pulmonary edema or a left ventricular aneurysm.

Dressler's syndrome (postmyocardial infarction syndrome) is manifested radiographically as enlargement of the cardiac silhouette by pericardial effusion. Pleural effusion (usually unilateral and on the left side) is common, and consolidation is present in a minority of patients.[20]

Occasionally, a left ventricular aneurysm can develop after myocardial infarction. A true aneurysm is most frequently located at the cardiac apex or on the anterior ventricular wall. On chest radiographs, the aneurysm appears as a focal bulge along the left border of the heart.[21] A thin rim of calcification is sometimes seen within the aneurysm. A false aneurysm can arise after left ventricular rupture secondary to acute transmural infarction.[22] Although most patients with cardiac rupture die immediately, in a small percentage the rupture is contained by the surrounding soft tissues. Chest films can be normal or can reveal a mass, most often along the posterior or diaphragmatic aspect of the heart.[22] Definitive diagnosis is made by MRI, CT, or echocardiography. Cross-sectional imaging can distinguish a false aneurysm, with its narrow neck, from a true aneurysm, which has a wide mouth communicating with the ventricular chamber.

Papillary muscle rupture is an unusual complication of myocardial infarction. Chest radiographs demonstrate a wide spectrum of findings, from no abnormality to marked cardiomegaly and pulmonary edema. Echocardiography or MRI can be performed to diagnose the abnormal mitral valve leaflets and to quantify the severity of mitral regurgitation.[23]

In patients with dilated cardiomyopathy or ischemic cardiomyopathy, the left ventricular ejection fraction is decreased. Left ventricular—and later biventricular—failure develops in most of these patients. The radiographic presentation can vary from a normal heart to diffuse globular enlargement, which may simulate a large pericardial effusion. Ventricular hypokinesis and dilatation of the left atrium and left ventricle are the findings at echocardiography.

Coronary artery calcification is an indicator of atherosclerosis, and the quantity of calcification correlates with the total atherosclerotic burden.[24] Coronary artery calcification can be identified by various imaging modalities, including radiography, fluoroscopy, and CT. Electron-beam CT has the greatest diagnostic accuracy for detection of coronary artery calcification.[24] In the past several years, electron-beam CT has been investigated for identification of coronary atherosclerosis. Evidence from several recent studies seems to support the use of electron-beam CT for risk stratification in asymptomatic persons and for diagnosis of coronary artery disease in patients with atypical chest pain.[25]

## Pericardial Disease

On lateral chest radiographs, the normal pericardium can be seen in many patients as a curved, linear opacity between the pericardial fat and the subpericardial fat. Because of their excellent contrast resolution, CT and MRI depict the pericardium more readily than plain radiographs.[26, 27]

Small pericardial effusions often are not seen on chest radiographs. As the quantity of pericardial fluid increases, the cardiac silhouette may acquire a "water bottle" or globular configuration (Fig. 11–5). The normal bulges and indentations of the cardiac borders may become obscured, and the contours of the heart may become blunted and featureless. Because the cardiac silhouette is enlarged in the presence of a pericardial effusion,[27] it may be difficult to distinguish pericardial effusion from cardiomegaly. Because the pericardium extends to the main pulmonary artery, a large pericardial effusion can obscure the hilar vessels, a finding not associated with cardiomegaly alone. Occasionally, pericardial effusion may be seen on a lateral chest radiograph as an opaque band between the pericardial fat and the subpericardial fat. This is known as the *fat pad sign* (see Fig. 11–5C). Although this sign is highly specific for pericardial effusion, its sensitivity is limited.

Echocardiography is more sensitive than plain radiography for the diagnosis of pericardial effusion.[28] When a pericardial effusion is suggested by clinical or radiographic findings, echocardiography can be used for more definitive evaluation. CT and MRI also can identify pericardial effusion (see Fig. 11–5D).[29]

Constrictive pericarditis may occur as a result of open heart surgery, radiation therapy, viral infection or tuberculosis, or hemopericardium.[30] The cardiac silhouette usually is normal or small, and the right heart border may be flattened.[31] The majority of these patients have a pericardial effusion, and a minority exhibit enlargement of the left atrium and azygos vein. In a small proportion of patients with pericardial constriction, calcification of the pericardium may be seen. Most often due to tuberculous pericarditis, such calcification is seen most readily along

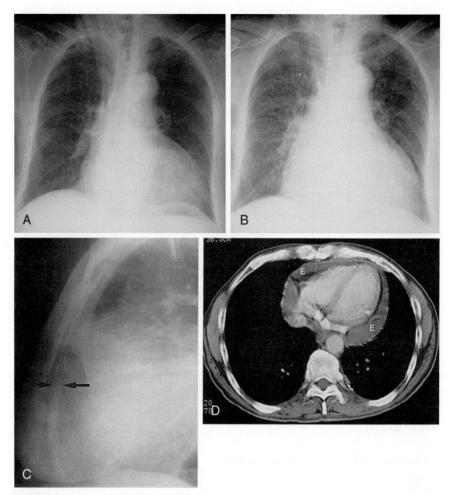

**Figure 11–5** ■ Pericardial effusion in a 52-year-old woman on hemodialysis. *(A)* Baseline frontal chest film. *(B, C)* Films performed 2 days later, just before dialysis. *(B)* The cardiac silhouette has increased in size. *(C)* The lateral view shows the "fat pad sign." There is a dense layer of fluid *(between arrows)* between the lucent epicardial and pericardial layers of fat. *(D)* Contrast-enhanced CT demonstrates a large pericardial effusion (E).

the anterior and inferior borders of the heart and in the atrioventricular and interventricular grooves (Fig. 11–6).

Because constrictive pericarditis and restrictive cardiomyopathy may have overlapping clinical presentations and findings, MRI and CT can be important for distinguishing the two diagnoses. Pericardial thickening of at least 4 mm is very sensitive and specific for constrictive pericarditis.[29] Ancillary findings of constrictive pericarditis include enlargement of the right atrium, inferior vena cava, and hepatic veins and a narrowed, "tubular" right ventricle. Although pericardial calcification and thickening indicate chronic pericardial inflammation and can be used to support the diagnosis of pericardial constriction, the diagnosis must be based on clinical criteria in addition to imaging findings.

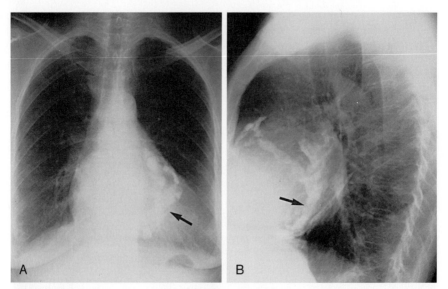

**Figure 11–6** ■ Calcific pericarditis in a patient with a history of tuberculosis. Frontal *(A)* and lateral *(B)* radiographs demonstrate dense calcium in the interventricular groove *(arrows)*.

When a mediastinal mass is identified on chest radiography, CT or MRI may be performed for more precise evaluation (Fig. 11–7). A pericardial cyst appears as a smooth, well-marginated, fluid-filled paracardiac structure. Because pericardial cysts are benign and generally asymptomatic, they may be clinically important only because cross-sectional imaging must be performed to differentiate a cyst from a solid mass. Echocardiography also can be used to make the diagnosis of pericardial cyst.

## Congenital Heart Disease in Adults

There are three groups of adults with congenital heart disease: (1) those who were treated in childhood, (2) those whose disease was diagnosed in childhood who did not receive surgical intervention, and (3) those whose disorder was not recognized until adulthood.

### Coarctation of the Aorta

In adults, focal postductal stenosis is the most common manifestation of coarctation. Chest radiographs may demonstrate a characteristic abnormal contour of the aortic arch known as the *figure 3 sign*, a double-bulge immediately above and below the region of the aortic knob (Fig. 11–8A).[32] Bilateral symmetric rib notching in an older child or adult is diagnostic of coarctation. In recent years, MRI has been used to evaluate coarctation of the aorta before and after surgical repair or angiography (Fig. 11–8B).[33] Because MRI is a noninvasive technique that provides complete anatomic and functional evaluation of the coarctation, it can usually be performed in place of diagnostic angiography.

### Left-to-Right Shunts

Ostium secundum atrial septal defect (ASD), the most common left-to-right shunt diagnosed in adult life, accounts for more than 40% of adult congenital heart

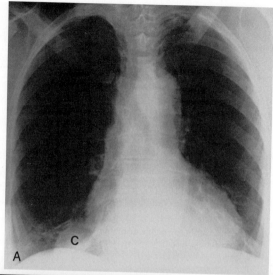

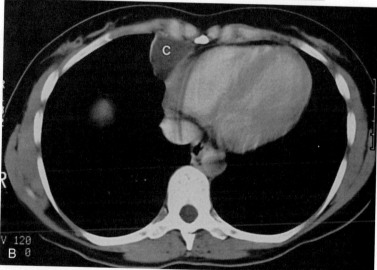

**Figure 11–7** ▪ Pericardial cyst (C). *(A)* Frontal chest film reveals a smoothly marginated round mass in the right cardiophrenic angle. *(B)* Contrast-enhanced CT demonstrates a well-circumscribed, thin-walled mass of fluid density.

defects.[34] Although the chest radiograph may be normal in a patient with a small shunt, the main pulmonary artery, peripheral pulmonary branches, right atrium, and right ventricle are enlarged (see Fig. 11–2A). Echocardiography can delineate the size and location of the ASD and of associated abnormalities such as mitral valve prolapse. MRI can be performed if echocardiography does not reveal the ASD (see Fig. 11–2B).

If a ventricular septal defect VSD is small, the chest film is normal. When the left-to-right shunt is large or there is secondary pulmonary hypertension, however,

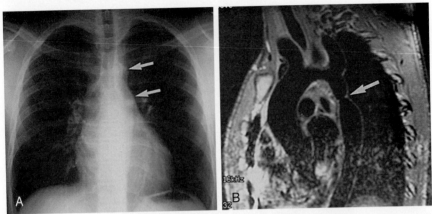

**Figure 11–8** ■ In a young man with hypertension, frontal chest radiograph *(A)* shows a "figure 3" sign *(arrows)* consistent with coarctation of the aorta. Rib notching is not seen in this film. *(B)* Oblique sagittal electrocardiographically gated spin echo MRI image demonstrates severe, discrete postductal narrowing of the aorta.

the pulmonary arteries, both ventricles, and the left atrium are enlarged. Echocardiography usually demonstrates the site of the defect. MRI is performed in certain cases to evaluate associated abnormalities or to define certain lesions, such as a supracristal VSD, which may be difficult to image by echocardiography.[35]

## ■ REFERENCES

1. Steiner RM, Gross G, Flicker S, et al: Congenital heart disease in the adult patient. J Thorac Imaging 1995;10:1–25.
2. Danza FM, Fusco A, Breda M: Ductus arteriosus aneurysm in an adult. AJR 1984;143:131–133.
3. West JB: Regional differences in gas exchange in the lung in erect man. J Appl Physiol 1962;17:893–898.
4. Kabala JE, Wilde P: Measurement of heart size in the anteroposterior chest radiograph. Br J Radiol 1987;60:981–986.
5. Milne ENC, Burnett K, Aufrichtig D, et al: Assessment of cardiac size on portable chest films. J Thorac Imaging 1988;3:64–72.
6. Higgins CB, Reinke RT, Jones WE, et al: Left atrial dimension on the frontal thoracic radiograph: A method for assessing left atrial enlargement. AJR 1978;130:251–255.
7. Carlsson E, Gross R, Hold RG: The radiological diagnosis of cardiac valvar insufficiencies. Circulation 1977;55:921–933.
8. Jefferson K, Rees S: Clinical Cardiac Radiology, 2nd ed. London: Butterworth's, 1980:3–24.
9. Murphy ML, Blue LR, Ferris EJ, et al: Sensitivity and specificity of chest roentgenogram criteria for right ventricular hypertrophy. Invest Radiol 1988;23:853–856.
10. Berdon WE, Baker DH: Plain film findings in azygos continuation of the inferior vena cava. AJR 1968;104:452–457.
11. Gutierrez FR, Moran CJ, Ludbrook PA, et al: Pulmonary arterial calcification with reversible pulmonary hypertension. AJR 1980;135:177–178.
12. Harrison MO, Conte, PJ, Heitzman ER: Radiological detection of clinically occult cardiac failure following myocardial infarction. Br J Radiol 1971;44:265–272.
13. Grainger RG: Interstitial pulmonary oedema and its radiological diagnosis. A sign of pulmonary venous and capillary hypertension. Br J Radiol 1958;31:201–217.
14. Higgins CB: Radiography of acquired heart disease. In Higgins CB (ed): Essentials of Cardiac Radiology and Imaging. Philadelphia: JB Lippincott, 1992:1–48.
15. Lasser A: Calcification of the myocardium. Hum Pathol 1983;14:824–826.
16. Follman DF: Aortic regurgitation. Identifying and treating acute and chronic disease. Postgrad Med 1993;93:83–90.
17. Green CE, Kelley MJ, Higgins CB: Etiologic significance of enlargement of the left atrial appendage in adults. Radiology 1982;142:21–27.

18. Gurney JW, Goodman LR: Pulmonary edema localized in the right upper lobe accompanying mitral regurgitation. Radiology 1989;172:397–399.
19. Stanford W, Galvin JR: The radiology of right heart dysfunction: Chest roentgenogram and computed tomography. J Thorac Imaging 1989;4:7–19.
20. Watanabe AM: Ischemic heart disease. *In* Kelly NW (ed): Essentials of Internal Medicine. Philadelphia: JB Lippincott, 1994:1511–1512.
21. Higgins CB, Lipton MJ: Radiography of acute myocardial infarction. Radiol Clin North Am 1980;18:359–368.
22. Higgins CB, Lipton MJ, Johnson AD, et al: False aneurysms of the left ventricle. Identification of distinctive clinical, radiographic, and angiographic features. Radiology 1978;127:21–27.
23. Kotler MN, Mintz GS, Panidis I, et al: Noninvasive evaluation of normal and abnormal prosthetic valve function. J Am Coll Cardiol 1983;2:151–173.
24. Wexler L, Brundage B, Crouse J, et al: Coronary artery calcification: Pathophysiology, epidemiology, imaging methods, and clinical implications. A statement for health professionals from the American Heart Association. Circulation 1996;94:1175–1192.
25. Rumberger JA, Sheedy PF, Breen JF, et al: Electron beam computed tomography and coronary artery disease: Scanning for coronary artery calcification. Mayo Clin Proc 1996;71:369–377.
26. Olson MC, Posniak HV, McDonald V, et al: Computed tomography and magnetic resonance imaging of the pericardium. Radiographics 1989;9:633–649.
27. Steiner RM, Rao VM: Radiology of the pericardium. *In* Grainger RG, Allison J (eds): Diagnostic Radiology. London: Churchill Livingstone, 1986:675–689.
28. Engel PJ: Echocardiography in pericardial disease. Cardiovasc Clin 1983;13:181–200.
29. Sechtem U, Tscholakoff D, Higgins CB: MRI of the abnormal pericardium. AJR 1986;147:245–252.
30. Vaitkus PT, Kussmaul WG: Constrictive pericarditis versus restrictive cardiomyopathy: A reappraisal and update of diagnostic criteria. Am Heart J 1991;122:1431–1441.
31. Carsky EW, Mauceri RA, Azimi R: The epicardial fat pad sign: Analysis of frontal and lateral chest radiographs in patients with pericardial effusion. Radiology 1980;137:303–308.
32. Chen JTT, Khoury M, Kirks DR: Obscured aortic arch on the lateral view as a sign of coarctation. Radiology 1984;153:595–596.
33. Von Schulthess GK, Higashino SM, Higgins SS, et al: Coarctation of the aorta: MR imaging. Radiology 1986;158:469–474.
34. Whittemore R, Wells JA, Castellsague X: A second generation study of 427 probands with congenital heart disease and their 837 children. J Am Coll Cardiol 1994;23:1459–1467.
35. Bremerich J, Reddy GP, Higgins CB: MRI of supracristal ventricular septal defects. J Comput Assist Tomogr 1999;23:13–15.

## ▪ RECOMMENDED READING

Boxt LM (ed): Radiol Clin North Am 1999;37:257–456.
Higgins CB (ed): Essentials of Cardiac Radiology and Imaging. Philadelphia, JB Lippincott, 1992.
Miller SW (ed): Cardiac Radiology. The Requisites. St. Louis, Mosby–Year Book, 1996.
Steiner RM, Levin DC: Radiology of the heart. *In* Braunwald E (ed): Heart Disease. A Textbook of Cardiovascular Medicine, 5th ed. Philadelphia: WB Saunders, 1997:204–239.

# Chapter 12

# Cardiac Catheterization and Coronary Angiography

*Mark J. Ricciardi* ■ *Nirat Beohar* ■ *Charles J. Davidson*

## ■ HISTORICAL PERSPECTIVE

In 1929, Werner Forssman performed the first human cardiac catheterization when he passed a urethral catheter from his left antecubital vein into the right side of his heart.[1] With the introduction of left heart catheterization by Zimmerman[2] and Limon Lason[3] and selective coronary arteriography by Sones in 1958,[4, 5] the modern era of mechanical approaches to coronary artery disease began. In 1968, Favalaro reported the first successful coronary bypass grafting operation,[6] and in 1977, Andreas Gruentzig performed the first human percutaneous balloon coronary angioplasty.[7, 8] Both revascularization techniques have had dramatic effects on survival and quality of life for patients with coronary artery disease.

## ■ INDICATIONS

Cardiac catheterization remains an indispensable diagnostic tool when used in combination with noninvasive evaluation to determine the presence and severity of diseases of the heart. Identification and assessment of coronary artery disease are the most common indications for cardiac catheterization in adults. The AHA/ACC guidelines for coronary angiography[9] are given in Table 12–1. These guidelines have recently expanded to include cardiac catheterization for evolving and recent myocardial infarctions.[10]

In patients with myocardial disease, cardiac catheterization can assess coronary anatomy, quantify the severity of diastolic and systolic dysfunction, help to differentiate myocardial restriction from constriction, and rule out associated valvular disease. Active myocarditis can be detected by myocardial biopsy, and cardiovascular response to acute pharmacologic intervention can be evaluated.

In patients with valvular heart disease, cardiac catheterization provides both confirmatory and complementary data to echocardiographic and nuclear studies and defines the extent of obstructive coronary disease.[11]

In congenital cardiac anomalies, cardiac catheterization may be necessary to provide hemodynamic information such as shunt size and pulmonary vascular resistance and to define coronary, great artery, and cardiac anatomy.

## ■ COMPLICATIONS

The risk of major adverse outcomes after coronary angiography is exceedingly small (Table 12–2).[12, 13] A proper history, physical examination (with special attention to the cardiorespiratory and vascular examination), and review of all laboratory, electrocardiographic (ECG), and imaging studies select out many persons at risk

Table 12–1

## Class I and II Indications for Coronary Angiography

**KNOWN OR SUSPECTED CORONARY DISEASE** (known: previous myocardial infarction, or coronary bypass surgery or percutaneous transcatheter angioplasty (PTCA); suspected: rest- or exercise-induced ECG abnormalities suggesting silent ischemia)

**Asymptomatic Patients**

*Class I indications:*
1. Evidence for high risk on noninvasive testing
2. Individuals in high-risk occupations (airline pilot, bus driver, etc.)
3. Following successful resuscitation from cardiac arrest
*Class II indications:*
1. Positive noninvasive test in patient not at high risk
2. Multiple risk factors for coronary artery disease
3. Prior myocardial infarction with positive noninvasive testing
4. After cardiac transplantation
5. After coronary artery bypass grafting or PTCA with positive ischemia
6. Before noncardiac surgery with positive noninvasive test

**Symptomatic Patients**

*Class I indications:*
1. Inadequate response to medical treatment
2. Unstable angina
3. Prinzmetal or variant angina
4. Canadian Cardiovascular Society functional class I or II angina (no or slight limitation with ordinary physical activity) associated with the following:
   a. Positive exercise test
   b. History of myocardial infarction or hypertension with ECG changes
   c. Side effects of medical therapy
   d. Occupational or lifestyle "need to know"
   e. Episodic pulmonary edema
5. Before major vascular surgery if angina is present or noninvasive positive
6. After resuscitation from cardiac arrest
*Class II indications:*
1. Any angina in the following groups:
   a. Female patients <40 yr with positive noninvasive test
   b. Male patients <40 yr of age
   c. Patients <40 yr of age with history of myocardial infarction
   d. Patients requiring major nonvascular surgery
2. Canadian Cardiovascular Society functional class III or IV angina (angina with minimal activity or at rest) that improves on medical therapy
3. Patients who cannot be risk stratified by other techniques

**ATYPICAL CHEST PAIN OF UNCERTAIN ORIGIN**

*Class I indications:*
1. When noninvasive stress test reveals high risk for coronary disease
2. Suspected coronary artery
3. Associated symptoms or signs of abnormal LV function or failure
*Class II indications:*
1. Patients in whom coronary disease cannot be excluded by noninvasive studies
2. Severe symptoms despite negative noninvasive tests

**ACUTE MYOCARDIAL INFARCTION**

**Acute, Evolving Myocardial Infarction***

*Class I indications:*
1. Within the first 6 hr in candidates for revascularization therapy (Original guidelines considered this a class II indication; recently revised to class I)[10]
*Class II indications:*
1. After intravenous thrombolytic therapy when PTCA is contemplated

*Table continued on following page*

Table 12–1

**Class I and II Indications for Coronary Angiography** *Continued*

**Completed Myocardial Infarction (after 6 hr and before discharge evaluation)**

*Class I indications:*
1. Recurrent episodes of ischemic chest pain
2. Suspected ruptured septum or acute mitral regurgitation with congestive heart failure
3. Suspected left ventricular pseudoaneurysm
*Class II indications:*
1. Thrombolytic therapy during evolving myocardial infarction period
2. Congestive heart failure and/or hypotension during intensive medical therapy
3. Recurrent ventricular tachycardia and/or ventricular fibrillation
4. Cardiogenic shock
5. Myocardial infarction due to coronary embolism

**Convalescent Myocardial Infarction (predischarge to 8 wk)**

*Class I indications:*
1. Angina at rest or with minimal activity
2. Congestive heart failure, recurrent ischemia, or ventricular arrhythmias
3. Positive noninvasive study
4. Non–Q wave infarction
*Class II indications:*
1. Mild angina
2. Asymptomatic and <50 yr of age
3. Need to return to unusually active or vigorous activity
4. History of myocardial infarction or angina for >6 mo before the current myocardial infarction
5. Thrombolytic therapy given during evolving phase

**VALVULAR HEART DISEASE**

*Class I indications:*
1. Before valve surgery in an adult with chest discomfort and/or ECG changes
2. Before valve surgery in a male patient ≥35 yr
3. Before valve surgery in postmenopausal women
*Class II indications:*
1. During left heart catheterization in men <35 yr of age or women >40 yr when aortic or mitral valve surgery is being considered
2. Multiple risk factors for coronary disease
3. Reoperation for valve surgery when previous angiography done more than 1 year previously
4. In infective endocarditis when coronary embolization occurs

**CONGENITAL HEART DISEASE**

*Class I indications:*
1. Signs or symptoms of angina
2. Suspected congestive coronary anomaly
3. Male patient >40 yr of age or postmenopausal woman
*Class II indications:*
1. In presence of a congenital lesion with high frequency of coronary anomalies

**MISCELLANEOUS**

*Class I indications:*
1. Disease of the aorta in whom the absence, presence, or extent of coronary disease will affect management
2. Left ventricular failure without obvious cause
3. Angina associated with hypertrophic cardiomyopathy in patients ≥35 years or postmenopausal female patients with angina
*Class II indications:*
1. Dilated cardiomyopathy
2. Recent blunt chest trauma
3. Male patients >35 yr of age or postmenopausal women to undergo cardiac surgery other than coronary bypass
4. Prospective transplant donors
5. Kawasaki disease (coronary aneurysm)

*Revised ACC/AHA task force guidelines indicate a clinical role (Class I) for PTCA during acute myocardial infarction (Circulation 1993;88:2987). See text for details.
Data from Ross J, Brandenburg RO, Dinsmore RE, and members of the Subcommittee Task Force on Coronary Angiography of the AHA/ACC: J Am Coll Cardiol 1987;10:935.

Table 12–2

**Complications of Coronary Angiography[12]**

| Complication | Incidence (%) |
|---|---|
| Death | 0.10 |
| Myocardial infarction | 0.06 |
| Stroke | 0.07 |
| Serious arrhythmia | 0.47 |
| Vascular complications | 0.46 |
| Contrast reactions | 0.23 |

for untoward events. The most commonly encountered complications relate to vascular access and radiographic contrast media.

The most common vascular complications are subcutaneous hematoma, pseudoaneurysm formation, arteriovenous fistula, retroperitoneal bleeding, and rectus sheath hematoma. All are more common in persons of advanced age, those who have an extreme body habitus or bleeding diathesis, and those who use anticoagulant or antiplatelet drugs. Great care must be taken at the time of arterial puncture to avoid vascular misadventures at the access site. With the femoral artery approach, the artery should be entered at a level two fingerbreadths below the inguinal ligament (which can be palpated in thin persons and is located on a plane between the anterior superior iliac crest and the cephalad aspect of the pubic bone). Patients with truncal obesity require careful palpation of the bony landmarks and fluoroscopic visualization of the femoral head, which marks the level of the inguinal ligament. The less commonly used percutaneous brachial and radial approaches also require great care to ensure successful puncture. Before using the radial artery, a positive Allen's test of ulnar artery patency should be demonstrated (whereby, after manual compression of both the radial and ulnar arteries during fist clenching, normal color returns to the relaxed hand after pressure over the ulnar artery is released). These smaller upper extremity arteries have historically been more prone to arterial access complications and are usually reserved for persons with severe lower extremity vascular disease. In some centers there has been a resurgence in the use of the radial artery for arterial access. The brachial cutdown is performed in a small percentage of patients and has the benefit of direct arterial visualization and arteriotomy closure. The higher risk of thromboembolism with upper extremity arterial access warrants bolus administration of low-dose intravenous or intraarterial heparin.

Nearly all cardiac catheterizations are performed via an arterial sheath through which catheters are placed for cardiac hemodynamics and imaging. Very important in avoiding complications at the site of arterial access is proper management of the arterial sheath once it is in place. Since sheath dwell times correlate with vascular access complication rates, all sheaths need to be removed as soon as possible. Hemodynamic and anticoagulation issues are addressed before the sheath is removed (the blood pressure must not be excessively low or high and persons recently exposed to heparin should have an activated clotting time [ACT] of less than 170 seconds). In the case of the femoral artery approach, adequate compression of the femoral artery against the femoral head (just cephalad to the puncture site) is adjusted according to the presence or absence of bleeding and the presence or absence of pulses distally. With upper extremity access, care must be taken to limit the time of arterial occlusion to ensure viability of the hand. Atropine should be immediately available to treat vasovagal reactions that may accompany arterial compression.

Contrast media–related renal toxicity occurs in 1.4% to 2.3% of patients who receive contrast media.[14] The major predictors of contrast-mediated renal insufficiency are (1) baseline renal dysfunction, (2) dehydration, (3) contrast volume used, (4) diabetes mellitus, and (5) congestive heart failure. Hydration with saline alone is considered the most effective preventive measure to avoid contrast-induced acute renal insufficiency as compared with mannitol and furosemide.[15] Using less than 30 ml of contrast for the entire procedure can also minimize renal dysfunction. Nonionic, low-osmolar contrast agents (such as iodixanol and iopamidol) reduce acute adverse hemodynamic and electrophysiologic effects and less frequently cause anaphylactic reactions. They reduce the risk of contrast-induced nephropathy in persons with diabetes mellitus and moderate baseline renal insufficiency but not in patients with normal renal function. Nonionic, low-osmolar contrast agents also cause less nausea and flushing than ionic, high-osmolar agents.

# ■ RELATIVE CONTRAINDICATIONS

The relative contraindications to cardiac catheterization are listed in Table 12–3. Patient issues that increase procedural risk should be ameliorated before catheterization unless the potential benefits outweigh the risk of foregoing catheterization. Persons at increased risk for whom special precautions are recommended are listed in Table 12–4.

# ■ CATHETERIZATION LABORATORY PROTOCOL

To best prepare for a safe and informative cardiac catheterization procedure, a standardized preoperative protocol should be followed. The following is a list of issues to be addressed before beginning the procedure:

Highlights of the technical aspects of the procedure, risks, and benefits should be fully explained.

Precatheterization evaluation should address (1) whether there is a history of cardiac catheterization (and if so, information about catheters used, difficulty with arterial access or coronary cannulation); (2) whether the patient has had coronary artery bypass grafting (CABG) (date, number of grafts, graft type, and vessels bypassed); (3) whether the patient has had percutaneous transcatheter angioplasty (PTCA) (the vessel and equipment); and (4) whether there is a history of diabetes mellitus, contrast medium reaction, chronic anticoagulation, renal insufficiency, peripheral vascular disease, stroke, or a bleeding diathesis. Physical examination is performed with special attention to volume status, cardiorespiratory examination, and peripheral circulation. Laboratory evaluation should include complete blood count, platelet count, blood urea nitrogen, creatinine, serum electrolytes, blood glucose, prothrombin time, and partial thromboplastin time

Table 12–3

**Relative Contraindications to Coronary Angiography**

| | |
|---|---|
| Unexplained fever, untreated infection | Digitalis toxicity |
| Severe anemia (Hb <8 g/dl) | Previous contrast allergy without pretreatment |
| Severe electrolyte imbalance | Active or recent stroke (≤ 1 mo) |
| Active bleeding | Progressive renal insufficiency |
| Uncontrolled systemic hypertension | Pregnancy |

Table 12–4

**Factors That Increase the Risk of Complications of Coronary Angiography**

Increased general medical risk
Age >70 yr
Complex congenital heart disease
Morbid obesity
General debility or cachexia
Uncontrolled glucose intolerance
Arterial oxygen desaturation
Severe chronic obstructive lung disease
Chronic renal insufficiency with creatinine >1.5 mg/dl
Increased cardiac risk
Known three-vessel coronary artery disease
Known left main coronary artery disease
NYHA functional class IV
Significant mitral or aortic valve disease or mechanical prosthesis
Low ejection fraction (<35%)
High-risk exercise treadmill test results (hypotension or severe ischemia)
Pulmonary hypertension
Pulmonary artery wedge pressure >25 mm Hg
Increased vascular risk
Anticoagulation or bleeding diathesis
Uncontrolled systemic hypertension
Severe peripheral vascular disease
Recent stroke
Severe aortic insufficiency

(if necessary), and baseline ECG. Chest films are not mandated unless indicated by the preoperative evaluation.

The patient should fast for at least 6 hours. All cardiac medicines, including aspirin (but not anticoagulants) should be continued, and intravenous anticoagulation should be continued when clinically indicated. Metformin (glucophage)-associated lactic acidosis can be precipitated by contrast nephropathy. If renal function is normal, metformin is discontinued at the time of, or prior to, angiography and reinstituted only after renal function is shown to be normal 48 hours subsequent to the procedure. Warfarin should be held for at least 48 hours before the procedure to ensure an INR less than 2.0. Patients at high risk for thromboembolism should be admitted for heparinization while the effects of oral anticoagulation wane.

Premedication includes oral or intravenous sedation (with anxiolytics and/or narcotics) and can include antihistamines, which may decrease the risk of allergic reactions and prolong sedation.

Patients known to have contrast allergy need either oral or intravenous prophylaxis for 24 hours before the procedure (Table 12–5).

Table 12–5

**Recommended Premedication for Known Contrast Allergy**

| Oral Regimen (12 hr and Immediately before Study) | Intravenous Regimen (12 hr and Immediately before Study) |
| --- | --- |
| Prednisone, 60 mg | Hydrocortisone, 100 mg |
| Diphenhydramine, 25–50 mg | Diphenhydramine, 25–50 mg |
| Cimetidine, 300 mg | Cimetidine, 300 mg |

Table 12–6

**Normal Intracardiac Pressures**

| Chamber | Pressure (mm Hg) |
|---|---|
| Right atrium | 3–5 |
| Right ventricle | 20–25/3–5 |
| Pulmonary artery | 20–25/10–15 |
| Pulmonary capillary wedge | 10–15 |
| Left ventricle | 100–140/10–15 |
| Aorta | 100–140/60–80 |

## ■ RIGHT HEART CATHETERIZATION

Balloon flotation catheters are the simplest and most widely used for hemody-namic evaluation. They afford easy entry into the right atrium, right ventricle, and pulmonary artery via the internal jugular, subclavian, brachial, or femoral veins.

### Pressure Measurement

Intravascular pressures are typically measured using a fluid-filled catheter attached to a pressure transducer. The venous pressure waveforms, which represent diastolic filling, have three positive deflections (called the *a, c,* and *v* waves) and two negative deflections (the *x* and *y* descents).

The *a* wave reflects atrial contraction and follows the ECG *p* wave. The *x* descent follows the *a* wave and represents relaxation of the atrium and downward pulling of the tricuspid annulus by right ventricular (RV) contraction. The *x* descent is interrupted by the *c* wave, which is caused by protrusion of the closed tricuspid valve into the right atrium. The second pressure peak is the *v* wave, which is caused by blood returning to the atrium from the periphery and reflects atrial compliance. The *y* descent follows the *v* wave and reflects tricuspid valve opening and right atrial (RA) emptying into the ventricle. (For normal intracardiac pressures and waveforms, see Table 12–6 and Figure 12–1, respectively.)

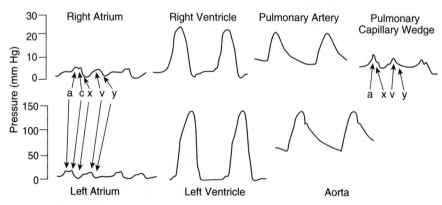

**Figure 12–1** ■ Representative right and left heart waveforms. See text for details.

## Cardiac Output

Volumetric flow or cardiac output (CO, expressed in liters per minute) can be measured by several methods. The Fick and thermodilution methods will be briefly discussed here. Other measures of CO include the indicator-dilution technique, angiographic CO, and the Doppler flow velocity method.

The Fick principle dictates that, in any circulation, the amount of an indicator substance in the blood leaving the circulation must equal the amount of that substance entering plus any amount added to the circulation during transit. The total amount of a substance passing any point in the circulation per unit of time is the product of its concentration and flow rate. CO by the Fick method[16] is calculated thus:

$$CO\ (l/min) =$$

$$\frac{O_2\ consumption\ (ml/min)}{A\text{-}V\ O_2\ difference\ (ml/100\ ml) \times O_2\text{-carrying capacity}\ (ml/100\ ml) \times 10}$$

$$= \frac{O_2\ consumption}{(Art\ sat\ -\ MV\ sat) \times Hb\ (g/100\ ml) \times 13.6}$$

where $(A\text{-}V)O_2$ is the difference in $O_2$ content between arterial and mixed venous blood, expressed as milliters of $O_2$ per 100 ml of blood. $O_2$-carrying capacity (ml/100 ml) is calculated by multiplying the hemoglobin (in g/100 ml) by 1.36.

The Fick method is the most accurate for assessing CO when the heart rate and rhythm are irregular (as in atrial fibrillation) or in low-output states. It is limited by the relatively cumbersome measurement of $O_2$ consumption. The Fick method tends to underestimate cardiac output in the presence of significant tricuspid regurgitation.

The thermodilution method requires injection of a bolus of liquid (saline or dextrose), the temperature of which differs from the body temperature, into the proximal port of the catheter. The resultant change in temperature in the liquid is measured by a thermistor mounted on the distal end of the catheter. CO is inversely related to the area under the thermodilution curve, plotted as a function of temperature versus time, with a smaller area indicating a higher CO. This method has become standard practice because it is easy to use. It is less accurate than the Fick method in the setting of irregular rhythm and low CO states.

Resistance to flow across both the pulmonary and systemic circuits can be calculated using pressure and output readings obtained at the time of right heart catheterization (Table 12–7).

## Intracardiac Shunts

Intracardiac shunts can be left to right (oxygenated blood from the left heart mixes with systemic venous blood), right to left (unoxygenated venous blood mixes with arterial blood), or mixed. The following terms are helpful in describing complex shunts and for shunt calculations (see Table 12–6):

*Effective flow* ($Q_{ef}$) is the quantity of systemically mixed venous blood that circulates through the lungs, is oxygenated, and then circulates through systemic capillaries.

*Recirculated systemic flow* ($Q_{rsf}$) is the amount of relatively desaturated, systemically mixed venous blood that recirculates directly into the aorta without being oxygenated by the lungs.

Table 12–7

**Commonly Used Hemodynamic Formulas**

| | | |
|---|---|---|
| Fick CO (l/min) | = | $\dfrac{\mathrm{V_{O_2}\ (ml/min)}}{\mathrm{(Art\text{-}MV\ O_2\ sat)}} \times \mathrm{Hb\ (mg/dl)} \times 13.6$ |
| SVR (Wood units) | = | $\dfrac{\mathrm{mAO\ (mm\ Hg)} - \mathrm{RA\ (mm\ Hg)}}{\mathrm{CO\ (l/min)}}$ |
| PVR (Wood units) | = | $\dfrac{\mathrm{mPA\ (mm\ Hg)} - \mathrm{mPCWP\ (mm\ Hg)}}{\mathrm{CO\ (l/min)}}$ |
| Qef (l/min) | = | $\dfrac{\mathrm{V_{O_2}\ (ml/min)}}{\mathrm{(PV_{O_2}\ sat} - \mathrm{MV_{O_2}\ sat)}}$ |
| Q recirculated systemic ($Q_{rsf}$, l/min) | = | $Q_s\ \mathrm{(l/min)} - Q_{ef}\ \mathrm{(l/min)}$ |
| Q recirculated pulmonary ($Q_{rpf}$, l/min) | = | $Q_p\ \mathrm{(l/min)} - Q_{ef}\ \mathrm{(l/min)}$ |
| Qp (l/min) | = | $\dfrac{\mathrm{V_{O_2}\ (ml/min)}}{\mathrm{(PV_{O_2}\ sat} - \mathrm{P_{AO_2}\ sat)}}$ |
| Qs (l/min) | = | $\dfrac{\mathrm{V_{O_2}\ (ml/min)}}{\mathrm{(Art\ O_2\ sat} - \mathrm{MV_{O_2}\ sat)}}$ |
| $MV_{O_2}$ sat (%) | = | $\dfrac{3\ \mathrm{SVC\ sat} + \mathrm{IVC\ sat}}{4}$ |
| % Left-to-right shunt | = | $\dfrac{Q_{rpf}\ \mathrm{(l/min)}}{Q_p\ \mathrm{(l/min)}}$ |
| % Right-to-left shunt | = | $\dfrac{Q_{rsf}\ \mathrm{(l/min)}}{Q_s\ \mathrm{(l/min)}}$ |

CO, cardiac output; $V_{O_2}$, oxygen consumption; Art, arterial; MV, mixed venous; sat, saturation (expressed as a fraction); Hb, hemoglobin (mg/dl); vol%, volume percent oxygen; SVR, systemic vascular resistance; mAO, mean aortic pressure; RA, right atrial pressure; PVR, pulmonary vascular resistance; mPA, mean pulmonary artery pressure; mPCWP, mean pulmonary capillary wedge pressure; Q, flow; Qs, systemic flow; Qef, effective flow; Qp, pulmonary flow; PV, pulmonary venous; SVC, superior vena cava; IVC, inferior vena cava.

*Recirculated pulmonary flow* ($Q_{rpf}$) is the quantity of fully saturated pulmonary venous blood that recirculates to the pulmonary artery without passing through the systemic capillaries.

*Total pulmonary flow* ($Q_p$) is the effective flow plus recirculated pulmonary flow.

*Systemic flow* ($Q_s$) is the effective flow plus recirculated systemic flow.

To quickly assess for the presence of left-to-right intracardiac shunting, serial $O_2$ saturation samplings are performed. A "stepup" in $O_2$ saturation indicates an abnormal increase in $O_2$ content between the chambers proximal and distal to the level of shunting. A significant left-to-right shunt is present when stepup is greater than 7% at the atrial level and greater than 5% at the ventricular or pulmonary level. The degree of shunting is reported in two ways: as a ratio of pulmonary to systemic flow ($Q_p/Q_s$) and percentage of shunt. $Q_p/Q_s > 1$ suggests left-to-right shunting; $Q_p/Q_s < 1$, right-to-left shunting. With bidirectional shunting, percentage of right-to-left and left-to-right shunt is reported.

## Evaluation of Stenotic Valvular Lesions

### Mitral Stenosis

Mitral stenosis (MS) causes a diastolic gradient between the left atrium and the left ventricle. The mean mitral valve gradient (MVG) depends upon the degree of MS, cardiac output, and the diastolic filling period (DFP). MVG can be measured directly from catheters placed in the left atrium and the left ventricle during diastole. More commonly, pulmonary capillary wedge pressure (PCWP) is used instead of the left atrial (LA) pressure. This requires a properly estimated wedge pressure using an end-hole catheter, fluoroscopic guidance, and/or confirmation by oxygen saturation (PCWP and LA saturations are >97%).

Mitral valve area (MVA) can be calculated thus using the Gorlin formula,[17]

$$MVA\ (cm^2) = \frac{1000 \times CO\ (l/min)}{37.7 \times \sqrt{MVG}\ (mm\ Hg) \times HR\ (beats/min) \times DFP\ (sec/beat)}$$

where MVA is mitral valve area, MVG, gradient across the mitral valve, and DFP, diastolic filling period.

Using the simplified formula of Hakki,[18]

$$MVA\ (cm^2) = \frac{CO\ (l/min)}{\sqrt{MVG}}$$

The MVA calculation can be erroneous in the setting of both low and high heart rates and concomitant mitral regurgitation. MS is severe when the MVA is less than approximately 1.2 cm$^2$.

## Aortic Stenosis

Like the MVG, the aortic valve gradient (AVG) depends upon the CO and severity of valvular stenosis. While the peak-to-peak gradient between aorta and left ventricle is commonly used to describe aortic stenosis (AS), it is a nonphysiologic measurement that is obtained from nonsimultaneous pressure tracings. The mean AVG, on the other hand, is physiologic and is the preferred measurement for providing information about severity of obstruction. In practice, the peak-to-peak gradient often closely matches the true mean gradient; however, it will not be accurate in cases of low-output states or irregular rhythms. The optimal method for obtaining AVG is to simultaneously measure aortic and ventricular pressures using catheters in each chamber.

Aortic valve area (AVA) can be calculated using the Gorlin formula[17]:

$$AVA = \frac{1000 \times CO\ (l/min)}{44.3 \times \sqrt{AVG}\ (mm\ Hg) \times HR\ (beats/min) \times SFP\ (sec/beat) \times SEP\ (sec/beat)}$$

where AVG is the aortic gradient, SFP, systolic filling period, and SEP, systolic ejection period.

Using the simplified formula of Hakki[18]:

$$AVA = \frac{CO\ (l/min)}{\sqrt{AVG}}$$

AVA calculations can be inaccurate in the presence of low or high heart rates, low CO, and significant aortic regurgitation. An AVA less than 1.0 cm$^2$ is consistent with severe AS; less than 0.75 cm$^2$ suggests critical AS.

## Restrictive and Constrictive Heart Disease

Both restriction and constriction are conditions of abnormal diastolic filling with relatively preserved systolic function. Diastolic dysfunction in restriction results from a noncompliant ventricular myocardium, whereas it is related to a thickened, noncompliant pericardium in constrictive heart disease. Abnormal filling in both conditions results in rapid early diastolic filling followed by a diastolic plateau (producing a "square root sign" [√] on ventricular filling tracings).

Even the most sophisticated hemodynamic analyses often fail to reliably differentiate the two conditions. In the majority of cases, clues from the clinical history, ECG, and chest film distinguish the two. For example, the presence of concomitant disease known to cause cardiac infiltration (e.g., amyloid), low voltage or conduction disease on ECG strongly favors the diagnosis of restriction in the appropriate hemodynamic setting. On the other hand, a history of pericardial disease or pathologic conditions known to affect the pericardium (tuberculosis, pericarditis, cancer, among others) in conjunction with pericardial calcium on chest films (or thickened pericardium on computed tomography [CT]) favors constrictive disease. When the history and simple diagnostic measures fail to clearly separate constriction from restriction, there are two invasive hemodynamic findings that are helpful: (1) Close matching of RV (RVEDP) and LV end-diastolic pressures (LVEDP) favors a constrictive process (RVEDP and LVEDP within 5 mm Hg). (2) Systolic pulmonary artery (PA) pressure greater than 60 mm Hg is rarely seen in constriction, whereas restrictive disease can result in PA pressures of 60 to 80 mm Hg (the reason for this difference in not known).

## Cardiac Tamponade

Cardiac catheterization is invaluable in establishing the hemodynamic importance of pericardial effusion. Cardiac tamponade is a condition in which pericardial fluid causes constraint and severely impaired filling, leading to hypotension, tachycardia, and diminished stroke volume.[19] Cardiac catheterization demonstrates several findings:

1. Elevated RA pressure with a characteristic preserved systolic $x$ descent and absence of or a diminutive diastolic $y$ descent (suggesting that RA emptying is impaired by compression of the right ventricle early in diastole).
2. Elevation and equalization of intrapericardial and RA pressures. The right ventricular (RV) diastolic pressure equals the intrapericardial and RA pressures and lacks the dip and plateau configuration of constrictive disease. Tamponade physiology occurs when the RV and LV filling is limited by the inability of the heart to distend adequately during diastole. If intrapericardial pressure is not elevated and RA and intrapericardial pressures are not virtually identical, the diagnosis of cardiac tamponade is questionable.
3. Exaggerated inspiratory elevation of RA pressure and depression of systemic pressure (pulsus paradoxus). Normally, inspiration increases venous return to the right heart, resulting in increased RV end-diastolic volume. The enlarged RV causes the interventricular septum to bulge into the LV, resulting in a slightly lower LV end-diastolic volume, stroke volume, and systolic blood pressure. In tamponade, the compression of the RV exaggerates leftward septal bulging and amplifies the reduction in systolic blood pressure during inspiration (> 10 mm Hg during quiet breathing).

## ■ CORONARY ARTERIOGRAPHY

Coronary arteriography is considered the reference standard for coronary artery imaging. It is the imaging modality of choice for establishing the presence or absence of coronary artery disease and for providing the most reliable information for making treatment decisions about medical therapy, angioplasty, or bypass surgery.

## Coronary Artery Anatomy

The heart is supplied by the left and right coronary arteries, which usually originate from the left and right sinuses of Valsalva, respectively.

## Coronary Dominance

The term *dominance* is applied to the artery that supplies the posterior diaphragmatic portion of the interventricular septum (the posterior descending artery [PDA]) and the diaphragmatic surface of the left ventricle (the posterior LV [PLV]). When these branches originate from the right coronary artery (RCA), the system is said to be *right dominant*; if they arise from the left circumflex artery (LCx), it is *left dominant* (the AV nodal artery also arises from the LCx in this case). Mixed or codominance occurs when these circulations are shared by the RCA and LCx. The coronary circulation is right dominant in approximately 85% of humans, left dominant in 8%, and codominant in 7%. Dominance, in the absence of coronary disease, has no particular clinical significance.

## Normal Coronary Anatomy (Fig. 12–2)

*The left main coronary artery (LMCA)* arises from the upper portion of the left sinus of Valsalva, is 3 to 6 mm in diameter and up to 10 mm long, and courses behind the right ventricular outflow tract before bifurcating into the left anterior descending (LAD) and LCx branches.

*The LAD artery* courses along the anterior interventricular groove toward the cardiac apex and gives off septal perforator and diagonal branches. In approximately a third of patients, the LMCA trifurcates, with a *ramus intermedius* arising between the LCx and LAD. This vessel supplies the free wall along the lateral aspect of the left ventricle.

*The LCx* originates at the bifurcation (or trifurcation) of the LMCA (or occasionally from a separate ostium of the left coronary sinus) and travels in the left atrioventricular groove. When dominant, the LCx gives rise to PDA, PLV, and frequently atrio-ventricular nodal arteries. A large LA branch arises proximally from the LCx in a third of people and gives rise to the sinus node artery. In disease states, it can be an important conduit for collateral flow to the RCA.

*The RCA* arises from the right coronary sinus at a point somewhat lower than the origin of the LCA from the left sinus. It travels first horizontally and then vertically, before going horizontally along the right atrioventricular groove toward the crux (a point on the diaphragmatic surface of the heart where the right atrioventricular groove, the left atrioventricular groove, and the posterior interventricular groove come together). The first branch of the RCA, the conus artery, can serve as a source of collateral circulation in patients with LAD occlusion. The sinus node artery originates from the proximal RCA in two thirds of patients and arises just distal to the conus artery. It supplies the sinus node, usually the right atrium, or both atria. Several small septal perforating arteries arise from the PDA and supply the lower third of the septum. As with the LAD, the right angle origin of the septal perforators helps to identify the PDA.

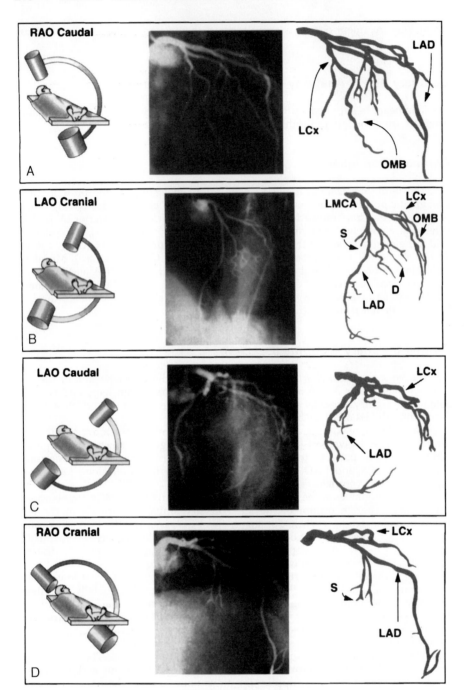

**Figure 12–2** ■ *See legend on opposite page*

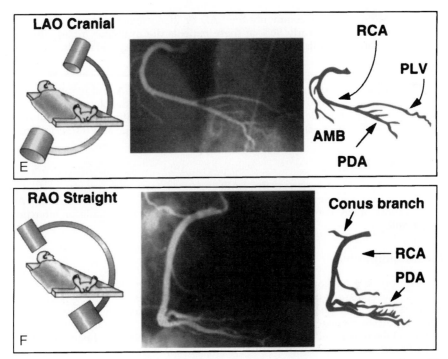

**Figure 12–2** ▪ Representative angiographic views of the left and right coronary systems are shown. The image intensifier position, as it relates to the patient, is used to describe the different views. *Left coronary artery views:* The RAO (right anterior oblique) caudal view shows the mid and distal left main (LM), the proximal left anterior descending (LAD), and most of the left circumflex (LCx) and obtuse marginal branches (OMB). The LAO (left anterior oblique) cranial view demonstrates the mid and distal LAD and its septal (S) and diagonal (D) branches, as well as the proximal LCx and its obtuse marginal branches. The LAO caudal or "spider" view shows the proximal LM and proximal LAD and LCx. The RAO cranial view demonstrates the mid and distal LAD and its S and D branches. *Right coronary artery views:* The LAO cranial view shows the body of the right coronary artery (RCA) and especially the "crux" or distal RCA bifurcation into the posterior left ventricular (PLV) and posterior descending artery (PDA) branches. The acute marginal branch (AMB) is also well seen. The RAO straight view also demonstrates the body of the RCA, the conus branch, and the mid and distal PDA. (From Bittle JA, Levin DC: Coronary arteriography. In Braunwald E (ed): Heart Disease: A Textbook of Cardiovascular Medicine, 5th ed. Philadelphia, WB Saunders, 1997.)

## Coronary Artery Anomalies

Knowledge of the commonly encountered coronary anomalies is essential to performing cardiac catheterization. Coronary anomalies are found on 1% to 1.5% of coronary angiograms[20] and are usually benign. The most common anomaly of coronary anatomy is separate origins for the LAD and LCx arteries (i.e., absence of the LMCA). This benign anomaly occurs in 0.4% to 1% of patients and may be associated with a bicuspid aortic valve. The second most common anomaly is the LCx arising from the RCA or from the right coronary sinus.

Of the clinically significant anomalies, the most common one is the LMCA or LAD arising from the right sinus of Valsalva or the RCA from the left sinus. A subset of these may course between the aorta and the pulmonary artery, predisposing to kinking and coronary insufficiency. In tetralogy of Fallot, the LAD arises from the RCA in 4% of patients.

The LMCA (and less commonly the LAD or RCA) sometimes originates from the pulmonary artery. Nearly 90% of these patients die in infancy unless there is left-to-right shunting with retrograde filling through coronary collaterals.

## Coronary Fistula

The majority of coronary artery fistulas involve the RCA and empty into the right ventricle, right atrium, or coronary sinus. Generally, the shunt is small and the patients asymptomatic. If the shunt is large, however, pulmonary hypertension, congestive failure, bacterial endocarditis, myocardial ischemia, and (rarely) rupture can occur.[21]

## Myocardial Bridging

In 5% to 12% of humans, the LAD descends from the epicardium to the submyocardium, where it is prone to systolic contraction and narrowing.[22] Although most of the coronary flow is diastolic, myocardial ischemia or infarction may result.

## Cineangiography

The primary aim of coronary angiography is lumen opacification of all segments of the epicardial coronary arteries and their branches (and any bypass grafts) in at least two orthogonal planes. Stenoses of the coronary arteries must be seen without foreshortening and without overlap of vessels. Coronary arteriography visualizes the major epicardial vessels and their second-, third-, and perhaps fourth-order branches.

### Terminology of Angiographic Views (see Fig. 12–2)

In most cardiac catheterization laboratories the x-ray tube is under the patient table and the image intensifier, with its coupled video and cinecamera, over the patient on a C-shaped arm. The angiographic projection defines the relationship between the image intensifier (II) and the patient. For example, if the II is oblique and on the patient's left, it is called *left anterior oblique* (LAO). In the caudal projection, the II is tilted toward the patient's feet. The degree of angulation of the II is noted in degrees (e.g., 45 degrees LAO, 20 degrees caudal).

### Angiographic Projections

The MCA can be considered to lie in one of two orthogonal planes. The LAD and PDA lie in the plane of the interventricular septum, and the RCA and LCx in the plane of the AV valves. Thus, the best angiographic projections to visualize these arteries in profile are the oblique views. The 60-degree LAO view looks down the plane of the interventricular septum. The 30-degree RAO looks down the plane of the AV valves, and the plane of the interventricular septum is seen en face.

Shortcomings caused by foreshortening and overlapping in the straight RAO and LAO views necessitate the addition of cranial or caudal angulation. Often, a combination of cranial or caudal and right and left oblique projections is used.

### Coronary Artery Bypass Graft Angiography

Coronary artery graft attrition and native vessel disease progression often warrant coronary and graft opacification in patients with coronary artery bypass grafts. Most aortocoronary grafts can be cannulated with a right Judkins catheter or specially designed left and right bypass catheters. Internal mammary catheters are also available for selective cannulation of the left and right internal mammary arteries. Views used to demonstrate the native vessels typically are also used for graft visualization. It is important to profile the proximal anastomosis to avoid misinterpreting poor catheter engagement as graft occlusion. The body of the graft should be seen from at least two projections. The distal anastomosis should be projected free of overlapping vessels, as it is frequently a site of stenosis. Graft occlusion must be proved by selective injection of the stump or supravalvular aortography. Unlike vein grafts, the body of the internal mammary artery is rarely affected by atherosclerosis.

## Pitfalls of Coronary Angiography

Most of the pitfalls in coronary angiography involve errors of omission whereby stenoses or anomalies are not appreciated. In this era of secondary prevention and life-prolonging coronary revascularization, failure to detect a patient's coronary disease puts him at a terrible disadvantage. Likewise, declaring coronary artery disease when none is present can lead to catastrophic medical and emotional sequelae. The most common angiographic pitfalls are listed next:

### Unrecognized LMCA Stenosis

The LMCA should be viewed in several projections with the vessel unobscured by the spine. Catheter pressure damping (a result of "wedging" into a stenosed vessel causing a damped waveform) and the absence of contrast reflux suggest the presence of ostial LMCA disease.

### Too Few Projections

Eccentric lesions and those obscured by overlap will go unnoticed unless enough projections are made.

### Inadequate Opacification

Inadequate opacification can result in streaming and give the impression of ostial stenosis, missing side branches, or thrombus. Most important, coronary stenosis may be over- or underestimated. Properly sized catheters and injection rates avoid this problem.

### Aorto-ostial Lesions

If an aorto-ostial lesion is suspected by partial ventricularization or pressure damping, injecting during withdrawal of the catheter from the ostium may be useful.

### Eccentric Stenoses

Eccentric stenoses may be missed if the short axis of the stenotic lumen is not projected (thus the need for orthogonal views).

### Failure to Recognize Occlusions

Occlusions at branch origins tend to escape detection and may be recognized only by late filling of the distal segment by collateral circulation.

## Catheter Tip–Induced Spasm

Catheter tip–induced spasm can occur at or within 1 cm of the catheter tip. It is caused by mechanical irritation and reflex contraction of the artery. Intracoronary or sublingual nitroglycerin should be given before the injection is repeated.

## Congenital Variants

Variations in the origin or distribution of the coronary branches may confuse the operator. It is useful to remember that acquired atherosclerotic coronary artery disease is far more common than unusual anatomic variants. Before an unusual vessel is accepted as a variant, an occlusion or large collateral channel should be ruled out.

## Superimposed Branches

Superimposition of branches may result in failure to recognize stenoses.

## Angiographic Assessment of Blood Flow and Lesion Quantification

Under stress conditions, normal coronary artery flow can increase three- to fourfold (coronary flow reserve of 3 to 4). With luminal diameter reductions of 50% (cross-sectional area reduction of 75%) the ability to normally increase coronary flow reserve is impaired (i.e., 50% or greater diameter narrowing is hemodynamically significant). A 70% diameter stenosis (90% cross-sectional area) makes it impossible to increase flow at all above resting level. A 90% diameter stenosis actually reduces antegrade blood flow.[23-25]

The capability of coronary angiography to quantify the degree of stenosis is limited by the fact that the image is a "lumenogram." Stenoses can be evaluated only by comparison to adjacent "reference segments," which are presumed to be disease free. The majority of arteries will have disease in the reference segment as well, however, in which case the degree of stenosis will be underestimated. In addition, vessel segments adjacent to areas of denser contrast (e.g., an overlying branch artery) are prone to perceptual artifact due to the Mach effect,[26] a consequence of the physiologic process of lateral inhibition. These neuroinhibitory interactions in the retina and central nervous system of the observer cause artery segments adjacent to the denser overlying artery to appear less dense and simulate stenosis.

To enhance quantification of vessel size, the absolute diameter of the coronary artery can be compared to the size of the diagnostic catheter. (Catheters are categorized by French size, the circumference expressed in millimeters. Each French number represents approximately 0.33 mm.) This approach to lesion quantification is limited by its dependence on visual estimation, which suffers from significant operator variability.[27] To overcome these limitations, digital calipers and quantitative coronary angiography (QCA) have been developed, as have several computer-assisted approaches to quantitative angiography.[28]

## Angiographic Assessment of Myocardial Blood Flow

The severity of the stenosis and the status of the microvasculature determine flow in the distal artery. The Thrombolysis in Myocardial Infarction (TIMI) study group first proposed a scheme for quantifying coronary perfusion (see later), which has proved useful in predicting outcome after myocardial infarction.[29] The TIMI Classification for Coronary Flow follows:

**Grade 0:** No perfusion. No antegrade flow of contrast is detected beyond the point of occlusion.

**Grade 1:** Penetration without perfusion. Contrast passes through the point of obstruction but antegrade flow fails to opacify the distal portion of the vessel at any time.

**Grade 2:** Partial perfusion. Contrast penetrates the point of obstruction but enters the distal vessel at a rate slower than that for nonobstructed arteries in the same patient.

**Grade 3:** Complete perfusion. Antegrade flow into the distal coronary bed is rapid and complete.

The mortality rate from myocardial infarction is lower in persons with TIMI grade 3 flow at 90 minutes after thrombolytic therapy than in those with less than TIMI 3 flow.[30]

TIMI frame count is also used to quantify angiographic coronary artery perfusion. An automated frame counter counts the number of cinefilm frames that elapse before the involved artery is opacified. Although TIMI frame count is more labor intensive, it is more objective and more reproducible, and correlates more closely with clinical outcomes than conventional methods.[31]

## Coronary Collateral Circulation

Collaterals usually cannot be demonstrated at coronary angiography unless the recipient vessel has developed at least 90% diameter stenosis. A common method of quantifying collateral filling is the Cohen and Rentrop grading system[32]:

**Grade 0:** No collaterals present.

**Grade 1:** Barely detectable collateral flow. Contrast medium passes through the collaterals but fails to opacify the recipient epicardial vessel at any time.

**Grade 2:** Partial collateral flow. Contrast medium enters but fails to completely opacify the target epicardial vessel.

**Grade 3:** Complete perfusion. Contrast enters and completely opacifies the target epicardial vessel.

The development and genetic manipulation of collateral formation in patients with obstructed coronary arteries is an area of intensive investigation. In some persons, collateral circulation is the only conduit for perfusion of certain myocardial territories. This very important "safety valve" for coronary obstruction has significant interpatient variability and can account for very different patient outcomes in both acute and chronic disease. In patients with total occlusions, regional LV contraction has been shown to be significantly better in segments supplied by adequate collaterals than in those with inadequate collateral circulation or none.

## Coronary Artery Spasm

Coronary spasm can play an important role in exercise-induced angina, unstable angina, acute myocardial infarction, and sudden death. Mechanisms of coronary vasospasm are varied and include abnormalities in release of nitric oxide, prostacyclin, thromboxane $A_2$, serotonin, and other endothelium-derived factors. Coronary spasm, in the absence of known atherosclerotic disease, is a well-documented potential cause of cardiac chest pain that often requires coronary arteriography for thorough evaluation (to rule out atherosclerotic narrowing and to establish the diagnosis). If provocative testing is contemplated, all vasodilators are withdrawn for at least 24 hours. Intravenous ergonovine maleate, a potent arterial vasoconstrictor with proven utility in diagnosing variant angina, is the provocative test of choice.[33] The ergonovine test is considered positive if focal spasm occurs and is associated with clinical symptoms and/or ECG ST segment changes. Induced coronary spasm is reversed by administering intracoronary nitroglycerin. The diagnostic yield of ergonovine testing depends on the population studied. Catheter tip–induced spasm should not be confused with vasospastic coronary disease.

## Abnormal Coronary Vasodilator Reserve

Some patients with angina and angiographically normal coronary arteries may have myocardial ischemia on the basis of abnormal vasodilator reserve. In these patients coronary blood flow fails to rise normally with pacing tachycardia or exercise, and the coronary vascular resistance increases abnormally.[34] A failure of small vessel coronary vasodilatation, inappropriate vasoconstriction at the arteriolar level, or functional abnormalities of capillary endothelial cells in releasing endothelium-derived relaxing factor have been postulated as pathophysiologic mechanisms. Routine coronary arteriography is poor at identifying this entity because only the epicardial vessels are visualized. Coronary flow reserve evaluation using special intracoronary Doppler flow wires can be used in this situation.

## Intravascular Ultrasonography

Although coronary angiography is considered the reference standard for coronary artery imaging, it detects only arterial disease that impinges on the luminal column of contrast medium. It reveals little else about the atherosclerotic plaque or the disease process itself. In contrast, intravascular ultrasonography (IVUS) provides tomographic assessment analogous to histologic cross sections and provides information about plaque morphology, vessel wall structure, and luminal and vessel area.[35, 36] IVUS offers the following advantages over angiography:

Clarification of angiographically equivocal or intermediate lesions. This is especially helpful with left main lesions, which can be difficult to quantitate with angiography.

Assessment of coronary stenoses before and after catheter-based coronary interventions. Balloon angioplasty is more likely to result in significant dissection if IVUS shows calcium adjacent to fibrous plaque. After balloon angioplasty, IVUS findings help to predict recurrence of stenosis. IVUS has also proven useful in ensuring adequate stent expansion and apposition to the vessel wall.

In cardiac transplant recipients, coronary artery disease is best studied by IVUS because of the diffuse nature of atherosclerosis that develops after transplantation.

## ■ LEFT VENTRICULOGRAPHY

Left ventriculography entails the opacification of the ventricle with contrast medium and is an important part of left heart catheterization. Indications for left ventriculography include assessment of LV size, wall motion abnormalities, overall systolic function (ejection fraction), and the presence and severity of mitral regurgitation.

## Assessment of Angiographic Cardiac Output

The angiographic stroke volume is the difference between end-diastolic volume (EDV) and end-systolic volume (ESV). The angiographic cardiac output can therefore be calculated as *(EDV − ESV) × Heart rate*. The inherent inaccuracies of calibrating angiographic volumes often make this method unreliable. In cases of valvular regurgitation or atrial fibrillation, angiographic cardiac output will not be accurate; however, for calculation of stenotic valve areas in patients with significant aortic and mitral regurgitation, the angiographic cardiac output is preferred over the Fick- or thermodilution-derived outputs.

## Segmental Wall Motion Analysis and Ejection Fraction

Biplanar assessment of LV wall motion provides an excellent means for assessing LV function. The segments of the left ventricle can be divided into anterobasal, anterolateral, apical, diaphragmatic, and inferobasal segments in the RAO view and into lateral, posterolateral, apical septal, and basal septal ones in the LAO view (Fig. 12–3). Wall motion is classified qualitatively as normal, mildly, moderately, and severely hypokinetic, akinetic (no systolic contraction), or dyskinetic (motion opposite to the rest of the ventricular wall in systole). Overall ejection fraction (the percentage of ventricular volume ejected during systole) is determined by computerized quantitative analysis. The most commonly used is the center line method of wall motion analysis, which uses end-diastolic and end-systolic contours to assess shortening fraction of the cardiac segments.

## Visual Assessment of Regurgitation

Valvular regurgitation can be assessed visually by determining the relative amount of contrast medium that opacifies the chamber proximal to the chamber injected. The original classification devised by Sellers[36] remains the standard in most catheterization laboratories:

**1+** Minimal regurgitant jet that clears rapidly with each beat.

**2+** Moderate opacification of proximal chamber, clearing with subsequent beats.

**3+** Intense opacification of proximal chamber, equal to that of the distal chamber.

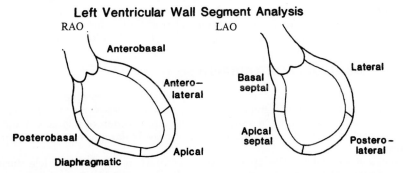

**Figure 12–3 ▪** The left ventricle, as viewed from the right anterior oblique (RAO) and left anterior oblique (LAO) views. This "biplanar" assessment allows for segmental analysis of ventricular function.

**4+** Intense opacification of proximal chamber, becoming more dense than the distal chamber. Opacification often persists over the entire series of images.

This scheme is often used to quantify mitral and aortic regurgitation. Mitral regurgitation is routinely assessed during ventriculography in the RAO view; aortic regurgitation is assessed during supravalvular aortography in LAO and RAO views. The main pitfall of this type of classification is that it does not control for different sized proximal chambers (e.g., mitral regurgitation of a given degree more completely opacifies a normal-sized left atrium than one that has undergone compensatory enlargement).

## Regurgitant Fraction

The regurgitant fraction (RF) provides a gross estimate of valvular regurgitation and, unlike visual assessment of regurgitation severity, uses angiographically derived volumes for quantification. The RF is that portion of the angiographic stroke volume that does not contribute to the net CO:

$$RF = \frac{RSV}{SV}$$

where *RSV* is regurgitant stroke volume (angiographic stroke volume − forward stroke volume), and *SV* is forward stroke volume.

The forward stroke volume is CO (as determined by the Fick or thermodilution method) divided by the heart rate. The thermodilution method should not be used in persons who have significant concomitant tricuspid regurgitation. A comparison of RF and regurgitation assessed visually follows:

RF less than 20% is equivalent to 1+ regurgitation.
RF between 21% and 40% is equivalent to 2+ regurgitation.
RF between 41% and 60% is equivalent to 3+ regurgitation.
RF greater than 60% is equivalent to 4+ regurgitation.

## Contraindications to Left Ventriculography

Ventricular opacification during ventriculography requires high-pressure injection of a significant volume of contrast medium (usually 40 ml) over a short time (usually 3 to 4 seconds). The osmolarity and vasodilatational effects of contrast introduced in this way can produce complications. Those at high risk for complications during left ventriculography include (1) severe symptomatic aortic stenosis, (2) severe congestive heart failure or angina at rest, (3) LV thrombus, especially if mobile or protruding into the LV cavity, and (4) left-sided endocarditis.

## ■ SUPRAVALVULAR AORTOGRAPHY

In 1929, Dos Santos and coworkers first described aortography[38] by direct needle puncture of the abdominal aorta. We now use peripheral arterial access, which, like ventriculography, requires high-pressure injection of a large volume of contrast over a short time. Indications for supravalvular (or root) aortography include these:

*Aortic Regurgitation.* The appearance of contrast in the left ventricle during supravalvular aortography confirms the diagnosis of AR.

*Coronary Artery Bypass Grafts:* When bypass graft location or number is not known or a "flush" proximal occlusion is suspected, supravalvular aortography can be used for nonselective graft opacification.

*Aortic Aneurysms:* Although a number of noninvasive techniques are now available, including transesophageal echocardiography, contrast CT, and magnetic resonance imaging (MRI), these modalities are not available everywhere and are sometimes contraindicated. Thoracic aortography therefore remains a widely used diagnostic tool for detecting aneurysms.

*Aortic Dissection.* Aortography can accurately identify aortic dissection by showing an intimal flap, opacification of the false lumen, and deformity of the true lumen. The choice of test (transthoracic or transesophageal echocardiography, CT, MRI, or aortography) depends on local expertise and the hemodynamic stability of the patient.

*Aortic Coarctation.* Aortography assumes an important role, as it can distinguish complete aortic interruption and hypoplastic aortic segment from the most common type of coarctation involving a stenosis at the site of the isthmus distal to the left subclavian artery. Again, centers with expertise in MRI can achieve similar diagnostic yield from that study.

## ■ SUMMARY

Invasive hemodynamic and radiographic contrast interrogation of the heart and related structures remain central to the evaluation of patients with cardiovascular disease. Many of the methods described in this chapter are the gold standard for cardiovascular assessment against which newer and less invasive tools are measured.

## ■ REFERENCES

1. Forssman W: Die Sondierung des rechlen Herzens. Klin Wochenschr 1929;8:2085.
2. Zimmerman HA, Scott RW, Becker ND: Catheterization of the left side of the heart in man. Circulation 1950;1:357.
3. Limon Lason R, Bouchard A: El cateterismo intracardico; Cateterizacion de las caridades izquierdas en el hombre intracaretanos. Arch Inst Cardiol Mexico 1950;21:271.
4. Sones FM Jr, Shirey EK, Prondfit WL, Westcott RN: Cinecoronary arteriography (abstract). Circulation 1959;20:773.
5. Sones FM Jr: Cine coronary arteriography. *In* Hurst JW, Logue RB (eds): The Heart, 2nd ed. New York: McGraw-Hill, 1970:377.
6. Favaloro RG: Saphenous vein autograft replacement of severe segmental coronary artery occlusion: Operative technique. Ann Thorac Surg 1968;5:334.
7. Gruntzig A, et al: Coronary transluminal angioplasty. Circulation 1977;56:II, 319.
8. Gruntzig A, Senning A, Siegenthaler WE: Non-operative dilation of coronary artery stenosis. Percutaneous transluminal coronary angioplasty. N Engl J Med 1979;301:61.
9. Ross J Jr, Pepine CJ, Brandenburg RO, et al: Guidelines for coronary angiography. A report of the American College of Cardiology/American Heart Association Task Force on Assessment of Diagnostic and Therapeutic Cardiovascular Procedures (Subcommittee on Coronary Angiography). J Am Coll Cardiol 1987;10:935.
10. Ryan TJ, Bauman WB, Kennedy JW, et al: Guidelines for percutaneous transluminal coronary angioplasty. A report of the AHA/ACC Task Force on Assessment of Diagnostic and Therapeutic Cardiovascular Procedures (Committee on Percutaneous Transluminal Coronary Angioplasty). Circulation 1993;88:2987–3007.
11. Roberts WC: Reasons for cardiac catheterization before cardiac valve replacement. N Engl J Med 1982;306:1291.
12. Davis K, Kennedy JW, Kemp HG, et al: Complications of coronary arteriography from the Collaborative Study of Coronary Artery Surgery (CASS). Circulation 1979;59:1105.
13. Johnson LW, Lozner EC, Johnson S, et al: Coronary arteriography 1984–1987: A report of the Registry of the Society for Cardiac Angiography and Interventions. I. Results and Complications. Cathet Cardiovasc Diagn 1989;17:5.
14. Shehadi WH: Contrast media adverse reactions: Occurrence, recurrence and distribution patterns. Radiology 1982;143:11.

15. Solomon R, Werner C, Mann D, et al: Effects of saline, mannitol, and furosemide on acute decrease in renal function induced by radiocontrast agents. N Engl J Med 1994;331:1416.
16. Fagard R, Conway J: Measurement of cardiac output: Fick principle using catheterization. Eur Heart J 1990;11:1.
17. Gorlin R, Gorlin SG: Hydraulic formula for calculation of the area of stenotic mitral valve, other cardiac valves, and central circulatory shunts. Am Heart J 1951;41:1.
18. Hakki AH: A simplified valve formula for the calculation of stenotic cardiac valve areas. Circulation 1981;63:1050.
19. Reddy PS, Curtis EI, O'Toole JD, Shaver JA: Cardiac tamponade: Hemodynamic observations in man. Circulation 1978;58:265.
20. Yamanaka O, Hoobs RE: Coronary artery anomalies in 126,595 patients undergoing coronary arteriography. Cathet Cardiovasc Diagn 1990;21:28.
21. Levin DC, Fellows KE, Abrams HL: Hemodynamically significant primary anomalies of the coronary arteries: Angiographic aspects. Circulation 1978;58:25.
22. Kramer JR, Kitazume H, Proudfit WL, Sones FM Jr: Clinical significance of isolated coronary bridges: Benign and frequent condition involving the left anterior descending artery. Am Heart J 1982;103:282.
23. Gould KL, et al: Physiologic basis for assessing critical coronary stenosis—instantaneous flow response and regional distribution during coronary hyperemia as measures of flow reserve. Am J Cardiol 1974;33:87.
24. Wilson RF, Marcus ML, White CW: Prediction of physiologic significance of coronary arterial lesions by quantitative lesion geometry in patients with limited coronary artery disease. Circulation 1987;75:723.
25. Uren NG, et al: Relation between myocardial blood flow and the severity of coronary artery stenosis. N Engl J Med 1994;330:1782.
26. Randall PA: Mach bands in cine coronary arteriography. Radiology 1978;129:65.
27. Gibson CM, Safian RD: Limitations of cineangiography—impact of new technologies for image processing and quantitation. Trends Cardiovasc Med 1992;2:156.
28. Gronenshild E, Jannsen J, Tijdent F: CAAS II—a second generation system for off-line and on-line quantitative coronary angiography. Cathet Cardiovasc Diagn 1994;33:61.
29. TIMI Study Group: The Thrombolysis in Myocardial Infarction (TIMI) trial: Phase I findings. N Engl J Med 1985;312:932.
30. The GUSTO Angiographic Investigators: The effects of tissue plasminogen activator, streptokinase, or both on coronary artery patency, ventricular function, and survival after acute myocardial infarction. N Engl J Med 1993;32:1615.
31. Gibson CM: TIMI frame count: A new standardization of infarct-related artery flow grade, and its relationship to clinical outcomes in TIMI-4 trial. Circulation 1994;90:I-220.
32. Cohen M, Rentrop P: Limitations of myocardial ischemia by collateral circulation during sudden controlled coronary artery occlusion in human subjects. Circulation 1986;74:469.
33. Heupler FA, et al: Ergonovine maleate provocative test for coronary arterial spasm. Am J Cardiol 1978;41:631.
34. Cannon RO III, Watson RM, Rosing DR, Epstein SE: Angina caused by reduced vasodilator reserve of small coronary arteries. J Am Coll Cardiol 1983;1:1359–1373.
35. Graham SP, Brands D, Sheehan H, et al: Assessment of arterial wall morphology using intravascular ultrasound in vitro and in patients. Circulation 1989;80:II-565.
36. Marco J, Fajadet J, Robert G, et al: Intracoronary ultrasound imaging: Initial clinical trials. Circulation 1989;80:II-374.
37. Sellers RD, Levy MJ, Amplatz K, Lillehei CW: Left retrograde cardioangiography in acquired cardiac disease: Technique, indications and interpretation in 700 cases. Am J Cardiol 1964;14:437.
38. Dos Santos R, Lamas AC, Pereira-Caldas J: Arteriografia da aorta e dos vasos abdominalis. Med Contemp 1929;47:93.

*Chapter* 13

# Nuclear Imaging in Cardiovascular Medicine

*Diwakar Jain* ■ *Barry L. Zaret*

Nuclear imaging techniques play an important role in the noninvasive evaluation of patients who are suspected to have coronary artery disease (CAD) or who have established disease.[1] A number of different radiopharmaceuticals and scintigraphic techniques are available that obtain important diagnostic and prognostic information about myocardial perfusion, metabolism, cardiac function, and myocardial necrosis in patients with cardiovascular disorders. In this chapter we briefly describe various cardiac nuclear imaging techniques, their applications in clinical practice, and recent developments in this field.

## ■ MYOCARDIAL PERFUSION IMAGING

Of the various techniques in nuclear cardiology, myocardial perfusion imaging is the most widely used.

### Physiologic Considerations

The basic lesion of CAD is narrowing of the lumen of a coronary artery due to deposition of atheromatous material in its walls. This complex process evolves slowly over several decades. Symptoms occur relatively late in the course of disease and appear only after significant narrowing of coronary arteries has already occurred. Coronary arterial narrowing interferes with myocardial perfusion downstream. With partial narrowing of the lumen, myocardial perfusion may be normal at rest but fails to increase appropriately during conditions of increased demand such as physical exertion or drug-induced vasodilatation. This phenomenon is the basis of myocardial perfusion imaging with physical or drug-induced stress in clinical practice.

### Radiotracers

Exercise myocardial perfusion imaging with thallium 201 ($^{201}$Tl) is the conventional imaging technique for the detection of CAD.[2] $^{201}$Tl behaves as potassium analogues do and enters the myocytes through $Na^+$-$K^+$-ATPase channels. The patient is "stressed" on a treadmill or bicycle during continuous electrocardiographic (ECG) and blood pressure monitoring, and 2 to 3 mCi of $^{201}$Tl is injected intravenously at peak exercise. Within the next few minutes, $^{201}$Tl is extracted from the blood pool by the myocardium, skeletal muscle, and several organs. Approximately 2% to 4% of the injected dose of $^{201}$Tl goes to the myocardium. Myocardial uptake is proportional to regional blood flow. Cardiac imaging is begun soon after the exercise. Myocardial segments perfused by narrowed coronary arteries or scarred from prior myocardial infarction (MI) show diminished tracer uptake on these images. [201]Tl shows continuous redistribution after the initial tissue extraction. Stress images are followed by redistribution images 2 1/2 to 4 hours later to detect reversibility in the segments that demonstrated stress-related perfusion abnormality. Perfusion abnormality due to ischemia reverses on redistribution images, whereas that due to scar remains unchanged. Sometimes, scar and ischemia affect the same segments in patients with a history of MI. This condition is characterized by partial reversibility of the perfusion abnormality. Stress [201]Tl imaging has a sensitivity of nearly 85% to 92% and specificity of 90% or better for the detection of CAD,[1, 3] although the redistribution of [201]Tl is somewhat unreliable and unpredictable. In a significant proportion of defects due to ischemia, [201]Tl redistribution may be incomplete.[4] Thus, standard stress-redistribution [201]Tl imaging may underestimate the true extent of myocardial ischemia or viability. A number of different strategies have been proposed to overcome this limitation.[5] A second injection of [201]Tl with the patient at rest, given on the same day or another day, appears to be the most satisfactory way of overcoming this limitation in certain cases.[4-7] Giving this second injection of [201]Tl routinely to all patients, regardless of the presence or absence of perfusion abnormalities on the stress images, is unnecessary and inadvisable.

Although [201]Tl has been in clinical use for nearly two decades, it has several limitations. It has a long physical half-life (approximately 3 days), which limits the dose that can safely be used without causing undue radiation exposure to the patient. Furthermore, [201]Tl emits low-energy photons (69 to 83 keV) that can easily be attenuated by the thoracic wall and the soft tissue lying anterior to the heart. Because the attenuation can be particularly troublesome in obese patients and women, a number of technetium 99m ([99m]Tc)–labeled myocardial perfusion agents have been developed. [99m]Tc has a shorter half-life (approximately 6 hours) and emits slightly higher-energy photons (140 keV), and its chemical structure allows it to be incorporated into a number of different chemicals or ligands, which can be used to study the anatomy, perfusion, and metabolism of various organs. [99m]Tc-labeled agents can be used in much higher doses and provide better-quality images. Three agents are approved by the FDA: sestamibi (Cardiolite, Du Pont Pharmaceuticals, N. Billenca, MA), teboroxime (Cardiotech, Bracco Inc., Princeton, NJ), and tetrofosmin (Myoview, Nycomed-Amersham Inc., Princeton, NJ).[8-11] Sestamibi and tetrofosmin, the two [99m]Tc-labeled agents in clinical use, are lipophilic cationic agents. They are taken up by the myocardium because of their lipophilia and positive charge. Their myocardial uptake is not mediated by the $Na^+$ $K^+$-ATPase pump. In the myocytes, these agents are localized mainly in the mitochondria. They are tightly bound to the myocardium and show little or no redistribution after initial cardiac uptake. Therefore, two separate injections are required for stress and for rest imaging. Teboroxime is a neutral compound and shows very rapid washout after initial myocardial uptake. Because of this drawback, this agent is not currently in clinical use. Another new [99m]Tc-labeled agent, N-Noet (Cis Bio International, France), is undergoing clinical evaluation but is not yet available for routine use.[12] Table 13–1 gives a summary of different myocardial perfusion imaging agents.

Other advantages of [99m]Tc-labeled agents are that first-pass imaging can also be carried out during injection of the radiotracer during stress and rest.[13] The images can also be gated to the ECG, a strategy that can provide information about left and right ventricular function. Thus, it is possible to obtain information about myocardial perfusion and cardiac function with a single test. Both [99m]Tc-sestamibi and [99m]Tc-tetrofosmin suffer from several limitations, however: excessive liver and gastrointestinal uptake can degrade the image quality, and relatively low first-pass myocardial extraction has the potential to produce underestimation of myocardial

Table 13–1

**Salient Features of Agents for Myocardial Perfusion Imaging**

| Agent | Physical Half-Life (hr) | Chemical Structure | Site of Myocellular Localization | Myocardial Retention | Redis-tribution | Main Route of Excretion |
|---|---|---|---|---|---|---|
| [201]Tl | 72 | Element | Cytosol | Good | Yes | Renal |
| [99m]Tc-sestamibi | 6 | Isonitrile | Mitochondria | Good | Minimal | Hepatobiliary |
| [99m]Tc-tetrofosmin | 6 | Diphosphine | Mitochondria | Good | None | Hepatobiliary/renal |
| [99m]Tc-N-Noet* | 6 | Dithio-carbamate | Sarcolemma | Good | Yes | Unknown |

*Not approved by FDA for routine clinical use.

ischemia. An ideal $^{99m}$Tc myocardial perfusion tracer should have little or no hepatic and gastrointestinal uptake and should have a high first-pass myocardial extraction that tracks myocardial blood flow linearly over a wide range.

## Instrumentation

Myocardial perfusion imaging can be done with a planar camera or a tomographic camera (single-photon emission computed tomography or SPECT). With a planar camera, images are made in three views: anterior, left anterior oblique, and left lateral (Fig. 13–1). For SPECT imaging, a series of 32 to 64 images are acquired in a 180- to 360-degree orbit around the heart. These images are processed much as CT images are, so left ventricular myocardium is displayed in a series of slices of varying thickness (Figs. 13–2, 13–3). Planar imaging equipment is simpler and less expensive than SPECT cameras, and imaging can be carried out at the bedside. SPECT cameras are available with one, two, or three heads. Double and triple heads reduce the imaging time. Although both techniques have comparable sensitivity for the detection of CAD, SPECT imaging, particularly with $^{99m}$Tc-labeled agents, affords better anatomic delineation of the perfusion abnormalities and better angiographic correlation. The SPECT images can be gated with ECG (gated SPECT), and left ventricular regional wall motion, thickening, and ejection fraction can be assessed from the same study. Thus, myocardial perfusion and function can be assessed from a single study. Since myocardial ischemia and left ventricular function are the two most important determinants of optimal therapy and short-term (and long-term) prognosis, gated SPECT perfusion imaging is currently the single most powerful diagnostic and prognostic modality in cardiovascular medicine. Because of these advantages, gated SPECT imaging is currently preferred over planar imaging. Soft tissue attenuation, another major source of artifacts in myocardial perfusion imaging, can potentially be corrected with an appropriate attenuation-correction program. This is discussed in more detail in the section on Interpretation of the Perfusion Images.

## Choice of Stress

Exercise stress testing is the preferred method—in the United States, treadmill exercise, and in Europe, bicycle exercise. When exercise first-pass imaging is planned, bicycle exercise should be used. Patient motion during treadmill exercise precludes the acquisition of any meaningful first-pass imaging data without the

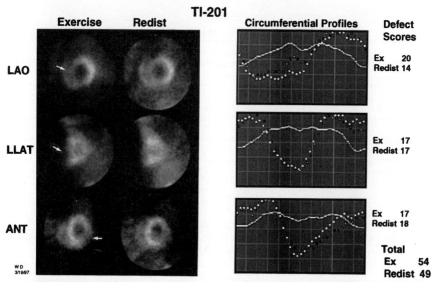

**Figure 13–1** ■ Standard three-view planar exercise (Ex) and redistribution (Redist) Tl 201 images and corresponding quantitative circumferential profiles of a 51-year-old man with a history of anterior wall MI. A large defect that involves the interventricular septum, anterior wall, and apex (*arrows*) is predominantly fixed with minimal reversibility in the apex. On the circumferential profiles (derived by plotting the average activity in 36 radial sectors of the myocardium after background subtraction), the solid white line corresponds to the normal reference value, the dotted white line represents the profile of stress images, and the dotted black line represents the profile of redistribution images. The defect scores represent the area between the patient's profile and the normal reference range and provides a quantitative estimate of the defect's size and reversibility. (LAO, left anterior oblique view; LLAT, left lateral view; ANT, anterior view.)

use of a complex motion-correction algorithm. Information about exercise capacity, changes in heart rate and blood pressure, adverse symptoms such as chest pain and undue fatigue, and ECG changes such as the magnitude and duration of ST-segment depression and arrhythmias are important clinically.

For patients who are unable to perform any kind of exercise because of severe peripheral vascular disease, musculoskeletal disorders, or pulmonary disease, pharmacologic agents can be used for myocardial perfusion imaging. Dipyridamole and adenosine are most widely used for this purpose.[14–16] Following intravenous administration, these agents cause marked coronary vasodilatation and can increase myocardial blood flow to 3 or 4 times the resting flow, although the increase is blunted in the myocardial segments that are perfused by narrowed coronary arteries. This produces flow heterogeneity and results in apparent perfusion abnormalities on the perfusion images. True ischemia is rare and occurs in association with severe CAD when collateral circulation contributes much to myocardial perfusion. Dipyridamole and adenosine may induce a coronary steal in such cases. At the cellular level, dipyridamole inhibits intracellular uptake of adenosine. Thus, adenosine is more direct-acting than dipyridamole and has more predictable effects on coronary blood flow.[16] Adenosine has an extremely short half-life, and its side effects are transient. Side effects are common with dipyridamole or adenosine infusion but generally are minor and self-limiting.[17] The most common side effects are nausea, headache, flushing of the face, and hypotension. Transient high-grade atrioventricular block can also occur with adenosine infusion. Chest pain occurs in

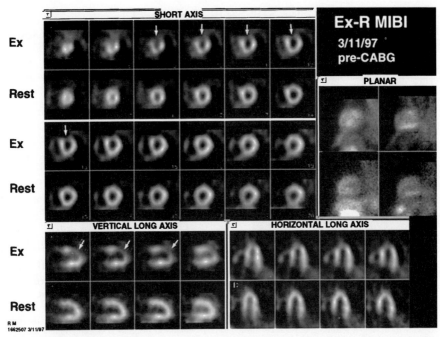

**Figure 13–2** ■ Exercise (Ex) and rest Tc 99m sestamibi images of a 63-year-old man with CAD who underwent three-vessel CABG 18 years earlier and presented with recurrent angina. The patient developed angina and 1-mm ST-segment depression on exercise. A moderate-sized area of perfusion abnormality involving the anterior wall (*arrows*) is reversible on rest imaging. On coronary angiography, the patient had severe disease of all three native vessels, the vein graft to the left anterior coronary artery was completely occluded, and the other two grafts were also diseased. The patient underwent repeat CABG. A follow-up exercise perfusion study 1 year later was normal.

approximately 25% of cases but is not specific for myocardial ischemia. The exact mechanism of dipyridamole- or adenosine-induced chest pain is not clear. Perhaps the drugs act directly on the pain receptors. ST segment depression is rare, but, when it occurs it is indicative of severe CAD. When possible, dipyridamole or adenosine infusion should be combined with low-level exercise.[18, 19] This reduces some of the adverse effects, such as hypotension and flushing, and also reduces radiotracer uptake in the liver and other splanchnic organs to improve image quality. Adding light exercise to adenosine infusion also improves sensitivity and specificity for the detection of CAD.[20] Theophylline derivatives, including caffeine, act as antagonists of dipyridamole and adenosine at the cellular level, and the patient should stop using them in preparation for dipyridamole or adenosine stress perfusion imaging. Aminophylline can be given intravenously if the side effects of dipyridamole are persistent and bother the patient. Because of the extremely short half-life, side effects of adenosine generally disappear on discontinuation of the infusion, and aminophylline is only very rarely required. Figure 13–3 is an example of markedly abnormal adenosine-[99m]Tc sestamibi study.

Intravenous dobutamine can also be used for stress imaging.[21] This acts by increasing heart rate and myocardial oxygen demand. It can be used when dipyridamole or adenosine is contraindicated, as for patients who have severe bronchopulmonary disease or congestive heart failure or who may not stop taking theophylline. Arbutamine is a dobutamine analogue that produces a greater chronotropic

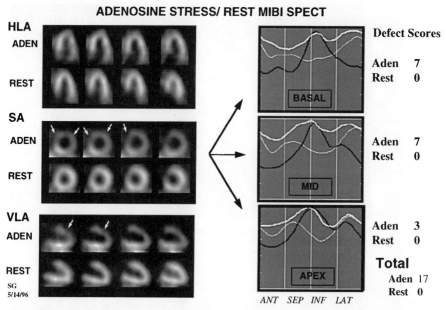

**Figure 13–3** ■ Adenosine stress (ADEN) and rest (REST) Tc 99m sestamibi SPECT images of an 80-year-old woman during a routine preoperative cardiovascular evaluation prior to knee replacement surgery. The patient developed chest pain and 2 mm of ST-segment depression during adenosine infusion. The images are displayed in standard horizontal long axis (HLA), short axis (SA), and vertical long axis (VLA) with circumferential profiles of the three representative short axis slices at apical, midventricular, and basal levels. The solid thin white line represents the normal reference range, the solid black line the myocardial activity in the stress images, and the bold white line the activity in the rest images. There is a large area of anterior, septal, and lateral ischemia (*arrows*) and transient stress-induced left ventricular dilatation. The defect scores represent the area between the patient's profile and the normal reference range and correspond to the percentage of the myocardium with abnormality. This is a high-risk, abnormal study. Coronary angiography showed a 99% left mainstem lesion and a 90% right coronary artery lesion. The patient underwent CABG followed by knee replacement surgery and had an uneventful postoperative course.

response than dobutamine, but its sensitivity and specificity for the detection of perfusion abnormalities are similar to those of dobutamine.[22] Table 13–2 lists various pharmaceuticals for myocardial perfusion imaging and their important characteristics. For myocardial perfusion imaging, adenosine or dipyridamole is preferred over dobutamine or arbutamine because they produce greater increases in myocardial blood flow and flow heterogeneity.

## Interpretation of the Perfusion Images

Interpretation of myocardial perfusion images requires experience, skill, and adequate understanding of cardiac physiology, pathology, and applied physics and awareness of the possible sources of artifacts. Both planar and SPECT imaging are prone to artifacts that are due to attenuation from the structures overlying the heart or near to it. Diaphragm and liver can attenuate the inferior wall. Women's breasts can also cause attenuation. Proximity of the liver to the inferior wall of the heart is another important source of artifacts. Tracer activity in the liver can result in artifactually higher counts in the inferior wall due to scattered counts. Conversely, during image reconstruction, oversubtraction of counts from the structures close to

Table 13–2

**Agents for Pharmacologic Stress Perfusion Imaging**

| Agent | Mode of Action | Effect on Heart Rate | Effect on Systolic Blood Pressure | Effect on Double Product |
|---|---|---|---|---|
| Dipyridamole | Coronary vasodilatation | Slight increase | Decrease | Minimal change |
| Adenosine | Coronary vasodilatation | Slight increase | Decrease | Minimal change |
| Dobutamine | Increased myocardial oxygen demand | Significant increase | Increase or no change | Increase |
| Arbutamine | Increased myocardial oxygen demand | Significant increase | Increase or no change | Increase |

the hot liver can result in artifactually lower counts in the inferior wall. SPECT imaging is prone to a variety of other artifacts, such as patient motion during imaging and tracer activity in the gut and other subdiaphragmatic structures. $^{99m}$Tc sestamibi and $^{99m}$Tc tetrofosmin produce high activity in the liver, gallbladder, and gut, particularly in rest and pharmacologic stress images. Sometimes, bowel loops with significant radiotracer activity may overlap the heart and substantially degrade image quality; in the worst case, they render the images uninterpretable. If bowel loops with radioactivity are seen to overlap the heart, image acquisition should be aborted and recommenced a few minutes later after repositioning the patient. Feeding fatty food before imaging does not enhance clearance of radiotracer from the liver. On the other hand, it can increase the amount of radioactivity in the gut because of dumping of gallbladder activity in the gut. Artifacts can also appear during various stages of processing of the raw data.

Great care is required to avoid misinterpreting the images because of these artifacts.[23] A number of techniques are currently under development for the correction of attenuation artifacts during SPECT imaging. Attenuation is nonuniform, being dependent on the density and thickness of the tissue around the heart. A three-dimensional spatial map of attenuation coefficients is obtained using an external transmission source. These attenuation maps are unique for each patient and are used to correct the emission images. This is a complex process, however, and still in a relatively early stage of development.[24, 25]

The perfusion images can be interpreted visually, but quantitative analysis is more reliable. Subtle abnormalities can be better appreciated with quantitative analysis, which can be performed with a simple circumferential analysis program or with a polar map. To obtain a circumferential profile, a region of interest is drawn around the cardiac contour, the myocardium is divided into 36 radial sectors, and the counts in these sectors are plotted and compared with the normal database (see Fig. 13–1). This approach can be used for planar and for SPECT images. In a polar plot, the short-axis myocardial slices from SPECT images are displayed as a series of concentric rings in a single display. The rings are displayed on a color scale, so that the myocardial segments with abnormally low radiotracer uptake are shown in a different color than the normal myocardium. Quantitative analysis can also provide an estimate of the extent or severity of myocardial ischemia, which is important if serial studies are used to follow the progress of disease. Quantitative analysis also minimizes the intra- and interobserver variability of the image interpretation.[23]

A systematic approach is required for comprehensive interpretation of myocardial perfusion studies. The raw images should be examined for any potential sources of artifacts. The patient's gender, body weight and habitus, the radiopharmaceutical and its dose, the interval between tracer injection and imaging, and the type of stress used should be taken into consideration while viewing the raw images. With [201]Tl, the lung fields should be examined for evidence of increased lung tracer uptake on stress images, an indicator of a high-risk study. The processed images should be interpreted qualitatively as well as quantitatively. Clinical history, pretest likelihood of CAD, details of stress testing, and ECG changes should be taken into consideration while performing the final interpretation.

## Clinical Applications of Myocardial Perfusion Imaging

### Detection of Coronary Artery Disease

Myocardial perfusion imaging is useful for establishing the diagnosis of CAD in patients who present with chest pain or when clinical suspicion of CAD is strong because of the presence of one or more risk factors. Myocardial perfusion imaging is an important noninvasive test for identifying who should be considered for further invasive studies. Adding myocardial perfusion imaging to exercise ECG increases the sensitivity and the specificity of the test for CAD.[26] The sensitivity and specificity of exercise ECG alone for CAD are 50% to 60% and 60%, respectively, whereas myocardial perfusion imaging has a sensitivity of 85% to 90% and specificity of 90% or better. Myocardial perfusion imaging has particular advantages over exercise ECG in patients with left ventricular hypertrophy, left bundle or such block, or another abnormality and those who are taking digoxin, as any of these could interfere with proper interpretation of ST segment changes on exercise. Myocardial perfusion imaging is an important and cost-effective gatekeeper for identifying who should undergo further invasive cardiac workup.[27] In a study of more than 4000 patients who underwent stress myocardial perfusion imaging for evaluation of CAD, the subsequent cardiac catheterization rates over a mean follow-up period of 9 months were 32% in those with reversible perfusion abnormality and only 3.5% in those without reversible perfusion abnormality.[28] Furthermore, in the reversible perfusion abnormality group, the cardiac catheterization rate was 60% for those with high-risk studies (reversible perfusion abnormality of the left anterior descending coronary artery territory, multiple areas of ischemia, or increased lung [201]Tl uptake) as compared with 9% for the remaining patients with reversible perfusion abnormalities. The findings of myocardial perfusion imaging were far more predictive of subsequent cardiac catheterization than were clinical and treadmill exercise ECG variables, alone or in combination, a fact that indicates the important role of stress myocardial perfusion imaging in the initial evaluation for suspected CAD.

### Risk Stratification

Information about the severity, location, and extent of myocardial ischemia is useful for risk stratification of patients known to have CAD. Large or multiple areas of perfusion abnormality identify patients at high risk for cardiovascular events on follow-up. Increased lung [201]Tl uptake and transient left ventricular dilatation on stress images are indicative of severe CAD and are predictive of poor prognosis.[29, 30] Both of these findings are due to transient left ventricular dysfunction during stress. The magnitude of ST depression on symptom-limited exercise testing does not correlate with the extent of ischemia on [201]Tl scintigraphy.[31] Of various clinical and laboratory variables, including ECG and coronary angiographic findings, myocardial perfusion imaging provides the most powerful prognostic information for all groups of patients with CAD. Patients with a negative myocardial perfusion study have an excellent prognosis and in several large clinical studies have been shown to have an annual cardiac event rate less than 1%.[32, 33] A normal myocardial perfusion study, even in the presence of angiographically documented CAD, is associated with excellent long-term prognosis and a very low incidence of cardiac events on follow-up.[34]

## Post–Myocardial Infarction Evaluation

Submaximal stress perfusion imaging is an established technique for risk stratification before hospital discharge of patients with uncomplicated MI.[35] Patients with fixed defects have a low incidence of adverse cardiac events, whereas those with reversible defects have a higher incidence. This test can be used to identify patients with recent MI who can benefit from cardiac catheterization and revascularization. The currently routine use of thrombolysis to reduce the infarct's size and subsequent identification of residual myocardial ischemia and appropriate treatment are largely responsible for substantial reductions in in-hospital mortality and 1-year mortality in recent years.

## Early Triage of Patients with Chest Pain of Unknown Origin

Resting myocardial perfusion imaging is being used increasingly for early triage of patients who have acute chest pain that arouses suspicion of myocardial ischemia but who exhibit no diagnostic ECG changes or enzymatic evidence of acute MI at presentation.[36, 37] Technetium $^{99m}$–labeled agents (tetrofosmin and sestamibi) are more suitable in this setting. These radiotracers can be injected soon after the patient presents to the emergency room. The images can be acquired after more detailed evaluation and stabilization of the patient. Because there is no significant redistribution, these images would reflect myocardial perfusion at the time of radiotracer injection and would not be affected by the subsequent treatment. Perfusion abnormalities in the absence of prior MI are indicative of an acute coronary syndrome and warrant admission to the coronary care unit and appropriate treatment. Absence of perfusion abnormalities points more toward a noncardiac cause of chest pain. Patients with negative resting perfusion images can undergo stress perfusion imaging within a short time to search for exercise-induced myocardial ischemia. This approach can significantly reduce the duration of the hospital stay and the number of admissions to the coronary care units and associated costs for the management of patients with chest pain of uncertain cause. Myocardial perfusion imaging is a potentially important tool for (the recently emerging) chest pain centers. Theoretically, in the context of acute chest pain suspected to be of cardiac origin, resting myocardial perfusion imaging may have some advantage over serial cardiac enzyme assays and other noninvasive tests, because myocardial perfusion imaging has the potential to identify acute MI and unstable angina, both of which warrant admission to the coronary care unit. Figure 13–4 shows a proposed scheme for the utilization of myocardial perfusion imaging in chest pain centers.

Serial myocardial perfusion imaging at rest has also been used to study the efficacy of thrombolytic agents in reducing the size of myocardial infarcts and the relationship between "area at risk" and final infarct size after various interventions.[38, 39] In these studies, $^{99m}$Tc sestamibi was injected as soon as possible into patients who presented with acute MI. Thrombolytic agents were administered next, without delay. Myocardial perfusion imaging was carried out several hours later, when the patient was more comfortable and stable and had received appropriate treatment. These images showed myocardial perfusion at the time of presentation, before any treatment was rendered. A second dose of $^{99m}$Tc sestamibi was injected 24 to 48 hours later, and these images showed myocardial perfusion after thrombolysis. The difference in the extent and severity of perfusion abnormalities

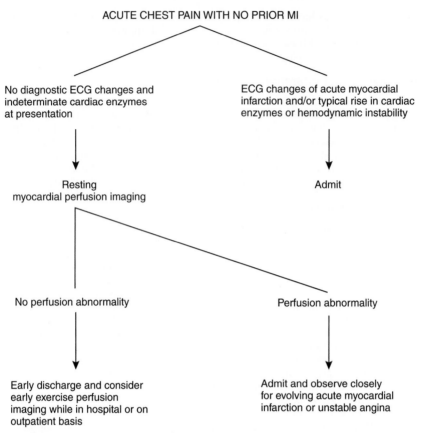

**Figure 13–4** ▪ A schematic representation of the proposed algorithm for early triage of patients who present with acute chest pain using myocardial perfusion imaging.

between these two sets of images was directly related to the efficacy of the treatment. These studies have greatly enhanced our understanding of the dynamics of myocardial salvage and functional recovery in patients with acute MI.

## Risk Stratification Prior to Noncardiac Surgery

Adverse cardiac events are an important cause of morbidity and mortality after noncardiac surgery, particularly in elderly patients and in those with known CAD or with risk factors for it.[40] Appropriate use of nuclear imaging techniques can significantly lower the incidence of this complication. The frequency of occurrence of adverse cardiac events in the perioperative period depends on a number of factors: the prevalence and severity of CAD and left ventricular dysfunction in this patient population and the nature and severity of hemodynamic stress during the perioperative period. Patients with a high prevalence of CAD (symptomatic or occult) and impaired left ventricular function are particularly vulnerable to cardiac events. Prolonged vascular surgery involving cross-clamping of the aorta, major shifts between intravascular and extravascular fluid compartments, and hypotension impose significant stress on the cardiovascular system and can result in arrhythmias, pulmonary edema, or MI in the perioperative period in patients with CAD. Patients with peripheral vascular disease have a high prevalence of CAD and are at a high risk for perioperative cardiac events. Even after peripheral vascular surgery, these patients continue to be at very high risk of morbidity and death from a cardiac event.[41] A number of studies have established the role of pharmaceutical stress perfusion imaging in identifying patients at high risk for perioperative cardiac events.[14, 42] Dipyridamole or adenosine is particularly suitable because of the inability of these patients to exercise (see Fig. 13–3). Abnormalities of dipyridamole perfusion imaging are predictive not only of perioperative morbidity and mortality but also of long-term mortality and morbidity.[43]

## Detection of Myocardial Viability

The impairment in left ventricular function and regional wall motion abnormalities in many patients with CAD may be reversible to some extent with proper utilization of revascularization procedures. Such interventions can improve left ventricular function, ameliorate symptoms of heart failure, and improve the prognosis, and they have the potential to avoid or delay cardiac transplantation for some patients with advanced heart failure. Identification of viable but dysfunctional myocardium that has the potential to recover contractility and left ventricular dynamics and distinguishing it from the irreversibly scarred myocardium that has no potential for recovery of function poses a major challenge in the practice of cardiology. Symptoms, clinical examination, ECG, and conventional techniques for functional assessment often are not helpful. A number of techniques, such as dobutamine echocardiography and magnetic resonance imaging, have been employed with varying success, but nuclear imaging techniques, both conventional perfusion imaging and positron emission tomography (PET), have played crucial roles in this field.[4] Myocardial uptake and retention or washout of perfusion tracers is dependent upon the structural and metabolic integrity of the myocytes. Rest-redistribution $^{201}$Tl imaging can be used to detect myocardial viability. Significant myocardial uptake on quantitative analysis (at least 50% greater uptake than in normal myocardial segments) or redistribution on delayed imaging is indicative of myocardial viability and predictive of functional improvement after revascularization in abnormal myocardial segments.[44] Resting $^{99m}$Tc sestamibi or $^{99m}$Tc tetrofosmin can also provide information about myocardial viability via a quantitative approach. Uptake of at least 50% of $^{99m}$Tc sestamibi or $^{99m}$Tc tetrofosmin in abnormal myocardial segments is predictive of myocardial viability.[45] Recent findings indicate a promising role for nitrate administration before injection of myocardial perfusion imaging tracers for the detection of myocardial viability. Viable myocardial segments with resting hypoperfusion show improvement in perfusion after nitrate administration, and this change is predictive of functional improvement after revascularization.[46] PET imaging techniques for myocardial viability are based on the demonstration of metabolic activity in the dysfunctional myocardial segments. This is described later in this chapter. Table 13–3 provides a summary of the indications for myocardial perfusion imaging and the best imaging techniques and radiotracers for each indication.

## ■ ASSESSMENT OF LEFT VENTRICULAR FUNCTION

Although a number of techniques—echocardiography, contrast ventriculography, magnetic resonance imaging—can be used to assess ventricular function, nuclear imaging techniques offer a distinct advantage in several clinical situations. With nuclear imaging techniques, left ventricular function can be assessed by first-pass imaging, equilibrium radionuclide angiocardiography, or gated SPECT.

Table 13–3

**Indications for Myocardial Perfusion Imaging and the Most Appropriate Techniques and Radiotracers**

| Indication | Technique | Radiotracer* |
|---|---|---|
| Detection of CAD | Exercise SPECT | $^{201}$Tl or $^{99m}$Tc tracers ($^{99m}$Tc tracers for women and overweight men) |
| Risk stratification with known CAD | Gated exercise-rest SPECT | $^{99m}$Tc tracers |
| Post-MI evaluation | Gated exercise-rest SPECT | $^{99m}$Tc tracers |
| Acute chest pain of uncertain origin | Gated rest SPECT | $^{99m}$Tc tracers |
| Evaluation before noncardiac surgery | Gated pharmacologic stress-rest SPECT | $^{99m}$Tc tracers |
| Detection of myocardial viability | Rest-redistribution SPECT or gated rest SPECT (preferably with nitrates) | $^{201}$Tl or $^{99m}$Tc tracers |

$^{99m}$Tc tracers: $^{99m}$Tc sestamibi or $^{99m}$Tc tetrofosmin.

## First-Pass Imaging

First-pass imaging is dynamic imaging of the passage of radioactive tracer from the superior vena cava to the right heart and lungs and then to the left heart after a bolus of tracer is injected into a peripheral vein. Right and left ventricular ejection fractions can be calculated from these data. An important advantage of the newer $^{99m}$Tc-labeled myocardial perfusion imaging agents is that dynamic first-pass imaging can be carried out during injection of these agents, either at rest or during exercise. Thus, information about perfusion and function can be obtained with a single injection of radiopharmaceutical.[13] The widespread use of $^{99m}$Tc-labeled myocardial perfusion imaging agents in current clinical practice has revived interest in first-pass imaging. Adding first-pass imaging provides incremental diagnostic and prognostic information to supplement the exercise perfusion findings.[47]

## Equilibrium Radionuclide Angiocardiography

Equilibrium radionuclide angiocardiography (ERNA) is performed by labeling the blood pool with $^{99m}$Tc pertechnetate, which, when injected after the administration of pyrophosphate, binds to red blood cells. The ECG-gated images of the heart are acquired in three standard views (anterior, left anterior oblique, left lateral) to assess the left ventricular wall motion and to calculate left ventricular ejection fraction. A time-activity curve reflecting the temporal changes in left ventricular volumes during the cardiac cycle can also be obtained from these images. From this curve, left ventricular ejection fraction can be calculated. The slopes of this curve during rapid ejection phase in systole and during the rapid filling phase in diastole provide the peak ejection and peak filling rates. Left ventricular ejection fraction (LVEF) is the most widely used index of left ventricular function. SPECT imaging can also be used with equilibrium radionuclide angiocardiography. This may provide a more detailed assessment of regional left ventricular function; however, so far, this technique has found only limited acceptance. With the wider acceptance of gated SPECT myocardial perfusion imaging, this is likely to become the most widely used technique for determining LVEF in patients with CAD.

In patients with CAD, LVEF is an important determinant of long-term prognosis.[48] Measurement of LVEF also has important therapeutic implications in patients with CAD. Progressive spontaneous deterioration of LVEF occurs with moderately impaired LVEF (<40%) due to ventricular remodeling. This process can be arrested by appropriate use of angiotensin-converting enzyme inhibitors.[49]

Serial LVEF monitoring is also useful for the prevention of overt heart failure in cancer patients undergoing chemotherapy with anthracyclines. Congestive heart failure is the most important complication of doxorubicin and other anthracycline derivatives. However, anthracycline-induced congestive heart failure is preceded by progressive deterioration in left ventricular function, which, in the initial stages is asymptomatic but nevertheless provides an opportunity for the prevention of overt heart failure by discontinuation of anthracyclines at an early stage with only a subclinical manifestation of left ventricular dysfunction. This requires a highly reliable, reproducible, and accurate technique for serial monitoring of left ventricular function. Because of its high reproducibility and accuracy, ERNA is ideal for detecting changes in LVEF early in the course of doxorubicin chemotherapy. In contrast, echocardiography provides an approximation of LVEF, which may be suboptimal for detecting early changes in that variable on serial studies. With the appropriate use of guidelines for performing serial ERNA in various subsets of patients, it is possible to reduce the incidence of doxorubicin-induced congestive heart failure from 20% to 2% to 3%.[50-53]

## Exercise Equilibrium Radionuclide Angiocardiography

ERNA can also be carried out during exercise. Initially this was used to detect CAD, but owing to widespread use of myocardial perfusion imaging, ERNA is rarely used these days for that purpose. ERNA has also been used for the risk stratification of patients known to have CAD. A significant drop in LVEF with exercise is indicative of poor prognosis despite preserved LVEF at baseline.[54] Currently, dynamic first-pass imaging during injection of $^{99m}$Tc tracers has largely replaced exercise ERNA.

## Left Ventricular Volumes and Pressure Volume Relations

From ERNA findings, absolute left ventricular end-diastolic, end-systolic, and stroke volumes can also be measured.[55] When the heart rate and blood pressure are known, it is possible to measure cardiac output and peripheral vascular resistance. Thus, a comprehensive assessment of hemodynamic status can be obtained with ERNA. Recently, ERNA has been used in conjunction with a forearm Doppler-based device for indirect measurement of the ascending aortic pressure, to study the pressure-volume based indices of left ventricular contractility.[56] This appears to be a promising technique for studying intrinsic left ventricular contractility and left ventricular contractile reserve.[57]

## Ambulatory Left Ventricular Function Monitoring

Ambulatory function monitoring is unique to nuclear imaging of the heart. A combination of ERNA plus Holter monitoring makes possible continuous ambulatory monitoring of left ventricular function over several hours.[58] This device uses a miniature radiation detector that is positioned on the chest after blood pool labeling with $^{99m}$Tc-pertechnetate and that monitors and records left ventricular blood pool activity on a modified Holter monitor. The technique has been used for studying the effects of "interventions" such as mental stress on left ventricular function and for detecting spontaneous changes in left ventricular function in patients with CAD.[59] Figure 13–5 shows LVEF, heart rate, and relative end-diastolic and end-systolic volume trends at baseline, all in response to mental stress and to exercise in a patient with chronic stable CAD. In response to two different forms of mental stress, this patient showed a significant drop in ejection fraction that was not

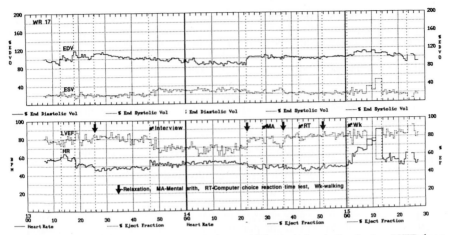

**Figure 13–5** ■ Continuous data trend over 2.5 hours of left ventricular ejection fraction (LVEF), heart rate (HR; *lower panel*), and relative end-diastolic (EDV) and end-systolic (ESV) volumes (*upper panel*) for a patient with chronic stable angina. The EF and HR are normal at baseline. After a period of stabilization, the patient underwent a psychological interview (Interview). This was accompanied by a minimal increase in HR, a significant fall in EF, and an increase in ESV. Mental arithmetic, another form of mental stress, produced similar changes. In contrast, computer choice reaction time, a nonstressful task, produced no changes in EF or HR. Walking resulted in an increase in HR but no change in EF.

accompanied by any symptoms or ST segment depression. A recent study indicates that mental stress–induced left ventricular dysfunction is predictive of adverse cardiac events in patients with chronic stable angina.[60] Figure 13–6 shows the incidence of adverse cardiac events over 1 year in CAD patients, with and without mental stress–induced left ventricular dysfunction. Spontaneous episodes of left ventricular dysfunction can be detected by ambulatory left ventricular function monitoring in patients with non–Q wave MI, unstable angina, and Q-wave MI treated with thrombolytic agents. Preliminary studies have shown, that, in patients with acute MI treated with thrombolytic agents, episodes of spontaneous left ventricular dysfunction are predictive of poor prognosis.[61]

## ■ MYOCARDIAL NECROSIS IMAGING

Technetium 99m pyrophosphate was used in the 1970s and 1980s for imaging acute myocardial necrosis, but, owing to several technical drawbacks, it is used very rarely these days. Indium 111 ([111]In)–labeled fraction of antibody (Fab) against cardiac myosin ([111]In antimyosin; Centocor) is highly selective for imaging the necrotic myocardium.[62] This has high sensitivity and specificity for diagnosing acute MI. [111]In antimyosin imaging can be used for confirming the diagnosis of acute MI in patients with atypical clinical presentations or when ECG changes are absent or unreliable for diagnosing acute MI.[63] Because of its slow clearance from the blood pool and slow localization in the necrotic myocardium, however, an interval of 24 to 48 hours is needed between [111]In antimyosin injection and imaging. This significantly limits the clinical utility of the technique for the detection of acute MI. It is more useful for diagnosing acute myocarditis and for detecting cardiac transplant rejection.[64–66] These conditions are characterized by diffuse myocardial uptake of [111]In antimyosin. Indium 111-antimyosin imaging is a potential alternative to endomyocardial biopsy, today the conventional technique for diagnos-

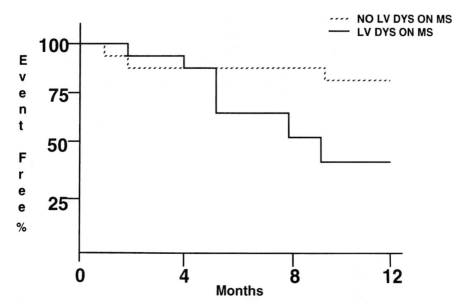

**Figure 13–6** ▪ Cardiac event-free survival rates for two groups of patients with chronic stable angina. One group had left ventricular dysfunction (*solid line*) in response to mental stress and the other group had no left ventricular dysfunction (*dotted line*) in response to mental stress. A significantly greater proportion of patients with mental stress–induced left ventricular dysfunction developed cardiac events over the next year. (Jain D, Burg MM, Soufer RS, Zaret BL: Prognostic significance of mental stress induced left ventricular dysfunction in patients with coronary artery disease. Am J Cardiol 1995;76:31–35.)

ing these conditions. It has also been used for evaluating doxorubicin cardiotoxicity.[51, 66] Most patients show abnormal myocardial uptake of [111]In antimyosin after receiving intermediate doses of doxorubicin, even in the absence of any fall in LVEF. An intense [111]In antimyosin uptake pattern after intermediate doses of doxorubicin, even with normal LVEF is, however, strongly predictive of an impending drop in LVEF and of congestive heart failure if doxorubicin therapy continues. Currently, [111]In antimyosin is no longer commercially available in the United States because of limited demand.

A new [99m]Tc-labeled agent, technetium Tc 99m glucarate, has been observed to be an infarct-avid agent. Glucaric acid is a simple six-carbon dicarboxylic acid sugar that can be labeled with [99m]Tc. It localizes in the infarcted myocardium as early as 2 to 4 hours after being injected and also clears rapidly from the blood pool. Experimental studies have shown that abnormal [99m]Tc glucarate uptake can be seen as early as 3 to 4 hours after the onset of MI. This may allow acute infarct imaging within a relatively short time and is potentially promising for use in chest pain centers.[67]

## ▪ POSITRON EMISSION TOMOGRAPHY

Positron emission tomography (PET) involves the use of positron-emitting isotopes ([11]C, [18]F, [13]N, [15]O). Positrons disintegrate into two gamma rays released 180 degrees apart that can be detected as coincident photons by an array of detectors placed around the patient. PET images have very high technical quality. The tracers have relatively short half-lives and a cyclotron is required on site to produce them. PET traces can be incorporated into a number of metabolic substrates (e.g., deoxyglucose, fatty acids, acetate, sympathomimetic amines) and are useful for studying the metabolic and adrenergic neuronal activity of the myocardium.[68] $^{15}$O-water and $^{13}$N-ammonia can be used for myocardial perfusion imaging. A major advantage of PET perfusion imaging is that, apart from a qualitative assessment, it can also provide accurate quantitative assessment of the regional myocardial blood flow per gram of myocardial tissue at rest and under various physiologic conditions. $^{18}$F-fluorodeoxyglucose ($^{18}$FDG) imaging is useful for studying myocardial viability. Chronically ischemic but viable myocardial segments preferentially take up $^{18}$FDG disproportionately as compared with regional perfusion. This is the classical paradigm for tissue viability with PET imaging. However, $^{18}$FDG imaging requires strict control of the metabolic milieu and is of limited value in patients who have diabetes or recently had an MI.

Recently, $^{18}$FDG imaging has been made possible through some alterations in the conventional SPECT cameras.[69] Dual-head cameras can also be used in coincidence imaging mode, similar to standard PET imaging. Alternatively, a high-energy collimator can be used for standard SPECT imaging of $^{18}$FDG. Although the quality of these images is suboptimal as compared with standard PET images, with further technologic advances $^{18}$FDG has the potential for wider use for studying myocardial viability and metabolic activity using commonly available instrumentation. Because $^{18}$FDG also localizes in various tumors, it is currently being used extensively for tumor imaging with either PET or modified SPECT cameras.

## ■ NEW RADIOTRACERS

A number of new radiotracers are in various stages of clinical development. Monoclonal antibodies to platelet glycoprotein IIb/IIIa and fibrin labeled with $^{111}$In or $^{99m}$Tc have been used for thrombus imaging.[70] Metaiodobenzylguanidine (MIBG) labeled with iodine 123 and parafluorobenzylguanidine labeled with $^{18}$F can be used for imaging cardiac sympathetic neuronal activity.[71, 72] In patients with congestive heart failure, there is activation of the sympathetic activity, and the extent of such activation correlates negatively with their prognosis. Thus, this technique has the potential to elucidate the mechanisms of various interventions in these patients. Fatty acids labeled with $^{123}$I, such as iodophenylpentadecanoic acid (IPPA) and 15-(p-iodophenyl)3R, S-methylpentadecanoic acid (BMIPP), have been used for studying regional myocardial fatty acid metabolism. This is useful for studying the extent of myocardial viability.[73] Monoclonal antibodies targeted against various components of atheromas are being developed for atheroma imaging.[74] In the future, it may become possible to radiolabel various adhesion molecules, interleukins, and other mediators of endothelial dysfunction, intimal injury, and atherogenesis in experimental models to elucidate the pathophysiologic mechanisms of these lesions.

## Conclusion

Radionuclide imaging techniques have greatly enhanced our understanding of cardiovascular physiology and pathology. These techniques have played a crucial role in the evaluation of patients known or suspected to have CAD and for optimal and cost-effective utilization of various therapeutic options. Myocardial perfusion imaging, the most important and most widely used nuclear imaging technique, provides important diagnostic and powerful prognostic information in men and women when used to evaluate suspected or known CAD or acute MI. New imaging techniques, radiopharmaceuticals, and imaging paradigms are emerging to meet the challenges of the changing practice of cardiovascular medicine.

# ■ REFERENCES

1. Zaret BL, Wackers FJT: Nuclear cardiology, (two parts). N Engl J Med 1993:329;775–783, 855–863.
2. Kaul S, Boucher CA, Newell JB, et al: Determination of the quantitative thallium imaging variables that optimize detection of coronary artery disease. J Am Coll Cardiol 1986:7:527–537.
3. Wackers FJT, Fetterman RC, Mattera JA, Clements JP: Quantitative planar thallium-201 stress scintigraphy: A critical evaluation of the method. Semin Nucl Med 1985;15:46–66.
4. Jain D, Zaret BL: Nuclear imaging techniques for the assessment of myocardial viability. Cardiol Clin 1995;13;43–57.
5. Wackers FJT: The maze of myocardial perfusion imaging protocols in 1994. J Nucl Cardiol 1994;1:180–188.
6. Dilsizian V, Rocco T, Freedman N, et al: Enhanced detection of ischemic but viable myocardium by the reinjection of thallium after stress-redistribution imaging. N Engl J Med 1990;323:141–146.
7. Kayden DS, Sigal S, Soufer R, et al: Thallium-201 for assessment of myocardial viability: Quantitative comparison of 24-hour redistribution imaging with imaging after reinjection at rest. J Am Coll Cardiol 1991;18:1480–1486.
8. Wackers FJT, Berman DS, Maddahi J, et al: Technetium-99m hexakis 2-methoxyisobutyl isonitrile: Human biodistribution, dosimetry, safety and preliminary comparison to thallium-201 for myocardial perfusion imaging. J Nucl Med 1989;30:301–311.
9. Hendel RC, McSherry B, Karimeddini M, Leppo JA: Diagnostic value of new myocardial perfusion agent, Teboroxime (SQ 30217), utilizing a rapid planar imaging protocol: Preliminary results. J Am Coll Cardiol 1990;16:855–861.
10. Jain D, Wackers FJT, Mattera J, et al: Biokinetics of $^{99m}$Tc-Tetrofosmin: Myocardial perfusion imaging agent: Implications for a one day imaging protocol. J Nucl Med 1993;34:1254–N1259.
11. Zaret BL, Rigo P, Wackers FJT, et al: Myocardial perfusion imaging with technetium-99m tetrofosmin: Comparison to thallium-201 imaging and coronary angiography in a phase III multicenter trial. Circulation 1995;91:313–319.
12. Fagret D, Marie PY, Brunotte F, et al: Myocardial perfusion imaging with technetium-99m-Tc NOET: Comparison with thallium-201 and coronary angiography. J Nucl Med 1995;36:936–943.
13. Iskandrian AS, Heo J, Kong B, et al: Use of technetium-99m isonitrile in assessing left ventricular perfusion and function at rest and during exercise in coronary artery disease and comparison with coronary angiography and exercise thallium-201 SPECT imaging. Am J Cardiol 1989;64:270–275.
14. Eagle KA, Singer DE, Brewster DC, et al: Dipyridamole-thallium scanning in patients undergoing vascular surgery: Optimizing preoperative evaluation of cardiac risk. JAMA 1987;257:2185–2189.
15. Miller DD, Stratmann HG, Shaw L, et al: Dipyridamole technetium 99m sestamibi myocardial tomography as an independent predictor of cardiac event–free survival after acute ischemic events. J Nucl Cardiol 1994;1:72–82.
16. Taillefer R, Amyot R, Turpin S, et al: Comparison between dipyridamole and adenosine as pharmacologic coronary vasodilators in detection of coronary artery disease with thallium 201 imaging. J Nucl Cardiol 1996;3:204–211.
17. Lette J, Tatum JL, Fraser S, et al: Safety of dipyridamole testing in 73,806 patients: The Multicenter Dipyridamole Safety Study. J Nucl Cardiol 1995;2:3–17.
18. Pennell DJ, Mavrogeni SI, Forbat SM, et al: Adenosine combined with dynamic exercise for myocardial perfusion imaging. J Am Coll Cardiol 1995;25:1300–1309.
19. Candell-Riera J, Santana-Boado C, Castell-Conesa J, et al: Simultaneous dipyridamole/maximal subjective exercise with $^{99m}$Tc-MIBI SPECT: Improved diagnostic yield in coronary artery disease. J Am Coll Cardiol 1997;29:531–536.
20. Samady H, Wackers F, Deman P, et al: Low level exercise combined with adenosine myocardial perfusion imaging improve image quality, diagnostic accuracy, and side effect profile (Abstract). Circulation 1997;96(Suppl):I–735.
21. Calnon DA, Glover DK, Beller GA, et al: Effects of dobutamine stress on myocardial blood flow, $^{99m}$Tc sestamibi uptake, and systolic wall thickening in the presence of coronary artery stenoses: Implications for dobutamine stress testing. Circulation 1997;96:2353–2360.
22. Shehata AR, Ahlberg AW, Gillam LD, et al: Direct comparison of arbutamine and dobutamine stress testing with myocardial perfusion imaging and echocardiography in patients with coronary artery disease. Am J Cardiol 1997;80:716–720.
23. Wackers FJ: Science, art, and artifacts: How important is quantification for the practicing physician interpreting myocardial perfusion studies? J Nucl Cardiol 1994;1:S109–117.
24. Barnden LR, Ong PL, Rowe CC: Simultaneous emission transmission tomography using technetium-99m for both emission and transmission. Eur J Nucl Med 1997;24:1390–1397.
25. Heller EN, DeMan P, Liu YH, et al: Extracardiac activity complicates quantitative cardiac SPECT imaging using a simultaneous transmission-emission approach. J Nucl Med 1997;38:1882–1890.

26. Beller GA, Gibson RS: Sensitivity, specificity and prognostic significance of noninvasive testing for occult or known coronary disease. Prog Cardiovasc Dis 1987;24:241–270.

27. Wackers FJ, Zaret BL: Radionuclide stress myocardial perfusion imaging: The future gatekeeper for coronary angiography (Editorial). J Nucl Cardiol 1995;2:358–359.

28. Bateman TM, O'Keefe JH, Dong VM, et al: Coronary angiographic rates after stress single photon emission computed tomographic scintigraphy. J Nucl Cardiol 1995;2:217–223.

29. Jain D, Lahiri A, Raftery EB: Lung thallium uptake on rest, stress and redistribution cardiac imaging: State-of-the-art review. Am J Card Imaging 1990;4:303–309.

30. Gill JB, Ruddy TD, Newell JB, et al: Prognostic importance of thallium uptake by the lungs during exercise in coronary artery disease. N Engl J Med 1987;317:1485–1489.

31. Taylor AJ, Sackett MC, Beller GA: The degree of ST-segment depression on symptom-limited exercise testing: Relation to the myocardial ischemic burden as determined by thallium-201 scintigraphy. Am J Cardiol 1995;75:228–231.

32. Iskander S, Iskandrian AE: Risk assessment using single-photon emission computed tomographic technetium-99m sestamibi imaging. J Am Coll Cardiol 1998;32:57–62.

33. Raiker K, Sinusas AJ, Wackers FJ, Zaret BL: One-year prognosis of patients with normal planar or single-photon emission computed tomographic technetium 99m labeled sestamibi exercise imaging. J Nucl Cardiol 1994;1:449–456.

34. Wahl JM, Hakki AH, Iskandrian AS: Prognostic implications of normal exercise Tl-201 images. Arch Intern Med 1985;145:253–256.

35. Gibson RS, Watson DD, Craddock GB, et al: Prediction of cardiac events after uncomplicated myocardial infarction: A prospective study comparing predischarge exercise thallium-201 scintigraphy and coronary angiography. Circulation 1983;68:321–336.

36. Varetto T, Cantalupi D, Altieri A, Orlandi C: Emergency room technetium-99m sestamibi imaging to rule out acute myocardial ischemic events in patients with nondiagnostic electrocardiograms. J Am Coll Cardiol 1993;22:1804–1808.

37. Heller GV, Stowers SA, Hendel RC, et al: Clinical value of acute rest technetium-99m tetrofosmin tomographic myocardial perfusion imaging in patients with acute chest pain and nondiagnostic electrocardiograms. J Am Coll Cardiol 1998;31:1011–1017.

38. Wackers FJT, Gibbons RJ, Verani MS, et al: Serial quantitative planar technetium-99m isonitrile imaging in acute myocardial infarction: Efficacy for noninvasive assessment of thrombolytic therapy. J Am Coll Cardiol 1989;14:861–873.

39. Jain D, Wackers FJT, Zaret BL: Radionuclide imaging techniques in the thrombolytic era: *In* Becker R (ed): Modern Era of Coronary Thrombolysis. Norwell, Mass: Kluwer Academic, 1994:195–218.

40. Jain D, Fleisher LA, Zaret BL: Diagnosing perioperative myocardial infarction in noncardiac surgery. Int Anesthesiol Clin 1992;30:199–216.

41. Farkouh ME, Rihal CS, Gersch BJ, et al: Influence of coronary heart disease on morbidity and mortality after lower extremity revascularization surgery: A population-based study in Olmstead county, Minnesota (1970–1987). J Am Coll Cardiol 1994;24:1290–1296.

42. Leppo JA: Preoperative cardiac risk assessment for noncardiac surgery. Am J Cardiol 1995;75:42D–51D.

43. Fleisher LA, Rosenbaum SH, Nelson AH, et al: Preoperative dipyridamole thallium imaging and Holter monitoring as a predictor of perioperative cardiac events and long term outcome. Anesthesiology 1995;83:906–917.

44. Ragosta M, Beller GA, Watson DD, et al: Quantitative planar rest-redistribution [201]Tl imaging in detection of myocardial viability and prediction of improvement in left ventricular function after coronary bypass surgery in patients with severely depressed left ventricular function. Circulation 1993;87:1630–1641.

45. Caner B, Beller GA: Are technetium-99m–labeled myocardial perfusion agents adequate for detection of myocardial viability? Clin Cardiol 1998;4:235–242.

46. He ZX, Verani MS, Liu XJ: Nitrate-augmented myocardial imaging for assessment of myocardial viability (Editorial). J Nucl Cardiol 1995;2:352–357.

47. Borges-Neto S, Shaw LJ, Kesler KL, et al: Prediction of severe coronary artery disease by combined rest and exercise radionuclide angiocardiography and tomographic perfusion imaging with technetium 99m-labeled sestamibi: A comparison with clinical and electrocardiographic data. J Nucl Cardiol 1997;4(3):189–194.

48. Lee KL, Proyer DB, Pieper KS, et al: Prognostic value of radionuclide angiography in medically treated patients with coronary artery disease: A comparison with clinical and catheterization variables. Circulation 1990;82:1705–1717.

49. The SOLVD Investigators: Effect of enalapril on mortality and the development of heart failure in asymptomatic patients with reduced left ventricular ejection fractions. N Engl J Med 1992;327:685–691.

50. Schwartz RG, McKenzie B, Alexander J, et al: Congestive heart failure and left ventricular dysfunction complicating doxorubicin therapy: Seven-year experience using serial radionuclide angiocardiography. Am J Med 1987;82:1109–1118.

51. Jain D, Zaret BL: Antimyosin cardiac imaging: Will it play a role in the detection of doxorubicin cardiotoxicity? (Editorial). J Nucl Med 1990;31:1970–1975.

52. Jain D, Wackers FJ, Welles L, Zaret BL: Reduced cardiotoxicity of liposomal doxorubicin (D99): A phase III single agent study in patients with metastatic breast cancer (MBC) (Abstract). J Am Coll Cardiol 1999;33(Suppl A):426A.

53. Mitani I, Jain D, Joska TM, et al: Doxorubicin induced congestive heart failure: Decreasing incidence with routine use of radionuclide angiocardiography (Abstract). J Nucl Cardiol 1999;6:S–97.
54. Bonow RP, Kent KM, Rosing DR, et al: Exercise-induced ischemia in mildly symptomatic patients with coronary artery disease and preserved left ventricular function: Identification of subgroups at risk of death during medical therapy. N Engl J Med 1984;311:1339–1345.
55. Massardo T, Gal RA, Grenier RP, et al: Left ventricular volume calculation using a count-based ratio method applied to multigated radionuclide angiography. J Nucl Med 1990;31:450–456.
56. Marmor A, Jain D, Cohen LS, et al: Left ventricular peak power during exercise: A noninvasive approach for assessment of contractile reserve. J Nucl Med 1993;34:1877–1885.
57. Marmor A, Jain D, Zaret BL: Beyond ejection fraction. J Nucl Cardiol 1994;1:477–486.
58. Zaret BL, Jain D: Monitoring of left ventricular function with miniaturized non-imaging detectors. In Zaret BL, Beller GA (eds): Nuclear Cardiology: State of the Art and Future Directions, 2nd ed. St. Louis: Mosby–Year Book, 1999:191–200.
59. Burg MM, Jain D, Soufer R, et al: Role of behavioral and psychological factors in mental stress induced silent left ventricular dysfunction in coronary artery disease. J Am Coll Cardiol 1993;22:440–448.
60. Jain D, Burg MM, Soufer RS, Zaret BL: Prognostic significance of mental stress induced left ventricular dysfunction in patients with coronary artery disease. Am J Cardiol 1995;76:31–35.
61. Kayden DS, Wackers FJ, Zaret BL: Silent left ventricular dysfunction during routine activity after thrombolytic therapy for acute myocardial infarction. J Am Coll Cardiol 1990;15:1500–1507.
62. Jain D, Crawley JCW, Lahiri A, Raftery EB: Indium-111 antimyosin images compared with triphenyl tetrazolium chloride staining in a patient 6 days after myocardial infarction. J Nucl Med 1990;31:231–233.
63. Jain D, Lahiri A, Raftery EB: Immunoscintigraphy for detecting acute myocardial infarction without electrocardiographic changes. Br Med J 1990;300,151–153.
64. Dec GW, Palacios I, Yasuda T, et al: Antimyosin antibody cardiac imaging: Its role in the diagnosis of myocarditis. J Am Coll Cardiol 1990;16:97–104.
65. Ballester M, Bordes R, Tazelaar HD, et al: Evaluation of biopsy classification for rejection: Relation to detection of myocardial damage by monoclonal antimyosin antibody imaging. J Am Coll Cardiol 1998;31:1357–1361.
66. Carrio I, Estorch M, Berna L, et al: Indium-111-antimyosin and iodine-123-MIBG studies in early assessment of doxorubicin cardiotoxicity. J Nucl Med 1995;36(11):2044–2049.
67. Narula J, Petrov A, Pak C, et al: Hyperacute visualization of myocardia ischemic injury: Comparison of Tc-99m glucarate, thallium-201 and indium-111-antimyosin. J Am Coll Cardiol 1994;23:317.
68. Schelbert HR: Positron emission tomography as a biochemical probe for human myocardial ischemia. In Zaret BL, Kaufman L, Dunn R, Berson A (eds): Frontiers of Cardiac Imaging. New York: Raven, 1993:53–70.
69. Sandler MP, Patton JA: Fluorine 18-labeled fluorodeoxyglucose myocardial single-photon emission computed tomography: An alternative for determining myocardial viability. J Nucl Cardiol 1996;3:342–349.
70. Straton JR, Ritchie JL: $^{111}$In-platelet imaging of left ventricular thrombi: Predictive value for systemic emboli. Circulation 1990;81:1182–1189.
71. Schofer J, Spielman R, Schuchert A, et al: Iodine-123 metaiodobenzylguanidine scintigraphy: A noninvasive method to demonstrate myocardial adrenergic nervous system integrity in patients with idiopathic dilated cardiomyopathy. J Am Coll Cardiol 1988;12:1252–1258.
72. Berry CR, Garg PK, DeGrado TR, et al: Para-[18F] fluorobenzylguanidine kinetics in a canine coronary artery occlusion model. J Nucl Cardiol 1996;3:119–129.
73. Matsunari I, Saga T, Taki J, et al: Kinetics of iodine-123-BMIPP in patients with prior myocardial infarction: Assessment with dynamic rest and stress images compared with stress thallium-201 SPECT. J Nucl Med 1994;35:1279–1285.
74. Narula J, Petrov A, Bianchi C, et al: Noninvasive localization of experimental atherosclerotic lesions with mouse/human chimeric Z2D3 F(ab')2 specific for the proliferating smooth muscle cells of human atheroma. Imaging with conventional and charge-modified antibody fragments. Circulation 1995;92:474–484.

# ■ RECOMMENDED READING

Beller GA: Clinical Nuclear Cardiology. Philadelphia: WB Saunders, 1995.
Gerson MC: Cardiac Nuclear Medicine, 3rd ed. New York: McGraw-Hill, 1997.
Iskandrian AS, Verani MS: New Developments in Cardiac Nuclear Imaging. Futura, 1998.
Jain D: Technetium-99m labeled myocardial perfusion imaging agents. Semin Nucl Med 1999;19:221–236.
Zaret BL, Beller GA (ed): Nuclear Cardiology: State of the Art and Future Directions, 2nd ed. St. Louis: Mosby–Year Book, 1999.

*Chapter* 14

# Cardiovascular Magnetic Resonance and X-Ray Computed Tomography

*Gerald M. Pohost* ▪ *Mark Doyle* ▪ *Robert W. W. Biederman*

Magnetic resonance (MR) and electron beam computed tomography (EBCT) are two relatively new advanced cardiac imaging technologies. EBCT scans a cross-sectional "slice" through the chest in a fraction of a second. It is widely used as a means of detecting calcium in the coronary arteries, which constitutes evidence of atherosclerotic disease. Currently, this application is controversial, since available data do not yet support the utility of EBCT-detected coronary artery calcium as a diagnostic or prognostic indicator of ischemic heart disease. EBCT has several other potential uses, which will be discussed later in this chapter.

MR methods are among the newest of the imaging technologies. While MR generates images with high resolution and high contrast and requires no contrast agent, most MR systems available today must be gated to acquire high-quality images that demonstrate cardiac contraction. Newer systems only recently available allow image acquisition at high speed, obviating electrocardiographic (ECG) synchronization. Nevertheless, gated studies offer superior resolution and image contrast, but either gated or real-time MR imaging (MRI) is best suited to visualize the heart and its contractile function. MR angiography (MRA) is excellent for evaluating the aorta and the peripheral arteries without contrast medium injection, and images can be acquired and displayed in three dimensions (3D). MR spectroscopy (MRS) allows assessment of the biochemical character of the myocardium by generating spectra from the hydrogen and the phosphorus nuclei. Phosphorus spectroscopy can generate spectra that show the relative concentrations of the two high-energy phosphates adenosine triphosphate (ATP) and phosphocreatine (PCr). A relative decrease in PCr relative to ATP indicates a myocardial insult such as ischemia.

## ▪ MAGNETIC RESONANCE METHODS

### Technology: The Principle of Nuclear Magnetic Resonance

When an atomic nucleus contains an odd number of subatomic particles (i.e., protons plus neutrons) it possesses a net positive electrical charge. Additionally, the nucleus can be visualized to spin around its north-south axis in a manner similar to the rotation of the earth. Basic physics dictates that, when an electrically charged object (in this case, the atomic nucleus) moves, it generates a magnetic field. MR takes advantage of this nuclear magnetism, since atomic nuclei, which possess an intrinsic magnetic field, can interact with external magnetic fields. Sensitive atomic nuclei placed within an extrinsic magnetic field will align either *with* or *against* that field. Quantum mechanical considerations indicate that, for any amount of such material, slightly more nuclei will align with the field than will be antialigned. Thus, material placed in an external magnetic field possesses a bulk magnetism of its own. The stronger the field is, the greater the number of nuclei that preferentially align. If the nucleus is disturbed, for example by a radiofrequency (RF) field, it will be displaced out of alignment with the extrinsic magnetic field. When the RF energy is terminated, the nuclei precess back to their original position of alignment. *Precession* is the "slow wobbling" phenomenon that is observed when, for example, a child's spinning top or a gyroscope is pushed out of alignment with the earth's gravitational field. In a similar manner, nuclei with intrinsic "spin" and a magnetic moment will precess if pushed out of alignment with the external magnetic field. The frequency of precession depends on the strength of the magnetic field and the nuclear characteristics of a given element. Incidentally, the RF field has to be applied at the precession frequency (i.e., at the resonance frequency for the system). Thus, the phenomenon of nuclear MR is manifested when a substance with magnetically sensitive nuclei (e.g., the nucleus of hydrogen—1 or the proton, phosphorus—31, fluorine—19, and sodium—23) is momentarily pulsed with RF energy at the resonance frequency. The nuclei of all of these atoms are naturally abundant and stable, (i.e., not radioactive). Currently, virtually all MRI images and MR angiograms are derived from the hydrogen nucleus. During the process of free precession (i.e., after termination of the RF field) the nuclei give off a detectable signal, which, in an MRI system, is what an RF antenna detects.[1]

The units of magnetic field strength are the gauss (G) and the tesla (T). The strength of the earth's magnetic field is on the order of 0.5 G. A typical commercial MR system useful for cardiovascular studies has a field strength of 15,000 G. It is customary to express field strength with nuclear MR (NMR) teslas (1 T = 10,000 G). Thus, 15,000 G is equivalent to 1.5 T.

## The Importance of Radio Waves or Radiofrequency

Spectra from NMR spectrometers and images for MRI devices are generated by RF pulses that perturb the alignment of the nuclear spins. Typical pulses reorient the net magnetism of the nuclear spins by 90 or 180 degrees, whereas faster and newer imaging techniques use pulses of shorter duration. After the RF pulse, the net magnetization precesses back into alignment with the extrinsic magnetic field. As they precess, they emit RF waves, which are detected by an antenna in the magnet. The frequency of these radio waves is characteristic for a given atomic nucleus and is affected by the chemical milieu. The detected radio waves are digitized and converted into signal peaks using the mathematical process known as *Fourier transformation* to produce a spectrum or an image. The chemical milieu can cause the location of a resonance peak to change, a phenomenon known as *chemical shift*. Thus, the three peaks of adenosine triphosphate (ATP) are located in different spectral positions, and the hydrogen nuclei of water and of fat are also in different spectral locations.

The time that it takes for the magnetic field intrinsic to the tissue to reorient and align with the extrinsic field after the RF pulse is a variable known as *relaxation time*. There are two relaxation times: T1 (or spin/lattice relaxation) is related to the time required for the net magnetization of the sample to realign with the extrinsic field; T2 (or spin/spin relaxation time) is related to the time required for the spins that were in phase after the RF pulse to become incoherent, or *to dephase*. It is the concentration of the nuclei and the relaxation times that contribute to the magnitude of a peak in the spectrum which in an image is reflected by the intensity of a structure. Other variables that affect signal intensity are sample motion and turbulence. These influences form the basis for MRA, a modality in which excellent contrast can be generated between a blood vessel and surrounding tissues.

## Instrumentation for Magnetic Resonance Studies

An MRI system consists of a large (typically cylindrical) superconducting magnet; a RF body coil that fits within the bore of the magnet; gradient coils that generate the weaker magnetic fields needed to create images; and an image-processing computer (Fig. 14–1). The large magnet contains a coil of niobium-titanium, which has very high electrical resistance at room temperature but essentially no resistance to electrical current when it is supercooled. Such supercooling takes place when the coils in the magnet are bathed in liquid helium. Permanent magnets and "open" magnets are also available for MRI; however, the high-field superconducting magnet is preferable for cardiac applications. The gradient coils are positioned within the magnet bore and are used to vary the magnetic field in a precisely controlled manner. They effect small differences in magnetic field related to the position of an organ or a portion of an organ within the magnet. Gradient coils are essential for imaging but not for spectroscopy. The cylindrical body RF coil fits concentrically within the bore of a cylindrical magnet and transmits and receives the radio waves needed to create a spectrum or an image. Naturally, a system so complex requires substantial computer control, RF amplifiers, and a vast

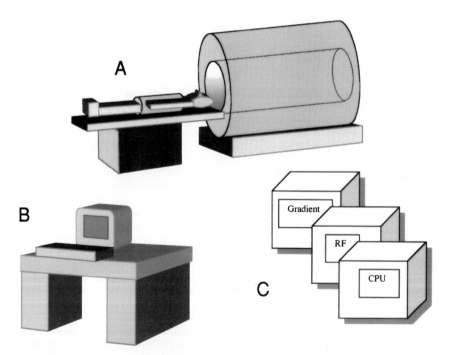

**Figure 14–1** ▪ Schematic diagram of components of a typical MRI system. *(A)* Scanner magnet and patient table. The table accommodates patient entry, exit, and positioning within the magnet bore. *(B)* The operator's console is remote from the scanner and affords control of scanner functions and incorporates an image and physiologic data viewing station. *(C)* Bulky hardware to power the scanner typically is located in a separate room. Components include gradient and radiofrequency power units and the controlling computer. RF, radiofrequency; CPU, central processing unit.

array of electronic components. Typically, an operator's console is placed in an adjacent room next to a window through which the operator of the MR system can watch the patient. This console provides a means for altering the acquisition methods or RF pulse sequences.

A spin echo image of the heart has high spatial resolution and "dark blood." A gradient echo pulse sequence typically generates images at higher speed with "bright blood." The dark-blood approach is ideal for assessing cardiac morphology; the bright-blood approach, for assessing ventricular function. When turbulence occurs in the bloodstream, the bright-blood approach demonstrates a reduction in brightness. Accordingly, with mitral or aortic regurgitation, for example, the regurgitant jet is dark owing to turbulence. The newest systems have higher-speed imaging capabilities and use acquisition approaches such as "echo-planar" and spiral imaging, which are capable of generating a cross-sectional image within 30 to 100 milliseconds. Both dark-blood and bright-blood imaging are performed with cardiac gating, to freeze heart motion at certain phases in the cardiac cycle. Typically, 20 frames are acquired in a gradient echo cine sequence. In this way both regional and global ventricular performance can be evaluated. A typical gradient echo sequence requires 10 to 20 seconds' acquisition time. Using echo-planar methods, snapshot images can be acquired throughout the cardiac cycle and then assembled in sequence in the computer. Such snapshot images require approximately 20 seconds to generate a cine loop that displays the entire heart and can be replayed repeatedly to allow evaluation of wall motion (Fig. 14–2).

MRI systems of the recent past consisted of a rather long cylindrical magnet, and as many as 5% of patients were unable to tolerate lying in such an enclosure owing to claustrophobia. Sometimes, claustrophobia is tolerable if the patient is removed from the magnet for a short while and then repositioned. Anxious patients known to be claustrophobic can be given a mild sedative such as a benzodiazepine. Most modern systems have shorter-bore magnets and are more "patient friendly." Also, with certain imaging sequences the system can be quite noisy; then, earplugs and headphones are used to damp the sound. Some patients, however, find the experience of having an MRI quite relaxing and sleep through the entire study. An intercom system is usually used to maintain verbal contact between system operator and patient.

## Current Applications

At this state of the technology, MRI and MRA are excellent for assessing global and regional left and right ventricular performance, for evaluating the abnormal morphology of congenital heart disease (Fig. 14–3), for characterizing myocardial tissue such as in arrhythmogenic myocardial dysplasia (Fig. 14–4), for assessing myocardial wall thickness and ventricular volumes in the cardiomyopathies and in valvular heart disease, for assessing the pericardium (particularly distinguishing constrictive pericarditis from restrictive myocardial disease; Fig. 14–5) for cardiac or paracardiac masses (Figs. 14–6, 14–7), for comprehensive evaluation of aortic dissection and aortic aneurysms, and for assessment of the larger arterial branches from the aorta, such as the carotids and iliofemorals, and (more recently) coronary arteries. MRI has the unique ability to acquire images of the heart in any tomographic plane the operator at the console selects. It is customary, however, to acquire imaging planes through the vertical long axis (two-chamber view), the horizontal long-axis (4-chamber view), and the short axis (see Fig. 14–2). Cardiac chamber size and myocardial wall thickness and mass are readily assessed from MR images. Chamber morphology, orientation, and relationships to the great vessels and other viscera are easily assessed. In addition, atrioventricular, venoatrial,

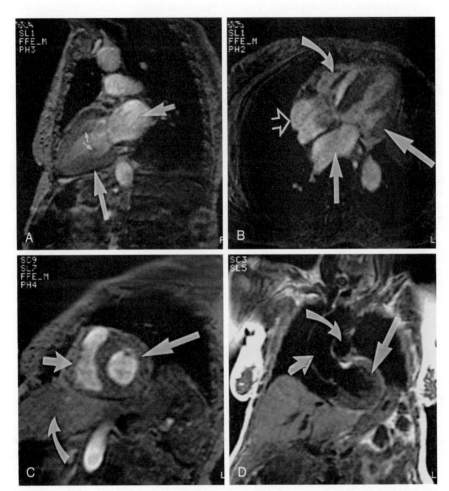

**Figure 14–2** ■ Gradient echo images of normal cardiac anatomy in four views. *(A)* The two-chamber view (left ventricle, *large arrow*; left atrium, *small arrow*; anterolateral and posteromedial papillary muscle, *smallest arrows*). *(B)* The four-chamber view (left ventricle, *large arrow*; left atrium, *small arrow*; right ventricle, *large curved arrow*; right atrium, *small open arrow*). *(C)* The short-axis view of the left and right ventricles (left ventricle, *large arrow*; right ventricle, *small arrow*; liver, *curved arrow*). *(D)* The coronal view (left ventricle, *large arrow*; ascending aorta, *curved arrow*; right pulmonary artery in cross section, *small curved arrow*).

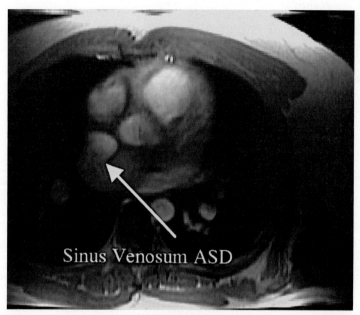

**Figure 14–3** ■ A 38-year-old white man referred because of syncope underwent an extensive workup, including transthoracic echocardiography and transesophageal echocardiography. An enlarged right atrium was noted. Right and left heart catheterization studies, where a "step up" was present retrospectively, and electrophysiology testing revealed no inducible abnormal tachycardias. On MRI spin echo imaging, an anomalous left upper pulmonary vein can be seen emptying into the high right atrium–superior vena cava junction as part of a sinus venosum atrial septal defect. Phase-velocity mapping of the aorta and pulmonary artery (not shown) yielded a Qp/Qs of 2.1 left-to-right shunt.

and ventriculoarterial connections can readily be defined. MRI can be used to reconstruct three-dimensional views of the heart when supported by the computer. Three-dimensional cardiac views can be rotated and viewed from any orientation on a computer screen. Such capability is ideal for assessing complex congenital heart disease.

## Ventricular Function

Both global and regional right and left ventricular function can be assessed using cine MRI (gradient echo) or other rapid acquisition sequences such as echoplanar imaging.[2] Ventricular volumes can be measured at end diastole and end systole using traditional area-length approaches from the long-axis images or using Simpson's rule with serial short-axis images.[3] Simpson's rule is the method of computing volumes of continuous objects by summing the areas of cross sections obtained at a discrete number of points and treating the gaps between sampled cross sections as if they were represented by the nearest cross-sectional view. In essence, the area is found by summing each cross-sectional area and multiplying it by the sum of the slice thickness and the interslice gap. The ejection fraction can be readily determined from the end-systolic and end-diastolic volumes. In addition to the geometrically simple left ventricle, the more irregularly shaped right ventricle can also be studied using a Simpson's rule approach with serial short-axis views from base to apex. The three-dimensional nature of MR images makes possible

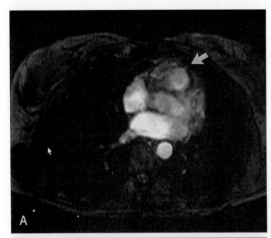

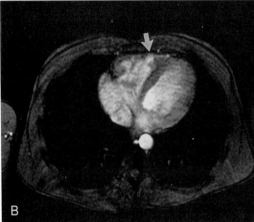

**Figure 14–4** ■ MRI was performed on a 36-year-old white woman referred for palpitations and tachycardia. ECG during the tachycardia suggested a possible right ventricular outflow tract lesion. *(A)* The multislice axial images (gradient echo) localized an area of out-pocketing and dyskinesia *(arrow)* to an area 1.5 cm below the pulmonic valve. This region was successfully ablated by radiofrequency pulse in the electrophysiology laboratory and the patient had no more episodes of tachycardia. *(B)* A 17-year-old black man suffered his first syncopal episode while playing basketball. He was referred for evaluation of idiopathic hypertrophic subaortic stenosis (IHSS). On gradient-echo imaging, there was no evidence of IHSS; however, the distal portion of the RV free wall was thinned and dyskinetic *(arrow)*, consistent with arrhythmogenic right ventricular dysplasia. Additionally, the RV function was mildly depressed globally while both the RV and LV were moderately dilated. The patient was referred for electrophysiology testing and underwent successful ablation of the electrophysiologic focus of the arrhythmia.

calculation of accurate right ventricular volumes and ejection fractions.[4] By evaluating size, shape, and the regional contractile ability of the left ventricle, lesions such as ventricular aneurysm and pseudoaneurysm, dilated hypertrophic cardiomyopathy, myocardial thinning, and remodeling can readily be detected. Since the myocardium is clearly visualized, it is easy to measure wall thickness and to evaluate wall thickening. Furthermore, myocardial mass can be measured.[5]

In addition to functional evaluation with conventional contrast imaging, two other methods are available for cardiovascular MR studies, phase-velocity mapping and RF tagging. Phase-velocity mapping is analogous to Doppler echocardiography. In phase-velocity mapping, the phase of the MR image is related to its velocity. Unlike Doppler echocardiography, it measures accurately (typically within 7%) in all three dimensions. Phase-velocity mapping has a plethora of applications, including blood flow and determination of stroke volume and cardiac output at the aortic valve. RF tagging provides MRI with a unique ability to more precisely evaluate regional myocardial function.[6] By using the appropriate pulse sequence, dark lines in a regular crisscross pattern can be embedded in the myocardium at the time of the ECG R wave. Since these lines move with the myocardium, its intrinsic motion

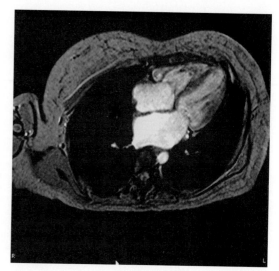

**Figure 14–5** ■ A diagnosis of restrictive cardiomyopathy was being considered for a 59-year-old white woman with dyspnea. The patient was referred for further evaluation. The four-chamber gradient-echo image reveals evidence of biatrial dilatation with normal-sized and functioning left and right ventricles compatible with restrictive cardiomyopathy.

can be visualized to assess true function without the confounding effect of myocardial through-plane motion[7] or remote muscle influences (tethering) (Fig. 14–8). Furthermore, changes in distance between intersections of RF grid lines can be tracked and regional strains, indices of rotation, and translation amounts calculated. Unlike tracking of material markers, RF tagging does not impede or influence myocardial dynamics, and it is completely noninvasive. It is likely that MRI is the most reliable means for assessing right and left ventricular function. MRI is three-dimensional, has excellent resolution and contrast without the risk of contrast medium, can evaluate aortic and pulmonic outflow, and can comprehensively evaluate regional function using a unique RF-tagging method.

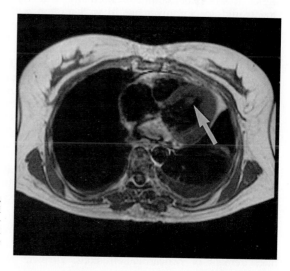

**Figure 14–6** ■ A previously healthy, 43-year-old white woman presented with a recent history of stroke. High-resolution spin echo images revealed an intracardiac mass attached to the septum (arrow).

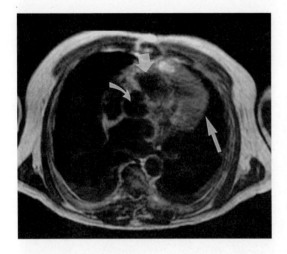

**Figure 14–7** ■ One week after coronary bypass grafting, a 75-year-old black man was referred with chest pain, dyspnea, and an abnormal cardiac silhouette on chest films. MRI revealed a paracardiac mass adjacent to the pericardium consistent with thrombus. The likely clinical scenario involved dehiscence of the distal saphenous vein graft that allowed a small leak that subsequently produced lung tamponade (mass, *long straight arrow*; right ventricular outflow tract, *small wide arrow*; aortic plane, *curved arrow*).

## Cardiomyopathies

Since MR can reliably evaluate the function of both ventricles by examining volumetric changes and changes in wall thickness, it can be used to determine the regional distribution of wall motion abnormality.[8, 9] Within a patient with dilated cardiomyopathy, the physician would expect to find both left and right ventricular involvement and homogeneously depressed left ventricular wall motion, except at the apex[10] (Fig. 14–9). In one with ischemic heart disease, inhomogeneous contractile function would be expected, function being poorest in the territories of previous myocardial infarction, and some degree of contractile dysfunction in regions of reduced perfusion secondary to tightly stenotic lesions but maintained viability. Recent reports suggest that dobutamine MRI can safely be used to assess myocardial viability (i.e., improved contractile function during infusion of low-dose dobutamine in regions that demonstrate asynergy at rest). Also, coronary artery disease can be diagnosed by using MRI to examine the deterioration in contraction with higher doses of dobutamine on normally or nearly normally contracting segments. One would see improvement in wall motion with low-dose dobutamine in the presence of viable but hypocontractile myocardium, but in a territory supplied by a critical stenosis, there would be deterioration of function at higher dobutamine doses as compared to rest.

A cardiomyopathic ventricle may be associated with hemochromatosis, a condition that MRI can readily diagnose. The iron that is localized in the myocardium and the liver generates a characteristic signal dropout pattern so that the liver and, in part, the myocardium become invisible. It has also been reported that, in sarcoidosis, one can visualize the granulomatous infiltrates that lead to ventricular dysfunction.

One cardiomyopathy that is well characterized by MRI is arrhythmogenic myocardial dysplasia. In this condition associated with life-threatening ventricular arrythmias, the right ventricle is involved with wall thinning and fat infiltration. The fatty infiltrate shows up as a bright signal on spin-echo MRI and regional wall motion dysfunction on gradient-echo images (see Fig. 14–4).

## Pericardial Disease

Naturally, such an imaging technology as MRI can readily visualize and allow measurement of pericardial effusions. Further, by using tissue characterization

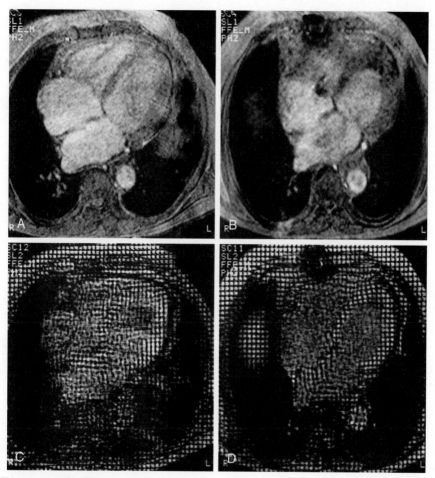

**Figure 14–8** ■ Images from a 69-year-old white man with a dilated cardiomyopathy referred for LV endoventricular circular patch plasty (Dor procedure). Four-chamber views on top row show (A) presurgical and (B) postsurgical LV reduction. Utilizing the radiofrequency myocardial tissue-tagging technique, the areas of greatest dysfunction (C) were identified and surgically excluded, allowing for normalization of LV size and geometry (D). The patient was able to resume premorbid activities.

methods it may be possible to evaluate fluid composition (i.e., to distinguish transudate from exudate). The problem of differentiating between constrictive pericarditis and restrictive cardiomyopathies is made easier by using MR methods, since the pericardium can be visualized and its thickness measured (see Fig. 14–5).[11] Under normal circumstance, pericardial thickness should not exceed 3 mm. Some reports suggest that restrictive physiology can be demonstrated by volumetric analysis using MRI.

## Valvular Disease

The application of MRI to assessing valvular disease is based on sensitivity to flow. With regurgitant or stenotic valves, there is loss of signal due to resultant

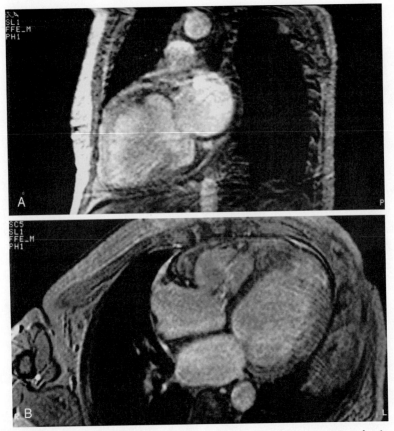

**Figure 14–9** ■ Idiopathic dilated cardiomyopathy in a 45-year-old white man. (*A*) Two-chamber view; (*B*) four-chamber view. His end-diastolic dimension was 78 mm, while the end-diastolic volume measured nearly 600 ml. His ejection fraction was 11%. He was referred for cardiac transplantation.

turbulence that on cine MR images (bright blood) appears as a black jet in the midst of the more laminar white blood (Fig. 14–10). With regurgitant lesions, there is a relationship between the size of the signal void, the size of the accepting chamber, the time over which the signal void persists, and the size and duration of persistence of the zone of proximal convergence (i.e., the region where blood converges uniformly and radially in the direction of a valve orifice that is small relative to the chamber from which it emanates).[12]

Another approach to assessing the severity of valve disease is known as *phase velocity mapping* and is similar to Doppler echocardiography. In contrast to anatomic images that are constructed from amplitude images corresponding to the number of hydrogen spins or concentration of hydrogen, phase velocity images are derived from data related to the phase of hydrogen spins passing through a given plane. Phase velocity mapping can be used to quantitate the flow rate and velocity of the blood. Stenotic valvular lesions are frequently characterized by velocities as high as or even higher than 8 m/sec (i.e., any velocity encountered in human valvular heart disease). To assess such velocities, the imaging device must have state-of-the-art hardware. Thus, MRI can be used to assess both regurgitant and stenotic

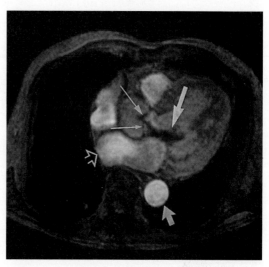

**Figure 14–10** ■ A 77-year-old white male presented with dyspnea, shortness of breath, and a diastolic murmur. On multislice axial images, a turbulent eccentric jet of aortic insufficiency *(long solid arrow)* is seen radiating from the anterolateral septal leaflet of the mitral valve. The LV end-diastolic and end-systolic dimensions were dilated, as were the aortic root and sinus of Valsalva. Although an Austin Flint murmur was not heard, there was evidence of LV inflow turbulence. The patient was referred for aortic valve replacement. *(Short solid arrow,* descending aorta; *open arrow,* left atrium; *thin arrows,* aortic valve leaflets.)

valvular disease. However, its ability to visualize normal valve tissue and associated abnormalities directly is somewhat limited as compared with echocardiography. From time to time, it is possible to make excellent images of a bicuspid or tricuspid aortic valve.

## Aortic and Peripheral Vascular Imaging

MRA has become an excellent approach for noninvasive imaging of the aorta, the cerebral vasculature, and the iliofemoral arterial system. Because signal is generated through the motion of blood, MRA requires no contrast agent, although such agents might serve to improve quality in the future. One of the most important applications of MRA is the detection and assessment of aortic disease. In fact, it is now recognized widely as the gold standard for diagnosis of aortic dissection and its extent and for the detection and sizing of aortic aneurysms. In dissection, intimal flaps and entry site can be identified, allowing for classification of the true and false lumen, differentiation between blood flow and clot in the pseudolumen, and involvement of branch vessels (Figs. 14–11, 14–12). The critical distinction between a DeBakey dissection type 1 or 2 and a type 3 lesion requires the high resolution that MRI can offer, permitting a high degree of confidence for surgical correction or medical management. Congenital anomalies of the aorta can also be identified, such as coarctation, arch interruption, and transposition.

The ability to image the cerebral arterial supply, including the carotids and vertebrals, has become routine in clinical practice and is rapidly being recognized as the best imaging strategy. Several studies indicate that catheter angiography is no longer the gold standard for carotid interrogations. Nonetheless, the Holy Grail of cardiology is the imaging of the coronary arteries. Substantial progress has been made toward this goal during the past decade, and with the newest instrumentation, imaging the proximal trunks of the coronary arteries is feasible. It has already been shown to be more accurate for the delineation of anomalous coronary arteries than x-ray angiography is (Fig. 14–13). More investigation is needed to refine coronary MRA. Such additions as the use of a blood pool contrast agent might improve the sensitivity and specificity as compared with catheter coronary angiog-

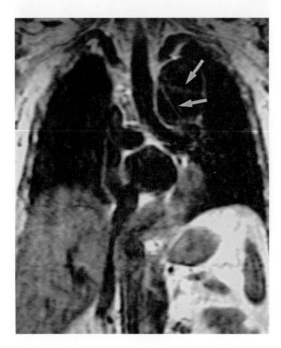

**Figure 14–11** ■ A 52-year-old white man presented with progressive chest pain and widened mediastinum on chest films. He was found to have a DeBakey I aortic aneurysm and underwent a composite graft limited to his ascending aorta. Follow-up MRI revealed progressive extension to the arch and descending aorta. The coronal image reveals a triluminal dissection *(arrows)*. The true lumen occupies a compressed and distorted space.

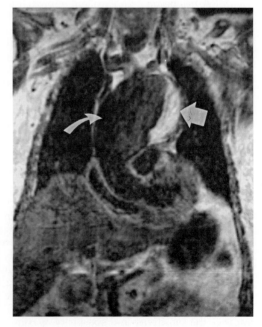

**Figure 14–12** ■ Coronal high-resolution spin echo images of a 72-year-old white man who had a markedly dilated ascending aortic aneurysm with unsuspected dissection *(curved arrow)* and localized thrombus *(wide arrow)*. The maximum intraluminal dimension is 100 mm. The patient elected not to have surgical correction.

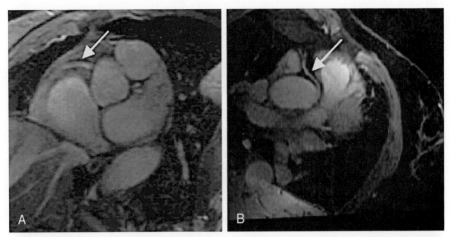

**Figure 14–13** ▪ After an inconclusive arteriogram, a 40-year-old black woman was referred for evaluation of an anomalous coronary artery. By cardiac catheterization, the course of the right coronary artery (RCA) as it originated from the proximal left anterior descending artery was unclear. An MRI fat suppression cine technique (A) suggested that the RCA may arise in the correct position (arrow); however, a slightly cranial view (B) revealed that the RCA (arrow) arises from the left coronary cusp to travel between the right ventricular outflow tract and the aorta before emerging anteriorly. This places the patient at a finite risk for sudden death. Treatment was surgical unroofing of the intracristal portion of the coronary artery.

raphy. A few investigators have even evaluated the potential for MR to characterize arterial plaque. Clinical determination of plaque vulnerability will probably emerge in the new millennium, since it is within the realm of possibility for this versatile technology.

## Future Applications

We are far from exhausting the potential of MR in applications to the cardiovascular system. It is now possible to obtain reasonably good images of the proximal coronary arteries, but substantial work is oriented toward myocardial perfusion imaging to generate images of perfusion patterns at rest and with stress or a stress equivalent (e.g., dipyridamole or adenosine vasodilators). At the present time, it appears that myocardial perfusion imaging can be performed using a bolus injection of a gadolinium chelate (i.e., MR contrast material). Using this approach has provided accuracies not significantly different from those obtained with the radiopharmaceuticals thallium-201 as the chloride and technetium-99m sestamibi or similar technetium-labeled compounds. Noteworthy recent investigations suggest that MRI gadolinium infusion may have a role in identifying myocarditis or pericarditis (Fig. 14–14). Another unique application is the assessment of myocardial energy metabolism using MR spectroscopy (MRS).

## ▪ COMPUTED TOMOGRAPHY

EBCT employs an electron gun and a fixed tungsten target, as opposed to a standard x-ray tube, to produce x-rays and permit rapid acquisition of tomographic images (Fig. 14–15). Typically, a series of transaxial images can be obtained in 100 msec with a scan slice thickness of 3 mm. Scans are usually acquired during

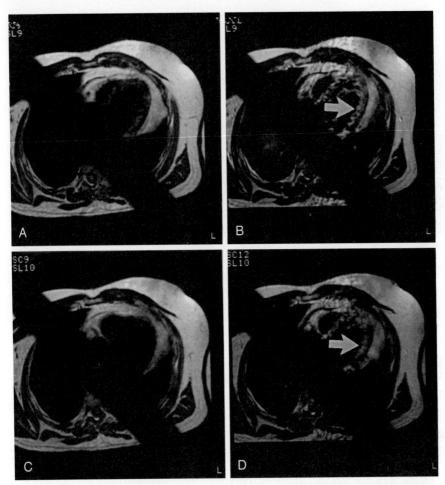

**Figure 14–14** ■ A 45-year-old white man had symptoms of LV dysfunction, chest pain, and no evidence of myocardial necrosis by laboratory findings. A paramagnetic agent (gadolinium DTPA) was infused, and, with a regional saturation slab applied (dark oblique band), myocardial enhancement was revealed. This suggested a myocardial inflammatory process consistent with myopericarditis (B, D). Note contrast enhancement of myocardium (arrow) with gadolinium as compared with the images without contrast (A, C). A and B show one slice; C and D, another.

breath holding, and acquisitions are triggered using the ECG signal to reduce the potentially blurring effect of heart motion.

There are several types of CT systems for cardiovascular diagnosis—conventional CT, helical CT, and EBCT. Conventional CT devices use a rotating x-ray source and a circular array of stationary detectors. Imaging time is typically much longer than is practical for cardiovascular purposes with conventional CT. If cardiac triggering were possible, it would still be impractical to acquire cardiac images in 2- to 5-second increments. The advent of helical CT permitted shorter acquisition times, which made cardiac imaging feasible. Helical CT is performed with the table continuously in motion during scanning, generating spiral or helical trajectories with better spatial resolution than conventional CT produces. The limita-

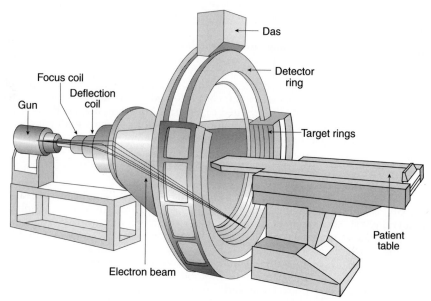

**Figure 14–15** ▪ Diagram of an electron beam computed tomographic imaging system. (Courtesy of Imatron.) (Das, digital amplification system.)

tion of conventional CT is that it cannot acquire images in a short time, and cardiac acquisitions must be coupled with a breath hold. EBCT is distinct from conventional and helical CT as neither scanner nor patient moves. An electron gun emits a 130-kV electron beam which is focused by electromagnetic coils and simultaneously deflected to stationary tungsten rings in which x-rays are generated. The produced x-ray is collimated through the patient to a high-grade crystal silicon photodiode detector. A series of detectors allow for high-resolution single-slice imaging in a temporal sequence consistent with cardiac motion. As with MRI, multiple planes can be obtained, but, unlike MRI, resolution is higher (on the order of 0.7 to 1.5 mm) owing to the higher contrast possible with x-ray imaging as compared with MRI.

One of the most important strengths of CT technology for cardiovascular imaging is its ability to generate volumetric images that represent three dimensions of data. A series of contiguous cross sections (tomographic sections) that are perpendicular to the long axis of the body can be obtained and, using retrospective reconstruction, provide a large volume of information. This allows evaluation of virtually any plane within the volume acquired. Conventional, spiral, or EBCT provides images superior to those of most other noninvasive methods. While previous generations of EBCT instruments have somewhat lower resolution than modern conventional CT imagers, recent improvements have refined EBCT so that its resolution is now comparable to that of conventional CT images. Another advantage of EBCT is that the shorter exposure times reduce the amount of radiation as compared with conventional CT. A consequence of less x-ray exposure is reduction in signal-to-noise ratio, particularly with cardiac imaging. Since scanning times are markedly reduced with EBCT, metallic scatter artifacts are considerably less prominent than with conventional or helical CT.

The major disadvantages of the CT techniques include the radiation exposure, particularly to the posterior structures of a supine patient (less with EBCT), and, because the relative densities of myocardium and the blood pool are nearly identical, there is an absolute need to administer radiopaque contrast medium. With regard to the first limitation, angiographic methods in the catheterization laboratory, coupled with interventional procedures, generate considerably more radiation exposure for patients and personnel. With regard to the second limitation, some patients may be allergic to radiopaque contrast medium, and, for patients who have borderline renal function, administration of contrast medium could precipitate renal failure. Finally, the osmotic load required to generate important diagnostic information could precipitate an episode of pulmonary edema in patients with congestive heart failure. Nevertheless, CT methods generate important diagnostic information.

## Present Applications

Many of the applications of EBCT are similar to those described for MRI: (1) coronary calcification/angiography, (2) assessment of the aorta and peripheral vasculature,[13] (3) assessment of cardiac chamber volumes and ventricular function,[14] (4) evaluation of pulmonary arteries, and (5) detection of cardiac masses. A number of studies have described the use of EBCT to assess right and left ventricular function. After intravenous administration of radiopaque contrast medium, serial images depict the cardiac chambers with good contrast between ventricular wall and ventricular blood pool. From such an acquisition, left and right ventricular ejection fractions and volumes can accurately be determined.

At present, the most common use[15] for EBCT is detecting coronary artery calcification, an indicator of atherosclerosis, an application for which MRI is unsuccessful. In view of the high speed of EBCT acquisition, the coronary arteries are virtually "frozen" in space, and the extent of calcification can be accurately assessed (Fig. 14–16). Although spiral CT can provide relatively fast (subsecond) acquisitions, the blurring effect due to cardiac motion could be problematic. Nevertheless, owing to the widespread availability of spiral CT scanners, in contrast to EBCT scanners, it would be desirable if spiral CT provided information comparable to that of EBCT. Advances in spiral CT technology should also allow it to be developed as a cardiac imaging tool.[16] While the application of EBCT to determining the extent of calcium has become somewhat of an industry, its true value as a predictor of functionally significant coronary artery disease and outcomes remains controver-

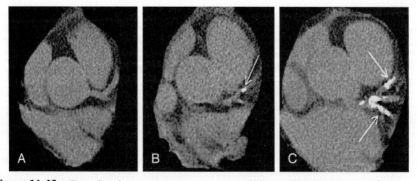

**Figure 14–16** ▪ Examples of progressive coronary artery calcification. Signal increases as the coronary intraluminal calcium burden rises *(arrows)*. Formal calcium scores can be quantified from the scans based on coronary artery calcification and density (Agaston algorithm). Although calcium is a well-accepted marker of atherosclerosis, the direct relation between calcium and prediction of clinical events is less conclusively established. (Courtesy of Imatron.)

sial.[17] It clearly indicates atherosclerosis but not its physiologic significance. The proponents of the application of EBCT maintain that it should become a routine study for risk assessment[18]; however, metaanalysis suggests that it is no better than the much less expensive ECG exercise test. Others suggest that plaque rupture, a common cause of coronary occlusion, is related to the lipid constituents of plaque (invisible to x-rays), not to the amount of calcium. At present, the role of EBCT coronary calcium score is uncertain although it does provide another, albeit expensive, means for risk assessment. This position has been supported by the American Heart Association. More data will be required to determine its actual utility.

Several approaches to coronary angiography by EBCT have been reported (Fig. 14–17). While the image quality is impressive, there is little anatomic and physiologic validation to support its use in current clinical practice.[19, 20] Moreover, at present, contrast medium injection is required.

## Aortic and Peripheral Vascular Disease

The thoracic and abdominal aorta can readily be evaluated using spiral CT after an injection of radiopaque contrast medium. Aortic aneurysms and dissections are defected and assessed. Where aortic MRI is not available, spiral or EBCT is preferred for diagnostic assessment. Like MRI, CT methods are useful for visualizing the internal flap and for determining the extent of branch vessel involvement. Whereas MRI is useful for differentiating between aortic aneurysm with mural

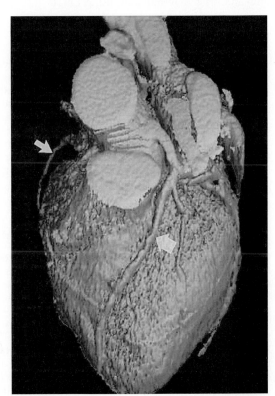

**Figure 14–17** ■ Three-dimensional electron beam computed tomography (EBCT) depicts the epicardium as well as the LAD *(thick arrow)* and the right coronary artery *(thin arrow)*. (*LAD,* left anterior descending artery; *RCA,* right coronary artery.) (Courtesy of Imatron.)

thrombus and dissection with thrombus in the pseudolumen, x-ray CT cannot readily make this distinction. If the aortic wall is calcified, the size of an aneurysm can be evaluated without contrast medium.

Both spiral and EBCT have been used to visualize the renal arteries for the diagnostic evaluation of patients with hypertension. Using contrast enhancement patterns, kidney volumes (including cortical and medullary) can be determined. The high speed of EBCT provides a means of examining renal blood flow and excretion. Although other branch vessels from the aorta can also be visualized, including the celiac, the superior and inferior mesenterics, the iliofemorals, the brachiocephalic, and the carotids and vertebral arteries, MRI is the preferred technique in the majority of patients.

## Cardiac Chamber Volumes, Ejection Fraction, and Mass

Like MRI, EBCT provides a means of evaluating heart function, including chamber volumes, ejection fraction, and myocardial mass. Of course, it is essential to use radiopaque contrast medium to define the inner borders of the cardiac chambers. High-resolution images can be generated that allow precise measurement of regional and global ventricular function. As with MRI, a series of short-axis ventricular tomographs approximately 1 cm thick are acquired. These slices can sample 10 to 20 or more images throughout the cardiac cycle. With a modification of Simpson's rule, ventricular volume and mass can be determined. Studies in both laboratory animals and humans demonstrate the reliability of left ventricular volume and mass determination using EBCT.

## Pulmonary Arteries

Pulmonary embolisms have been reliably identified using spiral CT, which, however, requires a breath hold for optimal imaging of the pulmonary arteries. EBCT requires no breath holding, which for patients with possible pulmonary embolism is a very difficult challenge. Both breath holding spiral CT and non–breath hold EBCT have been reported to have sensitivity on the order of 85% and specificity in the low 90% range with selection of a group with intermediate probability of disease by radionuclide ventilation perfusion scanning. Generally, the combination of ventilation-perfusion scanning followed by CT is the optimal strategy for detecting pulmonary embolism in a minimally invasive way.

## Pericardium and Cardiac Masses

The pericardium can be visualized by CT techniques as a line to 1 to 2 mm thick with radiodensity similar to that of myocardium. As with MRI, pericardial thickening and calcification can readily be visualized by spiral and EBCT, although the contrast between pericardium and myocardium is better on MRI. While pericardial diseases should be evaluated initially by two-dimensional echocardiography, both MRI and CT methods are useful for more comprehensive evaluation of patients for possible pericardial disease.

Clearly, intracardiac masses such as atrial myxomas and atrial and ventricular thrombi can be detected and evaluated by EBCT. Virtually any tumor within the heart or that compromises atrial or ventricular function can be assessed. Unfortunately, rhabdomyosarcomas and fibromas cannot be distinguished from myocardium on EBCT, since their density is equivalent to that of myocardium. Because of its T1 and T2 imaging parameters, MRI can frequently differentiate tumors from myocardium.

## ■ CONCLUSIONS

MRI and EBCT are the most advanced cardiovascular imaging technologies (Table 14–1). Both techniques have been available for clinical use since around 1980, and advances in both have been achieved throughout the years, but MRI has

Table 14–1

**MRI and EBCT: Respective Clinical Applications**

| | MRI | EBCT |
|---|---|---|
| **Cardiac morphology** | Excellent intrinsic soft tissue and blood contrast allows delineation of anatomic features with good resolution. No contrast medium required. | Requires contrast agent to delineate blood pool features but provides good anatomic depiction |
| **Cardiac function** | Excellent temporal and spatial resolution with any orientation allows optimal evaluation of contractile function. Radiofrequency tags provide further delineation of regional wall function. | Requires contrast agent to distinguish blood pool, limited angulation available, but three-dimensional images can be generated with good resolution. |
| **Coronary anatomy** | Breath-hold techniques allow coronary artery location to be traced to origin. | Contrast techniques allow coronary artery trajectory to be traced to origin. |
| **Coronary stenosis detection** | Limited ability at present to reliably detect stensosis due to decreased signal within the artery related to turbulence | Limited ability at present to detect stenosis, but some potential |
| **Myocardial perfusion** | Techniques being developed to detect myocardial perfusion | Techniques being developed to assess myocardial perfusion by tracking a bolus of radiopaque contrast |
| **Pericardial disease** | Allows differentiation between restrictive and constrictive disease (i.e., generally, myocardial vs. pericardial). "Gold standard" for assessing pericardial thickness. | Less able to distinguish between myocardium and pericardium |
| **Valvular assessment** | Can assess valve function and visualize turbulent flow to approximate the severity of regurgitation and stenosis | Unable to visualize turbulence; must rely on ancillary data (quantifying differences in stroke volumes between left and right ventricles) |
| **Metallic artifacts** | Signal void | Streak artifacts |
| **Cardiac massess** | Can be easily detected; may be a role for T1 and T2 tissue characterization | Can be identified after a contrast bolus |
| **Contrast agent** | Chelates of gadolinium and dysprosium with no known adverse effects | Iodinated contrast has many adverse effects: renal failure, anaphylaxis, pulmonary edema |
| **Angiography of the arterial system:** | No need for contrast agent, although early data suggest contrast markedly shortens acquisition time and further increases resolution | Radiopaque iodinated contrast agent required |
| Aorta | + + + + | + + + |
| Arch | + + + + | + + + |
| Carotids | + + + + | + + |
| Peripheral | + + + + | + + + |
| **Coronary calcification** | Not well visualized | Easily visualized without contrast administration |
| **Ionizing radiation** | No | Yes |

proven to be the more versatile, owing to its ability to use a number of contrast mechanisms, whereas EBCT methods rely only on x-ray attenuation. Both technologies have substantial clinical utility, however, and can often be used for similar diagnostic applications. When a facility has only MRI or only EBCT, it may be possible to use that modality as the primary diagnostic study. If the advances of the last decade are any indication, both techniques are poised for substantial breakthroughs in cardiovascular imaging for improving speed, resolution, and diagnostic accuracy.

## ■ REFERENCES

1. Pohost GM, and O'Rourke RA (eds): Basic Principles of Magnetic Resonance. Principles and Practice of Cardiovascular Imaging. Boston: Little, Brown (1990).
2. Cranney GB, Lotan CS, Dean L, et al: Left ventricular volume measurements using cardiac axis nuclear magnetic imaging: Validation by calibrated ventricular angiography. Circulation 1990;82:154–163.
3. Dell'Italia LJ, Blackwell GC, Pearce WJ, Pohost GM: Assessment of ventricular volumes using cine magnetic resonance in the intact dog. A comparison of measurement methods. Invest Radiol 1994;2:162–166.
4. Benjelloun H, Cranney GB, Kirk KA, et al: Interstudy reproducibility of biplane cine nuclear magnetic resonance measurements of left ventricular function. Am J Cardiol 1991;67:1413–1419.
5. Bottini PB, Carr AA, Prisant LM, et al: Magnetic resonance imaging compared to echocardiography to assess left ventricular mass in the hypertensive patient. Am J Hypertens 1995;8(3):221–228.
6. Young AA, Kramer CM, Ferrari VA, et al: Three-dimensional left ventricular deformation in hypertrophic cardiomyopathy. Circulation 1994;90:854–867.
7. Marcus JT, Gotte JW, DeWaal LK, et al: The influence of through-plane motion on left ventricular volumes measured by magnetic resonance imaging: Implications for image acquisition and analysis. J Cardiol Magn Reson 1999(1);1–6.
8. Semelka RC, Tomei E, Wagner S, et al: Interstudy reproducibility of dimension and functional measurements between cine magnetic resonance studies in the morphologically abnormal left ventricle. Am Heart J 1990;119:1367–1371.
9. Fujita N, Duerinckx AJ, Higgins CB: Variation in left ventricular wall stress with cine magnetic resonance imaging: Normal subjects versus dilated cardiomyopathy. Am Heart J 1993;125(5 Pt. 1):1337–1344.
10. Wallis DE, O'Connell JB, Henkin RE, et al: The value of echocardiographic regional wall motion abnormalities in dilated cardiomyopathies: A common finding and good prognostic sign. J Am Coll Cardiol 1984;4:674–670.
11. Friedrich MG, Strohm O, Schulz-Menger J, et al: Contrast media–enhanced magnetic resonance imaging visualizes myocardial changes in the course of viral myocarditis. Circulation 1998;97(18):1802–1809.
12. Fujita N, Chazouillers AF, Hartialla JJ: Quantification of mitral regurgitation by velocity encoding cine nuclear magnetic resonance imaging. J Am Coll Cardiol 1994;23:951–952.
13. Summers RM, Andrasko-Boutgeois J, Feuerstein IM, et al: Evaluation of the aortic root by MRI: Insights from patients with homozygous familial hypercholesterolemia. Circulation 1998;98(6):509–518.
14. Budoff MJ, Shavelle DM, Lamont DH, et al: Usefulness of electron beam computed tomography scanning for distinguishing ischemic from nonischemic cardiomyopathy. J Am Coll Cardiol 1998;32(5):1173–1178.
15. Schmermund A, Bailey KR, Rumberger JA, et al: An algorithm for noninvasive identification of angiographic three-vessel and/or left main coronary artery disease in symptomatic patients on the basis of cardiac risk and electron-beam computed tomographic calcium scores. J Am Coll Cardiol 1999;33(2):444–452.
16. Schmermund A, Bell MR, Lerman LO, et al: Quantitative evaluation of regional myocardial perfusion using fast x-ray computed tomography. Herz 1997;22(1):29–39.
17. Callister TQ, Raggi P, Cooil B, et al: Effect of HMG-CoA reductase inhibitors on coronary artery disease as assessed by electron-beam computed tomography. N Engl J Med 1998;339(27):1972–1978.
18. Woo P, Mao S, Wang S, Detrano RC: Left ventricular size determined by electron beam computed tomography predicts significant coronary artery disease and events. Am J Cardiol 1997;79(9):1236–1238.
19. Rumberger JA, Brundage BH, Rader DJ, Kondos G: Electron beam computed tomographic coronary calcium scanning: A review and guidelines for use in asymptomatic persons. Mayo Clinic Proc 1999;74(3):243–252.
20. Detrano RC, Wong ND, Doherty TM, et al: Coronary calcium does not accurately predict near-term future coronary events in high-risk adults. Circulation 1999;99(20):2633–2638.

## ■ RECOMMENDED READING

Detrano RC, Wong ND, Doherty TM, et al: Coronary calcium does not accurately predict near-term future coronary events in high-risk adults. Circulation 1999;99(20):2633–2638.

Manning WJ, Li W, Edelman RR: A preliminary report comparing magnetic resonance coronary angiography with conventional angiography. N Engl J Med 1993;328:828–832.

Martin ET, Fuisz AR, Pohost GM: Imaging cardiac structure and pump function. Cardiol Clin 1998;16(2):135–160.

Pohost GM, O'Rourke RA: Basic Principles of Magnetic Resonance. Principles and Practice of Cardiovascular Imaging. Little, Brown and Company, Boston, 1990.

Rumberger JA, Brundage BH, Rader DJ, Kondos G: Electron beam computed tomographic coronary calcium scanning: A review and guidelines for use in asymptomatic persons. Mayo Clin Proc 1999;74(3):243–252.

# Chapter 15

# Choosing Appropriate Imaging Techniques

*Robin L. Davisson* ■ *David J. Skorton*

The clinician who cares for patients known or suspected to have cardiovascular disease has an extremely large variety of diagnostic approaches from which to choose. Even in this high-technology era, the evaluation of such patients begins with the history and physical examination. After these initial data have been gathered, myriad laboratory examinations can be employed. With the exception of electrocardiography (ECG) and electrophysiologic examinations, most diagnostic procedures in current use fall into the category of imaging methods.[1, 2]

Chest roentgenography, the first imaging method available to clinicians, was followed by cardiac angiography, radionuclide methods, ultrasonography (US), and, more recently, computed tomography (CT), and magnetic resonance imaging (MRI). Our purpose in this chapter is to suggest a conceptual framework within which a busy clinician can choose wisely among the large and sometimes bewildering array of techniques available for imaging the heart and vascular system. The overriding theme of this discussion is that knowledge of the capabilities of the various methods and the specific diagnostic needs of a particular patient may lead to a logical decision about which diagnostic approach to pursue.

## ■ DECISION ELEMENTS IN THE CHOICE

### Goals of Imaging

The complete cardiovascular evaluation requires assessment of cardiac chamber anatomy and function in both systole and diastole, coronary arterial anatomy and function, valvular function, myocardial perfusion, myocardial biochemistry, and tissue characteristics. At the current state of development, imaging methods offer information on chamber anatomy and function, valvular function, and coronary anatomy that is often quantitatively precise and accurate. Today, information on coronary artery function and myocardial perfusion is based on qualitative, or at best semiquantitative, estimates of regional myocardial blood flow. Finally, scant data are available presently concerning myocardial biochemistry or tissue characteristics in the clinical setting.

### Determinants of Image Formation

The information available from the various imaging methods is based on different fundamental methods of image formation. Because of this, the information content of the methods differs and is sometimes complementary. Table 15–1 lists some physical and physiologic attributes that affect the information content of medical images.

Table 15–1

**Some Determinants of Image Intensity**

| Energy Form | Image Intensity Determinants |
| --- | --- |
| X-ray based methods | Density of tissue |
|   Plain film radiography | Local contrast (iodine) concentration |
|   Angiography | |
|   Computed tomography | |
| Ultrasound | Acoustic velocity |
| | Tissue density |
| | Tissue elasticity |
| | Contrast agent |
| Radionuclides | Tracer concentration (depends on biologic activity of ligand) |
| | Photon energy |
| Magnetic resonance methods | Proton (spin) density (i.e., water content) |
| | Nuclear magnetic resonance relaxation times |
| | Chemical shift |
| | Blood flow |
| | Contrast agent |

Skorton DJ, Brundage BH, Schelbert HR, Wolf GL: Relative merits of imaging techniques. *In* Braunwald E (ed): Heart Disease: A Textbook of Cardiovascular Medicine, 5th ed. Philadelphia: WB Saunders, 1997:349–359.

X-ray techniques, including chest roentgenography, fluoroscopy, cardiac angiography, and CT, rely on the different physical densities and atomic composition of tissues interposed between the x-ray source and the detector system. The contrast available in these images can be much improved by adding iodinated contrast agents like those commonly used in angiography. X-ray–based cineangiographic techniques offer fine spatial resolution and, therefore, the ability to define extremely small objects such as partially occluded coronary arterial lumens. The temporal resolution of angiographic methods is also excellent.

Radionuclide methods are perhaps the most versatile imaging approaches: what information is gathered depends on what radionuclide is used for labeling and on the physiologically relevant ligand to which the nuclide is linked. Modern cardiac radionuclide procedures are moving increasingly from the planar or projection mode to tomographic approaches, which greatly improve image contrast and anatomic specificity. *Planar* or *projection imaging* is an approach in which a radionuclide is inhaled by or injected into the patient and photons released during radionuclide decay are detected externally by a fixed camera. In tomography, photon data are gathered at many angles around the patient and integrated by computer to produce an image of the distribution of the radionuclide in a given "slice" of tissue.[3] This approach has improved the usefulness of radionuclide methods. In addition to contrast enhancement, tomography offers other advantages. For example, structures superimposed between the region of interest and the camera degrade planar images; this is improved with tomography.

The most widespread application of tomography in radionuclide imaging, single photon emission computed tomography (SPECT), uses thallium 201 or technetium 99m–labeled ligands (for myocardial perfusion) or [99mTc]-labeled red blood cells (for blood pool imaging). The spatial and temporal resolution of radionuclide methods is relatively poorer than those of conventional radiographic procedures, but the functional data are nonetheless extremely useful. The best resolution and greatest amount of quantitative information currently available by radionuclide imaging is obtained with positron emission tomography (PET).[4] As opposed to agents such as [201Tl] or [99mTc], positron-emitting radionuclides when they decay release a positively charged electron (positron). When the positron encounters an electron in nearby tissue both are annihilated, releasing two photons that travel in diametrically opposite directions. Simultaneous detection of the photons by a ring-like detector or by a modified gamma camera system[5] permits extremely accurate measurement of the distribution of the PET radionuclide within the slice of interest. PET scanning allows quantitative assessment of myocardial perfusion and evaluation of regional fuel substrate uptake and other metabolic variables in the myocardium. Unfortunately, the technology required for PET scanning is expensive, technically demanding, and not as widely available as that for SPECT imaging; however, with newer gamma camera configurations the cost will be reduced, and the availability and ease of use of these imaging agents should improve substantially.[5]

The preceding comments regarding projection and tomographic imaging are also applicable to methods of image formation other than radionuclide imaging. For example, chest roentgenography is another example of projection imaging, whereas CT is an example of tomography, in which x-rays are sent from an x-ray source, pass through the patient, and are detected on the opposite side of the patient. X-ray attenuation data from many such detections at varying angles are used to compute the CT image data.[6]

US evaluation of the heart (echocardiography) is among the most widely used techniques in cardiac diagnosis. US uses mechanical energy (sound) instead of the electromagnetic energy used in all other imaging methods.[3] Because of this, the attributes of US images are different from those of other imaging modalities. Spatial resolution is good and on the order of that obtainable with CT or MRI. Temporal resolution is generally superior to that of other techniques, particularly in M-mode echocardiographic applications.

The most recent addition to the clinician's diagnostic armamentarium is MRI. A complex technique whose image attributes depend on a variety of physical and physiologic variables (see Table 15–1), MRI has not yet made major inroads in clinical use for cardiovascular disease; however, the excellent spatial resolution, improving temporal resolution (of newer rapid-acquisition techniques), and broad range of information available from MRI make it likely that this approach to cardiac diagnosis will be used more in the near future.

## Logistics and Local Expertise

When choosing an imaging examination for a specific case, the clinician must make the best match between the constraints of the clinical situation and the methods available. Therefore, because they are portable, US methods, radionuclide scans, and chest roentgenography may be used in emergency settings and at the bedside, whereas angiography, CT, and MRI generally cannot be used in this setting.

A very important consideration in the choice of the imaging procedure is local expertise in the available methods. Particularly when two or more imaging techniques would gather approximately equally useful information, the relative expertise in use of each of the methods must be taken into account.

## Cost Effectiveness

Imaging methods vary greatly in the costs of the equipment, trained personnel, and other operational costs. At one end of the spectrum is US, the costs of which (for both the system and support personnel) are relatively modest. At the other end of the spectrum are MRI, CT, and PET, all of which cost much more to acquire and to operate. Between these two ends of the spectrum lie the other radionuclide techniques.

A more subtle measure of cost-effectiveness is the cost of the overall diagnostic workup for a given patient. A relatively expensive imaging method may in the long run prove cost-effective if it replaces other diagnostic techniques or gathers singularly useful data. For example, in one recent study,[7] coronary angiography was shown to be the most cost-effective initial test for coronary disease in a population at high risk. Unfortunately, historically, new technology introduced into medical practice has often been an addition to, and not a replacement for, other diagnostic modalities. Of the available imaging methods, MRI may have the best potential for broad application to the gamut of diagnostic goals. Unfortunately, at this time and in most medical centers, none of the commonly available techniques affords such broad diagnostic capability. Therefore, the clinician needs to focus narrowly on each particular patient and the specific diagnostic goals.

## ■ CAPABILITIES OF IMAGING METHODS BY DIAGNOSTIC GOAL

### Anatomy

Chest radiographs supply useful information on overall cardiac size and on the approximate sizes of individual cardiac chambers; however, quantitative measurements of chamber size from chest films are not very precise. Furthermore, no information is available on ventricular wall thickness or detailed coronary anatomy. Echocardiography supplies accurate information on the size of the left heart chambers and reasonably reliable information on the size of right heart chambers. Currently, transthoracic (TTE) and transesophageal echocardiography (TEE) offer extremely accurate information on the size and shape of all four cardiac chambers, the valvular apparatus, and the great vessels. Intravascular US permits high-resolution imaging of the coronary arterial system.[8]

Exquisitely accurate information on cardiac chamber anatomy can also be obtained with rapid CT[9] or MRI.[10] Because of the imaging attributes of these procedures, they are probably somewhat more accurate than echocardiography, although whether this degree of accuracy has clinical relevance is unclear. When echocardiographic imaging is difficult in a particular patient, CT or MRI should be considered.

Detailed definition of coronary arterial anatomy remains the purview of angiography and, to some extent, intravascular US. Relatively recent studies employing CT[11] and MRI[12, 13] suggest potential for direct noninvasive imaging of the details of coronary anatomy; these methods are at present investigational. Because of the strong (and increasing) emphasis on interventional catheter procedures in coronary disease, catheterization will likely continue to be an important method of assessing coronary anatomy far into the future.

Radionuclide methods supply some information on cardiac anatomy, particularly on the relative size of chambers, but do not offer the precision of higher-resolution tomographic methods such as US, CT, and MRI.

### Chamber and Valve Function

Modern imaging methods supply excellent information on left ventricular function by a variety of techniques.[14] Echocardiography, radionuclide techniques (equilibrium blood pool and first-pass imaging and ECG-gated perfusion studies), angiography, CT, and MRI all supply useful information on left ventricular chamber function. Echocardiography, CT, and MRI are capable of clearly delineating regional wall thickening and, thus, have at least a theoretical advantage over radionuclide methods and angiography. On the other hand, radionuclide methods, since they are based on measurement of radionuclide counts throughout the heart cycle (as an index of ventricular volume), are independent of geometric assumptions or measurements for the assessment of left ventricular function. Overall, from a clinical perspective, all of these methods probably supply equally useful information on left ventricular systolic function.

Left ventricular diastolic function is complex and difficult to measure. A variety of approaches to assessing diastolic function have been developed and are in clinical use to some extent.[15] Doppler echocardiographic methods permit assessment of diastolic function based usually on transmitral or other flow dynamics.[16] Other echocardiographic methods, as well as radionuclide blood pool scanning, MRI, and CT, may be used to assess diastolic function by determining ventricular filling dynamics or related parameters.[17, 18] There is no consensus at present on the optimal approach to assessing diastolic function.

Right ventricular function is more difficult to assess then left ventricular function, in part because the right ventricle, with its complex shape, defies the relatively simple geometric modeling that can be applied to the left ventricle. Angiographic and echocardiographic methods have been developed to assess right ventricular size and contractile function.[19] MRI[20] and CT[21] can supply useful information on right ventricular volume and function, but, because of their limited availability, they are not widely used for this application at present. Radionuclide methods are very useful in assessing right ventricular function,[22] even in abnormally shaped ventricles. Atrial function is one of the most difficult areas of chamber function to evaluate, but useful information can be obtained with echocardiography, CT, or MRI.[23]

## Myocardial Perfusion

The importance of myocardial perfusion as a diagnostic goal has inspired a large variety of approaches to determining perfusion or deriving an index of perfusion. Figure 15–1 shows conceptual approaches to the assessment of myocardial perfusion. Coronary angiography is still widely used to identify the clinical setting likely to lead to hypoperfusion by assessing the degree of coronary arterial stenosis. Based on abundant experimental evidence, it is accepted that resting coronary flow decreases after diameter stenosis is approximately 75% and that stimulated or hyperemic flow is limited at approximately 50% stenosis. Initially, these data were largely derived from animal experiments in which symmetric stenoses were produced in otherwise normal coronary arterial beds. Unfortunately, extrapolation from these stenosis data to humans, whose coronary disease is complex and diffuse, does not always offer reliable diagnostic information.[24, 25] Coronary flow reserve has been a helpful measure of the physiologic significance of coronary stenosis.[26] Coronary flow reserve may be defined as the potential for increase in flow in response to a hyperemic stimulus. Classically, the stimulus was transient occlusion of a coronary artery followed by release of the artery and measurement of hyperemic flow and its relation to resting flow.[25] Vasodilators such as adenosine and dipyridamole have also been used to produce hyperemia, with coronary flow reserve calculated as the ratio of peak flow to resting flow. Utilizing coronary flow reserve as an independent standard, intermediate grades of coronary diameter stenosis have been shown to be quite imperfect predictors of the functional significance of coronary arterial stenosis in some patients.[24, 25] Therefore, a variety of functional measures have been developed, ranging from intravascular measurement of coronary flow in the clinical setting with a catheter-tipped Doppler crystal[27] to measurements of microvascular transit utilizing angiographic "blush" or CT or

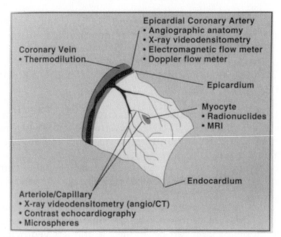

**Figure 15–1** ■ Some approaches to the assessment of coronary flow and myocardial perfusion. The illustration, a schematic cross-section of the left ventricular wall, indicates at which anatomic levels various methods are used to evaluate perfusion. At the level of the epicardial coronary arteries, angiographic anatomy is commonly used to identify hydraulically significant stenoses. X-ray videodensitometry and electromagnetic and Doppler flowmeters also may be used to assess perfusion at the level of the coronary arteries. (Some of these methods can be used only with an open chest). Coronary venous thermodilution methods afford some insight into global or regional perfusion. At the arteriolar/capillary level, x-ray videodensitometry, contrast echocardiography, and microspheres may be employed. Finally, radionuclide and MRI methods attempt to assess perfusion at the level of the myocyte. Angio, angiography. (Skorton DJ, Brundage BH, Schelbert HR, Wolf GL: Relative merits of imaging techniques. *In* Braunwald E (ed): Heart Disease: A Textbook of Cardiovascular Medicine, 5th ed. Philadelphia: WB Saunders, 1997:349–359.)

echocardiographic contrast transit.[28] Myocyte uptake of tracers such as thallium 201 or technetium 99m–labeled ligands or PET tracers and magnetic resonance contrast methods have also been used to measure myocardial flow. In present clinical practice, the most widely available techniques for directly assessing myocardial perfusion are thallium or $^{99m}$Tc-labeled molecules (such as sestamibi) used in perfusion radionuclide imaging. This category of imaging includes ECG-gated tomography,[29] which provides information on regional perfusion, regional wall motion, and ejection fraction.

An indirect approach to assessing perfusion deficits is to identify abnormalities in regional myocardial contraction related to hypoperfusion. This approach is the basis of exercise blood pool radionuclide scanning and of exercise or pharmacologic stress echocardiography. The goal is to identify new or increased regional wall motion disturbances during stress, which are indicators of hypoperfusion. In recent studies,[30, 31] stress echocardiography and stress radionuclide imaging have both been found efficacious in identifying hypoperfusion, in predicting prognosis, and in identifying potentially viable myocardium in ischemia.

In the future, other methods of assessing perfusion and viability will likely become available to the clinician. These will include contrast echocardiography,[28] the contrast agent being injected intravenously, and MRI,[32] probably utilizing magnetic resonance contrast agents.

## Myocardial Biochemistry

As knowledge of basic aspects of cardiovascular function in health and disease increases, clinicians will wish increasingly to evaluate the biochemical status of the myocardium at rest and with stress, particularly in patients with heart failure or acute or chronic ischemic heart disease. Some assessment of myocardial biochemistry has been afforded for decades by coronary venous lactate levels, which may be used to identify increases in myocardial anaerobic metabolism. This assessment, however, has required cardiac catheterization and was not very useful for assessing localized myocardial metabolism. The advent of PET has permitted direct evaluation of myocardial uptake of fuel substrates such as glucose. Other aspects of myocardial biochemistry, such as oxidative and fatty acid metabolism, can be assessed with PET.[33] Information on fatty acid and glucose metabolism can also be obtained with SPECT systems.[33] MRI, with nuclear magnetic resonance (NMR) spectroscopy, also holds the promise of evaluating myocardial bioenergetic status (e.g., levels of phosphocreatine and adenosine triphosphate).[33, 34] Routine myocardial biochemical evaluation by magnetic resonance spectroscopy is not currently available, and PET scanning with conventional, ring-type gantries is limited to a relatively small number of centers. Therefore, none of the currently available methods that is widely available permits comprehensive assessment of myocardial biochemistry in a manner that is helpful to the clinician.

## Tissue Characterization

A variety of cardiac disorders affect the gross or microscopic architecture or tissue composition of the myocardium or the blood vessel wall. In atherosclerotic coronary arteries, normal vessel wall structure is disrupted by fat deposition and calcification. After myocardial infarction or myocarditis, normal regions of myocardium are replaced by collagenous connective tissue. In hypertrophic cardiomyopathy, the regular, parallel arrangement of myofibrils is replaced by regions of myofibrillar disarray. In all of these clinical situations, assessment of anatomy (such as ventricular wall thickness) or function (such as regional myocardial contraction) suggests the disorder, but the clinician would be greatly aided by direct identification of scar, abnormal tissue architecture, or deposition of abnormal material. The attempt to demonstrate these tissue abnormalities has been termed *tissue characterization*, and a number of investigations have been performed with US,[35,] MRI,[36] and, to a lesser extent, CT[37] in attempts to characterize abnormal cardiac tissue.

The most extensive tissue characterization effort has employed US. Echocardiographers have long been aware that thickened, fibrotic, or calcified valvular tissue reflects US strongly, resulting in bright echoes on standard echocardiographic images. A large body of investigative literature has documented acoustic changes in ischemic, cardiomyopathic, fibrotic, and calcified tissue and in myocardium with amyloid deposition, myofibrillar disarray of hypertrophic cardiomyopathy, or other conditions.[38] Although promising, clinical use of US tissue characterization is currently limited to two applications: (1) visual recognition on standard echocardiograms of calcified valvular tissue and abnormally echogenic myocardium secondary to postinfarction scarring or amyloid or hypertrophic cardiomyopathy and (2) identification of atherosclerotic coronary arterial walls (with intravascular US).[39] Further investigation will determine whether more quantitative, objective means of US tissue characterization will be clinically useful.

A variety of changes in the physical state or composition of cardiac tissue will affect its nuclear magnetic resonance (NMR) properties.[36] This phenomenon is most likely related to induced changes in NMR relaxation times or other, complex, NMR image parameters. Acutely ischemic myocardium, fibrotic tissue, fatty deposition, and other myocardial abnormalities have been shown to alter NMR relaxation times or MRI appearance.[36, 40] Currently, these methods have not reached the stage of clinical utility, but they show great promise for the future.

CT images are affected by such abnormalities as calcification owing to differential attenuation of x-rays by the abnormal tissue. This phenomenon is responsible for the ability of CT to identify the presence and extent of coronary calcification, potentially useful information on the presence and severity of coronary atherosclerosis.[37, 41] CT cardiac tissue characterization is growing somewhat in clinical use, although, ultimately, its utility remains to be determined.

## ■ IMAGING OPTIONS IN SPECIFIC DISEASES

### Ischemic Heart Disease

Imaging methods are useful in assessing patients with ischemic heart disease by detecting coronary atherosclerosis, identifying acute changes in coronary flow and ischemia, delineating infarction and reperfusion, and detecting scar in chronically infarcted myocardium.

### Identification of Coronary Disease

Detecting atherosclerotic coronary artery disease and identifying its extent are key diagnostic challenges for clinicians. Both direct and indirect imaging approaches have been applied to detect and quantify coronary atherosclerosis.

Advanced coronary atheromas frequently calcify, and the detection of calcification can therefore be a marker for atherosclerosis. The sensitivity of CT for detection of calcium (because of its abnormal x-ray attenuation characteristics) has created widespread interest in screening for coronary calcification with CT. In some studies,[37, 41] CT has been shown to be a sensitive marker of coronary atherosclerosis.

Doppler echocardiographic methods have been used to identify abnormal flow patterns characteristic of severe coronary stenosis[42] but will not likely become mainstream methods of detecting coronary disease in the near future. CT and MRI may, in the future, permit noninvasive coronary angiography.[11–13]

Direct assessment of the extent and severity of coronary artery disease by selective coronary angiography will remain a mainstay of cardiac diagnosis for the foreseeable future. This is true because (1) the still unparalleled spatial resolution of coronary angiography affords imaging of even extremely stenotic lumina and (2) interest in interventional procedures done in the catheterization laboratory is increasing. Digital image-processing approaches, when applied to coronary arterial data, may increase the amount of information derived from these studies.[43]

Intravascular US permits high-resolution assessment of the coronary lumen and adjacent wall composition, including identification of components of the atheromatous plaque. In some regions where angiography predicted normal vessel status, intravascular US detected evidence of atherosclerotic disease.[44]

### Acute Ischemia

Evaluation of patients for suspected coronary disease often centers on the identification of reduced coronary flow or transient ischemia, particularly with exercise or pharmacologic stress. This strategy employs a variety of direct and indirect approaches using imaging techniques. Radionuclide scanning using [201]Tl- or [99m]Tc-labeled agents is capable of identifying decrements in regional myocardial perfusion produced by exercise stress or pharmacologic vasodilatation. These findings enhance the diagnostic value of exercise (treadmill) ECG studies.[45]

Identification of regional myocardial contraction abnormalities is an indirect approach to detecting acute ischemia. Exercise and pharmacologic stress echocardiography (the latter performed, for example, with dobutamine) and exercise radionuclide scanning are sensitive approaches to identifying acute myocardial ischemia and the extent of ischemic myocardium based on wall motion abnormalities. Local expertise may determine the technique of choice, but stress echocardiography and stress radionuclide methods are probably approximately equally sensitive for detecting acute myocardial ischemia. Because echocardiography permits precise measurement of regional wall thickening, assessment may be more complete with this approach. With ECG-gated SPECT radionuclide scanning, both perfusion and regional wall motion may be evaluated.[29] Stress imaging of regional contraction may also be done with CT or MRI, but this is not common practice at present.

## Acute Infarction

Imaging techniques for identification of acute myocardial infarction include the indirect approaches mentioned above: gated blood pool or SPECT radionuclide scanning and echocardiography to identify regional wall motion disturbances. If abnormal wall motion is persistent and is known to have become abnormal with an acute event, then a regional wall motion disturbance can confidently be attributed to myocardial infarction. If earlier study results are not available, it may be difficult to know how to interpret regional wall motion disturbances. The assessment of regional wall motion abnormalities by any technique is also rendered more difficult because of biological heterogeneity of contraction in normal subjects[46] and the fact that regional wall motion patterns appear to be somewhat dependent on loading conditions[47] and other factors. A wall motion disturbance may be caused by ischemia, infarction, or scar, leading to some difficulty in interpreting indirect studies of infarction based on regional wall motion disturbances.

Direct identification of acutely necrotic tissue can be accomplished with $^{99m}$Tc pyrophosphate scans and by using labeled monoclonal antimyosin-specific antibodies.[48] The relatively coarse spatial resolution of these techniques limits their ability to assess the details of infarct extent, but they play an important role in certain patients.

In conditions of chronic hypoperfusion or in the setting of acute myocardial infarction, the reversibility of abnormalities in perfusion or regional wall motion is of much interest to clinicians. Whether due to acute infarction, "stunning," or "hibernation," reversal of regional wall motion disturbance identified by any of a variety of imaging techniques will identify the viability of the involved myocardium.[49] Determination of viability by regional wall motion assessment with echocardiography or by perfusion assessment using $^{201}$Tl or technetium-based agents are probably about equally effective in clinical use. MRI may in the future play a role in the assessment of viability by demonstrating either abnormal regional contraction or contrast enhancement of the myocardium.[50]

At present, the independent standard most accepted for definitive determination of myocardial viability is metabolic imaging with PET. By combining scans of perfusion with assessment of fuel substrate uptake, viable myocardium can be distinguished from nonviable tissue.[51] In nonviable (necrotic) myocardium, both perfusion and fuel substrate uptake are diminished or absent; however, in viable myocardium, although perfusion may be greatly diminished, fuel substrate uptake is preserved and may even be enhanced (for example, because of increased glucose uptake with anaerobic glycolysis in ischemia).

Metabolic studies using MR spectroscopy and assessment of high-energy phosphate stores may in the future also prove helpful in identifying the viability of myocardium.

## Scar

The identification of collagenous replacement of myocardium due to the residua of acute infarction, myocarditis, or another cause is frequently of clinical interest. From early observations, echocardiographers have long been aware that chronically scarred myocardium not only fails to contract normally but is also thinner than normal in diastole. Scarred tissue at times may also be identifiable by echogenicity (brightness) greater than that of adjacent, normal tissue. Quantitative US tissue characterization seeks to make that determination more objective and reliable.

Radionuclide perfusion imaging is used to infer the presence of scar when regional perfusion persists after an acute ischemic episode. The accuracy of this approach depends in part on such variables as the severity of the perfusion deficit and the lack of redistribution.

## Valvular Heart Disease

The main goals of imaging-based diagnosis in valvular heart disease are assessment of valvular anatomy and function and determination of the function of the abnormally loaded ventricle. At present, echocardiography is the procedure of first choice, because it may be used to assess virtually all of the important parameters in a patient with valvular heart disease. The combination of high-resolution echocardiographic imaging and Doppler echocardiography permits complete assessment of most patients with valvular heart disease and guides decisions on medical, surgical, or catheter-based therapy. Angiography and cardiac catheterization sometimes may be needed, particularly in complex multivalvular disease, to assess chamber and great artery pressures and to define coronary artery anatomy. Furthermore, occasionally ventricular function is better assessed with radionuclide techniques, particularly when echocardiography is limited because of body habitus. Although CT and MRI are certainly capable of great accuracy in assessing ventricular function, at present they have secondary roles in the assessment of valvular heart disease. It should be noted that flow-sensitive MRI methods may give useful information somewhat analogous to that available with Doppler echocardiography, along with data on ventricular volumes.[52]

## Congenital Heart Disease

Evaluation of patients with congenital heart disease requires accurate delineation of cardiac anatomy, intracardiac and great vessel blood flow patterns, and ventricular and valvular function. Particularly because of the sometimes complex morphologic characteristics of congenital heart disease, high-resolution depiction of anatomy is paramount. Presently, echocardiography is the initial method of choice for evaluating the anatomy of the heart from fetal life through adulthood. Echocardiographic techniques, particularly with the inclusion of Doppler and transesophageal studies, often provide sufficiently accurate diagnostic information to allow the cardiologist to refer patients for surgery or catheter interventions without further diagnostic studies.[53]

Radionuclide studies, particularly first-pass angiography, are also useful in congenital heart disease because of their ability to accurately and noninvasively quantitate intracardiac shunts.[54]

The highest-resolution methods, CT and MRI, also offer useful information on congenital heart disease. In particular, MRI permits clear depiction of cardiac anatomy and of extracardiac conduits.[55]

## Cardiomyopathy

Echocardiography is capable of clearly differentiating among restrictive, hypertrophic, and dilated cardiomyopathies. Tissue characterization techniques, if they become clinically available, may help to determine specific causes of dilated cardio-myopathy; however, at present, echocardiography offers enough information to classify the cardiomyopathy and to direct initial clinical management. Radionuclide techniques also contribute to the assessment of left ventricular function (particularly when echocardiographic studies are difficult owing to body habitus) or right ventricular systolic function.

Cardiac catheterization still has a place in evaluating cardiomyopathies because of the need for detailed hemodynamic evaluation and knowledge of coronary artery status in certain patients and the need in some circumstances for endomyo-cardial biopsy. Assessment of cardiac biochemistry utilizing MRI spectroscopy or PET scanning may also be of use in future for patients with myocarditis or cardiomyopathy.

## Heart Trauma

Patients who have experienced chest trauma frequently have cardiovascular injuries, which range from aortic dissection to chordal rupture, myocardial contusion, hemopericardium, valvular avulsion, and coronary laceration. Transthoracic and transesophageal echocardiography and cardiac catheterization are frequently used in patients with acute trauma. In centers where they are available, CT and MRI may also be of use, but usually they cannot be deployed at the bedside in the emergency department. Technetium-99m pyrophosphate and antimyosin antibody imaging sometimes permit identification of acute myocardial contusion.

## Pericardial Disease

Echocardiography, CT, and MRI all permit excellent delineation of pericardial effusion. CT and MRI are likely superior to echocardiography for assessment of pericardial thickness. The sensitivity of CT to calcification may help to identify calcified constrictive pericardial disease. Doppler studies and volumetric curves derived from radionuclide data, CT, or MRI may prove useful in identifying restrictive (versus constrictive) physiologic processes.

## Infective Endocarditis

Echocardiography is sensitive to the valvular vegetations of endocarditis, and the advent of TEE has further enhanced this sensitivity.[56] Accordingly, echocardiography is the imaging technique of first choice for investigating suspected infective endocarditis. It can also be used to identify complications of endocarditis such as valvular insufficiency and chordal rupture, among others. CT and MRI may prove helpful in identifying these abnormalities and intracardiac abscesses.

Table 15–2 summarizes our opinion on the relative utility of the various cardiac imaging methods in specific patient groups.

## ■ IMAGING AND RESEARCH IN CARDIOVASCULAR DISEASE

One of the great challenges in clinical cardiology is to identify disorders before they are clinically manifested. A variety of longitudinal clinical studies of high-risk populations can help to identify the sensitivity of imaging techniques to early, preclinical changes in cardiac structure or function. Another approach to identifying preclinical disease and to understanding the place of a diagnostic technology in this identification is in the research setting, particularly by utilizing animal models.

Table 15–2

**Relative Usefulness of Imaging Methods
for Investigating Specific Cardiac Disorders**

| Disorder | CXR | Echo/ Doppler | Angio* | Radio- nuclides | RCT | MRI |
|---|---|---|---|---|---|---|
| Ischemia | + | + + + | + + + + | + + + | + + | + + |
| Valve disease | + + | + + + + | + + + + | + + | + + + | + + + |
| Congenital disorder | + + | + + + + | + + + + | + + | + + + | + + + + |
| Trauma | + + | + + + | + + + | + + | + + | + + |
| Cardiomyopathy | + | + + + + | + + + | + + | + + + | + + + |
| Pericardial disease | + | + + + | + + | 0 | + + + + | + + + + |
| Endocarditis | + | + + + + | + + | 0 | + + | + + + |
| Masses | 0 | + + + + | + + + | + | + + + + | + + + + |

0, no information; + + + +, maximum information; CXR, chest x-ray; echo, echocardiography (includes intravascular ultrasound); angio, angiography; RCT, rapid computed tomography; MRI, magnetic resonance imaging.
* Angio includes both imaging and hemodynamic evaluation.
Modified and updated from Skorton DJ, Brundage BH, Schelbert HR, Wolf GL: Relative merits of imaging techniques. In Braunwald E (ed): Heart Disease: A Textbook of Cardiovascular Medicine, 5th ed. Philadelphia: WB Saunders, 1997:349–359.

The pace of discovery in basic research is increasing, and imaging methods have an important place in this progress.

Recent advances in molecular genetics and the ability to generate genetically engineered animal models provide new opportunities for understanding mechanisms of human cardiac development and function in health and disease. A gene suspected of playing an important role in a particular cardiovascular state can be ablated ("knocked out" by gene targeting and homologous recombination), overexpressed, or modified. Understanding of the phenotypic consequences of genetic manipulation elucidates the mechanisms by which the gene of interest and its encoded protein function in vivo.

The mouse is the most widely used animal for such studies, since the techniques for genetic modification in vivo with this mammal are most advanced. Indeed, genetic alteration of loci thought to be responsible for cardiac development or function has led to numerous murine models of cardiac hypertrophy and cardiomyopathies.[57] Now the emphasis is shifting toward understanding the functional sequelae of these genetic modifications. Modern imaging methods for evaluating the heart in these tiny animals are powerful tools for this functional analysis. Here, we give two examples of recent applications of imaging methods to understanding the functional consequences of altered gene expression that are relevant to common cardiac conditions.

In one recent study, transgenic mice were generated that developed hypertension and cardiac hypertrophy secondary to ablation of a gene necessary for responses to atrial natriuretic peptide.[58] Using MRI to determine left ventricular mass in a fashion similar to that used in clinical imaging, these investigators demonstrated an excellent correlation between mass evaluated by MRI and at necropsy in these tiny left ventricles, which ranged in mass from 150 to 350 mg.

In another example, investigators used a high-frequency echocardiographic transducer to accurately assess left ventricular internal dimensions and fractional shortening and to estimate ejection fractions in mice that overexpressed the cardiac stimulatory G protein α subunit.[59] The development of cardiomyopathy over time was clearly demonstrated in this important murine model of chronic sympathetic stimulation. This study underscores the importance of being able to perform serial, noninvasive monitoring of a phenotype in the same animal to understand progression or regression of disease.

Both studies provide examples of how combining modern imaging techniques with new biologic modeling will vastly improve our understanding of the disease process. It is clear that modern imaging techniques are enormously versatile in assessment of the cardiovascular system. Insights into the mechanisms of cardiac disease gained through such studies will inform the use of similar imaging techniques to detect and monitor human cardiac diseases and to understand their genetic and other causes.

## Conclusion/Summary

A variety of imaging methods are available to clinicians, and the choices are increasing. In the assessment of anatomy and ventricular function, several methods produce similarly useful information, although higher-contrast tomographic techniques have some theoretical advantages over other approaches. Detailed evaluation of coronary anatomy remains the province of angiography and, increasingly, of intravascular US. Valvular function can be assessed well in most patients by echocardiography, although sometimes cardiac catheterization is still needed for pressure measurement. MRI may someday rival echocardiography for investigating valvular disease. Today, myocardial perfusion is most directly assessed with radionuclide methods, although US and MRI soon may produce helpful information. Evaluation of myocardial biochemistry may be accomplished with PET scanning in the few centers that have the capability. Since coincidence imaging with positron-emitting agents using more conventional gamma camera–like instruments is now available, this technique may come into wider use. Assessment of cardiac biochemistry by NMR spectroscopy and tissue characterization remain investigational.

Knowledge of the capabilities of the various imaging methods, local expertise, and the lowest cost and risk diagnostic algorithm will guide a logical approach to choosing of imaging methods for specific patient subgroups. For the foreseeable future, imaging will remain the predominant laboratory approach to cardiac diagnosis.

## ■ REFERENCES

1. Skorton DJ, Schelbert HR, Wolf GL, Brundage BH (eds): Marcus Cardiac Imaging, 2nd ed. Philadelphia: WB Saunders, 1996.
2. Pohost GM, O'Rourke RA: Principles and Practice of Cardiovascular Imaging. Boston: Little, Brown, 1991.
3. Collins SM, Skorton DJ (eds): Cardiac Imaging and Image Processing. New York: McGraw-Hill, 1986.
4. Schelbert HR: Blood flow and metabolism by PET. Cardiol Clin Nucl Cardiol 1994;12:303.
5. Srinivasan G, Kitsiou AN, Bacharach SL, et al: [18 F] fluorodeoxyglucose single photon emission computed tomography: Can it replace PET and thallium SPECT for the assessment of myocardial viability? Circulation 1998;97:843–850.
6. Hounsfield GN: Computed medical imaging. Nobel Lecture, December 8, 1979. J Comput Assist Tomogr 1980;4:665.
7. Patterson RE, Eisner RL, Horowitz SF: Comparison of cost-effectiveness and utility of exercise ECG, single photon emission computed tomography, positron emission tomography, and coronary angiography for diagnosis of coronary artery disease. Circulation 1995;91:54–65.
8. St Goar FG, Pinto FJ, Alderman EL, et al: Intracoronary ultrasound in cardiac transplant recipients. In vivo evidence of "angiographically silent" intimal thickening. Circulation 1992;85:979.
9. Feiring AJ, Rumberger JA, Reiter SJ, et al: Determination of left ventricular mass in dogs with rapid-acquisition cardiac computed tomographic scanning. Circulation 1985;72:1355.
10. Florentine MS, Grosskreutz CL, Chang W, et al.: Measurement of left ventricular mass in vivo using gated nuclear magnetic resonance imaging. J Am Coll Cardiol 1986;8:107.
11. Achenbach S, Moshage W, Ropers D, et al: Value of electron-beam computed tomography for the noninvasive detection of high-grade coronary-artery stenoses and occlusions. N Engl J Med 1998;339:1964–1971.
12. Pennell DJ, Bogren HG, Keegan J, et al: Assessment of coronary artery stenosis by magnetic resonance imaging. Heart 1996;75:127–133.

13. Manning WJ, Li W, Edelman RR: A preliminary report comparing magnetic resonance coronary angiography with conventional angiography. N Engl J Med 1993;328:828.
14. Rumberger JA, Behrenbeck T, Bell MR, et al: Determination of ventricular ejection fraction: A comparison of available imaging methods. The Cardiovascular Imaging Working Group. Mayo Clin Proc 1997;72:860–870.
15. Little WC, Downes TR: Clinical evaluation of left ventricular diastolic performance. Progr Cardiovasc Dis 1990;32:273.
16. Nishimura RA, Tajik AJ: Evaluation of diastolic filling of left ventricle in health and disease: Doppler echocardiography is the clinician's Rosetta Stone. J Am Coll Cardiol 1997;30:8–18.
17. Clements IP, Sinak LJ, Gibbons RJ, et al: Determination of diastolic function by radionuclide ventriculography. Mayo Clin Proc 1990;65:1007–1019.
18. Rumberger JA, Weiss RM, Feiring AJ, et al: Patterns of regional diastolic function in the normal human left ventricle: An ultrafast computed tomography study. J Am Coll Cardiol 1989;14:119.
19. Aebischer NM, Czegledy F: Determination of right ventricular volume by two-dimensional echocardiography with a crescentic model. J Am Soc Echocardiogr 1989;2:110.
20. Pattynama PMT, Lamb HJ, Van der Geest R, et al: Reproducibility of MRI-derived measurements of right ventricular volumes and myocardial mass. J Magn Reson Imaging 1995;13:53.
21. Reiter SJ, Rumberger JA, Feiring AJ, et al: Precision of measurements of right and left ventricular volume by cine computed tomography. Circulation 1986;74:890–900.
22. Rezai K, Weiss R, Stanford W, et al: Relative accuracy of three scintigraphic methods for determination of right ventricular ejection fraction: A correlative study with ultrafast CT. J Nucl Med 1991;32:429–435.
23. Vandenberg BF, Weiss RM, Kinzey J, et al: Comparison of left atrial volume by two-dimensional echocardiography and cine-computed tomography. Am J Cardiol 1995;75:754–757.
24. Heller LI, Cates C, Popma J, et al: Intracoronary Doppler assessment of moderate coronary artery disease: Comparison with [201]Tl imaging and coronary angiography. FACTS Study Group. Circulation 1997;96:484–490.
25. White CW, Wright CB, Doty DB, et al: Does the visual interpretation of the coronary arteriogram predict the physiological importance of a coronary stenosis? N Engl J Med 1984;310:819.
26. Marcus ML: The Coronary Circulation in Health and Disease. New York: McGraw-Hill, 1983:73–84, 254–266.
27. Wilson RF, Johnson MR, Marcus ML, et al: The effect of coronary angioplasty on coronary flow reserve. Circulation 1988;77:873–885.
28. Kaul S: Myocardial contrast echocardiography: 15 years of research and development. Circulation 1997;96:3745–3760.
29. Germano G, Berman DS (eds): Clinical Gated Cardiac SPECT. Armonk, NY: Futura Publishing Co, 1999.
30. Vanoverschelde JL, D'Hondt AM, Marwick T, et al: Head-to-head comparison of exercise-redistribution-reinjection thallium single-photon emission computed tomography and low dose dobutamine echocardiography for prediction of reversibility of chronic left ventricular ischemic dysfunction. J Am Coll Cardiol 1996;28:432–442.
31. Olmos LI, Dakik H, Gordon R, et al: Long-term prognostic value of exercise echocardiography compared with exercise [201]Tl, ECG, and clinical variables in patients evaluated for coronary artery disease. Circulation 1998;98:2679–2686.
32. Ramani K, Judd RM, Holly TA, et al: Contrast magnetic resonance imaging in the assessment of myocardial viability in patients with stable coronary artery disease and left ventricular dysfunction. Circulation 1998;98:2687–2694.
33. Valkema R, van Eck-Smit BL, van der Wall EE: Cardiac metabolism: A technical spectrum of modalities including positron emission tomography, single-photon emission computed tomography, and magnetic resonance spectroscopy. J Nucl Cardiol 1994;1:546–560.
34. Scholz TD, Grover-McKay M, Fleagle SR, Skorton DJ: Quantitation of the extent of acute myocardial infarction by phosphorus-31 magnetic resonance spectroscopy. J Am Coll Cardiol 1991;18:1380.
35. Pérez JE, Holland MR, Barzilai B, et al: Ultrasonic characterization of cardiovascular tissue. In Skorton DJ, Schelbert HR, Wolf GL, Brundage BH (eds): Marcus Cardiac Imaging, 2nd ed. Philadelphia: WB Saunders, 1996:606–627.
36. Johnston DL: Myocardial tissue characterization with magnetic resonance imaging techniques. Am J Cardiac Imaging 1994;8:140.
37. Budoff MJ, Georgiou D, Brody A, et al: Ultrafast computed tomography as a diagnostic modality in the detection of coronary artery disease: A multicenter study. Circulation 1996;93:898–904.
38. Takiuchi S, Ito H, Iwakura K, et al: Ultrasonic tissue characterization predicts myocardial viability in early stage of reperfused acute myocardial infarction. Circulation 1998;97:356–362.
39. Waller BF, Pinkerton CA, Slack JD: Intravascular ultrasound: A histologic study of vessels during life. The new "gold standard" for vascular imaging. Circulation 1992;85:2305–2310.
40. Scholz TD, Fleagle SR, Parrish FC, et al: Effect of tissue fat and water content on nuclear magnetic resonance relaxation times of cardiac and skeletal muscle. Magn Reson Imaging 1990;8:605–611.
41. Baumgart D, Schmermund A, Goerge G, et al: Comparison of electron beam computed tomography with intracoronary ultrasound and coronary angiography for detection of coronary atherosclerosis. J Am Coll Cardiol 1997;30:57–64.
42. Iliceto S, Marangelli V, Memmola C, et al: Transesophageal Doppler echocardiography evaluation

of coronary blood flow velocity in baseline conditions and during dipyridamole-induced coronary vasodilation. Circulation 1991;83:61.

43. Fleagle SR, Johnson MR, Wilbricht CJ, et al: Automated analysis of coronary arterial morphology in cineangiograms: Geometric and physiologic validation in humans. IEEE Trans Med Imag 1989;8:387–400.
44. Mintz GS, Painter JA, Pichard AD, et al: Atherosclerosis in angiographically "normal" coronary artery reference segments: An intravascular ultrasound study with clinical correlations. J Am Coll Cardiol 1995;25:1479–1485.
45. Botvinick EH: Stress imaging. Current clinical options for the diagnosis, localization, and evaluation of coronary artery disease. Med Clin North Am 1995;79:1025–1061.
46. Pandian NG, Skorton DJ, Collins SM, et al: Heterogeneity of left ventricular segmental wall thickening and excursion in two-dimensional echocardiograms of normal humans. Am J Cardiol 1983;51:1667–1673.
47. Weiss RM, Shonka MD, Kinzey JE, et al: Effects of loading alterations on the pattern of heterogeneity of regional left ventricular function (Abstract). FASEB J 1988;2:1494A.
48. Johnson LL: Imaging acute myocardial necrosis (monoclonal antibodies and technetium-99m pyrophosphate). In Skorton DJ, Schelbert HL, Wolf GL, Brundage BH (eds): Marcus Cardiac Imaging, 2nd ed. Philadelphia: WB Saunders, 1996:1012–1020.
49. Iskandrian AS, Heo J, Schelbert HR: Myocardial viability: Methods of assessment and clinical relevance. Am Heart J 1996;132:1226–1235.
50. Dendale P, Franken PR, Block P, et al: Contrast enhanced and functional magnetic resonance imaging for the detection of viable myocardium after infarction. Am Heart J 1998;135:875–880.
51. Tillisch J, Brunken R, Marshall R, et al: Reversibility of cardiac wall-motion abnormalities predicted by positron tomography. N Engl J Med 1986;314:884.
52. Hundley WG, Li HF, Willard JE, et al: Magnetic resonance imaging assessment of the severity of mitral regurgitation. Comparison with invasive techniques. Circulation 1995;92:1151–1158.
53. Tworetzky W, McElhinney DB, Brook MM, et al: Echocardiographic diagnosis alone for the complete repair of major congenital heart defects. J Am Coll Cardiol 1999;33:228–233.
54. Askenazi J, Ahnberg DS, Korngold E: Quantitative radionuclide angiocardiography: Detection and quantitation of left to right shunts. Am J Cardiol 1976;37;382.
55. Martinez JE, Mohiaddin RH, Kilner PJ, et al: Obstruction in extracardiac ventriculopulmonary conduits: Value of nuclear magnetic resonance imaging with velocity mapping and Doppler echocardiography. J Am Coll Cardiol 1992;20:338.
56. Lowry RW, Zoghbi WA, Baker WB, et al: Clinical impact of transesophageal echocardiography in the diagnosis and management of infective endocarditis. Am J Cardiol 1994;73:1089.
57. James JF, Hewett TE, Robbins J: Cardiac physiology in transgenic mice. Circ Res 1998;82:407–415.
58. Franco F, Dubois SK, Peshock RM, Shohet RV. Magnetic resonance imaging accurately estimates LV mass in a transgenic mouse model of cardiac hypertrophy. Am J Physiol 1998;274:H679–H683.
59. Iwase M, Uechi M, Vatner DE, et al: Cardiomyopathy induced by cardiac Gs alpha overexpression. Am J Physiol 1997;272:H585–H589.

## ■ RECOMMENDED READING

Blackwell GG, Pohost GM: The evolving role of MRI in the assessment of coronary artery disease. Am J Cardiol 1995;75:74D–78D.
Cox IJ: Development and applications of in vivo clinical magnetic resonance spectroscopy. Prog Biophys Molec Biol 1996;65:45–81.
Garcia MJ, Thomas JD, Klein AL: New Doppler echocardiographic applications for the study of diastolic function. J Am Coll Cardiol 1998;32:865–875.
Gilbert JC, Glantz SA: Determinants of left ventricular filling and of the diastolic pressure-volume relations. Circ Res 1989;64:827–852.
Skorton DJ, Brundage BH, Schelbert HR, Wolf GL: Relative merits of imaging techniques. In Braunwald E (ed): Heart Disease: A Textbook of Cardiovascular Medicine, 5th ed. Philadelphia: WB Saunders, 1997:349–359.
Thomas JD: Principles of imaging. In Fozzard HA, Haber E, Jennings RB, et al (eds): The Heart and Cardiovascular System: Scientific Foundations, 2nd ed. New York: Raven, 1991:625–668.

Chapter 16

# Electrophysiology of Cardiac Arrhythmias

*David J. Slotwiner* ▪ *Kenneth M. Stein*
*Steven M. Markowitz* ▪ *Suneet Mittal* ▪ *Marc Scheiner*
*David J. Christini* ▪ *Bruce B. Lerman*

The normal cardiac cycle is initiated by electrical events that precede cardiac contraction. Abnormalities in the initiation and propagation of cardiac impulses can produce a variety of arrhythmias. Our intent in this chapter is to introduce the cellular mechanisms responsible for normal impulse formation and conduction and to review the clinical consequences when these mechanisms are perturbed.

## ▪ CELLULAR ELECTROPHYSIOLOGY

### The Cardiac Action Potential

The cardiac action potential consists of five phases that are determined by channels that allow ions to flow passively down their electrochemical gradients plus a series of energy-dependent ion pumps (Fig. 16–1). Ion channels are protein tunnels that span the cell lipid membrane. By selectively permitting the passage of specific ions, they maintain the electrochemical cell membrane potential. Flow of a specific ion through a channel is dependent on gating of the channel and on the electrical and chemical concentration gradients of that particular ion. Ions will flow passively down a chemical gradient if the channel is gated open and will also be drawn toward their opposite charge.

$Na^+$ and $Ca^{++}$ channels consist of a single $\alpha$ subunit that contains six hydrophobic transmembrane regions (Fig. 16–2). The voltage-gated $K^+$ channel consists of four identical subunits, each containing a six-transmembrane-spanning unit similar to $Na^+$ and $Ca^{++}$ channels. The six transmembrane units, S1 to S6, form the core of the $Na^+$ and $Ca^{++}$ channels and most $K^+$ channels. At the amino-terminal region of the $K^+$ channel is a "ball-and-chain" structure that may block the passage of ions through the channel. The positively charged lysine and arginine residues on S4 serve as voltage sensors. Essential residues lining the channel pore are found at H5 (between S5 and S6). This peptide loop projects into the channel pore and affects the permeation properties of the channel.

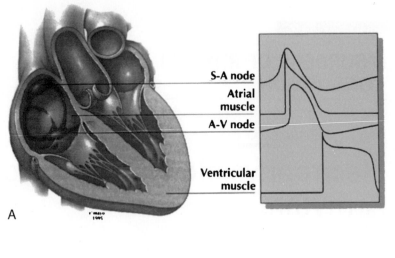

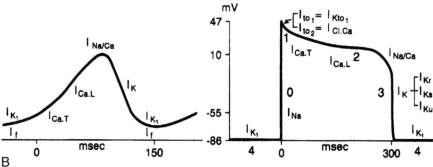

B

**Figure 16–1** ■ The human cardiac action potential. *A,* Action potential recorded from different regions of the heart. *B,* Principal currents responsible for the sinoatrial (S-A) nodal *(left)* and ventricular *(right)* action potential. (Ackerman M, Clapham D: Normal cardiac electrophysiology. *In:* Chien K [ed]: Molecular Basis of Cardiovascular Disease. Philadelphia: WB Saunders, 1999:281.)

Na$^+$, K$^+$, Ca$^{++}$, and Cl$^-$ are principally responsible for the membrane potential (Fig. 16–3). It is helpful to recall the equilibrium potential of these ions when considering the cardiac action potential (Table 16–1). The positive and negative values reflect the intracellular potential relative to a reference electrode. When a single type of ion channel opens, the membrane potential approaches the equilibrium potential of that ion. Thus, during diastole (phase 4) the cell membrane is impermeable to Na$^+$. However, K$^+$ diffuses freely out of the cell until the concentration gradient is balanced by the negative intracellular potential that attracts K$^+$. This balance represents the potassium electrochemical equilibrium potential ($E_K$). It is described by the Nernst equation

$$E_K = (RT/F) \ln [K^+]_O/[K^+]_I,$$

where $E_K$ is the K$^+$ equilibrium potential, $R$ is the gas constant, $T$ is the absolute temperature, $F$ is the Faraday number, $[K^+]_O$ is the extracellular K$^+$ concentration, and $[K^+]_I$ is the intracellular K$^+$ concentration.[1] Solving this equation for $E_K$ predicts

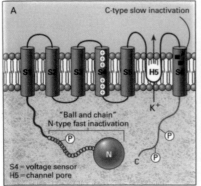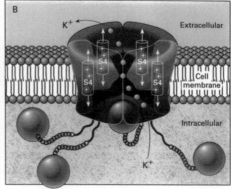

**Figure 16–2** ■ *A,* A subunit containing six transmembrane-spanning motifs, S1 through S6, that forms the core structure of Na$^+$, Ca$^{++}$, K$^+$ channels. The "ball-and-chain" structure at the N terminal of the protein is the region of a K$^+$ channel that participates in N-type "fast inactivation," occluding the permeation pathway. The circles containing plus signs in S4, the voltage sensor, are positively charged lysine and arginine residues. Key residues lining the channel pore (H5) are found between S5 and S6. Panel B shows four such subunits assembled to form a K$^+$ channel. (Ackerman MJ, Clapham DE: Ion channels—basic science and clinical disease. N Engl J Med 1997;336:1575.)

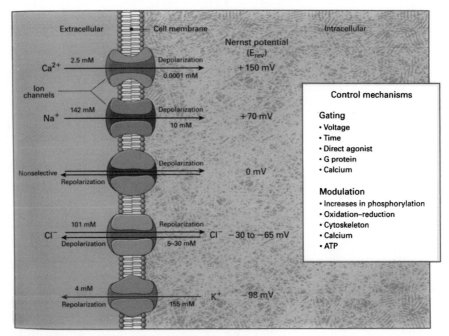

**Figure 16–3** ■ Physiology of ion channels. Five major types of ion channels determine the transmembrane potential of a cell. The concentrations of the primary species of ions (Na$^+$, Ca$^{++}$, Cl$^-$, K$^+$) are millimolar. The ionic gradients across the membrane establish the Nernst potentials (E$_{rev}$) of the ion-selective channels (approximate values are shown). Under physiologic conditions, Ca$^{++}$ and Na$^+$ ions flow into the cell and depolarize the membrane potential (that is they drive the potential toward the values shown for E$_{Ca}$ and E$_{Na}$), whereas K$^+$ ions flow outward to repolarize the cell toward E$_K$. Nonselective channels and Cl$^-$ channels drive the potential to intermediate voltages (0 mV and $-30$ to $-65$ mV, respectively). ATP, adenosine triphosphate. (Ackerman MJ, Clapham DE: Ion channels—basic science and clinical disease. N Engl J Med 1997;336:1575.)

## Table 16-1

### Summary of Transmembrane Currents

| Ion | Nernst Potential (mV) | Currents | Genes (Chromosomes) | Role in AP | Disease |
|---|---|---|---|---|---|
| Potassium | −98 | $I_f$—Inward "pacemaker" current (also carried by $Na^+$) | | Activated in nodal tissue polarization of membrane during phase 4 | |
| | | $I_{K1}$—Inward rectifier responsible for resting membrane potential | | Maintains phase 4 resting membrane potential; absent in sinus node | |
| | | $I_{Kur}$—Inward ultra-rapid rectifier | Kv1.4, Kv4.2/4.3 | Minor current of phase 1 repolarization | |
| | | $I_{Kr}$—Inward rapid rectifier | HERG (7q35-36) | Primary current of rapid phase 3 repolarization | LQT2 |
| | | $I_{Ks}$—Inward slow rectifier | KvLQT1 (11p15.5) | Contributes to late phase 3 repolarization | LQT1 |
| | | $I_{to1}$ ($=I_{Kto1}$)—Transient voltage-sensitive outward current | | Activated (by voltage) briefly during phase 1 rapid repolarization | |
| | | $I_{K(ACh)}$—Outward current | | Activated by muscarinic ($M_2$) receptors via GTP; important in nodal and atrial cells, where it may cause hyperpolarization and shortening of action potential duration | |
| | | $I_{K(Ado)}$—Outward current | | Appears identical in function to $I_{K(ACh)}$ but activated by adenosine | |
| | | $I_{K(ATP)}$—Outward current | | Blocked by ATP; activated during hypoxia (when ATP concentration low); shortens action potential during ischemia | |

| Ion | | Current | Gene | Function | Disease |
|---|---|---|---|---|---|
| Sodium | +70 | $I_{Na}$—Fast inward current carried by $Na^+$ through a voltage-gated channel | SCN5A (3p21-24) | Phase 0 | LQT3 |
| | | $I_{tn}$—Transient inward current | | Activated during phase 4 by release of $Ca^{++}$ from the sarcoplasmic reticulum; contributes to DADs | |
| | | $I_{Na\text{-}K\ pump}$—Bi-directional current | | Pumps 3 $Na^+$ out for 2 $K^+$ in producing small rectifier current. When this channel is blocked by digoxin the Na-Ca exchanger $I_{NaCa}$ takes over, resulting in intracellular $Ca^{++}$ overload | |
| | | $I_{NaCa}$—Outward current | | Exchanges 1 $Ca^{++}$ (into the cell) for 1 $Na^+$ (out of the cell) during intracellular $Na^+$ overload. During digoxin toxicity this may result in intracellular $Ca^{++}$ overload and triggered arrhythmias | |
| Calcium | +150 | $I_{Ca\text{-}L}$—Slow inward calcium current, blocked by dihydropyridines | | Active during phase 0 in nodal cells, phase 2 of atrial, ventricular, and His-Purkinje cells | |
| | | $I_{Ca\text{-}T}$—Transient inward current | | May contribute to phase 4 depolarization in sinus and His-Purkinje cells | |
| | | $I_{NaCa}$—Inward current | | Exchanges 1 $Ca^{++}$ (out of the cell) for 3 $Na^+$ (into the cell) during phase 2. During digoxin toxicity this may result in intracellular $Ca^{++}$ overload and triggered arrhythmias | |
| Chloride | −30 | $I_{Cl}$—Outward current | | Contributes to phase 3 repolarization; activated by adrenergic stimulation | |
| | | $I_{to2}$—Transient ($Ca^{++}$-activated) outward chloride current | | Activated briefly during phase 1 rapid repolarization | |

a transmembrane potential of $-96$ mV, close to that observed in normal atrial and ventricular myocytes. During phase 0, when the cell membrane is freely permeable to $Na^+$, the membrane potential approaches $+50$ mV (see Fig. 16–1). Typically, more than one channel type is open. The resulting membrane potential is determined by the balance of the competing currents.

Phase 0 marks the initiation of the action potential. Nodal cells are characterized by influx of $Ca^{++}$, whereas atrial, ventricular, and His-Purkinje cells depend on influx of $Na^+$. Initiation of each cardiac cycle depends on membrane depolarization initiated at the sinus node. In nodal cells, the pacemaker current, $I_f$, initiates each cycle. $I_f$ is activated by the polarization of phase 4 and carries a nonselective inward current comprised primarily of $Na^+$ and $K^+$ ions and a small $Ca^{++}$ current. $I_f$ causes slow depolarization of the nodal cell membranes during diastole until a threshold for firing is achieved. After initial local membrane depolarization by $I_f$, the upstroke of the nodal action potential is completed by a slow inward $Ca^{++}$ current. Two types of $Ca^{++}$ currents are present; the predominant slowly inactivating and dihydropyridine-sensitive L current ($I_{Ca-L}$) and rapidly inactivating T current ($I_{Ca-T}$; see Fig. 16–1, Table 16–1). Local membrane depolarization is propagated to neighboring cells via gap junction channels.

In "nonpacemaker" tissue, $I_f$ is absent. In these cells, phase 0 is triggered when the cell membrane is depolarized by adjacent cells. Once a sufficient proportion of a cell surface is depolarized and the cell reaches its activation threshold, the permeability or conductance of the cell surface membrane to $I_{Na}$ is markedly increased, allowing $Na^+$ to enter the cell and complete phase 0 depolarization. Blocking this inward current decreases the rate of change of the upstroke of the action potential (dV/dt) and slows conduction velocity.

Phase 1 consists of rapid membrane repolarization. This is achieved by inactivation of the inward $Na^+$ current and activation of $I_{to}$. $I_{to}$ consists of two currents: $I_{to1}$ is a voltage-activated outward potassium current and $I_{to2}$ is a calcium-activated chloride current. Phase 2, the plateau phase, may last as long as 100 msec and is characterized by a small change in membrane potential generated by $I_{Ca-L}$.

Rapid repolarization of the cell occurs during phase 3. $I_{Ca-L}$ is inactivated in a time-dependent fashion, thus decreasing the flow of cations into the cell. Simultaneously, several outward potassium currents, known as the *delayed slow* ($I_{Ks}$), *rapid* ($I_{Kr}$), and *ultrarapid* ($I_{Kur}$) *currents*, become active. This results in a net outward positive current and a negative transmembrane potential.

## ■ MECHANISMS OF ARRHYTHMIAS

### Automaticity

Rhythmic (pacemaker) activity is an inherent property of certain cell types. There is a normal hierarchy in the frequency of the initiated action potentials, the sinus node being the dominant pacemaker. More distal components of the conduction system may become the pacemaker because of enhanced or abnormal automaticity.

Under conditions of disease, the resting membrane potential can decrease, which can lead to spontaneous phase 4 depolarization in all cardiac cells.[2] Abnormal automaticity is defined as spontaneous impulse initiation in cells that are not fully polarized. The disturbances in the normal ionic balance that lead to abnormal automaticity may result from perturbations in various currents (e.g., reduction in $I_{K1}$). During the subacute phase (24 to 72 hours after coronary occlusion), automatic arrhythmias arise from the borders of the infarction.

Table 16–2

**Electropharmacologic Matrix***

|  | Reentry | Automaticity | cAMP-Triggered Activity |
|---|---|---|---|
| Catecholamine stimulation | Facilitates/no effect | Facilitates | Facilitates |
| Induction with rapid pacing | Facilitates/no effect | No effect | Facilitates |
| Overdrive pacing | Terminates/accelerates | Transiently suppresses | Terminates/accelerates |
| β-Blockade | No effect/rarely terminates | Terminates | Terminates |
| Vagal maneuvers | No effect† | Transiently suppresses | Terminates |
| Calcium channel blockade | No effect | No effect | Terminates |
| Adenosine | No effect | Transiently suppresses | Terminates |

*Automaticity refers to arrhythmias that arise from spontaneous phase 4 depolarization from nearly fully repolarized cells. Abnormal automaticity (which arises from cells with resting membrane potentials $\leq -60$ mV) is not included in this table, because it has not conclusively been shown to be a cause of clinical arrhythmias.

†An exception is intrafascicular reentry, which is sensitive to verapamil.

Lerman BB, Stein KM, Markowitz SM: Adenosine-sensitive ventricular tachycardia: A conceptual approach. J Cardiovasc Electrophysiol 1996;7:559.

## Clinical Correlates

A representative clinical example of an automatic rhythm is atrial or ventricular tachycardia (VT) that is precipitated by exercise in patients who have no structural heart disease. These forms of tachycardia are thought to represent adrenergically mediated automaticity, because programmed stimulation cannot initiate or terminate the arrhythmia whereas the tachycardia is induced with catecholamine stimulation and is sensitive to beta blockade (Table 16–2). This form of tachycardia is also suppressed momentarily (for as long as 20 seconds), but not terminated, by adenosine.[3]

The cellular mechanism governing automatic arrhythmias and their anatomic substrate are poorly delineated. Catecholamines modulate the rate of action potential initiation in automatic cells by increasing synthesis of cyclic adenosine monophosphate (cAMP) and alter the kinetics of $I_f$, so that it is activated at less negative membrane potentials.[4] Adenosine appears to attenuate $I_f$ through inhibition of cAMP synthesis, an antiadrenergic mechanism[5] similar to that mediated by vagal stimulation (Fig. 16–4).

## Triggered Activity

Oscillations of membrane potential in cardiac cells that occur during or after the action potential are called *afterdepolarizations*.[6] They are generally divided into two subtypes: early and delayed (EAD and DAD, respectively; Fig. 16–5). When an afterdepolarization achieves sufficient amplitude and the threshold potential is reached, a new action potential is evoked in what is known as a *triggered response*. This process may, under appropriate circumstances, become iterative, resulting in a sustained triggered rhythm (Fig. 16–6). Triggered activity differs fundamentally from abnormal automaticity in that abnormal automaticity depends on partial depolarization of the resting membrane potential.

### Early Afterdepolarizations and Arrhythmogenesis

An EAD can appear during the plateau phase (phase 2) or repolarization (phase 3) of the action potential (see Fig. 16–5). The distinction between phase-2

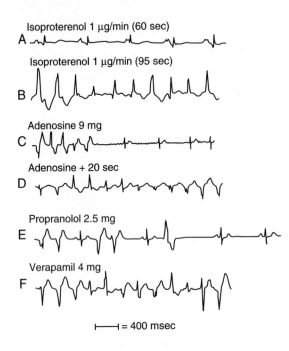

Isoproterenol 1 µg/min (60 sec)

A

Isoproterenol 1 µg/min (95 sec)

B

Adenosine 9 mg

C

Adenosine + 20 sec

D

Propranolol 2.5 mg

E

Verapamil 4 mg

F

⊢——⊣ = 400 msec

**Figure 16–4** ■ Initiation of idiopathic automatic ventricular tachycardia (VT) in a patient during isoproterenol infusion. *A*, Sinus rhythm recording 60 seconds after beginning isoproterenol infusion (1 µg/min). *B*, Sustained polymorphic VT identical to the patient's clinical arrhythmia) developed 95 seconds after initiation of isoproterenol infusion (1 µg/min). *C*, Adenosine transiently suppressed automatic VT (for approximately 5 seconds). This was followed by the emergence of multiform ventricular extrasystoles until sustained VT resumed (not shown). *D*, Resumption of automatic VT 20 seconds after initial effects of adenosine were demonstrated. *E*, Termination of automatic VT with propranolol. *F*, Lack of effect of verapamil on automatic VT. (Lerman BB: Response of nonreentrant catecholamine-mediated ventricular tachycardia to endogenous adenosine and acetylcholine. Circulation 1993; 87:382.)

**Figure 16–5** ■ Examples of *A*, phase 2 early afterdepolarization (EAD); *B*, Phase 3 EAD; *C*, delayed afterdepolarization (DAD). (Jalife J, Delmar M, et al: Basic Cardiac Electrophysiology for the Clinician. Armonk, NY: Futura, 1999.)

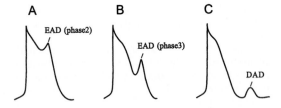

A

EAD (phase2)

B

EAD (phase3)

C

DAD

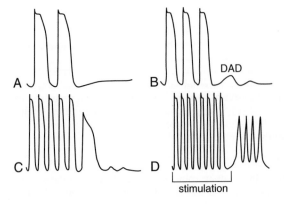

A

B

DAD

C

D

stimulation

**Figure 16–6** ■ Delayed afterdepolarization (DAD) and triggered activity resulting from inhibition of the Na-K pump. *A*, No DADs following rapid pacing. *B*, Single DADs but no sustained triggered activity following rapid pacing. *C*, One triggered beat following rapid pacing. *D*, Repetitive triggered activity following very rapid pacing. (Jalife J, Delmar M, Davidenko J, et al: Basic Cardiac Electrophysiology for the Clinician. Armonk, NY: Futura, 1999.)

## Common cellular mechanism of LQT

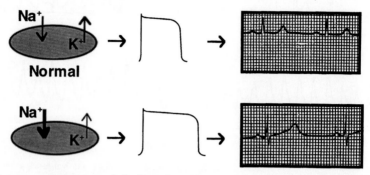

Increased Na current Delayed myocellular Long QT syndrome
or decreased K    repolarization

**Figure 16–7** ■ Molecular and cellular mechanisms of early afterdepolarization (EAD)–induced arrhythmias, such as that observed in the long QT syndrome. Gain of function mutations in cardiac sodium channel genes, or loss of function mutations in cardiac $K^+$ channel genes, leads to prolongation of the cardiac action potential. Abnormal myocellular repolarization and inhomogeneity of cardiac repolarization lead to QT prolongation. (Curran M, Sanguinetti M, Keating M. Molecular basis of inherited cardiac arrhythmias. *In* Chien K [ed]: Molecular Basis of Cardiovascular Disease. Philadelphia: WB Saunders Company, 1999:302–311.)

and -3 EAD is often based on the takeoff potential of the EAD (e.g., $< - 35$ mV for phase 2 and $\geq - 35$ mV for phase 3 or late EAD). Sometimes, both forms of EAD appear during the same action potential. Critical prolongation of repolarization, by a reduction in outward currents, an increase in inward currents, or a combination of the two, is normally required for the manifestation of EAD-induced ectopic activity (Fig. 16–7).[7] EAD are often potentiated by bradycardia or a pause, phenomena that further prolong repolarization.

### Clinical Correlates

A wide variety of drugs can produce EAD, EAD-related ectopic activity, or even a form of polymorphic VT known as *torsade de pointes* (Fig. 16–8).[8] These agents excessively prolong repolarization and include antiarrhythmic drugs of class Ia (quinidine and procainamide) and class III (sotalol, ibutilide) and a variety of noncardiac drugs, including antibiotics (e.g., erythromycin), pentamidine, and nonsedating antihistamines (e.g., terfenadine and astemizole).

One of the EAD-related arrhythmias studied most extensively is that associated with congenital long-QT syndrome. Although this is a rare disorder (incidence one in 10,000 births), it provides an opportunity to examine the effects of ion channel mutations on structure and function of these channels.

Initially, two distinct phenotypes of congenital long-QT syndrome were recognized. In 1957, Jervell and Lange-Nielsen (JLN) described the autosomal-recessive pattern of the congenital long-QT syndrome associated with congenital sensorineural hearing loss and recurrent syncope.[9] Several years later, an autosomal-dominant form of the disease manifested only as QT prolongation was described by Romano and Ward.[10, 11] Molecular genetics have now revealed at least six forms of the long-QT syndrome (LQT1 through LQT6).

Certain clinical features appear to be common to most forms of the congenital

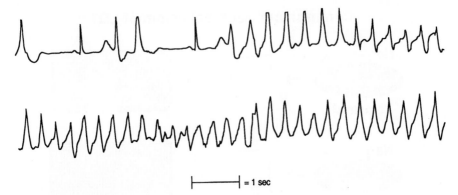

**Figure 16–8** ▪ Initiation of torsade de pointes following a "long-short" interval in a patient with the prolonged QT syndrome.

long-QT syndrome.[12] Most patients have a QT interval (corrected for heart rate) of 460 msec or greater.[13] The standard heart rate correction, according to Bazett's formula, is $QTc = QT/RR^{1/2}$, where $RR$ is the RR interval expressed in milliseconds.[14] A scoring system has been developed to assist in the diagnosis of the long-QT syndrome. It takes into account the QT interval and the patient's symptoms and family history (Table 16–3).[12, 15] The syndrome appears to be equally distributed between men and women. Early recognition and evaluation of the entire family is critical, since the 10-year mortality in untreated patients approaches 50%.

LQT1, the most common genotype, accounts for 30% to 50% of all cases. The

Table 16–3

**Diagnostic Criteria for Congenital Long-QT Syndrome**

| Finding | Points |
|---|---|
| **ECG** | |
| QTc (sec) | |
|   0.48 | 3 |
|   0.46–0.47 | 2 |
|   0.45 (men) | 1 |
| Torsade de pointes | 2 |
| T wave alternans | 1 |
| Notched T wave in three leads | 1 |
| Low heart rate for age | 0.5 |
| **Clinical history** | |
| Syncope | |
|   With stress | 2 |
|   Without stress | 1 |
| Congenital deafness | 0.5 |
| **Family history** | |
| Family members with confirmed long-QT syndrome | 1 |
| Unexplained sudden cardiac death before age 30 among immediate family | 0.5 |

Scoring: ≤1 point, low probability of long-QT syndrome; 2–3 points, intermediate probability; ≥4 points, high probability.

Used with permission from Ackerman MJ: The long QT syndrome: Ion channel diseases of the heart. Mayo Clin Proc 1998;73:250–269; and Schwartz PJ, Moss AJ, Vincent GM, et al: Diagnostic criteria for the long QT syndrome. An update. Circulation 1993;88:782–784.

responsible gene is located on the short arm of chromosome 11 and encodes the pore-forming α subunit (one of the two proteins) that controls $I_{Ks}$, the slowly activating delayed rectifier current. Defective $I_{Ks}$ is inactive, thus repolarization is prolonged and the patient predisposed to EAD.

The second subunit of $I_{Ks}$, the β subunit, is encoded by minK (located on chromosome 21), and mutations in this gene also result in prolonged QT secondary to defective $I_{Ks}$ and, thus, delayed repolarization (LQT5). Mutations in one allele of either the α or β subunit of $I_{Ks}$ appear to be expressed phenotypically as the Romano-Ward syndrome. Both subunits have been demonstrated in the stria vascularis of the inner ear of mice. Mutations in both alleles (homozygotes) for the α or β subunit are associated with the JLN phenotype.

Mutations in the gene encoding $I_{Kr}$ on chromosome 7 appear to be responsible for another autosomal-recessive form of the long-QT syndrome known as LQT2. At least 12 different mutations of this gene (HERG) have been described, all of which inactivate $I_{Kr}$ and result in prolonged phase 3 repolarization.

LQT3 has been linked to SCN5A, a gene on chromosome 3 that encodes $I_{Na}$, the current responsible for phase 0 rapid depolarization. LQT3 results from a channel that fails to inactivate appropriately. This causes continued inward $Na^+$ current (beyond phase 0) throughout the action potential, thus prolonging the action potential. Mexiletine, a selective $Na^+$ channel blocker, has been demonstrated to shorten the QTc in affected patients and may, therefore, have a therapeutic role.

The genotype and mutated ion channel of LQT4 remains unknown. It is clear that other loci are also responsible for the long-QT syndrome, and the designation LQT6 has been reserved for future genotypes of the syndrome not yet accounted for.

## Delayed Afterdepolarizations and Arrhythmogenesis

DAD are oscillations in membrane potential that occur after repolarization and during phase 4 of the action potential. In contrast to automatic rhythms which originate de novo during spontaneous diastolic depolarization, DAD are dependent on the preceding action potential. By definition, they do not occur in the absence of a previous action potential.

During the plateau phase of the normal action potential, $Ca^{++}$ enters the cell. The increase in intracellular $Ca^{++}$ triggers release of $Ca^{++}$ from the sarcoplasmic reticulum (SR), which effect further elevates intracellular $Ca^{++}$ and initiates contraction. Relaxation occurs through sequestration of $Ca^{++}$ by the SR. DAD arise when the cytosol becomes overloaded with $Ca^{++}$ and triggers $I_{Ti}$, a transient inward current (Fig. 16–9). $I_{Ti}$ is generated by the $Na^+$-$Ca^{++}$ exchanger ($I_{NaCa}$) and/or a nonspecific $Ca^{++}$-activated current.[16, 17] DAD can originate from Purkinje fibers and from myocardial, mitral valve, and coronary sinus tissues. Rapid pacing potentiates DAD, because more $Na^+$ (and $Ca^{++}$) enters the cell during rapid depolarization, furthering $Ca^{++}$ loading of the cell. Most experimental studies on triggered activity were performed under conditions of digoxin excess. By blocking the $Na^+$-$K^+$ pump, digoxin increases the concentration of intracellular $Na^+$. The high concentration of $Na^+$ stimulates the $Na^+$-$Ca^{++}$ exchanger that moves $Na^+$ out of the cell in exchange

**Figure 16–9** ■ Mechanism of DADs related to catecholamines and digoxin toxicity. Intracellular $Ca^{2+}$ overload triggers $I_{Ti}$, a depolarizing inward $Na^+$ current. $Ca_i$, inward $Ca^{++}$ current; $Na_i$, increased intracellular $Na^+$ concentration; $I_{Ti}$, depolarizing inward $Na^+$ current; SR, sarcoplasmic reticulum.

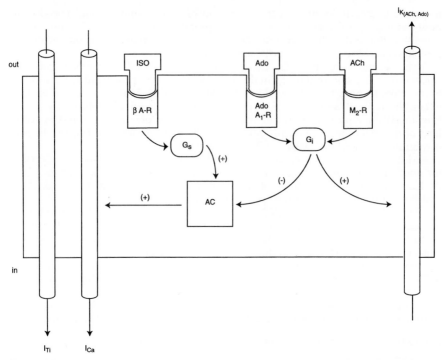

**Figure 16–10** ■ Schematic representation of the cellular model for adenosine. AC, adenylyl cyclase; ACh, acetylcholine; Ado, adenosine; $A_1$-R, adenosine $A_1$ receptor; β A-R, β-adrenergic receptor; ISO, isoproterenol; $G_s$, stimulatory G protein; $G_i$, inhibitory G protein; $M_2$R, muscarinic cholinergic receptor. (Lerman BB, Belardinelli L: Cardiac electrophysiology of adenosine. Basic and clinical concepts. Circulation 1991;83:1499.)

for allowing entry of $Ca^{++}$ into the cytosol. This results in intracellular $Ca^{++}$ overload and DAD. Beta-adrenergic stimulation, which is mediated by an increase in intracellular cAMP, also provokes DAD by increasing the inward $Ca^{++}$ current.

## Clinical Correlates

The prototypical clinical arrhythmia due to cAMP-mediated triggered activity (DAD-dependent) is idiopathic ventricular tachycardia (VT) arising from the right ventricular outflow tract (RVOT),[18] which segregates into two phenotypes, paroxysmal stress-induced VT and repetitive monomorphic VT (RMVT). These forms of arrhythmia represent polar ends of the spectrum of clinical VT secondary to cAMP-mediated triggered activity.[19] RMVT occurs during rest and is characterized by frequent ventricular extrasystoles, ventricular couplets, and salvos of nonsustained VT with intervening sinus rhythm. In contrast, paroxysmal stress-induced VT usually occurs during exercise or emotional stress and is a sustained arrhythmia. Common to both groups is the absence of structural heart disease, similar tachycardia morphology (left bundle branch block, inferior axis), and similar site of origin (RVOT), although the tachycardia occasionally originates from the left ventricle.[20] Overlap between these two subtypes of VT can be considerable.

Since activation of adenylyl cyclase and $I_{Ca-L}$ is critical for the development of cAMP-mediated triggered activity, the triggered arrhythmia would be expected to be sensitive to many electrical and pharmacologic stimuli, including beta blockade, calcium channel blockade (verapamil), vagal maneuvers, and adenosine (Fig. 16–10, Table 16–2). Termination of VT with adenosine is thought to be a specific response for identifying cAMP-mediated triggered activity due to DAD, since adenosine has no electrophysiologic effect in the absence of β-adrenergic stimulation and has no effect on digoxin-induced DAD or quinidine-induced EAD. Furthermore, adenosine has no effect on catecholamine-facilitated reentry that is due to structural heart disease.[21] The clinical effects of adenosine and verapamil on a patient with VT attributed to cAMP-mediated triggered activity are shown in Figure 16–11. While Ca$^{++}$ blockers may be helpful in the cardiac electrophysiology laboratory for determining the mechanism of a specific arrhythmia (Table 16–2), their use is *contraindicated* for treatment of most clinical forms of VT.

## Reentry

The normal cardiac impulse follows a predetermined path. It is initiated at the sinus node and is extinguished after it has activated the ventricles. Reentrant arrhythmias arise when the cardiac impulse circulates around an obstacle to initiate an independent, repetitive rhythm (Fig. 16–12). Reentry may be classified into several subtypes.

### Anatomic Reentry

In the anatomic model of reentrant arrhythmias, four prerequisites must be met to initiate reentry (see Fig. 16–12): (1) a predetermined anatomic circuit; (2) unidirectional block due to an extra stimulus occurs in one limb of the reentrant circuit; (3) slow conduction in a contiguous pathway of the circuit, allowing recovery of excitability of the previously refractory limb; and (4) wavelength of the impulse shorter than the length of the circuit (Fig. 16–13).[22]

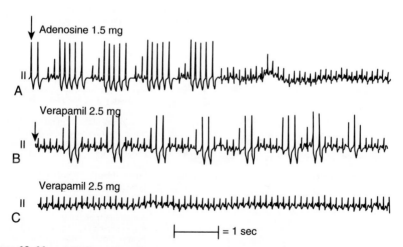

**Figure 16–11** ▪ *A*, ECG recording showing termination of incessant repetitive monomorphic ventricular tachycardia (VT) by adenosine. The vertical arrow indicates the completion of adenosine administration and a saline flush. *B*, Administration of verapamil during incessant repetitive monomorphic VT. Vertical arrow indicates completion of verapamil infusion. *C*, Termination of VT 100 seconds after verapamil administration. Surface lead II is shown. (Lerman BB, Stein K, Engelstein ED, et al: Mechanism of repetitive monomorphic ventricular tachycardia. Circulation 1995;92:421.)

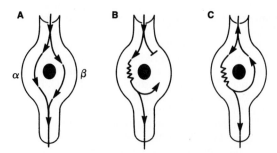

**Figure 16–12** ▪ Model of anatomic reentry. *A,* The impulse passes through a hypothetical conduit via two pathways, α and β, which meet at a common exit point. Since α and β have distinct refractory properties, a hypothetical extra stimulus could be blocked in β pathway and conduct slowly over α pathway and reenter β pathway retrogradely, *B. C,* This could result in sustained circus movement. (Prestowsky E, Klein G: Mechanism of tachycardia. *In* Prestowsky E, Klein G [eds]: Cardiac Arrhythmias: An Integrated Approach. New York: McGraw-Hill, 1994.)

The concept of wavelength is inherent in the anatomic model of reentry. The leading edge of the wave must encounter excitable tissue in which to propagate. Thus, the rotation *time* around the reentrant circuit must be longer than the recovery period of all segments of the circuit, and the *length* of the circuit must exceed the product of the conduction velocity and the recovery (or refractory) period of the tissue (see Fig. 16–13A). Interruption of the anatomic circuit at any point, by definition, interrupts reentry.

## Functional Reentry

The mechanisms of most reentrant arrhythmias confined to the atria or ventricles appear to be more complex than anatomic reentry. It has become apparent that reentry may be sustained, even in the absence of a specific anatomic circuit and in the absence of abnormal myocardium. This type of reentry is termed *functional.*

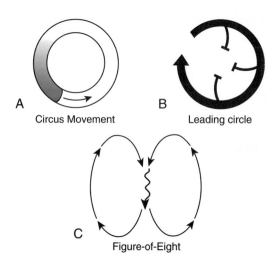

A
Circus Movement

B
Leading circle

C
Figure-of-Eight

**Figure 16–13** ▪ *A,* Circus movement reentry. The impulse (gray region) must be shorter than the entire length of the circuit (circle) and travel at a rate slow enough to allow separation of the impulse from its own refractory tail. This interval (depicted as white) is called the excitable gap. Reentry will be extinguished if the leading edge of the impulse (black) impinges upon its tail (gray). *B,* Model of leading circle reentry. Reentry follows the smallest possible circuit with tissue at the vortex remaining inexcitable. No anatomic barrier is present. *C,* Figure-of-eight reentry in anisotropic cardiac muscle. Two reentrant circuits rotate in opposite directions, sharing a central common pathway. (*A,* Jalife J, Delmar M, Davidenko J, et al: Basic Cardiac Electrophysiology for the Clinician. Armonk, NY: Futura, 1999.)

toward the region of depressed conduction, but the damaged cells are incapable of being excited and the action potential is unable to propagate any further. A small current is generated across the cells, however, and, if the distance across the gap is relatively small, current may reach the distal segment and bring those cells to threshold, where propagation of an action potential can be initiated. If propagation of current to the distal side of the gap is long enough delayed, the distal action potential may be reflected backward across the gap, reinitiating (or reflecting) an action potential.

## Clinical Correlates

Most clinical supraventricular and ventricular arrhythmias are due to reentry. In this section, we describe the most common reentrant arrhythmias. The surface electrocardiogram (ECG) provides important clues to the mechanism of reentrant tachycardias (Fig. 16–17). Supraventricular or narrow complex tachycardias due to AV node reentry or an accessory AV pathway typically have a short interval between the surface ECG P wave and the preceding R wave (denoted as the RP′ interval <50% of the RR interval). Conversely, supraventricular tachycardias (SVT) such as atrial tachycardias (including sinus node reentry), the atypical form of AV node reentry (discussed below), and the permanent form of junctional reciprocating tachycardia (a reentrant SVT due to a slowly conducting retrograde accessory pathway), demonstrate a long RP′ interval (≥50% of the RR interval). When evaluating wide complex tachycardia, dissociation of the surface ECG P waves from the QRS complexes supports the diagnosis of VT (Fig. 16–18). However, a 1:1 relationship between the P waves and QRS complexes may be observed in VT or SVT conducted with a wide QRS complex.

### Sinus Node Reentry

Sinus node reentry is a relatively infrequent cause of sustained supraventricular tachycardia (SVT) (1% to 3% of all symptomatic SVT).[24, 25] The P waves of tachycardia resemble those of sinus rhythm, and the tachycardia is mapped to the region of the sinus node. Clinically, it is characterized by relatively slow heart rates (typically 110 to 140 bpm), and it terminates in response to vagal maneuvers such as carotid sinus massage or Valsalva or to adenosine, $Ca^{++}$ channel blockers, or β-

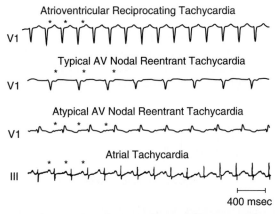

**Figure 16–17** ▪ Typical AV nodal reentrant tachycardia demonstrates a short RP′ interval on the surface ECG. Similarly, orthodromic AV reciprocating tachycardia is characterized by a short RP′ interval. Atrial tachycardias and atypical AV nodal reentrant tachycardia are characterized by a long RP′ interval.

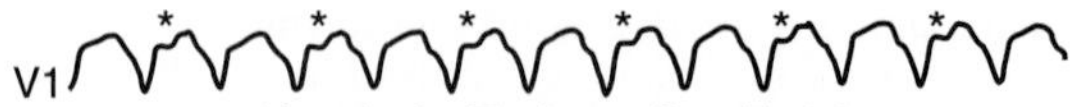

V1 [waveform]

Ventricular Tachycardia with 2:1
Retrograd Atrial Conduction

**Figure 16–18** ■ Dissociation of the P waves from the QRS complexes, or variable retrograde conduction to the atria, strongly supports the diagnosis of ventricular tachycardia. This is demonstrated in the figure. However, a 1:1 relationship of P waves to a wide complex tachycardia may be due to ventricular tachycardia with 1:1 retrograde conduction to the atria, or a supraventricular tachycardia with 1:1 antero-grade conduction to the ventricles in a patient with a preexisting bundle branch block.

adrenergic blockers. Radiofrequency catheter ablation provides a permanent cure for this arrhythmia.

### Intraatrial Reentry

Intraatrial reentrant tachycardias comprise a diverse group of arrhythmias that do not involve the sinus node. Reentrant arrhythmias may occur anywhere in the atria,[26, 27] and may affect persons with or without structural heart disease. Because areas of scar tissue may provide the substrate for reentry, they have been called *incisional reentrant tachycardias.*[26] Another common form of intraatrial reentry is atrial flutter (Fig. 16–19). The "typical" form of atrial flutter has a remarkably consistent rate of 250 to 300 bpm with propagation proceeding counterclockwise around the tricuspid valve annulus, down the free wall of the right atrium, and up the interatrial septum. When conduction proceeds up the interatrial septum, the caudocraniad activation inscribes the superiorly directed flutter waves (negative in the inferior leads) observed on the surface ECG. Clockwise, or "atypical," right atrial flutter (in the opposite direction) is less common.

Most intraatrial reentrant tachycardias are not responsive to adenosine, β-blockers, or Ca$^{++}$ channel blockers.[28] Over the past decade, electrophysiologists have made substantial progress in mapping and ablating reentrant atrial tachycardias. As with all reentrant arrhythmias, disruption of any part of the circuit terminates the tachycardia. For example, both the typical and atypical forms of flutter depend on a critical isthmus of slow conduction at the base of the right atrium. Creating a linear ablation lesion extending from the tricuspid valve annulus to the inferior vena cava blocks conduction across this isthmus and effectively eliminates tachycardia.

### AV Nodal Reentrant Tachycardia

Excluding atrial flutter and fibrillation, typical AV nodal reentrant tachycardia is the single most common form of SVT and accounts for nearly 50% to 60% of all sustained SVT in adults.[29, 30] Usually, it presents before age 40, and SVT rates

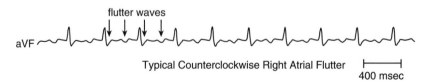

flutter waves

aVF

Typical Counterclockwise Right Atrial Flutter

400 msec

**Figure 16–19** ■ Typical counterclockwise right atrial flutter is characterized by 2:1 ventricular response and a ventricular rate of 150 beats per minute. Flutter waves on the surface ECG are usually negative in the inferior leads (II, III, aVF) as atrial activation proceeds down the right atrial free wall and up the interatrial septum, activating the interatrial septum and left atrium in a caudal to cranial sequence.

## AV NODE REENTRY

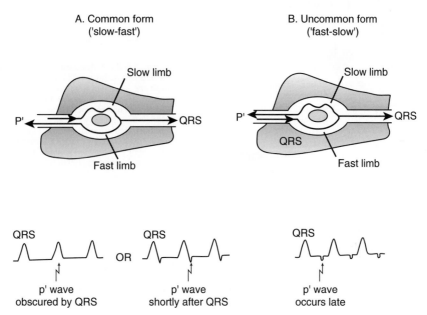

A. Common form
('slow-fast')

B. Uncommon form
('fast-slow')

QRS · p' wave obscured by QRS

OR

QRS · p' wave shortly after QRS

QRS · p' wave occurs late

**Figure 16–20** ■ Schematic drawing of AV nodal reentrant tachycardia. Illustrations depict two forms of supraventricular tachycardia due to reentry within the AV node. See text for details. (Benditt D, Reyes W, Gornick C, et al: Supraventricular tachycardias: Recognition and treatment. *In* Naccerelli G [ed]: Cardiac Arrhythmias: A Practical Approach. Mount Kisco, NY: Futura, 1991:135.)

typically range from 160 to 200 bpm but may vary greatly (from 100 to 300 bpm).[25] The reentrant circuit is limited to the peri-AV nodal region, with anterograde conduction proceeding over a "slow" pathway and retrograde conduction traversing a "fast" pathway (Fig. 16–20). In the usual case, the fast pathway has a longer refractory period than the slow pathway. Therefore, initiation of reentry occurs when a premature atrial beat is blocked in the fast pathway and is conducted along the slow pathway. By the time the impulse reaches the distal portion of the slow pathway, the retrograde fast pathway has regained excitability and is able to conduct the impulse to the atrium, perpetuating the arrhythmia by engaging and activating the slow anterograde pathway. The atypical form of AV nodal reentry activates these limbs in the opposite direction, anterograde conduction proceeding over the fast pathway and retrograde conduction across the slow pathway. As one would predict, the typical form of AV nodal reentry (with retrograde conduction up the fast pathway) is characterized by a short RP' interval on the surface ECG, whereas atypical reentry inscribes a long RP' interval (see Fig. 16–20). An electrophysiologic hallmark of AV nodal reentry is that neither the atria nor the ventricles are necessary parts of the reentrant circuit.

Adenosine is effective in terminating reentrant tachycardias that involve the AV node, and is mediated by activation of the outward $K^+$ current $I_{K(Ado, ACh)}$, which hyperpolarizes the AV node to about $-90$ mV and abbreviates the action potential. Adenosine can terminate tachycardia in either limb, but it occurs most often in the slow pathway.[31–33] Vagal maneuvers (carotid sinus massage or Valsalva) also

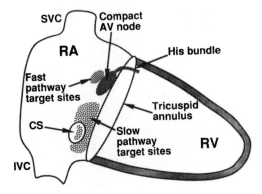

**Figure 16–21** ■ Anatomic positions of slow and fast pathways. The posterior position of the slow pathway, remote from the compact AV node, makes it the target of choice for radiofrequency catheter ablation. (Kalbfleisch S, Morady F: Catheter ablation of atrioventricular nodal reentrant tachycardia. *In* Zipes D, Jalife J [eds]: Cardiac Electrophysiology: From Cell to Bedside. Philadelphia: WB Saunders, 1995:1477.)

terminate AV nodal–dependent reentry by activating the same outward $K^+$ current $I_{K(Ado, ACh)}$.

The slow pathway is located in the region of the posteroseptal space of the interatrial septum and is readily amenable to catheter ablation (95% success rate; Fig. 16–21).[34] This location, remote from the compact AV node, minimizes the chance of AV node damage during ablation. Ablation of the fast pathway also effectively treats AV nodal reentry but carries a relatively high risk of complete heart block.

### Atrioventricular Reciprocating Tachycardia

Reentrant arrhythmias utilizing an accessory AV connection comprise the second most common form of regular, narrow-complex tachycardias (approximately 35% of SVT). Accessory pathways are composed of muscle bridges along the tricuspid and mitral valve annuluses that provide an abnormal electrical connection between the atria and ventricles.[35] The electrophysiologic properties of most accessory pathways resemble those of normal atrial tissue. Because the resting membrane potential is approximately −90 mV, typically, accessory pathways are insensitive to vagal maneuvers, adenosine, and $Ca^{++}$ channel blockers.

Most accessory pathways conduct in only one direction—retrograde from the ventricles to the atria—and are thus concealed during sinus rhythm (Fig. 16–22). Conversely, accessory pathways with anterograde conduction properties usually result in ventricular preexcitation (known as Wolff-Parkinson-White syndrome). During sinus rhythm conduction proceeds simultaneously down the AV node and the accessory pathway (Fig. 16–23). Preexcitation of the ventricles by the accessory pathway inscribes a delta wave that is visible on the surface ECG and that prolongs, or widens, the QRS complex. Typically, the PR interval is abbreviated (<120 msec) owing to rapid conduction over the accessory pathway. Orthodromic reciprocating tachycardia (antegrade conduction over the AV node and retrograde across the accessory pathway) accounts for 90% of reentrant arrhythmias in patients with Wolff-Parkinson-White syndrome. This arrhythmia may degenerate into atrial fibrillation; then, conduction would proceed anterograde over the accessory pathway. Atrial fibrillation in patients with the Wolff-Parkinson-White syndrome may precipitate ventricular fibrillation because of rapid conduction over the accessory pathway. A less common arrhythmia, antidromic reciprocating tachycardia (the anterograde limb being the accessory pathway and the retrograde limb the AV node), inscribes a wide QRS complex on the surface ECG.

Reentry utilizing an accessory pathway is initiated by an atrial or ventricular premature beat. For example, a premature atrial beat may encounter an accessory

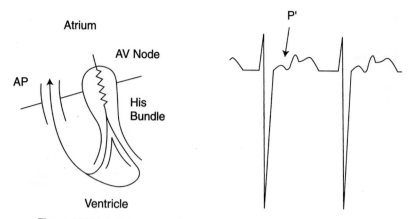

**Figure 16–22** ■ Schematic of orthodromic atrioventricular reentrant tachycardia.

pathway that has not recovered excitability from the previous beat and, thus, can conduct only over the AV node and through the His-Purkinje system. When the impulse reaches the ventricular input of the accessory pathway, it may engage the pathway, with conduction proceeding to the atrium, thus completing the reentrant circuit.

### Ventricular Reentrant Arrhythmias

Most ventricular arrhythmias occur in patients who have a history of myocardial infarction. Experimental evidence suggests that the mechanism of the tachycardia depends on the time since infarction. Within the first 30 to 60 minutes (early phase) after an acute myocardial infarction, the intracellular and extracellular milieus appear to favor reentrant ventricular arrhythmias, as does autonomic tone.[36] Automatic idioventricular rhythms with rates typically between 60 and 120 bpm are usually observed within the first 6 to 10 hours (delayed phase). After the relatively quiescent second phase, the third (and final) stage of ventricular arrhythmias (late phase) begins within 48 to 72 hours after infarction and is characterized by rapid, monomorphic tachycardias, owing to reentry arising in the periinfarct border zone. Inhomogeneous conduction of the periinfarction tissue creates regions

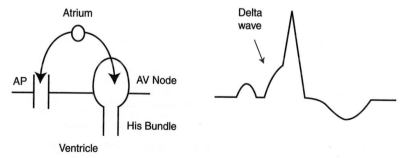

**Figure 16–23** ■ Schematic of Wolff-Parkinson-White syndrome with normal sinus rhythm beat. Conduction over the accessory pathway activates the ventricle simultaneously with conduction over the AV node. Preexcitation of the ventricles by the accessory pathway creates the delta wave visible on the surface ECG.

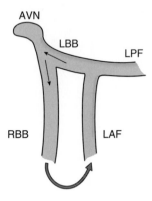

**Figure 16–24** ■ Model of bundle branch reentry. See text for explanation. AVN, AV node; LBB, left bundle branch; RBB, right bundle branch; LPF, left posterior fascicle; LAF, left anterior fascicle. (Jalife J, Delmar M, Davidenko J, et al: Basic Cardiac Electrophysiology for the Clinician. Armonk, NY: Futura, 1999.)

of slow and rapid conduction, causing anisotropic and figure-of-eight reentry. The risk of reentrant late-phase ventricular arrhythmias persists indefinitely after myocardial infarction and is thought to account for at least half of all deaths among myocardial infarction survivors. Electrophysiologic studies and endocardial mapping in humans have demonstrated that monomorphic VT that occurs late after a myocardial infarction is caused by areas of slow conduction and diastolic activation. The fact that these arrhythmias may be induced or terminated with pacing maneuvers supports the idea that a reentrant mechanism of the tachycardia originates from the border zone of the infarcted myocardium.

Another example of reentrant VT in patients with heart disease is bundle branch reentrant VT. This example of anatomic reentry is usually observed in patients with diseased His-Purkinje system function, complete or incomplete left bundle branch block during sinus rhythm, and nonischemic, dilated cardiomyopathy. The incidence of bundle branch reentry as the cause of sustained monomorphic VT ranges from less than 1% to 6%[25, 37] and most often bundle branch reentrant VT has a left bundle branch block–left superior axis morphology. Typically, it is initiated by a ventricular premature beat that follows a pause. The premature impulse blocks in the retrograde direction within the right bundle but conducts retrograde up the left bundle. When it reaches the His bundle it is able to engage the right bundle in the anterograde direction and then continues back to the left bundle (Fig. 16–24). It is important to recognize this form of tachycardia, since it is readily curable by radiofrequency catheter ablation of the right bundle.

## ■ REFERENCES

1. Ackerman MJ, Clapham DE: Ion channels—basic science and clinical disease. N Engl J Med 1997;336:1575–1586.
2. Surawicz B: Normal and abnormal automaticity. *In* Rosen MR, Janse MJ, Wit AL (eds): Cardiac Electrophysiology: A Textbook. Mount Kisco, NY: Futura, 1990:159–173.
3. Markowitz SM, Stein KM, Mittal S, et al: Differential effects of adenosine on focal and macroreentrant atrial tachycardia. J Cardiovasc Electrophysiol 1998;10(4):489–502.
4. DiFrancesco D, Angoni M, Maccaferri G: The pacemaker current in cardiac cells. *In* Zipes DP, Jalife J (eds): Cardiac Electrophysiology: From Cell to Bedside. Philadelphia: WB Saunders, 1995:96–103.
5. Belardinelli L, Shryock JC, Song Y, et al: Ionic basis of the electrophysiologic actions of adenosine on cardiomyocytes. FASEB J 1995;9:359–365.
6. Cranefield P, Aronson R: Cardiac Arrhythmias: The Role of Triggered Activity and Other Mechanisms. Mount Kisco, NY: Futura, 1988.
7. Roden DM, Lazzara R, Rosen M, et al: Multiple mechanisms in the long-QT syndrome. Current knowledge, gaps, and future directions. The SADS Foundation Task Force on LQTS. Circulation 1996;94:1996–2012.

8. Hohnloser SH, Singh BN: Proarrhythmia with class III antiarrhythmic drugs: Definition, electrophysiologic mechanisms, incidence, predisposing factors, and clinical implications. J Cardiovasc Electrophysiol 1995;6:920–936.
9. Jervell A, Lange-Nielsen F: Congenital deaf-mutism, functional heart disease with prolongation of the QT interval, and sudden death. Am Heart J 1957;54:59–68.
10. Romano C, Gemme G, Pongiglione R: Aritmie cardiache rare dell'eta'pediatrica. II. Accessi sincopali per fibrillazione ventricolare parossistica. Clin Pediatr (Bologna) 1963;45:656–683.
11. Ward OC: A new familial cardiac syndrome in children. J Irish Med Assoc 1964;54:103–106.
12. Ackerman MJ: The long QT syndrome: Ion channel diseases of the heart. Mayo Clin Proc 1998;73:250–269.
13. Keating MT: The long QT syndrome: A review of recent molecular genetic and physiologic discoveries. Medicine 1996;75:1–5.
14. Bazett HC: An analysis of the time-relations of electrocardiograms. Heart 1920;7:353–370.
15. Schwartz PJ, Moss AJ, Vincent GM, et al: Diagnostic criteria for the long QT syndrome. An update. Circulation 1993;88:782–784.
16. Luo CH, Rudy Y: A dynamic model of the cardiac ventricular action potential. II. Afterdepolarizations, triggered activity, and potentiation. Circ Res 1994;74:1097–1113.
17. Han X, Ferrier GR: Contribution of $Na^+$-$Ca^{2+}$ exchange to stimulation of transient inward current by isoproterenol in rabbit cardiac Purkinje fibers. Circ Res 1995;76:664–674.
18. Lerman BB, Belardinelli L, West GA, et al: Adenosine-sensitive ventricular tachycardia: Evidence suggesting cyclic AMP-mediated triggered activity. Circulation 1986;74:270–280.
19. Lerman BB, Stein K, Engelstein ED, et al: Mechanism of repetitive monomorphic ventricular tachycardia. Circulation 1995;92:421–429.
20. Lerman BB, Stein KM, Markowitz SM: Mechanisms of idiopathic left ventricular tachycardia. J Cardiovasc Electrophysiol 1997;8:571–583.
21. Lerman BB, Stein KM, Markowitz SM, et al: Catecholamine facilitated reentrant ventricular tachycardia: Uncoupling of adenosine's antiadrenergic effects. J Cardiovasc Electrophysiol 1999;10:17–26.
22. Jalife J, Delmar M, Davidenko J, et al: Basic Cardiac Electrophysiology for the Clinician. Armonk, NY: Futura, 1999.
23. Spach MS, Dolber PC, Heidlage JF: Influence of the passive anisotropic properties on directional differences in propagation following modification of the sodium conductance in human atrial muscle. A model of reentry based on anisotropic discontinuous propagation. Circ Res 1988;62:811–832.
24. Benditt D, Reyes W, Gornick C, et al: Supraventricular tachycardias: Recognition and treatment. In Naccerelli G (ed): Cardiac Arrhythmias: A Practical Approach. Mount Kisco, NY: Futura, 1991:135–176.
25. Josephson M: Clinical Cardiac Electrophysiology: Techniques and Interpretations, 2nd ed. Philadelphia: Lea & Febiger; 1993.
26. Lesh MD, Kalman JM: To fumble flutter or tackle "tach"? Toward updated classifiers for atrial tachyarrhythmias. J Cardiovasc Electrophysiol 1996;7:460–466.
27. Wu D, Amat-y-leon F, Denes P, et al: Demonstration of sustained sinus and atrial re-entry as a mechanism of paroxysmal supraventricular tachycardia. Circulation 1975;51:234–243.
28. Markowitz SM, Stein KM, Mittal S, et al: Mechanistic spectrum of adenosine-sensitive atrial tachycardia. J Am Coll Cardiol 1997;25:345A.
29. Josephson ME, Kastor JA: Supraventricular tachycardia: Mechanisms and management. Ann Intern Med 1977;87:346–358.
30. Wu D, Denes P: Mechanisms of paroxysmal supraventricular tachycardia. Arch Intern Med 1975;135:437–442.
31. DiMarco JP, Sellers TD, Lerman BB, et al: Diagnostic and therapeutic use of adenosine in patients with supraventricular tachyarrhythmias. J Am Coll Cardiol 1985;6:417–425.
32. Belhassen B, Glick A, Laniado S: Comparative clinical and electrophysiologic effects of adenosine triphosphate and verapamil on paroxysmal reciprocating junctional tachycardia. Circulation 1988;77:795–805.
33. Lerman BB, Greenberg M, Overholt ED, et al: Differential electrophysiologic properties of decremental retrograde pathways in long RP' tachycardia. Circulation 1987;76:21–31.
34. Calkins H, Yong P, Miller JM, et al: Catheter ablation of accessory pathways, atrioventricular nodal reentrant tachycardia, and the atrioventricular junction: Final results of a prospective, multicenter clinical trial. The Atakr Multicenter Investigators Group (see Comments). Circulation 1999;99:262–270.
35. Anderson RH, Becker AE, Brechenmacher C, et al: Ventricular preexcitation. A proposed nomenclature for its substrates. Eur J Cardiol 1975;3:27–36.
36. Scherlag BJ, el-Sherif N, Hope R, et al: Characterization and localization of ventricular arrhythmias resulting from myocardial ischemia and infarction. Circ Res 1974;35:372–383.
37. Caceres J, Jazayeri M, McKinnie J, et al: Sustained bundle branch reentry as a mechanism of clinical tachycardia. Circulation 1989;79:256–270.
38. Ackerman M, Clapham D: Normal cardiac electrophysiology. In Chien K (ed): Molecular Basis of Cardiovascular Disease. Philadelphia: WB Saunders, 1999:281–301.
39. Lerman BB: Response of nonreentrant catecholamine-mediated ventricular tachycardia to endogenous adenosine and acetylcholine. Evidence for myocardial receptor-mediated effects. Circulation 1993;87:382–390.

40. Lerman BB, Belardinelli L: Cardiac electrophysiology of adenosine. Basic and clinical concepts. Circulation 1991;83:1499–1509.
41. Prestowsky E, Klein G: Mechanism of tachycardia. *In* Prestowsky E, Klein G (eds): Cardiac Arrhythmias: An Integrated Approach. New York: McGraw-Hill, 1994.
42. Kalbfleisch S, Morady F: Catheter ablation of atrioventricular nodal reentrant tachycardia. *In* Zipes D, Jalife J (eds): Cardiac Electrophysiology: From Cell to Bedside. Philadelphia: WB Saunders, 1995:1477–1487.
43. Lerman BB, Stein KM, Markowitz SM: Adenosine-sensitive ventricular tachycardia: A conceptual approach. J Cardiovasc Electrophysiol 1996;7:559–569.

# Chapter 17

# Treatment of Cardiac Arrhythmias

*Davendra Mehta* ▪ *J. Anthony Gomes*

## ▪ TACHYARRHYTHMIAS

During the past decade, new diagnostic and therapeutic modalities have revolutionized the management of cardiac arrhythmias. Newly developed and approved drugs, and particularly radiofrequency catheter ablation therapy, have cured otherwise refractory and even life-threatening cardiac arrhythmias. Furthermore, catheter ablation has also helped us to better understand the pathophysiology of these arrhythmias. For the purpose of this chapter, cardiac arrhythmias are divided into tachyarrhythmias and bradyarrhythmias. Tachyarrhythmias are managed with antiarrhythmic drugs, radiofrequency catheter ablation, and implantable devices. Pacemakers are the main tool for managing bradyarrhythmias.

## ▪ SUPRAVENTRICULAR ARRHYTHMIAS

### Sinus Tachycardia

Pathologic sinus tachycardia is caused by extracardiac stresses such as fever, hypotension, anemia, thyrotoxicosis, hypovolemia, pulmonary emboli, shock, and increased cardiac demands secondary to myocardial infarction or congestive heart failure. Drugs such as atropine, caffeine, nicotine, isoproterenol, thyroid hormones, and aminophylline can cause sinus tachycardia. *Inappropriate sinus tachycardia* is defined as sinus tachycardia without any obvious cause.[1] It is a nonparoxysmal condition and usually presents as an inappropriately high resting sinus rate and markedly increased sinus rate after a minimal increase in activity. It is often accompanied by anxiety disorder and mitral valve prolapse syndrome. Although the mechanism remains undefined, imbalance between sympathetic and parasympathetic control is thought to be one of the contributing factors. For physiologic sinus tachycardia, the primary condition is treated, such as infections with antibiotics, hypotension with fluid replacement, and thyrotoxicosis with beta-blockers and antithyroid drugs. Management of inappropriate sinus tachycardia is more difficult. A beta-blocker is the first line of therapy and often results in control of sinus rate and associated symptoms. In patients with contraindications to beta-blockers, calcium channel blockers such as verapamil or diltiazem are useful. For those who do not respond to beta-adrenergic or calcium channel blockers, modification of the sinoatrial node with radiofrequency catheter ablation has been shown to produce at least short-term improvement.

### Sinus Node Reentry Tachycardia

Sinus node reentry accounts for 5% of supraventricular tachycardias and is usually associated with structural heart disease. The diagnosis is suggested by the presence of P waves, (which are similar but not identical to the sinus P waves) and abrupt termination of the tachycardia. The diagnosis is established by electrophysiologic studies.[2] Sinus node reentry tachycardia can be terminated by intravenous adenosine, verapamil, or beta-blockers. Calcium channel blockers and beta-blockers are effective in preventing recurrent episodes. Radiofrequency catheter ablation is very effective in treating sinus node reentry.[3] A permanent pacemaker usually is not required, as lesions in the area of the sinus node alter the node without affecting its automaticity. The risk of complete loss of sinus node function with radiofrequency catheter ablation is minimal.

## Atrial Tachycardia

Atrial tachycardias can be related to abnormal automaticity, reentry, or triggered activity.[4] The atrial rate of these tachycardias is usually between 150 and 200 bpm.[5] The morphology of the P wave depends on the site of origin of tachycardia. The P wave is usually located in the second half of the RR interval (long RP interval). These tachycardias are often associated with structural heart disease such as cardiomyopathy, cor pulmonale, or previous myocardial infarction. It is important to realize that persistent atrial tachycardia can induce cardiomyopathy. This should be considered when any patient presents with atrial tachycardia and dilated cardiomyopathy.[6] Treatment of tachycardia leads to complete recovery of left ventricular function. Digitalis intoxication should always be considered in patients with atrial tachycardia and atrioventricular (AV) block.[7] Management involves treatment of the underlying condition, such as heart failure, cor pulmonale, or digoxin intoxication. In patients with persistent tachycardia with fast ventricular rate, beta-blockers or calcium channel blockers can be administered to decrease ventricular rate. Class IA, IC, or III drugs can be used in an attempt to terminate the tachycardia (Table 17–1). The choice of drugs is based on left ventricular function; in patients with impaired left ventricular function, class 1A and 1C antiarrhythmic drugs should be avoided because of the high risk of proarrhythmia.

Table 17–1

**Vaughan-Williams Classification of Antiarrhythmic Drugs**

| Class I (Drugs That Predominantly Inhibit the Fast Sodium Channel) | Class II (Beta-Adrenergic Antagonists) |
| --- | --- |
| IA | Cardioselective |
| Procainamide | Metoprolol |
| Quinidine | Atenolol |
| IB | Acebutalol |
| Lidocaine | Nonselective |
| Mexiletine | Propranolol |
| IC | Nadolol |
| Flecainide | Pindolol |
| Propafenone | Timolol |
| **Class III (Primarily Act on Potassium Channels and Prolong Repolarization)** | **Class IV (Calcium Channel Antagonists)** |
| Used intravenously | Diltiazem |
| Ibutalide | Verapamil |
| Dofetalide | |
| Bretylium | |
| Used orally | |
| Sotalol (also has class II action) | |
| Amiodarone (also has class I, II, and IV action) | |

Sotalol is used when left ventricular function is normal or mildly impaired. Amiodarone is the drug of choice in the presence of moderate to severe left ventricular dysfunction. If no primary cause is identifiable, radiofrequency catheter ablation is the treatment of choice for recurrent atrial tachycardias.

## Reentrant Supraventricular Tachycardias

The three important causes of reentrant supraventricular tachycardia are AV nodal reentry, AV bypass tracts, and atrial tachycardias (see Chapter 16). These present as regular, narrow, complex tachycardia. Atrial flutter with 2:1 block should also be considered as the diagnosis when the ventricular rate is 140 to 160 bpm.

### Acute Management

Acute management involves a trial with a vagal maneuver. Valsalva's maneuver has been shown to be the most effective of all vagal maneuvers. Attempted with the patient lying supine and soon after the onset of supraventricular tachycardia, it is effective in 70% of patients.[8] Intravenous adenosine, verapamil, and diltiazem are used for acute termination. As adenosine has a half-life of 3 to 5 seconds, it has become the treatment of choice. It is given as a rapid bolus of 6 mg; if this fails, 12 mg more can be given.[9] Lower doses should be given to younger patients and those taking dipyridamole. Higher doses are needed for patients with slow circulation times or left-to-right shunting of blood, and to those receiving therapy with methylxanthines. Transient side effects include flushing, chest discomfort, breathing difficulty, and AV block. Adenosine should be avoided by patients with bronchial asthma because of the risk of bronchospasm. Instead, intravenous verapamil or diltiazem should be given. Adenosine can safely be used by patients taking other cardiac medications, such as digoxin, beta-blockers, calcium channel blockers, and angiotensin-converting enzyme (ACE) inhibitors. It is effective in terminating 98% of supraventricular tachycardias (SVT) caused by AV nodal reentry, and AV bypass tracts. Some atrial tachycardias also respond to adenosine. In patients with atrial flutter, adenosine is useful in diagnosis, as it increases AV block so that atrial flutter waves can be clearly identified.

### Chronic Suppression

Table 17–2 lists the drugs used for chronic suppression of SVT.[10] Digoxin by itself has a limited role in the management of SVT. For patients in whom the AV node is part of the reentrant circuit (AV nodal reentry and AV reentry tachycardia with accessory pathway), initial therapy is an AV node–blocking agent such as a beta-blocker or verapamil. Class I and III antiarrhythmic drugs are used only when patients fail to respond to AV node–blocking agents. For SVT that does not involve the AV node, AV nodal–blocking agents may slow the ventricular response, but they are not suppressive. In such patients, procainamide (class IB), flecainide (class IC), propafenone (class IC), amiodarone (class III), or sotalol (class III) are used to suppress the arrhythmia. The choice of appropriate therapeutic approach is made after detailed assessment of the clinical condition relative to the mechanism of arrhythmia and the presence or absence of heart disease. A class IC agent like flecainide is the treatment of choice for refractory SVT due to an accessory pathway, as its sodium channel–blocking action selectively blocks conduction in accessory pathway. Class III drugs, with their potassium channel–blocking action, which prolongs the atrial refractory period, are highly effective for suppression of atrial arrhythmias like atrial tachycardia, atrial flutter, and fibrillation.[11]

The Cardiac Arrhythmia Suppression Trial (CAST) and other antiarrhythmic trials have shown increased risk of ventricular proarrhythmia with the use of class

Table 17–2

## Medical Treatment of Supraventricular Tachycardia

**Acute Conversion (Intravenous)—for patients with normal renal and liver function only**

| | |
|---|---|
| Adenosine | 6 mg × 1; if ineffective, repeat 6 mg × 1 in another 5 minutes; repeat 12 mg × 1 in another 5 minutes if ineffective |
| Amiodarone | 150 mg over 10 minutes, then 1 mg/min × 6 hours, then 0.5 mg/min (re-bolus 150 mg if breakthrough arrhythmias occur); total loading dose of 6–12 g |
| Diltiazem | 0.25 mg/kg × 1; repeat in 15 minutes 0.35 mg/kg × 1 (total bolus dose can be up to 20–25 mg); then start infusion of 5–15 mg/hour |
| Esmolol | 500 μg/kg/min × 1; start 50 μg/kg/min; if ineffective, can repeat bolus in 5 minutes, then increase drip rate by an increment of 50 μg/kg/min |
| Metoprolol | 5 mg every 5 minutes up to 20 mg |
| Procainamide | 1 g infuse at a rate of no greater than 50 mg/min |
| Propranolol | 0.1–0.15 mg/kg bolus; repeat doses of 0.5–0.75 mg/kg every 1–2 minutes, up to a total of 5 mg |
| Verapamil | 2.5–5 mg over 2 minutes, then 5–10 mg in 15–30 minutes (repeat up to a cumulative dose of 20 mg) |

**Chronic Suppression (Oral)—for patients with normal renal and liver function only**

| | |
|---|---|
| Amiodarone | 100–400 mg daily |
| Atenolol | 25–200 mg daily |
| Diltiazem | 90–360 mg daily (in 3–4 divided doses if immediate release formulations are used and once daily if sustained formulations are used) |
| Flecainide | 50–150 mg twice daily |
| Metoprolol | 25–400 mg daily (in 2 divided doses if immediate release formulations are used and once daily if sustained formulations are used) |
| Procainamide | 500 mg–2000 mg twice daily (sustained formulation) |
| Propafenone | 150 mg–300 mg three times daily |
| Propranolol | 10–30 mg every 4–6 hours up to total of 160 mg/day |
| Sotalol | 40 mg–160 mg twice daily |
| Verapamil | 240–480 mg per day (in 3 divided doses if immediate release formulations are used and once daily if sustained formulations are used) |

I antiarrhythmic drugs in patients with a history of myocardial infarction.[12] Thus, for the treatment of supraventricular arrhythmias, class I antiarrhythmic agents must be restricted to patients with no history of myocardial infarction or left ventricular dysfunction. In patients with a history of coronary artery disease, myocardial infarction, left ventricular dysfunction, or ventricular hypertrophy, SVT is treated with a class III agent, sotalol or amiodarone, as these are less likely to lead to ventricular proarrhythmia and to increase the risk of death in a high-risk population. Given the option of long-term drug therapy and its potential toxicity or catheter ablation, which these days is very safe, the majority of patients prefer the latter.

## Radiofrequency Catheter Ablation

Radiofrequency catheter ablation now is the treatment of choice for long-term management of SVT. Most SVT, including AV nodal reentry tachycardia, AV reentry tachycardia due to accessory pathway, type 1 atrial flutter, intraatrial reentry tachycardia, and automatic atrial tachycardias are now curable by radiofrequency catheter ablation (Table 17–3). It has become the first line of therapy and is offered to all patients with SVT, as it is safe and cost-effective and eliminates the underlying arrhythmia mechanism with minimal risk of complications.

Catheter ablation involves application of radiofrequency current from an external generator via a catheter at the site of the accessory pathway, the slow AV nodal pathway, or the mapped site of atrial tachycardia, which produces coagulation necrosis by controlled heat production. Catheter ablation is performed during the electrophysiology study after the mechanism of SVT has been determined and the

Table 17–3

**Indications for Catheter Ablation of Supraventricular Tachycardia (SVT)**

**Conventional**

Drug-refractory SVT
Wolff-Parkinson-White syndrome with recurrent SVT or atrial fibrillation
High-risk WPW syndrome (short refractory period)
Women with childbearing potential

**Newer**

Any patient having an electrophysiology study for SVT
Young patients
Patient's occupation (e.g., bus driver, airline pilot)
Patient preference over medication

optimal site for ablation defined. As the application of radiofrequency energy to the heart produces very little discomfort, general anesthesia is not necessary. The majority (95%) of patients go home the day after catheter ablation. With AV nodal reentry tachycardias and AV reentry tachycardias, the success rate of radiofrequency catheter ablation is 95% to 98%, and in atrial tachycardias and atrial flutter, it is 70% to 80%. The incidence of complications with catheter ablation is less than 2% to 3%. Complications include right- or left-sided thrombus, thromboembolic events, cardiac tamponade, AV block, and vascular (bleeding or hematoma), and coronary artery spasm.[13]

## Catheter Ablation of Specific Tachycardias

### Atrioventricular Nodal Reentry Tachycardia

Catheter ablation is very successful in curing AV nodal reentry tachycardia, the commonest form of SVT. Ablation can be performed for the fast or the slow pathway. Fast-pathway ablation is performed in the AV node–His bundle region in the anterosuperior portion of the tricuspid annulus. Fast-pathway ablation results in prolongation of the PR interval and loss of retrograde conduction. There is a 5% risk of AV block. The preferred technique for modification of AV nodal function for cure of AV nodal reentry tachycardia is ablation of the slow pathway.[14] Ablation is guided anatomically between the ostium of the coronary sinus and the AV node. Application of radiofrequency current at slow pathway location results in transient junctional rhythm. Successful ablation of the slow pathway does not alter the PR interval or the retrograde VA conduction. The risk of complete heart block is less than 3%, significantly lower than that with fast-pathway ablation. Also, the long-term success of slow-pathway ablation is superior to that of fast-pathway ablation.

### Accessory Pathways

Accessory pathways can lead to orthodromic tachycardias, antidromic tachycardias, and atrial fibrillation with preexcitation. Preexcited atrial fibrillation is associated with significant risk of ventricular arrhythmias. Ablation of accessory pathways is curative for all associated arrhythmias and is one of the most gratifying invasive cardiac electrophysiologic procedures (Fig. 17–1).[15] After mapping of the atrioventricular ring, the catheter is positioned at the site of the pathway, and radiofrequency current is applied to cauterize the pathway selectively. For left-sided accessory pathways, ablation can be performed via either the femoral artery, using the retrograde approach by advancing the catheter across the aortic valve, or the transseptal approach. The choice of the approach is based on operator prefer-

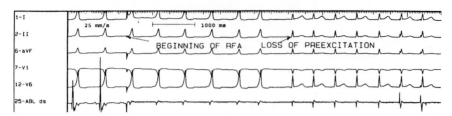

**Figure 17–1** ■ Surface and intracardiac ECGs in a patient with Wolff-Parkinson-White syndrome. Onset of radiofrequency current (RF) leads to normalization of QRS. PR interval increases and delta wave disappears.

ence; however, the transseptal approach is preferred for very young and elderly patients who are at higher risk for complications with the retrograde approach.[16] Right-sided accessory pathways can be ablated via the femoral vein or right internal jugular vein approach. The success rate for accessory pathway ablation is 95% to 98% and risk of recurrence 2% to 5%. Because of its safety and high success rate, catheter ablation should be offered to all patients with symptomatic Wolff-Parkinson-White syndrome.

## Atrial Tachycardia

Focal atrial tachycardia is the least common form of SVT. In 70% to 80% of the patients the atrial focus can be mapped and successfully ablated in the electrophysiology laboratory.[17] The site of ablation is identified as the site of earliest atrial activation during the tachycardia. Ablation is also successful in the majority of patients whose atrial tachycardia is attributable to a reentrant mechanism. This is identified by recording middiastolic potentials and entrainment mapping. For some patients with atrial tachycardia who cannot be cured by ablation of the focus, palliative ablation of the AV node and permanent pacemaker implantation controls symptoms. As with ablation of the focus, control of rapid ventricular response by AV nodal ablation and pacemaker implantation restores ventricular dysfunction in patients with tachycardia-induced cardiomyopathy. Catheter ablation is also successful in the majority of patients with sinus node reentry tachycardia. Interestingly, normal sinus node function is not affected by catheter ablation of sinus node reentry tachcyardia.

## Atrial Flutter

Atrial flutter can be terminated by electrical cardioversion, chemical cardioversion, or overdrive atrial pacing.[18] Low-energy shocks of 50 to 100 J are often successful in terminating atrial flutter. Chemical cardioversion can be attempted with oral class I agents. Rapid chemical cardioversion is now done with intravenous ibutalide, which is successful in converting 60% of patients with atrial flutter.[19] Typical or type 1 atrial flutter (defined by a 12-lead electrocardiogram [ECG] as "saw-tooth" or "picket-fence" pattern P waves in the inferior leads and positive P waves in lead V1) can also be terminated by overdrive atrial pacing.[18] Overdrive pacing is particularly useful immediately after cardiac surgery, as, postoperatively, patients have epicardial wires in the atria. Atrial pacing can be performed using transvenous pacing wire or an esophageal lead. Long-term medical therapy for atrial flutter is similar to that for atrial fibrillation and is discussed later. Patients with longstanding atrial flutter are at risk for thromboembolic complications albeit less than atrial fibrillation. Guidelines for anticoagulation for atrial flutter identical to those for atrial fibrillation.

It has been shown that type 1 (typical) atrial flutter is due to a macroreentrant circuit around the tricuspid valve ring.[20] Diagnosis is confirmed by a 20-electrode catheter placed around the tricuspid ring. The circuit is activated in counter clockwise direction with breakthrough anteriorly in the area of the His bundle then along the lateral wall anteroposteriorly, followed by right to left activation of the posterior tricuspid valve ring. The area of slow conduction in these patients is from posterolateral right atrial free wall to the low posteromedial (septal) right atrium. Conduction block between the low right atrium and the ostium of the coronary sinus is associated with termination of atrial flutter and long-term cure.[20] This is done by radiofrequency catheter ablation. Acute success with catheter ablation is achieved in approximately 80% of patients with type 1 atrial flutter. Atypical atrial flutter is due to clockwise circuit with breakthrough at the upper end of the crista terminalis or is related to multiple ill-defined circuits.[21] The former can be cured by ablation, but the latter is not amenable to catheter ablation and thus is treated medically or by catheter ablation of the AV node and placement of a permanent ventricular pacemaker.

## Atrial Fibrillation

Atrial fibrillation is the most common persistent arrhythmia seen in clinical practice. The prevalence increases dramatically with age. The overall prevalence of atrial fibrillation in persons older than 65 years is approximately 6%, and 85% of patients who have atrial fibrillation are older than 65 years.[22] In the elderly, it produces substantial morbidity. Nonvalvular atrial fibrillation is associated with a fourfold to fivefold increase in the risk of stroke and a moderate increase in mortality.[23] Thus, appropriate management of atrial fibrillation is important. Although risks associated with atrial fibrillation are identified, its appropriate management still is not clearly defined.

The severity of symptoms with atrial fibrillation is determined by ventricular rate, nature and extent of underlying heart disease, ventricular function (systolic *and* diastolic), and, at times, the precipitating cause. Symptoms commonly seen include irregular palpitations, chest discomfort, lightheadedness, and fatigue. Severe symptoms include heart failure, angina, and syncope. Stroke or systemic embolism may also be the initial presentation. At times, it remains asymptomatic and is discovered when medical advice is sought for an unrelated problem. In a patient with atrial fibrillation of new onset, careful clinical assessment is needed to detect any associated cardiac conditions, such as congestive heart failure, active myocardial ischemia, pericardial disease, significant valvular heart disease, hypertrophic cardiomyopathy, acute cor pulmonale, and preexcitation syndrome.

Management of atrial fibrillation involves control of ventricular rate, restoration of sinus rhythm, anticoagulation for the prevention of thromboembolic complications, and long-term treatment.[23] Correction of the underlying cardiac abnormality should be undertaken when feasible. For example, if acute pulmonary embolism is the cause of atrial fibrillation, anticoagulation will lead to a decrease in pulmonary pressure that will result in control of ventricular rate—and very often spontaneous conversion to sinus rhythm. Although drugs continue to be the mainstay of long-term management of atrial fibrillation, devices (pacemakers and defibrillators) and catheter-based interventions are presently being actively evaluated.

### Control of Ventricular Rate

Patients with hemodynamic compromise should undergo immediate electrical cardioversion.[24] Cardioversion is life saving for patients with Wolff-Parkinson-

White syndrome with preexcited atrial fibrillation who are at risk of ventricular fibrillation. AV node–blocking drugs can be detrimental to these patients. Verapamil shortens the refractory period of the accessory pathway and thus can precipitate ventricular fibrillation.

If the patient is stable, initial treatment is directed at relieving symptoms by slowing the ventricular rate by blocking the AV node with diltiazem, verapamil, beta-blockers, or digoxin. All of these agents can be administered intravenously. The choice of an agent is determined by the clinical situation; for patients with mild symptoms, beta-blockers might be adequate, whereas for patients with chronic lung disease and moderate symptoms, intravenous diltiazem is the drug of choice. In patients with heart failure, calcium channel blockers and beta-blockers should be used cautiously because of the risk of hypotension. Concomitant treatment of heart failure, lung disease, or chest infection, if present, is very important for the control of ventricular rate. Prolonged periods of fast ventricular rate can lead to tachycardia-induced cardiomyopathy. This diagnosis should always be considered in patients with dilated cardiomyopathy and chronic atrial fibrillation.[25] When medical treatment fails to control ventricular rate, radiofrequency catheter ablation of the AV node and implantation of a rate-adaptive ventricular pacemaker (VVIR) should be undertaken. Dual-chamber pacemakers with capabilities for mode switching to ventricular mode when the patient goes into atrial fibrillation are being used increasingly after catheter ablation of the AV node in patients with paroxysmal atrial fibrillation. In patients with tachycardia-induced cardiomyopathy, ablation of the AV node and pacemaker implantation restores left ventricular function. Following ablation of the AV node, as atrial fibrillation is still present, these patients are at risk for thromboembolic complications and thus need lifelong anticoagulation.

## Restoration of Sinus Rhythm

Restoration of sinus rhythm should be considered for "nonanticoagulated patients" with recent-onset (less than 48 hours) atrial fibrillation, especially when atrial fibrillation is associated with moderate symptoms. If performed within 48 hours, the risk of thromboembolic complications is minimal. Both electrical and chemical cardioversion are used. Direct current cardioversion is successful in 90% to 95% of patients. It is a safe procedure, but it does require intravenous sedation. Chemical cardioversion has become increasingly accepted. Intravenous ibutalide (Corvert) has aroused interest.[19] Its success is in the range of 60% to 70% in patients with recent-onset atrial fibrillation or atrial flutter. Intravenous ibutalide is associated with 3% to 5% risk of torsades de pointes, especially in patients with left ventricular dysfunction. Thus, close monitoring is essential for 3 to 4 hours after it is given.[19]

## Antithrombotic Therapy

**Persistent Atrial Fibrillation.** All patients with mitral valve disease and atrial fibrillation should receive an anticoagulant. Multivariate analysis of five large randomized, controlled trials in patients with nonvalvular atrial fibrillation has shown that six independent predictors of stroke are a history of (1) stroke or transient ischemic attacks, (2) diabetes, (3) hypertension, (4) congestive heart failure, or (5) myocardial infarction and (6) age above 75 years (Table 17–4).[26] In patients younger than 60 years who have none of these risk factors, risk of bleeding from long-term anticoagulation (0.5% per year) outweighs the risk of stroke. In patients older than 65 years who have associated risk factors, the risk of stroke outweighs the risk of bleeding, and thus oral anticoagulation should be undertaken. Recent trials have shown that an enlarged left atrium is still another risk factor.[26]

Table 17–4

**Atrial Fibrillation and Thromboembolism**

Risk Factors for Thromboembolic Complications of Atrial Fibrillation

| | |
|---|---|
| Rheumatic valvular disease | Diabetes |
| History of or current heart failure | Hypertrophic cardiomyopathy |
| History of stroke or transient ischemic attack | Hypertension |
| Echocardiographic systolic dysfunction | |

Recommendations for Antithrombotic Therapy

| | No Risk Factors | One or More Risk Factors |
|---|---|---|
| Age <65 years | Aspirin/no therapy | Warfarin |
| Age 65–75 years | Aspirin | Warfarin |
| Age >75 years | Warfarin | Warfarin |

**Paroxysmal Atrial Fibrillation.** Patients with short episodes of paroxysmal atrial fibrillation (less than 24 hours in duration) are at less risk of thromboembolic complications than those who have chronic atrial fibrillation. In the absence of the risk factors just cited, aspirin alone can be used. In the presence of risk factors, warfarin should be used, since episodes of atrial fibrillation, when associated with relatively slower ventricular rate, may be asymptomatic.

**Pericardioversion.** There is substantial risk of thromboembolic complications after chemical or electrical cardioversion. Patients with atrial fibrillation of more than 48 hours in duration should be anticoagulated for 3 to 4 weeks before and 2 to 3 weeks after cardioversion. Recent data show that patients whose left atrial appendage can be clearly seen at transesophageal echocardiography to be free of thrombi can safely undergo cardioversion without prior anticoagulation.[27] In the presence of risk factors, however, patients should be treated with anticoagulation therapy for 3 to 4 weeks before cardioversion.

## Maintenance of Sinus Rhythm

Atrial fibrillation begets atrial fibrillation. The longer the patient has been in atrial fibrillation the greater is the likelihood that he or she will remain in atrial fibrillation. When sinus rhythm is restored, only 30% to 50% of patients still maintain sinus rhythm 12 months later. Maintenance of sinus rhythm is affected by the duration of atrial fibrillation and the size of the left atrium.[28] Patients who have been in atrial fibrillation for less than 12 months have a better chance of maintaining sinus rhythm. The larger the left atrium is, the smaller is the chance of maintaining sinus rhythm after cardioversion. Drug therapy currently used to maintain sinus rhythm is far from ideal. Class IA, IC, and III drugs are used to maintain sinus rhythm (Table 17–5).[29] Proarrhythmia continues to be a major concern with all of these drugs, more so in patients with left ventricular dysfunction.[30] It is difficult to compare the efficacy of these drugs, as clinical trials have involved heterogeneous groups of patients whose left atrial sizes and durations of atrial fibrillation differed. Relative efficacy of these agents is shown in Table 17–5. Choice of drug is dependent on left ventricular function, the side effect profile, and the risk of proarrhythmia. A large, multicenter National Institutes of Health trial, Atrial Fibrillation Follow-up Investigation in Rhythm Management (AFFIRM), is presently under way to compare the efficacy of these agents in maintaining sinus rhythm. Preliminary results indicate that amiodarone is better than class I drugs for the maintenance of sinus rhythm at 1 year. An important caution for the use of antiarrhythmic drugs is that class IC drugs should be used only in patients with normal left ventricular function and no coronary artery disease.

Table 17–5

## Comparative Efficacy of Antiarrhythmic Drugs for Atrial Fibrillation to Maintain Sinus Rhythm

| Drug | Efficacy | Proarrhythmic Potential |
|------|----------|------------------------|
| Quinidine | + + + | + + + |
| Procainamide | + + | + + |
| Disopyramide | + + | + |
| Tocainide | 0 | – |
| Mexiletine | 0 | |
| Flecainide | + + + + | + + |
| Propafenone | + + + | + + |
| Amiodarone | + + + + | + (mainly bradycardia) |
| Sotalol | + + + | + |
| Ibutilide | + + | + + |
| Dofetalide* | + + + | + + |
| Beta-blockers | + | 0 |
| Verapamil | 0 | 0 |
| Digoxin | 0 | + |

*Recently approved by FDA for treatment of atrial fibrillation.

Several nonpharmacologic approaches have also been used. In patients with drug-resistant atrial fibrillation, surgical procedures such as maze and corridor operations have been shown to be successful in 70% to 80% of patients.[31] These involve creating multiple areas of block in the atria by surgical incisions and resuturing; however, the complexity of the surgical procedures restricts them to a few centers. Catheter-based corrective procedures are still experimental. Mapping and catheter ablation of sites in pulmonary veins has recently been reported to cure a certain group of patients with atrial fibrillation.[32] Dual-site atrial pacing has been shown to reduce the frequency of recurrent episodes. An atrial defibrillator might prove useful in a small group of patients with atrial fibrillation.

## Ventricular Arrhythmias

The management of ventricular arrhythmias has changed radically over the last 10 years, owing to better understanding of the proarrhythmic effect of antiarrhythmic drugs, large multicenter trials showing the beneficial effect of implantable cardioverter-defibrillators (ICD) on death rates, and the success of radiofrequency catheter ablation for certain monomorphic ventricular tachycardias. The management of asymptomatic ventricular premature beats and nonsustained ventricular tachycardia is less aggressive and is significantly affected by the presence of associated heart disease.

### Ventricular Premature Complexes

Asymptomatic ventricular premature beats in the absence of a cardiac abnormality do not need treatment. In patients with frequent ventricular premature beats of recent onset, every effort should be made to identify the cause.[33] Electrolyte disturbances, especially hypokalemia or hypomagnesemia, cardiac causes such as mitral valve prolapse, myocardial ischemia or infarction, cardiomyopathy, hypertensive heart disease, and persistent bradycardia are some of the important causes. Treatment of an identifiable reversible cause should be attempted before antiarrhythmic agents are used. In the presence of mitral valve prolapse, symptomatic ventricular premature beats are best treated with beta-blocker therapy. If beta-blockers[9] are contraindicated or ineffective, class I antiarrhythmic agents such as mexiletine, procainamide, flecainide, or propafenone are very effective, but they should not be given to patients with left ventricular dysfunction. In patients with recent myocardial infarction, lidocaine is used only for frequent premature beats that are producing hemodynamic compromise. Procainamide is used if lidocaine fails. Long-term suppression of asymptomatic ventricular premature beats with oral antiarrhythmic agents has not, however, been associated with improved survival. In the Cardiac Arrhythmia Suppression Trial (CAST), suppression of asymptomatic ventricular arrhythmias with type I antiarrhythmic agents was associated with increased mortality.[12] Similar results were seen with the pure class III agent d-sotalol.[34] Amiodarone, a class III agent with beta-blocking and calcium channel blocking properties, is highly effective in suppressing ventricular ectopy and has been shown not to increase mortality because of proarrhythmia. It has been associated with improved survival from arrhythmic death in the European and Canadian Myocardial Infarction Amiodarone Trials (EMIAT and CAMIAT, respectively).[35, 36] In patients with heart failure, the presence of ventricular premature beats is associated with higher total mortality but not increased mortality from arrhythmia. Class I antiarrhythmic agents should not be used to suppress ectopy as decreased left ventricular function is associated with increased risk of proarrhythmia. There is some evidence that amiodarone might be beneficial. The Group de Estudio de la Sobrevida en la Insuficiencia Cardiaca en Argentina (GESSICA) trial showed improved survival in heart failure patients treated with low-dose amiodarone, while, in the Amiodarone in Patients with Congestive Heart Failure and Asymptomatic Ventricular Arrhythmias (CHF-STAT) trial, use of amiodarone offered no benefit.[37, 38] Thus, the role of amiodarone in primary prevention of sudden death in patients with heart failure is not established.

## Nonsustained Ventricular Tachycardia

Nonsustained ventricular tachycardia is defined as three consecutive ventricular beats at a rate of at least 120 bpm lasting less than 30 seconds and that does not lead to hemodynamic compromise. Class I antiarrhythmic drugs have no role in the management of nonsustained ventricular tachycardia. As the CAST study showed, they may increase mortality because of their proarrhythmic effects.[12] Asymptomatic nonsustained ventricular tachycardia in patients with normal left ventricular function is not associated with poor long-term prognosis and, thus, does not need treatment either. In the presence of presyncope or syncope, patients with nonsustained ventricular tachycardia should undergo an electrophysiologic study to see if sustained ventricular tachycardia can be induced. Induction of sustained ventricular tachycardia is associated with increased risk of sudden death. In the presence of left ventricular dysfunction, nonsustained ventricular tachycardia is associated with increased mortality, especially in patients with coronary artery disease.[39] Thus, further risk stratification with an electrophysiologic study is indicated. Multicenter Automatic Defibrillator Implant Trial (MADIT) has shown that, in patients with nonsustained ventricular tachycardia, a history of myocardial infarction, a left ventricular ejection fraction no greater than 35%, and inducible sustained ventricular tachycardia that is not suppressed with procainamide on electrophysiologic studies, implantation of cardioverter-defibrillator when compared to conventional antiarrhythmic therapy was associated with significantly better long-term survival.[40] The prognostic significance of nonsustained ventricular tachycardia in patients with nonischemic cardiomyopathy has not been established. In the absence of symptoms, no intervention is presently undertaken. As ventricular tachycardia usually is not inducible at electrophysiologic study, symptomatic nonsustained ventricular tachycardia may be treated with amiodarone. Ongoing prospective studies are designed to compare the benefits of an implantable defibrillator and amiodarone in patients with nonsustained ventricular tachycardia and cardiomyopathy.

## Sustained Ventricular Tachycardia

**Antiarrhythmic Medications.** Antiarrhythmic drugs are the first-line therapy for acute management of ventricular arrhythmias. Lidocaine, procainamide, bretylium, and amiodarone are available in intravenous forms. The use of amiodarone for acute management has increased, as it is less proarrhythmic and intravenous therapy can be followed by oral therapy. Class I antiarrhythmics are no longer the first line of therapy for long-term management of sustained ventricular tachycardia, because their proarrhythmic effects increase mortality. Cardiac Arrest in Seattle: Conventional Versus Amiodarone Drug Evaluation (CASCADE) showed that amiodarone and the Electrophysiologic Versus Electrocardiographic Monitoring study (ESVEM) showed that sotalol, both class III antiarrhythmic agents, are associated with significantly better survival in patients with life-threatening ventricular arrhythmias than are class I antiarrhythmic drugs.[41, 42] Use of sotalol is limited by its beta-blocking properties. It cannot be used in patients with heart failure or significantly reduced left ventricular function. Amiodarone is the drug of choice for sustained ventricular arrhythmias and reduced left ventricular function. Class I antiarrhythmic drugs are added when amiodarone is only partially effective. Long-term therapy with amiodarone is associated with a significant incidence of side effects and thus requires close monitoring of thyroid, liver, and pulmonary functions. Large multicenter trials have shown lower total mortality rates with implantable cardioverter-defibrillators than with amiodarone[43], however, approximately 40% of patients with ventricular arrhythmias who have an implantable cardioverter-defibrillator need antiarrhythmic drugs in addition for recurrent ventricular tachycardia.

**Implantable Cardioverter Defibrillators.** The implantable cardioverter-defibrillator is considered a first-line therapy for patients with ventricular tachycardia and fibrillation, according to the joint guidelines of The American College of Cardiology and The American Heart Association.[44] Indications for the use of an implantable defibrillator are shown in Table 17–6. This is based on three recent, large multicenter trials. Antiarrhythmic Versus Implantable Defibrillator (AVID) compared an implantable defibrillator to amiodarone or sotalol; Cardiac Arrest Study Hamburg (CASH) compared defibrillator to amiodarone and metoprolol; and Canadian Implantable Defibrillator Study (CIDS) compared defibrillator to amiodarone. All three studies showed better survival with an implantable defibrillator than with medical therapy. Implantation of a modern defibrillator does not require thoracotomy as earlier models did. Like pacemakers, defibrillators are implanted under local anesthesia using a transvenous approach to place endocardial sensing and defibrillator leads. Over the years, the size of implantable defibrillators has become more acceptable, to the extent that all defibrillators are now implanted subcutaneously in the pectoral region. Perioperative mortality, even in high-risk patients with left ventricular dysfunction and heart failure, is less than 1%.

All new implantable defibrillators have programmable therapies with multiple algorithms of antitachycardia pacing (Fig. 17–2) and low-energy shocks, both of which are used to terminate ventricular tachycardia. High-energy shocks are programmed for ventricular fibrillation therapy. All defibrillators have backup ventricular pacing capabilities. Dual-chamber pacing has recently become available in the new generation of defibrillators. All defibrillators keep a record of events that allows complete analysis of arrhythmic events (Fig. 17–3). Diagnosis of ventricular

Table 17–6

## Indications for Implantable Cardioverter-Defibrillator Therapy*

**Class I (General Agreement That Treatment Is Beneficial, Useful, and Effective)**

1. Cardiac arrest due to VF or VT, not due to a transient or reversible cause
2. Spontaneous sustained VT
3. Syncope of undetermined origin with clinically relevant, hemodynamically significant sustained VT or VF induced at electrophysiology study when drug therapy is ineffective, not tolerated, or not preferred
4. Sustained VT with coronary disease, prior myocardial infarction, left ventricular dysfunction, and inducible VF or sustained VT at electrophysiology study that is not suppressible by a class I antiarrhythmic drug

**Class II (Conflicting Evidence About Efficacy/Usefulness)**

1. Cardiac arrest presumed to be due to VF when electrophysiology testing is precluded by other medical conditions
2. Severe symptoms attributable to sustained ventricular tachyarrhythmias while awaiting cardiac transplantation
3. Familial or inherited condition with a high risk for life-threatening ventricular tachyarrhythmias such as long QT syndrome or hypertrophic cardiomyopathy
4. Nonsustained VT with coronary artery disease, prior myocardial infarction, and left ventricular dysfunction, and inducible sustained VT or VF at electrophysiological study
5. Recurrent syncope of undetermined etiology in the presence of ventricular dysfunction and inducible ventricular arrhythmias at electrophysiological study when other causes of syncope have been excluded

**Class III (Evidence That Procedure/Treatment Is Not Effective and in Some Cases May Be Harmful)**

1. Syncope of undetermined cause in a patient without inducible ventricular tachyarrhythmia
2. Incessant VT or VF
3. VF or VT resulting from arrhythmias amenable to surgical or catheter ablation (e.g., atrial arrhythmias associated with Wolff-Parkinson-White syndrome, right ventricular outflow tract VT, idiopathic left ventricular VT, or fascicular VT)
4. VT due to transient reversible disorder (e.g., myocardial infarction, drugs, trauma, electrolyte disturbance)
5. Significant psychiatric illnesses that may be aggravated by ICD implantation or may preclude systemic follow-up.
6. Terminal illness with projected life expectancy ≤6 months
7. Patients with coronary artery disease with LV dysfunction and prolonged QRS duration in the absence of spontaneous or inducible sustained or nonsustained VT who are undergoing coronary bypass surgery
8. New York Heart Association class IV drug-refractory congestive heart failure in patients who are not candidates for cardiac transplantation

VT, ventricular tachycardia; VF, ventricular fibrillation; ICD, implantable cardioverter-defibrillator
*American College of Cardiology/American Heart Association Guidelines.

arrhythmia by current-generation devices is mainly by rate of the arrhythmia. The device can be activated by any arrhythmia that exceeds the programmed rate. An SVT with a rate exceeding the programmed rate for ventricular tachycardia will activate an implantable defibrillator to deliver pacing or shock. The newer generation of defibrillators can discriminate supraventricular and ventricular arrhythmias by sensing atrial and ventricular electrograms.

There has been an exponential increase in the number of patients with implantable cardioverter-defibrillators. Frequent shocks from an implantable defibrillator is a not uncommon cause for presentation to the emergency department. Management of these patients requires close cooperation between emergency room physicians, cardiologists, and electrophysiologists. The history of symptoms prior to shock and the assessment of the stored electrogram from the defibrillator memory are used to differentiate appropriate and inappropriate shocks.

**Radiofrequency Catheter Ablation for Ventricular Tachycardia.** Catheter abla-

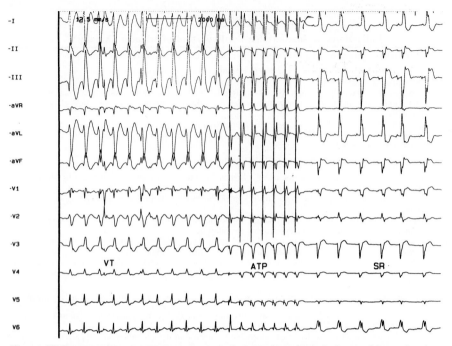

**Figure 17–2** ■ ECG shows termination of sustained ventricular tachycardia by overdrive pacing from implantable defibrillator. *VT,* venticular tachycardia; *ATP,* adenosine triphosphate; *SR,* sinus rhythm.

tion is useful in the management of certain cases of ventricular tachycardia (Table 17–7). It is the treatment of choice for idiopathic ventricular tachycardia when there is no other evidence of cardiac abnormality. The prerequisite for catheter ablation of ventricular tachycardia is precise localization of the critical area that is essential for maintaining ventricular tachycardia.[45, 46] This could be an area of slow conduction in a reentrant circuit or a focal area of abnormal automaticity or triggered activity. Ventricular tachycardia due to bundle branch reentry, which is usually seen

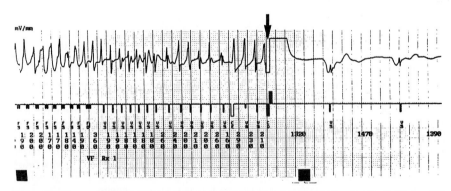

**Figure 17–3** ■ Retrieved ECG from implantable defibrillator in a patient with ventriclar fibrillation (VF) shocks shows termination of arrhythmia (*bold arrow*).

Table 17-7

**Ventricular Tachycardia: Indications for Catheter Ablation**

**Catheter Ablation Is Suggested First-Line Therapy**
  Idiopathic VT: right ventricular outflow tract tachycardia, fascicular tachycardias
  Bundle branch reentry in patients with cardiomyopathy (VT has left bundle branch
    block–like morphology)

**Catheter Ablation Should Be Considered**
  VT with coronary artery disease with multiple implantable cardioverter-defibrillator shocks
  Slow, incessant VT resistant to multiple medications

**No Data to Suggest Its Efficacy; Ablation Should Not Be Performed**
  Arrhythmogenic right ventricular dysplasia
  Dilated nonischemic cardiomyopathy

---

in patients with dilated cardiomyopathy and valvular heart disease, is amenable to catheter ablation. The right bundle is an essential part of the reentrant circuit; ablation of the right bundle is curative. In patients with structural heart disease such as coronary artery disease and cardiomyopathy, the substrate for reentrant ventricular tachycardia is less well-defined because of the large area of scarring and fibrosis; thus, it cannot always be eliminated by radiofrequency catheter lesions.[46] The first line of therapy for these patients is an implantable cardioverter-defibrillator. Catheter ablation is undertaken if the patient has recurrent episodes of monomorphic ventricular tachycardia that induce defibrillator shocks and that cannot be controlled by medical therapy.

## Specific Forms of Ventricular Tachycardia

**Idiopathic Ventricular Tachycardia.** Ventricular fibrillation and ventricular tachycardia sometimes occur without any underlying cardiac abnormality. For patients who present with ventricular fibrillation, detailed cardiac evaluation should be undertaken to rule out any underlying cardiac abnormality such as right ventricular dysplasia, hypertrophic cardiomyopathy, or intermittent long QT syndrome. Another cause of sudden cardiac death recently recognized is Brugada's syndrome. In affected patients with ventricular fibrillation, the 12-lead ECG shows right bundle branch block with ST segment elevation in right-sided chest leads. In the majority of patients with idiopathic ventricular fibrillation, electrophysiologic studies are normal. The risk of recurrence of idiopathic ventricular fibrillation is not firmly established. Implantable defibrillator therapy is the treatment of choice, as drug efficacy cannot be confirmed. Detailed assessment of all family members of patients who present with long QT syndrome and ventricular arrhythmias is important.[47] Two morphologies of idiopathic ventricular tachycardias are identified. A large proportion of ventricular tachycardias seen in patients with an apparently normal heart have left bundle branch block–like morphology with inferior frontal plane axis. The tachycardia originates from the right ventricular outflow tract, and the underlying mechanism of the tachycardia is thought to be triggered activity. It responds to adenosine, beta-blockers, and calcium channel blockers. Radiofrequency catheter ablation is curative for this form of ventricular tachycardia and is performed by mapping the focus of tachycardia in the right ventricular outflow tract. The second form of idiopathic ventricular tachycardia, also known as *fascicular tachycardia*, originates from the left posterior septum in the region of the posterior fascicle of the left bundle branch. Electrophysiologic features of this tachycardia suggest a reentrant mechanism, and the tachycardia can be terminated with intravenous verapamil. Medical therapy with calcium channel blocker and beta-blocker therapy is successful in suppressing the arrhythmia. As the arrhythmia is focal in origin, radiofrequency catheter ablation is frequently successful. As catheter ablation is safe and curative, it is now the treatment of choice for all symptomatic patients with "idiopathic" ventricular tachycardia.[45]

**Arrhythmogenic Right Ventricular Dysplasia.** Arrhythmogenic right ventricular dysplasia leads to ventricular tachycardias of right ventricular origin. Patients often have left bundle branch block–like tachycardias (right ventricular origin) with multiple morphologies with different axes. At times, it is familial in distribution. The diagnosis is suggested by the morphology of ventricular tachycardia and by right ventricular enlargement on echocardiography. Signal-averaged ECG are grossly abnormal. MRI of the heart shows fat deposition in the right ventricular wall. This is an important cause of potentially fatal arrhythmias in young adults and children who have an apparently normal left ventricle. Treatment modalities in these patients include medical therapy and use of an implantable defibrillator.

**Hypertrophic Cardiomyopathy.** Ventricular arrhythmias account for significant mortality in patients with hypertropic cardiomyopathy. The risk of sudden death is higher in association with a history of syncope or a history of "sudden death" in first-degree relatives, and in the presence of non-sustained ventricular tachycardia. An electrophysiology study can identify the risk of sudden death; however, the history of syncope is very specific. Amiodarone has been shown to reduce nonsustained ventricular tachycardia, but its role in decreasing sudden death is not well-established. Patients who have documented sustained ventricular tachycardia or positive electrophysiologic findings should have an implantable defibrillator.[48] Prophylactic use of an implantable defibrillator has been suggested for patients with hypertrophic cardiomyopathy who are at risk of sudden death. Dual-chamber pacemakers have been shown to reduce the symptoms and left ventricular outflow tract gradient, but whether they reduce the incidence of sudden cardiac death is not known.

**Torsades de Pointes.** Torsades de pointes describes polymorphic ventricular tachycardia with QRS complexes that progressively change in amplitude and morphology, with the appearance of a twisting axis around a point of depolarization. It is usually associated with long QT syndrome. In patients with acquired long QT syndrome, every effort must be made to identify the underlying cause. A complete drug history is essential, and any suspect drug should be eliminated. Intravenous magnesium is given first, followed by atrial or ventricular pacing. In patients with torsades who have a normal QT interval, antiarrhythmic drugs might be needed for recurrent arrhythmia. Lidocaine, mexiletine, phenytoin, and potassium channel openers have been tried. Antiarrhythmic drugs that prolong the QT interval, such as class IA (procainamide) and III (sotalol and amiodarone) drugs, can worsen the arrhythmia. In patients with congenital long QT syndrome, beta-blockers, stellate ganglionectomy, pacemakers, and implantable defibrillators have been used. In patients with long QT syndrome due to a defect in the sodium channel (LQT3), the sodium channel blocker mexiletine has been shown to normalize the QT interval,[49] but its effect on mortality is still being investigated. Asymptomatic family members should be screened.

# ■ BRADYARRHYTHMIAS

Management of bradyarrhythmias involves critical decisions about the placement of temporary or permanent pacemakers. Indications for the placement of pacemaker are based on the cause of the bradyarrhythmia.

## Temporary Cardiac Pacing

Transvenous or transcutaneous pacing is performed for the immediate management of life-threatening bradycardia. In the presence of syncope, hypotension, or heart failure, and when the underlying cause for bradycardia cannot immediately be corrected, a temporary pacemaker should be inserted. At times, persistent bradycardia can lead to ventricular arrhythmias. The placement of a pacemaker in these patients can suppress ventricular arrhythmia.

In patients with acute myocardial infarction, the decision to insert a temporary pacemaker depends on the location of the infarct and the presence of preexisting conduction system disease. The site of AV block in patients with inferior myocardial infarction is usually above the His bundle. The block is usually associated with a narrow QRS complex, and no hemodynamic compromise; it responds to intravenous atropine; and it is transient. A temporary pacemaker is inserted only when the heart rate is less than 40 bpm or there are symptoms of low cardiac output, associated angina, or ventricular irritability. In the presence of a stable escape rhythm and despite the presence of complete heart block, temporary pacing usually is not needed. AV conduction resumes in the majority of these patients, although it might take as long as 2 weeks. In patients with anterior myocardial infarction, AV block is usually due to a block below the level of the His bundle, the QRS complex is usually wide, and escape rhythms are slow and do not respond to atropine. These patients usually have large myocardial infarctions and associated pump failure. As progression to complete heart block contributes independently to morbidity and mortality, temporary pacing should be established promptly.[50] The availability of transcutaneous pacing systems has been associated with both increased indications for standby pacing and a decline in the need for transvenous pacing. Indications for transcutaneous patches are shown in Table 17–8. The transcutaneous pacemaker systems are suitable for providing standby pacing in acute myocardial infarction, especially for patients who do not require immediate pacing and who are at only moderate risk for progression to AV block, and who are at risk of complications of intravenous indwelling catheters. As transcutaneous pacing may be uncomfortable, especially when prolonged, it is intended to be prophylactic and temporary. A transvenous pacing electrode should be placed in patients who require ongoing pacing and in those with a 30% to 40% probability of requiring prolonged pacing.[51]

Antiarrhythmic drugs, beta-blockers, calcium channel blockers, digoxin, reserpine, and parasympathomimetic agents can lead to bradycardia, more so in patients with idiosyncratic reactions and conduction system disease. With these drugs, bradycardia may occur even at low blood levels. Temporary pacing may be required for the duration of the drug's action or until its effect is counteracted. If long-term therapy with these agents is needed, as with antiarrhythmic agents for ventricular arrhythmias, permanent pacing is indicated.

Prophylactic temporary pacing is needed in the cardiac catheterization laboratory when there is risk of complete heart block during the procedure. A pacing lead is inserted during right heart catheterization in patients with preexisting left bundle branch block. It is also used during certain interventions to the right coronary artery when there is risk of prolonged ischemia.

Although temporary cardiac pacing wires are inserted in the right ventricle, temporary dual-chamber pacing is preferred for patients with bradycardia and noncompliant ventricles (e.g., those with hypertrophic cardiomyopathy, heart failure, or sizable myocardial infarctions) and for hemodynamic compromise following cardiac surgery.[52]

## Permanent Cardiac Pacing

The indications for the insertion of permanent pacemakers in patients with *heart block and sinus node disease,* as recommended by the Joint Committee of

Table 17–8

### Indications for Placement of Transcutaneous Patches and Active (Demand) Transcutaneous Pacing Patches in Acute Myocardial Infarction*

**Class I** (Conditions for which there is evidence and/or general agreement that a given procedure or treatment is beneficial, useful, and effective)

    1. Sinus bradycardia (rate <50 bpm) with symptoms of hypotension (systolic blood pressure <80 mm Hg) unresponsive to drug therapy

    2. Mobitz type II second-degree AV block

    3. Third-degree heart block

    4. Bilateral BBB (alternating BBB, or RBBB and alternating left anterior fascicular block [LAFB], left posterior fascicular block [LPFB]), irrespective of time of onset.

    5. Newly acquired or age-indeterminate LBBB, and LAFBa, RBBB, and LPFBa

    6. RBBB or LBBB and first-degree AV block

**Class II** (Conditions for which there is conflicting evidence and/or a divergence of opinion about the usefulness/efficacy of a procedure or treatment)

**IIa:** (Weight of evidence/opinion is in favor of usefulness/efficacy)

    1. Stable bradycardia (systolic blood pressure >90 mm Hg, no hemodynamic compromise, or compromise responsive to initial drug therapy).

    2. Newly acquired or age-indeterminate RBBB

**IIb:** (Usefulness/efficacy is less well-established by evidence/opinion)

    1. Newly acquired or age-indeterminate first-degree AV block

**Class III** (General agreement that a procedure/treatment is not useful/effective and in some cases may be harmful)

    1. Uncomplicated acute MI without evidence of conduction system disease

*Recommendations for Temporary Transvenous Pacing in Acute Myocardial Infarction*

**Class I** (Conditions for which there is evidence and/or general agreement that a given procedure or treatment is beneficial, useful, and effective)

    1. Asystole

    2. Symptomatic bradycardia (includes sinus bradycardia with hypotension and type I second-degree AV block with hypotension not responsive to atropine)

    3. Bilateral BBB (alternating BBB or RBBB with alternating LAFB/LPFB), any age

    4. New or indeterminate age bifascicular block (RBBB with LAFB or LPFB, or LBBB) with first-degree AV block

    5. Mobitz type II second-degree AV block

**Class II** (Conditions for which there is conflicting evidence and/or a divergence of opinion about the usefulness/efficacy of a procedure or treatment)

**IIa** (Weight of evidence/opinion is in favor of usefulness/efficacy)

    1. RBBB and LAFB or LPFB (new or indeterminate)

    2. RBBB with first-degree AV block

    3. LBBB, new or age indeterminate

    4. Incessant VT, for atrial or ventricular overdrive pacing

    5. Recurrent sinus pauses (>3 seconds) not responsive to atropine

**IIb** (Usefulness/efficacy is less well-established by evidence/opinion)

    1. Bifascicular block of indeterminate age

    2. New or age-indeterminate isolated RBBB

**Class III**

    1. First-degree heart block

    2. Type I second-degree AV block with normal hemodynamics

    3. Accelerated idioventricular rhythm

    4. Bundle branch block or fascicular block known to exist before acute MI

---

AV, atrioventricular; LAFB, left anterior fascicular block; LBBB, left bundle branch block; LPFB, left posterior fascicular block; RBBB, right bundle branch block.

*American College of Cardiology/American Heart Association recommendations.

American College of Cardiology and the American Heart Association, are shown in Table 17–9.[44] It must be clearly understood that, despite these guidelines, the decision to insert a pacemaker is influenced by several additional factors. Before a pacemaker is implanted, reversible causes for bradycardia must be excluded (e.g., Lyme disease, hypervagotonia, drugs, metabolic or electrolyte imbalances). As a

### Table 17–9

### Indications for Placement of Permanent Pacemaker

**Indications for Permanent Pacing in Acquired Atrioventricular Block in Adults**

**Class I** (Conditions for which there is evidence and/or general agreement that a given procedure or treatment is beneficial, useful, and effective)

    1. Third-degree AV block at any anatomic level, associated with any one of the following conditions:

        a. Bradycardia with symptoms presumed to be due to AV block

        b. Arrhythmias and other medical conditions that require drugs that produce symptomatic bradycardia

        c. Documented periods of asystole 3.0 seconds (25) or any escape rate <40 beats per minute (bpm) in awake, symptom-free patients

        d. After catheter ablation of the AV junction

        e. Postoperative AV block that is not expected to resolve

        f. Neuromuscular diseases with AV block such as myotonic muscular dystrophy, Kearns-Sayre syndrome, Erb's dystrophy (limb-girdle), and peroneal muscle atrophy

    2. Second-degree AV block, regardless of type or site of block, with associated symptomatic bradycardia

**Class IIa** (Weight of evidence/opinion is in favor of usefulness/efficacy)

    1. Asymptomatic third-degree AV block at any anatomic site with average awake ventricular rates of 40 bpm or faster

    2. Asymptomatic type II second-degree AV block

    3. Asymptomatic type I second-degree AV block at intra- or infra-His levels found incidentally at electrophysiologic study performed for other indications

    4. First-degree AV block with symptoms suggestive of pacemaker syndrome and documented alleviation of symptoms with temporary AV pacing

**Class IIb** (Usefulness/efficacy is less well-established by evidence/opinion)

    1. Marked first-degree AV block (>0.30 second) in patients with LV dysfunction and symptoms of congestive heart failure in whom a shorter AV interval results in hemodynamic improvement, presumably by decreasing left atrial filling pressure

**Class III** (General agreement that a procedure/treatment is not useful/effective and in some cases may be harmful)

    1. Asymptomatic first-degree AV block

    2. Asymptomatic type I second-degree AV block at the supra-His (AV node) level or not known to be intra- or infra-His

    3. AV block expected to resolve and unlikely to recur

**Indications for Permanent Pacing in Chronic Bifascicular and Trifascicular Block**

**Class I**

    1. Intermittent third-degree AV block

    2. Type II second-degree AV block

**Class IIa**

    1. Syncope not proved to be due to AV block when other likely causes have been excluded, specifically ventricular tachycardia

    2. Incidental finding at electrophysiologic study of markedly prolonged HV interval (100 milliseconds) in asymptomatic patients

    3. Incidental finding at electrophysiologic study of pacing-induced infra-His block that is not physiologic

**Class IIb**

  None.

**Class III**

    1. Fascicular block without AV block or symptoms

    2. Fascicular block with first-degree AV block without symptoms

*Table continued on following page*

Table 17–9

**Indications for Placement of Permanent Pacemaker** *Continued*

**Indications for Pacing in Patients with Sinus Node Disease**

**Class I**
1. Sinus node dysfunction with documented symptomatic bradycardia, including frequent sinus pauses that produce symptoms. In some patients, bradycardia is iatrogenic and will occur as a consequence of essential long-term drug therapy of a type and dose for which there are no acceptable alternatives
2. Symptomatic chronotropic incompetence

**Class IIa**
1. Sinus node dysfunction occurring spontaneously or as a result of necessary drug therapy, with heart rate <40 bpm when a clear association between significant symptoms consistent with bradycardia and the actual presence of bradycardia has not been documented

**Class IIb**
1. In minimally symptomatic patients, chronic heart rate <30 bpm while awake

**Class III**
1. Sinus node dysfunction in asymptomatic patients, including those in whom substantial sinus bradycardia (heart rate <40 bpm) is a consequence of long-term drug treatment
2. Sinus node dysfunction in patients with symptoms suggestive of bradycardia that are clearly documented as not associated with a slow heart rate
3. Sinus node dysfunction with symptomatic bradycardia due to nonessential drug therapy

general principle, permanent pacing is performed for even asymptomatic complete heart block, alternating bundle branch block, or second-degree AV block with associated bundle branch block.

*Isolated first-degree AV block* is usually due to a delay in AV conduction as a result of enhanced vagal tone or drug therapy. Patients with a very long PR interval may develop symptoms secondary to delayed opening of the AV valves and thus benefit from dual-chamber pacing with physiologic AV delay. First-degree AV block with left or right bundle branch block, especially of recent onset, reflects infra-His conduction delay. This is an indication for placement of a permanent pacemaker as progression to higher-degree AV block is common.[53]

In *second-degree AV block* the level of block cannot be determined by ECG; however, in type I second-degree AV block with a normal QRS complex, the block is usually in the AV node and is not an indication for a pacemaker. Type II second-degree AV block, especially when associated with widening of the QRS complex, is usually infra-Hisian and is associated with conduction system disease. Thus, it is an indication for implantation of a permanent pacemaker.[44]

Symptoms in patients with *sinus node disease* can be due to tachycardia, bradycardia, or both. Patients might present with palpitations, weakness, dizziness, or syncope. About a third of patients with sick sinus syndrome have an associated AV conduction abnormality. A permanent pacemaker should be implanted only in the presence of a causal relationship between bradycardia and symptoms. Asymptomatic *sinoatrial exit block, sinus bradycardia,* and *sinus pauses* are not indications for pacing. In *tachycardia-bradycardia syndrome,* drugs might worsen bradycardia. Such patients are best managed with a permanent pacemaker and antiarrhythmic drugs.

Electrophysiologic evaluation of sinus node function can be performed in patients who are asymptomatic during detailed noninvasive monitoring, but it has poor sensitivity. Dual-chamber pacing is being used more and more for sick sinus syndrome, as a newer generation of pacemakers have the function of automatic mode switching whereby, with the onset of atrial arrhythmia, the pacemaker changes pacing mode from dual-chamber to ventricular.[54] In North America, about 46% of permanent pacemakers are implanted for sinus node disease. Indications for the use of permanent pacing in the management of patients with sick sinus syndrome are shown in Table 17–9.

*Neurally mediated syncope* is a form of vasovagal syncope that is reproduced by tilt-table testing. Symptoms can be very disabling. Therapy with beta-blockers, disopyramide, or mineralocorticoids, alone or in some combination, should be tried initially. For patients with drug-refractory symptoms and a significant bradycardia component during syncope, permanent dual-chamber pacemakers are used. Use of permanent pacemakers has been shown to reduce the incidence of syncope, although it cannot prevent all the symptoms, especially in patients with a prominent vasodepressor component. In patients with the cardioinhibitory type of carotid sinus hypersensitivity, permanent dual-chamber pacemakers reduce the incidence of syncope episodes. Dual-chamber pacing with a short PR interval has been shown to reduce the left ventricular outflow tract gradient. It has been shown that pacing with an optimal (short) AV interval leads to long-term hemodynamic and symptomatic improvement.

## ■ REFERENCES

1. Krahn AD, Yee R, Klein GJ, Morillo C: Inappropriate sinus tachycardia: Evaluation and therapy. J Cardiovasc Electrophysiol 1995;6:1124.
2. Gomes JA, Mehta D, Langan MN: Sinus node reentrant tachycardia. Pacing Clin Electrophysiol 1995;18:1045–1057.
3. Sanders WE Jr, Sorrentino RA, Greenfield RA, et al: Catheter ablation of sinoatrial node reentrant tachycardia. J Am Coll Cardiol 1994; 23;926–934.
4. Wellens HJJ, Brugada P: Mechanism of supraventricular tachycardia. Am J Cardiol 1988;62:10D–15D.
5. Haines DE, DiMarco JP: Sustained intra-atrial reentry tachycardia: Clinical, electrocardiographic and electrophysiologic characteristics and long-term follow-up. J Am Coll Cardiol 1990;15:1345–1354.
6. Gillette PC, Smith RT, Garson A, et al: Chronic supraventricular tachycardia: A curable cause of congestive cardiomyopathy. JAMA 1985;253:391–392.
7. Lown B, Marcus F, Levin HD: Digitalis and atrial tachycardias with block. N Engl J Med 1959;260:301–309.
8. Mehta D, Wafa S, Ward DE, Camm AJ: Relative efficacy of various physical manoeuvres in the termination of junctional tachycardia. Lancet 1988;28:1181–1185.
9. Malcolm AD, Garratt CJ, Camm AJ: The therapeutic and diagnostic cardiac electrophysiological uses of adenosine. Cardiovasc Drugs Ther 1993;7:139–147.
10. Basta M, Klein GJ, Yee R, et al: Current role of pharmacologic therapy for patients with paroxysmal supraventricular tachycardia. Cardiol Clin 1997;15:587–597.
11. Hohnloser SH, Woosley RL: Sotalol. N Engl J Med 1994;331:31–38.
12. Echt DS, Liebson PR, Mitchell LB, et al: Mortality and morbidity in patients receiving encainide, flecainide or placebo. The Cardiac Arrhythmia Suppression Trial. N Engl J Med 1991;324:781–788.
13. Hindricks G: The Multicentre European Radiofrequency Survey (MERFS): Complications of radiofrequency catheter ablation of arrhythmias. The Multicentre European Radiofrequency Survey (MERFS) investigators of the Working Group on Arrhythmias of the European Society of Cardiology. Eur Heart J 1993;14:1644–1653.
14. Jackman WM, Beckman KJ, McClelland JH, et al: Treatment of supraventricular tachycardia due to atrioventricular nodal reentry, by radiofrequency catheter ablation of slow-pathway conduction. N Engl J Med 1992;327:313–318.
15. Jackman WM, Wang XZ, Friday KJ, et al: Catheter ablation of accessory atrioventricular pathways (Wolff-Parkinson-White syndrome) by radiofrequency current. N Engl J Med 1991;324:1605–1611.
16. Saul JP, Hulse JE, De W, et al: Catheter ablation of accessory atrioventricular pathways in young patients: Use of long vascular sheaths, the transseptal approach and a retrograde left posterior parallel approach. J Am Coll Cardiol 1993;21:571–583.
17. Chen SA, Chiang CE, Yang CJ, et al: Sustained atrial tachycardia in adult patients: Electrophysiological characteristics, pharmacological response, possible mechanisms and effects of radiofrequency ablation. Circulation 1994;90:1262–1278.
18. Tucker KJ, Wilson C: A comparison of transesophageal atrial pacing and direct current cardioversion for the termination of atrial flutter: A prospective randomized clinical trial. Br Heart J 1993;69:530–538.
19. Ellenbogen KA, Stambler BS, Wood MA, et al: Efficacy of intravenous ibutilide for rapid termination of atrial fibrillation and atrial flutter: A dose-response study. J Am Coll Cardiol 1996;28:130–136.
20. Schwartzman D, Callans DJ, Gottlieb CD, et al: Conduction block in the inferior vena caval–tricuspid valve isthmus: Association with outcome of radiofrequency ablation of type I atrial flutter. J Am Coll Cardiol 1996;28:1519–1531.

21. Gomes JA, Santoni-Rugiu F, Mehta D, et al: Uncommon atrial flutter: Characteristics, mechanisms, and results of ablative therapy. Pacing Clin Electrophysiol 1998;21:2029–2042.
22. Kannel W, Abbott R, Savage D, McNamara P: Epidemiologic features of chronic atrial fibrillation: The Framingham Study. N Engl J Med 1982;17:1018–1022.
23. Wipf JE, Lipsky BA: Atrial fibrillation. Thromboembolic risk and indications for anticoagulation. Arch Intern Med 1990;150:1598–1603.
24. Morris JJ Jr, Peter RH, McIntosh HD: Electrical cardioversion of atrial fibrillation. Immediate and long-term results and selection of patients. Ann Intern Med 1966;65:216–231.
25. Geelen P, Goethals M, de Bruyne B, Brugada P: A prospective hemodynamic evaluation of patients with chronic atrial fibrillation undergoing radiofrequency catheter ablation of the atrioventricular junction. Am J Cardiol 1997;80:1606–1609.
26. [Investigators of five atrial fibrillation studies]: Risk factors for stroke and efficacy of antithrombotic therapy in atrial fibrillation: Analysis of pooled data from five randomized controlled trials. Arch Intern Med 1994;154:1449–1457.
27. Manning WJ, Silverman DI, Keighley CS, et al: Transesophageal echocardiographically facilitated early cardioversion from atrial fibrillation using short-term anticoagulation: Final results of a prospective 4.5-year study. J Am Coll Cardiol 1995;25:1354–1361.
28. Van Gelder IC, Crijns HJ, Van Gilst WH, et al: Prediction of uneventful cardioversion and maintenance of sinus rhythm from direct current electrical cardioversion of chronic atrial fibrillation and flutter. Am J Cardiol 1991;68:41–46.
29. Bolognesi R: The pharmacologic treatment of atrial fibrillation. Cardiovasc Drug Ther 1991;5:617–628.
30. Falk RH: Proarrhythmia in patients treated for atrial fibrillation or flutter. Ann Intern Med 1992;11:529–535.
31. Wellens HJ, Sie HT, Smeets JL, et al: Surgical treatment of atrial fibrillation. J Cardiovasc Electrophysiol 1998;9:S151–154.
32. Haissaguerre M, Jais P, Shah DC, et al: Spontaneous initiation of atrial fibrillation by ectopic beats originating in the pulmonary veins. N Engl J Med 1998;339:659–666.
33. Wang K, Hodges M: The premature ventricular complex as a diagnostic aid. Ann Intern Med 1992;117:766–770.
34. Waldo AL, Camm AJ, deRuyter H, et al: Effect of d-sotalol on mortality in patients with left ventricular dysfunction after recent and remote myocardial infarction. The SWORD Investigators. Survival with oral d-sotalol. Lancet 1996;348:7–12.
35. Cairns JA, Connolly SJ, Roberts R, Gent M: Randomised trial of outcome after myocardial infarction in patients with frequent or repetitive ventricular premature depolarisations: CAMIAT. Canadian Amiodarone Myocardial Infarction Arrhythmia Trial Investigators. Lancet 1997;349:675–682.
36. Julian DG, Camm AJ, Frangin G, et al: Randomised trial of effect of amiodarone on mortality in patients with left-ventricular dysfunction after recent myocardial infarction: EMIAT. European Myocardial Infarct Amiodarone Trial Investigators. Lancet 1997;349: 667–674.
37. Doval HC, Nul DR, Grancelli HO, et al: GESICA, Capital Federal, Argentina. Randomised trial of low-dose amiodarone in severe congestive heart failure. Lancet 1994; 344:493–498.
38. Singh SN, Fletcher RD, Fisher S, et al: Veterans Affairs congestive heart failure antiarrhythmic trial. CHF STAT Investigators. Am J Cardiol 1993; 72:99F–102F.
39. Buxton AE, Lee KL, DiCarlo L, et al: Nonsustained ventricular tachycardia in coronary artery disease: Relation to inducible sustained ventricular tachycardia. MUSTT Investigators. Ann Intern Med 1996;125:35–39.
40. Moss AJ, Hall WJ, Cannom DS, et al: Improved survival with an implanted defibrillator in patients with prior myocardial infarction, low ejection fraction and asymptomatic non-sustained ventricular tachycardia. N Engl J Med 1996;335:1933–1940.
41. Cardiac Arrest in Seattle: Conventional versus amiodarone drug evaluation (the CASCADE study). Am J Cardiol 1991;67:578–584.
42. The ESVEM Investigators: Determinants of predicted efficacy of antiarrhythmic drugs in the electrophysiologic study versus electrocardiographic monitoring trial. Circulation 1993;87:323–329.
43. The AVID Investigators: A comparison of antiarrhythmic drug therapy with implantable defibrillators in patients resuscitated from near fatal ventricular arrhythmias. N Engl J Med 1997;337:1576–1583.
44. Gregoratos G, Cheitlin MD, Conill A, et al: ACC/AHA Guidelines for Implantation of Cardiac Pacemakers and Antiarrhythmia Devices: Executive Summary—a report of the American College of Cardiology/American Heart Association Task Force on Practice Guidelines (Committee on Pacemaker Implantation). Circulation 1998;97:1325–1335.
45. Klein LS, Shih HT, Hackett FK, et al: Radiofrequency catheter ablation of ventricular tachycardia in patients without structural heart disease. Circulation 1992;85:1666–1674.
46. Stevenson WG, Khan H, Sager P, et al: Identification of reentry circuit sites during catheter mapping and radiofrequency ablation of ventricular tachycardia late after myocardial infarction. Circulation 1993;88:1647–1670.
47. Breithardt G, Wichter T, Haverkamp W, et al: Implantable cardioverter defibrillator therapy in patients with arrhythmogenic right ventricular cardiomyopathy, long QT syndrome, or no structural heart disease. Am Heart J 1994;127:1151–1158.
48. Almendral JM, Ormaetxe J, Martinez-Alday JD, et al: Treatment of ventricular arrhythmias in patients with hypertrophic cardiomyopathy. Eur Heart J 1993;14(Suppl J):71–72.

49. Splawski I, Timothy KW, Vincent GM, et al: Molecular basis of the long-QT syndrome associated with deafness. N Engl J Med 1997;336:1562–1567.
50. Goldberg RJ, Zevallos JC, Yarzebski J, et al: Prognosis of acute myocardial infarction complicated by complete heart block (the Worcester Heart Attack Study). Am J Cardiol 1992;69:1135–1141.
51. Klein LS, Miles WM, Heger JJ, Zipes DP: Transcutaneous pacing: Patient tolerance, strength interval relations and feasibility for programmed stimulation. Am J Cardiol 1988;62:1126–1131.
52. Shinbane JS, Chu E, DeMarco T, et al: Evaluation of acute dual-chamber pacing with a range of atrioventricular delays on cardiac performance in refractory heart failure. J Am Coll Cardiol 1997;30:1295–1300.
53. Barold SS: Indications for permanent cardiac pacing in first-degree AV block: Class I, II, or III? Pacing Clin Electrophysiol 1996;19:747–751.
54. Connolly SJ, Kerr C, Gent M, Yusuf S: Dual-chamber versus ventricular pacing: Critical appraisal of current data. Circulation 1996;94:578–583.

# ■ RECOMMENDED READING

Basta M, Klein GJ, Yee R, et al: Current role of pharmacologic therapy for patients with paroxysmal supraventricular tachycardia. Cardiol Clin 1997;15(4):587–597.

Cannom DS, Prystowsky EN: Management of ventricular arrhythmias: Detection, drugs, and devices. JAMA 1999;281:172–179.

Connolly SJ, Kerr C, Gent M, Yusuf S: Dual-chamber versus ventricular pacing: Critical appraisal of current data. Circulation 1996;94:578–583.

Ganz LI, Friedman PL: Supraventricular tachycardia. N Engl J Med 1995;332(3):162–173.

Gregoratos G, Cheitlin MD, Conill A, et al: ACC/AHA Guidelines for Implantation of Cardiac Pacemakers and Antiarrhythmia Devices: Executive Summary—a report of the American College of Cardiology/American Heart Association Task Force on Practice Guidelines (Committee on Pacemaker Implantation). Circulation 1998;97:1325–1335.

Pinski SL, Trohman RG: Implantable cardioverter-defibrillators: Implications for the nonelectrophysiologist. Ann Intern Med 1995;122:770–777.

Sarter BH, Callans DJ, Gottlieb GD, et al: Implantable defibrillator diagnostic storage capabilities: Evolution, current status, and future utilization. Pacing Clin Electrophysiol 1998;21:1287–1298.

Zipes DP, Jalife J: Cardiac Electrophysiology: From Cell to Bedside, 2nd ed. Philadelphia: WB Saunders, 1997.

*Chapter* 18

# Syncope

*Wishwa N. Kapoor*

Syncope is defined as sudden transient loss of consciousness associated with a loss of postural tone and spontaneous recovery that does not require electrical or chemical cardioversion. Syncope is common and can be disabling, and there are subsets of patients who are at high risk for sudden death. Furthermore, syncope has a large differential diagnosis and can often be difficult to evaluate.[1, 2] The purpose of this article is to review the recent findings on evaluation of syncope and to provide an approach to this problem using currently available diagnostic testing methods.

## ■ CAUSES

Causes of syncope can be divided into four broad categories (Table 18–1). The first and largest one consists of a wide variety of disorders that are associated with sudden transient hypotension and/or bradycardia. These entities are termed *neurally mediated* or *neurocardiogenic syndromes*.[3] The best example is vasovagal or vasodepressor syncope, which may be associated with pain, emotional stress, prolonged standing, or another stressor. Other entities include carotid sinus syncope, cough, defecation, micturition or swallow syncope, syncope in association with certain drugs such as nitroglycerin, and others (see Table 18–1). Syncope associated with certain cardiac disorders also may be due to neurocardiogenic mechanisms. Syncope occurs in patients with aortic stenosis, hypertrophic cardiomyopathy, supraventricular tachycardias, and paroxysmal atrial fibrillation.[4, 5]

The second large category is orthostatic hypotension, which has many causes, ranging from volume depletion and medications to diseases affecting the autonomic nervous system (Table 18–2).[6] Orthostatic hypotension after meals is another known cause of syncope in elderly persons. In this instance, systolic blood pressure drops, generally within 60 minutes after a meal.[7]

The third category is neurologic disorders, which infrequently cause syncope. The major group consists of migraines and transient ischemic attacks. Seizures may also be confused with syncope and are thus an important cause of loss of consciousness. Seizures may reflect temporal lobe epilepsy, unwitnessed grand mal seizures, or atonic seizures.

The fourth category is cardiac causes of syncope. These include disorders due to structural heart disease and those secondary to arrhythmias.

## Structural Heart Disease

A large group of cardiac disorders are associated with obstruction to the outflow tract of the left or right ventricle. Exertional syncope may occur when cardiac output is fixed and does not increase with exercise. The mechanism of exertional syncope in ventricular outflow obstruction is believed to be a neurally mediated response. An increase in ventricular systolic pressure without a corres-

Table 18–1

## Causes of Syncope

| | |
|---|---|
| **Neurally mediated syncope** | **Decreased cardiac output** |
| Vasovagal | Obstruction to flow |
| Situational | Obstruction to left ventricular outflow |
| Micturition | Aortic stenosis (hypertrophic cardiomyopathy) |
| Cough | Mitral stenosis |
| Swallow | Obstruction to right ventricular outflow |
| Defecation | Pulmonic stenosis |
| Carotid sinus syncope | Pulmonary edema, pulmonary hypertension |
| Neuralgias | Myxoma |
| High altitude | Other heart disease |
| Psychiatric disorders | Pump failure: myocardial infarction, coronary artery disease, |
| Others (exercise, selected drugs) | coronary spasm |
| **Orthostatic hypotension** | Tamponade, aortic dissection |
| **Neurologic diseases** | Arrhythmias |
| Migraines | Bradyarrhythmias |
| Transient ischemic attacks | Sinus node disease |
| Seizures | Second- and third-degree atrioventricular block |
| | Pacemaker malfunction |
| | Drug-induced bradyarrhythmias |
| | Tachyarrhythmias |
| | Ventricular tachycardia |
| | Torsades de pointes (e.g., associated with congenital long QT syndromes or acquired QT prolongation) |
| | Supraventricular tachycardia |

Table 18–2

## Causes of Orthostatic Hypotension

**Primary**
    Autonomic failure (idiopathic, Shy-Drager syndrome, Parkinson disease)
**Secondary**
    General medical disorders: diabetes, amyloidosis, renal failure, alcoholism
    Autoimmune disease: Guillain-Barré syndrome, collagen vascular disease (mixed connective tissue disease; rheumatoid arthritis; systemic lupus erythematosus); Eaton-Lambert syndrome
    Metabolic disease: Vitamin $B_{12}$ deficiency, porphyria, Fabry disease, Tangier disease
    Infections of the nervous system: syphilis, Chagas disease, human immunodeficiency virus, botulism, herpes zoster
    Central brain lesions: vascular lesion or tumors involving the hypothalamus and midbrain (i.e., craniopharyngioma, multiple sclerosis, Wernicke's encephalopathy
    Spinal cord lesions
    Familial dysautonomia
    Aging
**Drugs**
    Tranquilizers: phenothiazines, barbiturates
    Antidepressants: tricyclics, monoamine oxidase inhibitors
    Vasodilators: prazosin, hydralazine, calcium channel blockers
    Centrally acting hypotensive drugs: methyldopa, clonidine
    Adrenergic neuron blocking drugs: guanethidine
    Alpha-adrenergic blocking drugs: phenoxybenzamine, labetalol
    Ganglion-blocking drugs: hexamethonium, mecamylamine
    Angiotensin-converting enzyme inhibitors: captopril, enalapril, lisinopril

Adapted from Bannister SR (ed): Autonomic Failure, 2nd ed. Oxford: Oxford University Press, 1992.

ponding increase in aortic pressure may result in excessive stimulation of ventricular mechanoreceptors, leading to hypotension or bradycardia.

Syncope is a common manifestation of severe aortic stenosis (prevalence 42% in these patients). Syncope is prognostically important in the absence of valve replacement, since average survival is 2 to 3 years after its onset. Syncope in hypertrophic cardiomyopathy has a similar mechanism and is reported in as many as 30% of these patients.[8] In this entity, worsening obstruction due to increased contractility, decreased chamber size, or decreased afterload and distending pressures may result in stimulation of ventricular mechanoreceptors. The Valsalva maneuver and drugs such as digitalis may also precipitate hypotension and syncope. Additionally, ventricular tachycardias are commonly reported in patients with hypertrophic cardiomyopathy and are important causes of syncope.

Effort syncope is also common in pulmonary hypertension and pulmonary stenosis. Syncope is also a well-recognized feature of congenital heart diseases such as tetralogy of Fallot, patent ductus arteriosus, and interatrial septal defects in which patients may experience syncope with effort or crying due to sudden reversal of left-to-right shunt and a drop in arterial oxygen saturation.

Syncope is a known manifestation of pulmonary embolism and is more often associated with massive pulmonary embolism. Other causes of syncope include atrial myxomas and mitral stenosis. In elderly persons, myocardial infarction may present with syncope. The mechanism may be sudden pump failure or arrhythmia. Syncope has been reported with unstable angina and coronary artery spasm. It is also a rare manifestation of acute aortic dissection.

## Arrhythmias

Arrhythmias may lead to a sudden decrease in cardiac output that results in syncope or presyncope. Severe bradycardia may result in an inadequate compensatory increase in stroke volume. Tachycardias may lead to a decrease in diastolic filling and cardiac output, resulting in hypotension and syncope. Supraventricular tachycardias and paroxysmal atrial fibrillation may activate cardiac mechanoreceptors leading to syncope because of diminished cardiac volume and more vigorous ventricular contraction.[9]

Sick sinus syndrome, a disorder of sinoatrial impulse formation or conduction, is an important cause of syncope, especially in the elderly. Electrocardiographic (ECG) manifestations include sinus bradycardia, pauses, arrest, and exit block. Supraventricular tachycardia or atrial fibrillation may occur in association with bradycardia. Syncope is reported in 25% to 70% of patients with sick sinus syndrome.

Ventricular tachycardias, important causes of syncope, generally affect patients with structural heart disease. Syndromes of prolonged QT interval are associated with syncope when polymorphic ventricular tachycardia or torsades de pointes occur. These syndromes may be acquired, from drugs, electrolyte abnormalities, or central nervous system disorders. Drugs most often implicated include quinidine, procainamide, and disopyramide. Prolonged QT interval may also be congenital and may or may not be associated with deafness.

## How Often Are Causes of Syncope Identified?

Most of the literature on population-based studies of syncope was published in the early 1980s.[10–14] These studies show that the most common causes of syncope are vasovagal syncope, organic heart diseases, arrhythmias, orthostatic hypotension and seizures (Table 18–3). The studies in the 1980s showed that causes of syncope

Table 18–3

**Causes of Syncope**

| Cause | Prevalence (%) | |
|---|---|---|
| | Mean | Range |
| Vasovagal syncope | 18 | 8–37 |
| Situational syncope | 5 | 1–8 |
| Carotid sinus | 1 | ≤4 |
| Orthostatic hypotension | 8 | 4–10 |
| Medications | 3 | 1–7 |
| Psychiatric disorders | 2 | 1–7 |
| Neurologic disorders | 10 | 3–32 |
| Cardiac disease | | |
|     Organic heart disease | 4 | 1–8 |
|     Arrhythmias | 14 | 4–38 |
| Unknown | 34 | 13–41 |

went undetected in as many as 34% of patients; however, with the development of tilt-table testing, wider use of electrophysiologic testing, and attention to psychiatric illness, a much smaller proportion (about 10%) of patients have unexplained syncope today.

## ■ DIAGNOSTIC EVALUATION

Careful clinical assessment is the cornerstone of the evaluation for syncope. A careful initial history, physical examination, and ECG leads to the diagnosis of many of the causes of syncope or to potential causes that can be diagnosed by directed testing. There are three major clinical issues in patients who present with loss of consciousness.

1. *Does the Patient Have Syncope?* History is important is distinguishing syncope from other states of altered consciousness. Loss of consciousness lasting more than 5 minutes, confusion after the episode, and tonic-clonic motions are suggestive of seizures. Pallor and sweating are more likely to be associated with syncope, but someone must have witnessed the episode.

2. *Risk Stratification.* History of structural heart disease, especially congestive heart failure, history of ventricular arrhythmias, age older than 45 years, and an abnormal ECG have been associated with greater likelihood of diagnosis of arrhythmia or death in patients with syncope.[15] Thus, presence of these variables allows patients to be stratified at high or low risk for these outcomes.

3. *Using the History and Physical Examination to Plan Further Workup.* The history and physical examination help to identify causes of syncope or to suggest specific ones. Table 18–4 shows specific findings from the history and physical examination that are clues to specific causes of syncope (e.g., situational syncope, vasovagal syncope, orthostatic hypotension). Physical examination may also help with the diagnosis of various entities. Specific findings that are particularly helpful include orthostatic hypotension, cardiovascular signs, and the neurologic examination. Orthostatic hypotension is generally defined as a decline of 20 mm Hg or more in systolic blood pressure on assuming an upright position. This finding is commonly reported in elderly persons. Thus, the clinical diagnosis of orthostatic hypotension as a cause of syncope should include symptoms such as syncope and

Table 18–4

**Clinical Features Suggestive of Specific Causes**

| Reported Feature | Diagnostic Consideration |
|---|---|
| Sudden unexpected pain, unpleasant sight, sound, or smell | Vasovagal syncope |
| Micturition during or immediately after cough, swallow, defecation | Situational syncope |
| Neuralgia (glossopharyngeal or trigeminal) | Vasodepressor reaction or bradycardia |
| Arising from seated or lying position | Orthostatic hypotension |
| Prolonged standing at attention | Vasovagal |
| Exertion in a well-trained athlete | Neurally mediated |
| Changing position (from sitting to lying, bending, turning over in bed) | Atrial myxoma, thrombus |
| Exertion | Obstructive heart disease, coronary artery disease, neurally mediated |
| Head rotation, pressure on carotid sinus (as from tumor, shaving, tight collars) | Carotid sinus syncope |
| Vertigo, dysarthria, diplopia, other motor and sensory symptoms of brain stem ischemia | Transient ischemic attack, subclavian steal, basilar artery migraine |
| Arm exercise | Subclavian steal |
| Confusion after episode | Seizure |

dizziness in association with a decrease in systolic blood pressure on rising. Orthostatic hypotension is detected by measuring supine blood pressure and heart rate after the patient has been lying down at least 5 minutes. Standing measurements should be obtained immediately and for at least 2 minutes. Sitting measurements are not reliable for detecting orthostatic hypotension.

Cardiovascular findings that are helpful in patients with syncope are differences in pulse intensity and blood pressure in the two arms, which are suggestive of aortic dissection or subclavian steal syndrome. Generally, a blood pressure difference of 20 mm Hg or greater is needed to consider these entities. The cardiovascular examination should seek aortic stenosis, pulmonary hypertension, aortic dissection, atrial myxoma, idiopathic hypertrophic subaortic stenosis, and other cardiac diseases in the differential diagnosis.

Laboratory tests generally are not abnormal nor the results helpful in identifying the cause of syncope. Hypoglycemia, hypocalcemia, hyponatremia, or renal failure is observed in 3% of the patients, but they seem to be ones who have seizures rather than syncope. These abnormalities are often suspected clinically. Bleeding is generally diagnosed clinically and confirmed by a complete blood count or Hemoccult testing.

## Diagnostic Tests

Clinical assessment and ECG are the first steps in the evaluation of patients with syncope. If the initial assessment leads to a diagnosis (Fig. 18–1), treatment can start. Clinical assessment finding that are not diagnostic may nevertheless provide suggestive evidence for some of the causes of syncope (such as aortic stenosis). These findings can be further investigated with the diagnostic tests most likely to reveal those entities. In a large group of patients, however, a diagnosis is not established by initial clinical assessment and ECG. Then, further diagnostic testing is often in order. In this section, I review various diagnostic tests used for

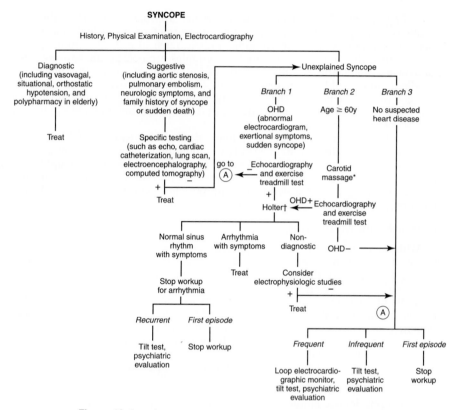

**Figure 18–1** ▪ The diagnosis of syncope. (OHD, organic heart disease.)

patients who have syncope, and later I provide an approach to diagnostic testing of patients with syncope.

## Cardiovascular Testing

### Twelve-Lead Electrocardiography

Although some 50% of patients who present with syncope have abnormal ECG findings,[10] most do not identify the cause of the syncope. Such findings include bundle branch block, old myocardial infarction, and left ventricular hypertrophy. In fewer than 5% of patients, the cause of syncope is identified from the initial ECG and a rhythm strip.[10] Since the ECG is a simple test that may allow the consideration of arrhythmias as a diagnosis, it is always recommended to investigate syncope.

### Prolonged Electrocardiographic Monitoring

Prolonged ECG monitoring or Holter monitoring is frequently used to seek arrhythmias in patients with syncope. The major problem with Holter monitoring is that arrhythmias so diagnosed often are not associated with symptoms. Studies have shown that during Holter monitoring only 4% of patients have symptoms concurrent with arrhythmia.[16] An additional 17% report symptoms though arrhythmias are not documented during monitoring; thus, arrhythmias are ruled out as a cause of symptoms. The vast majority of patients (approximately 79%) exhibit no symptoms during monitoring, which may show brief or no arrhythmia. In the absence of symptoms during monitoring, finding transient or no arrhythmias does not rule our arrhythmic syncope. Brief arrhythmias are nonspecific and are often found in asymptomatic, healthy persons. Additionally, because arrhythmias are episodic, failure to document one during 24-hour monitoring does not exclude them as a cause of syncope. When an arrhythmia is very likely a cause of syncope (especially in association with structural heart disease or an abnormal ECG), further diagnostic tests are in order.

Extending Holter monitoring to 72 hours does not increase the yield of symptom-producing arrhythmias. In one study of monitoring, the yield of brief arrhythmias was 14% during the first day, increased by 11% on the second day and by 4% more on the third day.[17] None of the arrhythmias found during the second or third day of monitoring was associated with symptoms, however. Thus, currently, Holter monitoring for more than 24 hours is not recommended.

## Loop or Event Monitoring

With the loop event technology, patients can now be monitored for prolonged periods of time, such as weeks to months. The advantage of loop monitors is that they can be activated after an episode of syncope and record 2 to 5 minutes of rhythm strip before being activated and 30 to 60 seconds afterward. Tracings are transmitted by telephone and are immediately available for interpretation. Studies of event monitoring show that approximately 8% to 20% of patients who have frequent recurrent syncope have arrhythmias with symptoms.[1, 2, 18] A similar proportion of patients report symptoms when there is no concurrent arrhythmia. Loop monitoring is useful when the likelihood of recurrence of syncope is high, as an arrhythmia can be "captured" during the monitoring period.

### Electrophysiologic Studies

Electrophysiologic studies are relatively safe for patients with syncope, but they are expensive and invasive. The associated risks are low but they include pulmonary embolism, cardiac perforation, arteriovenous fistula, and myocardial infarction (risk >3%). The most important finding of electrophysiologic testing in syncope is sustained monomorphic ventricular tachycardia. Other findings include evidence of conduction system disease, sinus node disease, and, sometimes, induction of supraventricular tachycardias.

The exact findings and criteria for establishing a cause based on electrophysiologic studies are controversial. Generally, the following results are considered positive in patients with syncope: (1) sustained monomorphic ventricular tachycardia; (2) markedly prolonged HV interval, longer than 90 msec; (3) corrected sinus node recovery time longer than 1000 msec; (4) spontaneous or induced infra-Hisian block; and (5) supraventricular tachycardia associated with hypotension during testing. The most important predictor of an abnormal electrophysiologic study is structural heart disease and/or an abnormal ECG.

A summary of electrophysiologic findings in syncope patients who had organic heart disease or an abnormal ECG show that 21% had ventricular tachycardia and 34% had bradycardia.[1, 2, 19, 20] On the other hand, in patients with normal hearts, only 1% had ventricular tachycardia and 10% had documented bradycardia. It should be noted that in these studies, approximately 14% of the patients had a dual diagnosis: ventricular tachycardia and bradycardia. The overall diagnostic yield of electrophysiologic studies is approximately 50% in patients with organic heart disease and about 10% in patients with no evidence of cardiac disease.

Patients with syncope and structural heart disease (such as myocardial infarction or congestive heart failure), patients with preexcitation syndrome (Wolff-

Parkinson-White syndrome), and those whose ECGs show evidence of conduction system disease or other abnormalities, are candidates for electrophysiologic studies when a cause of syncope cannot be determined by noninvasive means and when symptoms suggest an arrhythmia.

### Signal-Averaged Electrocardiography

Signal-averaged ECG (SAGE) detects low-amplitude signals (called *late potentials*). Late potentials have sensitivity of 73% to 89% and specificity of 89% to 100% for prediction of inducible ventricular tachycardia by electrophysiologic testing.[21] Although this test is widely utilized to evaluate syncope, the exact utility of SAGE is not clear. It is possible that this test could be used to determine the need for electrophysiologic testing when ventricular tachycardia is a possible diagnosis. In electrophysiologic testing, however, abnormalities other than ventricular tachycardia are often discovered. Therefore, SAGE is not likely to decrease or eliminate the need for electrophysiologic testing.

### Carotid Massage

Carotid sinus syncope is diagnosed in patients who have carotid sinus hypersensitivity as shown by the reproduction of symptoms during carotid sinus massage.[22] In patients with a hypersensitive response (see later) but no symptoms during carotid massage, carotid sinus syncope is still likely when (1) spontaneous episodes are related to activities that stretch the carotid sinus or (2) patients have a negative workup and recurrent syncope.

Carotid sinus massage is performed with the patient in a supine position and, if the vasodepressor variety of carotid hypersensitivity is suspected and the supine test results negative, is repeated in the sitting and standing positions. It is recommended that noninvasive ECG and blood pressure monitoring accompany carotid sinus massage. The cardioinhibitory variety of carotid sinus massage is defined as a sinus pause of at least 3 seconds upon carotid sinus massage. The vasodepressor variety is diagnosed when there is a decline of 50 mm Hg of systolic blood pressure during carotid sinus massage when the cardioinhibitory response is not present or is abolished with atropine or atrioventricular sequential pacing. Complications of carotid massage are rare. The prevalence of neurologic complications is less than 0.2%. For patients with cerebrovascular disease, it is recommended that the test be done after other diagnostic modalities have shown no evidence of another cause of syncope and carotid sinus syncope is considered likely.

### Echocardiography

An echocardiogram is generally needed to evaluate valvular heart disease when ventricular dysfunction is suspected or cardiac murmurs are detected on physical examination. Echocardiography in the absence of clinical evidence of organic heart disease does not generally reveal unexpected findings that identify the cause of syncope.[23] This test is not recommended for screening, but should be used in a directed manner and when clinical findings suggest or confirm cardiac disease.

### Exercise Testing

There is very little information in the literature on the use of exercise testing in patients with syncope. It is useful in patients who have exertional or postexertional syncope, with or without clinical structural heart disease. The yield of exercise stress testing in identifying the cause of syncope is less than 1%. Exercise testing is important in the diagnosis of coronary artery disease in patients with syncope, especially before electrophysiologic testing or tilt testing. In these circumstances, hypotension is a major concern because it should be avoided in patients with coronary artery disease. When cardiac disease is not suspected, this test generally is not needed.

### Upright Tilt Testing

The indications and techniques for tilt-table testing are shown in Table 18–5.[24] Upright tilt testing is used to provoke abnormal autonomic responses in patients with syncope. At least three different responses to upright tilt testing have been identified:

1. **Neurally mediated response.** Provocation of sudden hypotension and/or bradycardia, which is believed to provoke vasovagal reactions in the laboratory.
2. **Dysautonomic response.** Gradual decrease in systolic and diastolic blood pressure over the period of tilt-table testing.
3. **Postural orthostatic tachycardia syndrome.** Development of sinus tachycardia (with resulting hypotension) observed immediately on standing upright that persists throughout the test.

Most responses in patients with syncope are neurally mediated. In the remainder of this chapter, *positive upright tilt testing* refers to neurally mediated responses.

The mechanisms of the neurally mediated responses are controversial. It is generally believed that upright tilt testing leads to pooling of blood in the lower limbs and a resulting decrease in venous return. Normal compensatory responses to upright posture are reflex tachycardia and more forceful contraction of the ventricle. In persons susceptible to vasovagal syncope, this forceful ventricular contraction in the setting of the decreased ventricular volume may activate cardiac mechanoreceptors that produce reflex hypotension or bradycardia. It is also found that catecholamines released before the onset of syncope may be an important trigger for the activation of neurally mediated responses.

Tilt testing is generally performed using a footboard support.[24, 25] There are two broad categories of tilt testing protocols. One consists of passive tilt testing without the use of provocative drugs. The second is passive tilt testing with periods during which isoproterenol or another drug is utilized. Most laboratories in the

### Table 18–5

### Tilt-Table Testing: Indications and Techniques

| | |
|---|---|
| Indication | • Recurrent unexplained syncope |
| | • Single episode in high-risk patients (e.g., pilots) |
| Laboratory | • Quiet, dim lighting, comfortable temperature |
| | • 20–45 min supine equilibration period |
| Patient | • Fasting overnight or for several hours before procedure, parenteral fluid replacement (rarely) |
| | • Follow-up studies should be at similar times of day |
| Recordings | • Minimum of three ECG leads continuously recorded |
| | • Beat-to-beat blood pressure recordings using the least intrusive means (may not be feasible in children) |
| Table | • Footboard support |
| | • Smooth, rapid transitions (up and down) |
| Tilt angle | • 60–80 degrees (70 degrees becoming most common) |
| Tilt duration | • Initial drug-free tilt 30–45 min |
| | • Pharmacologic provocation—depends on agent |
| Pharmacologic provocation | • Isoproterenol (most common) |
| | • Nitroglycerin |
| Supervision | • Physician in attendance or nearby and immediately available |

ECG, electrocardiogram.
Modified from Benditt DG, Ferguson DW, Grubb BP, et al: Tilt table testing for assessing syncope. Reprinted with permission from the American College of Cardiology (Journal of the American College of Cardiology, 1996, Vol. 28, pp 263–275).

United States use isoproterenol as a provocative agent, but in Europe nitroglycerin is more common. Either agent can activate cardiac mechanoreceptors, but they do so by different actions. Isoproterenol may directly increase ventricular contractility; nitroglycerin may decrease venous return. The mechanism by which isoproterenol and nitroglycerin provoke neurally mediated responses is not well understood. Most tilt-table protocols use 60 to 80 degrees of tilt. The passive tilt-table protocols use 45 to 60 minutes of tilt duration. Tilt testing protocols using isoproterenol generally use 10 to 60 minutes of a passive phase, and, if an endpoint is not reached, the patient is placed supine and isoproterenol infusion is started. The dose of isoproterenol has varied between 1 and 5 µg/min, although most protocols currently use 1 to 3 µg/min infusion rates. Some protocols have used heart rate increases to develop an appropriate dose of isoproterenol. Before each increment in the isoproterenol infusion rate, patients are lowered to the supine position. While they are supine, isoproterenol infusion is increased and they are then tilted for another 10 to 15 minutes. The endpoints of tilt testing are the development of syncope or presyncope in association with hypotension or bradycardia.

The sensitivity of tilt testing is not well-studied, since there is no "gold standard" for diagnosis of vasovagal syncope. Sensitivity can be determined from small studies of patients with known vasovagal syncope which report positive rates of 67% to 83%.[26] Specificity of this test has varied.[25] With passive tilt testing, overall specificity is approximately 90%. With isoproterenol, the specificity appears to be somewhat lower—between 75% and 90%.[25, 27] The lower specificity may be due partly to the use of large doses of isoproterenol.[27, 28]

In patients with unexplained syncope, a positive response of 49% has been reported with the passive tilt testing protocol (range 26% to 90%).[25] With isoproterenol, positive responses in patients with unexplained syncope have been higher: 62% (range 39% to 87%).[25] Approximately two thirds of the responses with isoproterenol occurred during the infusion phase. About two thirds of the responses appeared to be cardioinhibitory, and the remainder were vasodepressor or mixed responses. The reproducibility of tilt testing is 65% to 85%, although some studies show a value as low as 35%.[25] A negative tilt test result is more often reproducible than a positive test.

In general, treatment is offered to patients with recurrent syncope. The recurrence rates after a single episode are low and treatment is not recommended. Table 18–6 shows treatments used for neurally mediated syncope. Currently, the most widely used treatments are beta blockers and salt and fludrocortisone. The vast majority of studies in neurally mediated syncope have reported on case series of patients who were treated and comparison has been made to either "tilt-negative" patients or those who received no treatment. Randomized controlled trials using

Table 18–6

**Common Therapies for Recurrent Vasovagal Syncope**

| Therapies | Dose (mg/day) |
|---|---|
| Beta-blockers | |
|   Atenolol | 25–200 |
|   Metoprolol | 50–200 |
|   Propranolol | 40–160 |
| Disopyramide | 200–600 |
| Fludrocortisone | 0.1–1 |
| Fluoxetine | 20–40 |
| Scopolamine patch | 1 patch every 3 days |
| Theophylline | 6–12 per kg body weight |

clinical endpoints such as recurrent syncope have been small and generally have not shown significant improvement in treated groups. Pacemakers may be considered for patients with frequent recurrence of syncope who do not respond to medications. Patients with significant bradycardia or sinus arrest are considered for pacemaker treatment.

## Neurologic Testing

Neurologic studies such as skull films, lumbar puncture, radionuclide scan, and cerebral angiography have not been useful in evaluating the cause of syncope. Electroencephalography (EEG) and computed tomography (CT) have been reported to show findings diagnostic of causes of syncope in 2% to 4% of patients who had unexplained syncope.[10] Almost all of these patients have subtle neurologic findings or symptoms consistent with seizure. Thus, currently, EEG and CT should be reserved for patients with symptoms compatible with seizure or suspicion of neurologic diseases that cause syncope.[29]

## Psychiatric Assessment

Several psychiatric illnesses can cause syncope: generalized anxiety disorder, panic disorder, major depression, somatization disorder, and alcohol and substance abuse disorders, among others. Except for somatization disorder, stress, anxiety, and depression may result in autonomic stimulation leading to neurally mediated responses. In recent studies, psychiatric illness has been diagnosed in 10% to 20% of patients who present with unexplained syncope.[30]

## ■ APPROACH TO THE EVALUATION OF PATIENTS WITH SYNCOPE

Figure 18–1 shows an approach to the evaluation of syncope. These decision points can be considered:

1. Approximately 50% of the patients have diagnostic findings on initial history, physical examination, and ECG. For them, a specific diagnosis can be made and therapy started. Examples include orthostatic hypotension, situational syncope, and vasovagal syncope diagnosed clinically.
2. History and physical examination may provide suggestive findings, such as evidence of aortic stenosis, symptoms compatible with pulmonary embolism, and others. In these instances, specific testing can be used to diagnose the entities under consideration and treatment can be initiated.
3. The remainder of the patients' syncope can be classified as unexplained. In such cases, three different branches can be proposed in using diagnostic testing in a directed manner:

Branch 1: Organic heart disease or abnormal ECG findings. In these patients, initial evaluation may consist of echocardiography and exercise testing to determine the extent of organic heart disease. In patients with ventricular dysfunction or evidence of coronary artery disease, evaluation should be directed toward detecting arrhythmias. When Holter monitoring, the test of first choice, shows arrhythmias with symptoms, treatment can be instituted. If no arrhythmia is found and the patient does not have symptoms during monitoring, electrophysiologic testing is recommended. Loop event monitoring may be useful in patients with recurrent episodes, either before electrophysiologic testing or when such studies are negative.

Branch 2: Advanced age. Carotid sinus massage should be considered in elderly patients, who are more likely to have carotid sinus syncope. Echo-

Table 18–7

**Indications for Hospital Admission in Patients with Syncope**

Indicated
  History of coronary artery disease, congestive heart failure, or ventricular arrhythmia
  Accompanying symptoms of chest pain
  Physical signs of significant valve disease, congestive heart failure, stroke, or focal neurologic disorder
  Electrocardiogenic findings: ischemia, arrhythmia (serious bradycardia or tachycardia), increased QT
    interval, bundle branch block
Often indicated
  Sudden loss of consciousness with injury, tachycardia, or exertional syncope
  Frequent spells, suspicion of coronary disease or arrhythmia (for example, use of medications
    associated with torsades de points)
  Moderate to severe orthostatic hypotension
  Age >70 years

Adapted from Linzer M, Yang E, Esters M, et al: Diagnosing syncope. Value of history, physical examination, and electrocardiography. Ann Intern Med 1997; 126(12):989–996.

cardiography and exercise testing are recommended for diagnosis of occult coronary artery disease. If evidence of heart disease is found, evaluation proceeds as in Branch 1.

Branch 3: No evidence of heart disease, clinically or after an evaluation. The most likely diagnoses in this case are neurally mediated syncope, psychiatric illnesses, and, rarely, brief arrhythmias such as bradycardias. For patients in this category who have recurrent syncope, tilt testing and psychiatric evaluation are recommended. If there is a strong clinical suspicion of arrhythmia as the cause of syncope, loop monitoring is recommended. Patients who have had only one episode of syncope can be followed closely without further diagnostic testing.

# ■ ADMISSION DECISIONS FOR PATIENTS WITH SYNCOPE

No studies have evaluated the admission decisions and guidelines for admitting patients with syncope. Patients should be admitted if a rapid diagnostic evaluation is needed, if there is concern for serious arrhythmias or sudden death, or if there is newly diagnosed cardiac disease such as aortic stenosis. Table 18–7 provides some of the indications for admission in patients with syncope,[1, 2] but studies are needed to develop more evidence-based indications.

# ■ REFERENCES

1. Linzer M, Yang E, Estes M, et al: Diagnosing syncope. Value of history, physical examination, and electrocardiography. Ann Intern Med 1997;126(12):989–996.
2. Linzer M, Yang E, Estes M, et al: Diagnosing syncope. Unexplained syncope. Ann Intern Med 1997;127(1):76–86.
3. Abboud FM: Neurocardiogenic syncope. N Engl J Med 1993;15:1117–1120.
4. Grech ED, Ramsdale DR: Exertional syncope in aortic stenosis. Am Heart J 1991;121:603–606.
5. Gilligan DM, Nihoyannopoulos P, Chan WL, Oakley CM: Investigation of a hemodynamic basis for syncope in hypertrophic cardiomyopathy. Use of head-up tilt test. Circulation 1992;85:2140–2148.
6. Bannister SR, Mathias CJ (eds): Autonomic Failure: A Textbook of Clinical Disorders of the Autonomic Nervous System, 2nd ed. Oxford: Oxford Medical Publishers 1992:1–20.
7. Vaitkevicius PV, Esserwein DM, Maynard AK, et al: Frequency and importance of postprandial blood pressure reduction in elderly nursing-home patients. Ann Intern Med 1991;115:865–870.
8. Nienaber CA, Hiller S, Spielmann RP, et al: Syncope in hypertrophic cardiomyopathy: Multivariate analysis of prognostic determinants. J Am Coll Cardiol 1990;15:948–955.

9. Brignole M, Gianfranchi L, Menozzi C, et al: Role of autonomic reflexes in syncope associated with paroxysmal atrial fibrillation. J Am Coll Cardiol 1993;22:1123–1129.
10. Kapoor W: Evaluation and outcome of patients with syncope. Medicine 1990;69:160–175.
11. Silverstein MD, Singer DE, Mulley A, et al: Patients with syncope admitted to medical intensive care units. JAMA 1982;248:1185–1189.
12. Martin GJ, Adams SL, Martin HG, et al: Prospective evaluation of syncope. Ann Emerg Med 1984;13:499–504.
13. Day SC, Cook EF, Funkenstein H, Goldman L: Evaluation and outcome of emergency room patients with transient loss of consciousness. Am J Med 1982;73:15–23.
14. Ben-Chetrit E, Flugeman M, Eliakim M: Syncope: A retrospective study of 101 hospitalized patients. Isr J Med Sci 1985;21:950–953.
15. Martin TP, Hanusa BH, Kapoor WN: Risk stratification of patients with syncope. Ann Emerg Med 1997;29(4):459–466.
16. DiMarco JP, Philbrick JT: Use of ambulatory electrocardiographic (Holter) monitoring. Ann Intern Med 1990;113:53–68.
17. Bass ES, Curtiss El, Arena VC, et al: The duration of Holter monitoring in patients with syncope: Is 24 hours enough? Arch Intern Med 1990;150:1073–1078.
18. Linzer M, Pritchett ELC, Pontinen M, et al: Incremental diagnostic yield of loop electrocardiographic recorders in unexplained syncope. Am J Cardiol 1990;66:214–219.
19. Kapoor WN, Hammill SC, Gersh BJ: Diagnosis and natural history of syncope and the role of invasive electrophysiologic testing. Am J Cardiol 1989;63:730–734.
20. DiMarco JP: Electrophysiologic studies in patients with unexplained syncope. Circulation 1987;75(Suppl 111):140–143.
21. Steinberg JS, Prystowsky E, Freedman RA, et al: Use of the signal averaged electrocardiogram for predicting inducible ventricular tachycardia in patients with unexplained syncope: Relation to clinical variables in a multivariate analysis. J Am Coll Cardiol 1994;23:99–106.
22. Strasberg B, Sagie A, Erdman S, et al: Carotid sinus hypersensitivity and the carotid sinus syndrome. Prog Cardiovasc Dis 1989;5:379–391.
23. Recchia D, Barzilai B: Echocardiography in the evaluation of patients with syncope. J Gen Intern Med 1995;10:649–655.
24. Benditt D, Ferguson D, Grubb B, et al: Tilt table testing for assessing syncope. J Am Coll Cardiol 1996;28(1):263–275.
25. Kapoor WN, Smith M, Miller NL: Upright tilt testing in evaluating syncope: A comprehensive literature review. Am J Med 1994;97:78–88.
26. Calkins H, Kadish A, Sousa J, et al: Comparison of responses to isoproterenol and epinephrine during head-up tilt in suspected vasodepressor syncope. Am J Cardiol 1991;67:207–209.
27. Natale A, Akhtar M, Jazayeri M, et al: Provocation of hypotension during head up tilt in subjects with no history of syncope or presyncope. Circulation 1995;92:54–58.
28. Kapoor WN, Brant NL: Evaluation of syncope by upright tilt testing with isoproteronol: A nonspecific test. Ann Intern Med 1992;116:358–363.
29. Davis TL, Freemon FR: Electroencephalography should not be routine in the evaluation of syncope in adults. Arch Intern Med 1990;150:2027–2029.
30. Kapoor WK, Fortunato M, Hanusa SH, Schulberg HC: Psychiatric illnesses in patients with syncope. Am J Med 1995;99:505–512.

## ■ RECOMMENDED READINGS

Benditt D, Ferguson D, Grubb B, et al: Tilt table testing for assessing syncope. J Am Coll Cardiol 1996;28(1):263–275.
Kapoor WN: Syncope and hypotension. *In* Braunwald E (ed): Heart Disease. A Textbook of Cardiovascular Medicine, 5th ed. Philadelphia: WB Saunders, 1997:863–875.
Linzer M, Yang E, Estes M, et al: Diagnosing syncope. Value of history, physical examination, and electrocardiography. Ann Intern Med 1997;126(12):989–996.
Linzer M, Yang E, Estes M, et al: Diagnosing syncope. Unexplained syncope. Ann Intern Med 1997; 127(1):76–86.

Chapter 19

# Pathophysiology of Heart Failure

*Ian F. Purcell* ■ *Philip A. Poole-Wilson*

Heart failure is a clinical entity diagnosed by doctors. It is initiated by abnormal function of the heart (often a reduction of muscle contraction). Death from heart failure is most often the result of a cardiac event such as an arrhythmia, ischemia of the heart muscle, or decompensated heart failure. Thus, the natural history of heart failure begins and ends with the heart, but almost all of the clinical characteristics of patients with heart failure result from persistent stimulation of interacting compensatory mechanisms in the heart, peripheral circulation, and body organs. The clinical manifestations and pathophysiologic mechanisms of heart failure should be considered consequences of a multisystem disease. Understanding of the pathophysiology of heart failure, particularly in terms of cellular and molecular biology, has advanced much in recent years, and in this chapter we summarize some of the important mechanisms that have emerged.

## ■ DEFINITION

Despite progress in understanding the pathophysiologic mechanisms of heart failure and the wide use of the term, there is not yet a universally accepted definition of the condition. Some examples of definitions are given in Table 19–1. Most are unsatisfactory because they emphasize one or another of the physiologic or biochemical features of heart failure. The symptoms of heart failure occur or predominate on exercise, so definitions based on observations at rest are inevitably flawed, and with modern treatment the classic physical signs of heart failure may be absent. Emphasis should not be placed on ventricular filling pressure, as it may be normal at rest, can be manipulated by diuretics, varies from moment to moment, and in chronic heart failure is poorly related to symptoms. Currently, a useful definition is "a clinical syndrome caused by an abnormality of the heart and recognized by a characteristic pattern of hemodynamic, renal, neural, and hormonal responses."[1] This definition recognizes two cardinal features of heart failure. The first is that an abnormality of the heart is the origin of heart failure. The second is that the systemic response to cardiac dysfunction is important in producing the clinical picture. This definition is sufficiently pragmatic to be used in clinical practice. For epidemiologic purposes, attempts have been made to formulate criteria

Table 19–1

### Some Definitions of Heart Failure

1933. A condition in which the heart fails to discharge its contents adequately. *Lewis*[45]

1950. A state in which the heart fails to maintain an adequate circulation for the needs of the body, despite a satisfactory filling pressure. *Wood*[46]

1980. A pathophysiological state in which an abnormality of cardiac function is responsible for the failure of the heart to pump blood at a rate commensurate with the requirements of the metabolizing tissues. *Braunwald*[47]

1985. A clinical syndrome caused by an abnormality of the heart and recognized by a characteristic pattern of hemodynamic, renal, neural, and hormonal responses. *Poole-Wilson*[1, 48]

1987. ... Syndrome ... which arises when the heart is chronically unable to maintain an appropriately high blood pressure without support. *Harris*[44]

1988. A syndrome in which cardiac dysfunction is associated with reduced exercise tolerance, a high incidence of ventricular arrhythmias, and shortened life expectancy. *Cohn*[49]

1989. ...Ventricular dysfunction with symptoms. *Unattributed*[48]

1993. Heart failure is the state of any heart disease in which, despite adequate ventricular filling, the heart's output is decreased or in which the heart is unable to pump blood at a rate adequate for satisfying the requirements of the tissues with function parameters remaining within normal limits. *Denolin et al.*[50]

1994. The principal functions of the heart are to accept blood from the venous system, deliver it to the lungs where it is oxygenated (aerated), and pump the oxygenated blood to all body tissues. Heart failure occurs when these functions are disturbed substantially. *Lenfant*[51]

1996. Abnormal ventricular function, symptoms or signs of heart failure (past or current), and heart failure on treatment (? with a favorable response to treatment). *European Society of Cardiology*[2, 48]

that identify patients with a varying degree of certainty. The Framingham study used such an approach. The guidelines of the European Society of Cardiology[2] are useful, because they require symptoms (or a doctor to diagnose heart failure), a demonstrable abnormality of the heart, and preferably, a favorable response to treatment. Such criteria can be applied in epidemiologic studies.

Clinically, heart failure can usefully be categorized as acute heart failure, chronic heart failure, or circulatory collapse. Since heart failure is a dynamic condition, one disorder may in time progress to a different clinical state. The pathophysiologic mechanisms of acute and chronic heart failure are not distinct, and the conditions may be thought of as different points on a continuum.

So-called high-output or circulatory heart failure may eventually result in damage or reduced function of the heart secondary to volume overload. It is associated with neurohormonal activation, but this entity should not be regarded as heart failure per se because the original abnormality is not in the heart itself (Table 19–2).

Table 19–2

### Causes of Cardiac Failure

| Causes of "High-Output Cardiac Failure" | General Causes of True Cardiac Failure |
| --- | --- |
| Anemia | Myocardial disease (largest group, |
| Thyrotoxicosis | includes coronary artery disease, |
| Beriberi | which is the cause underlying 70% of |
| Arteriovenous fistula | all cases of cardiac failure) |
| Cirrhosis of the liver | Arrhythmia |
| Paget's disease | Pericardial disease |
| Pregnancy | Valvular disease |
| Renal cell carcinoma | Congenital heart disease |

Physicians have used many other terms. Thus, there are forward and backward failure, right-sided and left-sided failure, high-output and low-output failure, and—currently fashionable—systolic and diastolic heart failure. These phrases can be useful clinical shorthand, but often they are misleading in terms of understanding the disease process, are the inheritance from old and incorrect concepts, or are merely unnecessary words. For example, the commonest cause of right-sided heart failure (by which is meant a pattern of clinical findings) is left ventricular dysfunction; that way lies confusion.

## Systolic or Diastolic Abnormality?

Systolic dysfunction is defined simply as abnormal systolic ventricular contraction, which is often diagnosed by measurement of ejection fraction. Rigid definitions of systolic dysfunction based on a measurement of ejection fraction and a cutoff value that identifies which subjects have heart failure have been applied. This is problematic, because measures of ventricular contraction and volumes are not bimodal but are normally distributed in the population. Thus, some patients' conditions will be incorrectly defined, regardless of what cutoff point is chosen.[3] Moreover, a definition of systolic failure that relies rigidly on a single global parameter of cardiac function lacks sensitivity, as abnormal systolic function in heart failure may be regional or manifested only at maximal exercise.

Diastolic dysfunction can be most simply described as increased resistance to ventricular filling. Diastole may be divided into four phases: isovolemic relaxation, early filling, late filling, and atrial systole. Abnormality of any diastolic event may affect the end-diastolic volume and pressure, depending on the heart rate. Abnormal diastolic function is difficult to quantify because diastolic function changes with age and is influenced by ventricular loading conditions, systolic function, and heart rate. Furthermore, there is no clear physical definition of what "resistance to filling" represents. Diastolic heart failure should be suspected in patients who have the symptoms of heart failure, normal heart size, and evidence of myocardial hypertrophy or cardiac ischemia. Diastolic heart failure may occur in as many as 50% of patients with heart failure in the community, and it is common in elderly persons. It is important to identify, since the diagnosis has therapeutic implications. Evidence of prolonged or incoordinate isovolemic relaxation of the left ventricle and reduced mitral Doppler E-wave amplitude with a relative increase in the corresponding A-wave support the diagnosis of diastolic heart failure. Diastolic heart failure may respond to treatment that reduces ventricular load, improves ventricular relaxation, increases compliance, and reduces subendocardial ischemia, such as beta blockers (which also prolong diastolic filling time), nitrates, and other vasodilators. In practice, systolic and diastolic heart failure often coexist, and the two are distinguished only with difficulty.

## ■ CAUSES OF HEART FAILURE

Heart failure is the final common result of almost any insult to cardiac function, though the nature of progression to heart failure depends on the cause. The general causes of heart failure can be categorized as arrhythmia, pericardial disease, valvular disease, congenital heart disease, and myocardial disease (see Table 19–2). The largest group, myocardial disease, may be due to coronary artery disease, hypertension, drugs, or intrinsic myocardial disease. The term *cardiomyopathy* should be reserved for intrinsic cardiac muscle disease in the absence of coronary artery disease, hypertension, valvular disease, congenital heart disease, and pericardial disease. Idiopathic dilated cardiomyopathy, as its name implies, is enlargement

Table 19–3

### Causes of Dilated Cardiomyopathy

**Familial cardiomyopathies**
**Genetic cardiomyopathies**
**Infectious causes**
  Bacteria
  Fungi
  Parasites (trypanosomiasis, toxoplasmosis, schistosomiasis, trichinosis)
  Rickettsiae
  Spirochetes
  Viruses (coxsackievirus, adenovirus, human immunodeficiency virus)
**Toxins**
  Alcohol
  Cocaine
  Heavy metals (cobalt, lead, mercury)
  Carbon monoxide or hypoxia
**Drugs**
  Chemotherapeutic agents (bleomycin, doxorubicin, busulfan)
  Antibiotics and antivirals (chloroquine, zidovudine)
  Antipsychotics
**Metabolic disorders**
  Endocrine disease (diabetes mellitus)
  Nutritional deficiencies (selenium, thiamine)
  Storage disease (hemochromatosis, Refsum's disease, Fabry's disease)
**Autoimmune and collagen vascular diseases** (sarcoidosis, systemic lupus
  erythematosus, rheumatoid arthritis, Churg-Strauss syndrome)
**Peripartum cardiomyopathy**
**Neuromuscular disorders** (muscular dystrophies, Friedreich's ataxia)

of the heart of no known cause. It occurs in approximately 3% of patients with heart failure and is familial in 25% of cases, and genetic abnormalities have been described recently. Dilated cardiomyopathy is characterized by an enlarged left ventricle (left ventricular end-diastolic dimension greater than 2.7 cm/m$^2$ body surface area) and ejection fraction less than 45% or M-mode fractional shortening of less than 30%. Dilated cardiomyopathy is the end point of many different pathologic insults (Table 19–3). Hypertrophic cardiomyopathy is a cardiac condition characterized by hypertrophy of nondilated left and/or right ventricles in the absence of a cardiac or systemic stimulus to hypertrophy. Molecular genetic analysis has revealed that hypertrophic cardiomyopathy is an autosomal-dominant disorder that results from mutations in genes encoding sarcomeric proteins.[4, 5] The culprit genes identified so far code for beta-myosin heavy chain (β-MHC), myosin light chains 1v and 2v, cardiac troponins I and T, alpha-tropomyosin, myosin-binding protein C, and actin. Restrictive cardiomyopathy is characterized by a stiff, non-compliant ventricle with abnormal ventricular filling. Causes of restrictive cardiomyopathy are listed in Table 19–4.

## Coronary Artery Disease

In numerical terms, heart failure today is largely a manifestation of coronary artery disease, which is the underlying cause in 70% of cases.[6] Myocardial ischemia may also produce altered functional states distinct from heart failure known as *hibernation, stunning,* and *ischemic preconditioning* (Table 19–5). Some of the consequences of ischemia lead to abnormal cardiac function (Table 19–6).

Table 19–4

**Causes of Restrictive Cardiomyopathy**

| Diastolic dysfunction associated with fibrosis | Storage disorders |
|---|---|
| Aging | Endomyocardial disorders |
| Hypertrophy | Endomyocardial fibrosis |
| Ischemia | Hypereosinophilic syndrome |
| Scleroderma | Carcinoid |
| **Infiltrative disorders** | Metastases |
| Amyloidosis | Radiation |
| Sarcoidosis | |
| Inborn errors of metabolism | |
| Neoplasms | |

# ■ THE FAILING HEART: FROM ORGAN TO MOLECULE

A substantial body of information is now available on the cellular and molecular abnormalities in heart failure. Most of the findings are descriptive, and it is often unclear whether the changes observed are the cause of heart failure or are associated with heart failure. It is now apparent that, in spite of the fact that heart failure is caused by a wide range of disparate conditions, a number of common features characterize failing heart muscle (Table 19–7).

## Ventricular Chamber Size, Shape, and Remodeling

Cardiac chambers have the capacity to alter their size and shape in response to chronic changes in hemodynamic load. In general, systolic failure is accompanied by ventricular chamber enlargement without a compensatory increase in wall thickness. Cardiac dilatation may occur suddenly, for example after myocardial infarction or acute severe valvular regurgitation, or may occur gradually as part of a process known as *remodeling*. In the context of coronary artery disease, remodeling was described by Mitchell and coworkers as "left ventricular enlargement and distortion of regional and global ventricular geometry occurring after myocardial infarction."[7] The first changes of postinfarction remodeling are thinning and stretching of the infarcted area (infarct expansion). Myocardial thinning is mediated at a microscopic level by myocyte slippage, myocyte cell lengthening, and alterations in the intercellular matrix. Later, eccentric hypertrophy of noninfarcted myocardium, progressive left ventricular dilatation, and increased chamber sphericity develop. Remodeling is associated with cardiac rupture, development of heart failure, and increased mortality. The process may be progressive, even in the absence of further cardiac ischemia, and can produce heart failure many months after the original

Table 19–5

**Definitions of Myocardial Stunning, Hibernation, and Ischemic Preconditioning**

**Stunning:** Transient and reversible contractile dysfunction following ischemia despite restored coronary flow

**Hibernation:** Persistent but potentially reversible contractile dysfunction due to episodes of reduced coronary perfusion or associated with limited coronary reserve

**Ischemic preconditioning:** Resistance of myocardium to sustained ischemia conferred by transient sublethal periods of ischemia

## Table 19–6

### Features of the Various Mechanisms Whereby Ischemia Affects the Myocardium

| Ischemic Mechanism | Normal | Acute Ischemia | Infarction | Acute Stunning | Hibernating | Ischemic Preconditioning |
|---|---|---|---|---|---|---|
| Blood supply | Normal | Reduced | Episode of prolonged occlusion | Transient prior reduction then restoration | Chronic reduction, may be modest at rest but repetitively reduced under stress | Recurrent brief episodic reduction |
| Resting contractile function | Normal | Normal | Nil | Impaired | Impaired | Normal |
| Function under stress | Normal | Impaired | Nil | Impaired | Impaired | Preserved |
| Metabolic activity (PET scanning) | Normal: Low [18F]-fluorodeoxyglucose (FDG) uptake relative to perfusion | — | Low perfusion and 18F-FDG uptake | — | 18F-FDG uptake high relative to perfusion | — |
| Radionucleotide perfusion features | Normal | Reduced | Nil | — | Reduced but may improve with delayed reinjection techniques ± nitrates | — |
| Echo features with dobutamine stress | Normal | Impaired contractility with high-dose dobutamine | No contraction | — | Some transient improvement in contractility at low doses | — |
| Histologic features | Normal | — | Scarring and fibrosis | May be normal histologically | Spectrum from myofibril loss to cell matrix changes and scarring | — |
| Biochemical features | Normal | Rise in inorganic PO$_4$ and adenosine from ATP breakdown seen during ischemia | Nil or minimal metabolic activity | Increased cytosolic calcium | Downregulated ATP demand | Reduced ATP demand under stress protein C activated |
| Response to further ischemia | — | May proceed to infarction (or one of the other syndromes) | — | May become hibernating | Eventually proceeds to infarction | Decreased infarct size |
| Response to revascularization | — | Normalized | No effect | Normalized | Potential full or partial recovery | Normalized |

From Fox KF, Cowie MR, Wood DA, et al: New perspectives on heart failure due to myocardial ischaemia. Eur Heart J 1999;20:256–262, with permission.

Table 19–7

**Abnormalities in Failing Myocardium**

Loss of muscle
Incoordinate contraction and abnormal timing of contraction
Extracellular changes
  Fibrosis
  Altered extracellular architecture
  Altered shape and size of ventricle
  Slippage of cells
  Altered fiber orientation
Cellular changes
  Change of cell structure: Loss of intracellular matrix, hypertrophy, ? hyperplasia
  Change of cell function, systolic and/or diastolic
  Molecular: Calcium release and/or uptake, response of contractile proteins to calcium

myocardial infarct. Remodeling also occurs in other cardiovascular diseases such as hypertension and valvular disease, but the associated changes tend to be global rather than regional.

## Myocyte Loss—Necrosis and Apoptosis

Cardiac contraction is impaired when the proportion of viable myocytes in the ventricular muscle is reduced. The commonest cause of macroscopic myocyte necrosis is myocardial infarction. Animal studies have determined that after myocardial infarction cardiogenic shock will ensue when 40% of left ventricular myocardium is lost. More gradual cell death is better tolerated because of compensatory hypertrophy of remaining myocytes. Microscopic areas of necrotic myocyte loss have been seen in postmortem specimens from patients with connective tissue disease, particularly scleroderma.

Apoptosis is increasingly recognized as a cause of myocyte loss in normal cardiac development, ischemia/reperfusion injury, myocardial infarction, and heart failure. Evidence for myocyte apoptosis in heart failure has accumulated from several animal and human sources. Animal and human cardiac myocytes in culture undergo apoptosis in response to a variety of stimuli, including hypoxia, nitric oxide, and tumor necrosis factor alpha. In dogs and in models of pressure overload hypertrophy in rodents, cardiac myocyte apoptosis is increased in heart failure induced by pacing and chronic ischemia. In failing human hearts, levels of apoptotic cells are increased as compared with controls. Much remains to be determined about the importance of apoptosis in heart failure. Importantly, the true incidence of apoptosis in failing myocardium is still unknown, since results with different detection methods have varied from 0.2% to 35%[8, 9] and the role of apoptosis in the causation of heart failure is currently unproved. If the higher rates of apoptosis are correct, then cell replacement would be necessary to account for the natural history of heart failure as it is observed clinically. It is generally believed that cardiac myocytes cease to divide soon after birth and that enlargement of the heart is the result of cell hypertrophy (that is, the myocyte is a terminally differentiated cell). This view is currently being challenged, particularly in pathologic states marked by cardiac hypertrophy. Approximately 20% of myocardial cells in the human heart have two nuclei (multinucleate), so it is possible that cells could form from cell separation and from mitosis.

## Myocyte Size, Shape, and Intercellular Connections

In response to increased hemodynamic load, myocytes may become hypertrophic (increased in size). The classic teaching is that pressure overload leads to concentric hypertrophy, that is, a thickened ventricular wall without an increase in cavity size. In concentric hypertrophy, the myocyte cross-sectional area increases to a greater extent than cell length, a phenomenon that suggests parallel deposition of sarcomeres. Volume overload gives rise to eccentric hypertrophy (cavity enlargement without a corresponding increase in wall thickness). In eccentric hypertrophy the increase is predominantly in myocyte length, a finding that suggests serial deposition of myocytes. Cardiac hypertrophy is associated with activation of gene transcription, which makes possible myocyte growth (Table 19–8).

Myocyte slippage is thought to underlie the chamber dilatation seen in cardiac remodeling and other forms of ventricular dilatation. Myocyte disarray is a characteristic microscopic feature of hypertrophic cardiomyopathy but can also be found in myocardial hypertrophy of any cause, in ischemic heart disease, and even in normal, healthy hearts.

Gap junctions are membrane proteins that permit transfer of low-molecular-weight molecules between adjacent myocytes. The key protein in a gap junction, a connexon, is made up of six connexins. Gap junctions are abnormally distributed on myocytes from ischemic, hypertrophic, and failing ventricles.[10, 11] Abnormal connexon distribution may alter contractile function and contribute to electrical instability.

## The Interstitium in Failing Hearts

The collagen interstitial matrix has multiple functions in heart muscle (Table 19–9). Collagen turnover is regulated by matrix metalloproteinases (MMP) and tissue inhibitors of metalloproteinase (TIMP), which, respectively, degrade and inhibit degradation of collagen. Both MMP and TIMP are upregulated in failing ventricular muscle.[12] Whatever the cause, failing hearts show a net increase in interstitial fibrillar collagen content. Collagen accounts for 4% of the weight of normal ventricular muscle, but in failing hearts it can constitute more than 25%, causing progressive functional impairment. Twofold to threefold collagen excess impairs diastolic relaxation, and fourfold or greater excess affects systolic contraction. In failing hearts, collagen synthesis is stimulated by the renin-angiotensin-aldosterone system via the proliferative effects of angiotensin II and aldosterone. Increased expression of MMP may lead to destruction of the fibrillar collagen

---

Table 19–8

**Transcriptional Changes of Cardiac Hypertrophy**

| Time | Transcriptional Event |
| --- | --- |
| 30 min | Immediate early genes c-*fos*, c-*jun*, Erg-1, c-*myc*, Hsp70 |
| 6–12 hr | β-myosin heavy chain, skeletal α-actin |
| | β-tropomyosin, atrial natriuretic peptide |
| | β-Na-K-ATPase |
| 12–24 hr | Myosin light chain 2, cardiac α-actin |
| >24 hr | Increased RNA |
| | Increased protein |
| | Increased sarcomerogenesis |
| | Increased cell size |

Table 19–9

**The Role of Collagen in the Myocardium**

Transmit force
Maintain alignment of myocytes and muscle bundles
Prevent overdistention of myocardium
Support intramural coronary arteries
Store energy in systole (which contributes to relaxation)
Determine shape and architecture of the heart (? memory of cardiac structure)
Repair myocardial damage and respond to stress (reactive)

matrix that runs perpendicular to cardiac myocytes. This can result in myocyte slippage that causes ventricular thinning as part of the remodeling process.

# ■ MYOCYTE FUNCTION IN HEART FAILURE

Isolated myocytes from failing human hearts show differences in contractile function as compared with myocytes from normal hearts, including reduced responsiveness to inotropic drugs and a negative force-frequency response. Abnormalities in important intracellular processes are known to occur in failing human myocytes, a fact that may explain these contractile changes. The changes are summarized schematically in Figure 19–1. In general, the action potential is prolonged, the duration of contraction is increased, and both the rate of contraction and the rate of relaxation are reduced.

## Adrenergic Receptors

Two major classes of adrenergic receptors (AR) are present in the human heart: $\alpha$-AR and $\beta$-AR. These are divided, respectively, into subclasses known as $\alpha_1$- and $\alpha_2$-AR and $\beta_1$-, $\beta_2$-, and $\beta_3$-AR, and a putative cardiostimulatory $\beta_4$-AR. The receptor $\alpha_2$-AR is not found in significant amounts in human heart and does not appear to have a significant role in heart failure. In contrast, $\alpha_1$-AR is involved in the induction of myocardial hypertrophy, and stimulation of this receptor is associated with arrhythmias. In heart failure the density of $\alpha_1$-AR is slightly increased.

With heart failure come significant changes in $\beta_1$-AR and $\beta_2$-AR function and downstream effects. First, $\beta_1$-AR number is downregulated in failing hearts.[13] The extent of this downregulation correlates with the severity of heart failure and is independent of its cause. Because $\beta_2$-AR number is not downregulated, as many as 40% of all $\beta$-AR in failing hearts may be $\beta_2$-AR, as compared with 20% in normal hearts. Second, $\beta_1$- and $\beta_2$-AR are uncoupled from their signal transduction pathways by phosphorylation-induced desensitization.[14] Third, the inhibitory G protein $G_i$ is upregulated.[15] Fourth, adenylyl cyclase activity and myocardial tissue levels of cyclic adenosine monophosphate (cAMP) are decreased in the failing human heart.[16] A functional role for the cardiodepressant $\beta_3$-AR has been suggested in heart failure because it appears to be more resistant to downregulation than the stimulatory $\beta_1$- and $\beta_2$-AR and may assume relatively more importance in the failing heart.

Desensitization of $\beta$-AR in heart failure is related to chronic sympathetic overstimulation. The extent of $\beta$-AR desensitization correlates with increased plasma norepinephrine levels, and many of the features of $\beta$-AR subsensitivity may be induced in animals by long-term administration of catecholamine. Since catecholamine stimulation of $\beta_1$- and $\beta_2$-AR enhances systolic contraction and

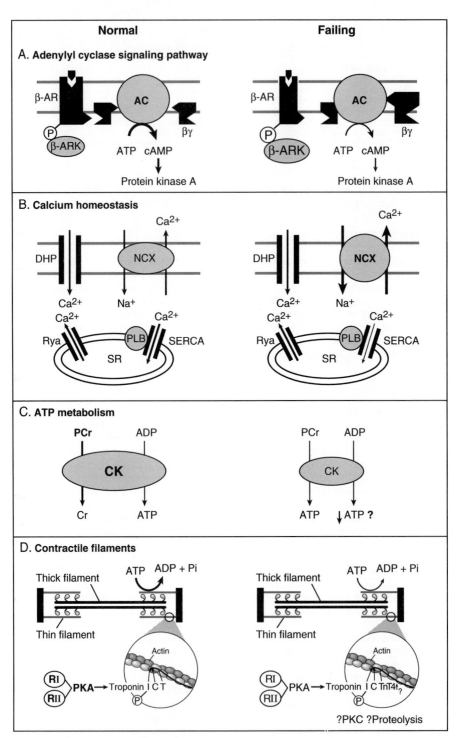

**Figure 19–1** ■ *See legend on opposite page*

diastolic relaxation, subsensitivity of these receptors contributes to the contractile abnormalities seen in failing hearts and to the blunted response to catecholamine inotropic agents. The changes in receptors in the myocardium are not uniform from apex to base or from epicardium to endocardium.

## Calcium Homeostasis

Alterations in some of the key proteins involved in calcium homeostasis suggest that abnormal myocyte calcium handling plays an important role in heart failure. In failing human hearts, activity of the sarcoplasmic reticulum (SR) $Ca^{2+}$ pump (SERCA2), phospholamban, and SR calcium release channels are reduced while activity of the sarcolemmal $Na^+/Ca^{2+}$ exchanger is increased.[17–19] There is no change in calsequestrin, and if any change in L-type calcium channels occurs, that is not known.[20] The net effect of alterations in calcium-handling proteins appears to be to prolong the calcium transient but reduce its amplitude and to increase diastolic levels of calcium. This, in turn, would be expected both to reduce the force of systolic contraction and to impair diastolic relaxation.

## Myocardial Energy Metabolism in the Failing Heart

There are two important high-energy phosphate compounds in the heart: adenosine triphosphate (ATP), which provides chemical energy directly for excitation and contraction in myocytes, and phosphocreatine (PCr), which is involved in ATP production via transfer of its high-energy phosphate group to adenosine diphosphate (ADP) in a reaction catalyzed by creatine kinase. Investigation by phosphorus 31 nuclear magnetic resonance (NMR) spectroscopy has suggested that myocardium is ATP deficient in rodents with severe heart failure. Direct determination of ATP content from heart muscle has failed to show a difference, and noninvasive assessment of failing human hearts has not shown a consistent reduction in high-energy phosphate. There is evidence, from experiments using heart muscle samples from patients with dilated cardiomyopathy and from noninvasive NMR spectroscopy in patients with heart failure of various causes, that creatine kinase content and activity, PCr content, and the PCr-ATP ratio are all reduced in the failing heart.[21, 22] This points to a state of reduced energy reserve in heart failure.

---

**Figure 19–1** ■ Adrenergic receptors, calcium homeostasis, adenosine triphosphate (ATP) metabolism, and contractile proteins in nonfailing and failing myocardium.

(A) The number of $\beta_1$-AR is reduced in failing heart muscle (indicated in the figure by decreased size); activity of β-AR kinase (β-ARK) is increased (indicated by increased size in the figure), leading to phosphorylation-mediated receptor inhibition; inhibitory G protein (βγ) is increased; and adenylyl cyclase (AC) activity is reduced. This results in reduced production of cAMP and decreased activation of protein kinase A.

(B) In failing myocardium, the protein content of the L-type calcium channel (DHP) and the calcium release channel (Rya) are unaltered. The increased threshold of activation of Rya is shown by a greater distance between DHP and Rya in the Failing Myocardium panel. Uptake of calcium by the $Ca^{2+}$-ATPase of the sarcoplasmic reticulum (SERCA) is reduced, but extrusion of $Ca^{2+}$ by the sarcolemmal $Na^+$-$Ca^{2+}$ exchanger (NCX) is increased.

(C) Phosphocreatine (PCr) content, PCr-ATP ratio, and creatine kinase (CK) content and activity are all reduced in failing myocardium. The question of reduced ATP content in failing hearts is unresolved.

(D) Myofilament ATPase activity is reduced in failing hearts. Troponin I phosphorylation by PKA is decreased via downregulation of subunits RI and RII. The occurrence of altered troponin T (TnT) isoform expression, troponin proteolysis, and altered protein kinase C (PKC) function in heart failure is not defined. (Adapted from Mittman C, Eschenhagen T, Scholz H: Cellular and molecular aspects of contractile dysfunction in heart failure. Cardiovasc Res 1998;39:267–275, with permission from Elsevier Science.)

Functionally, this may contribute to the reduced contractile reserve exhibited by failing hearts.

## Cardiac Contractile Proteins

The basic contractile unit of heart muscle is the sarcomere. Cardiac contraction occurs by shortening of the sarcomere that is mediated by complementary sliding of interdigitating myosin and actin filaments driven by ATP hydrolysis. Actin and myosin interaction is regulated by the thin filament troponin complex acting with tropomyosin in response to the $Ca^{2+}$ concentration in the myofilament space. Maximum ATPase and peak isometric force are reduced in myofibrillar preparations from patients with heart failure, whereas calcium sensitivity may be increased over that of healthy hearts. These differences must follow from contractile protein alteration. Two MHC genes, α and β, are expressed in human heart. Downregulation of β-MHC mRNA has been demonstrated in hypertrophic and failing human ventricles,[23, 24] but the proportion of β-MHC expressed at a protein level is not altered in hypertrophy or heart failure. There are two myosin light chains: myosin light chain 1 (MLC1), the essential light chain, and myosin light chain 2 (MLC2), the regulatory light chain. Two genes for MLC1 are expressed in the heart: the atrial (MLC1A) and the ventricular (MLC1V) isoforms.[25] In hypertrophic and failing human ventricles, there is reexpression of the fetal isoform MLC1A, which correlates with increased velocity of unloaded shortening of muscle fibers and with clinical severity of heart failure.[26] There is no evidence for altered actin, tropomyosin, or troponin C isoform expression in human heart failure. There is no change in troponin I (TnI) isoform expression in cardiac disease, but phosphorylation of TnI by protein kinase A (PKA), an effect of β-AR stimulation, is reduced in myocardial samples from patients with end-stage cardiac failure due to downregulation of PKA regulatory subunits.[27, 28] This would be expected to increase myofilament calcium sensitivity. In isolated rat heart preparations, selective degradation of TnI is associated with reduced $Ca^{2+}$ sensitivity in myocardial ischemia/reperfusion injury (stunning). There are as yet no human data that demonstrate selective TnI degradation in stunning or hibernation, but this phenomenon has been reported in myocardial samples from patients with dilated cardiomyopathy.[29]

Four troponin T isoforms (TnT1 to TnT4), which are produced by alternative splicing of a single gene transcript, have been demonstrated at protein level in human heart. Reexpression of the fetus-associated isoform TnT4 has been reported in failing human heart muscle and correlated in degree with the depression of maximum myofibrillar ATPase and clinical indicators of disease severity.[30, 31] This finding has not been consistently reproduced by other groups.[32, 33]

## Oxidative Stress

Under normal circumstances 3% to 5% of oxygen taken up by a cell undergoes univalent reduction, a process that produces free radicals. Free radicals are balanced by antioxidant enzymes and antioxidant compounds. Oxidative stress occurs when an excess of free radicals is not balanced by antioxidant activity. There is evidence for increased oxidative stress and free radical activity in heart muscle in both animal and human studies of hypertrophy and heart failure. In addition, noninvasive markers of lipid and arachidonic acid peroxidation caused by oxidative stress are increased after myocardial infarction and ischemia/reperfusion, and with diabetes mellitus or heart failure.[34-37] Free radicals have many potential toxic effects on the myocardium: reduction of high-energy phosphates, depressed contractile

Table 19–10

**Vasoactive and Growth Mediators in Heart Failure**

| Constrictors | Dilators | Growth or Apoptotic Factors |
|---|---|---|
| Norepinephrine | Natriuretic peptides | Insulin |
| Renin/angiotensin II | Atrial natriuretic peptide, BNP | Tumor necrosis factor-α, interleukin-1β |
| Vasopressin | Prostaglandin $E_2$ and metabolites | Growth hormone |
| Neuropeptide Y | Nitric oxide | Angiotensin II |
| Endothelin | Dopamine | Catecholamines |
| | Calcitonin gene-related peptide | Nitric oxide |
| | Adrenomedullin | Cytokines |
| | Vasoactive intestinal peptide | Oxygen radicals |
| | | Chemokines |
| | | Inflammatory cytokines |
| | | Immunomodulatory cytokines |

function, ultrastructural damage, apoptosis, and reduced transcription of contractile protein genes.

# ■ THE BODY RESPONSE IN HEART FAILURE

Neuroendocrine, vasoactive, and cytokine systems are activated in heart failure and contribute to disease development and progression. Vasoactive and growth mediators in heart failure are listed in Table 19–10.

## Sympathetic Activity in Heart Failure

Sympathetic overstimulation is an early feature of heart failure that precedes activation of the renin-angiotensin-aldosterone system. Plasma and urinary norepinephrine values are elevated (secondary to "spill-over" from sympathetic nerve terminals rather than to adrenal overactivity) to degrees that correlate directly with the clinical severity of heart failure and inversely with the patient's prognosis.[38] The trigger for sympathetic overactivity is not completely understood. It may come from the arterial baroreflex, ergoreceptors, or a cardiopulmonary reflex, all abnormal early in heart failure. The consequences of sympathetic overstimulation are listed in Table 19–11.

Table 19–11

**Consequences of Sympathetic Overactivity in Chronic Heart Failure**

| Cardiac | Renal | Peripheral Vessels |
|---|---|---|
| ↓ β-AR number and function | ↑ Tubular absorption of sodium | Vasoconstriction |
| Myocyte hypertrophy | Activation of renin-angiotensin-aldosterone system | Hypertrophy of smooth muscle cells |
| Myocyte necrosis, apoptosis | ↓ Response to natriuretic factors | |
| Myocardial fibrosis | ↑ Vascular resistance | |
| ↓ Norepinephrine stores | | |
| ↓ Sympathetic innervation | | |
| Arrhythmias | | |
| Impaired and incoordinate contraction | | |

Table 19–12

**Consequences of Renin-Angiotensin-Aldosterone Overactivation in Chronic Heart Failure**

| Cardiac | Peripheral |
|---|---|
| Positive inotrope in atrial muscle | Arterial constriction (afterload) |
| Diastolic dysfunction | Venous constriction (preload) |
| Arrhythmias | Regional blood flow redistribution |
| Subendocardial ischemia | Increased norepinephrine release |
| Myocyte necrosis | Glomerular efferent constriction |
| Hypertrophy | Vasopressin release |
| Remodeling | Aldosterone release |
| | Vascular hypertrophy |
| | Sodium retention |

## Renin-Angiotensin-Aldosterone System

Activation of the renin-angiotensin-aldosterone system is well-recognized in heart failure, where it has an important role in producing both the peripheral changes and progressive ventricular impairment. In heart failure, renin release is stimulated by reduced renal blood flow, enhanced sympathetic activity, and hyponatremia, and by diuretics, prostaglandins, and vasopressin. Increased renin activity leads to increased production of angiotensin II, which in the context of heart failure has many actions in addition to vasoconstriction (Table 19–12). In addition to the hormonal effects of circulating angiotensin II, components of the renin-angiotensin-aldosterone system are present in the heart, blood vessels, kidneys, brain, and adrenal glands, where angiotensin II may function as a paracrine or an autocrine hormone, independent of the circulating hormone.

## Increased Peripheral Resistance in Heart Failure

Increased systemic vascular resistance is a cardinal feature of heart failure. Initially, this was attributed simply to the effects of sympathetic activity and circulating angiotensin II; however, inhibition of α-AR and angiotensin II does not completely or rapidly induce vasodilatation.[39] Multiple factors are now known to contribute to the increased peripheral vascular resistance of chronic heart failure (Table 19–13).

Table 19–13

**Causes of Increased Peripheral Resistance in Chronic Heart Failure**

**Reduced skeletal muscle mass**
**Anatomic alterations**
  Thickened capillary basement membrane
  Vascular remodeling (smooth muscle hyperplasia and proliferation)
  Endothelial cell edema
  Microvascular infarction
**Vasoconstriction**
  Sodium-calcium exchange
  Neuroendocrine activation (norepinephrine, angiotensin II, vasopressin, endothelin, neuropeptide Y)
  Reduced response to nitric oxide (mediated by oxygen free radicals and other interactions)
**Failure of vasodilatation**
  Altered response to accumulated metabolites

Table 19–14

**Inflammatory Mediators Elevated in Heart Failure**

| | |
|---|---|
| Soluble CD14 receptor | Interleukin 8 |
| Tumor necrosis factor α | Interleukin 10 |
| Soluble tumor necrosis factor receptor 1 | Interferon γ |
| Soluble tumor necrosis factor receptor 2 | Intracellular adhesion molecule 1 |
| Interleukin 1β | Expression of a leukocyte-adhesion molecule 1 |
| Interleukin 6 | |

## Inflammatory Mediators in Chronic Heart Failure

Cytokine activation is a well-recognized feature of chronic heart failure (Table 19–14). A functional role for cytokine activation in heart failure is suggested by two findings. First, cytokine levels in peripheral blood correlate with the clinical severity of heart failure.[40] Many of the features of chronic heart failure may be produced by the known effects of these molecules: impaired myocardial contraction, myocyte apoptosis, oxygen free radical production, peripheral and pulmonary edema, reduced peripheral blood flow, and β-AR uncoupling. Among patients with heart failure, a syndrome of cachexia associated with metabolic and immune dysfunction and with poor prognosis is recognized.[41, 42]

## ■ ORIGIN OF SYMPTOMS IN HEART FAILURE

There is little relation between left ventricular function (as measured by ejection fraction) and exercise capacity in heart failure.[43] The symptoms and signs of heart failure are listed in Table 19–15. Symptoms correlate better with changes in circulatory, pulmonary, and skeletal muscle function (Table 19–16). Symptom severity in heart failure may be graded according to the New York Heart Association classification (Table 19–17). The muscle hypothesis suggests that many of the symptoms of heart failure, and the progression of the symptoms, are related to the activation of ergoreceptors in skeletal muscle. This activity is relayed in turn to the central nervous system.

Table 19–15

**Symptoms and Signs of Heart Failure**

**Symptoms**
Fatigue
Dyspnea (exertional, orthopnea, paroxysmal nocturnal dyspnea)
Swelling (lower limbs, abdomen)
**Signs**
Tachycardia >90 bpm
Systolic blood pressure <90 mm Hg
Jugular venous distention
Abnormal hepatojugular reflex
Abnormal apex beat (displaced, sustained, dyskinetic, or enlarged)
Third heart sound
Inspiratory crackles on lung auscultation
Edema (peripheral, ascites)

Table 19–16

### Origin of Symptoms in Chronic Heart Failure

**Circulation**
  ↓ Blood flow to skeletal muscle
  ↑ Production of metabolites in skeletal muscle
  Altered response to metabolites in skeletal muscle
**Lungs**
  ↑ Stiffness of lungs due to raised venous pressure and lymphatic distention
  ↑ Left atrial pressure
  ↑ Physiologic dead space
  ↑ Respiratory rate
  Diaphragmatic weakness
**Skeletal muscle**
  Rest atrophy
  Ischemic atrophy
  Ergoreceptor activation

## ■ AN INTEGRATED VIEW OF THE PATHOGENESIS OF HEART FAILURE

The initial changes in cardiac failure can be considered an adaptive response to reduced cardiac contractility that is probably perceived systemically as a drop in blood pressure.[44] In evolutionary terms, the initial response was designed to cope with blood loss or flight from a predator, short-lived stresses on cardiac performance. In heart failure, the low-output state or cardiac stress is chronic. This leads to persistence of the invoked compensatory mechanisms, which have harmful effects on the heart, circulation, and other organs. The ensuing clinical syndrome of heart failure is dominated by the systemic response. For example, inadequate cardiac output causes reduced renal blood flow, which leads directly to enhanced sodium and water retention and to activation of the sympathetic and renin-angiotensin systems. In consequence, release of aldosterone and vasopressin causes vasoconstriction and further water retention. These metabolic and vascular changes result in elevated venous pressure, increased capillary pressure, and, ultimately, peripheral edema, one of the cardinal signs of heart failure. The short-term and long-term effects of the compensatory mechanisms in heart failure are summarized in Table 19–18 and Figure 19–2. Progression of heart failure is then characterized by multiple interactions between the systemic and cardiac responses and changes in the heart muscle itself. These pathophysiologic interactions lead to spirals of declining cardiac function and progressive systemic disease (Fig. 19–3). A major difficulty in clinical cardiology is determining which mechanisms are predominant and at which moments in the natural course of heart failure. That knowledge is a

Table 19–17

### New York Heart Association Classification of Cardiac Function

**Class I**   No limitation. Ordinary physical activity does not cause undue fatigue, dyspnea, or palpitation.
**Class II**  Slight limitation of physical activity. Such patients are comfortable at rest. Ordinary physical activity results in fatigue, dyspnea, palpitation, or angina pectoris.
**Class III** Marked limitation of physical activity. Although patients are comfortable at rest, less than ordinary activity will lead to symptoms.
**Class IV**  Inability to carry on any level of physical activity without discomfort. Symptoms suggestive of congestive failure are present even at rest. With any physical activity, increased discomfort is experienced.

Table 19-18

## Short-Term and Long-Term Responses to Impaired Cardiac Performance

| Response | Short-Term Effects* | Long-Term Effects† |
|---|---|---|
| Salt and water retention | Augments preload | Causes pulmonary congestion, anasarca |
| Vasoconstriction | Maintains blood pressure for perfusion of vital organs (brain, heart) | Exacerbates pump dysfunction (afterload mismatch); increases cardiac energy expenditure |
| Sympathetic stimulation | Increases heart rate and ejection | Increases energy expenditure |
| Sympathetic desensitization | —— | Spares energy |
| Hypertrophy | Unloads individual muscle fibers | Leads to deterioration and death of cardiac cells; cardiomyopathy of overload |
| Capillary deficit | —— | Leads to energy starvation |
| Mitochondrial density | Increase in density helps meet energy demands | Decrease in density leads to energy starvation |
| Appearance of slow myosin | —— | Increases force, decreases shortening velocity and contractility; is energy-sparing |
| Prolonged action potential | —— | Increases contractility and energy expenditure |
| Decreased density of sarcoplasmic reticulum calcium-pump sites | —— | Slows relaxation; may be energy-sparing |
| Increased collagen | May reduce dilatation | Impairs relaxation |

*Short-term effects are mainly adaptive and occur after hemorrhage and in acute heart failure.
†Long-term effects are mainly deleterious and occur in chronic heart failure.
From Katz AM: Mechanisms of disease: Cardiomyopathy of overload a major determinant of prognosis in congestive heart failure. N Engl J Med 1990;322:100–110. Copyright © 1990 Massachusetts Medical Society. All rights reserved.

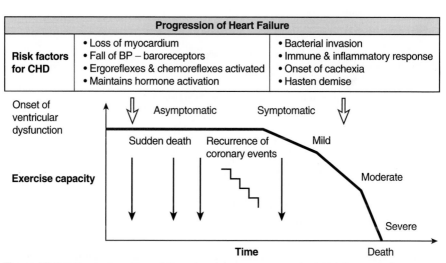

**Figure 19–2** ■ Progression of heart failure. A patient may progress, after initial damage to the myocardium, to ever worsening heart failure that results in death. Alternatively, life may be limited by a lethal arrhythmia (*closed arrows*). A further event, such as a coronary event or repeated exposure to a toxic substance, may lead to step changes in ventricular function (*stepped line*). There is often a prolonged period of asymptomatic ventricular dysfunction before the onset of cardiac failure. At this stage, cardiac and systemic compensatory mechanisms are sufficient to maintain the patient's functional status. Studies carried out at peak exercise may, however, reveal a reduced functional reserve. Initially, the progression of heart failure is determined by the neurohumoral response, but, in severe heart failure, the inflammatory response and the immune system are activated. CHD, coronary heart disease; BP, blood pressure.

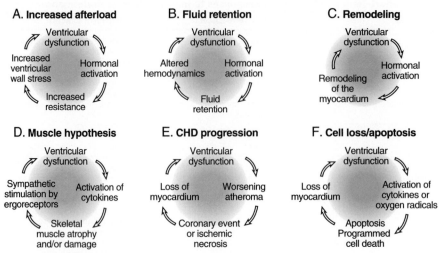

**Figure 19–3** ■ Spirals of heart failure. Many spirals with positive feedback have been described to explain the progression of heart failure. Each of these spirals represents one system in the body which may go awry and be the determining feature of progression at one moment in the natural history of any individual patient. CHD, coronary heart disease.

prerequisite for improved treatment based on selective and targeted application of current drugs.

# ■ REFERENCES

1. Poole-Wilson P: Heart failure. Med Int 1985;2:866–871.
2. The Task Force on Heart Failure of the European Society of Cardiology: Guidelines for the diagnosis of heart failure. Eur Heart J 1995;16:741–751.
3. McDonagh TA, Morrison CE, Lawrence A, et al: Symptomatic and asymptomatic left-ventricular systolic dysfunction in an urban population. Lancet 1997;350:829–833.
4. Watkins H, Seidman JG, Seidman CE: Familial hypertrophic cardiomyopathy: A genetic model of cardiac hypertrophy. Hum Mol Genet 1995;4:1721–1727.
5. Bonne G, Carrier L, Richard P, et al: Familial hypertrophic cardiomyopathy: From mutations to functional defects. Circ Res 1998;83:580–593.
6. Gheorghiade M, Bonow R: Chronic heart failure in the United States. A manifestation of coronary artery disease. Circulation 1998;97:282–289.
7. Mitchell G, Lamas G, Vaughan D, Pfeffer M: Left-ventricular remodeling in the year after 1st anterior myocardial infarction—A quantitative analysis of contractile segment lengths and ventricular shape. J Am Coll Cardiol 1992;19:1136–1144.
8. Olivetti G, Abbi R, Quaini F, et al: Apoptosis in the failing human heart. N Engl J Med 1997;336:1131–1141.
9. Narula J, Haider N, Virmani R, et al: Apoptosis in myocytes in end-stage heart failure. N Engl J Med 1996;335:1182–1189.
10. Peters NS, Green CR, Poole-Wilson PA, Severs NJ: Reduced content of connexin 43 gap junctions in ventricular myocardium from hypertrophied and ischemic human hearts. Circulation 1993;88:864–875.
11. Severs N: Gap junction alterations in the failing heart. Eur Heart J 1994;15 (Suppl D):D53–57.
12. Thomas CV, Coker ML, Zellner JL, et al: Increased matrix metalloproteinase activity and selective upregulation in LV myocardium from patients with end-stage dilated cardiomyopathy. Circulation 1998;97:1708–1715.
13. Bristow MR, Ginsburg R, Umans V, et al: Beta 1- and beta 2-adrenergic-receptor subpopulations in nonfailing and failing human ventricular myocardium: Coupling of both receptor subtypes to muscle contraction and selective beta 1-receptor down-regulation in heart failure. Circ Res 1986;59:297–309.
14. Hausdorff WP, Caron MG, Lefkowitz RJ: Turning off the signal: Desensitization of beta-adrenergic receptor function [erratum published in FASEB J 1990;4(12):3049]. FASEB J 1990;4:2881–2889.

15. Feldman AM, Cates AE, Veazey WB, et al: Increase of the 40,000-mol wt pertussis toxin substrate (G protein) in the failing human heart. J Clin Invest 1988;82:189–197.
16. Feldman MD, Copelas L, Gwathmey JK, et al: Deficient production of cyclic AMP: Pharmacologic evidence of an important cause of contractile dysfunction in patients with end-stage heart failure. Circulation 1987;75:331–339.
17. Schwinger RH, Bohm M, Schmidt U, et al: Unchanged protein levels of SERCA II and phospholamban but reduced $Ca^{2+}$ uptake and $Ca^{2+}$-ATPase activity of cardiac sarcoplasmic reticulum from dilated cardiomyopathy patients compared with patients with nonfailing hearts. Circulation 1995;92:3220–3228.
18. Nimer LR, Needleman DH, Hamilton SL, et al: Effect of ryanodine on sarcoplasmic reticulum $Ca^{2+}$ accumulation in nonfailing and failing human myocardium. Circulation 1995;92:2504–2510.
19. Flesch M, Schwinger RH, Schiffer F, et al: Evidence for functional relevance of an enhanced expression of the $Na^+$-$Ca^{2+}$ exchanger in failing human myocardium. Circulation 1996;94:992–1002.
20. Meyer M, Schillinger W, Pieske B, et al: Alterations of sarcoplasmic reticulum proteins in failing human dilated cardiomyopathy. Circulation 1995;92:778–784.
21. Ingwall JS, Kramer MF, Fifer MA, et al: The creatine kinase system in normal and diseased human myocardium. N Engl J Med 1985;313:1050–1054.
22. Neubauer S, Horn M, Pabst T, et al: Contributions of 31P-magnetic resonance spectroscopy to the understanding of dilated heart muscle disease. Eur Heart J 1995;16 (Suppl O):115–118.
23. Lowes B, Minobe W, Abraham W, et al: Changes in gene expression in the intact human heart. J Clin Invest 1997;100:2315–2324.
24. Nakao H, Minobe W, Roden R, et al: Myosin heavy chain expression in human heart failure. J Clin Invest 1997;100:2362–2370.
25. Price K, Littler W, Cummins P: Human atrial and ventricular myosin light-chain subunits in the adult and during development. Biochem J 1980;191:571–580.
26. Schaub MC, Hefti MA, Zuellig RA, Morano I: Modulation of contractility in human cardiac hypertrophy by myosin essential light chain isoforms. Cardiovasc Res 1998;37:381–404.
27. Bodor GS, Oakeley AE, Allen PD, et al: Troponin I phosphorylation in the normal and failing adult human heart. Circulation 1997;96:1495–1500.
28. Zakhary DR, Moravec CS, Stewart RW, Bond M: Protein kinase A (PKA)-dependent troponin-I phosphorylation and PKA regulatory subunits are decreased in human dilated cardiomyopathy. Circulation 1999;99:505–510.
29. Margossian S, Caulfield J, Slayter H: Activation of a protease during idiopathic dilated cardiomyopathy. J Mol Cell Cardiol 1994;26:S50.
30. Anderson PAW, Malouf NN, Oakeley AE, et al: Troponin T isoform expression in humans. A comparison among normal and failing heart, fetal heart and adult and fetal skeletal muscle. Circ Res 1991;69:1226–1233.
31. Saba Z, Nassar R, Ungerleider R, et al: Cardiac troponin T isoform expression correlates with pathophysiological descriptors in patients who underwent corrective surgery for congenital heart disease. Circulation 1996;94:472–476.
32. Solaro J, Powers F, Gao L, Gwathmey J: Control of myofilament activation in heart failure. Circulation 1993;87(Suppl VII):VII-38–VII-43.
33. Mesnard-Rouiller L, Mercadier J-J, Butler-Brown G, et al: Troponin T mRNA and protein isoforms in the human left ventricle: Pattern of expression in failing and control hearts. J Mol Cell Cardiol 1997;29:3043–3055.
34. Mallat Z, Philip I, Lebret M, et al: Elevated levels of 8-iso-prostaglandin $F_{2alpha}$ in pericardial fluid of patients with heart failure: A potential role for in vivo oxidant stress in ventricular dilatation and progression to heart failure. Circulation 1998;97:1536–1539.
35. Reilly MP, Delanty N, Roy L, et al: Increased formation of the isoprostanes $IPF_{2alpha}$-1 and 8-epi-prostaglandin $F_{2alpha}$ in acute coronary angioplasty: Evidence for oxidant stress during coronary reperfusion in humans. Circulation 1997;96:3314–3320.
36. Delanty N, Reilly MP, Pratico D, et al: 8-epi $PGF_{2alpha}$ generation during coronary reperfusion. A potential quantitative marker of oxidant stress in vivo. Circulation 1997;95:2492–2499.
37. Davi G, Ciabattoni G, Consoli A, et al: In vivo formation of 8-iso-prostaglandin $F_{2alpha}$ and platelet activation in diabetes mellitus: Effects of improved metabolic control and vitamin E supplementation. Circulation 1999;99:224–229.
38. Cohn JN, Levine TB, Olivari MT, et al: Plasma norepinephrine as a guide to prognosis in patients with chronic congestive heart failure. N Engl J Med 1984;311:819–823.
39. Drexler H, Banhardt U, Meinertz T, et al: Contrasting peripheral short-term and long-term effects of converting enzyme inhibition in patients with congestive heart failure. A double-blind, placebo-controlled trial. Circulation 1989;79:491–502.
40. Torre-Amione G, Kapadia S, Benedict C, et al: Proinflammatory cytokine levels in patients with depressed left ventricular ejection fraction: A report from the Studies of Left Ventricular Dysfunction (SOLVD). J Am Coll Cardiol 1996;27:1201–1206.
41. Anker SD, Ponikowski P, Varney S, et al: Wasting as independent risk factor for mortality in chronic heart failure. Lancet 1997;349:1050–1053.
42. Anker SD, Chua TP, Ponikowski P, et al: Hormonal changes and catabolic/anabolic imbalance in chronic heart failure and their importance for cardiac cachexia. Circulation 1997;96:526–534.

43. Franciosa JA, Park M, Levine TB: Lack of correlation between exercise capacity and indexes of resting left ventricular performance in heart failure. Am J Cardiol 1981;47:33–39.
44. Harris P: Congestive heart failure: Central role of the arterial blood pressure. Br Heart J 1987;58:190–203.
45. Lewis T: Diseases of the Heart. London: Macmillan, 1933.
46. Wood P: Diseases of the Heart and Circulation. London: Eyre and Spottiswoode, 1950.
47. Braunwald E: Clinical manifestations of heart failure. *In* Braunwald E (ed): Heart Disease: A Textbook of Cardiovascular Medicine. Philadelphia: WB Saunders, 1988:471–484.
48. Poole-Wilson P: Chronic heart failure: Definition, epidemiology, pathophysiology, clinical manifestations and investigations. *In* Julian D, Camm A, Fox K, et al (eds): Diseases of the Heart. London: WB Saunders, 1996:467–482.
49. Cohn J: Is neurohormonal activation deleterious to the long term outcome of patients with congestive heart failure? J Am Coll Cardiol 1988;12:547–548.
50. Denolin H, Kuhn H, Krayenbuehl H, et al: The definition of heart failure. Eur Heart J 1983;4:445–448.
51. Lenfant C: Report of the task force on research in heart failure. Circulation 1994;90:1118–1123.

# ▪ RECOMMENDED READING

Clark A, Poole-Wilson P, Coats A: Exercise limitation in chronic cardiac failure: Central role of the periphery. J Am Coll Cardiol 1996;28:1092–1102.
Harris P: Evolution and the cardiac patient. Cardiovasc Res 1983;17:313–319, 373–378, 437–445.
Mittmann C, Eschenhagen T, Scholz H: Cellular and molecular aspects of contractile dysfunction in heart failure. Cardiovasc Res 1998;39:267–275.
Niebauer J, Volk HD, Kemp M, et al: Endotoxin and immune activation in chronic heart failure: A prospective cohort study. Lancet 1999;353:1838–1842.
Solaro RJ, Rarick HM: Troponin and tropomyosin: Proteins that switch on and tune in the activity of cardiac myofilaments. Circ Res 1998;83:471–480.
Weber K: Extracellular matrix remodeling in heart failure. Circulation 1997;96:4065–4082.

# Chapter 20

# Treatment of Congestive Heart Failure

*Stephen S. Gottlieb*

The goals of heart failure treatment include both symptomatic improvement and prolongation of life. These goals are not necessarily concordant. Related to this problem is the fact that the immediate results of an intervention may be very different from the long-term effects. Those who treat heart failure, therefore, must understand the immediate and long-term desires of each particular patient and the immediate and long-term consequences of the therapy. The result is an uncomfortable one: use of acute treatments known to have adverse consequences over the long-term and long-term treatments that are counterintuitive. Fortunately, however, congestive heart failure has been thoroughly investigated in multiple large studies that demonstrate the several consequences of many of our standard interventions.

## ■ INITIAL WORKUP

The terms *systolic dysfunction* and *congestive heart failure* are often (and inappropriately) used interchangeably. Half of all patients with heart failure do not have systolic dysfunction. Since treatment of systolic dysfunction is different from the treatment of other causes of heart failure, assessment of left ventricular function is essential when a patient presents with heart failure. If systolic dysfunction is the cause of the heart failure, proper treatment can be based on the results of well-controlled studies. (Most investigators of heart failure limit themselves to this particular group of patients.) For heart failure without systolic dysfunction, however, few studies provide guidance. The rest of this chapter refers to systolic dysfunction unless stated otherwise.

## Determining Whether Dyspnea Is the Result of Congestive Heart Failure

The initial diagnostic dilemma in many patients with dyspnea is whether the symptoms have a cardiac or a pulmonary cause. If pulmonary function tests are abnormal and there is left ventricular dysfunction, it may be difficult to determine the cause of the symptoms. Physical findings such as wheezing can be nonspecific. Certainly, rales, orthopnea, and paroxysmal nocturnal dyspnea suggest a cardiac cause, and chronic hypoxia suggests a pulmonary cause, but fluid overload can be secondary to right-sided or left-sided failure. Even experienced clinicians are often fooled. If there is any question about the cause of the symptoms, pulmonary artery catheterization should be considered.

Similarly, it may be difficult to determine whether dyspnea in a patient with heart failure is secondary to deconditioning or to continued volume overload and poor cardiac function. Proper treatment may depend on the results of right heart catheterization. Many clinicians feel that such intervention is necessary only for severe symptoms, but findings are more likely to affect treatment when the cause of the symptoms is in question.

## Reversible Causes of Systolic Dysfunction

In addition to assessment of cardiac function, initial evaluation includes ruling our reversible causes of systolic dysfunction. Ischemic heart disease must always be considered, and the perceived risk of atherosclerosis should determine which tests, if any, are needed to rule out coronary artery disease. Although many cardiologists perform cardiac catheterization on every patient with heart failure, a young patient without risk factors or clinical evidence of ischemia can probably be assessed by an exercise tolerance test. This is especially true if another cause, such as ethanol abuse, can be identified. Similarly, a patient without ischemic symptoms who is not a surgical candidate need not undergo catheterization. It should be noted, though, that assessment of myocardial viability and exercise-induced ischemia may be useful even in some patients with very poor contractility at rest.

Echocardiography is helpful for identifying some causes of heart failure, such as valvular disease. The importance of mitral regurgitation, however, may be difficult to evaluate. Mitral regurgitation is common in patients with dilated ventricles, and it may be impossible to determine whether the valvular disease is primary or secondary. In the setting of poor contractility, however, surgical correction of either primary or secondary mitral regurgitation carries great risk. While increasing numbers of surgeons are willing to undertake mitral valve repair or replacement, the proper role of mitral valve surgery in patients with poor systolic function remains uncertain.

The possibility that nonischemic cardiomyopathy is caused by thyroid abnormalities, hemochromatosis, or complications of human immunodeficiency virus (HIV) infection can usually be eliminated simply by blood tests. Treatment of these disorders is straightforward, but resultant cardiomyopathies may persist despite treatment of the underlying problem. Nutritional abnormalities and ethanol abuse should also be considered as potential causes of reversible cardiomyopathy.

## Myocardial Biopsy

The detection of myocarditis rarely affects treatment. Since there are no randomized controlled studies that support the use of immunosuppressive therapy and immunosuppression entails considerable risk, immunosuppressive therapy is not prescribed by most clinicians. Thus, a diagnosis of myocarditis usually does not affect treatment, although that diagnosis might have prognostic implications because it suggests the potential for rapid changes (positive or negative) in the patient's condition. If the expected prognosis will affect the clinical management, myocardial biopsy might be indicated.

When the clinician suspects reversible disease that can be diagnosed by myocardial biopsy (such as sarcoidosis, hemochromatosis, or amyloidosis) and treatment would be affected by the findings, biopsy is indicated. Biopsy may also identify giant cell myocarditis, a rare entity generally believed to carry a poor prognosis. Since immunosuppression may be considered for these patients, biopsy could be appropriate in a patient who has symptoms of recent onset, a rapid downhill course, and no obvious cause of heart failure.

## Follow-up Assessments of Cardiac Function

Once the cause of heart failure has been determined, further assessments are needed only when there are questions about the patient's status. Thus, repeat echocardiograms or gated blood pool scans are rarely needed when a patient has known systolic dysfunction and persistent symptoms. A slight increase or decrease in ejection fraction adds little to a physician's clinical judgment and should not be the basis for a change in therapy. Occasionally, repeat assessment is necessary to rule out the possibility of normalization of cardiac function (at which point treatment might be cautiously withdrawn) or marked deterioration in function.

# ■ DIURETICS

Diuretic medications (Table 20–1), the primary treatment for early symptomatic relief of congestive heart failure, produce rapid and dramatic improvements in patients with exacerbations or newly diagnosed disease. In addition, they are needed for long-term relief of symptoms. Potential long-term adverse consequences, however, mandate that they not be the only treatment for patients with systolic dysfunction.

## Fluid Restriction

The best means of keeping patients euvolemic would be to avoid the causes of fluid and sodium retention. Reducing sodium intake can decrease the need for high doses of diuretics and should be encouraged for all patients, but fluid restriction is rarely beneficial. Although the hyponatremia and fluid overload associated with congestive heart failure make fluid restriction appealing, such an approach is rarely successful. First, the drive to drink water is strong, and it is virtually impossible to successfully restrict a patient's fluid intake. Second, diuresis can be successful without fluid restriction. Third, chronic hyponatremia rarely causes problems, and excessive hyponatremia can be successfully treated by modifying the diuretic regimen. In patients with congestive heart failure, only the combination of diuresis and angiotensin-converting enzyme (ACE) inhibition has been demonstrated to reverse hyponatremia.

## Extent of Diuresis

The most common clinical problem related to diuretics is underutilization of the drugs. Hospitalized patients who are treated for pulmonary edema are often discharged with marked fluid overload and prescribed doses of diuretics that are inadequate to continue diuresis. Such patients frequently return to the hospital because of repeated exacerbations. The absence of rales should not be taken as evidence of adequate diuresis. Assessment of total body fluid (as evidenced by peripheral edema, ascites, and sacral edema) is easy and can determine whether more diuresis is indicated. Controversy still surrounds whether treatment should be guided by pulmonary artery catheter determination of optimal pulmonary capillary wedge pressure, but it is nevertheless clear that adequate diuresis is essential and can be guided by clinical endpoints.

Another common obstacle to proper utilization of diuretic medications is fear of large doses. Patients with severe heart failure and evidence of renal dysfunction often need doses that clinicians perceive to be extremely high; daily dosing with 200 mg of furosemide is not uncommon. Despite the frequent need for diuretics in high concentrations, furosemide need not necessarily be given by the intravenous route to induce clinically important diuresis. Oral dosing may produce the desired result, even in markedly fluid-overloaded persons. This is important because successful outpatient diuresis can save money, prevent iatrogenic complications, and

Table 20–1

## Comparison of Diuretic Medications, Listed According to Site of Action

| Diuretic | FENa+ (Max) (%) | Dosage (mg/day) | Onset of Action | | Duration of Action | | Peak Oral Effect (hr) | Comments |
|---|---|---|---|---|---|---|---|---|
| | | | Oral (hr) | IV (min) | Oral (hr) | IV (hr) | | |
| **Ascending Loop of Henle** | | | | | | | | |
| Furosemide | 20–25 | 40–400 | 1 | 5 | 6 | 2–3 | 1–3 | |
| Bumetanide | 20–25 | 1–5 | 0.5 | 5 | 6 | 2–3 | 1–3 | |
| Torsemide | 20–25 | 10–200 | 1 | 10 | 6–8 | 6–8 | 1–3 | |
| Ethacrynic acid | 20–25 | 50–100 | 0.5 | 5 | 6–8 | 3 | 2 | High ototoxicity risk, but (unlike other loop diuretics) can be used in sulfa-allergic patient |
| **Early Distal Tubule** | | | | | | | | |
| Metolazone | 5–8 | 2.5–20 | 1 | — | 12–24 | — | 2–4 | Greatest potential for potassium loss; also slight actions in proximal tubule |
| Chlorthalidone | 5–10 | 25–200 | 2 | — | 24–48 | — | 6 | Ineffective when GFR <30 |
| Hydrochlorothiazide | 5–8 | 25–100 | 2 | — | 12 | — | 4 | Ineffective when GFR <30 |
| Chlorothiazide | 5–8 | 500–1000 | 1 | 15–30 | 8 | — | 4 | Ineffective when GFR <30 |
| **Late Distal Tubule** | | | | | | | | |
| Spironolactone | 2 | 25–100 | 48–72 | — | 48–72 | — | 1–2 days | Efficacy depends on aldosterone presence in patient |
| Triamterene | 2 | 75–300 | 2 | — | 12–16 | — | 6–8 | |
| Amiloride | 2 | 5–10 | 2 | — | 24 | — | 6–16 | |
| **Proximal Tubule** | | | | | | | | |
| Acetazolamide | 4 | 250–375 | 1 | 30–60 | 8 | 3–4 | 2–4 | Efficacy limited by metabolic acidosis (side effect) |

IV, intravenous; FENa+ (Max, %), maximal natriuretic effect (maximum fractional excretion of filtered sodium).
Adapted from Gottlieb SS: Diuretics. In Hosenpud JD, Greenberg B (eds): Congestive Heart Failure: Pathophysiology, Differential Diagnosis, and Comprehensive Approach to Management. New York: Springer-Verlag, 1993.

improve a patient's quality of life. Outpatient diuresis, however, demands close follow-up to ensure success and prevent deadly electrolyte abnormalities. Although the data suggest that most edematous patients should be given a trial of oral diuretics, for some intravenous dosing is necessary. When immediate diuresis is necessary because of severe decompensation and pulmonary edema, the more rapid onset of intravenous diuretics may be essential.

## Diuretic Combinations

It is often difficult to produce effective diuresis in patients with severe heart failure. The physiologic stimulus to retain fluid may be strong enough to overwhelm the diuretic actions of any single agent. Thus, potent diuretics (e.g., loop diuretics) may be rendered ineffective by distal reabsorption. In contrast, agents that act distally, such as the potassium-sparing drugs, may not be potent enough to produce the desired results. In such cases, synergistic effects by combining diuretics can have many beneficial consequences.

The combination of loop diuretics and metolazone has proven to be particularly potent.[1] With this combination, effective diuresis may be produced when other interventions have failed. It may take days to see the results of the addition of metolazone, however, because of the pharmacokinetics of the drug. It is also important to realize that the hypokalemia that results from combined use of loop diuretics and metolazone may be profound; these patients' serum potassium concentrations need to be watched especially carefully. The other useful method of combining diuretics is to add a potassium-sparing agent to the regimen. Not only does this potentiate the diuretic actions of the original regimen, but it also prevents extreme potassium loss and simplifies electrolyte management.

Spironolactone is not a potent diuretic, but a recent study (RALES) shows a better survival rate for patients who received relatively small doses.[2] Spironolactone conserves potassium and magnesium and can be synergistic when combined with other diuretic medications. However, other effects may be even more important. For example, spironolactone may affect fibrosis formation in hearts of patients with cardiomyopathy and may exert direct effects on the sodium-potassium pump. Further investigation is needed.

## Disease Refractory to Diuretics

Some patients require inotropic therapy to produce acute diuresis. Agents such as dobutamine and milrinone often lead to diuresis in patients with worsening renal function secondary to cardiac dysfunction. Anecdotes continue to support the use of low-dose dopamine in patients whose renal function is limited by severe heart failure. Although few studies document increased renal perfusion and increased urine output with low doses of dopamine (2 to 3 $\mu$g/kg/min),[3, 4] its use is commonplace—and not unreasonable.

When all else fails, ultrafiltration may improve fluid status. In some patients, the result is long lasting, and treatment need not be continued once euvolemia is restored. Perhaps the many effects of diuresis on cardiac performance and neurohormones explain the reports of long-term benefits of this intervention.[5]

Since improving volume status is so important for treating the symptoms of congestive heart failure, chronic dialysis can be considered for volume control, not only for renal failure. Some euvolemic patients develop renal failure; their renal function is maintained only with fluid overload. Since dialysis can markedly improve the quality of life for such patients, its use is appropriate if the patient agrees to it.

## Adverse Effects

There is no doubt that diuretics, though essential for symptomatic relief and to decrease cardiac distension, have adverse consequences; electrolyte depletion, neurohormonal activation, and renal failure can ensue. While potentially harmful, these side effects can be overcome with other interventions. For example, ACE inhibitors and spironolactone can prevent potassium and magnesium depletion. In the rare instances when it is necessary, potassium replacement can also be given.

Diuretics lead to activation of the renin-angiotensin, sympathetic, and other neurohormonal systems, processes that have the potential for immediate and long-term repercussions (see later). These problems should not prevent adequate use of diuretic medications, however; they can generally be blocked with ACE inhibitors, beta-blockers, or aldosterone antagonists.

The physician must always be alert when combining agents with opposing actions. Treatment of congestive heart failure usually includes both potassium-wasting and potassium-sparing agents. The results may be unpredictable, and patients must be followed carefully to ensure that neither hypokalemia nor hyper-kalemia develops.

Slight increases in serum creatinine and blood urea nitrogen (BUN) concentrations should be expected (and tolerated) to achieve adequate diuresis. Diuretic-induced increases in serum creatinine concentrations can be worrisome, but they can usually be resolved by slowing the rate of diuresis. It may also be advisable to limit the use of angiotensin-converting enzyme inhibitors while aggressively diuresing a patient. The patients who develop renal failure with ACE inhibition are usually depleted of intravascular sodium and volume.[6] Giving ACE inhibitors after the patient is euvolemic may prevent the renal failure that occasionally occurs when patients are prescribed ACE inhibitors during active diuresis.

## ▪ ANGIOTENSIN-CONVERTING ENZYME INHIBITORS
(Table 20–2)

The long-term effects of ACE inhibitors on both symptoms and mortality are clear. Not only has their survival benefit been consistently demonstrated in patients with systolic dysfunction,[7, 8] but ACE inhibitors increase exercise tolerance, decrease hospitalization rates, and improve other indices reflective of symptoms. This information has been widely disseminated, and therapeutic ACE inhibition is now appropriately widespread. Concerns persist, however: are these agents being used to their greatest benefit?

Table 20–2

**Therapeutic Doses of Angiotensin-Converting Enzyme Inhibitors**

| Drug | Dosage |
|------|--------|
| Captopril | 25–50 mg t.i.d. |
| Enalapril | 10–20 mg b.i.d. |
| Lisinopril | 20–40 mg q.d. |
| Monopril | 20–40 mg q.d. |
| Ramipril | 5–10 mg b.i.d. |
| Quinapril | 20 mg b.i.d. |

These recommendations for final doses are based on doses used in heart failure studies.

## Dosing

The commonly used doses of ACE inhibitors are lower than those studied that demonstrated benefit. Patients in SOLVD reached mean daily enalapril doses of 16.6 mg, and the severely ill CONSENSUS patients received average doses of 18.4 mg. Nevertheless, enalapril and lisinopril (both have equivalent daily dosing) are frequently prescribed in doses of 2.5 or 5 mg per day.

The ATLAS (Assessment of Treatment with Lisinopril and Survival) trial enrolled 3164 heart failure patients to address the issue of dosing. Patients were randomized to receive either 2.5 to 5 or 32.5 to 35 mg of lisinopril daily. The patients who received the higher doses had better outcomes. Although the decreased mortality of 8% was not significant, the combination of mortality and frequency of hospitalization was significantly improved—by 12% in patients who received the higher doses.

The doses with demonstrated efficacy are also doses that were tolerated in multiple studies of patients who ranged from being severely ill to relatively asymptomatic. It is therefore important to explore the reasons physicians frequently are reluctant to prescribe these doses. Understanding the effects of ACE inhibition and the ways to prevent adverse consequences should lead to more effective use of these agents.

## Adverse Effects

Patients with heart failure often have low blood pressures, but the evidence seems clear that asymptomatic hypotension should not limit use of these agents. Indeed, ACE inhibitors often do not decrease the blood pressure of patients with heart failure; indeed, they may even increase it. It should be remembered, however, that blood pressure drops when ACE inhibition is combined with intravascular depletion. Thus, patients who do not tolerate these agents when they are being actively diuresed may tolerate them after their condition has stabilized. A slight liberalization of fluid status might also help patients with symptomatic hypotension who are taking ACE inhibitors.

The other factor that often limits dosing of ACE inhibition is renal dysfunction. Contrary to many physicians' assumptions, preexisting kidney disease does not increase the risk of renal deterioration (Fig. 20–1).[9] ACE inhibitors may cause renal

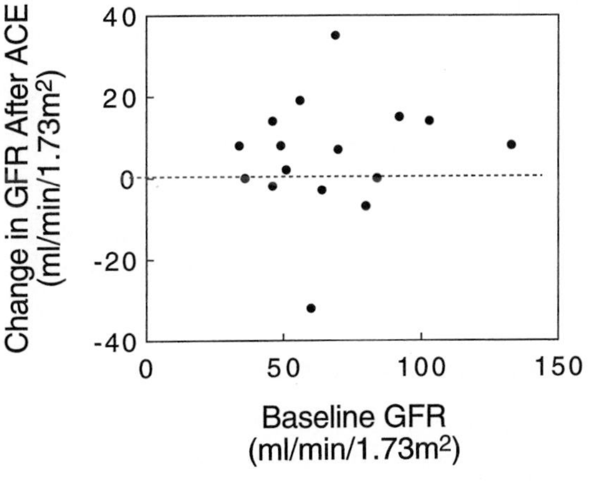

**Figure 20–1** ■ The baseline glomerular filtration rate (GFR) as it relates to the percentage change in GFR after ACE inhibition. There was no relation between baseline renal function and the change in GFR. (Gottlieb SS, Robinson S, Wier MR, et al: Determinants of the renal response to ACE inhibition in patients with congestive heart failure. Am Heart J 1992;124:131–136.)

dysfunction in a small percentage of persons with any baseline kidney function (especially those with renal artery stenosis), and this complication should be carefully sought during initiation of ACE inhibition. However, deterioration of serum creatinine status is usually the result of intravascular depletion, and a change in fluid status usually permits initiation and upward titration of these agents in patients who at first appear intolerant. Effective ACE inhibition can be achieved in the overwhelming majority of patients.

Hyperkalemia may accompany ACE inhibition. Often, this is because of continued potassium supplementation, either by prescription or by ingestion of potassium through salt substitutes or foods rich in potassium. Before the drug is blamed and discontinued, therefore, a careful dietary history must be taken.

Angioedema, neutropenia, and other clear contraindications to ACE inhibitors are infrequent. Other side effects, such as cough and rash, are often ascribed to these agents, even though it may be difficult to distinguish a side effect from a concomitant condition. Furthermore, these conditions are often tolerated well and are not necessarily cause for discontinuation of medications known to be effective. Nevertheless, at times these side effects are severe enough to warrant discontinuation of an ACE inhibitor. At that time, other agents can be tried.

## ■ OTHER VASODILATORS

### Angiotensin II Blockers

Angiotensin II receptor blockers are approved for hypertension, and their effects on the renin-angiotensin axis suggest that they might exert beneficial effects in patients with heart failure. At present, however, they have not been sufficiently evaluated in these patients to allow clear determination of their efficacy. In contrast to ACE inhibitors, which increase bradykinin concentrations in addition to preventing angiotensin II production, the angiotensin II receptor blockers work on only a single system. Bradykinin presumably causes some of the adverse side effects attributed to ACE inhibitors such as cough, but they may also provide some of the benefits. Since the importance of the bradykinin effects of ACE inhibitors is unknown, angiotensin II blockers should not be considered their therapeutic equivalent in patients with congestive heart failure.

The data comparing ACE inhibitors and angiotensin II blockers are contradictory. The Evaluation of Losartan in the Elderly (ELITE) trial was designed to compare the renal effects of the angiotensin II blocker losartan and captopril in older persons.[10] Although the primary endpoint was negative, a beneficial effect on mortality was seen. However, this was a small study, not powered to look at mortality, and the relevance and statistical validity of the finding are unclear. Indeed, a similar-sized study of another angiotensin II blocker showed a possible increase in mortality.[11] The results of ELITE II were recently reported. Patients who received captopril had a statistically insignificant improved survival as compared to patients who received losartan. Multiple studies are now looking at the impact of angiotensin II blockers, both in addition to and instead of ACE inhibitors. At present, however, angiotensin II receptor blockers must be considered second-line treatment of heart failure, to be used only when ACE inhibitors are truly contraindicated.

### Hydralazine and Nitrates

The other treatment for ACE-intolerant patients is the combination of hydralazine and nitrates. This combination appeared to improve survival in the Vasodilator–Heart Failure Trial (V-HeFT).[12] Although clearly not as good as ACE inhibitors,[13] these drugs may also improve symptoms and exercise tolerance. Daily doses up to 300 mg have been prescribed, but nausea often limits how much a patient will tolerate. Long-term side effects, such as a lupus syndrome, are much less frequent. Unfortunately, hydralazine has a short half-life and must be given three or four times daily to be effective. For this reason, its utility has been limited.

In patients with severe disease, however, hydralazine may be effective when given in addition to ACE inhibitors. This has not been widely investigated, but the decreased afterload induced by hydralazine may be particularly beneficial in patients with mitral regurgitation. Furthermore, patients with advanced disease may be more willing to take this medicine as frequently as necessary.

Nitrates can also be effective for symptomatic relief. Such medications should always be prescribed with an appreciation of the tolerance that patients can develop. Thus, patients should receive nitrates to prevent the most important symptoms. For some, a single dose of isosorbide dinitrate (10 to 40 mg) before sleep may prevent orthopnea and paroxysmal nocturnal dyspnea. Others benefit from longer-acting preparations taken before activities during the day. Sublingual nitroglycerin can also be helpful before unaccustomed exertion. When tailored to the individual patient, nitrates can improve the quality of life.

## Calcium Channel Blockers

Most calcium channel blockers have negative inotropic properties and have been shown to have adverse consequences when given to patients with congestive heart failure. These drugs are appealing because of their benefit in treating anginal symptoms, a condition common in patients with heart failure. However, studies after myocardial infarction consistently show that patients with poor ventricular function have worse survival rates when given calcium channel blockers. Similarly, studies in patients with heart failure suggest that the older calcium channel–blocking agents, such as nifedipine, diltiazem, and verapamil, produce a worse outcome.

Other calcium channel–blocking agents have been advocated for use in the treatment of heart failure. For example, amlodipine and felodipine have been evaluated in patients with heart failure; however, the results are equivocal. One study of amlodipine found no overall benefit when it was given to heart failure patients but improved survival in patients with nonischemic cardiomyopathy.[14] In contrast, a study of felodipine found no benefit in any group of patients.

Routine use of any calcium channel blocker is not indicated at present. It is possible, however, that these agents can be used without adverse consequences to treat other conditions, such as hypertension. Ongoing studies should elucidate proper use of these drugs in patients with heart failure.

## ■ BETA BLOCKERS

Recent studies conclusively support the concept that chronic beta blockade can improve cardiac function, decrease symptoms, and prolong survival for at least some patients with heart failure. Despite meta-analyses suggesting symptomatic and mortality benefits from long-term use of beta blockers, the "paradox" of giving a negative inotrope to patients with heart failure made physicians understandably reluctant to use them. In light of recent large-scale randomized studies demonstrating benefit on hospitalization rates and mortality[15–17] (Fig. 20–2), prescription of beta blockade for heart failure is rapidly increasing. These drugs are difficult to use, however, and there are many misconceptions about their actions and their

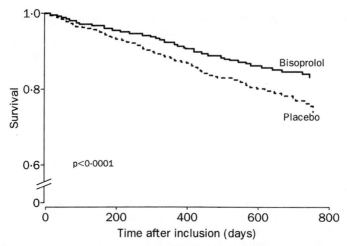

**Figure 20–2** ■ Mortality rates for patients randomized to placebo and bisoprolol in the CIBIS-II study. Patients randomized to bisoprolol had a 34% improvement in survival. (CIBIS II Investigators and Committees: The Cardiac Insufficiency Bisoprolol Study II [CIBIS II]: A randomized trial. Lancet 1999;353:9–13.)

proper use in patients with heart failure. There is no doubt that, used incorrectly, they can lead to exacerbations of heart failure and death. Used properly, they can produce long-lasting benefits.

## Method of Administration

Beta blockers should be given only to patients who are euvolemic, optimally treated with other medications, and stable. Proper institution of these agents is by slow titration (Table 20–3). Starting doses are minuscule but the evidence suggests that the final dose should be higher.[18] Indeed, in the MERIT trial, final daily doses were 200 mg of metoprolol XL, although treatment was initiated with either 12.5 or 25 mg and the dose was doubled weekly or biweekly. Similarly, the carvedilol and bisoprolol studies started treatment with extremely low doses and slowly titrated to effective beta-blocking doses.

Titration of beta-blocking agents should be performed cautiously and carefully. With each increase in dose, patients must be evaluated to ensure safety. For approximately the first month, the goal is not a positive effect; rather, the physician is acting to prevent deterioration. Fluid retention may occur, and increased diuretic doses may be needed temporarily. If there is clinical deterioration and evidence of worsening cardiac function, the usual weekly or biweekly titration should be extended. Bradycardia or heart block may limit dosing in some patients and pacemaker placement may be considered.

If the patient's condition deteriorates with institution of beta blockade, the dose may have to be decreased. Occasional patients even require temporary inotropic support. Slower titration can be considered when the initial effect is adverse. These caveats refer to all beta blockers used for heart failure, including carvedilol, metoprolol, and bisoprolol.

## Controversies

Debate persists about whether beta blockers are beneficial in the most severely ill patients. Anecdotal evidence suggests that such patients can respond—and that

Table 20–3

## Regimen for Initiation of Beta Blockade for Congestive Heart Failure*

Stabilize patient's condition:
  Diuretics
  Maximal ACE inhibition
  Digoxin
Evaluate
  Euvolemic
  No bradycardia unless pacemaker
    present
  No heart block unless pacemaker
    present
Step 1
  Carvedilol                3.125 mg b.i.d.
  Metoprolol XL             12.5 mg q.d. (can start with step 2 in NYHA class II)
  Metoprolol                6.25 mg b.i.d. (can start with step 2 in NYHA class II)
  Bisoprolol                1.25 mg q.d.
Step 2
  Carvedilol                6.25 mg b.i.d.
  Metoprolol XL             25 mg q.d.
  Metoprolol                12.5 mg b.i.d.
  Bisoprolol                2.5 mg q.d.
Step 3
  Carvedilol                12.5 mg b.i.d.
  Metoprolol XL             50 mg q.d.
  Metoprolol                25 mg b.i.d.
  Bisoprolol                3.75 mg q.d.
Step 4
  Carvedilol                25 mg b.i.d.
  Metoprolol XL             100 mg q.d.
  Metoprolol                50 mg b.i.d.
  Bisoprolol                5 mg q.d.
Step 5
  Carvedilol                If weight >85 kg, 50 mg b.i.d.
  Metoprolol XL             150 mg q.d. (can skip to step 6 if very stable)
  Metoprolol                75 mg b.i.d.
  Bisoprolol                7.5 mg q.d.
Step 6
  Metoprolol XL             200 mg q.d.
  Metoprolol                100 mg b.i.d.
  Bisoprolol                10 mg q.d.
*Cautions*
Between each step (every 1–2 wk):
  If no increased CHF symptoms and no increase in weight, proceed to next step.
  If no increased symptoms but increased fluid weight, increase diuretics and check patient in 1 week.
    When back to baseline, proceed to next step.
  If symptoms and weight increase, increase diuretics and check patient in 1 week. When back to
    baseline, proceed to next step.
  With slight increase in symptoms and no weight gain, make no change and check patient in 1 week.
    When back to baseline, proceed to next step.
  For marked increase in symptoms, stop drug.
  For symptomatic bradycardia, decrease dose of beta blocker.
  For heart block, decrease dose of beta blocker.

*Doses are based on clinical experience with each drug for treatment of congestive heart failure.

they have the most to gain. They are, however, also the patients for whom a slight temporary exacerbation can lead to further deterioration and death. At present, the data on treating these patients are inconclusive. The survival studies CIBIS II and MERIT enrolled patients with a wide range of disease severity, but the number of patients with New York Heart Association class IV symptoms enrolled in these and other studies is small. When the sickest patients are to be given a trial of beta blockers, it should be done with careful monitoring by very experienced physicians

The consequences of the differences among beta blockers are also unclear. There have been theoretical concerns about beta selectivity, other vasodilatory properties, and even antioxidant effects. The initial very positive data observed with the use of carvedilol even led some investigators to question whether the beneficial effects were class specific or drug specific. As markedly positive findings on metoprolol and bisoprolol were revealed, however, the "generalizability" of the benefits of beta blockade became apparent. Nevertheless, relatively few beta-blocking agents have been evaluated for heart failure, and use of drugs that have not been tested should be discouraged. While metoprolol, carvedilol, and bisoprolol should all be considered effective, studies comparing these agents and evaluating their use in severely ill patients are ongoing. The findings should provide the information necessary to further refine the proper use of beta blockers for heart failure.

## ■ DIGOXIN

Digoxin is used with varying frequency from nation to nation, undoubtedly because of ambiguous data on its efficacy. The consequences of using digoxin were recently clarified by the Digitalis Investigation Group (DIG) in a Veterans Administration study of 6800 patients whose ejection fractions were less than 45%.[19] There was no effect on mortality in this study: survival curves were identical for patients who took digoxin and those who received placebo.

Even though it had no effect on mortality, in DIG, digoxin decreased the overall hospitalization rate by 6% and the rate of hospitalization for heart failure by 28%. This improvement is consistent with previous studies, which showed that patients whose digoxin was withdrawn had more exacerbations of heart failure.[20] The use of digoxin to improve symptoms therefore appears appropriate. Furthermore, unlike other positive inotropic agents, digoxin can be given for symptom relief without fear that it will have long-term adverse effects.

Unfortunately, the narrow therapeutic window of digoxin leads to frequent toxicity. For example, declining renal function might lead to accumulation of digoxin in a patient who has tolerated a particular dose without any problem. The result might be bradyarrhythmia, tachyarrhythmia, nausea, or vision disturbances. One reason for the high prevalence of digoxin toxicity is the poor correlation between serum concentration and toxicity. Digoxin produces adverse effects at different concentrations in different persons, often at concentrations within the "therapeutic range." This obviously decreases the utility of serum digoxin concentrations.

Routine measurement of digoxin concentrations is not warranted because the optimal concentration is no known. Furthermore, it is not even known whether high or low concentrations are preferable. Many studies demonstrate that low digoxin concentrations have beneficial neurohormonal actions. The long-term symptomatic benefit observed with digoxin might be secondary to these effects rather than to the positive inotropic effects that occur at higher ("therapeutic") concentrations.

While elevated serum digoxin concentrations can support the diagnosis of digoxin toxicity, routine monitoring of the concentration is expensive and not necessary. It appears wiser to treat patients with doses that are unlikely to cause toxicity and to check concentrations only when there is a clinical question.

# ■ POSITIVE INOTROPES

## Long-Term Use

No controlled studies support the use of positive inotropes for long-term treatment of congestive heart failure. Although anecdotal findings of uncontrolled studies suggest that intermittent use of dobutamine or milrinone may be beneficial, controlled studies are negative.[21] Furthermore, trials of oral inotropes such as milrinone[22] and vesnarinone[23] have demonstrated increased mortality, especially in the sickest patients. Although immediate inotropic therapy benefits patients with decompensated heart failure, long-term dosing cannot be justified except in very rare instances when there is absolutely no alternative.

The analogy with beta blockers strongly supports the conclusion that inotropic therapy should be used only acutely. Just as initially beta blockers have adverse consequences, it is not surprising that catecholamines (such as dobutamine) and phosphodiesterase inhibitors (such as milrinone) may be useful acutely to improve symptoms, increase renal perfusion (and diuresis), and permit time for other treatments to be effective. The long-term improvement in contractility and survival associated with beta blockers suggests, however, that long-term inotropic therapy leads to decreased contractility, more rapid progression of disease, and increased risk of death. The studies of oral inotropes confirm this conclusion.

At present, widespread use of chronic or intermittent infusion therapy of positive inotropes is inappropriate and not supported by data. It is conceivable that these agents are suitable for occasional patients who are willing to accept long-term risks because no other intervention will relieve debilitating symptoms. Long-term therapy with inotropic drugs should be used only when both doctor and patient understand that refractory symptoms might be treated at the cost of more rapid progression of the disease.

## Short-Term Use

Early hospital treatment of patients with congestive heart failure is very different from long-term treatment. Since the most common cause of hospitalization is volume overload (which increases pulmonary vascular pressure and exacerbates symptoms), interventions that enhance diuresis can help. In some patients, inotropic therapy with dobutamine or milrinone is very useful for this purpose. In others, short-term inotropic therapy may improve cardiac function until long-term interventions can be instituted or causes of acute deterioration reversed. In still other patients, a short course of inotropic therapy appears to interrupt a downward spiral, and it may produce a prolonged effect.

There is little reason to use phosphodiesterase inhibitors routinely for acute inotropic therapy. Dobutamine is far less expensive than milrinone and is effective for most patients. While milrinone has been advocated because of the possibility that it more efficiently improves contractility, with less cardiac oxygen consumption, the importance of such a benefit has not been documented. Physicians should remember, however, that tolerance to dobutamine can develop because of downregulation of the beta receptors. For the same reason, rapid weaning from this agent can cause deterioration in some patients for whom a slower wean can be successful. At times a phosphodiesterase inhibitor is useful. For example, some patients appear to respond better to a phosphodiesterase inhibitor. Furthermore, the combination of milrinone and dobutamine may be effective for refractory symptoms.

## ■ ARRHYTHMIAS

Despite recent improvements in treatment of congestive heart failure, the mortality rate remains high. The unexpected death of patients who appear to be doing well are particularly troubling. Although such deaths are frequently attributed to primary ventricular arrhythmias, other causes, such as pulmonary embolus, ischemia, and infarction, undoubtedly also contribute to the overall mortality. Furthermore, bradyarrhythmias may be the cause of a substantial number of sudden deaths.[24] Nevertheless, ventricular arrhythmias are often seen in patients with congestive heart failure and clearly cause sudden death in some. This fact has prompted a search for treatments to prevent arrhythmia-related deaths.

The adverse consequences of conventional antiarrhythmic agents have led to a marked decrease in their use. They have negative inotropic actions that might exacerbate heart failure (the underlying cause of the arrhythmias) and have the potential to be proarrhythmic. Agents such as quinidine and procainamide are being prescribed less and less, even for atrial fibrillation.[25] Other interventions are more promising, although the best way to prevent sudden death is still controversial.

### Amiodarone

The evidence for amiodarone's efficacy is inconclusive, and, as a result, there is much variation in its use. It is clearly excellent for treating atrial arrhythmias and is being used more and more as the safest and most reliable antiarrhythmic for the maintenance of sinus rhythm in patients with heart failure. It is often recommended to prevent ventricular arrhythmias and sudden death. There are even suggestions that amiodarone might improve cardiac function and thus improve both symptoms and survival rates in the belief that all patients with heart failure should receive this medication.

Unfortunately, findings of controlled studies have not been as positive as we once hoped. Two large, randomized, and rigorous studies came to opposite conclusions about amiodarone. The Argentine GESICA study found a 28% reduction in mortality,[26] whereas the Veterans Administration–sponsored Survival Trial of Antiarrhythmic Therapy in Congestive Heart Failure (CHF-STAT) reported an adverse trend in survival.[27] Many attempts have been made to explain the conflicting results, but the reasons remain unclear.

The side effects of amiodarone can be clinically important, difficult to identify, and, possibly, a partial explanation of the worse outcomes in some studies. Particularly problematic is pulmonary toxicity, both acute and chronic, which can go undiagnosed in patients with heart failure who complain of dyspnea, with devastating results. Pulmonary function tests should be performed at least yearly in patients who are taking amiodarone, and pulmonary toxicity should be considered when any patient's symptoms are exacerbated. The physician must also remember to search for other side effects, such as thyroid and skin abnormalities.

Amiodarone continues to be studied in patients with heart failure, but the proper use of this agent has yet to be determined. Although it cannot be recommended for routine use in patients with heart failure, it is the drug of choice if an antiarrhythmic agent is to be used for either atrial or ventricular arrhythmias.

## Implantable Defibrillators

Data supporting the use of implantable defibrillators in patients with heart failure are accumulating. Indications are strongest for patients with ischemic heart disease or previous infarction, for whom inducibility on electrophysiologic testing predicts high risk of death and who appear to benefit from defibrillation.[28] However, the predictability of inducibility in patients with nonischemic cardiomyopathy has not been proven. Similarly, patients with heart failure who do not have "inducible electrophysiologic findings" may still experience sudden death, and the appropriate use of implantable defibrillators in these patients is unknown.

Implantable defibrillators are being used increasingly in patients with heart failure (and both inducible and noninducible electrophysiologic studies) who present with syncope and symptomatic ventricular arrhythmias. Such patients are at particularly high risk, and oral antiarrhythmic agents have limited benefit. Thus, physicians have anticipated that the data will show benefit, and they have acted accordingly. Some investigators even believe that survival will increase if all patients with heart failure receive implantable defibrillators. These devices could prevent both bradyarrhythmic and tachyarrhythmic deaths. This hypothesis is being tested in the ongoing NIH-sponsored Sudden Cardiac Death in Heart Failure Trial (SCD-HeFT).

## ■ ANTICOAGULATION

### Warfarin

The use of warfarin, aspirin, and other antiplatelet agents in patients with heart failure has been debated. Clots can form in large, poorly contracting ventricles, and there is concern that these clots may embolize, causing cerebrovascular accidents. Unfortunately, the use of anticoagulants in heart failure patients has been tested only in retrospective studies. Although these studies suggest that anticoagulation might be beneficial, further investigations are limited by the realistic concern that patients who are prescribed anticoagulants in uncontrolled reports are healthier. This would then explain their better outcome.

Since the side effects of warfarin are not negligible, many physicians are very concerned about prescribing an agent that might cause harm when its benefit is not clear. At present, there are no accepted recommendations on anticoagulation in patients with poor cardiac function and normal sinus rhythm.

For some other groups of patients anticoagulation is clearly indicated. For example, patients with atrial fibrillation and cardiac disease experienced fewer events when they took effective therapeutic doses of warfarin.[29] Since the atrial fibrillation patients with congestive heart failure are at particularly high risk of embolism, they should be given warfarin unless contraindications are strong. The warfarin dose should be adjusted so that the INR remains between 2.0 and 3.0.

### Aspirin

Even more problematic is the use of aspirin in patients with heart failure. The benefits of aspirin in ischemic heart disease are well-documented, and many patients with heart failure receive them after a myocardial infarction or another ischemic episode.

There are suggestions, however, that aspirin might counteract some of the beneficial effects of ACE inhibitors. Aspirin can decrease kidney function in heart failure patients, whose renal perfusion may depend on prostaglandins. Other adverse hemodynamic actions can result from vasoconstriction. Aspirin also inhibits bradykinin production, antagonizing the effects of ACE inhibitors on bradykinin. The role of bradykinin in heart failure is not known, nor is there evidence that bradykinin contributes to the beneficial effects of ACE inhibitors. Thus, whether the actions of aspirin are detrimental to patients who have heart failure or are taking ACE inhibitors is not clear.

It is possible that clopidogrel or ticlopidine will prove to have useful antiplatelet actions without adversely affecting prostaglandins or bradykinin. Such a benefit remains theoretical, however, and the cost of these agents mandates proof before their widespread use. Until such a study is completed, patients with ischemic heart disease should take aspirin. Theoretical concerns cannot overpower the known and considerable benefit for patients who have already had bypass surgery or a myocardial infarction. Prophylactic use of aspirin in patients with heart failure but without known ischemic heart disease is inappropriate, however.

The routine pharmacologic treatment of congestive heart failure is shown in Table 20–4, based on major heart failure survival trials (Table 20–5).

## ■ TRANSPLANTATION

Cardiac transplantation is now a routine and accepted option for patients with severe heart failure that is refractory to medical therapy. One-year survival in many programs approaches 90%, a rate far superior to that expected for patients with severe disease. Furthermore, patients' symptoms can improve enough to allow them to return to work and function independently. The indications for cardiac transplantation are shown in Table 20–6.

The clinical outcome for patients who survive transplantation suggests important benefit.[30] Four fifths of patients who survive the initial hospitalization have no activity limitations at 1 year. Considering that these patients were generally New York Heart Association class III or IV before the transplant, this is a dramatic benefit. These same patients continue to be affected by their disease, however; only 27% have returned to work full time.

The reason for low employment rates are many, but in large part they can be explained by complications of the transplant. Despite improving survival rates, the risks of transplantation remain considerable: rejection and infectious complications are most worrisome during the first year, and coronary artery disease and neoplasms become more prevalent with time. Indeed, 42% of patients who survive the

---

Table 20–4

**Routine Pharmacologic Treatment of Congestive Heart Failure— Current Practice**

| | |
|---|---|
| Proven therapy | |
|   Angiotensin-converting enzyme inhibitors | Lisinopril, 20–40 mg; captopril, 25–50 mg t.i.d.; enalapril, 10–20 mg b.i.d.; or equivalent |
|   Diuretics | Furosemide as needed or other diuretics |
|   Digoxin | 0.125–0.25 mg |
|   Beta blockers | Metoprolol, carvedilol, or bisoprolol |
|   Spironolactone | 25 mg |
| Therapy beneficial to certain patients | |
|   Warfarin | |
|   Amiodarone | |
|   Aspirin | |

All of these medications should be considered for all patients with heart failure.

Table 20–5

**Major Heart Failure Survival Trials**

| Trial (Acronym) | Drug | Patients (N) | Goal Daily Dose (mg) | Improvement |
|---|---|---|---|---|
| **ACE Inhibitors** | | | | |
| CONSENSUS[8] | Enalapril vs. placebo in advanced disease | 253 | 40 | 27% |
| SOLVD-treatment[7] | Enalapril vs. placebo | 2569 | 20 | 16% |
| SOLVD-prevention[39] | Enalapril vs. placebo | 4228 | 20 | No effect on mortality; hospitalizations decreased |
| V-HeFT-II[13] | Hydralazine/ isosorbide dinitrate vs. enalapril | 804 | Enalapril: 20 Hydralazine: 300 Nitrates: 160 | With enalapril 28% |
| **Vasodilators** | | | | |
| PRAISE[14] | Amlodipine vs. placebo | 1153 | 10 | No change, but possible subgroup effect in non-ischemics |
| VHeFT-III[40] | Felodipine vs. placebo | 450 | 10 | No effect |
| V-HeFT | Hydralazine/ nitrates vs. prazosin vs. placebo | 642 | Hydralazine: 300 Nitrates: 160 Prazosin: 20 | Improvement with hydralazine/ nitrates |
| **Inotropes** | | | | |
| VEST[23] | Vesnarinone vs. placebo | 3833 | 30 and 60 | Increased mortality |
| PROMISE[22] | Milrinone vs. placebo | 1088 | 40 | Increased mortality |
| DIG[19] | Digoxin vs. placebo | 6800 | Dose varies | No effect on mortality; hospitalizations decreased |
| **Beta Blockers** | | | | |
| CIBIS-II[17] | Bisoprolol vs. placebo | 2647 | 10 | 34% |
| MERIT-HF[16] | Long-acting metoprolol vs. placebo | 3991 | 200 | 34% |
| **Amiodarone** | | | | |
| GESICA[26] | Amiodarone vs. placebo | 516 | 300 | 28% |
| CHF-STAT[27] | Amiodarone vs. placebo | 674 | 300 | No effect |
| **Spironolactone** | | | | |
| RALES | Spironolactone vs. placebo | 1663 | 25 | 30% |

ACE, angiotensin-converting enzyme; vs., versus.

Table 20–6

**Indications for Heart Transplantation**

**Definite**
  Volume of oxygen use <10 ml/kg/min
  NYHA class IV
  History of recurrent hospitalization for congestive heart failure
  Refractory ischemia with inoperable coronary artery disease and left ventricular ejection fraction <20%
  Recurrent symptomatic ventricular arrhythmias
**Probable**
  Volume of oxygen use <14 ml/kg/min
  NYHA class III or IV
  Recent hospitalizations for congestive heart failure
  Recurrent "high-grade" ectopy with family history of sudden death
  Unstable angina not amenable to coronary artery bypass grafting or percutaneous transluminal
    coronary angioplasty with left ventricular ejection fraction <30%
**Inadequate**
  Volume of oxygen use >14 ml/kg/min
  NYHA class I or II
  Left ventricular ejection fraction <20%
  Stable, exertional angina with left ventricular ejection fraction >20%

Adapted from Miller LW, Kubo SH, Young JB, et al: Report of the Consensus Conference on Candidate Selection for Heart Transplantation—1993. J Heart Lung Transplant 1995;14:562–571.

initial hospitalization are rehospitalized in the first year. Furthermore, important chronic diseases such as renal failure, hypertension, and diabetes often develop. It is not easy for a patient to undergo a cardiac transplantation.

Considering both the risks of transplantation and the limited availability of hearts, patients whose prognosis is very poor *and* symptoms severe should be selected for transplantation. While any patient with congestive heart failure is at increased risk of dying, the severity of the disease is directly related to the risk of mortality. For this reason, mortality benefits can be assumed only for the sickest patients. Since, by itself, a low ejection fraction does not portend a particularly poor prognosis, for patients with minimal symptoms a transplant may not improve survival.

It is apparent that a cardiac transplant can improve the quality of life only for patients with severe symptoms. Given the morbidity associated with transplantation, some assurance that the patient will benefit is mandatory. Partially for this reason, it is common to evaluate symptoms objectively by performing an exercise test with metabolic monitoring. Peak oxygen consumption gives excellent documentation of limitation of activity, and a low peak oxygen consumption (below approximately 14 ml/kg/min) indicates marked limitation of function. The physician evaluating a patient with heart failure must also remember that deconditioning can lead to continued symptoms of dyspnea and fatigue. Distinguishing between symptoms of heart failure and of deconditioning can be extremely difficult, and, often, only time makes the diagnosis evident.

Physicians must continually assess patients with heart failure. Those who have substantially improved need to be removed from transplant lists, and those who initially appeared to be "too healthy" may have deteriorated. Although it may be stressful to inform a patient that a transplant is no longer needed, transplanting a heart into a healthy patient benefits no one.

It is also unwise to offer transplants to patients whose risk of complications from the procedure is great.[31] Patients with end organ damage, such as fixed pulmonary hypertension, hepatic failure, renal failure, or peripheral vascular disease, are at high risk. Similarly, because brief episodes of noncompliance can have devastating effects, patients who lack social support and the ability to follow medical regimens carefully should not receive transplants. Transplantation is miraculous for some patients, but used inappropriately it can cause irrevocable harm.

## ■ MECHANICAL INTERVENTIONS

### Left Ventricular Assist Devices (LVAD)

A mechanical heart substitute that could be permanently implanted would be ideal for patients with end stage heart disease. The small supply of hearts available for transplantation and the complications inherent with immunosuppression severely limit the number of patients who can benefit from transplantation. Recent advances in technology, including thrombosis prevention and miniaturization, have brought the possibility of widespread use of ventricular assist devices closer to reality.[32] At present, however, such devices are being used chiefly as a bridge to transplantation and for temporary circulatory support (Fig. 20–3).

LVADs are placed with an outflow conduit sewn in to the apex of the left ventricle after removal of an adequate size plug. The inflow conduit is then placed

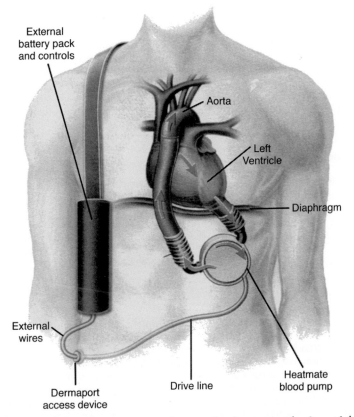

**Figure 20–3** ■ Placement of the inflow and outflow cannulas, the pumping chamber, and the external controls in wearable left ventricular assist devices. (Adapted from Goldstein DJ, Oz MC, Rose EA: Medical progress: Implantable left ventricular assist devices. N Engl J Med 1996:78:966–999.)

into the ascending aorta, and the LVAD is implanted in the abdomen outside the peritoneum. Ventricular assist devices can permit end organ perfusion in patients whose own hearts cannot perform adequately.

In the setting of myocardial infarction, acute myocarditis or inability to wean from cardiopulmonary bypass, short-term interventions might provide time for recovery from the insult. Thus, intraaortic balloon pumps and extracorporeal devices might be useful. In patients with chronic heart failure, however, implantable devices such as the Novacor and the Heartmate can lead to decreased symptoms, improved organ function, and even improved mobility and functioning.

Today, most assist devices are intended as a bridge to transplantation. With such support patients can even be sent home until a donor organ becomes available. With the long lists of transplantation candidates and the long waits that even very ill hospitalized patients experience, mechanical support has become essential to sustaining life until an organ is available. Furthermore, the normal cardiac output provided by the device can reverse long-term problems such as organ failure, anorexia, and muscle weakness and improve the outcome when transplant surgery is performed.

Ultimately, it is possible that these devices will be alternatives to transplantation rather than mere bridges. In some patients they afford opportunity for cardiac remodeling, and, after enough time, might successfully be removed. For the many patients who cannot receive a transplant because of medical reasons or lack of an organ, moreover, permanent use would be life saving. The outcome for patients randomized to receive a left ventricular assist device or conventional therapy is already being evaluated in a well-designed NIH-sponsored trial.

Certain risks of LVAD placement—whether short term or long term—must be considered. Placement of an LVAD is major surgery, and bleeding and infections are not uncommon complications. While right-sided heart failure may occur because of pulmonary vasoconstriction, the risks of thromboembolism are surprisingly low. The resolution of the clotting problem has raised hopes that a reliable mechanical heart substitute will be soon available.

## Ventriculectomy

Much excitement was generated by the ventriculectomy work of Batista. Despite very high mortality rates and no controlled studies, the idea of decreasing the size of the ventricle, and thus improving its function, appealed to many transplant surgeons. At this point, however, no "controlled data" on the efficacy of this major surgery are available. Considering the obvious high risk of the ventriculectomy operation, it remains purely investigational and should not be used instead of conventional therapy.

## Mitral Valve Repair

One aspect of ventriculectomy surgery that likely has produced much of the observed beneficial effect is correction of mitral regurgitation. Patients with severe heart failure often have marked mitral regurgitation caused by annular dilatation. The regurgitation can seriously exacerbate the underlying problem, causing increased pulmonary pressures and decreased forward flow. If a patient can tolerate the operation, the benefits of surgically decreasing backward flow are obvious.

Previously, the risk of such surgery was felt to be too high for patients with left ventricular dysfunction. Indeed, because the ejection fraction can be markedly increased by mitral regurgitation, the true extent of myocardial dysfunction is difficult to assess in patients with mitral regurgitation, and patients with extremely poor myocardial function are less likely to survive the surgery or experience substantially improved cardiac performance. However, a few surgeons are now reporting excellent outcomes by correcting mitral regurgitation with mitral annuloplasty, even in patients with severe congestive heart failure and left ventricular dysfunction.[33] Factors that portend a better outcome with this surgery need to be understood before mitral annuloplasty becomes an accepted treatment for patients with severe heart failure.

## Pacemaker

Many investigators have been intrigued by the idea that pacemakers can be used to increase cardiac output in patients with heart failure. Trials of decreasing the atrioventricular delay, optimizing the location of the pacing lead, and using biventricular or left ventricular pacing have reported varying degrees of success. Review of these reports reveals some promising modalities, but it also emphasizes the need to assess interventions carefully in well-designed and controlled studies.

A prolonged atrioventricular delay can lead to ineffectual atrial contraction, and the benefit of synchronous atrial and ventricular contraction can be substantial. Some investigators, however, have believed that a particularly short atrioventricular delay might be beneficial, even for patients who otherwise have no need for a pacemaker. While initial uncontrolled data were promising, the benefit of optimizing the atrioventricular delay has not been borne out by controlled studies.

More promising have been findings that suggest that left ventricular or biventricular pacing might be beneficial for patients with left bundle branch block or other conduction abnormalities. The contraction wave in such patients may not permit optimal efficiency. Small mechanistic studies have been promising, and larger clinical studies are now under way.

## ■ NURSING INTERVENTIONS

One of the most important interventions that can be used to treat patients with heart failure is close follow-up and treatment of problems before major decompensations develop. This is the thinking behind many nursing interventions now in use. Managed care has realized that preventing hospitalizations by close follow-up can both save money and make patients feel better.

The optimal means of close follow-up is not known. Many studies report benefit from combined interventions; frequent nursing visits, ready access to knowledgeable physicians, education, diet modification, and social work help are often tried in combination.[34] Close follow-up with frequent home nursing visits, transtelephonic monitoring, and heart failure clinics have all been tried and appear to be successful (usually in uncontrolled trials). Personnel used have ranged from qualified nurses with heart failure expertise to lesser trained persons who ask a few key (scripted) questions.

Howsoever it is done, addressing fluid overload before it progresses to pulmonary edema and ensuring that patients are prescribed medications proven to be beneficial (and that they are taking these medications) will prevent heart failure exacerbations and hospitalizations. Expenditures on outpatient care inevitably reduce costs overall.

## ■ EXERCISE

Exercise intolerance is often the result of decreased muscle tone, which in turn is the result of deconditioning, anorexia, and malnutrition. While the decreased cardiac output and increased ventricular and pulmonary pressures initially limit exercise for patients with heart failure, improvement in cardiac performance does not lead to immediate return of normal capabilities. Indeed, the old idea that patients with heart failure should not exercise rendered medically treated patients incapable of improving their functional status. Presently, it is clear that steady exercise will improve muscle (and perhaps vascular) function and enhance the quality of life.

Many studies have shown that formal exercise programs increase oxygen consumption and exercise tolerance. Unfortunately, the applicability of these reports is suspect. Often, motivated young patients are studied, and compliance of sicker and elderly patients may be different. Furthermore, it is not clear whether the cost associated with these programs is necessary. Formal cardiac programs with monitoring enhance patients' confidence, but they are expensive. In addition, it has never been demonstrated that they improve the safety of exercising.

Another unanswered question is whether exercise must be aerobic. Traditionally, isometric exercise was prohibited for heart failure patients. Physicians were concerned that the increased afterload induced by the exercise would be detrimental, but this theory has not been tested. At present, one must conclude that aerobic exercise should be encouraged in whatever setting is possible.

## ■ METABOLIC INTERVENTIONS

### Coenzyme $Q_{10}$

The hypotheses behind the use of coenzyme $Q_{10}$ in patients with congestive heart failure are varied. It is reputedly an antioxidant, and supplementation is said to prevent lipid peroxidation. Perhaps more interesting is its role in electron transfer within the respiratory chain, with consequent potential to affect oxidative phosphorylation. Coenzyme $Q_{10}$ has captured the imagination of many patients and, despite its expense, is much used.

There are few controlled trials testing the impact of coenzyme $Q_{10}$ in heart failure, and results of those are conflicting. The studies are small, however, and it is possible that some groups of patients benefit. At the present time, the risks of using coenzyme $Q_{10}$ appear to be few, but its benefit is questionable. Physicians and patients should be aware that the high doses that have been used in the trials are expensive for such an unproven therapy.

### Nutrition

Functional capacity depends on the nutritional status of patients, and cachexia is associated with increased risks of mortality and morbidity. For example, patients with less muscle mass have less functional capacity. Whether cachexia causes the poor outcome or merely reflects the severity of disease is not clear, however. A number of investigational approaches are addressing this issue by attempting to improve nutrition and prevent the effects of cachexia.

The simplest means of improving nutrition would be to provide supplements. Good nutrition should be encouraged in all patients, but there is no evidence that this can have a major impact on patients with heart failure. Other interventions, such as anabolic hormones, are being investigated. Growth hormone and other anabolic steroids could, theoretically, improve both cardiac and peripheral muscle function. Another approach to improving nutritional status would be to prevent cachexia. Since cytokines such as tumor necrosis factor alpha (TNF-α) can cause anorexia and other potential adverse effects, their antagonism might improve nutrition. Although the importance of nutrition is clear, it is not clear whether addressing it as a primary problem will improve the status of patients with heart failure.

# ■ INVESTIGATIONAL NEUROHORMONAL ANTAGONISTS

## Antagonists with Renal Actions

Investigation of the cause of water retention in patients with heart failure has long focused on neurohormonal activation. Thus, it is not surprising that various neurohormonal antagonists are being studied as possible effective and safe diuretics. For example, a number of arginine vasopressin antagonists are being investigated to determine whether they might increase urine flow while increasing serum sodium concentration.

The possible importance of adenosine as a regulator of renal function is also being investigated. Plasma adenosine concentrations are increased in patients with congestive heart failure, and adenosine has been shown to decrease renal blood flow (by increasing vasoconstriction in resistance arteries) in these patients. Since adenosine antagonists may increase both glomerular filtration rate and urine flow in healthy persons, investigation into their possible effects as diuretic agents with beneficial effects on renal function is ongoing.[35]

The natriuretic peptides may also benefit patients with heart failure. Either by giving atrial natriuretic peptide or brain natriuretic peptide or by preventing degradation with neutral endopeptidase inhibitors, these agents may improve diuresis. In short-term studies, the natriuretic peptides have proven to be effective diuretics[36, 37]; however, they may not be effective over the long term or for persons with persistent ANP stimulation.[38]

## Antagonists with Vasodilator Activity

The natriuretic peptides are also effective vasodilators when given acutely. Tolerance may develop, however, and, thus, long-term hemodynamic effects of natriuretic peptides are unknown. Interestingly, agents that combine NEP inactivation and ACE inhibition are being investigated as therapeutic agents. The arginine vasopressin antagonists may also lead to vasodilatation, and the importance of such actions is being evaluated.

The endothelins are a family of vasoactive peptides that have a variety of cardiac and neurohormonal actions. They affect not only the renin-angiotensin-aldosterone axis, prostaglandins, and nitric oxide but also cell proliferation. Endothelin concentrations are elevated in patients with heart failure, but the hemodynamic and cardiac effects of endothelin receptor antagonists are not known.

Different endothelin receptors have different actions. $ET_a$ receptors are located in vascular smooth muscle, where stimulation can lead to vasoconstriction, but also in myocardial cells, where stimulation increases contractility. In contrast, $ET_b$ receptor stimulation causes vasodilatation via nitric oxide release, but it can also cause vasoconstriction. Both $ET_a$-specific antagonists and nonspecific antagonists are being evaluated. Thus far, they have been shown to improve hemodynamic parameters. Whether antagonism of the cardiac receptors will have beneficial or detrimental long-term effects, however, is not known.

## Cytokines

The cytokine most studied in patients with heart failure is TNF-$\alpha$, which acutely decreases contractility, an effect that can be reversed by TNF-binding proteins. Interestingly, the failing heart produces it and high circulating concentrations are seen in patients with heart failure. Perhaps more important than its acute effects, however, are its chronic effects. It can cause anorexia, but there is also evidence that TNF might cause inflammation and consequent detrimental chronic effects. TNF has even affected remodeling in some studies. It is possible that the usual progressive deterioration of heart failure can be interrupted by antagonizing cytokines.

## ▪ CONCLUSION

The treatment of congestive heart failure demands close follow-up, attention to detail, and listening to the patient. Fortunately, careful studies have guided us to effective treatment of these patients, and the questions that remain can and must also be addressed in ways that lead to evidence-based medicine. Physicians should learn from these studies how to treat patients with medicines proven to be effective at appropriate doses. The treatments can affect symptoms or mortality, but the physician should understand the impact of any treatment on both.

## ▪ REFERENCES

1. Channer KS, McLean KA, Lawson-Matthew P, Richardson M: Combination diuretic treatment in severe heart failure: A randomized controlled trial. Br Heart J 1994;71:146–150.
2. Pitt B, Zannad F, Reme WJ, et al: The effect of spironolactone on morbidity and mortality in patients with severe heart failure. Randomized Aldactose Evaluation Study Investigators. N Engl J Med 1999;341:709–717.
3. Pabico RC, Rogal GJ, McKenna BA, et al: Renal effects of dobutamine and dopamine in congestive heart failure. In Puschett JB, Greenberg A: Diuretics III: Chemistry, Pharmacology, and Clinical Applications. New York, Elsevier Science, 1990:302–312.
4. Vargo DL, Brater DC, Rudy DW, Swan SK: Dopamine does not enhance furosemide-induced natriuresis in patients with congestive heart failure. J Am Soc Nephrol 1996;7:1032–1037.
5. L'Abbate A, Emdin M, Piacenti M, et al: Ultrafiltration: A rational treatment for heart failure. Cardiology 1989;76:384–390.
6. Hricik DE: Captopril-induced renal insufficiency and the role of sodium balance. Ann Intern Med 1985;103:222–223.
7. The SOLVD Investigators: Effect of enalapril on survival in patients with reduced left ventricular ejection fractions and congestive heart failure. N Engl J Med 1991;325:293–302.
8. The CONSENSUS Trial Study Group: Effects of enalapril on mortality in severe congestive heart failure: Results of the Cooperative North Scandanavian Enalapril Survival Study (CONSENSUS). N Engl J Med 1987;316:1429–1434.
9. Gottlieb SS, Robinson S, Weir MR, et al: Determinants of the renal response to ACE inhibition in patients with congestive heart failure. Am Heart J 1992;124;131–136.
10. Pitt B, Segal R, Martinez FA, et al: Randomised trial of losartan versus captopril in patients over 65 with heart failure (Evaluation of Losartan in the Elderly Study, ELITE). Lancet 1997;349:747–752.
11. Tsuyuki RT, Yusuf S, Rouleau JL, et al: Combination neurohormonal blockade with ACE inhibitors, angiotensin II antagonists and beta-blockers in patients with congestive heart failure: Design of the Randomized Evaluation of Strategies for Left Ventricular Dysfunction (RESOLVD) pilot study. Can J Cardiol 1997;13:1166–1174.
12. Cohn JN, Archibald DG, Ziesche S, et al: Effect of vasodilator therapy on mortality in chronic congestive heart failure. Results of a Veterans Administration Cooperative Study. N Engl J Med 1986;314:1547–1552.
13. Cohn JN, Johnson G, Ziesche S, et al: A comparison of enalapril with hydralazine-isosorbide dinitrate in the treatment of chronic congestive heart failure. N Engl J Med 1991;325:303–310.
14. Packer M, O'Connor CM, Ghali JK, et al: Effect of amlodipine on morbidity and mortality in severe chronic heart failure. Prospective Randomized Amlodipine Survival Evaluation Study Group. N Engl J Med 1996;335:1107–1114.
15. Packer M, Bristow MR, Cohn JN, et al: Effect of carvedilol on morbidity and mortality in chronic heart failure. N Engl J Med 1996;334:1349–1355.
16. MERIT Investigators: Effect of metoprolol CR/XL in chronic heart failure: Metoprolol CR/XL Randomized Intervention Trial in Congestive Heart Failure. Lancet 1999;353:2001–2007.
17. CIBIS II Investigators and Committees: The cardiac insufficiency bisoprolol study II (CIBIS-II): A randomized trial. Lancet 1999;353:9–13.

18. Bristow MR, O'Connell JB, Gilbert EM, et al: Dose-response of chronic beta-blocker treatment in heart failure from either idiopathic dilated or ischemic cardiomyopathy. Circulation 1994;89:1632–1642.
19. The Digitalis Investigation Group: The effect of digoxin on mortality and morbidity in patients with heart failure. N Engl J Med 1997;336:525–533.
20. Packer M, Gheorghiade M, Young JB, et al: Withdrawal of digoxin from patients with chronic heart failure treated with angiotensin-converting-enzyme inhibitors. RADIANCE Study. N Engl J Med 1993;329:1–7.
21. Packer M: The development of positive inotropic agents for chronic heart failure: How have we gone astray? J Am Coll Cardiol 1993;22(4 Suppl A):119A–126A.
22. Packer M, Carver JR, Rodeheffer RJ, et al: Effect of oral milrinone on mortality in severe chronic heart failure. N Engl J Med 1991;325:1468–1475.
23. Cohn JN, Goldstein SO, Greenberg BH, et al: A dose-dependent increase in mortality with vesnarinone among patients with severe heart failure. Vesnarinone Trial Investigators. N Engl J Med 1998;339:1810–1816.
24. Luu M, Stevenson W, Stevenson L, et al: Diverse mechanisms of unexpected cardiac arrest in advanced heart failure. Circulation 1989;80:1675–1680.
25. Flaker GC, Blackshear JL, McBride R, et al: Antiarrhythmic drug therapy and cardiac mortality in atrial fibrillation. The Stroke Prevention in Atrial Fibrillation Investigators. J Am Coll Cardiol 1992;20:527–532.
26. Doval HC, Nul DR, Grancelli HO, et al: Randomised trial of low-dose amiodarone in severe congestive heart failure. Grupo de Estudio de la Sobrevida en la Insuficiencia Cardiaca en Argentina (GESICA). Lancet 1994;344:493–498.
27. Singh SN, Fletcher RD, Fisher SG, et al: Amiodarone in patients with congestive heart failure and asymptomatic ventricular arrhythmia: Survival Trial of Antiarrhythmic Therapy in Congestive Heart Failure. N Engl J Med 1995;333:77–82.
28. Moss AJ, Hall WJ, Cannom DS, et al: Improved survival with an implanted defibrillator in patients with coronary disease at high risk for ventricular arrhythmia. Multicenter Automatic Defibrillator Implantation Trial. N Engl J Med 1996;335:1933–1940.
29. Adjusted-dose warfarin versus low-intensity, fixed-dose warfarin plus aspirin for high-risk patients with atrial fibrillation: Stroke Prevention in Atrial Fibrillation III randomised clinical trial. Lancet 1996;348:633–638.
30. Brann WB, Bennett LE, Keck BM, Hosenpud JD: Morbidity, functional status, and immunosuppressive therapy after heart transplantation: An analysis of the Joint International Society for Heart and Lung Transplantation/United Network for Organ Sharing Thoracic Registry. J Heart Lung Transplant 1998;17:374–382.
31. Miller LW, Kubo SH, Young JB, et al: Report of the Consensus Conference on Candidate Selection for Heart Transplantation—1993. J Heart Lung Transplant 1995;14:562–571.
32. Goldstein DJ, Oz MC, Rose EA: Medical progress: Implantable left ventricular assist devices. N Engl J Med 1998;339:1522–1533.
33. Bach DS, Bolling SF: Improvement following correction of secondary mitral regurgitation in end-stage cardiomyopathy with mitral annuloplasty. Am J Cardiol 1996;78:966–969.
34. Rich MW Beckham V, Wittenberg C, et al: A multidisciplinary intervention to prevent the readmission of elderly patients with congestive heart failure. N Engl J Med 1995;333:1190–1195.
35. Gottlieb SS, Skettmo SL, Wolff A, et al: Effects of BG 971 (CUT-124), an A1-adenosine antagonist, and furosemide on glomerular filtration rate and natriuresis in patients with congestive heart failure. J Am Coll Cardiol 2000;35:56–59.
36. Rademaker MT, Fitzpatrick MA, Charles CJ, et al: Comparison of chronic neutral endopeptidase inhibition and furosemide in an ovine model of heart failure. J Cardiovasc Pharmacol 1996;27:439–446.
37. Conte G, Bellizzi V, Cianciaruso B, et al: Physiologic role and diuretic efficacy of atrial natriuretic peptide in health and chronic renal disease. Kidney Int 1997;59 (Suppl): S28–32.
38. De Zeeuw D, Janssen WMT, de Jong PE: Atrial natriuretic factor: Its (patho)physiological significance in humans. Kidney Int 1992;41:1115–1133.
39. The SOLVD Investigators: Effect of enalapril on mortality and the development of heart failure in asymptomatic patients with reduced left ventricular ejection fractions. N Engl J Med 1992;327:685–691.
40. Cohn JN, Ziesche S, Smith R, et al: Effect of the calcium antagonist felodipine as supplementary vasodilator therapy in patients with chronic heart failure treated with enalapril: V-HeFT III. Circulation 1997;96:856–863.

# ■ RECOMMENDED READING

Konstam MA, Dracup K, Baker DW, et al: Heart Failure: Evaluation and Care of Patients with Left Ventricular Systolic Dysfunction. Clinical Practice Guideline No. 11. AHCPR publication No. 94-0612. Rockville, Md: Agency for Health Care Policy and Research, 1994.

*Chapter* 21

# Congenital Heart Disease

*Julien I. E. Hoffman*

Considering the complexity of the embryonic development of the heart, it is not surprising that major developmental anomalies of the cardiovascular system occur in 10% to 20% of fetuses. Most anomalies are associated with chromosomal abnormalities and have a high mortality rate early in pregnancy; so these account for only 5% to 8% of congenital heart disease (CHD) in the neonate. A few congenital anomalies are associated with single gene defects, for example, Holt-Oram (hypoplasia of the radius, and atrial [ASD] or ventricular septal defect [VSD]) and Noonan (webbed neck, short stature, ptosis, pulmonic stenosis, and hypertrophic cardiomyopathy) syndromes. Most of the rest are due to the interplay of genetic abnormalities with environmental factors or chance, although a few are attributable to teratogens like alcohol, lithium, and retinoic acid.

At birth, about 3% of term infants have a tiny muscular VSD; almost all of these close spontaneously by age 1 year, and few pose clinical problems. Another 2% to 3% have a bicuspid, but not stenotic, aortic valve. These seldom cause problems in childhood, but they can calcify or degenerate in middle age or late adult life. About 1% of live-born children have classic types of CHD: left-to-right shunts in 60% to 70%, obstructive lesions without shunts in about 15%, and right-to left shunts in 20% to 25%, who are usually cyanotic.[1] A fourth group has become prominent, namely, congenital lesions of the coronary artery origins (Table 21–1).

## ■ LEFT-TO-RIGHT SHUNT LESIONS

### Pretricuspid Shunts

Shunting occurs left to right across the atrial defect or through the anomalous pulmonary veins when the right ventricle becomes more distensible than the left ventricle a few weeks after birth (Fig. 21–1). With a large shunt (pulmonary blood flow more than twice systemic blood flow), the right atrium and ventricle become enlarged and hyperactive. Clinically this is manifested by a large excursion and rapid pulsation over the lower left sternal border (due to the large stroke volume) and is demonstrated by imaging techniques and increased pulmonary arterial markings on chest x-ray films. No murmur occurs across the atrial defect because low flow velocity across a large opening does not cause turbulence, but the large pulmonary blood volume causes a moderately loud systolic pulmonic ejection murmur. A tricuspid mid-diastolic rumble may also be heard. Pulmonary arterial

Table 21–1

## Incidence of Congenital Heart Disease

| Lesion | Incidence* per Million Live Births (% of All CHD)‡ | Relative Frequency in Adults |
|---|---|---|
| **A. Left-to-right shunts** | | |
| 1. Pretricuspid | | |
| Atrial septal defect | 563 (9) | Common |
| Atrioventricular septal defect (partial) | 84 (5) | Uncommon |
| Partial anomalous pulmonary venous connection | ? | |
| 2. Postricuspid | | |
| Ventricular septal defect | 2267 (38) | Common |
| Patent ductus arteriosus | 471 (8) | Common |
| Atrioventricular septal defect (complete) | 200 (3) | Rare |
| **B. Pure obstructive lesions** | | |
| Pulmonic stenosis | 404 (7) | Common |
| Aortic stenosis | 284 (5) | Common |
| Coarctation of the aorta | 332 (6) | Common |
| **C. Right-to-left shunts (cyanotic)** | | |
| Transposition of the great arteries | 327 (5) | Very rare |
| Tetralogy of Fallot | 311 (5) | Rare + |
| Persistent truncus arteriosus | 86 (1) | Rare |
| Hypoplastic left heart (aortic, mitral atresia) | 230 (4) | Very rare |
| Hypoplastic right heart (tricuspid, pulmonary atresia) | 171 (3) | Rare |
| Double-inlet left ventricle (single ventricle) | 87 (1) | Rare + |
| Double-outlet right ventricle | 79 (1) | Rare |
| Total anomalous pulmonary venous connection | 53 (1) | Rare |
| **D. Coronary artery anomalies** | | |
| Left main coronary artery from pulmonary artery | ? | Rare |
| Left main coronary artery from right sinus of Valsalva | ? | Rare |
| Right main coronary artery from left sinus of Valsalva | ? | Rare |

*Median incidence from several studies of the incidence of CHD.
‡Figures in parentheses are percentages of the lesions shown in the table; excludes miscellaneous lesions and combinations of several lesions.
Rare+, rare in adults but still more common than other rare forms of CHD.

pressures are usually normal (see Fig. 21–1C), so pulmonic closure is not loud; however, the increased right ventricular output produces the characteristic wide, fixed, split, second heart sound that must always be sought. In ostium primum defects (partial AVSD), there may be a murmur of mitral incompetence and sometimes of a small VSD.

Patients with a secundum ASD or partial anomalous pulmonary veins are usually asymptomatic. For this reason, their lesions may not be diagnosed in childhood, and those with an ASD are one of the largest groups of patients with CHD seen by adult cardiologists. If a large ASD is not closed, the patient may develop congestive heart failure or pulmonary vascular disease, usually after 20 years of age.[2] Late onset of mitral incompetence can occur, as can thrombosis of large pulmonary arteries. Patients with a large ASD are at risk of severe atrial arrhythmias, and a few suffer stroke from paradoxical embolism. Therefore, any patient with a large ASD (i.e., one that causes right ventricular dilatation) needs prophylactic closure, either surgically or by one of the experimental catheter-inserted closure devices.

A patient with a small ASD is probably at risk only from paradoxical embolism. Catheter closure of the ASD may someday be the recommended treatment for these.

Patients with partial AVSD usually develop severe arrhythmias or congestive

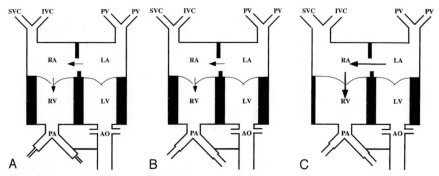

**Figure 21–1** ▪ Diagram to show why pulmonary arterial pressures are low with a large left-to-right atrial shunt. *(A)* At birth, both ventricles are equally thick and have similar distensibilities. Thus even with a large ASD, the shunt is small *(short, thin arrow)*. *(B)* After 1 to 2 weeks, pulmonary vascular resistance and pressure have fallen, but the ventricles still have similar thickness and distensibility. The shunt remains small. *(C)* After a few months, the right ventricular (RV) wall has become thinner than the left ventricular (LV) wall, and the RV is now more distensible. Therefore, in diastole the RV can accept more blood than can the LV, and a large shunt *(longer, thicker arrow)* occurs in association with the low pulmonary arterial (PA) pressure. In other words, in an ASD, the shunt is pulled from the left (LA) to the right atrium (RA), whereas, in a VSD, the shunt is pushed from LV to RV. (Note that, with a big ASD, there is no pressure gradient between the atria to push the blood across the defect.) SVC, IVC, superior and inferior vena cava; PV, pulmonary vein; AO, aorta.

heart failure early in adult life and need surgical repair, which usually has low operative mortality and produces fairly good long-term results. Mitral valve reoperations may be needed later, however.

## Post-tricuspid Shunts

The degree of shunting and its effect on heart and lungs depend on the size of the defect between the two circulations and the pulmonary vascular resistance. If the defect is small (e.g., VSD or patent ductus arteriosus (PDA) smaller than 3 mm in diameter), there is only a small left-to-right shunt (Fig. 21–2A, B). The patient has no symptoms. Apart from the distinctive murmur, the heart and lungs are normal on clinical, radiologic, and electrocardiographic (ECG) examination. The echocardiogram confirms the small shunt, normal right ventricular and pulmonary arterial systolic pressures, and normal chamber sizes.

If the defect is large (i.e., about the diameter of the aortic annulus), the left-to-right shunt is huge once pulmonary vascular resistance decreases (Fig. 21–2C, D) and right ventricular and pulmonary arterial systolic pressures are systemic. Most of these patients have severe congestive heart failure in early infancy. Both left and right ventricles are hyperactive (increased rapid excursion of the ventricle) because of the huge stroke volumes and are dilated and hypertrophic on clinical examination and by chest radiography, ECG, and echocardiography. The pulmonic component of the second heart sound is loud because of pulmonary arterial hypertension. The large diastolic flow across the mitral valve produces a mid-diastolic rumble at the apex. With complete atrioventricular septal defect (AVSDc) (also termed *endocardial cushion defect* or *common atrioventricular canal*), because of the associated left-to-right atrial shunt there is often a mid-diastolic rumble over the tricuspid valve as well, and the second heart sound has the wide, fixed, split characteristic of ASD. Chest films show not only cardiomegaly but a marked increase in pulmonary

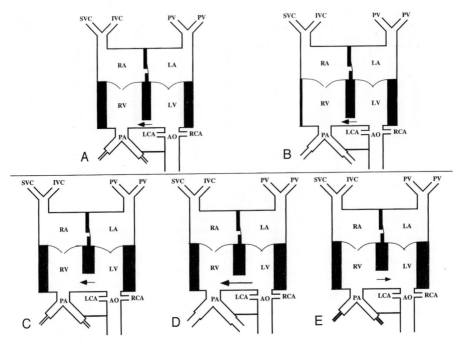

**Figure 21–2** ■ Diagram of effects of size of defect and pulmonary vascular resistance on posttricuspid left-to-right shunt, exemplified by a VSD. With a small VSD, there is a small shunt at birth *(A)* and at any later age *(B)*. With a large VSD, because soon after birth *(C)* the pulmonary vascular resistance is high (indicated by narrow peripheral pulmonary arteries), the shunt is small *(short arrow)*. After several weeks *(D)*, the lower pulmonary vascular resistance (wider peripheral vessels) allows a large shunt (long arrow). *(E)* A secondary rise in pulmonary vascular resistance (narrower and thicker peripheral vessels) may eventually cause a right-to-left shunt. SVC, IVC, superior and inferior vena cava; PV, pulmonary vein; RA, LA, right and left atrium; RV, LV, right and left ventricle; PA, pulmonary artery; AO, aorta; LCA, RCA, left and right coronary artery.

vascular markings secondary to widening of the peripheral pulmonary arteries from the increased flow.

Defects of intermediate size produce moderate left-to-right shunts and pulmonary arterial systolic pressures less than half of systemic levels. Symptoms vary from mild fatigue and dyspnea on exertion to moderate congestive heart failure. The left ventricle, with its increased stroke volume, is hyperactive, dilated, and hypertrophic. The right ventricle can be (1) normal with PDA, and pulmonary arterial pressures can be low when the shunt does not pass through the right ventricle, (2) hyperactive and moderately dilated in the VSD with low pulmonary arterial pressures because the shunt goes from the left to the right ventricle and then to the pulmonary artery, or (3) forceful and hypertrophic with either lesion if there is pulmonary hypertension. The second heart sound may be loud, and a soft mid-diastolic murmur may be audible at the apex. Pulmonary vascular markings are moderately increased.

If pulmonary vascular resistance is high, there is only a small left-to-right shunt—and, sometimes, none—no matter how large the defect (see Fig. 21–2E); there may even be right-to-left shunting. The left ventricle is normal, but the right ventricle has a forceful lift owing to right ventricular systolic hypertension. Pulmonic closure is very loud, and there may be an early systolic ejection click. There is no middiastolic rumble, but there may be in early diastole a high-pitched blowing murmur of pulmonic incompetence along the left sternal border (Graham Steele murmur). The chest radiograph shows a rounded and enlarged right ventricle and large central pulmonary arteries with sparse narrow peripheral arteries ("tree in winter" appearance). The ECG shows pure right ventricular hypertrophy. The site of the defect is shown by echocardiography.

These features are common to all posttricuspid shunts. Each lesion, however, has certain distinctive differences, discussed below.

## Ventricular Septal Defect

After infancy, about 85% of VSD are perimembranous (i.e., in the region of the membranous septum just under the aortic and tricuspid valves), and another 5% to 10% are in the muscular septum. At both sites, spontaneous closure is common. A few are in inlet VSD, under the tricuspid valve; these are always large, never close spontaneously, and need surgical closure early in infancy. Others are in the outflow tract, just below the pulmonary valves. These are called *supracristal* or *doubly committed subarterial defects*. Because this defect leaves the aortic valve cusp (noncoronary or sometimes right coronary cusp) unsupported, the cusp prolapses into the defect and partly occludes it so that the left-to-right shunt is small even though the VSD is usually large. There is a tendency for progressive prolapse of the valve cusp and aortic insufficiency; eventually, the cusp may be damaged and need replacement. This site for the VSD occurs in about 5% of whites and blacks but in about 35% of Chinese and Japanese. Because of the risk of aortic valve damage with this lesion, in every patient with VSD it is essential to localize the defect by careful echocardiographic investigation.

A tiny VSD (smaller than 2 mm diameter) has a soft, high-pitched systolic murmur localized to the lower left sternal border. A small VSD has a typical harsh, loud systolic murmur, usually pansystolic and heard best at the left lower sternal border but occasionally ejection in type. It may be heard at the upper left sternal border if the VSD is in the outflow tract, but this is not a reliable sign. The first heart sound is obscured by the murmur. The patient with a medium-sized or large VSD has the same typical harsh pansystolic murmur; the size of the VSD and the amount of shunting must be judged not on the murmur but on the activity of the heart and the precordium. With a large VSD and high pulmonary vascular resistance, the systolic murmur becomes soft and short because there is little left-to-right shunting across a large defect and a right-to-left shunt across the VSD produces little or no murmur.

Because about 70% of VSD, even large ones, close spontaneously, initial treatment is conservative. Small defects warrant only prophylaxis against infective endocarditis. Larger, symptomatic defects usually respond to digoxin, diuretics, afterload reduction, and maintenance of normal hemoglobin concentration. The few patients in whom therapy fails have surgical closure of the VSD, an operation with very low operative mortality and excellent outcome. Patients often exhibit clinical improvement about 1 year of age. This change may be due either to a decrease in VSD size or to early pulmonary vascular disease, and it is cause for concern and investigation. A few patients have large shunts and low pulmonary arterial pressures with minimal symptoms if any. If their defects do not close spontaneously in a few years, the VSD should be closed surgically to preserve optimal ventricular function.

## Patent Ductus Arteriosus

Persistent patent ductus arteriosus has a typical continuous "machinery" or "train in a tunnel" murmur usually heard best below the left clavicle. The size of the PDA and the amount of shunting are determined, not from the continuous murmur but from the loudness of the second heart sound, and evidence of left ventricular dilatation and hypertrophy on clinical, radiologic, ECG, and echocardiographic examination. The defects are usually closed to prevent heart failure and pulmonary vascular disease (with big shunts) and infective endocarditis (with small shunts). Defects smaller than 5 mm in diameter are closed at cardiac catheterization by coils or other devices, or sometimes by thoracoscopic procedures. Large defects are closed surgically by open thoracotomy. Outcome after surgery is essentially normal.

## Complete Atrioventricular Septal Defect

Because complete AVSD combines atrial- and ventricular-level shunting as well as mitral and tricuspid regurgitation, it has the features of both a VSD (above) and a secundum ASD. There is marked right atrial and biventricular enlargement and murmurs consistent with mitral and tricuspid regurgitation and a ventricular septal defect. The huge volume load on both ventricles produces severe congestive heart failure in early infancy, independent of any decrease in pulmonary vascular resistance. The major diagnostic feature is a left superior axis deviation of the QRS complex, between $-60°$ and $-180°$, with a counterclockwise frontal plane loop. Echocardiography demonstrates the ASD and VSD and the common atrioventricular valve shared by the mitral and tricuspid orifices.

Most of these patients have huge volume loads early in life and develop congestive heart failure—and often pulmonary vascular disease—by a few months after birth. They do not survive long without surgery. Surgery involves closing the atrial and ventricular defects and repairing the cleft atrioventricular valves. Late valve problems or even reoperation is relatively common, and complete atrioventricular block may occur.

## Pulmonary Vascular Disease

Anyone with a large left-to-right shunt (alone or in addition to a right-to-left shunt) may develop pulmonary vascular disease. If pulmonary arterial pressure is high, the small pulmonary arteries become thicker owing to increased smooth medial muscle that extends farther down the vascular tree than is normal for children.[3, 4] The high pulmonary blood flow produces abnormal shear forces on the endothelial cells. A local elastase is activated that damages the internal elastic lamina of the small pulmonary arteries.[5] Endothelial dysfunction is followed by aggregation of platelets and macrophages with release of cytokines, which pass into the media. They induce the smooth muscle cells to transform into fibroblast-like cells that migrate into and thicken the intima, thus narrowing the lumen. These cells secrete a hyalinized, collagen-like material that eventually replaces them. Finally, the small arteries become occluded. Growth of new pulmonary arteries after birth is also inhibited, so that not only are the small arteries narrowed or occluded, but eventually there may be as few as a third the normal number.

These changes begin during the first year of life except in ASD, when they are rare before age 20 years. Once the changes start, they are progressive, although surgical closure of the defect before age 2 years may prevent newly formed vessels from being damaged.

As pulmonary vascular disease progresses, the pulmonary vascular resistance rises and the left-to-right shunt is reduced and finally becomes a right-to-left shunt (Eisenmenger's syndrome). At this stage, closure of the defect is dangerous. Even if the patient survives surgery, the high fixed pulmonary vascular resistance cannot allow increased flow out of the right ventricle with increased venous return (as in exercise). Thus, if there is no defect to allow decompression of the right ventricle, acute right ventricular dilatation, heart failure, or fatal arrhythmias can occur. Furthermore, the increased right ventricular muscle mass demands a high volume of myocardial blood flow, so any decrease in aortic pressure can cause acute right ventricular failure and arrhythmias. At this stage, only lung transplantation avails. These patients are cyanotic, but often do well until the third or fourth decades.[6] Death is either sudden (presumably from arrhythmia) or the result of congestive heart failure in the majority, but a few die from hemoptysis or brain abscess. Death during pregnancy is common, and affected women are advised against becoming pregnant.[7, 8]

## ■ OBSTRUCTIVE LESIONS

### Valvar Pulmonic Stenosis

In a few patients, pulmonic stenosis (PS) is severe in utero, the right ventricle is usually hypoplastic, and the patient is cyanotic because the small right ventricle cannot accept the whole venous return, some of which shunts right to left across the foramen ovale. Early relief of the obstruction by surgery or balloon valvotomy is effective. Most of these patients, however, have more moderate stenosis. They have varying degrees of right ventricular hypertrophy which produces a forceful lift at the left lower sternal border and typical changes in the ECG and chest films. The pulmonic component of the second heart sound is delayed (wide split second heart sound) and may be softer than normal, but the split varies during respiration. There is usually at the upper left sternal border an early systolic ejection click that may vary with respiration; this click is associated with poststenotic dilatation of the pulmonary artery. There is a characteristic harsh ejection murmur. As the stenosis becomes more severe, it takes the right ventricle longer to eject its stroke volume, so that the murmur gets longer and its peak shifts toward the second sound. The frequency of the murmur increases, because flow velocity must be higher to force the normal stroke volume through a narrowed orifice. These changes give reliable estimates of severity, which can be confirmed by echocardiography. Sometimes, secondary infundibular hypertrophy increases the obstruction. Those with substantial right ventricular hypertrophy can have the valve opened by balloon valvotomy, which is as effective as surgery and has replaced it (unless the valve is dysplastic). Long-term results are excellent.

### Valvar Aortic Stenosis

A few children have severe aortic stenosis in utero, their left ventricle is hypoplastic, and they become critically ill soon after birth. Valvotomy by open operation or balloon valvotomy may help, but in some the left ventricle is so small that a single ventricle repair (Norwood operation) is needed. The majority are asymptomatic. They have a typical ejection murmur that may be maximal anywhere between the apex and the upper right sternal border. There is in the same region an early systolic ejection click that does not vary with respiration. The second heart sound is usually normal, but for reasons that are not clear the first heart sound is soft if the stenosis is severe. Left ventricular hypertrophy may be palpable and visible on ECG, but palpation, murmur, and the ECG are all unreliable for determining severity. Inversion of T waves in left chest leads with exercise predicts severity, but false-negative results occur. The only effective noninvasive test is echocardiography, which should be done at least yearly to follow these patients. Annual exercise testing may also be warranted.

Balloon valvotomy can be done effectively if there is not much associated aortic incompetence, and it has the advantage of easy repeatability. Unfortunately, the aortic valve is usually bicuspid or monocuspid, and recurrence of the obstruction after valvotomy is the rule. Eventually, the valve may have to be replaced because of calcification or severe aortic incompetence. It is usually replaced with an aortic homograft, sometimes by a mechanical valve, and, with increasing frequency today, by the Ross procedure, in which the native pulmonary valve is moved to the aorta and a homograft is used in place of the pulmonary valve. Early surgical results for all of these are good, but fewer than 25% of patients go 25 years without having another valvotomy, valve replacement, congestive heart failure, or infective endocarditis (which is more common after than before valvotomy).

Bicuspid aortic valves without stenosis, the commonest congenital heart lesion, may be asymptomatic for many decades but carry the risk of infective endocarditis. Most eventually calcify and become obstructive, often over 1 to 2 years, or deteriorate and produce aortic incompetence.

## Subaortic Stenosis

Occasionally there is a membranous, fibrous, or fibromuscular ring just below the aortic valve, a lesion that can be isolated or associated with other lesions, especially VSD. There is often associated aortic incompetence, perhaps because of damage from the high-velocity jet through the stenosis. Clinically, these lesions resemble valvar aortic stenosis, and echocardiography is needed to distinguish them. Balloon valvotomy is less useful than in valvar stenosis, and surgical excision may be needed. Complete removal of the obstruction is difficult because the stenosis involves the septal leaflet of the mitral valve, and recurrences are common.

## Supravalvar Aortic Stenosis

Supravalvar stenosis is rare and often is associated with Williams syndrome (infantile hypercalcemia, mental retardation, elfin facies). The stenosis may resemble an hourglass or be long and diffuse; it can narrow coronary ostia. The features resemble those of valvar aortic stenosis but with no ejection click. Frequently, systolic blood pressure is about 15 mm Hg higher in the right arm than in the left one because of the direction of the jet coming through the stenosis. When the lesion is severe, surgical repair is indicated.

## Coarctation of the Aorta

Coarctation of the aorta is a localized narrowing of the aorta just beyond the left subclavian artery. Some infants have critical obstruction with congestive heart failure and shock and need early removal of the obstruction. Most are asymptomatic, although some have congestive heart failure and a few have intermittent claudication. The main features are hypertension in the upper body with decreased pulses and pressures in the legs. Often, diastolic pressures are similar in arms and legs but systolic pressures differ markedly. Most patients have palpable collateral arteries around the scapula. Left ventricular hypertrophy is evident clinically and on ECG. A systolic or continuous murmur is heard best in the middle of the back, and sometimes, for unknown reasons, there is a mid-diastolic rumble at the apex even though there is no mitral stenosis. On chest films, the ascending aorta is dilated, as is the descending aorta below the constricted site of the coarctation; the hourglass pattern shows up as the 3 sign on plain films and the E sign on barium swallow. Confirmation by echocardiography should include demonstration of delayed acceleration of flow in the descending aorta by Doppler study.

Coarctation frequently is missed in childhood, and it accounts for a large proportion of adult patients with CHD. If it goes untreated, patients die prematurely from congestive heart failure, cerebral vascular accidents (especially subarachnoid hemorrhage), infective endocarditis, rupture of the aorta, or premature coronary artery disease.[9] Some experts treat the coarctation by balloon dilatation, but others, who are concerned about the small risks of early aortic rupture or late aneurysm formation, resect the narrowed region surgically. About 50% of these patients have a bicuspid aortic valve and need prophylaxis against infective endocarditis, even after successful repair of the coarctation.

## ■ RIGHT-TO-LEFT SHUNTS (CYANOTIC HEART DISEASE)

The commonest right-to-left shunts are transposition of the great arteries (d-TGA) and tetralogy of Fallot (with or without pulmonary atresia), which each account for 4% to 5% of classical CHD. Then there are double-outlet right ventricle (DORV), tricuspid atresia, pulmonary atresia with intact ventricular septum, truncus arteriosus, total anomalous pulmonary venous connection (TAPVC), single ventricle, hypoplastic left heart syndromes, and a collection of rarities. The relative frequency of these lesions is shown in Table 21–1, and the main ones are diagrammed in Figure 21–3.

These lesions have four main physiologic presentations:

1. Some have greatly decreased pulmonary blood flow because little blood enters the pulmonary arteries; examples are tricuspid or pulmonary atresia, severe tetralogy of Fallot or single ventricle with pulmonic stenosis, and severe Ebstein anomaly (downward displacement of one or two tricuspid valve leaflets into the right ventricle, resulting in a small right ventricle, tricuspid regurgitation, and usually a right-to-left atrial shunt). Because little or no blood passes directly from right ventricle to pulmonary arteries, pulmonary blood flow depends on the ductus arteriosus, which in these lesions is narrow and closes soon after birth. These infants are deeply cyanotic, acidotic, and hypoglycemic and die soon unless surgery is done to increase pulmonary blood flow. The heart is quiet to feel, although there may be a forceful right ventricular impulse. The chest x-ray shows oligemic lung fields.

    An important subgroup includes those with TGA. Pulmonary blood flow is normal, but, because the pulmonary artery arises from the left ventricle, it receives blood that has already been oxygenated. Only the small amount of systemic venous blood that crosses the ductus arteriosus and the foramen ovale can be oxygenated. Affected children are physiologically similar to those already described, but, on chest films the pulmonary vascular markings are normal or even slightly increased.

2. Some have left-to-right shunts, in addition, and have greatly increased pulmonary blood flow. Examples are transposition of the great arteries with VSD, truncus arteriosus, single ventricle without pulmonic stenosis, and total anomalous pulmonary venous return without obstruction. These children usually present in congestive heart failure with minimal cyanosis and hyperactive hearts from the large stroke volumes, and on chest films the lung fields are plethoric.

3. Some infants have total anomalous pulmonary venous connection with obstruction of pulmonary venous return. They have pulmonary edema and decreased pulmonary blood flow. The edema produces marked tachypnea

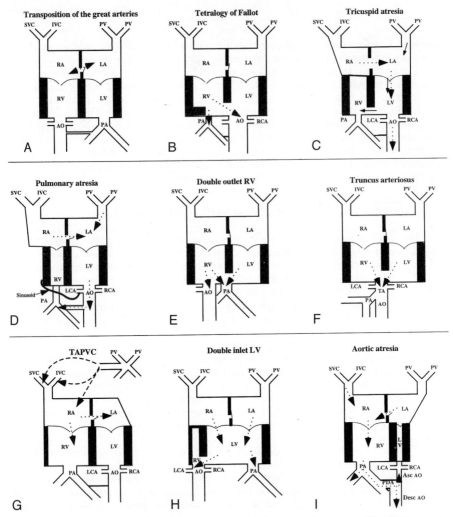

**Figure 21–3** ▪ Forms of cyanotic heart disease. *(A) d*-Transposition of the great arteries, showing small bidirectional atrial shunt and closing ductus arteriosus (PDA). *(B)* Tetralogy of Fallot with severe infundibular pulmonary stenosis and small pulmonary annulus and arteries. Other patients have complete pulmonary atresia. *(C)* Tricuspid atresia with small right ventricle. Small arrows show that pulmonary blood flow is less profuse than systemic flow *(large arrows)*. These arrows do not indicate the saturations of the bloodstreams. *(D)* Pulmonary atresia with an intact ventricular septum. Right ventricle is small but hypertrophic (owing to suprasystemic systolic pressure). About half of these patients have sinusoids conducting blood from the right ventricle to one or both coronary arteries. Pulmonary blood flow comes via the ductus arteriosus. *(E)* One form of double outlet right ventricle (DORV) with pulmonary artery related to the VSD. Only one coronary artery is shown, for clarity. *(F)* Truncus arteriosus, in which aorta, pulmonary arteries, and coronary arteries all come off a single great artery at the base of the heart. There is a VSD. *(G)* Total anomalous pulmonary venous connection in which all the pulmonary veins join to form a single venous trunk, which enters the heart via the superior vena cava, inferior vena cava (usually via the portal vein), or the right atrium, directly or via the coronary sinus. All systemic flow has to pass from right (RA) to left atrium (LA) through the foramen ovale. *(H)* The most common form of single ventricle, a double inlet left ventricle. There is no true right ventricle, only a rudimentary outflow tract chamber that receives blood from the single ventricle through a bulboventricular foramen and conducts it to a levo-transposed aorta. *(I)* The most common form of hypoplastic left heart with aortic atresia. The left ventricle is tiny or may be absent. All systemic blood comes via the ductus arteriosus, including coronary arterial blood, which flows retrograde through a very hypoplastic ascending aorta. SVC, IVC, superior and inferior vena cava; PV, pulmonary vein; RA, LA, right and left atrium; RV, LV, right and left ventricle; AO, aorta; PA, pulmonary artery; RCA, LCA, right and left coronary artery; Asc, ascending; Desc, descending.

and retractions, basal rales, and classical edema on chest films. Early relief of the obstruction is life saving.

4. A few patients who would otherwise be in group 2 (increased pulmonary blood flow) have moderate pulmonic stenosis that prevents gross hyperperfusion of the lungs; examples are (1) TGA with a VSD and PS or (2) a single ventricle with some PS. Patients are cyanotic but are not in congestive heart failure. They are most likely of all persons with cyanotic heart disease to survive into adult life without treatment.

## ■ CORONARY ARTERIAL ANOMALIES

Although rare, coronary artery anomalies are potentially fatal but are treatable if diagnosed. There are many variations, but three are the most important.[10]

**1. Anomalous origin of the left coronary artery from the pulmonary artery.** The right coronary artery comes normally from the right sinus of Valsalva, but the left one comes from the pulmonary artery, usually the main stem. There is no problem during fetal life, because both arteries supply blood at normal pressures and with similar oxygen saturations. After birth, when pulmonary vascular resistance decreases, the left ventricle cannot be perfused from the low-pressure left coronary artery, but it receives some blood from collaterals from the right coronary artery. The low pulmonary arterial pressure diverts some of the collateral flow into the pulmonary artery (coronary steal). Perfusion of the left ventricle becomes inadequate, and an anterolateral infarction occurs after a few weeks of age. These patients usually present with congestive heart failure in infancy, but some are asymptomatic until adult life. When this condition is diagnosed in an adult—after investigation of ischemic symptoms or accidentally—the patient should be treated, because sudden death is common. The best treatment is surgical implantation of the anomalous artery into the aortic root.

**2. Anomalous origin of the left coronary artery from the right sinus of Valsalva.** In the commonest congenital coronary anomaly, the left coronary artery may reach the left ventricle by passing through the ventricular septum, behind the aorta, running over the right ventricular outflow tract, or passing between the aorta and the main pulmonary artery. The last configuration is cause for concern, because it often leads to sudden death. Patients at risk are almost always adolescent athletes. They may have warning episodes of ischemic pain, faintness, or syncope during or just after strenuous exercise, but the first episode may end in sudden death. Why symptoms do not occur at an earlier age is not known. Not only is the distal course of the artery abnormal, but its proximal intramural course through the aortic wall may be narrowed and a flap of tissue may partly cover the ostium. There are usually no distinguishing physical findings or ECG changes. Echocardiography may show the abnormal course of the artery, but false-negative findings have been reported. The safest diagnostic test is imaging by ultrafast computed tomography (CT) or magnetic resonance imaging, although coronary angiography—performed by an experienced cardiologist—is also useful. Treatment by surgical implantation into the left sinus of Valsalva is curative.

**3. Anomalous origin of the right coronary artery from the left sinus of Valsalva.** In this lesion, which is only about one tenth as common as the anomaly of the left coronary artery, the right coronary arteries always run between the two great vessels and may show narrowing of their aortic intramural portion and a flap over the origin. The signs and symptoms are those described earlier for anomalous origin of the left coronary artery from the right sinus of Valsalva, and diagnosis is made by the imaging tests described earlier. Surgical treatment to reimplant the artery is warranted.

## Principles of Treatment

Medical treatment of cyanotic heart disease is never curative. Most infants with serious congenital heart disease can have "corrective" surgery within the first few weeks or months of life. Waiting too long (more than 2 to 3 months) risks severe pulmonary vascular disease for patients with voluminous pulmonary blood flow.

For the few cyanotic patients whose lesion is inoperable, it is important to prevent iron deficiency anemia, which can lead to cerebral thrombosis because of the increased rigidity of iron-deficient red blood cells. On the other hand, if the hematocrit rises over 65%, the increased viscosity of blood not only predisposes to thromboses but also reduces oxygen delivery to tissues.[11] Some patients need periodic phlebotomy with volume replacement by saline or albumin solution.[12] Apart from thromboses, these patients are at risk for brain abscess because some organisms in the bloodstream escape being filtered in the lungs. Unexplained fever and headache, even without neurologic signs, are indications for computed tomography of the head. Bleeding problems, especially nosebleeds, may follow thrombocytopenia secondary to platelet consumption from low-grade thromboses or to erythropoietic overcrowding of the bone marrow. Precautions against bleeding may be necessary during surgery.

## Transposition of the Great Arteries

TGA is the most common type of cyanotic heart disease (see Table 21–1). By definition, this kind of *transposition* means that the aorta comes from the right ventricle and the pulmonary artery from the left ventricle; the ventriculoarterial connections are discordant. Because the aorta is usually to the right and anterior to the pulmonary artery, the term *d-TGA* is used, where *d* stands for *dextro*. About two thirds have only a small PDA and a foramen ovale; the remainder have a VSD, with or without pulmonic stenosis (Fig. 21–3A). The former group are treated immediately after birth by balloon atrial septostomy to open up the atrial septum and then, within 1 to 6 weeks, by complete repair. Originally, the repair was by Mustard or Senning procedure, in which an atrial baffle was placed to direct systemic venous blood to the left ventricle and thence to the lungs and to direct the pulmonary venous return to the right ventricle and thence to the aorta. Mortality was negligible, but the operation fell out of favor. The extensive atrial suture lines led to atrial arrhythmia (often severe atrial flutter or fibrillation) or else damaged the sinus node, so that, by 10 years after surgery, fewer than 50% of the patients were still in sinus rhythm. Furthermore, many patients developed right ventricular dysfunction and tricuspid incompetence, which, because of the atrial baffle, caused pulmonary venous hypertension. Surgeons therefore began to treat these patients with an "arterial switch." Moving the aorta and pulmonary arteries is relatively easy, but the coronary arteries have to be detached from the aortic root and implanted into the pulmonic root (now the new aortic root). This maneuver is not always easy, and many of the complications of surgery are due to early or late myocardial ischemia. To date, 10- to 15-year follow-up after the arterial switch shows excellent results, though occasionally supravalvar pulmonic or aortic stenosis develops at the suture line and some patients need coronary artery bypass surgery.

Infants with d-TGA and a VSD have early congestive heart failure with minimal cyanosis, and unless pulmonary blood flow and pressure are reduced before age 3 months, irreversible pulmonary vascular disease develops. They can usually be repaired, with little risk, by an arterial switch.

A few patients with d-TGA have VSD and PS (usually subpulmonic). Because the pulmonary vessels are protected by the PS, patients have neither congestive heart failure nor pulmonary vascular disease and so account for a fair proportion of the untreated cyanotic patients who present to adult clinics. Patients whose PS is not resectable are not candidates for an arterial switch, because they would then be left with subaortic stenosis. Options are (1) an atrial baffle with closure of the VSD and (2) some form of complex intraventricular tunneling to lead blood from the left ventricle to the aorta, combined with an extracardiac conduit to lead blood from the right ventricle to the pulmonary artery.

## Tetralogy of Fallot

Tetralogy of Fallot has the best "untreated natural history" of any cyanotic heart disease and, so, is the most common form of untreated cyanotic heart disease seen in adult clinics. The abnormality consists of a large VSD, right ventricular outflow tract obstruction due to infundibular and sometimes valvar PS, an overriding aorta, and right ventricular hypertrophy (see Fig. 21–3B). The right ventricular outflow tract is narrowed, and sometimes the main points of obstruction are a small pulmonary annulus and small peripheral pulmonary arteries, often with peripheral stenoses. The extent of obstruction varies greatly.

Definitive treatment is resection of the hypertrophic infundibular muscle, opening of stenotic valvar commissures, cutting across and patching of a small annulus, and closure of the VSD. At one time, this was preceded by a palliative systemic artery–pulmonary artery shunt, but, today, initial complete repairs can almost always be done before age 6 months. Results of surgery are good but not perfect. A small residual VSD is more a nuisance than a severe problem; however, many patients with annular patches have marked pulmonic incompetence, with resulting right ventricular dilatation. When the incompetence is severe or produces congestive heart failure, a homograft or prosthetic pulmonary valve needs to be inserted.

After surgery some patients develop complete atrioventricular block and then need a pacemaker. Of more concern are sequelae of ventricular tachycardia or (occasionally) sudden death. Prediction of the risk of sudden death is poor; the best predictor is a QRS duration longer than 0.18 seconds plus marked pulmonic incompetence, but many without these abnormalities die suddenly. Prophylactic antiarrhythmic agents have not been useful.

One variant of tetralogy has associated pulmonary atresia. Initially, pulmonary blood flow is maintained through a ductus arteriosus, but the patient soon needs an aortopulmonary shunt for better flow. Because the right ventricle is of normal size, a conduit from RV to pulmonary artery can establish pulmonary blood flow. The principal problem is that the pulmonary arteries are usually small and may supply only parts of the lungs, the remainder being supplied by large collaterals from the aorta. Often, the surgeon can detach these collaterals from the aorta and create anastomoses to the native pulmonary arteries; the procedure is termed unifocalization. These collaterals often have stenoses, and postoperative balloon dilatation with stent placement is often needed.

A second variant is marked by absense of the pulmonary valve, and affected patients have a classic to-and-fro "sawing wood" murmur at the base. Because the infundibular stenosis usually is not severe, they are only mildly cyanotic. Some infants have massively dilated main and branch pulmonary arteries that obstruct airways and cause early death. The remainder usually do quite well. Surgical repair involves closing the VSD, resecting the infundibular stenosis, and, usually, inserting a pulmonary valve.

## Tricuspid Atresia

Systemic venous return passes from right to left atrium across a foramen ovale and then into the left ventricle. From there, in most patients blood passes into the aorta and across a VSD into the hypoplastic right ventricle and then to the lungs (Fig. 21–3C). Pulmonary blood flow is usually decreased because of restriction to flow through the VSD, and, often, neonates depend on the patent ductus arteriosus for their main pulmonary blood flow. Even when initially the VSD is big, it may become smaller with time, or the patient may develop infundibular PS, so the trend is toward increasing cyanosis. Diagnostic findings are a large right atrial P wave, short PR interval, and left superior axis QRS deviation on ECG, a chest film with decreased pulmonary vascular markings and a small heart (like an apple on a stalk), and the absence of a connection between the right atrium and right ventricle on the echocardiogram.

Treatment is initially to relieve severe hypoxemia by increasing pulmonary blood flow by dilating the ductus arteriosus with prostaglandin $E_1$ and then to create a systemic-pulmonary shunt. Because this shunt increases the already elevated left ventricular volume, if left alone for many years it will produce a dilated cardiomyopathy. Therefore, the shunt is closed and replaced with a bidirectional Glenn shunt (superior vena cava connected to both pulmonary arteries) at about 6 months of age. At 2 to 4 years of age or later, the inferior vena caval return is directed to the pulmonary arteries, usually by an intraatrial or extracardiac conduit, so that all the systemic venous drainage bypasses the right ventricle and drains by gravity into the pulmonary vascular bed. This complete repair is termed the *Fontan* or *Fontan-Kreuzer procedure*. Because of the gravity drainage, it is essential that pulmonary vascular resistance be low and that left ventricular and mitral valve function be normal. Similar repairs are done for a variety of cardiac lesions with only one ventricle: single ventricle, aortic or mitral atresia and hypoplastic left ventricle, AVSD with a hypoplastic ventricle, among others. This type of repair, which leaves only one pumping ventricle, is often termed a *single-ventricle repair*.

A few patients with tricuspid atresia have TGA, and most of their left ventricular blood goes directly to the lungs; aortic blood comes indirectly from the left ventricle via the VSD and the right ventricle. Early congestive heart failure with minimal cyanosis and pulmonary vascular disease is the rule. Banding the pulmonary artery before age 3 months protects the pulmonary vessels so that a Glenn shunt can be done a few months later.

## Problems After Bidirectional Glenn and Fontan-Kreuzer Procedures

The bidirectional Glenn shunt improves saturation, but some cyanosis persists and possible problems from chronic cyanosis may occur (see earlier). The shunt may be effective for many years, but, eventually, oxygen saturation decreases, because, as children grow, a greater proportion of total venous return comes from the lower body and bypasses the lungs. A more serious problem is that some of these patients develop arteriovenous fistulas in the lungs, so that an increasing amount of pulmonary blood flow bypasses the alveoli. Shunting the inferior vena cava blood into the lungs causes regression of these fistulas, and cyanosis disappears. Even in the best Fontan-Kreuzer procedures, however, deterioration may occur after 10 to 20 years, with atrial arrhythmias, progressive mitral valve incompetence, and the development of protein-losing enteropathy. At times, the only effective therapy for these problems may be cardiac transplantation.

## Pulmonary Atresia with Intact Ventricular Septum

Pulmonary atresia with an intact ventricular septum is an extreme form of pulmonic stenosis, and initially all blood to the lungs comes via the ductus arteriosus. The right ventricle is hypoplastic despite suprasystemic systolic pressures, and, often, large sinusoids go from the right ventricle to the coronary arteries (see Fig. 21–3D); at times, all the coronary flow comes from these sinusoids. Multiple coronary arterial stenoses develop. Treatment consists of valvotomy, an aortopulmonary shunt, or both. With sinusoid-dependent coronary blood flow, reduction of right ventricular pressure must be avoided. Sometimes a bidirectional Glenn operation is done, to be followed by a Fontan-Kreuzer procedure, but the results are frequently poor.

## Double-Outlet Right Ventricle

A group of diseases are marked by both great arteries arising from the right ventricle; the obligatory VSD may be at any of several sites. If the aorta arises from the right ventricle near the VSD, the patient resembles one with a large VSD and is not cyanotic. Treatment is closure of the VSD so that left ventricular blood passes into the aorta. If the VSD is below the pulmonary artery (see Fig. 21–3E) or remote from both arteries, a variety of procedures can be done, depending on the exact anatomy. Sometimes, a long intracardiac tunnel can be placed to connect the left ventricle to the aorta without obstructing outflow from the right ventricle to the pulmonary artery. At other times, the VSD is closed so that the left ventricle ejects into the pulmonary artery, as in TGA, and an atrial baffle is then done to return systemic venous blood to the pulmonary artery. In other repairs, various forms of intracardiac tunnels and extracardiac conduits are placed.

## Truncus Arteriosus

In this lesion, the base of the heart gives off a large arterial trunk from which the aorta, coronary arteries, and pulmonary arteries arise (Fig. 21–3F), and there is a large VSD. Affected children have early and severe congestive heart failure and may develop pulmonary vascular disease by 3 months of age. Treatment is removal of the pulmonary arteries from the aorta, patching of the resulting aortic hole, closure of the VSD, and creation of a conduit from the RV to the pulmonary arteries. Because the pulmonary arteries are big, the conduit can be quite large, but it will have to be replaced as the child grows and several times during adult life.

## Total Anomalous Pulmonary Venous Connection

Usually, all the pulmonary veins join behind the heart to form a common pulmonary venous trunk which connects to the superior vena cava (supracardiac, prevalence 55%), the coronary sinus or right atrium (cardiac, 25%), or the portal vein (infracardiac, 20%; see Fig. 21–3G). There may be obstruction to the common pulmonary venous drainage in the supracardiac or cardiac types, but the obstruction always occurs in the infracardiac type. Infants with obstructed drainage present soon after birth with intense cyanosis and pulmonary edema and need early surgical repair, which is done by anastomosing the left atrium to the common pulmonary vein. The procedure is usually successful, but sometimes the infant develops stenoses of the pulmonary veins that are difficult to treat. Those forms of anomalous connection without obstruction behave as ASDs with a large shunt and minimal cyanosis. They often have congestive heart failure in the first year of life and can develop pulmonary vascular disease if their lesion is left untreated. When the lesion is diagnosed, surgical repair is usually successful.

## Single Ventricle

A group of lesions fall under the heading of *single* ventricle. Most common is the double-inlet single left ventricle from which the pulmonary artery arises (see Fig. 21–3H). The aorta comes off a rudimentary right ventricle that receives blood through a bulboventricular foramen. There may or may not be PS. Without PS, congestive heart failure develops early, and early pulmonary arterial banding is needed to prevent pulmonary vascular disease and prepare the child for staged single-ventricle repair. With PS often comes marked cyanosis, and a small systemic-pulmonary shunt is needed until the child is old enough to tolerate a single-ventricle repair. A few patients have only moderate PS and moderate cyanosis, and do quite well for a time without treatment. Consequently, they are seen fairly often in adult cardiology clinics.

## Hypoplastic Left Heart Syndromes

All forms of hypoplastic left heart syndrome have a hypoplastic left ventricle, most commonly with aortic (and with or without mitral) atresia (see Fig. 21–3I). Flow to the aorta comes from the right ventricle via the pulmonary artery and ductus arteriosus. Infants present early with congestive heart failure and often have arterial pulses that wax and wane as the ductus arteriosus narrows and widens. Without treatment, most die before 1 month of age. Surgical treatment is cardiac transplantation or the Norwood procedure, in which the diminutive ascending aorta is anastomosed to the main pulmonary artery, in effect creating a truncus arteriosus. The peripheral pulmonary arteries are disconnected from the main pulmonary artery and connected to the aorta or one of its branches by a conduit. A few months later, staged single-ventricle repair is carried out.

## Corrected Transposition of the Great Arteries (l-TGA)

With corrected TGA (l-TGA), abnormal looping of the cardiac tube causes the right atrium to connect to the mitral valve and anatomic left ventricle, the latter being connected to the pulmonary artery. The left atrium is connected by a tricuspid valve to the anatomic right ventricle, which ejects blood into the aorta. The aorta usually lies anterior and to the left, producing a characteristic straight segment at the left upper heart border on chest films and giving rise to the term l-TGA, where *l* refers to *levo-*. As described, because both atrioventricular and ventriculoarterial connections are discordant, systemic venous blood enters the lungs and oxygenated blood enters the aorta, thus, the term *physiologically corrected transposition*. Most of these patients have a VSD, many have PS as well, and impaired atrioventricular conduction is common. The presentation may mimic simple VSD or tetralogy of Fallot. Because the pulmonic stenosis is usually subvalvar and often due to accessory mitral valve tissue, and because the RV outflow tract is posterior, surgical repair is difficult. Many of these patients with balanced shunts attend adult clinics. One of the characteristic physical findings is a loud aortic second sound heard best at the upper left sternal border because of the abnormal aortic position. About 2% of them develop complete atrioventricular block each year. The ECG shows prominent Q waves in the right chest leads, a finding that often leads to the misdiagnosis of anterior myocardial infarction.

## Ebstein Anomaly

Ebstein anomaly is relatively rare. The septal leaflet of the tricuspid valve arises from the ventricular septum below the tricuspid annulus, so that part of the

Table 21–2

**Types of Congenital Heart Disease in Adults**

**Without Surgery**

1. Asymptomatic
   a. Potentially unimportant: Small VSD, PDA, mild PS
   b. Potentially important: ASD, bicuspid aortic valve, coarctation of the aorta
2. Symptomatic
   a. Moderately large left-to-right shunts in patients from underdeveloped countries
   b. Cyanotic heart disease (e.g., tetralogy of Fallot, single ventricle with pulmonic stenosis, d-TGA with VSD and PS, Ebstein anomaly, tetralogy of Fallot with absent pulmonary valve)
   c. Eisenmenger syndrome (pulmonary vascular disease)

**With Prior Surgery**

1. Small residual lesions: small VSD, minor PS, mild mitral, pulmonic, aortic, or tricuspid incompetence
2. Major residual lesions: marked pulmonic, aortic, and mitral incompetence, significant RV or LV outflow tract obstruction
3. Prosthetic valves, conduits
4. Single-ventricle repair: tricuspid atresia, single ventricle, aortic atresia
5. Two-ventricle repair with systemic right ventricle: d-TGA with atrial baffle, l-TGA
6. Coronary artery problems after arterial switch for TGA

VSD, ventricular septal defect; PDA, patent ductus arteriosus; PS, pulmonic stenosis; ASD, atrial septal defect; d-/l-TGA, dextro-/levo-transposition of the great arteries; RV/LV, right/left ventricular.

right ventricle is included in the right atrium. With very deep displacement of the valve there is tricuspid incompetence and a right-to-left atrial shunt. Patients often have a gigantic right atrium, demonstrable by chest radiography and may have severe atrial arrhythmias. Those with mild lesions are asymptomatic. Severe lesions shorten life. Surgical procedures involve repair or replacement of the tricuspid valve, resection of the redundant part of the right atrium, and, sometimes, procedures to ablate arrhythmogenic foci.

## Presentation in Adult Life

Which patients will be seen in adult clinics? They may be divided into those who earlier had surgery and those who did not (Table 21–2). How do they differ from children with similar forms of CHD? Children who have a severe form of CHD either will have been operated on early in life or will have died. If they become adults with minor lesions, regardless of whether they had previous surgery, their outcomes are likely to be almost normal, and except for appropriate prophylaxis against infective endocarditis, including good dental hygiene, they need little special attention. Those with more major lesions have problems specific to those lesions, but there are certain problems that they all share (Table 21–3).

Table 21–3

**Effects of Congenital Heart Disease in Adults**

| Medical | Socioeconomic |
| --- | --- |
| Arrhythmias | Employment |
| Ventricular dysfunction and congestive heart failure | Exercise |
| Infective endocarditis | Life insurance |
| Sudden death | Health insurance |
| Pregnancy and contraceptive complications | |

Atrial arrhythmias become more prevalent with age, particularly in persons with a large right atrium (secondary to a previous ASD or Ebstein anomaly) or who have had atrial surgery (e.g, atrial baffle in d-TGA). Atrial flutter and fibrillation are common, and restoration of sinus rhythm, sometimes with good anticoagulation, may be necessary. It may be difficult to prevent recurrences, and many medications may need to be explored.

Ventricular arrhythmias occur with previous ventriculotomy, or even just with chronic ventricular hypertrophy. These may also be difficult to treat. Sudden death is assumed to be due to such arrhythmias, but we can do little to prevent it.

Chronic ventricular hypertrophy is associated with myocardial scarring and biochemical changes that add to the risks of surgery and often work against the expected improvement after a volume or pressure load has been removed by surgery.

Infective endocarditis is rare after surgery in those with complete repairs and no residua. Morris and colleagues observed a cumulative incidence of endocarditis of less than 2.5% over 30 years in most major treated forms of CHD.[13] The notable exception was aortic stenosis, whose 30-year cumulative risk was 20%.

Pregnancy is usually tolerated well after successful cardiac surgery or when the lesion is mild or moderate.[8, 14, 15] Severe obstructive lesions should be treated before a woman becomes pregnant, but some have even needed emergency valvotomy during pregnancy, which can usually be done with balloon catheterization to avoid surgery, anesthesia, and their effects on the fetus. Cyanotic patients have reduced fertility, but, when they become pregnant, mothers are usually at little increased risk, although fetal mortality is higher than normal. Those at greatest risk during pregnancy are patients with pulmonary vascular disease; most series report high mortality rates for these mothers, so avoidance of pregnancy—and if necessary sterilization—have been recommended. Most women with CHD can take usual contraceptive measures, although estrogen preparations, with their risk of thrombosis, are contraindicated for women with pulmonary vascular disease and after single-ventricle repairs, when thrombosis in the slow-flowing venous channels is a risk. Women with artificial valves should probably avoid intrauterine contraceptive devices because of the risk of bacteremia and infective endocarditis.

Socioeconomic problems become important in adults with CHD. Employers often discriminate against them, especially when health insurance is an issue. Even when it is not, employers may be unwilling to risk frequent sick leave absences. For most of these subjects exercise is recommended at a level that they are comfortable with. Several recent publications give some guidance about the levels of exercise that can safely be undertaken.[16, 17]

Many of these subjects are denied life insurance or can obtain it only at very high premiums. A lot depends on what the cardiac problem is, and some insurance companies give certain patients with adequately corrected defects or minor lesions life insurance at little increase in price. There are big differences between the policies of different companies, and it is worthwhile for applicants to explore several.[18-20]

A more serious problem, health insurance, varies from country to country but is most serious in the United States. Children are usually covered by some form of Medicare, Medicaid, or Children's Medical Services, but coverage may not remain in effect after childhood. Many people get their health insurance through their employer (a problem alluded to earlier). It is difficult to know what to do for many of these patients who cannot buy a comprehensive insurance plan.

## ■ REFERENCES

1. Hoffman JIE: Incidence of congenital heart disease. I. Postnatal incidence. Pediatr Cardiol 1995;16:103–113.

2. Shah D, Azhar M, Oakley CM, et al: Natural history of secundum atrial septal defect in adults after medical or surgical treatment: Historical prospective study. Br Heart J 1994;71:224–228.
3. Heath D, Edwards JE: The pathology of pulmonary hypertensive disease. A description of six grades of structural changes in the pulmonary artery with special reference to congenital cardiac septal defects. Circulation 1958;18:533–547.
4. Reid LM: Structure and function in pulmonary hypertension. New perceptions. Chest 1986;89:279–288.
5. Rabinovitch M: It all begins with EVE (endogenous vascular elastase). Isr J Med Sci 1996;30:803–808.
6. Saha A, Balakrishnan KG, Jaiswal PK, et al: Prognosis for patients with Eisenmenger syndrome of various aetiology. Int J Cardiol 1994;45:199–207.
7. Bitsch M, Johansen C, Wennevold A, et al: Eisenmenger's syndrome and pregnancy. Eur J Obstet Gynecol Reprod Biol 1988;28:69–74.
8. Perloff J, Koos B: Pregnancy and congenital heart disease: The mother and the fetus. In Perloff JK, Child JS (eds): Congenital Heart Disease in Adults. Philadelphia: WB Saunders, 1998:144–164.
9. Reifenstein GH, Levine SA, Gross RE: Coarctation of the aorta. A review of 104 autopsied cases of the "adult type," 2 years of age or older. Am Heart J 1947;33:146–168.
10. Hoffman JIE: Congenital anomalies of the coronary vessels and the aortic root. In Emmanouilides GC, Allen HD, Riemenschneider TA, Gutgesell HP (eds): Moss and Adams' Heart Disease in Infants, Children and Adolescents. Baltimore: Williams & Wilkins, 1995:769–790.
11. Rosenthal A, Nathan DG, Marty AT, et al: Acute hemodynamic effects of red cell volume reduction in polycythemia of cyanotic congenital heart disease. Circulation 1970;42:297–308.
12. Perloff JK, Rosove MH, Sietsema KE, et al: Cyanotic heart disease: A multisystem disorder. In Perloff JK, Child JS (eds): Congenital Heart Disease in Adults. Philadelphia: WB Saunders, 1998:199–226.
13. Morris CD, Reller MD, Menashe VD: Thirty-year incidence of infective endocarditis after surgery for congenital heart defect. JAMA 1998;279:599–603.
14. Pitkin RM, Perloff JK, Koos BJ, et al: Pregnancy and congenital heart disease. Ann Intern Med 1990;112:445–454.
15. Mendelson MA: Congenital heart disease and pregnancy. Clin Perinatol 1997;24:467–482.
16. Mitchell JH, Haskell WL, Raven PB: Classification of Sports: 26th Bethesda Conference. Recommendations for determining eligibility for competition in athletes with cardiovascular abnormalities. J Am Coll Cardiol 1994;24:864–866.
17. Kaplan S, Perloff JK: Exercise and athletics before and after cardiac surgery or interventional catheterization. In Perloff JK, Child JS (eds): Congenital Heart Disease in Adults. Philadelphia: WB Saunders, 1998:189–198.
18. Truesdell SC, Skorton DJ, Lauer RM: Life insurance for children with cardiovascular disease. Pediatrics 1986;77:687–691.
19. Allen HD, Gersony WM, Taubert KA: Insurability of the adolescent and young adult with heart disease. Report from the Fifth Conference on Insurability, October 3–4, 1991, Columbus, Ohio. Circulation 1992;86:703–710.
20. Celermajer DS, Deanfield JD: Employment and insurance for young adults with congenital heart disease. Br Heart J 1992;69:539–543.

# ▪ SUGGESTED READING

Emmanouilides GC, Allen HD, Riemenschneider TA, Gutgesell HP (eds): Moss and Adams' Heart Disease in Infants, Children and Adolescents. Baltimore: Williams & Wilkins, 1995.
Perloff JK, Child JS: Congenital Heart Disease in Adults. Philadelphia: WB Saunders, 1998.

# CORONARY ARTERY DISEASE

*Chapter* 22

# Pathogenesis of Atherosclerosis

*Prediman K. Shah*

Atherosclerotic vascular disease is the leading cause of death in the United States and in much of the industrialized world, and it is rapidly gaining the same dubious distinction in the developing world.[1] Atherosclerosis involves the development of a plaque composed of variable amounts of connective tissue matrix (collagen, proteoglycans, glycosaminoglycans), vascular smooth muscle cells, lipoproteins, calcium, inflammatory cells (chiefly monocyte-derived macrophages, T lymphocytes, and mast cells), and new blood vessels (neoangiogenesis). The precise cause and pathogenesis of atherosclerosis are incompletely understood, but an emerging paradigm suggests that atherosclerosis may reflect a chronic inflammatory response to vascular injury caused by a variety of agents that activate or injure endothelium and promote lipoprotein infiltration, lipoprotein retention, and lipoprotein oxidation.[2]

## ▪ SITES OF PREDILECTION FOR ATHEROSCLEROSIS

Atherosclerosis involves the aorta and the large- and medium-sized elastic and muscular arteries of the heart, brain, kidneys, and extremities, and it predisposes such organs to ischemic injury (Table 22–1, Fig. 22–1). The sites of predilection for atherosclerosis appear to be characterized by increased influx or prolonged retention of lipoproteins, evidence of endothelial activation with expression of leukocyte adhesion molecules, and low shear stress. Changes in flow alter the expression of genes that have elements in their promoter regions that respond to shear stress. For example, the genes for intercellular adhesion molecule 1 (ICAM-1), platelet-derived growth factor beta (PDGF-β chain, and tissue factor in endothelial cells have these elements, and their expression is increased by reduced shear stress.[2–4] Alterations in blood flow appear to be critical in determining which arterial sites are prone to develop lesions.[4] Specific arterial sites, such as branches, bifurcations, and curvatures, cause characteristic alterations in blood flow, including decreased shear stress and increased turbulence. Rolling and adherence of monocytes and T cells occur at these sites as a result of upregulation of adhesion molecules on both the endothelium and the leukocytes. At these sites, specific molecules form on the endothelium that are responsible for the adherence, migration, and accumulation of monocytes and T cells. Such adhesion molecules, which act as receptors for

Table 22–1

### Key Steps in Atherogenesis

Endothelial injury with increased infiltration of atherogenic lipoproteins at sites of low or oscillating shear stress

Subendothelial retention and modification of atherogenic lipoproteins (LDL/VLDL), LDL oxidation, glycation, aggregation

Endothelial activation with increased mononuclear leukocyte (inflammatory cell) adhesion, chemotaxis, and subendothelial recruitment

Subendothelial inflammatory cell activation with lipid ingestion through monocyte scavenger receptor expression resulting in foam cell formation

Inflammatory cell (monocyte-macrophage) proliferation

Migration to intima and proliferation of medial/adventitial smooth muscle cells/myofibroblasts in response to growth factors released by activated monocytes with matrix production and formation of fibrous plaque and fibrous cap

Abluminal plaque growth with positive (outward) arterial adventitial remodeling preserving lumen size in early stages; later, plaque growth or negative remodeling results in luminal narrowing

Neoangiogenesis due to angiogenic stimuli produced by macrophages and other arterial wall cells (vascular endothelial growth factor [VEGF], interleukin 8)

Death of foam cells by necrosis/apoptosis leading to necrotic lipid core formation

Rupture of fibrous cap or endothelial erosion, exposure of thrombogenic substrate and arterial thrombosis

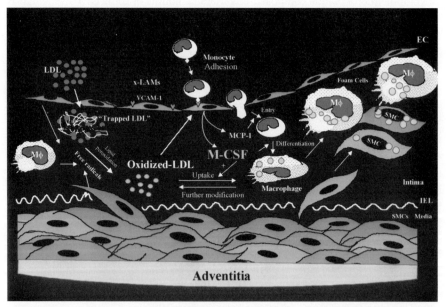

**Figure 22–1** ■ Schematic description of the various postulated steps in the initiation and progression of an atherosclerotic plaque (see Table 22–1 and text for details). LDL, low-density lipoprotein; VCAM, vascular cell adhesion molecule; x-LAMs, leukocyte adhesion molecules; M-CSF, macrophage colony–stimulating factor; MCP-1, monocyte chemotactic protein; Mϕ, monocyte-derived macrophages; EC, endothelial cell; SMC, smooth muscle cell; IEL, internal elastic lamina.

glycoconjugates and integrins on monocytes and T cells, include several selectins, intercellular adhesion molecules, and vascular cell adhesion molecules.[2-4] Molecules associated with the migration of leukocytes across the endothelium, such as platelet endothelial cell adhesion molecules, act in conjunction with chemoattractant molecules generated by the endothelium, smooth muscle, and monocytes (such as monocyte chemotactic protein 1, osteopontin, and modified low-density lipoprotein [LDL]) to attract monocytes and T cells into the artery.[2-4] Flow-mediated upregulation of various adhesion molecules and inflammatory genes is controlled by shear stress–responsive elements that are present in the promoter regions of genes like ICAM-1, PDGF-β, and tissue factor.[2-5] Chemokines may be involved in the chemotaxis and accumulation of macrophages in fatty streaks.[6] Activation of monocytes and T cells leads to upregulation of receptors on their surfaces, such as the mucinlike molecules that bind selectins, integrins that bind adhesion molecules of the immunoglobulin superfamily, and receptors that bind chemoattractant molecules. These ligand-receptor interactions further activate mononuclear cells, induce cell proliferation, and help define and localize the inflammatory response at the sites of lesions.

In genetically modified mice that are deficient in apolipoprotein E (and have hypercholesterolemia), ICAM-1 is constitutively increased at lesion-prone sites long before the lesions develop.[4] In contrast, vascular cell adhesion molecule 1 (VCAM-1) is absent in normal mice but is present at the same sites as ICAM-1 in mice with apolipoprotein E deficiency.[4] Mice that lack any ICAM-1, P-selectin, CD18, or combinations of these molecules, have reduced atherosclerosis in response to lipid feeding. Proteolytic enzymes may cleave adhesion molecules so that, in situations of chronic inflammation, it may be possible to measure the "shed" molecules in plasma as markers of a sustained inflammatory response to help patients at risk for atherosclerosis or other inflammatory diseases.[2, 7]

## ■ KEY ROLE OF ENDOTHELIAL ACTIVATION/DYSFUNCTION AND INJURY IN ATHEROGENESIS (Tables 22–2, 22–3)

Several studies have suggested that one of the earliest steps in atherogenesis is endothelial activation or injury or dysfunction with infiltration and retention of atherogenic lipoproteins (predominantly those that contain apo B) in the subendothelial space of the vessel wall.[8]

Various factors that may contribute to endothelial activation or the development of endothelial injury or dysfunction that predisposes to atherosclerosis include

Table 22–2

**Manifestations of Endothelial Dysfunction in Atherosclerosis**

Reduced vasodilator and increased vasoconstrictor capacity
  Enhanced oxidant stress with increased inactivation of nitric oxide
  Increased expression of endothelin
Enhanced leukocyte (inflammatory cell) adhesion and recruitment
  Increased adhesion molecule expression (ICAM, VCAM)
  Increased chemotactic molecule expression (MCP-1, interleukin 8, osteopontin)
Increased prothrombotic and reduced fibrinolytic phenotype
  Increased tissue factor expression and reduced nitric oxide bioavailability
  Increased plasminogen activator inhibitor expression
Increased growth-promoting phenotype
  Reduced nitric oxide bioavailability
  Increased endothelin expression

Table 22–3

**Factors Contributing to Endothelial Dysfunction**

Dyslipidemia and atherogenic lipoprotein modification
  Elevated LDL, VLDL, lipoprotein(a)
  LDL modification (oxidation, glycation)
  Reduced high-density lipoprotein
Increased oxidant stress: hypertension, diabetes, smoking
Estrogen deficiency
Hyperhomocysteinemia
Advancing age
Genetic predisposition
Infections

risk factors such as elevated and modified LDL/VLDL cholesterol; reduced high-density lipoprotein (HDL) cholesterol, oxidant stress caused by cigarette smoking, hypertension, and diabetes mellitus; genetic alterations; elevated plasma homocysteine concentrations; infectious microorganisms such as herpesviruses and *Chlamydia pneumoniae*; estrogen deficiency; and advancing age.[9] Endothelial activation and injury or dysfunction may be manifested in: (1) increased adhesiveness of the endothelium to leukocytes or platelets, (2) increased permeability, (3) change from an anticoagulant to a procoagulant phenotype, (4) change from a vasodilator to a vasoconstrictor phenotype, and (5) change from a growth-inhibiting phenotype to a growth-promoting one through elaboration of cytokines. Abnormal vasomotor function has been one of the best studied manifestations of endothelial dysfunction in subjects who either have established atherosclerosis or are at risk for it. Normal healthy endothelium produces nitric oxide from arginine through the action of a family of enzymes known as *nitric oxide synthases*.[9] Nitric oxide acts as a local vasodilator by increasing smooth muscle cell cyclic guanosine monophosphate (cGMP) levels while at the same time inhibiting platelet aggregation and smooth muscle cell proliferation.[9] In persons at risk, a reduced vasodilator response to endothelium-dependent vasodilator stimuli, or even a paradoxical vasoconstrictor response to such stimuli, has been observed in large vessels and in the microcirculation, even in the absence of structural abnormalities in the vessel wall.[9] These abnormal vasomotor responses have been attributed to reduced bioavailability of endothelium-derived relaxing factor(s)(specifically, nitric oxide) owing to rapid inactivation of nitric oxide by oxidant stress or excessive generation of asymmetric dimethylarginine and/or increased production of vasoconstrictors such as endothelin.[9, 10]

## ■ HYPERCHOLESTEROLEMIA AND MODIFIED LOW-DENSITY LIPOPROTEINS (see Fig. 22–1)

One of the major contributors to endothelial injury is LDL cholesterol. When LDL is modified by processes such as oxidation, glycation (in diabetes), aggregation, association with proteoglycans, or incorporation into immune complexes, it is capable of inducing endothelial dysfunction.[11] Subendothelial retention of LDL particles results in progressive oxidation and its subsequent internalization by macrophages through the scavenger receptors.[11, 12] The internalization leads to the formation of lipid peroxides and facilitates the accumulation of cholesterol esters, resulting in the formation of foam cells. The degree to which LDL is modified can vary greatly.[11] Once modified and taken up by macrophages, LDL activates the foam cells. In addition to its ability to injure these cells, modified LDL is chemotactic for other monocytes and can upregulate the expression of genes for macrophage colony–stimulating factor (MCSF) and monocyte chemotactic protein derived from endothelial cells.[11–13] Thus, it may help to expand the inflammatory response by stimulating the replication of monocyte-derived macrophages and the entry of new monocytes into lesions. Oxidized LDL is present in lesions of atherosclerosis in animals and in humans.[11] In animal models of hypercholesterolemia, antioxidants can reduce the size of atherosclerotic lesions.[11] Antioxidants increase the resistance of human LDL to oxidation ex vivo in proportion to the vitamin E content of the plasma. Vitamin E intake is inversely correlated with the incidence of myocardial infarction, and vitamin E supplementation reduced coronary events in a preliminary clinical trial, whereas beta carotene produced no benefit.[14, 15]

Sustained inflammatory response stimulates migration and proliferation of smooth muscle cells that accumulate in the areas of inflammation to form an intermediate fibroproliferative lesion that thickens the artery wall.

## ■ VASCULAR REMODELING IN ATHEROSCLEROSIS
(see Table 22–1)

Several experimental and clinical studies have demonstrated that progressive accumulation of plaque in the vessel wall can lead to progressive enlargement of the entire vessel through expansion of the adventitia (positive remodeling) that helps to minimize luminal narrowing.[16] Eventually, failure of further remodeling in the face of continued plaque growth can result in luminal narrowing; alternatively, luminal narrowing may result from adventitial constriction or contraction (negative remodeling).[16]

## ■ THE INFLAMMATORY AND IMMUNE RESPONSE IN ATHEROSCLEROSIS (Table 22–1, Fig. 22–1)

The inflammatory and immune response in atherosclerosis consists of accumulation of monocyte-derived macrophages and specific subtypes of T lymphocytes at every stage of the disease.[17, 18] The fatty streak, the earliest type of lesion and common in infants and young children, consists of monocyte-derived macrophages and T lymphocytes.[17, 18] Continued inflammation results in increased numbers of macrophages and lymphocytes, which both migrate from the blood and multiply in the lesion. Activation of these cells leads to the release of proteolytic enzymes, cytokines, chemokines, and growth factors, which can induce further damage and eventually lead to focal necrosis.[19] Necrosis and/or apoptosis of foam cells results in the formation of the necrotic lipid core in the plaque. Thus, cycles of accumulation of mononuclear cells, migration and proliferation of smooth muscle cells, and formation of fibrous tissue lead to further enlargement and restructuring of the lesion, so that it becomes covered by a fibrous cap that overlies a core of lipid and necrotic tissue, resulting in the formation of an advanced and complicated plaque.

The inflammatory response can also affect lipoprotein transfer in the vessel wall. Inflammatory mediators such as tumor necrosis factor alpha, interleukin 1, and MCSF increase binding of LDL to endothelium and smooth muscle and increase the transcription of the LDL receptor gene.[2] After binding to scavenger receptors in vitro, modified LDL initiates a series of intracellular events that include the induction of proteases and inflammatory cytokines.[2] Thus, a vicious circle of inflammation, modification of lipoproteins, and further inflammation can be maintained in the artery by the presence of these lipids.

Monocyte-derived macrophages are present in various stages of atherogenesis and act as scavenging and antigen-presenting cells. They produce cytokines, chemokines, growth-regulating molecules, metalloproteinases, and other hydrolytic enzymes. The continuing entry, survival, and replication of monocytes/macrophages in lesions depend in part on growth factors such as MCSF and granulocyte-macrophage colony–stimulating factor (GM-CSF), whereas interleukin 2 is involved in a similar manner for T lymphocytes.

Activated macrophages and lesional smooth muscle cells express class II histocompatibility antigens such as HLA-DR that allow them to present antigens to T lymphocytes.[2, 20] The fact that atherosclerotic lesions contain both CD4 and CD8 T cells implicates the immune system in atherogenesis.[2, 20] T-cell activation after antigen processing results in production of various cytokines such as interferon gamma and tumor necrosis factor alpha and beta, which can further enhance the inflammatory response.[2] Among the antigens presented are oxidized LDL and heat shock protein 60, which may participate in the immune response.[21]

Macrophages, T cells, and endothelial and smooth muscle cells in the atherosclerotic lesions express CD 40 ligand and its receptor, which may play a role in atherogenesis by regulating the function of inflammatory cells.[22, 23] The antiatherogenic effect of CD 40–blocking antibodies in the murine model of atherosclerosis suggests that CD 40 may play an important role in atherogenesis.[22, 23]

Platelet adhesion and mural thrombosis are ubiquitous in the initiation and generation of the lesions of atherosclerosis in animals and humans.[2] Platelets can adhere to dysfunctional endothelium, exposed collagen, and macrophages. When activated, platelets release their granules, which contain cytokines and growth factors that, together with thrombin, may contribute to the migration and proliferation of smooth muscle cells and monocytes.[24] Activation of platelets leads to the formation of free arachidonic acid, which can be transformed into prostaglandins such as thromboxane $A_2$ (one of the most potent vasoconstricting and platelet-aggregating substances known) or into leukotrienes, which can amplify the inflammatory response.

Angiotensin II, a potent vasoconstrictor, may also contribute to atherogenesis by stimulating the growth of smooth muscle, increasing oxidant stress, inducing LDL oxidation, and a pro-inflammatory response.[2, 25] Elevated plasma homocysteine concentrations, resulting from enzymatic defects or vitamin deficiency, may also facilitate atherothrombosis by inducing endothelial dysfunction with a reduction in vasodilator capacity and enhanced prothrombotic phenotype and smooth muscle cell replication.[26] Hyperhomocysteinemia is associated with an increased risk of atherosclerosis of the coronary, peripheral, and cerebral arteries.[26] Trials are under way to determine whether reduction of plasma homocysteine levels by vitamins such as folic acid and vitamins $B_6$ and $B_{12}$ can reduce atherothrombotic events in humans.[27]

## ■ POTENTIAL ROLE OF INFECTION IN ATHEROTHROMBOSIS
(Tables 22–4, 22–5)

Several recent reports have suggested that certain infectious organisms, such as cytomegalovirus, *Chlamydia pneumoniae*, and *Helicobacter pylori* may contribute to inflammation and, thus, to atherogenesis or plaque disruption and thrombosis in the presence of preexisting atherosclerosis.[28–34] Increased titers of antibodies to these organisms have been used as predictors of further adverse events in patients who have had a myocardial infarction. Organisms, particularly *C. pneumoniae*, have been identified in atheromatous lesions in coronary arteries and in other organs obtained at autopsy. The case for *C. pneumoniae* is of particular interest, since in both hypercholesterolemic rabbits and genetically hyperlipidemic mice acceleration of atherosclerosis with *C. pneumoniae* infection has been demonstrated. In addition,

Table 22–4

**Pathogens Implicated in Atherosclerosis and Thrombosis**

| Viruses | Bacteria |
|---|---|
| Herpesvirus | *Chlamydia pneumoniae* |
| Cytomegalovirus | *Helicobacter pylori* |
| | *Porphyromonas gingivalis?* |

findings from pilot clinical trials of anti-*Chlamydia* macrolide antibiotics have raised the intriguing possibility that such therapy may reduce the risk of recurrent coronary events.[29, 33] Studies in vitro have suggested that *C. pneumoniae* can trigger proatherogenic events such as foam cell formation, procoagulant activity, and metalloproteinase activity in monocytes, probably mediated by its heat shock protein 60 (HSP 60).[28, 30] Molecular antigenic mimicry between certain *Chlamydia* antigens and myosin has raised the possibility that such antigenic mimicry may also be involved in immune-mediated vascular and myocardial injury.[34] Large-scale clinical trials are currently under way to more clearly define the role of *Chlamydia* infection in atherothrombosis. Although there is no direct evidence that these organisms can cause the lesions of atherosclerosis, it is nevertheless possible that infection, combined with other risk factors, may contribute to atherogenesis or destabilization of preexisting atherosclerotic lesions in some patients.

## ■ ANGIOGENESIS IN ATHEROSCLEROSIS (Table 22–1)

Angiogenesis or neovascularization is an essential process that supports chronic inflammation and fibroproliferation, processes involved in atherogenesis. Several studies have demonstrated increased neoangiogenesis in atherosclerotic lesions, and hypercholesterolemia has been shown to increase adventitial neovascularity in porcine arteries before an atherosclerotic lesion develops.[35] Proinflammatory chemokines such as interleukin 8 and other angiogenic growth factors such as vascular endothelial growth factor (VEGF) have been demonstrated in atherosclerotic lesions, where they may contribute to angiogenesis.[35] Recent preliminary data demonstrating an inhibitory effect of angiostatin in murine model of atherosclerosis suggests the potential proatherogenic role for angiogenesis.[36]

## ■ PLAQUE INSTABILITY AND VULNERABILITY, PLAQUE RUPTURE, PLAQUE EROSION, AND THROMBOSIS
(Table 22–6, Fig. 22–2)

Thrombosis complicating atherosclerosis is the mechanism by which atherosclerosis leads to acute ischemic syndromes of unstable angina, non-q and q-wave

Table 22–5

**How Infections May Contribute to Atherothrombosis**

Direct infection of the vascular wall with endothelial injury and inflammatory cell recruitment and activation (*Chlamydia pneumoniae*, herpesvirus, cytomegalovirus)

Immune-mediated vascular injury through molecular mimicry (*Chlamydia pneumoniae*)

Remote infections with systemic activation of the inflammatory response (*Helicobacter pylori*, *Porphyromonas gingivalis*)

Table 22–6

**Determinants of Vulnerability to Plaque Disruption**

| | |
|---|---|
| Large lipid core | Reduced collagen and smooth muscle cell |
| Thin fibrous cap | content |
| Increased number and activity of inflammatory cells: | Increased neovascularity |
| macrophages, T cells, mast cells | |

myocardial infarction, and many cases of sudden cardiac death.[37, 38] In most cases, coronary thrombosis is the result of uneven thinning and rupture of the fibrous cap, often at the shoulders of a lipid-rich lesion where macrophages enter, accumulate, and are activated and where apoptosis may occur.[37, 38] Thinning of the fibrous cap may result from (1) elaboration of metalloproteinases such as collagenases, gelatinases, elastases, and stromelysins,[37, 38] which in turn may be stimulated by oxidized LDL, cell-cell interaction such as activated T cells, mast cell–derived proteases, oxidant radicals, and infectious agents[37, 38] and/or (2) increased smooth muscle cell death and reduced matrix production.[37, 38] These changes may also be accompanied by the production of tissue factor procoagulant and other hemostatic factors that further increase the possibility of thrombosis.[37, 38] Thrombosis may also occur on a proteoglycan-rich matrix without a large lipid core, and in such cases evidence of superficial endothelial erosion is found.[39] This plaque erosion may account for thrombosis in a relatively larger proportion of young victims of sudden death, particularly women and smokers.[39] The precise molecular basis for these plaque erosions is not clear, although endothelial desquamation through activation of basement membrane–degrading metalloproteinases may be involved.[40]

Plaques with a large lipid core, active inflammatory infiltration, and a thinned-out fibrous cap are therefore considered vulnerable or unstable. They may be particularly difficult to identify because, in the absence of flow-limiting stenoses, they may not produce symptoms and may thus escape detection by stress testing, and even angiography.[37, 38] Macrophage accumulation may be associated with increased plasma concentrations of both fibrinogen and C-reactive protein, two markers of inflammation thought to be early signs of atherosclerosis.[41] Elevated CRP levels have been associated with increased risk of adverse cardiac events in patients with symptomatic vascular disease and in asymptomatic subjects at risk for vascular disease.[41]

## ■ SUMMARY AND CONCLUSIONS

Atherosclerosis is a complex disease process that involves lipoprotein influx, lipoprotein modification, increased prooxidant stress, and inflammatory, angiogenic, and fibroproliferative responses intermingled with extracellular matrix and lipid accumulation, the entire process resulting in the formation of an atherosclerotic plaque. Endothelial dysfunction is common in atherosclerosis and often is manifested as a reduced vasodilator or enhanced vasoconstrictor phenotype that contributes to luminal compromise. Thrombosis resulting from plaque rupture or superficial erosion complicates atherosclerosis and often results in abrupt luminal occlusion with resultant acute ischemic syndromes. Infectious agents may contribute to the inflammatory response and thus to destabilization of lesions. Better understanding of the pathophysiology of atherosclerosis is providing novel directions for its prevention and treatment.

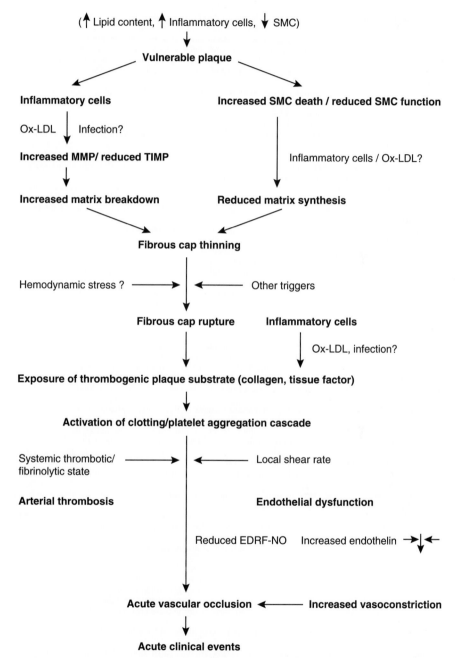

**Figure 22–2** ▪ Schematic description of the postulated key steps involved in plaque rupture and thrombosis.

# ■ REFERENCES

1. Breslow JL: Cardiovascular disease burden increases, NIH funding decreases. Natl Med 1997;3:600–601.
2. Ross R: Atherosclerosis: An inflammatory disease. N Engl J Med 1999;340:115–126.
3. Nagel T, Resnick N, Atkinson WJ, et al: Shear stress selectively upregulates intercellular adhesion molecule-1 expression in cultured human vascular endothelial cells. J Clin Invest 1994;94:885–891.
4. Nakashima Y, Raines EW, Plump AS, et al: Upregulation of VCAM-1 and ICAM-1 at atherosclerosis-prone sites on the endothelium in the ApoE-deficient mouse. Arterioscler Thromb Vasc Biol 1998;18:842–851.
5. Springer TA, Cybulsky MI: Traffic signals on endothelium for leukocytes in health, inflammation, and atherosclerosis. In Fuster V, Ross R, Topol EJ (eds): Atherosclerosis and Coronary Artery Disease (Vol. 1). Philadelphia: Lippincott-Raven, 1996:511–538.
6. Boisvert WA, Santiago R, Curtiss LK, Terkeltaub RA: A leukocyte homologue of the IL-8 receptor CXCR-2 mediates the accumulation of macrophages in atherosclerotic lesions of LDL receptor-deficient mice. J Clin Invest 1998;101:353–363.
7. Hwang S-J, Ballantyne CM, Sharrett AR, et al: Circulating adhesion molecules VCAM-1, ICAM-1, and E-selectin in carotid atherosclerosis and incident coronary heart disease cases: The Atherosclerosis Risk in Communities (ARIC) study. Circulation 1997;96:4219–4225.
8. Napoli C, D'Armiento FP, Mancini FP, et al: Fatty streak formation occurs in human fetal aortas and is greatly enhanced by maternal hypercholesterolemia: Intimal accumulation of low density lipoprotein and its oxidation precede monocyte recruitment into early atherosclerotic lesions. J Clin Invest 1997;100:2680–2690.
9. Kinlay S, Ganz P: Role of endothelial dysfunction in coronary artery disease and implications for therapy. Am J Cardiol 1997;80:111–161.
10. Lerman A, Edwards BS, Hallett JW, et al: Circulating and tissue endothelin immunoreactivity in advanced atherosclerosis. N Engl J Med 1991;325:997–1001.
11. Steinberg D: Low density lipoprotein oxidation and its pathobiological significance. J Biol Chem 1997;272:20963–20966.
12. Rajavashisth TB, Andalibi A, Territo MC, et al: Induction of endothelial cell expression of granulocyte and macrophage colony–stimulating factors by modified low-density lipoproteins. Nature 1990;344:254–257.
13. Leonard EJ, Yoshimura T: Human monocyte chemoattractant protein-1 (MCP-1). Immunol Today 1990;11:97–101.
14. Stephens NG, Parsons A, Schofield PM, et al: Randomised controlled trial of vitamin E in patients with coronary disease: Cambridge Heart Antioxidant Study. Lancet 1996;347:781–786.
15. Omenn GS, Goodman GE, Thornquist MD, et al: Effects of a combination of beta carotene and vitamin A on lung cancer and cardiovascular disease. N Engl J Med 1996;334:1150–1155.
16. Gibbons GH, Dzau V J: The emerging concept of vascular remodeling. N Engl J Med 1994;330:1431–1438.
17. Jonasson L, Holm J, Skalli O, et al: Regional accumulations of T cells, macrophages, and smooth muscle cells in the human atherosclerotic plaque. Arteriosclerosis 1986;6:131–138.
18. van der Wal AC, Das PK, Bentz van de Berg D, et al: Atherosclerotic lesions in humans: In situ immunophenotypic analysis suggesting an immune mediated response. Lab Invest 1989;61:166–170.
19. Falk E, Shah PK, Fuster V: Pathogenesis of plaque disruption. In Fuster V, Ross R, Topol EJ (eds): Atherosclerosis and Coronary Artery Disease (Vol. 2). Philadelphia: Lippincott-Raven, 1996:492–510.
20. Hansson GK, Jonasson L, Seifert PS, Stemme S: Immune mechanisms in atherosclerosis. Arteriosclerosis 1989;9:567–578.
21. Wick G, Romen M, Amberger A, et al: Atherosclerosis, autoimmunity, and vascular-associated lymphoid tissue. FASEB J 1997;11:1199–1207.
22. Schonbeck U, Mach F, Sukhova GK, et al: Regulation of matrix metalloproteinase expression in human vascular smooth muscle cells by T lymphocytes: A role for CD40 signaling in plaque rupture? Circ Res 1997;81:448–454.
23. Mach F, Schonbeck U, Sukhova GK, et al: Reduction of atherosclerosis in mice by inhibition of CD40 signalling. Nature 1998;394:200–203.
24. Bombeli T, Schwartz BR, Harlan JM: Adhesion of activated platelets to endothelial cells: Evidence for a GPIIbIIIa-dependent bridging mechanism and novel roles for endothelial intercellular adhesion molecule 1 (ICAM-1), (α) v (β) 3 integrin, and GPIb α. J Exp Med 1998;187:329–339.
25. Chobanian AV, Dzau VJ: Renin angiotensin system and atherosclerotic vascular disease. In Fuster V, Ross R, Topol EJ (eds): Atherosclerosis and Coronary Artery Disease (Vol. 1). Philadelphia: Lippincott-Raven, 1996:237–242.
26. Verhoef P, Stampfer MJ: Prospective studies of homocysteine and cardiovascular disease. Nutr Rev 1995;53:283–288.
27. Omenn GS, Beresford SAA, Motulsky AG: Preventing coronary heart disease: B vitamins and homocysteine. Circulation 1998;97:421–424.
28. Libby P, Egan D, Skarlatos S: Roles of infectious agents in atherosclerosis and restenosis: An assessment of the evidence and need for future research. Circulation 1997;96:4095–4103.

29. Gupta S, Leatham EW, Carrington D, et al: Elevated *Chlamydia pneumoniae* antibodies, cardiovascular events, and azithromycin in male survivors of myocardial infarction. Circulation 1997;96:404–407.
30. Shah PK: Plaque disruption and coronary thrombosis: New insight into pathogenesis and prevention. Clin Cardiol 1997;20:38–44.
31. Muhlestein JB, Anderson JL, Hammond EH, et al: Infection with *Chlamydia pneumoniae* accelerates the development of atherosclerosis and treatment with azithromycin prevents it in a rabbit model. Circulation 1998;97:633–636.
32. Hu H, Pierce GN, Zhong G: The atherogenic effects of chlamydia are dependent on serum cholesterol and specific to *Chlamydia pneumoniae*. J Clin Invest 1999;103:747–753.
33. Gurfinkel E, Bozovich G, Daroca A, et al: Randomised trial of roxithromycin in non–Q wave coronary syndromes: ROXIS Pilot Study. ROXIS Study Group [see comments]. Lancet 1997;350:404–407.
34. Bachmaier K, Neu N, de la Maza LM, et al: *Chlamydia* infections and heart disease linked through antigenic mimicry. Science 1999;283:1335–1339.
35. Folkman J: Angiogenesis in cancer, vascular, rheumatoid and other diseases. Nature Med 1995;1:27–31.
36. Moulton KS, Heller E, Konerding MA, et al: Angiogenesis inhibitor endostatin or TNP-470 reduces intimal neovascularization and plaque growth in apolipoprotein E deficient mice. Circulation 1999;99:1726–1732.
37. Lee RT, Libby P: The unstable atheroma. Arterioscler Thromb Vasc Biol 1997;17:1859–1867.
38. Shah PK: Role of inflammation and metalloproteinases in plaque disruption and thrombosis. Vasc Med 1998;3:199–206.
39. Burke AP, Farb A, Malcom GT, et al: Coronary risk factors and plaque morphology in men with coronary disease who died suddenly. N Engl J Med 1997;336:1276–1282.
40. Rajavashisth TB, Xu XP, Jovinge S, et al: Membrane type 1 matrix metalloproteinase expression in human atherosclerotic plaques: Evidence for activation byproinflammatory mediators. Circulation 1999;99:3103–3109.
41. Ridker PM, Cushman M, Stampfer MJ, et al: Inflammation, aspirin, and the risk of cardiovascular disease in apparently healthy men. N Engl J Med 1997;336:973–979.

# ■ RECOMMENDED READING

Gibbons GH, Dzau VJ: The emerging concept of vascular remodeling. N Engl J Med 1994;330:1431–1438.
Kinlay S. Ganz P: Role of endothelial dysfunction in coronary artery disease and implications for therapy. Am J Cardiol 1997;80:111–161.
Libby P, Egan D, Skarlatos S: Roles of infectious agents in atherosclerosis and restenosis: An assessment of the evidence and need for future research. Circulation 1997;96:4095–4103.
Ross R: Atherosclerosis: An inflammatory disease. N Engl J Med 1999;340:115–126.
Shah PK: Role of inflammation and metalloproteinases in plaque disruption and thrombosis. Vasc Med 1998;3:199–206.
Springer TA, Cybulsky MI: Traffic signals on endothelium for leukocytes in health, inflammation, and atherosclerosis. *In* Fuster V, Ross R, Topol EJ (eds): Atherosclerosis and Coronary Artery Disease (Vol. 1). Philadelphia: Lippincott-Raven, 1996:511–538.
Steinberg D: Low density lipoprotein oxidation and its pathobiological significance. J Biol Chem 1997;272:20963–20966.

# Chapter 23

# Coronary Blood Flow and Myocardial Ischemia

*Robert J. Henning* ▪ *Ray A. Olsson*

Over the past 40 years, increasingly sophisticated physiologic studies in conscious experimental animals and, more recently, in humans, have determined which physical factors determine coronary flow under physiologic conditions. Findings of recent studies at the cellular and molecular levels provide new insights into the mechanisms underlying the control of myocardial perfusion and the complex responses to coronary insufficiency. Several earlier reviews of coronary physiology[1-3] remain useful. This review focuses on newer developments, emphasizing myocardial ischemia and the body's adaptive responses to it.

## ▪ PHASIC CORONARY FLOW

Instantaneous flow through the epicardial coronary arteries and veins varies throughout the cardiac cycle in a way that reflects the interaction of aortic perfusion pressure and the action of the intramyocardial pump. Under basal conditions, flow through arteries supplying the left ventricle is antegrade throughout the cardiac cycle, but the flow rate is substantially higher in diastole (Fig. 23–1A). Owing to differences in flow rates and the longer duration of diastole, 60% to 80% of coronary flow occurs during diastole. The inflation of an intraaortic balloon during diastole as a means of augmenting coronary perfusion exploits this peculiarity of the coronary circulation. The lower flow rate in systole, when perfusion pressure is actually higher than during diastole, reflects the effect of the intramyocardial pump.

---

**Figure 23–1** ▪ Phasic flow patterns in epicardial coronary arteries of conscious, instrumented dogs. *(A)* Normal dog. From above downward, curves are electrocardiogram (ECG), flow in the left anterior descending (LDCF) and circumflex (LCCF) branches of the left coronary artery, aortic root pressure (ABP), left ventricular pressure (LVP) and end-diastolic pressure (LVEDP), and cardiac output (CO). Note that coronary blood flow is predominantly in diastole. Mean flow rate in systole is lower than in diastole. Arrows indicate the momentary decrease in coronary flow caused by atrial systole. *(B)* Phasic flow pattern of the right coronary arteries of conscious dogs. From top to bottom, curves are aortic pressure (AP, mm Hg), right coronary flow (RCF, mL/min), and cardiac output (CO, L/min). The left panel is a normal dog, the center and right panels are from dogs with congenital pulmonic stenosis. Note that, in normal dogs, systolic flow rate in the right coronary artery is higher than in a left coronary branch (compare with panels A and D) and that pulmonic stenosis decreases the systolic component of total flow in proportion to the degree of right ventricular systolic overload *(center and right)*. *(C)* Phasic flow pattern in a dog with idiopathic hypertrophic subaortic stenosis. From above downward, the curves are aortic pressure (ABP), circumflex coronary flow (LCCF), and cardiac output (CO). Note that backflow early in systole results in net negative flow in this portion of the cardiac cycle. *(D)* Phasic flow patterns in a coronary artery and a coronary vein of an anesthetized, open-chest dog. From above downward, curves are flow in the left anterior descending coronary artery (LAD) and great cardiac vein (GCV) and pressures in the aorta and great cardiac vein. Note that, whereas coronary arterial inflow is predominantly diastolic, venous outflow is predominantly systolic. (Reprinted from American Journal of Cardiology, Vol. 79, pages 2 to 9, Abrams J: Role of endothelial dysfunction in coronary artery disease. Copyright 1997, with permission from Excerpta Medica, Inc.)

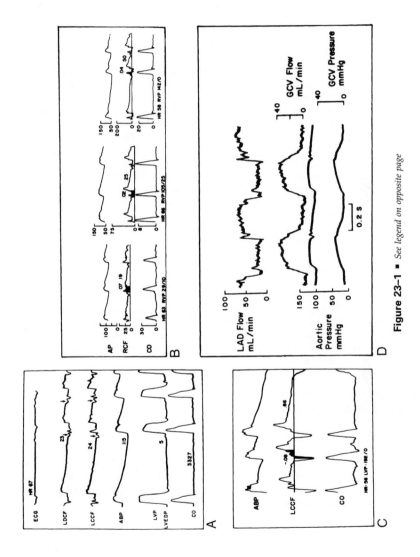

**Figure 23–1** ■ *See legend on opposite page*

Cardiac contraction does not simply throttle forward flow. Rather, it pumps blood "backward" from the depths of the myocardial wall, opposing forward flow in the epicardial arteries. Increasing myocardial contractility can cause retrograde flow during systole. This is evidence for an intramyocardial pump rather than a throttle effect, which would only reduce flow to zero.

Unlike the human coronary system, the right coronary artery of the dog supplies only the right ventricle and thus provides additional information about the influence of chamber pressure on phasic coronary flow patterns. Systolic flow rate in the right coronary artery is higher than in the left coronary branches (Fig. 23–1B, *left*), a fact that probably reflects the lower intramyocardial pressures developed in the wall of the right ventricle. Additional evidence for the importance of the intramyocardial pump comes from records of phasic coronary flow in dogs with congenital pulmonic stenosis and idiopathic hypertrophic subaortic stenosis. The flow pattern of the right coronary artery of dogs with pulmonic stenosis resembles that of the left coronary branch in that right coronary flow during systole decreases as right ventricular pressure increases (Fig. 23–1B, *center* and *right*). Similarly, there is substantial retrograde systolic flow in the left coronary branches of dogs with idiopathic hypertrophic subaortic stenosis (Fig. 23–1C). As a generalization, any stimulus that increases contractile force can cause systolic backflow, for example, administration of norepinephrine or dobutamine. Cardiac contraction also determines the timing of the coronary venous outflow of the left ventricle, which is almost entirely systolic (Fig. 23–1D).

Basal resistance in the coronary circulation is higher than in any other organ as the result of myogenic contraction of coronary smooth muscle in response to the distending force exerted by intracoronary pressure. The coronary circulation exhibits a high degree of autoregulation, which is the ability of the resistance vessels to adjust myogenic tone over a wide range of perfusion pressures to maintain a relatively constant perfusion rate (Fig. 23–2). Perfusion pressures below about 40 to 60 mm Hg exhaust the capacity of the resistance vessels to autoregulate. Below that limit, flow is proportional to perfusion pressure. As Figure 23–2 illustrates, autoregulatory tone is higher in the epicardial than in the endocardial arteries, which explains why the endocardium is particularly vulnerable to ischemia at low coronary perfusion pressures.

## ■ MYOCARDIAL ENERGY METABOLISM AND CORONARY PERFUSION

The constant activity of the beating heart demands a higher oxygen consumption for the left ventricle (5 to 10 ml/min/100 g of myocardium under basal conditions) than the brain (4 ml/min/100 g) or skeletal muscle (0.2 ml/min/100 g). Such measurements derive from the Fick principle, which allows calculation of the metabolic rate (MR) of a substance from measurements of blood flow rate (Q) and the concentrations of the substance in arterial and venous blood, respectively (Ca and Cv):

$$MR = Q(Ca - Cv)$$

Positive MR values indicate uptake of the substance, and negative values indicate release. In the case of the left ventricle, the composition of blood in the coronary sinus represents the venous drainage of the entire left ventricle; consequently, the calculation is straightforward. This approach to measuring oxygen consumption by the right ventricle and interventricular septum is not practical because of difficulty obtaining representative samples of venous blood from these structures. The coro-

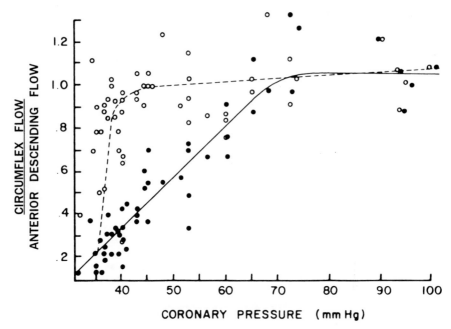

**Figure 23–2** ▪ Coronary autoregulation and autoregulatory reserve. Radiomicrosphere measurements of regional myocardial blood flow in the subendocardial *(closed circles)* and subepicardial *(open circles)* layers of the left ventricle supplied by the left circumflex branch of a dog, normalized by expressing as a fraction of flow in the corresponding regions supplied by the normally perfused left anterior descending branch. Controlled constriction of the circumflex branch reduced perfusion pressure. Autoregulatory reserve in the epicardium is high, flow being independent of pressure above 40 mm Hg. By contrast, autoregulatory reserve in the subendocardium is lower, flow becoming pressure dependent at about 70 mm Hg. (Reprinted from American Journal of Cardiology, Vol. 79, pages 2 to 9, Abrams J: Role of endothelial dysfunction in coronary artery disease. Copyright 1997, with permission from Excerpta Medica, Inc.)

nary venous drainage of the right ventricle consists of a number of small veins that drain into the right atrium. Owing to the difficulty of sampling blood from many small vessels, there is no evidence that each vein has the same oxygen content. Similarly, thebesian veins in the central portion of the interventricular septum drain directly into the cavity of the right ventricle. Oxygen consumption can, however, be measured in the right ventricle and interventricular septum by measuring blood flow with radiomicrospheres and arterial and venous oxygen content by reflectance spectroscopy. Oxygen consumption in the interventricular septum is similar to that of the left ventricular free wall, and that in the right ventricle is somewhat less, probably reflecting the lower workload of that chamber.[4]

The combination of high oxygen use and high basal coronary resistance causes a high transcoronary oxygen extraction of 60% to 80%. Thus, coronary sinus blood has the lowest oxygen content of any venous blood in the body, typically 5 ml/100 ml or less, and it changes very little when flow increases. The coronary venous $PO_2$, which is in the range of 20 mm Hg, is at an inflection point in the hemoglobin oxygen saturation curve. As a consequence, further oxygen extraction is limited by a disproportionate increase in thermodynamic work that is needed to dissociate oxyhemoglobin.

Since myocardial oxygen extraction is already near maximal at rest, an increase in coronary flow rate is the predominant response to increased oxygen use. Basal coronary flow is 50 to 100 ml/min/100 g and can increase as much as sixfold. Over

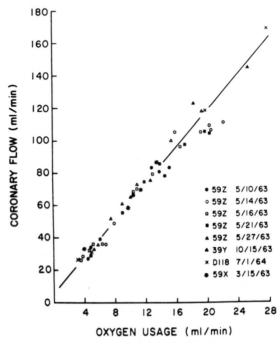

**Figure 23–3** ▪ Relationship between coronary flow and myocardial oxygen consumption in conscious dogs with various degrees of exertion. (Reprinted from American Journal of Cardiology, Vol. 79, pages 2 to 9, Abrams J: Role of endothelial dysfunction in coronary artery disease. Copyright 1997, with permission from Excerpta Medica, Inc.)

this physiologic range, coronary flow closely parallels oxygen use (Fig. 23–3). Hypoxia and ischemia are very potent stimuli to coronary vasodilatation. A 20- to 30-second coronary occlusion causes maximum coronary vasodilatation during the ensuing postischemic reactive hyperemia response.

The heart is not fastidious with respect to carbon sources for metabolism; lipids, organic acids, and glucose serve equally well as substrates. Studies of substrate metabolism by the human heart show that the oxidation of free fatty acids accounts for about two-thirds of myocardial oxygen consumption.

## Heterogeneity of Myocardial Perfusion and Metabolism

The average values of myocardial blood flow and metabolism over large volumes of myocardium conceal the marked heterogeneity of both regional myocardial blood flow (RMBF) and metabolism observed at the level of the perfusion fields of individual resistance vessels. It is now clear that regions of low RMBF and metabolism can coexist with areas of high RMBF and metabolism.

The first evidence of flow heterogeneity came from studies using the indicator dilution technique. Mathematical analysis of coronary venous outflow time-concentration curves established that RMBF varies over at least a 10-fold range. Measurements of RMBF by radiomicrosphere deposition also indicate heterogeneity of RMBF of three sorts. There is a *transmural gradient of perfusion*; flow to the subendocardium is 20% to 40% greater than that to the subepicardium. Second, there is *spatial heterogeneity* of flow within those layers; flow varies from region to region by an amount larger than the analytical error of the method for measuring RMBF. Because the large number of perfusion fields included in a tissue sample tends to "average out" the variability between individual perfusion fields, the range of values is narrower than that estimated by the indicator dilution technique, as little as threefold in tissue samples weighing 200 mg or more. Third, there is *temporal heterogeneity* of RMBF. Consecutive injections of radiomicrospheres labeled with different isotopes show that flow to a particular part of the left ventricle varies over time. At the level of the individual perfusion field, such a result suggests that the arteriole oscillates between open and closed states, the so-called "twinkling phenomenon."

Variability in local partial pressure of oxygen ($PO_2$), as measured by polarographic microelectrodes inserted into the myocardium, provided the first evidence that myocardial metabolism, like RMBF, may be heterogeneous. Further evidence of metabolic heterogeneity came from measurements of oxyhemoglobin saturation in intramyocardial venules by means of reflectance spectroscopy of frozen samples of heart muscle. These measurements showed that venous saturation varied widely from vein to vein, between zero and 60%. Average saturation was lower in the subendocardium, probably because of the greater workload of that layer. Correlations of RMBF with the rate of [³H]deoxyglucose uptake in samples of dog left ventricle (weighing an average of 83 mg) show that (1) RMBF varied from sample to sample over a 25-fold range and (2) glucose uptake paralleled RMBF, suggesting that high-flow regions have a higher metabolic rate.[5] Low-flow regions did not accumulate adenosine and therefore were not ischemic. Capillary density, mitochondrial density, and the activities of glycolytic and citric acid cycle enzymes were uniform, evidence that the low-flow areas had the potential for recruitment in the event of an increase in cardiac workload. Reducing coronary flow caused adenosine to accumulate in high-flow regions, evidence that a lower-flow reserve makes these areas vulnerable to ischemia. A drawback to the experimental measurement approach is that it characterizes the heart at a single point in time. Such "snapshots" do not answer a critical question: *Are the regional differences in RMBF and metabolism static, or do they oscillate over time?* The combination of a fixed pattern of flow heterogeneity and the vulnerability of high-flow regions could explain the patchy distribution of pathologic changes observed in hibernating myocardium (see later).

Thus, it appears that regions of low flow and metabolism normally coexist with regions of high flow and metabolism in the same heart. Whether regional heterogeneity of metabolism reflects heterogeneity of contractile function is not known.

## Regulation of Coronary Flow[6–8]

Coronary flow regulation may be conveniently thought of as consisting of two factors, a background of high myogenic vasoconstrictor tone opposed by endogenous vasodilators (see also Chapter 4). Type L voltage-gated calcium channels are important mediators of vasoconstrictor tone. Blockade of the $I_{CaL}$ current might account for the coronary vasodilator action of calcium entry blockers. For some time it was thought that adenosine, formed by the breakdown of adenosine triphosphate (ATP), could account for the control of coronary flow, but it is now clear that control is the result of the interaction of a number of autacoids (Table 23–1). Nitric oxide and adenosine appear to be the most important autacoids in the coronary circulation.

Endothelial cells generate the endogenous vasodilator nitric oxide in response to pulsatile stress, the force exerted by flowing blood. Activation of endothelial cell receptors for substances such as acetylcholine and bradykinin also stimulates nitric

Table 23–1

**Humoral Regulation of Coronary Blood Flow**

| Vasoactive Agent | Source | Direct Effect on Coronary Arteries | Mechanism |
|---|---|---|---|
| Norepinephrine | Adrenergic nerve fibers | Constriction<br>Dilatation | α-Adrenergic activation<br>β-Adrenergic activation |
| Epinephrine | Adrenal gland and sympathetic nerve fibers | Constriction<br>Dilatation | α-Adrenergic activation<br>β-Adrenergic activation |
| Dopamine | Adrenergic nerve fibers | Dilatation | Dopaminergic receptors |
| Angiotensin | Systemic circulation | Constriction | Angiotensin I receptors |
| Adenosine | Breakdown of adenosine triphosphate | Dilatation | Adenosine $A_2$ receptors |
| Histamine | Mast cells and basophils | Constriction<br>Dilatation | Histamine H1 receptors<br>Histamine H2 receptors |
| Prostacyclin | Vascular endothelium | Dilatation | Prostacyclin receptors |
| Thromboxane $A_2$ | Vascular endothelium and platelets | Constriction | Thromboxane $A_2$ receptors |
| Bradykinin | Vascular endothelium | Dilatation | Bradykinin $B_2$ receptors |
| Serotonin | Aggregating platelets | Constriction | Serotonin $S_1$ receptors |

Adapted from Feliciano L, Henning RJ: Coronary artery blood flow: Physiologic and pathophysiologic regulation. Clin Cardiol 1999;22:775–786.

oxide production and vasodilatation. Nitric oxide is a highly reactive free radical gas that, through the activation of a guanylate cyclase having a haem prosthetic group, initiates a protein phosphorylation cascade catalyzed by a cyclic guanosine-monophosphate (cGMP)–dependent protein kinase that ultimately leads to vasodilatation. This nitric oxide pathway is an appropriate target for drug therapy. The activity of nitrovasodilators depends on the release of nitric oxide. Phosphodiesterase inhibitors such as sidenafil (Viagra) amplify the nitric oxide signal by preserving cGMP. Inhibitors of nitric oxide synthase raise basal coronary tone and modify vasomotor responses such as autoregulation, suggesting a role for nitric oxide in the setting of basal tone and in mediating vasodilatation under physiologic conditions.

Three hydrolytic processes generate adenosine in the heart, from: (1) intracellular adenosine monophosphate (AMP) by a cytosolic 5'-nucleotidase, (2) S-adenosyl-homocysteine by the action of a specific hydrolase, and (3) extracellular nucleotides released from adrenergic nerve terminals by the action of cell surface ATP/ADPases and an ecto-5'-nucleotidase. Most cells take up adenosine avidly and incorporate it into the cellular adenylate pool, particularly coronary endothelial cells, which act as a "metabolic barrier" to the movement of adenosine across the endothelium. Consequently, adenosine levels in the coronary venous effluent are less than those of the cardiac interstitium. The activation of adenosine $A_{2A}$ receptors coupled to adenylate cyclase initiates a cAMP-dependent protein phosphorylation cascade that culminates in vasodilatation.

The activation of outward potassium currents in coronary smooth muscle cells appears to be an important event in coronary vasodilatation initiated by nitric oxide, adenosine, and prostanoids. Outward potassium currents hyperpolarize the myocyte cell membrane, raising the threshold for the $I_{CaL}$ that generates vasoconstrictor tone. The various mediators act on different potassium channels.[9] Nitric oxide increases the open probability of the potassium channels' carrying the large-conductance $Ca^{2+}$-activated ($I_{K,Ca}$) and delayed rectifier ($I_{kdrf}$) currents, but adenosine activates the channel carrying the gliburide-sensitive ($I_{KATP}$) current. Prostanoids may stimulate either $I_{K,Ca}$ or $I_{kdrf}$. Redundancy of these effector systems ensures coronary artery regulation should one system fail.

Nitric oxide and adenosine act at different levels in the coronary microcirculation: Whereas adenosine acts at the level of the true resistance vessels with diameters smaller than 100 μm, nitric oxide acts at larger preresistance vessels. Small imbalances between myocardial oxygen supply and demand probably generate adenosine, which causes dilatation of the resistance vessels. The resulting increases of flow and pulsatile shear stress on the endothelium of preresistance vessels generate nitric oxide, thus amplifying the adenosine signal. Although nitric oxide and adenosine are important in the regulation of coronary flow, neither one is essential. Experimental evidence indicates that the loss of one mechanism induces compensation by others. Mice that lack the gene for either endothelial nitric oxide synthase or adenosine $A_{2A}$ receptor have normal basal coronary tone and postischemic reactive hyperemia responses.

Endothelium-dependent coronary regulation becomes important in diseases such as the hyperlipidemias, atherosclerosis, and diabetes mellitus, which have in common decreased responsiveness to endothelium-dependent vasodilatation.[10] Each of the several explanations advanced to account for decreased vasodilator reserve in these diseases enjoys partial support. Proposed mechanisms include destruction of nitric oxide through increased production of superoxide, interference with G protein–mediated signal transduction by oxidized lipids, decreased membrane fluidity, and depletion of the nitric oxide synthase substrate cofactor tetrahydrobiopterin. Some clinical trials show that long-term dietary supplementation of L-arginine, which is important in the formation of nitric oxide, improves endothelium-dependent vascular responsiveness.

The coronary arteries are richly innervated with automatic fibers, and both parasympathetic and sympathetic divisions participate in the regulation of coronary flow. Whereas vagal and β-adrenergic receptor activation cause vasodilatation, α-adrenergic receptor activation causes vasoconstriction. Vasodilatation due to the stimulation of cardiac sympathetic efferent nerves is principally a consequence of increased cardiac contractility and metabolism rather than a direct effect on the coronary vessels. Blockade of coronary α-adrenergic receptors has little effect on coronary flow, indicating that those receptors do not participate in the setting of basal resistance. However stimuli such as exercise do not usually cause maximum coronary vasodilatation, in part because exercise increases α-adrenergic coronary vasoconstrictor tone. The increase in adrenergic tone during exercise is not transmural; rather, it selectively involves subepicardial vessels and serves to prevent shunting of blood away from the subendocardium. The release of neuropeptides such as vasoactive intestinal peptide from nerve terminals as co-transmitters along with the classic neurotransmitters also contributes to vasomotor control.

## Myocardial Ischemia[11–13]

The heart is extremely vulnerable to ischemia because it depends heavily on aerobic metabolism for energy production. For example, the occlusion of a major coronary branch in an experimental animal causes deterioration of indices of global function, such as left ventricular end-diastolic pressure (LVEDP) and the rate of change of left ventricular pressure with time (dP/dt), in as few as three to five beats and complete loss of regional contractile function in less than 1 minute. Cell death is not immediate, however; necrosis requires at least 15 minutes of cell ischemia. The adaptive response to ischemia is complex and, depending on the *degree* and the *duration* of hypoperfusion, can be either deleterious or cardioprotective. The past decade has seen important progress in understanding the pathogenesis of the ischemic syndromes. Angina pectoris is probably the most familiar clinical manifestation of myocardial ischemia. Either coronary occlusion of short duration or transient global hypoperfusion can produce reversible contractile dysfunction lasting hours to days after the restoration of perfusion, a phenomenon called *myocardial stunning*. Subtotal obstruction leading to chronic coronary insufficiency produces chronic, reversible contractile dysfunction (*myocardial hibernation*). Paradoxically, just a few minutes of coronary occlusion can protect the heart from a subsequent occlusion long enough to cause infarction, a phenomenon known as *ischemic preconditioning*. Chronic, progressive coronary obstruction serves as a stimulus to the development of *coronary collateral* vessels that preserve perfusion of potentially ischemic myocardium.

## Angina Pectoris[14, 15]

Adenosine release from ischemic myocardium was once thought to be simply a marker of ischemia and thus coincidental to ischemic chest pain. The observation that patients receiving adenosine for perfusion scintigraphy experienced chest pain resembling angina pectoris suggested that adenosine is actually the trigger for the angina. Subsequent work showed that infusions of adenosine into peripheral arteries are algogenic, causing pain in the perfusion field of the recipient artery. Intracoronary administration of adenosine to patients with stable angina induces chest pain similar in location and quality to that of the patient's angina but without electrocardiographic evidence of ischemia. Adenosine receptor blockade alleviates that pain and diminishes the pain patients experience with strenuous exercise. The activation of $A_1$ adenosine receptors on sympathetic fibers initiates the pain signal, which travels centrally and ultimately projects to the right and left cerebral cortex. Failure of intracoronary administration of adenosine to cause pain for a heart transplant recipient is additional evidence of the importance of the cardiac nerves. Similarly, patients with diabetic neuropathy are less sensitive to the algogenic effect of adenosine and tend to have less severe angina.

The severity and duration of myocardial ischemia probably separate patients who have ischemia without chest pain (silent ischemia) from those with angina pectoris. Electrocardiographic and hemodynamic monitoring of patients with obstructive coronary artery disease suggests that episodes of silent ischemia tend to be shorter (less than 3 minutes) and cause smaller hemodynamic changes than do attacks of angina. Nevertheless, ischemia severe enough to cause infarction without chest pain is not rare.

## Prinzmetal's Vasospastic Angina[16]

Prinzmetal's vasospastic angina differs from classical angina in that it occurs without an increase in myocardial oxygen demand and is associated with ST segment changes. Coronary spasm in these patients does cause myocardial ischemia as determined from coronary sinus blood flow measurements and radionuclide scintigraphy. On average, patients with vasospastic angina are younger than those with classic angina. Most have a fixed coronary artery obstruction proximal to the site of spasm. A fixed stenosis and vasospasm are additive risk factors. Between attacks of vasospastic angina, angiography may show little or no narrowing at the site of coronary spasm. Nevertheless, intravascular ultrasonography often shows evidence of atherosclerosis at the vasospastic sites. During the acute phase of Prinzmetal's angina, which lasts about 6 months, the risk of infarction is 5% to 20%

and of sudden death 2% to 10%. Subsequently, symptoms tend to improve and the risk of cardiac events decreases.

The trigger for vasospasm is indeterminate; indeed, conflicting evidence suggests that the trigger may differ from patient to patient. An association with cigarette smoking—and, in a substantial number of patients, coexisting Raynaud phenomenon or migraine—suggests that vasospastic angina may be one facet of a spastic vasculopathy. Provocative tests using intracoronary infusions of ergonovine maleate, a stimulant of α-adrenergic and serotonin receptors, are useful in establishing the diagnosis. Ergonovine provocation does not identify the trigger for vasospasm, however, because blockers of α-adrenergic, serotonin, or thromboxane receptors are ineffective as prophylaxis against vasospasm. Attacks precipitated by cold or hyperventilation suggest that coronary vasospasm may be neurogenic. Acetylcholine can also precipitate focal coronary spasm, a response different from the diffuse narrowing it causes in patients who have endothelial dysfunction. Nitrates and/or calcium channel–blocking agents can be effective both in treating an acute attack and as prophylaxis.

## Myocardial Stunning[11-13]

Myocardial stunning describes "the *mechanical dysfunction* that persists after *coronary occlusion and reperfusion* despite the absence of *irreversible damage* and . . . return of *normal or near-normal coronary perfusion.*"[10] The broad spectrum of stunned myocardium ranges from the response to a single short-lived occlusion that produces no necrosis to a zone of stunned myocardium surrounding a subendocardial infarct. Currently, the oxyradical hypothesis and the calcium hypothesis are the favored explanations for the pathogenesis of stunning (Fig. 23–4). The two hypotheses are complementary rather than mutually exclusive. The oxyradical hypothesis proposes that reperfusion generates reactive oxygen species such as the hydroxyl radical that indiscriminately attack almost any of the proteins and lipids in the cardiac cell, including ion pumps in the sarcolemma and contractile proteins. Administration of antioxidants before or during the interval of ischemia, but not after reperfusion has begun, blunts stunning. Thus, stunning is but one facet of reperfusion injury, and it occurs immediately after perfusion is restored. The calcium hypothesis proposes that stunning reflects blunting of the calcium sensitivity of the contractile proteins. Clinically, stunning may occur whenever the heart

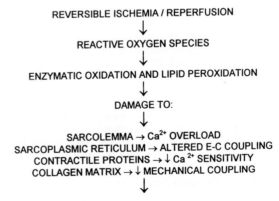

**Figure 23–4** ▪ Proposed pathophysiologic mechanisms that lead to myocardial stunning. E-C, excitation-contraction.

REVERSIBLE ISCHEMIA / REPERFUSION
↓
REACTIVE OXYGEN SPECIES
↓
ENZYMATIC OXIDATION AND LIPID PEROXIDATION
↓
DAMAGE TO:
↓
SARCOLEMMA → $Ca^{2+}$ OVERLOAD
SARCOPLASMIC RETICULUM → ALTERED E-C COUPLING
CONTRACTILE PROTEINS → ↓ $Ca^{2+}$ SENSITIVITY
COLLAGEN MATRIX → ↓ MECHANICAL COUPLING
↓
MECHANICAL DYSFUNCTION

suffers sublethal ischemia, as from unstable angina, exercise-induced ischemia, angioplasty, myocardial infarction treated with thrombolysis, or cardiac surgery.

## Myocardial Hibernation[11–13, 17]

Hibernation is chronic, reversible contractile dysfunction in the setting of coronary artery disease. Put another way, hibernation is an adaptive reduction of energy expenditure in response to a reduction of energy supply, a perfusion-contractility mismatch, and it represents the preservation of viability rather than necrosis in the dysfunctional segment. The definition of hibernation does not specifically include ischemia because there is neither consensus about the precise meaning of that term nor convincing evidence that coronary flow to hibernating myocardium is actually reduced to levels below the rather broad range called normal. If we define ischemia as a level of perfusion that cannot support contractile function, then hibernating myocardium meets the definition even when blood flow is in the normal range. On the other hand, if we define ischemia as a level of perfusion that stimulates anaerobic metabolism (as indicated by increased glucose uptake or lactate release), such biochemical evidence may be absent despite depressed myocardial contractility.

Early in the era of coronary bypass grafting, abnormalities of wall motion were attributed to infarction and scarring of the myocardium. It soon became evident, however, that, for a subset of patients, revascularization improved regional wall motion, a finding that could only mean that the myocardium was viable but dysfunctional. Currently, preoperative evaluation of candidates for coronary bypass surgery uses improvement in wall motion in response to an infusion of dobutamine as a means of identifying hibernating myocardium. Several nuclear imaging procedures are also useful for identifying hibernating myocardium. They include the delayed uptake of thallium 201 ($^{201}$Tl), uptake of technetium 99m ($^{99m}$Tm)-sestamibi that is at least 50% that of a myocardial segment with normal contractility, and the uptake of radiolabeled substrates such as carbon 11 ($^{11}$C) acetate or fluorine 18 ($^{18}$F) fluorodeoxyglucose. Imaging by positron emission tomography is ideally suited to the study of substrate uptake, but that technique is not widely available in the United States.

Clinically, it may be difficult to discriminate between myocardium undergoing hibernation and myocardium undergoing repeated stunning secondary to a stenotic coronary lesion that provides adequate perfusion at rest but not during exercise.

Histopathologic examination of samples of hibernating myocardium from patients undergoing revascularization detects structural changes in the myocytes and the interstitial space.[13] Glycogen stores increase, and mitochondria vary in size and are fewer in number. There may be disorganization of sarcomeres, cytoskeletal proteins, and the sarcoplasmic reticulum. Extracellular matrix proteins increase, and there may be reparative fibrosis. The morphologic and biochemical markers of apoptosis are demonstrable. Although the phenotype of a hibernating myocyte may resemble that of a fetal myocyte, the cells do not express fetal proteins, so the morphologic changes represent degeneration rather than dedifferentiation. The changes in myocyte structure are reversible, although restoration of contractile function may take weeks or months and is not necessarily complete. The delayed functional recovery of patients undergoing revascularization probably reflects the time necessary for cellular remodeling to occur. The time for recovery of contractile function is proportional to the severity of the histopathologic changes

## Ischemic Cardiomyopathy

Ischemic cardiomyopathy describes arteriosclerotic heart disease that produces severe myocardial dysfunction and clinical manifestations indistinguishable from those of primary dilated myocardiopathy. Later revisions of the definition include previous myocardial infarction or significant (greater than 70%) coronary stenosis and myocardial dysfunction out of proportion to the size of the infarction and the amount of coronary artery disease. Myocardial stunning and hibernation may account for this disparity. Symptoms of heart failure dominate the clinical picture. Patients with ischemic cardiomyopathy have increased activity of the renin-angiotensin and sympathetic nervous systems. The pathologic findings are those of hibernation and infarction. Histochemical studies of tissue samples show preservation of the enzymes of glycolysis and depletion of the enzymes of fatty acid oxidation.

Patients with ischemic cardiomyopathy have a poorer prognosis than those with dilated cardiomyopathy because the risks of ischemic events and of the cardiomyopathy are additive. Different trials place mortality rates between 5% and 50% per year, depending on the degree of ventricular dysfunction, the mass of infarcted or hibernating myocardium, arrhythmias, hypertension, and the patient's age. Treatment goals are (1) reduction of myocardial ischemia/hibernation, (2) modulating the activity of the renin-angiotensin system with angiotensin-converting enzyme inhibitors or angiotensin receptor blockers, and (3) blunting sympathetic stimulation with β-adrenergic receptor antagonists.

## Ischemic Preconditioning[10, 14]

Studies in experimental animals show that an interval of coronary occlusion too brief to cause infarction reduces the size of the infarct caused by a subsequent lethal occlusion, an effect called *ischemic preconditioning*. Consistent with the idea that adenosine released during ischemia was the stimulus for cardioprotection, later work showed that an intracoronary infusion of adenosine affords as much cardioprotection as does ischemia. Substances other than adenosine released from ischemic myocardium may also serve as stimuli to preconditioning, however. For example, ischemia causes neurotransmitter release from myocardial adrenergic terminals, and intracoronary administration of an α-adrenergic agonist induces preconditioning. Indeed, a number of agonists acting at receptors coupled to G proteins induce pharmacologic preconditioning, and antagonists acting at those receptors can prevent it. Muscarinic, opioid, bradykinin, and angiotensin receptor agonists are examples. Mitogens such as fibroblast growth factors 1 and 2 also precondition the myocardium, as can physical stimuli such as myocardial stretch. Preconditioning also occurs elsewhere than the heart, for example in skeletal muscle and brain. A reduction of infarct size is not the only index of the cardioprotection preconditioning affords; during reperfusion, preconditioned hearts have fewer arrhythmias and recovery of contractility is better.

The mechanism(s) that serve to precondition the myocardium are incompletely understood. One model with substantial support is that proposed by Downey (Fig. 23–5). Adenosine released during ischemia activates $A_1$ adenosine receptors coupled to phospholipase C (D?) via a pertussis toxin–sensitive G protein. The diacylglycerols generated by hydrolysis of phospholipids initiate a protein phosphorylation cascade through the activation of protein kinase C (PKC), probably the ε-isoform and perhaps the η-isoform. The substrates in that cascade are indeterminate, but they probably include sarcolemmal (and mitochondrial?) $K_{ATP}$ channels, tyrosine kinases, and protein phosphatase 2A. In any event, the $K_{ATP}$ channel appears to play an important role. Drugs that open $K_{ATP}$ channels, such as cromakalim can induce preconditioning, and, conversely, drugs that block $K_{ATP}$ channel opening, such as glibenclamide can prevent preconditioning. The Downey model may be only part of the story: there is evidence[15] that mitogenic peptides such as acidic

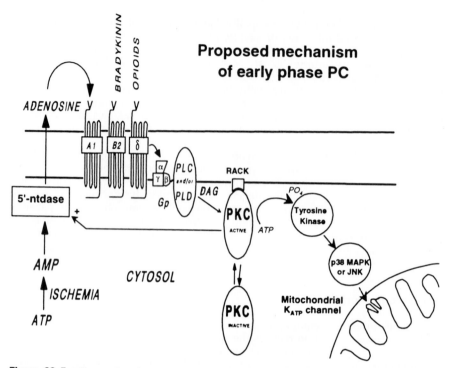

**Figure 23–5** ■ Proposed mechanism of ischemic preconditioning. A1 = adenosine A1 receptor, B2 = bradykinin B2 receptor, δ = delta opioid receptor, PLC = phospholipase C, PLD = phospholipase D, DAG = diacylglycerol, Gp = guanosine regulatory protein, 5′-ntdase = 5′-nucleotidase, PKC = protein kinase C, PO$_4$ = phosphate, AMP = adenosine monophosphate, ATP = adenosine triphosphate, MAPK = mitogen activated protein kinase, JNK = c-Jun N-terminal kinase, K$_{ATP}$ = adenosine triphosphate–activated potassium channel, PC = preconditioning, RACK = receptor for activated C-kinase. See text for discussion. (Courtesy of Dr. James M. Downey, University of South Alabama.) (Reprinted from American Journal of Cardiology, Vol. 79, pages 2 to 9, Abrams J: Role of endothelial dysfunction in coronary artery disease. Copyright 1997, with permission from Excerpta Medica, Inc.)

and basic fibroblast growth factors are expressed early in the course of cardiac ischemia and, when infused directly into heart muscle, are cardioprotective. Mitogenic peptides might not only participate in immediate cardioprotection but might also initiate the second window of protection (see later).

The cardioprotection provided by preconditioning is transitory, lasting only 1 to 2 hours. One explanation[16] is that preconditioning ischemia leads rapidly to the expression of insulin-like growth factor II (IGF-II), a peptide that binds to the insulin receptor and, like insulin itself, is cardioprotective. The expression of IGF-binding protein 5, which inhibits the cardioprotective effect of IGF-II, follows shortly thereafter and may serve as the "off" signal for preconditioning.

Many questions about the details of preconditioning remain unanswered. Preconditioning absolutely depends on an interval of reperfusion after the brief occlusion, but what happens during reperfusion is not clear. It is not clear either which PKC isoform(s) are important, nor whether there are PKC substrates other than K$_{ATP}$ channels that participate in preconditioning. Animal models are the main source of information about preconditioning, but because of important species differences, it is difficult to know which animal models best represent the human myocardium.

There is now evidence for preconditioning of human myocardium. Patients undergoing coronary angioplasty have greater ST segment elevation and report more chest pain during the first balloon inflation than during subsequent inflations. Preinfarction angina appears to be cardioprotective, reducing infarct size as assessed by the severity of electrocardiographic and enzyme changes, in-hospital mortality, and complications. Patients with coronary artery disease who undergo sequential exercise stress tests separated by a rest period have delayed-onset angina in the second test because of the "warmup" phenomenon.

## Delayed Preconditioning or the "Second Window of Protection"

Although the immediate protection afforded by an interval of preconditioning ischemia disappears after 1 to 2 hours, cardioprotection reappears 24 hours later and lasts up to 3 days. The mechanism of the late protection is unknown, but it probably differs from the immediate preconditioning response. The delay is long enough to bring into play factors such as gene expression and protein synthesis, which means that the second window of protection could involve the expression of more than one protein. The release of signaling molecules such as tumor necrosis factor, mitogens, and cytokines during reperfusion could serve as the stimulus to the second window of protection.

## Coronary Collaterals[17–19]

The coronary arteries are not end arteries. Rather, there are two types of coronary collateral vessels that differ in size, structure, and location within the ventricular wall. One type is the interarterial collateral vessels that extend from one epicardial coronary branch to another. Such vessels contain a muscular coat. The second type are tubes of endothelial cells the size of capillaries or slightly larger that are distributed throughout the ventricular wall but especially in the subendocardium, where they form a plexus. The extent of collateralization differs significantly between species. Normal human and pig hearts have only a few rudimentary collateral vessels, but the dog has a more developed collateral system. Ischemia is a powerful stimulus to coronary collateral formation. In dogs, a coronary constriction sufficient to abolish coronary reserve without affecting basal flow rate will, over 4 to 5 days, stimulate collateral growth that prevents myocardial infarction when the constricted artery is completely occluded. Although native collaterals are sparse in the human coronary circulation, competent collateral circulation to myocardium can support normal contractile activity. In large part, perfusion via collateral arteries explains why single-vessel coronary artery disease is relatively benign. In this instance, ischemia and contractile dysfunction appear only when disease in the donor artery curtails collateral flow to the myocardium.

The development of a collateral circulation involves two processes, enlargement of existing epicardial collateral arterioles by "recapitulated vasculogenesis" and budding off of new subendocardial collaterals by angiogenesis. The remodeling of epicardial coronary collateral vessels is a dynamic process that depends on local factors such as wall stress and an inflammatory response in the collateral vessel that leads to lysis of the extracellular matrix, proteolysis of the internal elastic membrane, apoptosis of smooth muscle cells, and, finally, proliferation of endothelial and smooth muscle cells. At least five peptide growth factors (vascular endothelial growth factor, acidic and basic fibroblast growth factors, platelet-derived growth factor, and insulin-like growth factor) regulate the structural changes.

Although collateral development is a response to ischemia, the two are not causally related. Collateral arterial growth occurs in epicardial vessels remote from the ischemic zone and continues after the ischemia is relieved. Because the evolving collateral is physically separated from the ischemic zone it is not clear what signal initiates collateral vessel development. In the case of angiogenesis, the release of cytokines from the surrounding tissues as part of the inflammatory response to ischemia seems to be an important stimulus.

## ■ REFERENCES

1. Feigl EO: Coronary physiology. Physiol Rev 1983:63:1–205.
2. Olsson RA, Bünger R, Spaan JAE: Coronary circulation. *In* Fozzard HA, Haber E, Jennings RB, et al (eds): The Heart and Cardiovascular System: Scientific Foundations. New York: Raven 1991: 1393–1425.
3. Spaan JAE (ed): Coronary Blood Flow. Dordrecht: Kluwer Academic Publishers, 1991.
4. Weiss HR, Sinha AK: Regional oxygen saturation of small arteries and veins in the canine myocardium. Circ Res 1978;42:119–126.
5. Loncar R, Flesche CW, Deussen A: Coronary reserve of high- and low-flow regions of the dog heart left ventricle. Circulation 1998;98:262–270.
6. Muller JM, Davis MJ, Chilian WM: Integrated regulation of pressure and flow in the coronary microcirculation. Cardiovasc Res 1996;32:668–678.
7. Chilian WM: Coronary microcirculation in health and disease: Summary of an NHLBI workshop. Circulation 1997;95:522–528.
8. Feigl EO: Neural control of coronary blood flow. J Vasc Res 1998;35:85–92.
9. Sylven C: Mechanisms of pain in angina pectoris—a critical review of the adenosine hypothesis. Cardiovasc Drugs Ther 1993;7:745–759.
10. Crea F, Gaspardone A: New look at an old symptom: Angina pectoris. Circulation 1997;96:3766–3773.
11. Crea F, Kaski JC, Maseri A: Key references on coronary spasm. Circulation 1994;89:2442–2446.
12. Kloner RA, Bolli R, Marban E, et al: Medical and cellular implications of stunning, hibernation and preconditioning: An NHLBI workshop. Circulation 1998;97:1848–1867.
13. Heusch G, Ferrari R, Hearse DJ, et al: Myocardial hibernation—questions and controversies. Cardiovasc Res 1997;36:301–309.
14. Wijns W, Vatner SE, Camici PG: Hibernating myocardium. N Engl J Med 1998;339:173–181.
15. Elsasser A, Schlepper M, Klovekorn WP, et al: Hibernating myocardium: An incomplete adaptation to ischemia. Circulation 1997;96:2920–2931.
16. Downey JM, Cohen MV: Signal transduction in ischemic preconditioning. Adv Exp Med Biol 1997;430:39–55.
17. Ping P, Zhang J, Qiu Y, et al: Ischemic preconditioning induces selective translocation of protein kinase C isoforms ε and η in the heart of conscious rabbits without subcellular translocation of total protein kinase C activity. Circ Res 1997;81:404–414.
18. Schaper W, Ito WD: Molecular mechanisms of coronary collateral vessel growth. Circ Res 1996;79:911–919.
19. Schaper W, Schaper J: Collateral Circulation: Heart, Brain, Kidney, Limbs. London: Kluwer Academic Publishers, 1993.

## ■ SUGGESTED READINGS

Abrams J: Role of endothelial dysfunction in coronary artery disease. Am J Cardiol 1997;79(12B):2–9.
Berne RM, Rubio R: Coronary circulation. *In* Berne RM, Sperelakis S (eds): Handbook of Physiology. Section 2: The Cardiovascular System, Vol. 1. Bethesda: American Physiological Society, 1979.
Feliciano L, Henning RJ: Coronary artery blood flow: Physiologic and pathophysiologic regulation. Clin Cardiol 1999;22:775–786.
Ganz P, Braunwald E: Coronary blood flow and myocardial ischemia. *In* Braunwald E (ed): Heart Disease, A Textbook of Cardiovascular Medicine, 5th ed. Philadelphia: WB Saunders, 1997:1161–1183.
Marcus M: Metabolic regulation of coronary blood flow. *In* Marcus M (ed): The Coronary Circulation in Health and Disease. New York: McGraw-Hill, 1983.
Maseri A: Role of coronary artery spasm in symptomatic and silent myocardial ischemia. J Am Coll Cardiol 1987;9(2):249–262.
Ross R: The pathogenesis of atherosclerosis: A perspective for the 1990's. Nature 1993;362:801–809.
Vane JR, Anggard EE, Bottling RM: Regulatory functions of the vascular endothelium. N Engl J Med 1990;323:27.

Chapter 24

# Risk Factors and Prevention, Including Hyperlipidemias

*Antonio M. Gotto, Jr.* ▪ *John Farmer*

Coronary artery atherosclerosis had long been considered to be a chronic progressive disease in which clinical management was limited solely to reducing symptoms by improving the balance between coronary flow and myocardial oxygen demand, with minimal survival benefits. Advanced coronary artery disease (CAD) had previously been managed by mechanical methods using either coronary artery bypass grafting or percutaneous transluminal angioplasty. These procedures gained widespread use without being verified by the rigorous placebo-controlled prospective trials that are required of most pharmacologic agents.

The past decade has seen major advances in the diagnosis and management of established atherosclerosis, and these benefits have been extended to persons with either preclinical atherosclerosis or simply with a significant risk factor profile. These advances have improved the ability to alter the risk factor profile in patients with CAD or at risk for its development. Antihypertensive medication such as the calcium channel blockers, angiotensin-converting enzyme (ACE) inhibitors, and angiotensin receptor blockers have been refined and lack many of the adverse metabolic side effects that hampered the use of previously available agents. Additionally, the advent of the 3-hydroxy-3-methylglutaryl coenzyme A (HMG CoA) reductase inhibitors (or statins) has revolutionized the ability to control dyslipidemia. Pharmacologic advances have been coupled with improvements in diagnostic modalities that have enhanced the ability to identify patients with preclinical disease and to modify the clinical course before an ischemic event.

## ▪ EPIDEMIOLOGY AND THE RISK FACTOR CONCEPT

Age-adjusted death rates for coronary atherosclerosis have been declining dramatically during the past three decades.[1] The absolute number of events is increasing, however, but with a shift to older individuals, and atherosclerosis remains the single most common cause of death in the United States. Approximately 1 million Americans suffer an acute myocardial infarction (MI) each year; this situation represents a major clinical and economic burden. Approximately 50 to 100 billion dollars per year is expended in medical interventions and lost wages.[2] Public health measures have been directed at patients who are considered to be at risk for development of overt coronary atherosclerosis because of a number of conditions that have been statistically linked to the incidence of atherosclerosis.

CAD represents a syndrome with many underlying causes, thus rendering a single approach to the therapy of at-risk patients problematic. The concept of risk factor management has evolved on the basis of epidemiologic studies that link a number of potential factors with the subsequent development of CAD. Epidemiology is a descriptive science, however, and factors that are statistically related to CAD either may be nonmodifiable or may simply exist as a marker of risk rather

**437**

than a condition involved in the distinct pathogenesis of atherosclerosis. Stamler has established criteria for assessing the etiologic significance of epidemiologic associations.[3]

1. *Strength of the association.* Relative risk expresses the statistical risk when the ratio of the incidence of the disease is tabulated to compare individuals exposed to the trait versus those not exposed.
2. *Gradation.* Gradation determines if the relative risk increases with enhanced exposure to the trait being studied.
3. *Time sequence.* Exposure to the risk factor must precede development of the disease in a temporal relation that is compatible with clinical or pathologic observations.
4. *Consistency.* The relative risk should be demonstrated to be increased in different populations under variable circumstances.
5. *Independence.* The persistence of the increased relative risk should be independent and additive to other traits known or suspected to be involved in disease etiology.
6. *Predictive capacity.* The risk factor should be demonstrated to predict disease incidence rates in other independent populations.
7. *Coherence.* The risk factor should demonstrate a plausible pathogenic mechanism by which the trait functions as an etiologic agent.

## ■ RISK FACTORS

### Modifiable Risk Factors

#### Hypertension

Elevations of both systolic and diastolic blood pressure have been correlated with increased morbidity and mortality due to various cardiovascular conditions including cerebrovascular accident, sudden cardiac death, aortic dissection, congestive heart failure, and acute MI. Meta-analysis of a large number of prospective intervention trials in hypertensive patients has demonstrated a consistent and graded correlation between blood pressure and risk for MI. This correlation has been strengthened by the demonstration of clinical benefit accruing after reduction of blood pressure. The magnitude of clinical benefit in morbidity and mortality of acute MI as it relates to hypertension control has, however, been less than anticipated from the epidemiologic relationships between blood pressure and coronary atherosclerosis. Analysis of the Multiple Risk Factor Intervention Trial (MRFIT) database estimated that 32% of all acute ischemic coronary mortality could be related to prevalence of diastolic blood pressure readings exceeding 80 mm Hg.[4] The majority of clinical trials did not achieve this degree of clinical benefit in MI after antihypertensive therapy, and this failure has been ascribed to a number of potential problems associated with therapeutic interventions, including induced adverse metabolic or electrolyte effects associated with certain classes of antihypertensive agents. Additionally, concern has been raised that overzealous lowering of blood pressure in patients with ostial lesions, extensive CAD, or diastolic abnormalities may result in decreased coronary perfusion and a potential J-shaped relation between blood pressure reduction and mortality. However, the Hypertensive Optimization Trial did not demonstrate an increase in mortality with aggressive lowering of blood pressure.[5] Additionally, regression of left ventricular hypertrophy is not necessarily achieved with all classes of antihypertensive agents, although newer drugs such as the ACE inhibitors, angiotensin receptor blockers, calcium blockers, and beta blockers all clearly reduce left ventricular mass. Modification of blood pressure has clearly been demonstrated to decrease all-cause mortality, and although trials involving alterations of CAD event rates may be less than optimal, blood pressure modification should be a cornerstone of preventive measures.

## Tobacco Use

The use of tobacco products has been associated with a number of adverse health outcomes including chronic obstructive pulmonary disease, carcinoma, and coronary atherosclerosis. Epidemiologic studies have estimated that 170,000 cardiovascular deaths in the United States could be attributed to the use of tobacco products.[6] However, the mechanism by which tobacco use is associated with increased cardiovascular risk has not been completely elucidated. Tobacco is associated with decreases in high-density lipoprotein (HDL) cholesterol of up to 5 mg/dl (0.13 mmol/l), and cessation of tobacco smoking restores HDL cholesterol levels to presmoking levels. Endothelial dysfunction, which is believed to be the first step in the pathogenesis of atherosclerosis, is exacerbated by the use of tobacco products and results in a tendency toward both vasoconstriction and reduction in the endothelial production of prostacyclin, which acts as not only a vasodilator but also an antiplatelet agent.[7] Oxidation of low-density lipoprotein (LDL) is a prerequisite for recognition, binding, and uptake by the monocyte-macrophage system and results in subsequent generation of foam cells. Increased oxidant stress is associated with increased risk for atherosclerosis, and the use of tobacco products has been associated with an increased level of oxidized LDL, which has been demonstrated histologically within the atherosclerotic plaque.[8, 9] In addition to the ways in which cigarette smoke affects lipid handling and platelet function, a number of other hemostatic parameters are adversely altered after ingestion of cigarette smoke. The disturbance in endothelial function also results in an imbalance between thrombotic and fibrinolytic factors. The dysfunctional endothelium has been demonstrated to reduce the production of tissue plasminogen activator (tPA) and increase plasminogen activator inhibitor (PAI-I), resulting in decreased ability to lyse a coronary thrombus.

The association of tobacco smoke with atherosclerosis has been prospectively verified in the Atherosclerosis Risk in Communities (ARIC) study, which analyzed the relation between tobacco smoke and the intimal medial thickness of the carotid artery as assessed by serial ultrasound examinations.[10] An increase in the intimal medial thickness of 50% was associated with the current use of tobacco smoke during the 36-month follow-up period. The impact of tobacco use on intimal medial thickness was more significant when combined with associated risk factors such as diabetes or hypertension.

The association of CAD and tobacco use represents a major modifiable risk factor, and cessation of smoking should be a major goal of preventive measures.

## Obesity

Clinical guidelines to the identification and evaluation of obesity have been published.[11] Obesity is defined as a body mass index of 30 kg/m² or greater when body mass index is defined as the weight in kilograms divided by the square of the height in meters. Overweight is defined as a body mass index of 25 to 29.9 kg/m². Obesity is believed to be a multifactorial, chronic disease that results from the interaction of genetic and nongenetic factors including a number of environmental causes. Epidemiologic studies have demonstrated that overweight or obese adults, as characterized by a body mass index of greater than 25 kg/m², have enhanced susceptibility to a number of cardiovascular problems including abnormal glucose tolerance, hypertension, dyslipidemia, and atherosclerosis. More importantly, clinical trials have demonstrated that achievement of ideal body weight may improve an individual's lipid profile, blood pressure, and glucose tolerance. Approximately

20% of the population in the United States may be considered to be overweight.[12] Increasing interest has focused on the localization of fat as a major determinant of the subsequent risk of the development of atherosclerosis. The male pattern of obesity is characterized by truncal adiposity and may be either estimated by the waist-hip circumference ratio or measured by computed tomography. The waist-hip ratio is associated with increased cardiovascular risk when it is in excess of 0.95 in men and 0.8 in women.

The mechanism by which truncal obesity conveys increased cardiovascular risk is complex but is clearly associated with a number of metabolic abnormalities including dyslipidemia and hyperinsulinemia. In addition to the abnormal metabolic profile associated with truncal obesity, a number of hemostatic abnormalities have also been correlated with increased truncal adiposity, including elevated levels of fibrinogen and PAI.

Randomized clinical trials of weight loss have also demonstrated an improvement in blood pressure, dyslipidemia, and hyperglycemia.[13] Limited evidence also shows that improvement in the waist-hip ratio decreases blood pressure in nonhypertensive but overweight individuals. Dyslipidemia is common in patients who are overweight and is generally characterized by increased levels of triglycerides and reduced levels of HDL associated with an increased number of small, dense LDL particles. Randomized clinical trials using lifestyle interventions have shown improvement in the lipid profile, which is especially beneficial if associated with weight loss. Lifestyle and pharmacotherapy studies of patients with type II diabetes have demonstrated improvement in fasting insulin and blood glucose levels and resultant hemoglobin A1C.

The treatment of obesity may involve a number of approaches including diet, behavior modification, increased physical activity, surgery, and pharmacologic therapies. Dexfenfluramine hydrochloride and fenfluramine hydrochloride were voluntarily withdrawn from the market because of their potential association with induced valvular abnormalities. Sibutramine hydrochloride has been approved by the Food and Drug Administration for weight loss and has been associated with maintenance of an induced decrease in body weight. Despite the complexities of definitely establishing an independent relation between increased body weight and its distribution to coronary atherosclerotic event rates, patients should be encouraged to increase physical activity and maintain a serious effort to achieve ideal body weight in a sustained manner.

## Diabetes

Both type I and type II diabetes are associated with increased cardiovascular risk, and a number of epidemiologic trials have demonstrated vascular disease to be the major cause of morbidity and mortality in diabetic subjects.[14] In addition to the abnormal carbohydrate metabolism in patients with diabetes, a number of other risk factors including obesity, dyslipidemia, and hypertension are frequently linked with diabetes in risk factor clustering. Diabetes is a prevalent condition in the United States. Approximately 16,000,000 individuals fulfill the diagnostic criteria, with the vast majority of diabetic persons classified as having type II. Moreover, a number of individuals may not satisfy strict criteria for the diagnosis of diabetes but have peripheral insulin resistance with either normal or minimally elevated glucose levels with associated hyperinsulinemia. Elevated insulin levels have been determined to be an independent cardiac risk factor for vascular disease and may be involved in the pathogenesis of hypertension because of stimulation of vascular smooth muscle cell growth, as well as sympathetic activation and increased sodium reabsorption by the renal tubules.[15] Diabetes is a major cardiac risk factor, and diabetic individuals who suffer an acute MI have significantly increased morbidity and mortality compared with nondiabetic persons. Women with diabetes lose the gender-mediated cardioprotection and have a higher post-MI complication rate.

Treatment of diabetes as a means to decrease complications of atherosclerosis remains controversial. The Diabetes Control and Complications Trial (DCCT) examined the role of intensive insulin treatment in a relatively young and presumably low-risk patient population. Because of the young age and relatively benign risk factor profile of the enrolled subjects, the incidence of cardiovascular events was too low to establish a definite statistical relation.[16] Additionally, the United Kingdom Prospective Diabetes Study Group evaluated the efficacy of intensive glucose control in a complex protocol with either sulfonylureas or insulin therapy compared with conventional treatment and were unable to demonstrate definite clinical benefit in macrovascular complications in patients with type II diabetes.[17]

Dyslipidemia is common in diabetic persons and is frequently characterized by borderline elevations of triglyceride levels associated with low levels of HDL cholesterol and increased levels of small, dense LDL. Although weight loss, exercise, and glycemic control may improve the lipid abnormalities in diabetic persons, the values may not normalize. Prospective lipid-modifying trials involving only diabetic individuals have not been performed, but retrospective subgroup analysis of the Scandinavian Simvastatin Survival Study and Helsinki Heart Study have shown beneficial trends in diabetic subjects enrolled in these major trials.[18, 19] Despite the lack of definite evidence in controlled clinical trials, most experts recommend aggressive metabolic interventions in diabetic patients, with optimization of blood pressure, body weight, dyslipidemia, and exercise levels in an attempt to decrease subsequent risk for coronary atherosclerosis.[20]

The American Diabetes Association has issued recommendations regarding categories of risk and lipid goals of therapy in individuals with non–insulin-dependent diabetes mellitus (NIDDM) (Table 24–1). The more stringent lipid goals

Table 24–1

**Categories of Risk and Treatment Decisions Based on Baseline Lipid Levels, mg/dl (mmol/l), in Non–Insulin-Dependent Diabetes Mellitus**

| Risk | LDL-C | HDL-C | Triglyceride |
|------|-------|-------|--------------|
| Higher | ≥130<br>(3.36) | <35<br>(0.91) | ≥400<br>(4.52) |
| Borderline | 100–129<br>(2.59–3.36) | 35–45<br>(0.91–1.16) | 200–399<br>(2.26–4.52) |
| Lower | <100<br>(2.59) | >45<br>(1.16) | <200<br>(2.26) |

| | Medical Nutrition Therapy | | Drug Therapy | |
|---|---|---|---|---|
| | Initiation Level | LDL-C Goal | Initiation Level | LDL-C Goal |
| With CAD, PVD, or CVD | >100<br>(2.59) | ≤100<br>(2.59) | >100<br>(2.59) | ≤100<br>(2.59) |
| Without CAD, PVD, and CVD | >100<br>(2.59) | ≤100<br>(2.59) | ≥130*<br>(3.36) | ≤100<br>(2.59) |

*For diabetic patients with one or more CAD risk factors (low HDL-C [<35 mg/dl], hypertension, smoking, family history of CVD, or microalbuminaria or proteinuria), some authorities recommend an LDL-C goal ≤100 mg/dl.

Caveats: (1) Medical nutrition therapy should be attempted before starting pharmacologic therapy. (2) Because diabetic men and women are considered to have equal CAD risk, age and sex are not considered risk factors.

LDL-C, low-density lipoprotein cholesterol; HDL-C, high-density lipoprotein cholesterol; PVD, peripheral vascular disease; CAD, coronary artery disease; CVD, cardiovascular disease.

Adapted from American Diabetes Association: Management of dyslipidemia in adults with diabetes. American Diabetes Association. Diabetes Care 1999;22(1):S56–59.

in primary prevention for patients with NIDDM reflect the greater risk for heart disease observed in these patients than in those in the general population who qualify for primary prevention.

## Physical Activity

Decreased physical activity is frequently associated with a number of cardiac risk factors including dyslipidemia and abnormal glucose tolerance. Maintenance of an increased level of physical exertion has been demonstrated to result in improvement of the risk factor profile. The impact of regular physical exercise has also been correlated with a decreased rate of cardiovascular complications in epidemiologic studies. The MRFIT demonstrated that physically active subjects who maintained moderate physical activity had an approximate 27% reduction in cardiovascular complications when compared with a sedentary control group.[21] The impact of exercise on cardiovascular risk factors is a function of either the duration or intensity of the level of activity.[22] The duration of physical activity as determined by the number of kilometers run per week and the intensity in a 12-km run has been analyzed in a large cohort of male and female athletes. Improvement in the lipid profile and blood pressure levels was demonstrated, and exercise has been associated with an increase in HDL cholesterol. The level of increase appears to be more closely correlated with the distance run per week rather than with intense, short bursts of speed. Long-distance runners have a significantly greater rise in HDL cholesterol when compared with subjects who ran less than 16 km/week. Physical activity should be encouraged for patients at risk for coronary atherosclerosis because of the demonstrable improvement in a number of cardiac risk factors and clinical event rates.

## Dyslipidemia

### Classification of Lipoproteins

Dyslipidemia is clearly a major modifiable risk factor for CAD, although an isolated serum cholesterol level has minimal predictive value in the individual patient, because cholesterol is distributed in a number of lipoprotein fractions that have variable clinical impact on cardiovascular risk. Dyslipidemia can currently be classified using sophisticated molecular biologic and genetic techniques. The Fredrickson classification, however, which provides a readily obtainable and clinically useful classification, still has utility for practicing physicians (Table 24–2).

Table 24–2

**Fredrickson Classification of the Hyperlipidemias**

| Phenotype | Elevated Lipoprotein(s) Level | Elevated Lipid Levels | Plasma TC | Plasma TG | Relative Frequency (%)* |
|-----------|-------------------------------|-----------------------|-----------|-----------|-------------------------|
| I | Chylomicrons | TG | N to ↑ | — | <1 |
| IIa | LDL | TC | ↑ ↑ | N | 10 |
| IIb | LDL and VLDL | TG, TC | ↑ ↑ | ↑ ↑ | 40 |
| III | IDL | TG, TC | ↑ ↑ | ↑ ↑ ↑ | <1 |
| IV | VLDL | TG, TC | N to ↑ | ↑ ↑ | 45 |
| V | VLDL and chylomicrons | TG, TC | ↑ to ↑ ↑ | ↑ ↑ ↑ ↑ | 5 |

*Percentages of patients in the United States with hyperlipidemia.

TC, total cholesterol; TG, triglyceride; N, normal; LDL, low-density lipoprotein; VLDL, very low-density lipoprotein; IDL, intermediate-density lipoprotein.

Adapted from International Lipid Information Bureau. The ILIB Lipid Handbook for Clinical Practice. New York: ILIB, 1995:29.

Plasma lipoproteins are responsible for the transport of lipids within the vascular compartment and are complex water-soluble particles. The circulating lipoproteins may be identified and subsequently classified by various techniques including density ultracentrifugation, electrophoretic mobility, and analysis of the chemical constituents on the surface of these particles. The major circulating lipoproteins are chylomicrons, chylomicron remnants, very low-density lipoprotein (VLDL), LDL, HDL, and lipoprotein(a).

**Chylomicron and Chylomicron Remnants.** Chylomicrons are large particles formed from the exogenous ingestion of fatty constituents in the diet. The density of these particles is less than 0.95 g/ml for chylomicrons and 1.006 g/ml for chylomicron remnants. Chylomicrons have a diameter ranging from 800 to 5000 nm and have no electrophoretic mobility. Chylomicron remnants, which normally are rapidly cleared from the circulation, are incompletely hydrolyzed particles that have a diameter greater than 300 nm and that also remain at the origin during electrophoretic studies.

**Very Low-Density Lipoprotein.** VLDL carries endogenously produced triglycerides and has a density of less than 1.006 g/ml and a particle diameter ranging between 300 and 800 nm. VLDL is produced by the liver and migrates in the prebeta region when subjected to an electrical field. Intermediate-density lipoprotein (IDL) particles are formed from incomplete catabolism of VLDL and are also triglyceride rich. The density of these particles ranges from 1.006 to 1.019 g/ml, with a diameter of 250 to 350 nm. IDL particles migrate in the broad beta region.

**Low-Density Lipoprotein.** LDL carries the bulk of circulating cholesterol, and its main component is cholesteryl ester. The density of this highly atherogenic particle ranges from 1.019 to 1.063 g/ml, with a diameter of 180 to 280 nm. LDL migrates in the beta region.

**High-Density Lipoprotein.** HDL carries mainly cholesteryl ester and is believed to be protective in cardiovascular disease because of a number of potential mechanisms including reverse cholesterol transport. HDL is a small particle with a density ranging between 1.063 and 1.210 g/ml, with a diameter of 50 to 90 nm. HDL migrates in the alpha region.

**Lipoprotein(a).** Lipoprotein(a) may be described as an LDL particle that is linked by a disulfhydryl group to a large hydrophilic glycoprotein termed *apo (a)*. Apo (a) has structural homology with plasminogen and has been linked to the presence and severity of atherosclerosis.[23] Lipoprotein(a) is distributed with a skewed distribution in Asians and whites, with the majority of individuals having a level of less than 10 mg/dl (0.26 mmol/l). Blacks demonstrate a more gaussian distribution of this particle.[24] Lipoprotein(a) lacks serine protease activity but has been demonstrated to bind to plasminogen receptors, thus potentially having a role not only in lipid metabolism but also in the inhibition of fibrinolysis.

### Clinical Dyslipidemia

**Conditions Associated Primarily with Hypercholesterolemia.** The Fredrickson classification is not an etiologic classification, nor does it consider levels of HDL cholesterol and lipoprotein(a) or differentiate between primary and secondary dyslipidemias (Tables 24–3 and 24–4). A practical approach to the management and classification of dyslipidemias is to consider the dyslipidemia on the basis of the abnormal lipid fraction, which may be relatively easily obtained from routine lipid determinations in the clinical laboratory (elevated cholesterol, elevated triglycerides, or low HDL cholesterol level). Pure hypercholesterolemia is characterized by a number of primary and secondary dyslipidemias that include conditions acquired by both genetic factors and sedentary lifestyle and poor dietary habits.

*Familial Hypercholesterolemia.* Familial hypercholesterolemia occurs with a gene frequency of approximately 1 in 500 individuals in the United States and thus

Table 24–3

### Selected Causes of Primary Dyslipidemia

| | |
|---|---|
| **Hypercholesterolemia** | **Primary combined hyperlipidemias** |
| Heterozygous familial hypercholesterolemia | Familial combined hyperlipidemia |
| Homozygous familial hypercholesterolemia | Type III hyperlipidemia |
| Familial defective apo B-100 | **Primary hypertriglyceridemia** |
| Polygenic hypercholesterolemia | Familial hypertriglyceridemia (type IV or V |
| **Disorders of high-density lipoprotein** | hyperlipidemia) |
| **metabolism** | Familial chylomicronemia |
| Familial hypoalphalipoproteinemia | Lipoprotein lipase deficiency |
| Lecithin: cholesterol acyltransferase deficiency | Apo C-III deficiency |
| Familial apo A-I/C-III deficiency | |
| Tangier disease, fish-eye disease | |
| Apo A-I$_{Milano}$ (A-I variant) | |

represents one of the more common genetic abnormalities in whites. Familial hypercholesterolemia has been demonstrated to be a genetic disorder involving decreased production or function of the LDL receptor. Familial hypercholesterolemia is transmitted as an autosomal disorder and may involve abnormalities in the synthesis, transport, or clustering of the LDL receptor within the coated pit. The end result, however, is a reduced capacity to clear circulating LDL and other lipoproteins containing apo B or apo E from the circulation. Individuals who are heterozygous for familial hypercholesterolemia have a reduction of 50% of the circulating LDL receptors, which results in an approximate doubling of LDL cholesterol. Even in the heterozygous state, familial hypercholesterolemia is associated with a significantly increased risk for the development of CAD, which typically develops by the age of 50 years in men and 60 years in women. The condition is generally diagnosed by the determination of increased circulating LDL without another genetic or secondary cause, coupled with a family history of premature atherosclerosis. Corneal arcus and tendinous xanthomas may also be present but are not necessary for the diagnosis.

Homozygous familial hypercholesterolemia is a rare condition and occurs only in approximately one per million persons in the United States. Affected individuals have no functioning LDL receptors, and the diagnosis may be made from umbilical cord blood. Individuals with this condition have extremely elevated LDL cholesterol levels, documented to be as high as 1200 mg/dl (31.04 mmol/l). Premature exten-

Table 24–4

### Selected Causes of Secondary Dyslipidemia

| | | |
|---|---|---|
| ↑ Low-density lipoprotein cholesterol | Hypothyroidism<br>Nephrotic syndrome<br>Chronic liver disease | Cholestasis<br>Dysglobulinemia<br>Anorexia nervosa |
| ↑ Triglycerides | Excessive alcohol consumption<br>Obesity<br>Pregnancy<br>Diabetes mellitus<br>Hypothyroidism<br>Chronic renal failure<br>Beta blockers | Diuretics<br>Exogenous estrogens<br>(oral administration)<br>Isotretinoin<br>Cushing syndrome<br>Oral contraceptives |
| ↓ High-density lipoprotein cholesterol | Physical inactivity<br>Smoking<br>Diabetes mellitus | Obesity<br>Hypertriglyceridemia |

sive coronary and peripheral atherosclerosis is the rule, and acute MI has been documented at less than 1 year of age.

*Polygenic Hypercholesterolemia.* Polygenic hypercholesterolemia has a complex etiology involving a genetic predisposition coupled with dietary increases in the intake of saturated fat and cholesterol.[25] The prevalence of polygenic hypercholesterolemia is unknown, but 1 to 5% of the population of the United States is thought to be affected. The associated dyslipidemia is less severe than in heterozygous familial hypercholesterolemia, although drug and dietary therapy may be required for normalization of the lipid profile.

*Familial Combined Hyperlipidemia.* Familial combined hyperlipidemia is relatively common and may be noted in 1% of the population in the United States but with increased prevalence in persons with atherosclerosis.[26] The genetic defect is transmitted in an autosomal dominant manner and is thought to be clinically manifested by hepatic overproduction of apo B-100–containing lipoproteins. Apo B-100 is distributed in VLDL, IDL, and LDL; thus, the clinical presentation of familial combined hyperlipidemia may be elevated cholesterol levels, elevated triglyceride levels, or a combined defect. Distinguishing this condition from other genetic disorders characterized by increased LDL cholesterol levels may be difficult, although tendinous xanthomas are uncommon with this disorder.

*Familial Defective Apo B-100.* Familial defective apo B-100 is characterized by inability to clear from the circulation the lipoproteins that carry this surface apoprotein.[27] The LDL receptor is normal in number and function but is unable to recognize apo B-100 because of a structural abnormality in the binding domain, which results in decreased recognition and clearance by the apo B/E receptor. Familial defective apo B-100 is less common than heterozygous familial hypercholesterolemia and has a gene prevalence of approximately 1 in 700.

**Conditions Associated Primarily with Decreased Levels of HDL Cholesterol.** Total and LDL cholesterol levels are related to risk for CAD in a continuous, graded curvilinear fashion.[28] Elevated HDL cholesterol level is associated with a decreased risk for atherosclerosis, although the mechanism is complex and multifactorial. LDL, when ineffectively cleared from the plasma compartment, is believed to be associated with deposition of cholesterol in the vascular wall. Oxidative modification of LDL and recognition by the monocyte-macrophage cellular elements results in the formation of foam cells. Decreased levels of HDL cholesterol have been associated with increased cardiovascular risk in a number of epidemiologic studies, although there are exceptions to this rule, as manifested by several genetic conditions associated with low HDL cholesterol but no apparent increased risk of premature CAD (see Table 24–3). The Framingham Heart Study demonstrated that both men and women whose HDL cholesterol levels fell below 35 mg/dl (0.91 mmol/l) had an eightfold relative increase in the incidence of symptomatic coronary atherosclerosis compared with subjects whose HDL cholesterol levels were greater than 65 mg/dl (1.68 mmol/l).[29] The benefit conferred by HDL is multifactorial and may include reverse cholesterol transport, by which HDL acts as a mediator for removal of cholesterol from peripheral tissues to the liver. Additionally, cholesterol can be transferred into apo B–containing particles (VLDL and LDL) using the cholesteryl ester transport protein. HDL has also been demonstrated to increase the half-life of prostacyclin, to stimulate endothelial repair, and to have potential roles in triglyceride metabolism.

Hypoalphalipoproteinemia may occur in up to 5% of the general population and is characterized by a primary decrease in circulating HDL cholesterol levels associated with normal levels of total cholesterol, LDL cholesterol, and triglycerides. Reductions in circulating levels of HDL may also be associated with various drugs (e.g., beta blockers, progesterone, and others) and other conditions such as the use of tobacco products or diets rich in polyunsaturated fats. Thus, exclusion of remediable secondary causes of low HDL cholesterol levels should be made before assigning a genetic origin to the disorder.

Several genetic disorders associated with low levels of HDL cholesterol are not clearly correlated with a significant increased risk for premature CAD. Tangier disease is a rare autosomal recessive disorder that has been demonstrated to be secondary to increased catabolism of HDL, apo A-I, and apo A-II.[30] The increased catabolic activity of HDL may be associated with enhanced reverse cholesterol transport and may partially explain the lack of a definite association with an increased prevalence of coronary atherosclerosis. Lecithin:cholesterol acyltransferase (LCAT) deficiency is a familial disorder that results in increased circulating cholesterol levels and a decrease in cholesteryl ester, which is associated with alteration of the structural components of circulating lipoproteins. HDL does not undergo maturation in this condition, and the levels are generally decreased.

**Conditions Associated Primarily with Hypertriglyceridemia.** The role of hypertriglyceridemia as an independent risk factor in coronary atherosclerosis remains controversial (see Table 24–3).[31] Early univariate analysis of clinical and angiographic trials established a strong relation between the presence of CAD and elevated levels of triglycerides. However, use of multivariate analysis has tended to minimize the potential independent role of hypertriglyceridemia as a cardiac risk factor when obesity, sedentary lifestyle, diabetes, hypertension, and low HDL cholesterol levels are considered. The use of multivariate analysis for statistical correlation has been questioned when analyzing risk factors that are metabolically interrelated. Catabolism of the triglyceride-rich VLDL via activation of lipoprotein lipase results in the rapid transfer of surface lipids into HDL and thus renders the statistical application of multivariate analysis problematic. Additionally, chemical determination of triglyceride levels lacks precision, and intervariability and intravariability in the measurements are considerable. Concern has also been raised about using the determination of triglycerides after a 15-hour fast. Patients with established CAD have been demonstrated to exhibit postprandial lipemia when subjected to a standardized oral fat load, implicating the potential role of cytotoxic triglyceride-rich remnant particles in the pathogenesis of atherosclerosis. Triglyceride values are also elevated in a multitude of clinical conditions without a predictable impact on risk.

Hypertriglyceridemia may be associated with genetic and nongenetic conditions. Sedentary lifestyle, obesity, and glucose intolerance are frequently associated with mild to moderate elevations of triglycerides that may often be returned to normal by hygienic measures. Triglyceride values are also elevated in the insulin resistance syndrome, which is characterized by truncal obesity, hypertension, clotting abnormalities, and dyslipidemia (predominantly involving high triglycerides and low HDL cholesterol levels).

Some genetic dyslipidemias have been associated with markedly elevated triglyceride levels that demonstrate a variable impact on cardiovascular risk. Familial hyperchylomicronemia (type I hyperlipidemia) is a rare disorder that is associated with dramatically elevated levels of triglycerides.[32] Type I hyperlipidemia is due to absence of the key enzyme in triglyceride metabolism, lipoprotein lipase, or its naturally occurring activator (apo C-II). The diagnosis is often made in infancy during evaluation for recurrent bouts of pancreatitis. Cutaneous manifestations are common and include eruptive xanthomas. Lipemia retinalis may also occur with severe hypertriglyceridemia. Familial chylomicronemia is associated with severe dyslipidemia and is refractory to management with the usually available pharmacologic agents. Dietary fat should be restricted to less than 10% of total calories and delivered in the form of short- and medium-chain triglycerides, which are absorbed directly into the portal vein instead of being reconstituted as chylomicrons within the lacteals of the gastrointestinal (GI) lymphatic syndrome.

Dysbetalipoproteinemia (type III hyperlipidemia) is inherited as a genetic abnormality involving apo E and is clinically manifested in individuals homozygous for apo E2/E2.[33] The gene for this disorder is relatively common but requires interaction with environmental factors to become clinically manifested. Dysbetalipoproteinemia is diagnosed in about 1 in 5000 persons in the United States. Patients with type III hyperlipidemia have a reduced capacity to clear apo E2–containing particles from the circulation, and lipoproteins bearing these apoproteins tend to accumulate in the plasma after a fatty meal.[34] The disorder should be suspected when levels of both cholesterol and triglycerides are elevated (for triglycerides, approximately 300 mg/dl [3.39 mmol/l]) and are roughly equal, but the precise diagnosis requires sophisticated testing with determination of apo E isoforms. Dysbetalipoproteinemia is often controllable with dietary restriction of fat but may require pharmacologic therapy in the form of fibrates or statins.

Familial endogenous hypertriglyceridemia presents as elevated VLDL levels and is classified in the Fredrickson classification as being type IV. Triglyceride levels in this condition generally are between 200 and 500 mg/dl (2.26 to 5.65 mmol/l), and HDL cholesterol value is often decreased. Premature atherosclerosis is not a clear feature of this disease, but attempts should be made to normalize the triglyceride levels.

Familial combined hyperlipidemia, which is due to hepatic overproduction of apo B–containing particles, may also present as pure hypertriglyceridemia, with treatment frequently directed against the elevated VLDL fraction.

**Secondary Dyslipidemias.** A full discussion of secondary causes of dyslipidemia is beyond the scope of this chapter. Before a diagnosis of primary dyslipidemia may be ventured, however, secondary causes of dyslipidemia must be precluded. For the purposes of testing for secondary dyslipidemias, the presentations of dyslipidemia may be divided into three categories: category 1, increased total cholesterol and normal triglyceride values; category 2, increased total cholesterol and increased triglyceride levels; and category 3, increased total cholesterol and increased triglyceride levels when the triglyceride level is three to five times higher than the cholesterol level and the plasma looks lipemic. Figures 24–1 to 24–3 provide algorithms to evaluate dyslipidemia in each of these categories, and Table 24–4 lists selected common causes of secondary dyslipidemias.

### National Cholesterol Education Program Guidelines

The National Cholesterol Education Program (NCEP) has established guidelines for the diagnosis of dyslipidemia and recommendations involving dietary and pharmacologic therapies in an attempt to decrease cardiovascular risk. Because the process of atherosclerosis is believed to begin relatively early in life, the NCEP recommends that all adults older than 20 years have a lipoprotein determination performed at least once every 5 years. Diagnostic and therapeutic recommendations differ, depending on whether interventions are being used in primary or secondary prevention. Primary prevention is directed at persons without clinical disease, and secondary includes those with clinical evidence of atherosclerosis. This distinction is somewhat arbitrary, because patients without symptomatic disease may nevertheless have significant atherosclerotic plaque.

The NCEP has recommended the establishment of the risk factor profile that consists of LDL cholesterol level and six other positive risk factors and one negative risk factor (Table 24–5). These other positive risk factors include the following:

1. Advancing age—Although nonmodifiable, advancing age is associated with increased cardiovascular morbidity and mortality, and men 45 years or older or women 55 years or older are considered to be at increased risk.
2. Positive family history of atherosclerosis—Atherosclerosis is considered to be a risk factor when documented in the family history to be manifested at

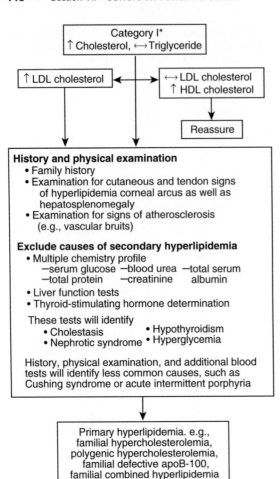

**Figure 24–1** ■ Algorithm to evaluate dyslipidemias in patients with increased total cholesterol and normal triglyceride levels. Usually polygenic, multifactorial causes.* (Gotto AM, Carlson LA, Illingworth DR, Thompson GR: Clinician's Manual on Hyperlipidemia, 5th ed. London: Science Press, 1998:38.)

a premature age, which is defined as documented MI or sudden cardiac death without a known noncardiac cause occurring before the age of 55 years in the individual's father or first-degree male relative or before the age of 65 years in the individual's mother or other female first-degree relative.

3. Current use of tobacco products.

4. Hypertension—Hypertension is defined as untreated blood pressure equal to or exceeding 140/90 mm Hg or the concomitant use of antihypertensive agents.

5. Low HDL cholesterol level—HDL cholesterol defined as less than 35 mg/dl (0.91 mmol/l) is associated with an increased risk.

6. Diabetes mellitus.

Elevated HDL cholesterol level is generally associated with decreased risk for premature atherosclerosis and is thus considered to be a negative risk factor when

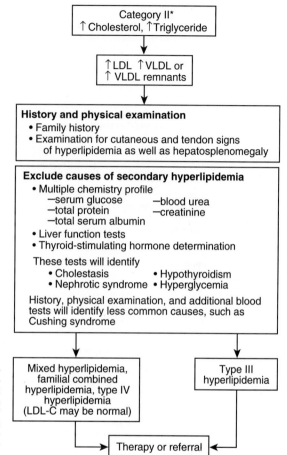

**Figure 24–2** ■ Algorithm to evaluate dyslipidemias in patients with increased total cholesterol and increased triglyceride levels. Establishment of a specific cause is usually difficult.* (Gotto AM, Carlson LA, Illingworth DR, Thompson GR: Clinician's Manual on Hyperlipidemia, 5th ed. London: Science Press, 1998:39.)

the HDL cholesterol level exceeds 60 mg/dl (1.55 mmol/L), thus allowing one risk factor to be subtracted from the total.

High risk, defined as a net of two or more CAD risk factors, leads to more vigorous intervention in primary prevention in adults without evidence of CAD. Advancing age (defined differently for men and women) is treated as a risk factor because rates of CAD are higher in the elderly than in the young and in men than in women of the same age. Obesity is not listed as a risk factor because it operates through other risk factors that are included (hypertension, hyperlipidemia, decreased HDL cholesterol level, and diabetes mellitus), but it should be considered a target for intervention. Physical inactivity is similarly not listed as a risk factor, but it too should be considered a target for intervention, and physical activity is recommended as desirable for the majority of individuals.

**Priority Groups for Cholesterol Screening.** Because of the current health care environment, universal lipid screening of patients may be considered impractical or economically unfeasible. However, selective screening of high-risk individuals should be undertaken. The patient population who should be considered for selec-

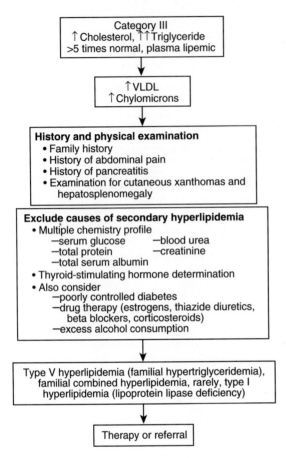

**Figure 24–3** ■ Algorithm to evaluate dyslipidemias in patients with increased triglyceride levels when the triglyceride levels are three to five times greater than the cholesterol level and the plasma looks lipemic. (Gotto AM, Carlson LA, Illingworth DR, Thompson GR: Clinician's Manual on Hyperlipidemia, 5th ed. London: Science Press, 1998:40.)

tive screening may be divided into four priority groups in a manner that complements the NCEP guidelines (Table 24–6).

**Primary Prevention.** The NCEP has established lipid goals for primary prevention and has designated a total cholesterol value of less than 200 mg/dl (5.17 mmol/l) as desirable. Cholesterol levels determined to be between 200 and 239 mg/dl (5.17 to 6.18 mmol/l) are considered to be borderline high, and greater than

Table 24–5

**Other Risk Factors in Evaluating Coronary Artery Disease Risk**

| Positive risk factors | Low HDL-C (<35 mg/dl [0.91 mmol/l])* |
|---|---|
| Age | Diabetes mellitus |
| Family history of coronary artery disease | Negative risk factor |
| Hypertension | HDL-C ≥60 mg/dl (1.55 mmol/l)*† |
| Current tobacco use | |

*Confirmed by measurements on several occasions.
†If the high-density lipoprotein cholesterol (HDL-C) level is ≥60 mg/dl (1.55 mmol/l), subtract one risk factor (because high HDL-C levels decrease coronary artery disease risk).

Table 24–6

**Priority Groups for Cholesterol Screening**

**Highest priority**
Patients with coronary artery disease or peripheral vascular disease and younger than 65 years.
Patients with clinical evidence of hypercholesterolemia
Those with family history of hyperlipidemias, premature coronary artery disease, or other
atherosclerotic diseases
Patients with diseases that affect lipid metabolism (e.g., diabetes, hypothyroidism, and renal
failure)
**Medium to high priority**
Those known to have two or more of the following risk factors: smoking, hypertension, obesity,
male sex
**Medium to low priority**
Those known to have a single risk factor
**Low priority**
Other adults

Adapted from Gotto AM, Carlson LA, Illingworth DR, Thompson GR: The Clinician's Manual on Hyperlipidemia, 5th ed. London: Science Press, 1998:28.

240 mg/dl (6.21 mmol/l) is considered elevated. The determination of the lipid levels for risk stratification is arbitrary, but large-scale epidemiologic studies such as the MRFIT have identified an approximate doubling in the relative risk for an MI as the cholesterol level increases from 200 to 240 mg/dl (5.17 to 6.21 mmol/l). However, there is considerable overlap between patients with and without documented atherosclerosis when total cholesterol level is considered, and approximately 20% of acute MIs occur in persons with cholesterol levels less than 200 mg/dl (5.17 mmol/l), emphasizing the potential importance of the assessment of lipid subfractions such as HDL cholesterol.[35]

After a patient's risk factor profile and lipid status are established, further evaluation is determined by the total risk factor score (Table 24–7). Patients who are clinically free of manifestations of atherosclerosis and who have an acceptable risk factor profile including normal total and HDL cholesterol levels require no specific intervention, although instruction in dietary approaches to risk reduction using the Step I diet should be offered. The risk factor profile and cholesterol level should be reassessed in 5 years. Patients whose cholesterol level falls in the borderline range but is associated with a normal HDL cholesterol level and less than two other risk factors should also be instructed about dietary therapy and other hygienic measures as a means to reduce the risk for the subsequent development of coronary atherosclerosis. These individuals should be increasingly monitored, however, and the risk factor and lipid profile should be reassessed in 1 to 2 years.

Table 24–7

**Initial Classification Based on Total and High-Density Lipoprotein
Cholesterol Levels**

| | |
|---|---|
| **Total cholesterol** | |
| Desirable blood cholesterol level | <200 mg/dl (5.17 mmol/l) |
| Borderline-high blood cholesterol level | 200–239 mg/dl (5.17–6.18 mmol/l) |
| High blood cholesterol level | ≥240 mg/dl (6.21 mmol/l) |
| **HDL-C** | |
| Low levels of HDL-C | <35 mg/dl (0.91 mmol/l) |

HDL-C, high-density lipoprotein cholesterol.

A full lipid analysis with determination of LDL cholesterol level is recommended for patients with low HDL cholesterol level plus two or more other risk factors if the cholesterol value is high or borderline elevated (Table 24–8). LDL cholesterol level is considered to be desirable if less than 130 mg/dl (3.36 mmol/l). LDL cholesterol level exceeding 160 mg/dl (4.14 mmol/l) is considered to be elevated in primary prevention, with a borderline level between 130 and 159 mg/dl (3.36 to 4.11 mmol/l). A desirable LDL cholesterol value should be managed with dietary measures similar to those for the general population. LDL cholesterol level in the borderline elevated range but with fewer than two other risk factors should also receive hygienic interventions using diet and exercise, and the lipoprotein analysis should be repeated in 1 year. Individuals who have a borderline elevated LDL cholesterol range and who have two or more risk factors or elevated LDL cholesterol levels should have a repeat analysis within 2 months, coupled with an attempt to lower LDL to a more desirable range.

**Secondary Prevention.** Secondary prevention is considered to stratify the patient into a group with increased risk for recurrent atherosclerosis, and a more aggressive approach is recommended. Cholesterol levels fall during a number of acute illnesses, including MI, thus potentially rendering a lipid determination in the periinfarction period to be falsely low. Lipid values obtained within the first 12 hours of an acute MI are generally reliable, however, and may be used for risk stratification purposes. Additionally, patients whose levels are elevated after 12 hours may be considered to have had significantly higher levels of LDL cholesterol before the acute event and are at increased risk because of the potential for underlying genetic causes of dyslipidemia.[36] In the presence of CAD, a therapeutic goal of 100 mg/dl (2.59 mmol/l) has been recommended. An LDL cholesterol level exceeding 100 mg/dl (2.59 mmol/l) should be addressed by complete clinical examination including evaluation for secondary and genetic causes of dyslipidemia,

## Table 24–8

### Treatment Decisions Based on Low-Density Lipoprotein Cholesterol Levels*

| Dietary Therapy | Initiation Level | LDL-C Goal |
|---|---|---|
| Without CAD and with fewer than two other risk factors | ≥160 mg/dl (4.14 mmol/l) | <160 mg/dl (4.14 mmol/l) |
| Without CAD and with two or more other risk factors | ≥130 mg/dl (3.36 mmol/l) | <130 mg/dl) (3.36 mmol/l) |
| With CAD | >100 mg/dl (2.59 mmol/l) | ≤100 mg/dl (2.59 mmol/l) |

| Drug Treatment | Consideration Level | LDL-C Goal |
|---|---|---|
| Without CAD and with fewer than two other risk factors | ≥190 mg/l (4.91 mmol/l) | <160 mg/dl (4.14 mmol/l) |
| Without CAD and with two or more other risk factors | ≥160 mg/dl (4.14 mmol/l) | <130 mg/dl (3.36 mmol/l) |
| With CAD | ≥130 mg/dl† (3.36 mmol/l) | ≤100 mg/dl (2.59 mmol/l) |

*In men younger than 35 years and premenopausal women with LDL-C levels 190–219 mg/dl (4.91 mmol/l), drug therapy should be delayed except in high-risk patients such as those with diabetes.

†In patients with CAD and LDL-C levels 100–129 mg/dl, the physician should exercise clinical judgment in deciding whether to initiate drug treatment.

LDL-C, low-density lipoprotein cholesterol; CAD, coronary artery disease.

with potential treatment options being determined by the response to nonpharmacologic therapy.

### Treatment

**Nonpharmacologic.** Lifestyle approaches to patients either at risk for the development of CAD or with established atherosclerosis should always be used initially and continued even with subsequent initiation of pharmacologic therapy. Reduction of dietary intake of calories and saturated fat should be used as a means to maintain ideal body weight and reduce circulating total and LDL cholesterol. Dietary therapy should be coupled with a regular exercise program, which may need to be monitored for patients with known atherosclerosis. Dietary therapy should be the cornerstone of preventive efforts, and a judicious diet should be begun by all patients. Benefits of diet have been demonstrated in several clinical trials and affect potentially not only the lipid profile but also glucose metabolism and elevated blood pressure.

The NCEP has used the Step I and Step II diets for both primary and secondary prevention (Table 24–9). In primary prevention, when an individual has fewer than two other risk factors, dietary intervention is recommended if the LDL cholesterol level exceeds 160 mg/dl (4.14 mmol/l). In primary preventive efforts that are accompanied by two or more risk factors, a more aggressive approach is used and diet is initiated at an LDL cholesterol level of 130 mg/dl (3.36 mmol/l). Secondary prevention uses the initial institution of dietary therapy to decrease LDL cholesterol levels below 100 mg/dl (2.59 mmol/l).

The Step I diet has been recommended for the general population and is composed of less than 30% of the total calories originating from fat, with 8% to 10% of total calories being accounted for by saturated fat. Cholesterol intake is limited to less than 300 mg/day, and no more than 15% of total calories should be from monounsaturated fat intake. Polyunsaturated fat should be no more than 10% of total calories. Caloric restriction should also be used in an attempt to maintain a desirable weight. If dietary therapy has proved to be ineffective in reaching the goals, progression to a Step II diet is recommended.

In primary prevention, the Step I diet should be followed for at least 3 months before institution of a more rigorous dietary approach. The Step II diet uses a reduction in total cholesterol intake to less than 200 mg/day and restricts saturated fat to less than 7% of total calories, with recommendations for other dietary constituents being similar to the Step I diet. In patients with documented atherosclerosis, a Step I diet is generally inadequate to achieve the proposed therapeutic

Table 24–9

**Dietary Therapy of High Blood Cholesterol Levels**

| Nutrient | Recommended Intake | |
|---|---|---|
| | Step I Diet | Step II Diet |
| Total fat | 30% or less of total calories | |
| Saturated fatty acids | 8–10% of total calories | <7% of total calories |
| Polyunsaturated fats | Up to 10% of total calories | |
| Monounsaturated fats | Up to 15% of total calories | |
| Carbohydrates | 55% or more of total calories | |
| Protein | Approximately 15% of total calories | |
| Cholesterol | <300 mg/day | <200 mg/day |
| Total calories | To achieve and maintain desirable weight | |

goals and a Step II diet is generally recommended as initial therapy. A Step I diet may generally achieve a 5% to 7% reduction in total circulating cholesterol, with the institution of a Step II diet accounting for an additional 5% to 13% reduction. Dietary therapy should be monitored in terms of both compliance and achievement of goals. The continuation of dietary therapy as the sole intervention should be a function of the presence or severity of other risk factors, documented CAD, and extent of dyslipidemia. An adequate trial of diet requires at least a 6-month period before consideration of the initiation of pharmacologic therapy. Because of the demonstrated efficacy of lipid modification in secondary prevention, however, some physician groups have endorsed a shorter trial of diet alone in patients with CAD, beginning drug therapy concurrently with diet in most instances of secondary prevention.[37]

The institution of pharmacologic therapy after inadequate response to dietary therapy in the achievement of established goals should not be taken lightly because of the potential long-term adverse effects of drug therapy and drug-drug interactions. In primary prevention, although dietary therapy may be recommended for at least 6 months, patients with severe underlying genetic conditions such as familial hypercholesterolemia or extensive documented atherosclerosis may benefit from earlier institution of pharmacologic agents because of a presumed more beneficial risk-benefit ratio in severely affected individuals. Interventional standards have been established for both primary and secondary prevention, depending on the lipid level and associated risk factors (see Table 24–8). In primary prevention with fewer than two other risk factors, pharmacologic therapy should be considered if the LDL cholesterol level exceeds 190 mg/dl (4.91 mmol/l), with the target goal for dietary efficacy for LDL cholesterol level established at 160 mg/dl (4.14 mmol/l). Primary prevention associated with a more significant risk factor profile (more than two associated risk factors) should have pharmacologic therapy considered at a level of 160 mg/dl (4.14 mmol/l), with the established goal being to lower cholesterol level to less than 130 mg/dl (3.36 mmol/l). In secondary prevention, pharmacologic therapy should be considered if the LDL cholesterol level exceeds 130 mg/dl (3.36 mmol/l), with the goal being established to lower LDL to less than 100 mg/dl (2.59 mmol/l). Clinical judgment should be used, and in younger patients (men < 35 years of age) or premenopausal women with an LDL cholesterol level between 190 and 220 mg/dl (4.91 to 5.69 mmol/l) and no other significant risks for coronary atherosclerosis, pharmacologic therapy may potentially be delayed.

Pharmacologic therapy may be optimized by using pharmacologic agents whose main effect is directed against the predominant lipid abnormality (elevated total and LDL cholesterol level or abnormalities predominantly involving triglycerides and HDL cholesterol). Table 24–10 summarizes available drug choices based on the dyslipidemia presented.

### Pharmacologic Agents with a Predominant Effect on LDL Cholesterol

*Bile Acid Resins.* The bile acid resins are quartenary ammonium salts, with cholestyramine and colestipol being the currently available agents. The efficacy, mechanism of action, and side effect profile of the two currently available resins are basically similar. The bile acid sequestrants interrupt the enterohepatic circulation of the cholesterol-rich bile acid pool by binding the negatively charged bile salts in the GI tract, thus increasing fecal loss of cholesterol. The increased fecal loss results in a reduction in intrahepatic cholesterol, which stimulates the subsequent upregulation of the apo B/E receptor, resulting in increased removal of LDL from the plasma compartment. The GI loss of cholesterol generally exceeds the clearance of LDL from the plasma, resulting in a decrease in intrahepatic cholesterol and a secondary stimulus of the rate-limiting enzyme in cholesterol synthesis, HMG CoA reductase, and thus a secondary blunting of the long-term effects of the bile acid

Table 24–10

**Summary of Drug Choices for Diet-Resistant Dyslipidemia**

| Dyslipidemia (Fredrickson Phenotype[s]) | Drug Therapy |
|---|---|
| Elevated LDL-C (type II-A)* | **First Choice**<br>Resin (cholestyramine, colestipol)<br>Statin (atorvastatin, cerivastatin, fluvastatin, lovastatin, pravastatin, simvastatin)<br>**Second Choice**<br>Fibrate (clofibrate, gemfibrozil, fenofibrate, bezafibrate, ciprofibrate) |
| Elevated triglyceride (types IV and V)† | Fibrate (clofibrate, gemfibrozil, fenofibrate, bezafibrate, ciprofibrate)<br>Nicotinic acid |
| Elevated LDL-C and triglyceride (types II-B and III)‡ | Nicotinic acid<br>Fibrate (clofibrate, gemfibrozil, fenofibrate, bezafibrate, ciprofibrate)<br>Statin (atorvastatin, cerivastatin, fluvastatin, lovastatin, pravastatin, simvastatin) |
| Isolated low HDL-C§ | Nicotinic acid |

*Nicotinic acid or higher-dose statin therapy may be of use in individuals with familial defective apo B-100.
†For individuals with type I hyperlipidemia (hyperchylomicronemia), drug therapy is ineffective if lipoprotein lipase is absent.
‡For individuals with type II-B hyperlipidemia (elevated LDL-C and very low-density lipoprotein triglyceride levels), combination therapy with fibrate and statin may be warranted but is not approved by the Food and Drug Administration because of the 1–5% risk of muscle toxicity with this combination. Type III hyperlipidemia is managed by dietary fat restriction and fibrate therapy.
§Fibrates may also be used to raise HDL-C levels but are more efficacious with associated hypertriglyceridemia. Some experts recommend lowering LDL-C level with statin therapy in these patients in order to improve the LDL:HDL ratio.
LDL-C, low-density lipoprotein cholesterol; HDL-C, high-density lipoprotein cholesterol.

resin monotherapy due to increased cholesterol production. Cholestyramine can be given up to a maximum of 24 g/day, and colestipol may be given to a maximum of 30 g/day. The bile acid resins are not palatable and are generally mixed in various vehicles to improve compliance, although a caplet has been devised. Patients who are able to tolerate a maximum dose of the bile acid sequestrants may expect to achieve an LDL cholesterol reduction of 15% to 30%. HDL cholesterol levels are generally not significantly altered by the bile acid resins, although a modest increase of 3% to 5% may be achieved. Plasma VLDL levels are generally not affected by the bile acid resins, although in individuals who are prone to hypertriglyceridemia, an increase in circulating triglycerides may be demonstrable. The use of the bile acid resins has decreased because of the availability of more efficacious and palatable agents. The major side effects of bile acid sequestrants relate to various GI complaints including constipation, nausea, and other nonspecific GI symptoms. Additionally, bile acid resin therapy is complicated because these agents are nonspecific binders and thus have the potential to interfere with the absorption of a number of commonly coadministered cardiovascular drugs such as digoxin, betablockers, thiazides, coumadin, and other agents.

*HMG CoA Reductase Inhibitors.* The availability of the statins has revolutionized the treatment of dyslipidemia because of the potency and tolerability of these agents. The currently available agents, in the order of their commercial release, are lovastatin, pravastatin, simvastatin, fluvastatin, atorvastatin, and cerivastatin. The HMG CoA reductase inhibitors have various structural characteristics and may also be differentiated by lipophilicity or metabolic fates; however, they seem to share a common mechanism of action. HMG CoA reductase is the rate-limiting enzyme in the synthesis of cholesterol, and the statins partially inhibit its activity. The resultant reduction in intrahepatic cholesterol synthesis stimulates the upregulation of the apo B/E receptor, thus allowing increased clearance from the circulation of circulating lipoproteins, which carry these apolipoproteins on their surface. The more lipophilic agents may have a direct intrahepatic effect on the synthesis or release of apo B–containing particles. The efficacy of the statins is considerable, and decreases in LDL cholesterol level ranging from 20% to 60% have been demonstrated with the various agents. The major impact on cholesterol levels occurs with the initial dose, with a relative flattening in the dose-response curve as the dosing of the statins is increased.

The currently demonstrable side effects of the statins appear to be minimal. Major concern was voiced early about the potential induction of cataracts, as noted in trials involving earlier inhibitors of cholesterol synthesis. Extensive studies using slit-lamp evaluations early in the clinical trials of the statins demonstrated no increase in lens opacities, and routine surveillance is currently no longer recommended.

The main side effects of the class relate to hepatic and muscular toxicity. Significant liver toxicity has been defined as elevations in levels of transaminase enzymes that exceed three times the upper limits of normal. The induced elevation in transaminases has been generally determined to be reversible after discontinuation of the drug, and fatal hepatic necrosis is extremely rare and has not been definitely associated with statin therapy. The large-scale Extended Clinical Evaluation of Lovastatin (EXCEL) demonstrated that the incidence of significant elevations of levels of transaminases was less than 1% when the usual clinically administered dose of lovastatin was given.[38] Liver toxicity associated with statin therapy is somewhat dose dependent, but clinical trials have demonstrated this to be an uncommon phenomenon, with significant transaminitis generally occurring with a less than 30% incidence. It is recommended, however, that liver enzyme values be monitored early in the course after the initiation of statin therapy or in patients thought to be at increased risk because of concomitant administration of potentially hepatotoxic drugs or preexisting liver disease. Rhabdomyolysis, defined as creatine kinase elevations in excess of 1000 international units with a compatible clinical presentation, occurs in approximately 0.1% of patients receiving statin monotherapy, although the risk may be increased when statins are coadministered with a fibric acid derivative, nicotinic acid, cyclosporine, or erythromycin. The mechanism involved in the statin-induced rhabdomyolysis has not been definitely determined but had been hypothesized to be secondary to inhibition of synthesis of intermediate compounds that are also generated using the cholesterol biosynthetic pathway. Ubiquinone-deficient muscle cell mitochondria with a secondary alteration of normal cellular metabolism had been hypothesized as a potential mechanism. However, biopsy findings in dyslipidemic patients treated with simvastatin revealed no alteration of the skeletal muscle concentration of high-energy phosphates or ubiquinone levels.[39]

### Pharmacologic Agents Predominantly Affecting Triglycerides and HDL

*Nicotinic Acid.* Nicotinic acid is a vitamin that acts as a cofactor in the intermediary metabolism of carbohydrates. Deficiency states of nicotinic acid result in pellagra, but when nicotinic acid is used as a drug at pharmacologic doses, a hypolipidemic effect can be demonstrated. Nicotinic acid has a complex mechanism of action that results in significant decreases in all circulating lipoproteins with the exception of chylomicrons. Nicotinic acid is the only commonly used pharmacologic agent that has been able to effect reductions in circulating levels of lipoprotein(a).

Nicotinic acid exerts its hypolipidemic effect via a peripheral action on the release of free fatty acids from adipose tissue. Free fatty acids form the major lipid component of VLDL, and reduced delivery of these compounds to the liver alters the synthetic capacity. Nicotinic acid also decreases release of newly synthesized

VLDL from the liver into the circulation. VLDL is the initial compound in the lipid cascade, and its reduction results in a subsequent decrease of all other intermediates including the end product LDL. Nicotinic acid is generally used at a dosing range between 1.5 and 5 g/day and may be expected to reduce LDL cholesterol by up to 20%. Triglyceride levels will decline by 20% to 50%, and there is generally a significant rise in HDL cholesterol levels of up to 35%. The use of nicotinic acid has been hampered by its side effect profile, which ranges from mild clinical irritations to life-threatening fulminant hepatic necrosis.[40] Cutaneous dilatation results in the common flushing and pruritus that are seen early in the administration of nicotinic acid. The flushing is prostaglandin mediated and may be blunted by pretreatment with aspirin. Nicotinic acid is also associated with a number of GI complaints, including reactivation of peptic ulcer disease. Metabolic abnormalities associated with administration of nicotinic acid include hyperuricemia, which may be associated with the precipitation of gouty arthritis and worsening of glucose tolerance. The most serious side effect associated with the use of nicotinic acid is fulminant hepatic necrosis. Mild elevations of liver enzyme levels may be found in up to 5% of individuals who receive nicotinic acid, but transaminitis is not an absolute indication for cessation of therapy, although close clinical monitoring is warranted.

*Fibric Acid Derivatives.* The currently available fibric acid derivatives in the United States are clofibrate, gemfibrozil, and fenofibrate, although a number of other agents are available worldwide.

The fibric acid derivatives have a complex mechanism of action, but the main hypolipidemic effect is secondary to the stimulation of lipoprotein lipase, with resultant increased catabolism of VLDL. Fibric acid derivatives also have peripheral effects, however, with a secondary decrease of free fatty acids, which may decrease VLDL synthesis.

Gemfibrozil has the largest clinical experience in the United States, and the efficacy at the generally administered dose of 1200 mg/day results in a decline in triglycerides of 20% to 50%, with an associated increase in HDL cholesterol level of 10% to 15%. The effects of gemfibrozil on LDL are variable and depend on the preexistent triglyceride levels and activity of the apo B/E receptor. LDL cholesterol level may decline by approximately 10% to 15% if the receptor activity is normal. Gemfibrozil has, however, been demonstrated to affect the composition of LDL particles beneficially, with a shift from the more atherogenic small dense LDL to a larger buoyant and presumably less atherogenic form. Fibric acids may also exert beneficial clinical effects by altering a number of hemostatic factors including PAI-I, platelet activity, and fibrinogen.[41]

The adverse effects of the fibric acid derivatives are generally mild and do not require cessation of therapy. The most common side effects of the fibrates are a mild, nonspecific GI symptom complex including dyspepsia and nausea. Fibrates have been associated with an increased prevalence of gallstones, although this has not been definitely correlated with other agents. Hepatic and muscle toxicity are uncommon with fibrate monotherapy, although combination therapy with other agents such as the statins may increase their incidence.

## Nonmodifiable Risk Factors

### Age

The ability to identify people at increased risk for coronary atherosclerosis, coupled with improved diagnostic and therapeutic modalities, has resulted in a marked decrease in age-adjusted morbidity and mortality for CAD. The decline in mortality has resulted in a shift in first cardiac event to an older age group. The first coronary event now occurs in patients older than 65 years in 80% of cases, and the attributable risk for coronary atherosclerosis increases significantly with age.[3] The role of risk factor modification in an elderly cohort has been controversial because of the impression that risk factor modification is of little or no benefit in patients with established atherosclerosis at an older age. However, clinical trials involving modification of both hypertension and dyslipidemia have proved these measures to be efficacious. Antihypertensive therapy in the Systolic Hypertension in the Elderly Program (SHEP) reduced cardiovascular events by 32% in a large-scale clinical trial.[42]

Hypolipidemic therapy has been demonstrated to be effective in subgroup analysis of the statin trials. The Scandinavian Simvastatin Survival Study and the Long-Term Intervention with Pravastatin in Ischaemic Disease (LIPID) trial demonstrated benefit for both men and women older and younger than 65 years, up to age 70.[43, 44] Patients should not be excluded from risk factor modification purely on the basis of chronologic age. A person who has reached 65 years of age has approximately an additional 17-year average life span. The early lipid trials did not show a significant separation in survival or freedom from cardiac events for approximately the first 3 years of therapy; thus, an estimation of physiologic age and life expectancy is required before initiation of drug therapy. However, the more recent clinical trials using statin therapy showed a relatively early (< 1 year) separation between patients randomized to drug therapy or placebo; these findings argue for a more aggressive position in patients believed to be at significant risk for the development of an acute event.

## Gender

Significant gender differences in morbidity and mortality due to atherosclerosis exist and are a function of age. Premenopausal women have a significantly lower incidence of acute MI when compared with age-matched men. In the postmenopausal years, however, LDL cholesterol levels begin to rise significantly in women and subsequently exceed the average level found in the male population. The rise in LDL cholesterol levels is accompanied by an increase in cardiac event rates after a lag period. Women tend to have the same modifiable risk factors as men, although diabetes appeared to confer a greater risk in women than men and diabetic women lose the protection associated with gender.

## Family History

Genetic syndromes have been demonstrated to confer increased risk for the subsequent development of cardiovascular disease, and atherosclerosis tends to aggregate in families. The family history has been demonstrated to be a significant independent variable for the development of symptomatic atherosclerosis, even when controlling for the classic risk factors. Obesity, hypertension, dyslipidemia, and diabetes all have a genetic component, and the family history should be carefully analyzed in an attempt to identify clustering of risk factors. Hypolipidemic and antihypertensive therapy should be individualized to minimize a negative impact on other metabolic parameters. For instance, hypertensive patients with truncal obesity have been demonstrated to respond adequately to ACE inhibition, with improvement in insulin sensitivity combined with blood pressure control without exerting a potential negative effect on lipid or coagulation parameters.

## Other Risk Factors

### Hemostatic

The recognition that acute MI is associated with an occlusive intracoronary thrombus has stimulated evaluation of the potential role of coagulation factors as modulators of risk for CAD. Epidemiologic studies have clearly demonstrated elevations of fibrinogen, factor VII, and factor X to be associated with increased risk for coronary atherosclerosis.[45] Evaluation of fibrinogen is complicated in large-scale epidemiologic studies because of the number of confounding factors that may influence the circulating levels in an individual. Despite these limitations, elevated fibrinogen level appears to be associated with a twofold to fourfold increased relative risk of developing CAD when the subjects are divided into quintiles and compared between the upper and lower groups.[46] The fibric acid derivatives have been demonstrated to lower fibrinogen, whereas the response to statin therapy is less predictable. Levels of PAI are elevated in high-renin hypertensive, diabetic, and dyslipidemic patients. Elevated levels of PAI-I have been demonstrated to be a risk for reinfarction, and this compound may be lowered by either statins or fibric acid derivatives, ACE inhibitors, or angiotensin receptor blocker.

## Homocystine

Homocystinuria is a rare autosomal recessive disorder that is associated with significant vascular abnormalities. Elevated levels of homocystine have been established as an independent risk factor for stroke and coronary atherosclerosis.[47] The Physicians' Health Study demonstrated that individuals with elevated homocystine levels had a significant increase in the 5-year risk of MI when compared with matched controls. Elevated homocystine levels may be treated with folate and $B_{12}$ supplementation, and ongoing trials are examining the potential benefit of vitamin supplementation in reduction of risk from coronary atherosclerosis.

## Type A Personality

The role of stress and personality type in risk stratification for coronary atherosclerosis remains controversial. Type A personality, which is associated with increased stress and competition, has been demonstrated to be an independent risk factor in the Western Collaborative Group Study, with a doubling of the rate of MI.[48] The 20-year follow-up of the Framingham Heart Study also demonstrated an increase in risk for angina but could not determine an increase in fatal MI, which was compatible with the MRFIT. The mechanism by which a type A personality may pose increased risk for CAD has not been definitely determined but may relate to increased levels of catecholamines, hypertension, or platelet abnormalities.

## Low Circulating Levels of Antioxidants

Oxidation of LDL has been demonstrated to be required for enhanced uptake and recognition by the monocyte-macrophage system via the scavenger receptor. In vitro studies have demonstrated alteration of foam cell generation after administration of a number of antioxidants and have stimulated interest in the potential role of antioxidant therapy in decreasing CAD risk. Numerous observational epidemiologic studies have demonstrated an inverse relationship between vitamin E intake and coronary events. These include the Health Professionals Follow-up Study and the Nurses Health Study, which were extremely large-scale epidemiologic trials that demonstrated that increased intake of vitamin E was associated with lower overall coronary risk.[49, 50] However, these studies have the same potential confounding problems associated with all large-scale observational trials. The Cambridge Heart Antioxidant Study (CHAOS) administered variable doses of vitamin E (400 and 800 IU) to survivors of an acute MI.[51] The coronary event rate was decreased, but this was not associated with an improvement in total mortality.

## ■ SUMMARY

During the past decade, major advances have been made in the identification of patients with preclinical atherosclerosis. Increased diagnostic ability has enabled clinicians to institute preventive measures before the advent of an ischemic event. Risk factor modification is continually being refined, and the ability to alter blood pressure, dyslipidemia, and other factors believed to be involved in the process of atherosclerosis has dramatically improved efforts in both primary and secondary prevention.

## ■ REFERENCES

1. Rosamund WD, Chambless LE, Folsom AR, et al: Trends in the incidence of myocardial infarction and in mortality due to coronary heart disease, 1987 to 1994. N Engl J Med 1998;339:861–867.
2. American Heart Association: Heart and Stroke Facts: 1998 Statistical Supplement. Dallas: American Heart Association, 1997.
3. Stamler J: Epidemiology, established risk factors, and the primary prevention of coronary artery disease. In Chatterjee K, Cheitlin MD, Karliner J, et al (eds): Cardiology: An Illustrated Text Reference. Philadelphia: JB Lippincott, 1991:7.2–7.36.
4. Stamler J: Epidemiology to establish risk factors in the primary prevention of coronary artery disease. In Parmley WW, Chaterjee K (eds): Cardiology, Vol. 2. Philadelphia: JB Lippincott, 1987;1:1–41.
5. Hansson L: Effects of intensive blood pressure lowering and low dose aspirin in patients with hypertension: Principle results of the Hypertension Optimal Treatment (HOT) randomized trial. Lancet 1988:351:1755–1762.
6. Centers for Disease Control: Cigarette smoking—attributable to mortality and years of potential life lost, United States, 1990. MMWR Morb Mortal Wkly Rep 1993;42:645–649.
7. Pittilo RM: Cigarette smoking and endothelial injury: A review in tobacco smoking and atherosclerosis. New York: Plenum Publishing Corp, 1989.
8. Harats D: Cigarette smoking renders LDL susceptible to peroxidated modification and enhanced metabolism by macrophages. Atherosclerosis 1989;79:242–245.
9. Meade TW, Imeson J, Stirling Y: Effects of changes in smoking and other characteristics of clotting factors in the risk of ischemic heart disease. Lancet 1987;2:986–988.
10. Howard G, Wagenknecht LE, Burke GL, et al: Cigarette smoking and the progression of atherosclerosis: The Atherosclerosis Risk in Communities (ARIC) Study. JAMA 1998;279(2):119–124.
11. Executive summary of the clinical guidelines on the identification, evaluation and treatment of overweight and obesity in adults. Arch Intern Med 1998;158(17):1855–1867.
12. National Institutes of Health Consensus Development Panel on the Health Implications of Obesity. Ann Intern Med 1985;103:1073–1077.
13. Rexrode KM, Manson JE, Hennekens CH: Obesity and cardiovascular disease. Curr Opin Cardiol 1996;11(5):490–495.
14. Wilson PW: Diabetes mellitus and coronary artery disease. Am J Kidney Dis 1998;32(5 Suppl 3):S89–100.
15. Reaven GM: Pathophysiology of insulin resistance in human disease. Physiol Rev 1995;75:473–486.
16. The DCCT Research Group: Effective and intensive insulin management of macrovascular events and risk factors in the Diabetes Control and Complications Trial. Am J Cardiol 1995;75:894–903.
17. UK Prospective Diabetes Study Group: Effect of intensive blood-glucose control with sulphonylureas or insulin compared with conventional treatment and risk of complications in patients with Type II diabetes. U.K. Prospective Diabetes Study. Lancet 1998;352(9131):837–853.
18. Pyorala K, Pedersen TR, Kjekshus J, et al: Cholesterol lowering with simvastatin improves prognosis of diabetic patients with coronary artery disease. A subgroup analysis of the 4S study. Diabetes Care 1997;20(4):614–620.
19. Koskinen P, Manttari M, Manninen V, et al: Coronary heart disease incidence in NIDDM patients in the Helsinki Heart Study. Diabetes Care 1992;15(7):820–825.
20. American Diabetes Association: Management of dyslipidemia in adults with diabetes. American Diabetes Association. Diabetes Care 1999;22(1):S56–59.
21. Leon AS, Connett J: Physical activity and 10.5 year mortality in the Multiple Risk Factor Intervention Trial. Int J Epidemiol 1991;20:690–694.
22. Williams PT: The relationship of heart disease risk factors to exercise quantity and intensities. Arch Intern Med 1998;158(3):237–245.
23. Rankinen T, Vaisanen S, Mercuri M, Rauramaa R: Apolipoprotein(a), fibrinopeptide A and carotid atherosclerosis in middle-aged men. Thromb Haemost 1994;72(4):563–566.
24. Rotimi CN, Cooper RS, Marcovina SM, et al: Serum distribution of lipoprotein(a) in African Americans and Nigerians: Potential evidence for a genotype-environmental effect. Genet Epidemiol 1997;14(2):157–168.
25. Grundy SM: Multifactorial etiology of hypercholesterolemia: Implications for prevention of coronary heart disease. Arterioscler Thromb Vasc Biol 1991;11:1619–1626.
26. Kwiterovich PO: Genetics and molecular biology of familial combined hyperlipidemia. Curr Opin Lipidol 1993;4:133–136.
27. Myant NB: Familial defective apoprotein B100: A review including some comparisons with familial hypercholesterolemia. Atherosclerosis 1993; 104:1–12.

28. Neaton JD, Blackburn H, Jacobs D, et al: Multiple Risk Factor Intervention Trial Research Group. Serum cholesterol level and mortality findings for men screened in the Multiple Risk Factor Intervention Trial. Arch Intern Med 1992;152:1490–1500.
29. Gordon T, Castelli WP, Hjortland MC: High density lipoprotein as a protective factor against coronary artery disease: The Framingham Study. Am J Med 1997;62:707–712.
30. Schaefer EJ, Blum CB, Levy RI: Metabolism of high density lipoprotein apoproteins in Tangier disease. N Engl J Med 1978;299:905–910.
31. Gotto AM: Triglyceride as a risk factor for coronary artery disease. Am J Cardiol 1998;82(9A):22Q–25Q.
32. Chit A, Brunyell JD: Chylomicronemia syndrome. Adv Intern Med 1991;37:249–265.
33. Feussner G, Piesch S, Dopmeyer J, Fischer C: Genetics of Type III hyperlipoproteinemia. Genet Epidemiol 1997;14(3):283–287.
34. Orth M, Wahl S, Hanisch M, et al: Clearance of postprandial lipoproteins in normolipemics: Role of the apolipoprotein E phenotype. Biochim Biophys Acta 1996;1303(1):22–30.
35. Kannel WB: Range of serum cholesterol values in the population developing coronary artery disease. Am J Cardiol 1995;76(9 Suppl):69C–77C.
36. Ryan TJ, Anderson JL, Antman EM, et al: ACC/AHA guidelines for the management of patients with acute myocardial infarction. A report of the American College of Cardiology/American Heart Association Task Force on Practice Guidelines (Committee on Management of Acute Myocardial Infarction). J Am Coll Cardiol 1996;28(5):1328–1428.
37. Grundy SM, Balady GJ, Criqui MH, et al: When to start cholesterol-lowering therapy in patients with coronary heart disease. A statement for healthcare professionals from the American Heart Association Task Force on Risk Reduction. Circulation 1997;95:1683–1685.
38. Bradford RH, Schear CL, Chremos AN: Expanded Clinical Evaluation of Lovastatin (EXCEL) study results. I. Efficacy in modified plasma lipoproteins and adverse event profile in 8,245 patients with moderate hypercholesterolemia. Arch Intern Med 1991;151:43–50.
39. Laaksonen R: The effect of simvastatin treatment on natural antioxidants in low-density lipoproteins and high-energy phosphates and ubiquinone in skeletal muscle. Am J Cardiol 1996;77(10):851–854.
40. Rader JI, Calvert RJ, Habcock JN: Hepatic toxicity of unmodified and time-released preparations of niacin. Am J Med 1992;92:77–81.
41. Andersen P, Smith P, Seljeflot I: Effects of gemfibrozil on lipids and hemostasis after myocardial infarction. Thromb Haemost 1990;63:174–179.
42. SHEP Cooperative Research Group: Prevention of stroke by antihypertensive drug therapy in older persons with isolated systolic hypertension: Final results of the Systolic Hypertension in the Elderly Program (SHEP). JAMA 1991;265:3255–3261.
43. Scandinavian Simvastatin Survival Study Group: Randomised trial of cholesterol lowering in 4444 patients with coronary heart disease: The Scandinavian Simvastatin Survival Study (4S). Lancet 1994;344:1383–1389.
44. The Long-Term Intervention with Pravastatin in Ischaemic Disease (LIPID) Study Group: Prevention of cardiovascular events and death with pravastatin in patients with coronary heart disease and a broad range of initial cholesterol levels. N Engl J Med 1998;339(19):1349–1357.
45. Miller GJ: Hemostasis and cardiovascular risk: The British and European experience. Arch Pathol Lab Med 1992;116:1318–1322.
46. Ernst E: Plasma fibrinogen, an independent cardiovascular risk factor. J Intern Med 1990;227:365–369.
47. Clarke R, Daly L, Robinson K: Hyperhomocysteinemia, an independent risk factor for vascular disease. N Engl J Med 1991;324:1149–1153.
48. Eaker ED, Abbott RD, Kannel WB: Frequency of uncomplicated angina pectoris in Type A compared to Type B persons (The Framingham Study). Am J Cardiol 1989;63:1042–1045.
49. Rimm EB, Stampfer MJ, Ascherio A, et al: Vitamin E consumption and the risk of coronary heart disease in men. N Engl J Med 1993;328(20):1450–1456.
50. Stampfer MJ, Hennekens CH, Manson JE, et al: Vitamin E consumption and the risk of coronary disease in women. N Engl J Med 1993;328(20):1444–1449.
51. Stephens NG, Parsons A, Schofield PM, et al: Randomised controlled trial of vitamin E in patients with coronary disease: Cambridge Heart Antioxidant Study (CHAOS). Lancet 1996;347(9004):781–786.

# ▪ RECOMMENDED READING

Downs JR, Clearfield M, Weis S, et al, for the AFCAPS/TexCAPS Research Group: Primary prevention of acute coronary events with lovastatin in men and women with average cholesterol levels. Results of AFCAPS/TexCAPS. JAMA 1998;279:1615–1622.
Levy RI, Fredrickson DS: Diagnosis and management of hyperlipoproteinemia. Am J Cardiol 1968;22(4):576–583.
National Cholesterol Education Program: Second report of the expert panel on detection, evaluation and treatment of high blood cholesterol in adults (Adult Treatment Panel II). Circulation 1994;89:1329–1445.

Sacks FM, Pfeffer MA, Moye LA, et al, for the Cholesterol and Recurrent Events Trial Investigators: The effect of pravastatin on coronary events after myocardial infarction in patients with average cholesterol levels. N Engl J Med 1996;335(14):1001–1009.

Shepherd J, Cobbe SM, Ford I, et al, for the West of Scotland Coronary Prevention Study Group: Prevention of coronary heart disease with pravastatin in men with hypercholesterolemia. N Engl J Med 1995;333(20):1301–1307.

Witztum JL: Drugs used in the treatment of hyperlipoproteinemias. *In* Hardman JG, Limbird LE, Molinoff PB, et al (eds): Goodman and Gilman's The Pharmacologic Basis of Therapeutics, 9th ed. New York: McGraw-Hill, 1996:875–898.

*Chapter* <u>25</u>

# Acute Myocardial Infarction

*James A. de Lemos* ▪ *Christopher P. Cannon* ▪ *Peter H. Stone*

In the second half of the 20th century, progress in the prevention and treatment of acute myocardial infarction (MI) led to a 50% reduction in mortality from acute MI. Advances have been made in all components of acute MI management, from primary and secondary prevention to prehospital care, acute reperfusion therapy, adjunctive medical therapy, and management of complications. Despite this progress, however, acute MI remains the most common cause of death in industrialized nations; in addition, whereas mortality rates have been falling, the incidence of new infarction has not declined in concert. As a result, the long-term effects of coronary artery disease (CAD) are becoming more important as our population grows older.

The practice of cardiology, perhaps more than any other area of medicine, has been transformed by the results of large, prospective, randomized trials. Our current use of thrombolytic therapy, primary angioplasty, aspirin, beta blockers, and angiotensin-converting enzyme (ACE) inhibitors is supported by strong evidence from clinical trials.

## ▪ OVERVIEW OF PATHOPHYSIOLOGIC MECHANISMS

During the past two decades, our understanding of the pathophysiologic mechanisms responsible for acute MI has continued to evolve (see Chapters 22 and 23). In the mid- to late 1970s, episodic coronary vasospasm was thought to be responsible for the development of unstable angina and acute MI. In the mid- to late 1980s and mid-1990s, plaque rupture and subsequent thrombus formation was considered paramount and coronary vasoconstriction was considered inconsequential. The different acute coronary syndromes were perceived as points on a single continuum of plaque rupture and thrombus formation (Fig. 25–1). The continuum ranges from stable plaque, asymptomatic or causing stable angina, through a ruptured plaque with little or no thrombus (often asymptomatic), to a ruptured plaque with moderate thrombus leading to partial coronary occlusion (unstable angina and non–ST-segment-elevation MI), to a ruptured plaque with extensive thrombus and complete occlusion of the artery (ST-elevation MI). In the mid- to late 1990s, however, this two-component pathophysiologic model of the acute coronary syndromes was acknowledged as inadequate for some patients. In a minority of patients, for example, superficial plaque erosion, rather than plaque rupture, may be the precipitating event. In addition, evidence from atherectomy samples indicates that in some patients with unstable angina and non–Q wave MI, their disease manifestation may be due to a rapid cellular proliferation of the atherosclerotic plaque itself, with little contribution from either major thrombus formation or vasoconstriction. These three mechanisms (plaque disruption, thrombus formation, and rapid cellular proliferation) may also be closely interrelated in a given patient, with substantial contribution from each.

Angiographic studies have consistently shown that MI more commonly devel-

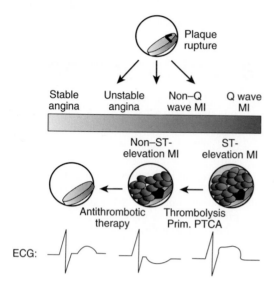

**Figure 25–1** ■ The spectrum of acute coronary syndromes. The various clinical syndromes of coronary artery disease can be viewed as a spectrum, ranging from cases with stable angina to those with acute ST-elevation myocardial infarction (MI). Across the spectrum of the acute coronary syndromes, atherosclerotic plaque rupture leads to coronary artery thrombosis: In acute ST-elevation MI, complete coronary occlusion is present. In those with unstable angina or non–Q wave MI, a flow-limiting thrombus is usually present. In patients with stable angina, thrombus is rare. PTCA, percutaneous transluminal coronary angioplasty; ECG, electrocardiogram. (Adapted from Cannon CP: Optimizing the treatment of unstable angina. J Thrombol 1995;2:205–218.)

ops from lesions associated with minor (<70%) rather than severe (≥70%) luminal narrowing. Basic research has demonstrated pathobiologic differences between those lesions that cause unstable angina and MI, on the one hand, and those that cause stable angina and restenosis after percutaneous transluminal coronary angioplasty (PTCA), on the other. Ultrasound studies have shown that lesions that lead to acute coronary syndromes tend to be associated with positive vessel remodeling, in which the entire vessel, including the external elastic lamina, is enlarged to accommodate the growing, lipid-rich plaque. Lesions associated with stable angina and restenosis after angioplasty, conversely, tend to be associated with negative vessel remodeling. These lesions typically have smaller plaque area, but constriction of the external elastic lamina leads to both a smaller lumen and a smaller overall vessel diameter.

Much work has been done to identify the factors that contribute to plaque erosion or rupture. The vulnerable atherosclerotic plaque has been characterized as having a dense lipid-rich core and a thin protective fibrous cap. The molecular factors that govern formation and breakdown of the extracellular matrix appear to regulate integrity of this protective fibrous cap. In active atherosclerotic lesions, inflammatory cells predominate at the shoulder region of the vulnerable plaque; local release of cytokines from these inflammatory cells contributes to weakening of the fibrous cap at this critical site. When the plaque ruptures, platelets adhere and aggregate, thrombin is activated, and the fibrin clot forms, leading to myocardial ischemia or infarction (Fig. 25–2).

## ST-Elevation Versus Non–ST-Elevation Myocardial Infarction

Experience with thrombolytic therapy has identified important differences in the pathophysiologic mechanisms underlying different types of acute MI and has dramatically improved mortality in certain subsets of patients. Patients whose acute MI is manifested by ST-segment elevation experience a substantial benefit from thrombolytic therapy, whereas those whose MI is not associated with ST-segment elevation do not. Angiographic studies have shown that this difference is due to

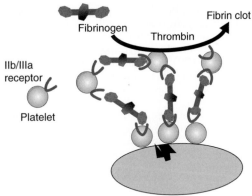

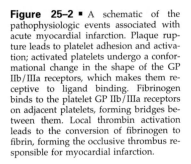

**Figure 25–2** ■ A schematic of the pathophysiologic events associated with acute myocardial infarction. Plaque rupture leads to platelet adhesion and activation; activated platelets undergo a conformational change in the shape of the GP IIb/IIIa receptors, which makes them receptive to ligand binding. Fibrinogen binds to the platelet GP IIb/IIIa receptors on adjacent platelets, forming bridges between them. Local thrombin activation leads to the conversion of fibrinogen to fibrin, forming the occlusive thrombus responsible for myocardial infarction.

the initial status of the infarct-related artery: Patients with ST-segment elevation exhibit 100% occlusion of the artery, whereas patients without ST-segment elevation exhibit a severely stenotic but nevertheless patent coronary artery (see Fig. 25–1). Thus, one can classify patients with ST-elevation MI versus non–ST-elevation MI on the basis of their pathophysiology and on their response to administration of acute reperfusion therapy.

## Q Wave Myocardial Infarction Versus Non–Q Wave Myocardial Infarction

As opposed to the distinction of ST-elevation versus non–ST-elevation MI, the determination of Q wave versus non–Q wave MI can be made only retrospectively and is a less useful classification in the early hours of patient care. Untreated, most patients with ST-elevation MI evolve a transmural infarction and develop Q waves on the surface electrocardiogram (ECG). With successful reperfusion therapy, however, many patients with ST elevation have necrosis limited to the subendocardial regions and do not develop Q waves. Patients without ST elevation at baseline generally do not develop Q waves, because infarction is limited to subendocardial regions.

## ■ DIAGNOSIS OF ACUTE MYOCARDIAL INFARCTION

### History

Taking a careful history is the most important initial diagnostic step in a patient with suspected acute MI. Most patients complain of chest pain, which resembles classic angina pectoris, and describe a severe, pressure-type pain in the midsternum, often radiating to the left arm, neck, or jaw. The pain may be distinguished from angina by its intensity, duration (>30 minutes), and failure to resolve with nitroglycerin administration. The pain may be accompanied by dyspnea, diaphoresis, nausea, vomiting, and profound weakness.

Particular attention should be given to the quality of pain, its variation with respiration and position, and whether it is similar to prior anginal episodes in quality, because characterization of the pain may help to distinguish it from other conditions that also cause chest discomfort. Aortic dissection, for example, typically causes a tearing pain, boring through to the back. Pulmonary embolism is usually accompanied by pleuritic pain, shortness of breath, and occasionally hemoptysis. Pericardial pain is also usually pleuritic and frequently changes with position, such that the patient may feel better sitting forward. The pain of pericarditis may radiate to the left shoulder or trapezius ridge. Not infrequently, inferior wall myocardial infarction (IMI) masquerades as indigestion or nausea rather than chest pain. Differentiating this from cholecystitis, peptic ulcer, and mesenteric ischemia by history alone may be very difficult, and a high index of suspicion for MI is necessary.

Many patients, particularly the elderly, present with atypical symptoms, which include dyspnea, indigestion, unusual locations of pain, agitation, altered mental status, profound weakness, and syncope. Furthermore, infarction may be silent in more than 25% of cases. This occurs more frequently in diabetic patients, as a result of the neuropathy that accompanies long-standing diabetes mellitus.

## Physical Examination

The physical examination findings are usually unremarkable in patients with uncomplicated acute MI. The objective of the initial examination should be to narrow the differential diagnosis and assess the stability of the patient. A focused examination can help to eliminate diagnoses such as pericarditis, pneumothorax, pulmonary embolus, and aortic dissection, which may mimic acute MI. It can also preclude aortic (or mitral) stenosis, which may complicate patient care. In addition, hemodynamic and mechanical complications of acute MI can often be detected by careful attention to physical findings.

Patients with acute MI often appear pale, cool, and clammy; in many cases, they are in obvious distress. Elderly patients, in particular, may be agitated and incoherent. Patients with cardiogenic shock may be confused and listless. Blood pressure and pulses should be checked in both arms, because a diminished pulse or decreased blood pressure in the left arm would divert the focus of the diagnostic workup toward aortic dissection. Cardiac examination should focus on eliciting murmurs and rubs. A pericardial rub, although often difficult to hear, suggests that pericarditis may be the cause of a patient's chest discomfort.

A brief survey for signs of congestive heart failure (CHF) should be performed. Cool extremities or impaired mental status suggests decreased tissue perfusion; elevated jugular venous pressure and moist rales on chest examination suggest elevated cardiac filling pressure. A careful examination of the peripheral circulation can detect peripheral or cerebral vascular disease, which in itself increases the likelihood of CAD.

## Electrocardiographic Findings (See Chapter 8)

The 12-lead ECG remains the most important initial diagnostic step in patients with suspected MI. Patients reporting to the emergency room with chest pain should have a 12-lead ECG performed immediately. If ST-segment elevation is seen and there are no contraindications to nitrates, a single sublingual nitroglycerin tablet should be given while patient assessment continues. If chest pain and ST elevation resolve completely with sublingual nitroglycerin, a diagnosis of coronary vasospasm (Prinzmetal variant angina) or possibly spontaneous reperfusion of a thrombotic coronary occlusion is suggested. Persistent ST elevation is virtually diagnostic of occlusive thrombus, and immediate reperfusion therapy should be administered to all patients who are candidates. ST-segment elevation suggestive of MI should be distinguished from that of pericarditis and the normal early repolarization variant. In pericarditis, ST elevation is usually diffuse and may be associated with depression of the PR segment. In the early repolarization variant, the contour of the elevated ST segment is concave rather than convex. Patients with prior transmural infarction and aneurysm formation may have persistent ST elevation, but this is generally associated with the presence of Q waves.

The presence of new, or presumed new, left bundle branch block (LBBB) in the setting of chest pain is suggestive of a large anterior infarction, and these patients should be considered for reperfusion therapy as well. Patients with LBBB of undetermined age present a diagnostic dilemma, and either emergency echocardiography (to look for an anterior wall motion abnormality) or cardiac catheterization should be considered. In patients with a preexisting LBBB, alternative methods are needed to make the diagnosis of acute MI, because ECG findings are not sufficiently reliable to guide therapy.

ST-segment depression, as opposed to ST elevation, is suggestive of subendocardial ischemia. Downsloping ST-segment depression is a more specific finding than upsloping depression or T-wave inversion. Unfortunately, many other conditions cause ST- and T-wave changes that can mimic those of ischemia, including left ventricular (LV) hypertrophy, electrolyte and metabolic disorders, and drug effects. Comparison with a patient's prior ECGs is particularly helpful for determining whether the ST- and T-wave changes seen represent new ischemic changes. In non–ST-elevation MI, a gradient of risk exists from ST depression to T-wave inversion to a normal ECG. Although normal ECG findings in the setting of chest pain do not preclude the diagnosis of MI, particularly in the high-lateral circumflex artery distribution, they make the diagnosis suspect. Importantly, patients with normal ECG findings in the setting of chest pain have an excellent short-term prognosis.

## Serum Cardiac Markers

Many new serum markers for myocardial necrosis have been developed. Measurements of cardiac troponin T (cTNT) and I have become routine, and rapid whole blood assays for myoglobin, CK-MB, and cTNT are now available and promise to facilitate point-of-service detection of acute MI in the emergency room.

### CK/CK-MB

Most published definitions of MI still require two of the following criteria to make the diagnosis of MI: typical chest pain, ECG evidence of infarction, and elevation of levels of serum creatine kinase (CK) or its myocardial isoform (CK-MB). Although CK is a sensitive marker of myocardial necrosis and assays for this marker are universally available, CK is present in adult skeletal muscle and consequently can rise with muscle trauma and injury. CK-MB is more specific for cardiac tissue, although it is also present in small amounts in skeletal muscle and other organs. CK-MB measured by mass assay (ng/ml) is more sensitive than older activity assays and allows for detection of small elevations in CK-MB without elevation in overall CK. These minor CK-MB elevations have been associated with adverse long-term cardiac events, particularly after percutaneous coronary intervention (PCI). Because CK and CK-MB are now often reported in different units, determining appropriate relationships between the two can be difficult. In general, if CK-MB (ng/ml) is greater than 2.5% of total CK (IU/ml), then a myocardial source of necrosis should be suspected. CK and CK-MB are detectable 3 to 6 hours after the onset of chest pain, peak at approximately 18 hours, and return to normal in approximately 3 days (Fig. 25–3). After successful thrombolysis, CK and CK-MB levels usually peak in less than 12 hours.

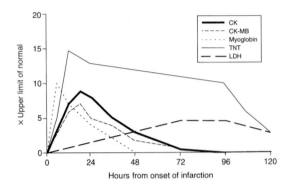

**Figure 25–3** ■ Time course of serum marker release in acute myocardial infarction. See text for details. CK, creatine kinase; CK-MB, myocardial isoform of CK; TNT, troponin T; LDH, lactate dehydrogenase. (Antman EM: General hospital management. *In*: Julian DG, Braunwald E [eds]: Management of Acute Myocardial Infarction. Philadelphia: WB Saunders, 1994:63.

## Cardiac Troponin T and I

The cardiac troponins are contractile proteins of approximately 22 kd that are released in response to MI. Like CK and CK-MB, these enzymes are detectable 3 to 6 hours after the onset of chest pain and peak at approximately 14 to 20 hours (see Fig. 25–3). They are unique, however, in that their levels remain elevated for up to 8 to 14 days (7 to 10 for cTNI, 10 to 14 for cTNT). This prolonged detection window makes troponins ideal for late diagnosis of infarction and has eliminated the role of lactate dehydrogenase (LDH) and its isoforms for this purpose. Because cTNT and cTNI are not found in adult skeletal muscle, they are highly specific for myocardial injury and are ideal markers for confirming the diagnosis of MI in difficult cases. Although cTNT and cTNI levels appear to provide similar information for most patients, in the setting of renal failure, cTNT level is often nonspecifically elevated, and in this situation, cTNI should be measured. Few data define the use of serial troponin measurements in a "rule-out MI" strategy.

In addition to their diagnostic utility, cTNT and cTNI levels have been investigated as predictors of mortality in both MI and unstable ischemia without infarction. Of interest, in patients with unstable angina (no infarction by CK-MB or ECG criteria), even minor elevations in cTNT and cTNI levels appear to be predictive of increased mortality.

## Myoglobin

Myoglobin is a small cytosolic molecule (17.8 kd) that is rapidly released from ischemic muscle and promptly cleared by the kidneys. Serum levels of myoglobin rise earlier than other available markers, and elevated levels can be detected as soon as 2 hours after the onset of chest pain (average 3 hours). Myoglobin peaks at approximately 6 hours and returns to normal levels within 18 to 24 hours (see Fig. 25–3). Widespread use of serum myoglobin determinations for the detection of MI has been limited by concerns about poor cardiac specificity and the fact that rapid assays have only recently become available. Skeletal muscle trauma (including even intramuscular injections) and renal failure can raise serum myoglobin levels in a nonspecific fashion. Nevertheless, myoglobin remains perhaps the most useful *early* marker owing to its rapid release and renal clearance: It is more sensitive than CK-MB for detecting MI within the first few hours after presentation, and in patients presenting to an emergency room *with chest pain*, specificity is similar to CK-MB.

A strategy using a combination of cardiac serum markers might prove to be more effective than serial measurements of a single marker. For example, the combination of an early myoglobin measurement(s) (at 3 to 6 hours), followed by either cTNI or cTNT determination at a later time (12 to 24 hours), would maximize the relative strengths of each marker and might prove to be a more time- and cost-effective strategy than current CK- and CK-MB–based protocols.

## Echocardiography

Portable echocardiography can help to confirm myocardial ischemia or MI in patients with nondiagnostic ECGs, particularly in situations in which rapid assays for serum markers are not available. In our experience, this is particularly useful when LBBB of undetermined duration is present or when it is necessary to distinguish pericarditis or early repolarization from acute MI. Transmural ischemia is almost always associated with hypokinesis or akinesis of the subtended myocardial segments. Therefore, absence of regional or global wall motion abnormalities argues strongly against transmural MI. Most but not all patients with subendocardial ischemia also have regional wall motion abnormalities. Transesophageal echocardiography (TEE) should be considered when suspicion of aortic dissection arises. In expert hands, TEE has greater than 90% sensitivity for the diagnosis of aortic dissection.

## Myocardial Contrast Echocardiography

Myocardial contrast echocardiography (MCE) is an emerging technology that holds great promise for the diagnosis of MI and the assessment of the efficacy of reperfusion therapies. Contrast is provided by microbubbles composed of gases surrounded by a liquid; these bubbles are small enough to pass through the capillaries and therefore can provide an image of tissue-level blood flow, yielding information similar to that obtained from radioactive microspheres. Current contrast agents include sonicated serum albumin and lipid-encapsulated fluorocarbons. When contrast is injected into the coronary arteries at the time of cardiac catheterization for acute MI, the risk area for myocardial necrosis can be accurately delimited. A follow-up study performed soon after reperfusion therapy can provide an assessment of microvascular and tissue-level reperfusion that cannot be determined by coronary angiography alone. For example, even when normal (TIMI grade 3) epicardial flow is restored after acute MI, myocardial (microvascular) reperfusion may be inadequate; this finding is associated with an adverse prognosis.

Additionally, myocardial contrast can enhance endocardial resolution and improve the assessment of regional and global function. This should be particularly helpful in the substantial number of patients who have technically limited echocardiograms. Widespread application of MCE awaits development of agents that can provide adequate tissue resolution when injected intravenously (IV). Second-harmonic imaging has improved resolution considerably and should allow wall motion to be assessed via IV injection; determination of myocardial perfusion, however, still requires intracoronary injection of contrast at this time.

## Radionuclide Imaging

New high-resolution agents, such as $^{99m}$Tc-sestamibi and $^{99m}$Tc-tetrofosmin, are now available for myocardial perfusion imaging. These radionuclides, unlike thallium-201, do not redistribute after their initial deposition. This property allows these agents to be given by IV injection during an episode of suspected ischemic pain, with imaging performed after stabilization or therapy. The images obtained provide a snapshot of myocardial perfusion at the time the tracer was injected.

This strategy may be a particularly useful means of excluding ischemia as a cause of prolonged chest pain in patients with a nondiagnostic ECG. In addition, like MCE, this imaging modality permits quantification of the area of myocardium at risk from an ischemic insult. Because of the resources and personnel required, widespread use of this technology in the emergency room is limited to select centers with very active nuclear cardiology practices.

## ■ THERAPY FOR ACUTE MYOCARDIAL INFARCTION

### Reperfusion Therapy for ST-Elevation Myocardial Infarction

#### Thrombolytic Therapy

The benefits of thrombolytic therapy for acute ST-elevation MI are related to the early achievement of infarct-related artery (IRA) patency. Early, successful coronary reperfusion limits infarct size, decreases LV dysfunction, and improves survival. In a combined analysis of six angiographic studies,[1] patients who achieved normal (TIMI grade 3) antegrade flow at 90 minutes had the lowest mortality (3.6%), patients with slow (TIMI grade 2) antegrade flow had an intermediate mortality of 6.6%, and patients with no flow or only a trickle of flow (TIMI grade 0 or 1 flow) had the highest mortality of 9.5% (p< 0.00001) (Fig. 25–4). A patent IRA not only optimizes blood flow to enhance regional myocardial function but also limits LV dilatation and dysfunction and reduces electrical instability after MI.

Time is a critical determinant in the success of any thrombolytic regimen. Patients who are treated within 1 hour from the onset of chest pain have an approximately 50% reduction in mortality, whereas those presenting more than 12 hours after onset of symptoms derive little if any benefit from thrombolysis. For each hour earlier that a patient is treated, there is an absolute 1% decrease in mortality, which translates into an additional 10 lives saved per 1000 treated. Figure 25–5 illustrates the crucial time dependence of administration of thrombolytic therapy.

Thrombolysis has been shown to reduce mortality in numerous placebo-con-

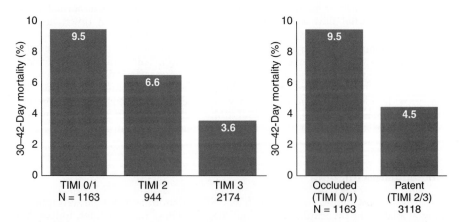

**Figure 25–4** ■ Relationship between TIMI flow grade (*left*) and patency (*right*) at 90 minutes and subsequent mortality in more than 4000 patients from the GUSTO, TIMI, TAMI, and German thrombolytic trials. The association between flow grade and mortality is highly statistically significant (p<0.00001). (Adapted from Cannon CP, Braunwald E: GUSTO, TIMI, and the case for rapid reperfusion. Acta Cardiol 1994;49:1–8).

**Figure 25–5** ■ Absolute reduction in 35-day mortality versus delay from symptom onset to randomization and treatment among 45,000 patients with ST-segment elevation or left bundle branch block myocardial infarction treated with thrombolytic therapy. Patients are grouped on the basis of time from symptom onset to randomization (0–1, 2–3, 4–6, 6–12, and 12–24 hours), and the numbers of patients in each group are shown. (Fibrinolytic Therapy Trialists' [FTT] Collaborative Group: Indications for fibrinolytic therapy in suspected acute myocardial infarction: Collaborative overview of early mortality and major morbidity results from all randomized trials of more than 1000 patients. Lancet 1994;343:311–322).

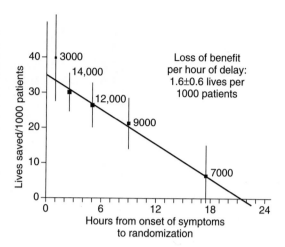

trolled trials using streptokinase, anistreplase (APSAC), and tissue plasminogen activator (tPA). These benefits have been shown to persist through 10 years of follow-up. The Fibrinolytic Therapy Trialists' overview of all the large placebo-controlled studies showed a 2.6% absolute reduction in mortality for patients with ST-elevation MI treated within the first 12 hours after the onset of symptoms.[2] In prospective trials, the benefit of treatment between 6 and 12 hours after the onset of symptoms is greater with tPA than with streptokinase. Patients presenting with LBBB and a clinical history strongly suggestive of acute MI also derive a large benefit from thrombolysis. However, those without ST-segment elevation or LBBB do not benefit from thrombolysis and indeed may be harmed.[3]

### Selection of an Appropriate Thrombolytic Regimen

All of the thrombolytic (fibrinolytic) agents currently available and under investigation are plasminogen activators. They all work enzymatically, directly or indirectly, to convert the single-chain plasminogen molecule to the double-chain plasmin, which has potent intrinsic fibrinolytic activity. Highlights of differences in dosing, pharmacokinetics, recanalization rates, and cost are shown in Table 25–1.

Given the importance of rapid reperfusion, one would expect that a more aggressive thrombolytic regimen, which achieves a higher rate of early infarct-related patency, would be associated with lower mortality. tPA was observed in the TIMI 1 trial to achieve reperfusion of occluded coronary arteries by 90 minutes in nearly twice as many patients as streptokinase and thus is a potentially superior agent.[4]

The results of the GUSTO trial[5] are presented in Figure 25–6. This study directly compared four thrombolytic regimens: "accelerated" or "front-loaded" tPA and concomitant IV heparin, streptokinase with IV heparin, streptokinase with subcutaneous heparin, and a combination of tPA and streptokinase with IV heparin. The accelerated tPA and heparin regimen achieved the highest 90-minute infarct-related artery patency and was associated with the lowest mortality. Although there was a small excess of hemorrhagic stroke in patients treated with tPA compared with streptokinase, the net clinical benefit (death or disabling stroke) still favored tPA (nine fewer deaths or disabling strokes per 1000 patients treated with tPA). Other complications of acute MI, including allergic reactions, CHF, cardiogenic shock, and atrial and ventricular arrhythmias, were less frequent with tPA as well.

## Table 25–1

### Thrombolytic Agents in Current Clinical Use

| | Alteplase | Reteplase | Streptokinase | Anistreplase (APSAC) |
|---|---|---|---|---|
| Fibrin-selective | +++ | ++ | – | – |
| Half-life | 5 min | 15 min | 20 min | 70 min |
| Dose | 15-mg bolus; then 0.75 mg/kg over 30 min; then 0.5 mg/kg over 60 min (max 100 mg total dose) | Two 10-unit bolus doses given 30 min apart | 1.5 million units over 30–60 min | 30 units as slow bolus over 5 min |
| Adjunctive heparin | Yes | Yes | No | No |
| Possible allergy | No | No | Yes | Yes |
| TIMI grade 2/3 flow (90 min) | 80% | 80% | 60% | 60% |
| TIMI grade 3 flow (90 min) | 55–60% | 60% | 32% | 43% |
| Cost | +++ | +++ | + | +++ |

APSAC, anisoylated plasminogen streptokinase activator complex.

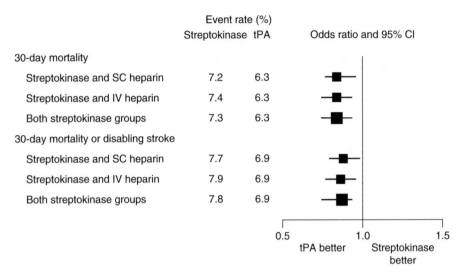

**Figure 25–6** ■ Primary results of the GUSTO trial, displaying odds ratios and 95% confidence intervals (CI) for reduction for mortality and net benefit (death or disabling stroke) in the group assigned to accelerated tissue plasminogen activator (tPA) versus the streptokinase groups. (The GUSTO Investigators: An international randomized trial comparing four thrombolytic strategies for acute myocardial infarction. N Engl J Med 1993;329:673–682).

The majority of studies indicate that accelerated tPA with IV heparin is currently the most effective therapy for achieving early reperfusion and enhanced survival in acute MI, but it is also substantially more expensive and is associated with more intracranial hemorrhage (ICH). Reteplase is a new double-bolus agent that was shown to have efficacy and risk similar to those of accelerated tPA in the GUSTO III trial[6]; importantly, it is easier to administer than tPA, a factor that could prevent dosing errors and possibly decrease "door-to-needle" time. Preliminary reports from the ASSENT II[7] and In TIME II[8] trials demonstrated that two new *single*-bolus agents, TNK-tPA and lanoteplase, were equivalent to tPA in terms of efficacy. TNK-tPA was also equivalent in terms of ICH, whereas lanoteplase was associated with a small but significant increase in ICH over tPA.

The cost-benefit ratio favors tPA and reteplase (and possibly TNK-tPA or lanoteplase) in patients presenting early after symptom onset with a large area of injury (e.g., acute anterior MI) and a low risk of ICH. In groups with smaller potential for survival benefit and a greater risk for ICH, streptokinase appears to be the agent of choice, particularly in view of the cost. Additional considerations include avoiding readministration of streptokinase or anistreplase to patients for at least 4 years (preferably indefinitely) because of a high prevalence of potentially neutralizing antibodies and because of a risk of anaphylaxis on reexposure to these drugs.

### Current Guidelines for Thrombolysis

Thrombolytic therapy is indicated for patients presenting within 12 hours of symptom onset if they have ST-segment elevation (or new LBBB), provided they have no contraindications to thrombolytic therapy (Table 25–2). Less clear are the indications in patients who are older than 75 years, those who can be treated only later than 12 to 24 hours after the onset of acute MI, and those who are hypertensive

Table 25–2

**Contraindications to Thrombolytic Therapy**

| Absolute Contraindications | Relative Contraindications |
|---|---|
| Active internal bleeding | Blood pressure consistently >180/110 mm Hg |
| History of CNS hemorrhage | History of stroke or TIA at any time in past |
| Stroke of any kind within the past year | Known bleeding diathesis |
| Recent head trauma or CNS neoplasm | Proliferative diabetic retinopathy |
| Suspected aortic dissection | Prolonged CPR |
| Major surgery or trauma within 2 wk | Prior exposure to SK or APSAK |
| | Pregnancy |

CNS, central nervous system; SK, streptokinase; APSAC, anisolylated plasminogen streptokinase activator complex (anistreplase); TIA, transient ischemic attack; CPR, cardiopulmonary resuscitation.

but present with high-risk MI. Patients should not be treated if the time to treatment exceeds 24 hours or if they present with only ST-segment depression.

### Limitations of Thrombolytic Therapy

Current thrombolytic regimens achieve patency (TIMI grade 2 or 3 flow) in approximately 80% of patients but complete reperfusion (TIMI grade 3 flow) in only 50% to 60% of cases. As described earlier, incomplete reperfusion is associated with a poor prognosis. In addition, even after successful thrombolysis, a 10% to 20% risk of reocclusion is present. Reocclusion and reinfarction are associated with a two- to threefold increase in mortality.[9]

Bleeding is the most common complication of thrombolytic therapy; major hemorrhage, as defined by the TIMI criteria, occurs in 5% to 15% of patients. ICH is the most devastating of the bleeding complications, causing death in the majority of patients affected and almost universal disability in survivors. In major clinical trials, ICH has occurred in 0.5% to 0.9% of patients; in clinical practice, where higher-risk patients are treated, rates are likely to be higher.

### Thrombolytic Therapy for Non–ST-Elevation Myocardial Infarction

Because thrombolytic therapy is beneficial in the treatment of patients with acute ST-elevation MI, it was hoped that it might have a role in the other acute ischemic syndromes. In the TIMI 3B trial,[3] 1473 patients with unstable angina or non–Q wave MI were randomized to receive either tPA or a placebo, in addition to conventional therapy. No difference was noted in the primary endpoint of death, postrandomization infarction, or recurrent ischemia through 6 weeks. The incidence of death or MI was actually higher in the tPA arm, and in addition, tPA was associated with a 0.55% incidence of ICH. These results have been corroborated by a meta-analysis of all previous smaller trials of thrombolytic therapy in unstable angina and non–ST-elevation MI, in which no benefit of thrombolytic therapy was observed. Thus, in the presence of anticoagulant, antiplatelet, and antiischemic therapy, the addition of tPA does not improve clinical outcome and thus is not indicated in unstable angina or non–Q wave MI.

The proposed mechanism for the adverse effect of thrombolysis in unstable angina and non–ST-elevation MI is that the thrombolytic agents themselves have prothrombotic effects. Thrombolysis is known to activate platelets, increase fibrino-peptide A, and expose clot-bound thrombin, which is enzymatically active and can lead to clot formation. Because most patients with unstable angina and non–ST-elevation MI have a patent culprit artery, these prothrombotic forces can lead to progression of the thrombus to 100% occlusion, thereby creating an MI, as was observed in TIMI 3B. As such, the focus of therapy in non–ST-elevation MI is antithrombotic therapy.

## Rescue Percutaneous Coronary Intervention

Because failure of thrombolytic therapy is associated with increased morbidity and mortality, rescue PCI is frequently performed in an attempt to improve outcomes in these high-risk patients. Data to support this practice are limited to observational studies and a single small randomized trial.[10] With the exception of patients who arrive in the catheterization laboratory in shock, rescue PCI is associated with high success rates, and the aggregate of data suggests that it may improve morbidity and mortality in patients with thrombolytic failure. Unfortunately, our ability to noninvasively identify patients in whom thrombolytic therapy has failed is limited and leads to unnecessary cardiac catheterization in some instances. Improvement in noninvasive detection of failed thrombolysis will allow more careful trials of rescue PCI to be performed. Whether patients with partial reperfusion (TIMI grade 2 flow) benefit from rescue PCI is not yet clear, and additional studies are needed in this area as well.

## Primary Percutaneous Coronary Intervention

An alternate method of achieving coronary reperfusion is the use of immediate or primary PCI, without concomitant administration of thrombolytic therapy. Initial randomized trials and a meta-analysis[11] have shown that primary PTCA appears to be more beneficial in reducing death or MI than administration of a thrombolytic agent (Table 25–3). The relative benefits of primary PCI seem greatest in patients at highest risk, including those with cardiogenic shock, right ventricular (RV) infarction, large anterior MI, and increased age (partly because of an increased ICH rate with thrombolytic therapy). However, as with thrombolysis, rapid time to treatment is paramount to success. In addition, operator and institutional experience seem to be critical to realize the full benefit of primary PCI. The superb procedural and clinical results observed in single-institution studies have not been replicated in larger trials and registries. A more recent development is the use of primary stenting for acute MI. Despite initial concerns, stenting appears to be safe even in the thrombus-rich environment of acute MI; further study is needed to determine whether a strategy of primary stenting is superior to one of primary PTCA with "bail-out" stenting.

Table 25–3

**PTCA Versus Thrombolysis Meta-Analysis**

|  | PTCA | Thrombolytic Therapy | Odds Ratio (95% CI) |
|---|---|---|---|
| Mortality |  |  |  |
|  | 4.0% | 5.9% (streptokinase) | 0.66 (0.29–1.50) |
|  | 5.0% | 7.2% (accelerated tPA) | 0.68 (0.42–1.08) |
|  | 4.4% | 6.5% (total) | 0.66 (0.46–0.94) |
| Death + nonfatal MI |  |  |  |
|  | 5.6% | 13.0% (streptokinase) | 0.40 (0.21–0.75) |
|  | 8.7% | 12.0% (accelerated tPA) | 0.70 (0.48–1.08) |
|  | 7.2% | 11.9% (total) | 0.58 (0.44–0.76) |

PTCA, percutaneous transluminal coronary angioplasty; CI, confidence interval; tPA, tissue plasminogen activator; MI, myocardial infarction.

Adapted from Weaver WD, Simes RJ, Betriu A, et al: Comparison of primary coronary angioplasty and intravenous therapy of myocardial infarction. A quantitative review. JAMA 1997;278:2093–2098.

## Use of Platelet Glycoprotein IIb/IIIa Inhibitors as Adjuncts to Primary Percutaneous Coronary Intervention

There is growing experience using platelet glycoprotein (GP) IIb/IIIa inhibitors (discussed later) as adjuncts to PCI in patients with ST-elevation MI, either as primary treatment or as rescue after failed thrombolytic therapy. The EPIC trial included an acute MI subgroup of 64 patients who underwent either primary or rescue PTCA.[12] Abciximab use was associated with a significant reduction in the combined rate of death, reinfarction, or need for revascularization at 30 days (26.1% vs 4.5%), and in recurrent ischemic events at 6 months (47.8% vs 4.5%). These findings were largely replicated in the subsequent RAPPORT trial,[13] in which patients with acute MI who received abciximab and primary PCI had a 30-day risk of death, reinfarction, or emergent revascularization that was approximately half that of the control group. At 6 months, however, there was no significant difference in the combined rate of death, MI, or target-vessel revascularization. In the setting of rescue PCI, preliminary results from a nonrandomized evaluation of 387 patients in the GUSTO III trial showed a greater than 60% reduction in 30-day mortality (9.8% vs 3.7%) in patients who received adjunctive abciximab for their rescue PTCA.[14]

Although primary PCI, particularly when performed with adjunctive GP IIb/IIIa inhibition, is an excellent reperfusion option in dedicated centers that can perform interventional procedures quickly and expertly, given current logistic and financial constraints, most patients will continue to be treated initially with thrombolytic therapy. Efforts should be made to transfer patients with contraindications to thrombolytic therapy, and those who appear to have failed to improve with thrombolysis, to centers that can perform emergent angioplasty. Consideration should be given to starting GP IIb/IIIa inhibitors before transfer of those patients without obvious bleeding risks.

## Reduced-Dose Thrombolysis Plus GP IIb/IIIa Inhibition: A Promising Investigational Strategy

Preclinical studies have suggested that the use of GP IIb/IIIa receptor inhibitors with thrombolytic agents may accelerate reperfusion and reduce the risk of reocclusion. The combination of a *reduced-dose* thrombolytic agent and a GP IIb/IIIa receptor blocker has been evaluated in the TIMI 14 trial, a phase II dose-ranging and confirmation trial.[15] Four regimens were compared: accelerated alteplase (control), full-dose abciximab with reduced doses of alteplase, abciximab with reduced doses of streptokinase, and abciximab. The optimal dose of tPA to be used in combination with full-dose abciximab was 50 mg, given as a 15-mg bolus and a 35-mg infusion over 60 minutes. This regimen was associated with substantial improvement in vessel patency and TIMI grade 3 flow at both 60 and 90 minutes. Major hemorrhage and ICH were similar between the combination tPA and abciximab and tPA control groups. A number of smaller ongoing trials and a planned large phase III trial will further explore the potential role of GP IIb/IIIa receptor inhibitors with reduced doses of fibrinolytic agents in patients with acute ST-elevation MI. It is hoped that combination therapy will enhance fibrinolysis and reduce reocclusion, with acceptable bleeding risks. In fact, because trials of GP IIb/IIIa inhibitors to date have shown no increase in the incidence of ICH compared with heparin, it is possible that the combination of a reduced-dose fibrinolytic plus a GP IIb/IIIa receptor inhibitor and low-dose heparin may be associated with reduced rates of ICH.

## Antithrombotic Therapy

In addition to achieving reperfusion in patients with acute ST-elevation MI, it is essential to provide adjunctive therapy to maintain coronary artery patency. After rapid treatment and early restoration of IRA patency for ST-elevation MI, reocclusion of the artery or its clinical correlate, reinfarction, can reverse the benefits of early patency. As such, both reocclusion and reinfarction become important targets for antithrombotic therapy after thrombolytic therapy. In addition, as described earlier, for non–ST-elevation MI, antithrombotic medications are the primary focus of therapy.

## Aspirin

In the setting of acute ST-elevation MI, aspirin has been shown to decrease reocclusion by more than 50%, reinfarction by nearly 50%, and mortality by 25%.[16] In patients with unstable angina or non–ST-elevation MI, aspirin reduces the risk of death or recurrent MI by more than 50% (Fig. 25–7). Aspirin should be given immediately on presentation (or preferably in the ambulance) and continued as an oral dose of 162 to 325 mg daily. After MI, aspirin also reduces subsequent cardiac events, a secondary prevention benefit that has now been observed to persist for as long as 4 years of follow-up.[17] Thus, aspirin has had a dramatic effect in reducing adverse clinical events and constitutes primary therapy for all acute coronary syndromes.

## Glycoprotein IIb/IIIa Receptor Inhibitors

The appreciation that aspirin is a relatively weak antiplatelet drug has led to the development of a class of drugs that inhibit platelet aggregation by binding to the platelet GP IIb/IIIa receptor. By preventing the final common pathway of platelet aggregation, fibrinogen-mediated cross-linkage, these agents are much more potent than aspirin and inhibit platelet aggregation in response to all types of stimuli. Three GP IIb/IIIa inhibitors are currently approved by the Food and Drug Administration (FDA), abciximab and eptifibatide for use in PCI and tirofiban and eptifibatide for unstable angina/non–ST-elevation MI (Table 25–4). In addition, as

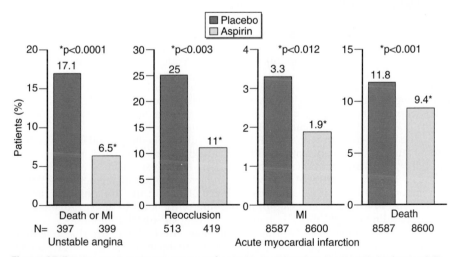

**Figure 25–7** ■ Benefit of aspirin in patients with unstable angina and acute myocardial infarction (MI). In unstable angina, the incidence of death or MI is reduced by more than 50%. In acute MI, aspirin reduces reocclusion of the infarct-related artery, reinfarction, and mortality. (Cannon CP: Optimizing the treatment of unstable angina. J Thrombol 1995;2:205–218).

Table 25–4

### Glycoprotein IIb/IIIa Inhibitors in Current Clinical Use

|  | Abciximab | Tirofiban | Eptifibatide |
|---|---|---|---|
| Dose | Bolus: 0.25 mg/kg<br>Infusion: 0.1 µg/kg/min | Bolus: 0.4 µg/kg/min<br>for 30 min<br>Infusion: 0.1 µg/kg/min | Bolus: 180 µg/kg over<br>1–2 min<br>Infusion: 2µg/kg/min |
| Mechanism of action | Fab fragment of monoclonal<br>antibody | Nonpeptide | Cyclic heptapeptide |
| Plasma half-life | 10–30 min | 2 hr | 2–3 hr |
| Duration of action | 4–10 days | 4 hr | 4 hr |
| Indications | Coronary interventions | Unstable angina/NQMI | Coronary interventions<br>Unstable angina/NQMI |
| Cost | + + + + | + + | + + |

NQMI, non–Q wave myocardial infarction.

noted earlier, several agents are being evaluated as adjuncts to either full- or reduced-dose thrombolytic therapy.

Abciximab, the Fab fragment of the monoclonal antibody, binds tightly to the GP IIb/IIIa receptor, leading to an antiplatelet effect that lasts much longer than the infusion period. Although this may lead to improved efficacy when compared with other agents, if bleeding occurs, discontinuing the drug does not reverse the antiplatelet effect immediately; in this circumstance, platelet transfusion should be given to reduce the level of platelet inhibition. The peptide and peptidomimetic inhibitors (e.g., tirofiban and eptifibatide) are competitive inhibitors of the GP IIb/ IIIa receptor. Thus, the level of platelet inhibition is directly related to the drug level in the blood. Because both inhibitors have short half-lives, the antiplatelet activity reverses after a few hours when the drug infusion is stopped and thus provides a potential benefit for avoiding bleeding complications. On the other hand, for prolonged antiplatelet effect, the drug needs to be given IV for a longer period.

### Use of GP IIb/IIIa Inhibition in Unstable Angina and Non–Q Wave Myocardial Infarction

Two agents, tirofiban and eptifibatide, are currently FDA approved for the treatment of unstable angina and non–Q wave MI. In the PRISM-PLUS trial, the combination of tirofiban, heparin, and aspirin reduced the rate of death, MI, or recurrent refractory ischemia at 7 and 30 days by more than 25%, without an increase in major hemorrhage.[18] Eptifibatide was studied in the PURSUIT trial, involving 10,948 patients with unstable angina and non–Q wave MI. Eptifibatide plus heparin and aspirin significantly reduced the rate of death or MI at 30 days from 15.7% to 14.2%, compared with heparin and aspirin alone.[19]

The major concern with the GP IIb/IIIa inhibitors is the potential for bleeding. Some studies suggested that GP IIb/IIIa inhibitors are associated with increased bleeding, but careful evaluation has suggested that excessive bleeding is more associated with excessive heparinization and prolongation of the activated partial thromboplastin time (aPTT) and less with use of the GP IIb/IIIa inhibitors. Use of lower doses of heparin and careful monitoring of the level of anticoagulation will avoid bleeding complications in patients receiving GP IIb/IIIa inhibitors.

Thrombocytopenia is the other major side effect of GP IIb/IIIa inhibition. Platelet counts less than 100,000 occur in approximately 1% to 2% of patients treated with GP IIb/IIIa inhibitors, and platelet counts less than 50,000 occur in less than 0.5% of patients. The mechanism by which thombocytopenia occurs is not well understood. Fortunately, it is nearly always reversible, with platelet counts returning to normal after a few days.

## Heparin

In acute ST-elevation MI, heparin is also an important adjunctive agent to decrease reocclusion after administration of tPA. Although no difference in IRA patency is seen at 90 minutes, patency is higher between 18 hours and 5 days in patients randomized to receive IV heparin, so that the benefit of heparin would seem to be a result of decreased reocclusion rather than enhanced thrombolysis. Furthermore, long-term patency rates are highest in patients who are effectively anticoagulated, with an aPTT of greater than 2 times control or greater than 60 seconds; a target range of 50 to 70 seconds appears to be optimal. After streptokinase or anistreplase (APSAC) administration, the role of heparin is less clear. Patients treated with streptokinase and IV or subcutaneous heparin in the GUSTO I trial had similar infarct-related artery patency at 90 minutes and 24 hours, but those receiving IV heparin had significantly higher patency at 5 to 7 days (84% vs 72%, p = 0.04).[20] Nonetheless, overall mortality and the rate of clinical reinfarction were the same between these two groups. Therefore, IV heparin may be considered optional in streptokinase-treated patients. Subcutaneous heparin has been shown to be of no benefit in preventing reinfarction or death.

In unstable angina and non–ST-elevation MI, heparin is an important component of primary therapy. In a meta-analysis,[21] treatment with aspirin and heparin lowered the risk of death or MI by 33%, compared with treatment with aspirin alone. These data support the use of aspirin plus heparin in acute coronary syndromes.

## Low-Molecular-Weight Heparin

A major advance in the use of heparin has been in the development of low-molecular-weight heparin (LMWH) agents. These agents are created by depolymerization of standard, unfractionated heparin and selection of those fragments with lower molecular weight. As compared with unfractionated heparin, which has nearly equal anti-IIa and anti-Xa activity, LMWH agents have increased ratios of anti-IIa to anti-Xa activity: either 1:2 (dalteparin) or 1:3 (enoxaparin or nadroparin). LMWH has several potential advantages over standard, unfractionated heparin: First, LMWH inhibits both factor IIa (thrombin) and factor Xa, thereby inhibiting both thrombin activity and its generation. LMWH also induces a greater release of tissue factor pathway inhibitor than standard heparin and is not neutralized by platelet factor 4. From a safety perspective, LMWH does not increase capillary permeability (which may lead to fewer bleeding complications) and most recently has been found to have a lower rate of thrombocytopenia and osteoporosis. Finally, the high bioavailability and reproducible anticoagulant response of LMWH allows for subcutaneous administration without monitoring of the coagulation system. This factor alone represents a major clinical improvement over unfractionated heparin.

In two large trials of patients with unstable angina or non–Q wave MI, enoxaparin, a LMWH with a 1:3 anti-IIa/anti Xa ratio, lowered the incidence of death, MI, or recurrent ischemia by approximately 15%, compared with standard unfractionated heparin.[22] In separate trials, no difference was found when dalteparin, a LMWH with a ratio of 1:2, was compared with unfractionated heparin. These results suggest that (1) enoxaparin appears to represent an improvement over standard unfractionated heparin in terms of clinical efficacy and (2) the LMWH agents cannot be considered interchangeable members of a single class of drugs. At this time, enoxaparin is the only LMWH indicated for the treatment of unstable angina or non–Q wave MI. It should be administered with aspirin, at a dose of 1 mg/kg subcutaneously twice per day. Studies are also in progress to determine if

LMWH is of value in the setting of ST elevation MI treated with thrombolytic therapy.

## Direct Thrombin Inhibitors

Direct thrombin inhibitors have also undergone extensive evaluation, although with less promising results. One such agent is the anticoagulant hirudin, which binds in a 1:1 relationship to thrombin, the last step in the coagulation cascade. In the TIMI 9B trial, although hirudin reduced the rate of recurrent MI following thrombolytic therapy, there was no difference in the primary endpoint, death, MI, or severe CHF/shock, at 30 days.[23] Hirudin was compared with unfractionated heparin in more than 12,000 patients across the full spectrum of acute coronary syndromes in the GUSTO IIB trial. There was a reduction in reinfarction (5.4% vs 6.3%, p = 0.04) but only a trend toward reduction in death or MI at 30 days (8.9% vs 9.8%, p = 0.06).[24] Other direct thrombin inhibitors have also been tested, and again, only modest or no improvements have been observed compared with heparin. Therefore, these agents are not recommended for routine use in patients with acute coronary syndromes.

## Warfarin/Oral Anticoagulation

Results from a number of clinical trials suggest that warfarin monotherapy appears to be at least as effective as aspirin for secondary prevention after MI. In several circumstances, the benefit or potential benefit with warfarin therapy exceeds that of aspirin. First, warfarin is superior to aspirin in preventing systemic emboli in patients with atrial fibrillation. In addition, warfarin has beneficial effects in reducing systemic emboli in post-MI patients with documented LV dysfunction. Because of a substantial risk of systemic embolization after a large anterior MI, even if thrombus is not visible on echocardiography, we recommend 3 to 6 months of warfarin therapy in these patients, if they are suitable candidates for anticoagulation.

Studies have also evaluated the combination of warfarin and aspirin after MI. Neither fixed-dose warfarin nor low-dose warfarin titrated to an International Normalized Ratio (INR) of approximately 1.5 appears to be superior to monotherapy with either agent alone, and the combination is associated with excess bleeding risk.[25] Thus, warfarin is a suitable alternative to aspirin as monotherapy after MI, but no evidence currently supports a combination regimen of warfarin plus aspirin.

## Clopidogrel

Clopidogrel, like its sister drug ticlopidine, is a thienopyridine derivative that inhibits platelet aggregation, increases bleeding time, and reduces blood viscosity. The two agents achieve their antiaggregatory action by inhibiting the binding of adenosine diphosphate (ADP) to its platelet receptors. Clopidogrel has been tested for secondary prevention in patients with either recent MI, stroke, or documented peripheral arterial disease and has been shown to reduce the incidence of MI by approximately 20% compared with aspirin.[26] Based on these findings, the FDA approved clopidogrel, at a dose of 75 mg once daily, for secondary prevention of vascular events among patients with symptomatic atherosclerosis. Whether clopidogrel provides additive benefit to aspirin is not yet known. Further studies are needed to determine the circumstances under which clopidogrel should be used instead of or in addition to aspirin and GP IIb/IIIa inhibitors. At present, our recommendation is to use clopidogrel as secondary prevention in patients who cannot take aspirin and to consider its use in combination with aspirin for patients with recurrent cardiac or vascular events on aspirin. Clopidogrel is also being used with aspirin in patients who have undergone coronary stent implantation.

## Antiischemic Therapy

### Beta Blockers

Beta blockers function as competitive antagonists to the β-adrenergic receptors on cell membranes. Selective $\beta_1$ antagonists act at receptor sites found primarily in the myocardium, inhibiting catecholamine-mediated increases in cardiac contractility and nodal conduction rates. $\beta_2$ receptors are found mainly in vascular and bronchial smooth muscle, and inhibition at these receptor sites can lead to vasoconstriction and bronchospasm. Beta blockers exert their beneficial effect in the acute coronary syndromes by preventing catecholamine-mediated $\beta_1$ activation and thus decreasing contractility and heart rate, so that the balance between oxygen supply and demand is improved. These drugs also exert an antiarrhythmic effect, as evidenced by an increase in the threshold for ventricular fibrillation (VF) in animals and a reduction in complex ventricular arrhythmias in humans. Finally, beta blockers may prevent plaque rupture by reducing the mechanical stresses imposed on the plaque.

Beta blockers were among the first therapeutic interventions used to limit the size of acute MI. Administration of a beta blocker very early after onset of acute MI decreases infarct size, recurrent MI, and mortality. When beta blockers are used in conjunction with thrombolytic therapy, they provide incremental benefit, particularly if they can be administered early after the onset of infarct symptoms.[27] Tabulation of the results from the available studies indicates a highly significant reduction of approximately 30% in the incidence of sudden death and a nonsignificant reduction of only about 12% in the incidence of nonsudden death (Fig. 25–8).[28] The fact that beta blockers are particularly effective in reducing sudden death and in reducing mortality among patients with complex ventricular ectopy at baseline again suggests that beta blockers exert much of their beneficial effect by reducing the frequency and severity of arrhythmias. In addition, they appear to decrease the risk of cardiac rupture significantly.

It is striking that the long-term mortality benefits of the beta blockers extend to most members of this class of agents. There does not seem to be a significant difference between agents with or without cardioselectivity. The presence of intrinsic sympathomimetic activity reduces the benefit considerably, however, and these agents should not be used in MI (Fig. 25–9). Reduction in heart rate appears to be

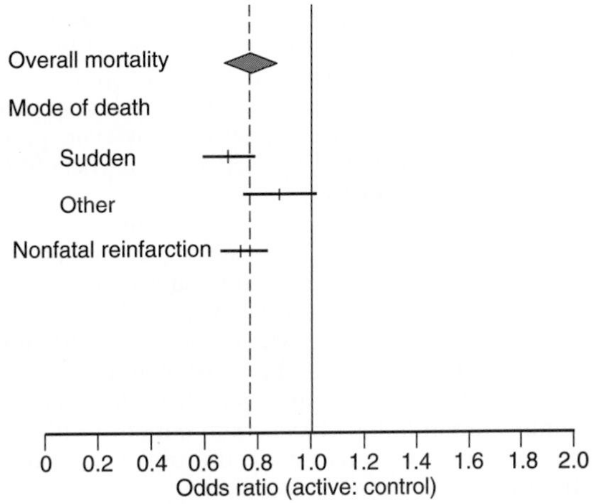

**Figure 25–8** ▪ Sudden death, other death, and nonfatal reinfarction in long-term beta-blocker trials that reported these endpoints separately: odds ratios, together with approximate 95% confidence ranges. (Yusuf S, Peto R, Lewis J, et al: Beta-blockade during and after myocardial infarction: An overview of the randomized trials. Prog Cardiovasc Dis 1985;27:335–371).

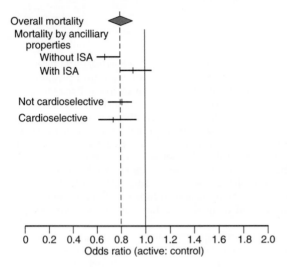

**Figure 25–9** ▪ Mortality in long-term beta-blocker trials, by ancillary properties of agent tested: odds ratios, together with approximate 95% confidence intervals. ISA, intrinsic sympathomimetic activity. (Yusuf S, Peto R, Lewis J, et al: Beta-blockade during and after myocardial infarction: An overview of the randomized trials. Prog Cardiovasc Dis 1985;27:335–371).

a critical feature associated with the protective effect of beta blockers. Indeed, there is a significant relationship between the magnitude of heart rate reduction observed and the magnitude of reduction in mortality.

In addition to the early benefits of beta blockers, these agents, when given long term, significantly reduce the incidence of nonfatal reinfarction. As observed for mortality, there is also a significant relationship between the magnitude of reduction in heart rate and the reduction in nonfatal recurrent MI. The magnitude of benefit from long-term beta blocker use is also dependent on patients' risk of mortality associated with their index MI. Post hoc analyses from the Beta Blocker Heart Attack Trial (BHAT)[29] indicate that those MI victims without electrical or mechanical complications experienced only a 6% relative benefit from the use of propranolol. MI victims with electrical complications experienced a 52% relative benefit, and those with mechanical complications experienced a 38% relative benefit. Considering the low cost of routine beta-blocker use, and its substantial benefit, such therapy has a very favorable cost-effectiveness ratio and represents one of the few bargains left in contemporary cardiology practice.

The side effects from prolonged beta-blocker use have generally been minor and are similar to those with placebo. In studies that report it, the incidence of heart failure is slightly but significantly higher in patients receiving a beta blocker than in those receiving placebo.[28] However, patients with a history of mild or moderate CHF actually experience greater benefit from β-blockade than do patients without a history of CHF.

Thus, beta blockers remain a cornerstone of therapy for acute MI. Treatment should be initiated IV, especially if it can be administered within 12 hours of symptom onset. We recommend using IV metoprolol in 2.5- to 5-mg boluses, given 5 minutes apart up to a total dose of 15 mg. IV therapy should be followed by continuous oral therapy: Metoprolol (25 to 100 mg bid to qid) and atenolol (25 to 100 mg qd to bid) are the most commonly used preparations. The American College of Cardiology/American Heart Association (ACC/AHA) guidelines for the administration of beta blockers to patients with acute MI are noted in Table 25–5.[30] Beta-blockers are consistently useful for secondary prevention following MI and should be maintained indefinitely.

Table 25–5

## Recommendation for Administration of Beta Blockers

*Class I* (conditions for which there is evidence and / or general agreement that treatment is beneficial, useful, and effective):

Patients without a contraindication to beta-blocker therapy who can be treated ≤12 hr of onset of MI, irrespective of administration of concomitant thrombolytic therapy

Patients with continuing or recurrent ischemic pain

Patients with tachyarrhythmias, such as atrial fibrillation with rapid ventricular response

As secondary prevention to all patients who can tolerate beta-blocker therapy

*Class IIa* (conditions for which there is conflicting evidence but the weight of evidence is in favor of usefulness and efficacy): patients with non–Q wave MI

*Class IIb* (conditions for which beneficial effects are less well established, but weight of evidence favors their use): patients with moderate or severe left ventricular failure or other contraindications to beta-blocker therapy, provided they can be clearly monitored

*Class III* (conditions for which evidence suggests treatment is not useful and may be harmful): none

MI, myocardial infarction.

Ryan TJ, Anderson JL, Antman EM, et al: ACC / AHA guidelines for the management of patients with acute myocardial infarction: A report of the American College of Cardiology/ American Heart Association Task Force on Practice Guidelines (Committee on Management of Acute Myocardial Infarction). J Am Coll Cardiol 1996;28:1328–1428.

## Nitrates

The clinical effects of nitrates are mediated through several distinct mechanisms. The first of these is dilatation of large coronary arteries and arterioles with redistribution of blood flow from epicardial to endocardial regions. Nitroglycerin provides an exogenous source of nitric oxide in vascular endothelium, facilitating coronary vasodilatation even when damaged endothelium is unable to generate endogenous nitric oxide owing to CAD. It is important to emphasize that these coronary vasomotor effects may either increase or decrease collateral flow. Second, peripheral venodilation leads to an increase in venous capacitance and a substantial decrease in preload, and thus reduces myocardial oxygen demand. Nitrates are consequently of particular value in treating patients with LV dysfunction and CHF. Third, peripheral arterial dilation, typically of a modest degree, may decrease afterload. In addition, nitrates have been shown to relieve dynamic coronary constriction, including that induced by exercise. Nitrates may also have an inhibitory effect on platelet aggregation, although the clinical significance of this finding is unclear.

Early studies demonstrated that nitrates may be of value to reduce infarct size and improve regional myocardial function when administered early in the course of acute MI. A meta-analysis of these earlier studies before the acute reperfusion era indicated that nitrates reduced the odds of death after acute MI by 35%.[31] However, it should also be noted that use of nitroprusside was found in early studies actually to exacerbate MI by causing a coronary steal phenomenon. Thus, nitroprusside should not be used in acute MI.

Studies have investigated the use of nitrates in the setting of routine use of thrombolytic therapy and aspirin. The GISSI-3 trial[32] randomly assigned 19,394 patients to a 24-hour infusion of nitroglycerin, followed by topical nitroglycerin (10 mg daily) for 6 weeks, or placebo. There was a nonsignificant reduction in mortality at 6 weeks in the group randomly assigned to nitrate therapy alone, compared with the control group (6.5% vs 6.9%). GISSI-3 also evaluated lisinopril in a similar fashion; 6-week mortality was reduced slightly. At both 6-week and at 6-month follow-up, the combined use of lisinopril and nitrates led to a greater reduction in mortality when compared with no nitrate therapy or lisinopril alone. The ISIS-4 trial[33] compared 28-day treatment of controlled-release oral isosorbide mononitrate with placebo control in 58,050 patients with suspected MI. Nitrate therapy led to a minor reduction in 35-day mortality compared with the control group (7.34% vs 7.54%; p = NS). In both the GISSI-3 and ISIS-4, the power to detect potential beneficial effects of routine nitrate therapy was reduced by the extensive early use (>50%) of off-protocol nitrates in patients in the control group.

A review of evidence from all pertinent randomized clinical trials does not support routine use of *long-term* nitrate therapy in patients with uncomplicated acute MI. However, it is reasonable to use nitroglycerin for the first 24 to 48 hours in patients with acute MI and recurrent ischemia, CHF, or hypertension. IV administration is recommended in the early stage of acute MI because of its immediate onset of action, ease of titration, and the opportunity for prompt termination in the event of side effects.

## Calcium Channel Blockers

The calcium channel blockers in current use fall into three main groups: dihydropyridines, of which nifedipine is the prototype; benzothiapines, of which diltiazem is the only member; and phenylalkylamines, of which verapamil is the only member. All of these agents block the entry of calcium into cells via voltage-sensitive (L type) calcium channels. In vascular smooth muscle cells, this blocking action causes coronary and peripheral vasodilation. In cardiac tissue, it leads to depression of myocardial contractility, cardiac pacemaker function, and atrioventricular (AV) nodal conduction. The differences between the three classes of calcium channel blockers relate to differences in their primary sites of actions.

### Dihydropyridines

Dihydropyridine calcium channel antagonists can be viewed as almost pure vasodilators. They dilate resistance vessels in both the peripheral and coronary beds and improve coronary blood flow. Although dihydropyridine-type calcium channel blockers may reduce oxygen demand by reducing blood pressure and wall stress, their action is countered by a reflex increase in heart rate, making the overall effect on oxygen demand unpredictable. This factor causes nifedipine alone, for example, to be potentially dangerous in the setting of acute MI. The addition of a beta blocker can prevent reflex tachycardia, however, and the combination of these two agents can be extremely effective.

Short-acting preparations of nifedipine appear to be responsible for most of the problems associated with this class of drugs, and there is no indication to use short-acting nifedipine in contemporary practice. Rapid hemodynamic fluctuations frequently occur, particularly in elderly patients, with potentially serious adverse consequences. Sustained-release preparations, on the other hand, appear to avoid these rapid hemodynamic changes and are safe when properly used. Amlodipine, a third-generation dihydropyridine agent, causes less reflex tachycardia than other dihydropyridines and usually has a neutral effect on heart rate.

Early studies that investigated dihydropyridine calcium channel blockers for the early treatment of MI found no benefit for these agents (Fig. 25–10). These agents were studied in particular because they could be safely combined with beta blockers without a concern for excessive reduction in myocardial contractility or bradycardia. The available formulation of dihydropyridines in this early era consisted of short-acting nifedipine, and this agent was found to be actually detrimental when used without a beta blocker to blunt the reflex sympathetic activity. Although nifedipine, when combined with a beta blocker, was found to reduce symptomatic manifestations of acute MI, this agent has been uniformly unsuccessful in reducing either mortality or the rate of reinfarction (see Fig. 25–10). Sustained-release dihydropyridine preparations do, however, remain useful for treating hypertension in the setting of acute MI, as long as they are used in combination with a beta blocker.

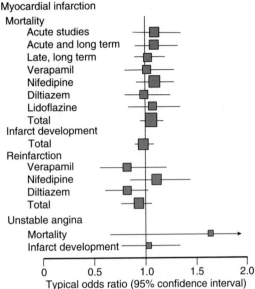

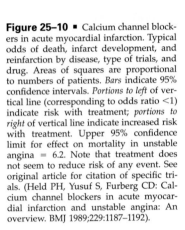

**Figure 25–10** ■ Calcium channel blockers in acute myocardial infarction. Typical odds of death, infarct development, and reinfarction by disease, type of trials, and drug. Areas of squares are proportional to numbers of patients. *Bars* indicate 95% confidence intervals. *Portions to left* of vertical line (corresponding to odds ratio <1) indicate risk with treatment; *portions to right* of vertical line indicate increased risk with treatment. Upper 95% confidence limit for effect on mortality in unstable angina = 6.2. Note that treatment does not seem to reduce risk of any event. See original article for citation of specific trials. (Held PH, Yusuf S, Furberg CD: Calcium channel blockers in acute myocardial infarction and unstable angina: An overview. BMJ 1989;229:1187–1192).

### Verapamil and Diltiazem

Verapamil and diltiazem can be considered together because their net pharmacologic effect is that of slowing the heart rate and, to some extent, reducing myocardial contractility, thereby reducing myocardial oxygen demand. Of the two agents, verapamil has greater negative inotropic and chronotropic effects. These agents have been given to patients as secondary prevention after stabilization of an index MI. A pooled analysis[34] indicated that verapamil and diltiazem had no effect on mortality following acute MI, but that they did significantly reduce the rate of reinfarction (6.0% vs 7.5%; p < 0.01). This effect seems to be similar for the two agents.

Although trials of verapamil showed no overall mortality benefit, subgroup analyses indicated that immediate-release verapamil, when initiated several days after acute MI in patients who were not candidates for a beta blocker, may reduce the incidence of reinfarction and death, *provided LV function is preserved and there is no clinical evidence of heart failure.* Verapamil is detrimental in patients with heart failure or bradyarrhythmias during the first 24 to 48 hours after acute MI.

Data from the Multicenter Diltiazem Postinfarction Trial (MDPIT) and the Diltiazem Reinfarction Study (DRS)[35, 36] suggest that patients with non–Q wave MI or those with Q wave infarction, preserved LV function, and no evidence of heart failure may also benefit from treatment with immediate-release diltiazem. In the DRS, patients were treated with either diltiazem (90 mg every 6 hours) or placebo initiated 24 to 72 hours after the onset of MI, and continued for 14 days.[36] There was no difference in mortality, but diltiazem reduced the rate of reinfarction and refractory postinfarction angina by almost 50%. In the MDPIT trial groups,[35] patients were treated with either diltiazem (240 mg/day) or placebo 3 to 15 days after the MI onset and were monitored for a mean of 25 months. Again, there was no difference in mortality between the two treatment arms. A significant bidirectional interaction was observed between diltiazem and the presence of CHF during the index MI (Fig. 25–11): Diltiazem significantly reduced cardiac events in patients

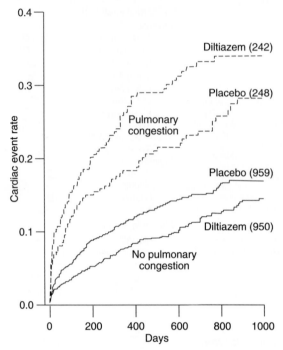

**Figure 25–11** ■ Diltiazem-treated patients with pulmonary congestion had a higher rate of cardiac events than patients receiving placebo; diltiazem-treated patients without pulmonary congestion had a lower rate of cardiac events than patients receiving placebo. The values in parentheses are numbers of patients. (Multicenter Diltiazem Postinfarction Trial Research Group: The effect of diltiazem on mortality and reinfarction after myocardial infarction. N Engl J Med 1988;319: 385–392).

with an ejection fraction (EF) greater than 40% and no evidence of pulmonary congestion, and increased cardiac events in patients with either a reduced EF or pulmonary congestion. The results of MDPIT may have been confounded by the use of beta blockers in more than 50% of patients in both the diltiazem and placebo groups. Furthermore, both studies were conducted in an era when aspirin use was less prevalent than it is today, so that further uncertainty is raised about the relevance of their findings for contemporary management of acute MI. Of particular clinical importance is the detrimental mortality effect of diltiazem in patients with LV dysfunction.

It should be emphasized that no studies have compared the efficacy of verapamil or diltiazem versus a beta blocker. Beta blockers more consistently reduce both mortality and reinfarction and should be recommended for those patients who can tolerate such medication. Verapamil or diltiazem may be a reasonable alternative for those patients who cannot tolerate a beta blocker but who can tolerate one of the calcium channel blockers—for example, patients with severe chronic obstructive pulmonary disease (COPD) or asthma. It should be noted, however, that many patients who cannot tolerate a beta blocker because of concern of excessive bradycardia or CHF may experience similar complications from diltiazem or verapamil. The current ACC/AHA recommendations for calcium channel blockers in the setting of acute MI are presented in Table 25–6.

Table 25–6

**Recommendation for Use of Calcium Channel Blockers**

*Class I* (conditions for which there is evidence and / or general agreement that treatment is beneficial, useful, and effective): none.

*Class IIa* (conditions for which there is conflicting evidence, but the weight of evidence is in favor of usefulness and efficacy): Verapamil or diltiazem may be given to patients in whom beta blockers are ineffective or contraindicated (i.e., bronchospastic disease) for relief of ongoing ischemic or control of a rapid ventricular response with atrial fibrillation after acute MI in the absence of CHF, LV dysfunction, or AV block.

*Class IIb* (conditions for which beneficial effects are less well established, but weight of evidence favors their use): in non–ST-segment-elevation MI, diltiazem may be given to patients without LV dysfunction, pulmonary congestion, or CHF. It may be added to standard therapy after the first 24 hr and continued for 1 yr.

*Class III* (conditions for which evidence suggests treatment is not useful and may be harmful): Short-acting nifedipine is generally contraindicated in routine treatment. Diltiazem and verapamil are contraindicated in patients with acute MI and associated LV dysfunction or CHF.

MI, myocardial infarction; CHF, congestive heart failure; LV, left ventricular; AV, atrioventricular.
Ryan TJ, Anderson JL, Antman EM, et al: ACC / AHA guidelines for the management of patients with acute myocardial infarction: A report of the American College of Cardiology/ American Heart Association Task Force on Practice Guidelines (Committee on Management of Acute Myocardial Infarction). J Am Coll Cardiol 1996;28:1328–1428.

## Angiotensin-Converting Enzyme Inhibitors

ACE inhibitors have become a mainstay in the treatment of acute MI because they prevent the deleterious LV chamber remodeling that may occur after MI and because they may prevent the progression of vascular pathology. The LV dysfunction associated with acute MI leads to a reduction in cardiac output and blood pressure, which is compensated by an increase in the renin-angiotensin-aldosterone system as well as an increase in sympathetic tone. These effects lead to salt and water retention as well as vasoconstriction, which in turn further dilate the LV and cause progressive LV dysfunction. This vicious cycle can be interrupted by ACE inhibitors, which block the increased renin-angiotensin activity and thereby prevent the progressive dilatation and dysfunction. The overview by the ACE Inhibitor Myocardial Infarction Collaborative Group,[37] which included observations of almost 100,000 patients with acute MI treated within 36 hours of the onset of chest pain, found a 7% reduction in 30-day mortality when ACE inhibitors were given to all patients with acute MI, with most of the benefit observed in the first week. The absolute benefit was particularly large in some high-risk groups, such as those in Killip class II or III (23 lives saved per 1000 patients) and those with an anterior MI (11 lives saved per 1000 patients).[37] ACE inhibitor therapy also reduced the incidence of nonfatal CHF (14.6% vs 15.2%, p = 0.01) but was associated with an excess of persistent hypotension and renal dysfunction. In the overview, more than 85% of the lives saved attributed to ACE inhibitor therapy occurred in the anterior MI subgroup, which represented 37% of the overall population.

As opposed to aspirin and reperfusion strategies, it is not crucial to introduce the ACE inhibitor in the hyperacute phase of acute MI. ACE inhibitor therapy is still of benefit when administered at any time after MI, although benefit is lessened if therapy is delayed by days or weeks. The benefits of ACE inhibition appear to be class specific, with little difference between agents. The current recommendations for use of ACE inhibitors for acute MI are shown in Table 25–7.

Of note, ACE inhibitors may also protect against progression of atherosclerosis and the development of MI by their antiproliferative and antimigratory effects on smooth muscle cells, neutrophils, and mononuclear cells, by enhancing endogenous fibrinolysis, and by improving endothelial dysfunction. Studies suggest that pa-

Table 25–7

**ACC/AHA Guidelines for Use of Angiotensin-Converting Enzyme Inhibitors for Acute Myocardial Infarction**

*Class I* (conditions for which there is evidence and/or general agreement that treatment is beneficial, useful, and effective):
  Patients within first 24 hr of MI with ST segment elevation in ≥2 anterior leads or with CHF
  Patients with MI and EF <40% or with CHF and systolic dysfunction during and after convalescence
*Class IIa* (conditions for which there is conflicting evidence, but the weight of evidence is in favor of usefulness and efficacy)
  All other MI patients within first 24 hr
  Asymptomatic patients with EF 40–50% and prior MI
*Class IIb* (conditions for which beneficial effects are less well established, but weight of evidence favors their use): patients recently recovered from MI with normal or mildly abnormal LV function
*Class III* (conditions for which evidence suggests treatment is not useful and may be harmful): none

MI, myocardial infarction; CHF, congestive heart failure; EF, ejection fraction; LV, left ventricular.
Ryan TJ, Anderson JL, Antman EM, et al: ACC/AHA guidelines for the management of patients with acute myocardial infarction: A report of the American College of Cardiology/American Heart Association Task Force on Practice Guidelines (Committee on Management of Acute Myocardial Infarction). J Am Coll Cardiol 1996;28:1328–1428.

tients treated with ACE inhibitors experience fewer MIs and episodes of unstable angina not related to hemodynamic effects and ventricular remodeling. Further studies are in progress to determine the role of such therapy in routine secondary prevention.

## Magnesium

Magnesium appears to protect myocytes from calcium-mediated reperfusion injury and, in experimental models, improves recovery of contractile function as long as it is given before or contiguous with reperfusion. Other potential beneficial effects of magnesium include inhibition of free radical injury, reduction of heart rate and blood pressure, coronary vasodilation, and even platelet inhibition. Randomized clinical trials have yielded conflicting evidence for the effects of magnesium. The LIMIT-2 trial[38] and a meta-analysis of seven prior randomized clinical trials[39] suggested that IV magnesium reduced mortality from 20% to 50%. Enthusiasm was subsequently tempered by the publication of the ISIS-4 trial,[33] which showed no benefit of magnesium therapy in 58,050 patients. Considerable controversy has arisen over these conflicting results, with some investigators arguing that the negative results in the ISIS-4 trial were a result of the delayed administration of magnesium, after the window for myocyte protection had closed. To resolve this controversy, the National Heart, Lung and Blood Institute (NHLBI) is sponsoring a large multicenter trial of *early* magnesium therapy for high-risk patients with ST-elevation MI, called the Magnesium in Coronaries (MAGIC) trial.

## ■ IN-HOSPITAL MANAGEMENT AFTER ACUTE MYOCARDIAL INFARCTION

### Risk Factor Modification

Correction of modifiable risk factors is essential for the treatment of patients who have suffered an MI. The benefits of aggressive risk factor modification are profound and are in fact more dramatic than those with any of the expensive treatment strategies described in this chapter. Risk factor modification, including lipid-lowering therapy, is discussed in detail in Chapter 24.

# Risk Stratification

Risk stratification in acute MI actually should begin the moment a patient arrives in the emergency room and should continue through hospital discharge and beyond. When a patient is first seen, history, physical examination, ECG, and serum marker information are rapidly integrated, both to arrive at a diagnosis and to estimate a patient's a priori risk for adverse outcome. For example, older age, female sex, presence of diabetes, and history of prior MI or CHF all are associated with increased risk. In addition, tachycardia or bradycardia, hypotension, and evidence of CHF are markers for increased risk that are easily obtained from a focused examination. The ECG provides incremental predictive power, in addition to distinguishing ST-elevation from non–ST-elevation MI. An anterior location of infarction (or an inferior infarction with RV extension or anterior ST depression) and greater ST deviation are associated with larger infarcts and increased risk. Finally, elevated serum markers at presentation, even in patients with known ST elevation, predict an increased risk for mortality.

Patients initially undergo triage on the basis of the presence or absence of ST-segment elevation on the presenting ECG (Figs. 25–12 and 25–13). Subsequent risk stratification steps should focus on identifying patients at risk for electrical, mechanical, and ischemic complications and on selecting those patients who will

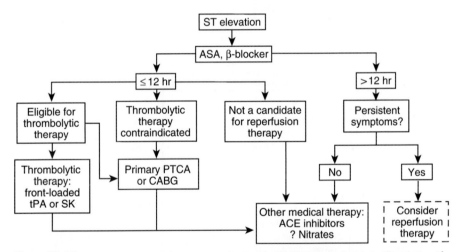

**Figure 25–12** ■ Recommendations for treatment of patients with ST-segment elevation. All patients with ST-segment elevation on the electrocardiogram should receive aspirin (ASA), beta-adrenoceptor blockers (in the absence of contraindications), and an antithrombin (particularly if tissue-type plasminogen activator [tPA] is used for thrombolytic therapy). The role of GP IIb/IIIa inhibitors in the setting of thrombolytic therapy is under active investigation. Whether heparin is required in patients receiving streptokinase (SK) remains a matter of controversy; the small additional risk for intracranial hemorrhage may not be offset by the survival benefit afforded by adding heparin to SK therapy. Patients who are treated within 12 hours and who are eligible for thrombolytics should expeditiously receive either accelerated-dose TPA or SK or be considered for primary percutaneous transluminal coronary angioplasty (PTCA) or stenting. Primary PTCA (or stenting) is also to be considered when thrombolytic therapy is absolutely contraindicated. Coronary artery bypass graft (CABG) may be considered if the patient is less than 6 hours from onset of symptoms. Individuals treated after 12 hours should receive the initial medical therapy noted earlier and, on an individual basis, may be candidates for reperfusion therapy or angiotensin-converting enzyme (ACE) inhibitors (particularly if left ventricular function is impaired). (Ryan TJ, Anderson JL, Antman EM, et al: ACC/AHA guidelines for the management of patients with acute myocardial infarction: A report of the American College of Cardiology/American Heart Association Task Force on Practice Guidelines [Committee on Management of Acute Myocardial Infarction]. J Am Coll Cardiol 1996;28:1328–1428).

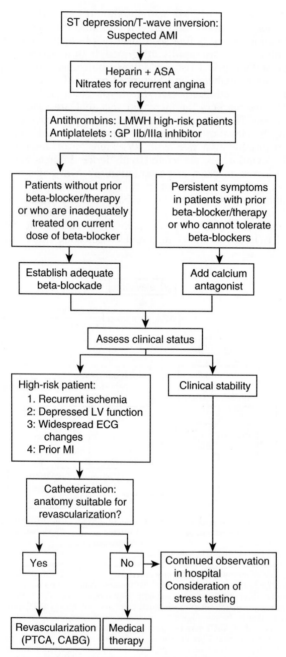

**Figure 25–13** ▪ *See legend on opposite page*

benefit most from particular therapies, such as revascularization (see Fig. 25–13). It should be remembered that with many therapies, absolute risk reduction is highest in those patients at greatest risk; therefore, the higher the risk for an individual patient, the more aggressive the care should be.

## Left Ventricular Function

LV function is the single most important determinant of long-term survival after MI; for example, patients with significant LV dysfunction (LVEF ≤ 40%) after MI have a 5-year mortality exceeding 25%. In addition, patients with LV dysfunction and multivessel CAD derive significant benefit from surgical revascularization. Because of the importance of LV function to risk assessment, almost all patients should have an EF measurement after an acute MI. Because reversible LV dysfunction, termed *myocardial stunning,* may follow an ischemic insult, initial measurements may significantly underestimate true LV function. Therefore, unless clinically indicated because of CHF, suspected valvular heart disease, or pericardial effusion, measurement of EF can be deferred until approximately 5 to 7 days after MI. Although echocardiography, contrast ventriculography, and radionuclide angiography all are reliable methods for assessing LVEF, echocardiography has the advantage of providing structural information as well. Contrast ventriculography should be considered for patients in whom acute mitral regurgitation is strongly suspected, because transthoracic echocardiography may underestimate the amount of regurgitation.

## Routine Coronary Angiography and Revascularization After Thrombolytic Therapy

As opposed to rescue PCI for failed thrombolysis, routine adjunctive PCI after thrombolysis is a much more controversial strategy. In the mid- to late 1980s, several studies evaluated the role for routine immediate or delayed angioplasty after thrombolytic therapy. The TIMI 2A trial found no benefit in mortality, reinfarction, or IRA patency in patients randomized to an early invasive strategy (*immediate* catheterization and PTCA for suitable lesions) after thrombolysis; in fact, complications were significantly increased in the invasive arm and there was a trend toward worse clinical outcomes.[40] The TIMI 2B trial was a larger trial comparing a *delayed* invasive versus conservative strategy (catheterization and PTCA for spontaneous or inducible ischemia only) after administration of tPA, heparin, and aspirin. No differences in mortality or recurrent infarction were noted between the two strategies at 1 year and 3 years of follow-up, despite the fact that revasculariza-

---

**Figure 25–13** ■ Recommendations for treatment of patients with acute myocardial infarction (AMI) without ST elevation. All patients without ST elevation should be treated with an antithrombin (heparin or low-molecular-weight heparin [LMWH]) and aspirin (ASA). In high-risk patients, the addition of GP IIb/IIIa to aspirin and heparin or the substitution of LMWH for unfractionated heparin should be considered. Nitrates should be administered for recurrent episodes of angina. Adequate beta-adrenoceptor blockade should then be established; when this is not possible or contraindications exist, a calcium antagonist (verapamil or diltiazem) can be considered. High-risk patients should undergo triage to cardiac catheterization with plans for revascularization if they are clinically suitable; patients who are clinically stable can be treated more conservatively, with continued observation in the hospital and consideration of a stress test to screen for myocardial ischemia that can be provoked. LV, left ventricular; ECG, electrocardiographic; PCTA, percutaneous transluminal coronary angioplasty; CABG, coronary artery bypass graft. (ISIS-4 Collaborative Group: ISIS-4: Randomized factorial trial assessing early oral captopril, oral mononitrate, and intravenous magnesium sulphate in 58,000 patients with suspected acute myocardial infarction. Lancet 1995;345:669–685).

tion rates were twice as high in the invasive arm.[41] Other investigators similarly found no role for routine immediate or delayed angioplasty after successful thrombolysis.

Since these trials were published, dramatic advances in interventional cardiology have taken place. Intracoronary stenting has significantly decreased the incidence of abrupt vessel closure after PTCA, the need for emergency coronary artery bypass grafting (CABG) for failed PTCA, and the need for target-vessel reintervention due to restenosis. Glycoprotein IIb/IIIa inhibitors have further decreased complications after both elective and emergent procedures. In addition, the management of vascular access sites has changed in parallel. Today's sheaths are smaller and removed earlier after PCI; less heparin is used during procedures; and new percutaneous closure devices have been developed to reduce local bleeding complications. These factors have combined to improve procedural efficacy and reduce complications and have rekindled enthusiasm among interventional cardiologists to perform adjunctive PCI after thrombolysis.

Preliminary results from the PACT trial support the *safety* of immediate PCI in the setting of thrombolytic therapy.[42] In this study, patients were randomized to either reduced-dose tPA or to placebo and then were taken *immediately* to cardiac catheterization, where angioplasty was performed unless TIMI grade 3 flow was found. Patients receiving tPA before catheterization had higher initial rates of TIMI grade 3 flow than those receiving placebo (32.8% vs 14.8%); after PCI, TIMI flow grade was similar between the two groups, indicating that tPA administration did not adversely impact procedural outcomes. Most importantly, there were no significant differences in bleeding or recurrent ischemic complications, suggesting that angioplasty could be safely performed immediately after a reduced dose of tPA. Despite the early promise of this study, the benefits of an early invasive approach after thrombolytic therapy need to be confirmed in studies enrolling larger numbers of patients; in addition to addressing safety, clinical trials will need to demonstrate reduced reocclusion rates, improved LV function, or decreased mortality.

At present, our recommendation is to reserve cardiac catheterization after *successful* thrombolytic therapy for patients with spontaneous or inducible ischemia or those with significantly reduced LV function (with "viable" myocardium). In addition, it may be reasonable to perform catheterization in other high-risk patients who may benefit from revascularization, including those with prior MI and those with significant ventricular arrhythmias.

## Coronary Angiography and Revascularization After Non–ST-Elevation Myocardial Infarction

Patients with non–ST-elevation (non–Q wave) MI have lower initial mortality rates than patients with ST-elevation MI but have higher recurrent ischemia and reinfarction rates, such that outcomes at 1 year are similar. This has prompted many clinicians to follow an aggressive approach to catheterization and revascularization. However, few data support that such an aggressive approach reduces the incidence of death or nonfatal reinfarction.

Advocates of the invasive approach note that definitive management can be accomplished in several days: Angiography can identify the 10% to 15% of patients with normal coronary arteries (who could be discharged home), as well as the 5% to 10% of patients with severe left main or three-vessel CAD who benefit from CABG; in the remaining patients who need revascularization, it can be carried out expeditiously and patients can return home rapidly.

With a more conservative approach using vigorous medical therapy, particularly in patients who have never previously received antianginal medication, unstable angina may quickly "cool off." If patients remain symptom free on medical therapy after beginning to ambulate, they may be treated conservatively. Treadmill exercise testing, with or without adjunctive imaging, may further help to define patient care. If the pattern of angina remains unstable or if ECG changes suggest ongoing ischemia, then coronary angiography is warranted.

Two large trials have prospectively compared the initial invasive versus conservative strategies. The TIMI 3B trial[3] found that both the early invasive and early conservative strategies led to a similar incidence of serious adverse outcomes, and thus both strategies are suitable for patients with these acute ischemic syndromes. However, because nearly two thirds of patients required catheterization despite aggressive medical treatment, the early invasive arm could be viewed as a more expeditious strategy for unstable angina and non–Q wave MI. The recent VANQWISH (V.A. Non–Q-Wave Infarction Strategies in-Hospital) trial compared invasive and conservative approaches in patients with non–Q wave MI and found no significant difference in the primary endpoint of death or nonfatal MI during a 12- to 44-month follow-up.[43] However, significantly more deaths occurred in patients assigned to the invasive compared with the conservative strategy at hospital discharge and at 1 year. Much of the early hazard in the invasive group was explained by a very high (13.4%) perioperative mortality in patients receiving CABG; although this has been a point of criticism, similarly high perioperative mortality rates have been reported by other investigators in high-risk patients with recent MI.

Thus, balancing TIMI 3B and VANQWISH, one must individualize the approach on the basis of patient characteristics and local expertise in PCI and CABG. In a broad group of patients with unstable angina and non–ST-elevation MI, in whom PCI can be carried out with low complication rates, an invasive strategy may be considered appropriate and more expeditious than an early conservative strategy. This invasive strategy may be particularly appropriate in patients who are at high risk for cardiac complications— that is, those who have ST-segment depression, those who have prior manifestations of CAD, or those who are older.[44] In patients with more severe infarction, in populations with a higher frequency of multivessel disease requiring CABG, and at hospitals where complication rates are higher, a more conservative approach may be more appropriate. Given the importance of this issue, trials are currently ongoing to reexamine the relative benefits of invasive versus conservative strategies in this patient population in the current era of GP IIb/IIIa inhibition and coronary stenting.

## Conservative Management Strategies

As described earlier, a conservative diagnostic strategy is indicated for most patients after successful thrombolysis for ST-elevation MI and for many patients with non–ST-elevation MI. This strategy consists of noninvasive determination of LV function and a modified exercise tolerance test (ETT) (with or without nuclear imaging) before discharge. Patients who complete a submaximum ETT without evidence of ischemia should subsequently have a symptom-limited ETT 4 to 6 weeks later before returning to full activity.

## ▪ COMPLICATIONS OF ACUTE MYOCARDIAL INFARCTION

### Infarct Expansion and Remodeling

After a large MI, particularly if it involves the anterior wall and apex of the LV, the infarct area may expand and cause thinning of the necrotic myocardium.

Over weeks to months, the LV may dilate and assume a more globular shape. This process, termed *LV remodeling*, has been associated with an increased risk for the development of LV dysfunction, heart failure, and death. Factors that have been found to favorably affect remodeling include use of the ACE inhibitors (described earlier) and establishment of a patent infarct-related artery. Indeed, one of the purported benefits of late reperfusion is improved tissue healing and prevention of adverse LV remodeling.

## Recurrent Ischemia and Infarction

After successful thrombolysis, reocclusion of the infarct artery and subsequent reinfarction may occur in up to 10% to 15% of patients by hospital discharge and 30% of patients by 3 months, a complication associated with a two- to threefold increase in mortality.[9] As described earlier, thrombolytic therapy itself may create a prothrombotic state that promotes reocclusion. Reocclusion rates after primary PCI are similarly high, although this complication may be reduced by the use of adjunctive stenting and GP IIb/IIIb inhibition. Recurrent infarction may be difficult to diagnose, particularly if it occurs within the first 24 to 48 hours after MI, when levels of cardiac enzymes remain elevated from the index event. Recurrent ST elevation or a new peak in CK-MB or myoglobin is highly suggestive of MI. Recurrent ischemia without infarction is also a frequent complication after MI. Because patients with postinfarction angina are at high risk for recurrent MI, in general, cardiac catheterization should be performed with a goal of target-vessel revascularization.

## Cardiogenic Shock

When cardiogenic shock occurs after MI, it is most commonly due to infarction of 40% or more of the LV. Other, less common causes include septal rupture, free wall rupture, acute mitral regurgitation, and RV infarction. Cardiogenic shock is characterized by tissue hypoperfusion, hypotension, low cardiac output, and elevated filling pressures. Patients who develop shock tend to be older, with a history of prior MI or CHF. Even in the modern era, the prognosis of cardiogenic shock is dismal, with mortality rates of at least 70%.

Given the poor prognosis of cardiogenic shock, early aggressive care is indicated. Invasive hemodynamic monitoring with a Swan-Ganz catheter can help to confirm the cause of shock in difficult cases and to tailor appropriate pressor and vasodilator therapy. The intraaortic balloon pump (IABP) has been used with success in patients with cardiogenic shock after MI; this device is of particular value in patients with mechanical complications such as acute mitral regurgitation or septal rupture, when its use can be lifesaving. The IABP augments cardiac output by creating a low-resistance zone for LV outflow and enhances coronary blood flow by inflating during diastole and increasing coronary perfusion pressure.

Dopamine and dobutamine are the pharmocologic agents most commonly used to treat cardiogenic shock. These positive inotropic agents increase heart rate and cardiac output by stimulating cardiac $\beta_1$-adrenergic receptors; they differ in that dobutamine is also a $\beta_2$ agonist and therefore causes peripheral vasodilation. For this reason, dobutamine may be a more physiologically appropriate drug to use in cardiogenic shock. In patients with severe hypotension, however, this effect may be undesirable. IV vasodilators such as nitroprusside and nitroglycerin may also be used to reduce systemic vascular resistance and increase cardiac output, provided the patient has sufficient blood pressure to tolerate these agents. Agonists of the $\alpha_1$-adrenergic receptor, such as norepinepherine and neosynepherine, should be used only when refractory hypotension is present and other options have been exhausted.

Unfortunately, although the treatments described earlier for cardiogenic shock may be helpful, they are temporizing measures and have not been shown to improve survival. Reperfusion and, in particular, revascularization appear to improve survival in selected patients. Although data are limited, emergent PCI and even CABG seem to be superior to thrombolytic therapy for patients with cardiogenic shock: In centers appropriately equipped, emergent catheterization and revascularization is the treatment of choice. In other centers, consideration should be given to placement of an IABP and transfer to a center that can perform urgent intervention.

## Right Ventricular Myocardial Infarction

RV infarction is a frequent complication of IMI and is almost always caused by proximal occlusion of the right coronary artery. The diagnosis should be suspected in patients with IMI and unsuspected hypotension, particularly when it occurs after small doses of nitrates. Patients usually have jugular venous distention but have clear lungs unless significant LV infarction is present as well. A right-sided ECG should be performed in all patients with IMI, because ST elevation of 0.1 mV or greater in $V_4R$ is sensitive and specific for the diagnosis of RV infarction. The hemodynamic profile is one of elevated right-sided filling pressures with reduced cardiac output, findings similar to those of pericardial tamponade. In patients without ECG evidence of RV infarction, therefore, echocardiography (or placement of a pulmonary artery catheter) is indicated to distinguish between the two diagnoses.

The hemodynamic derangements of RV infarction can be improved by expansion of intravascular volume with normal saline. In patients with severe RV infarction, many liters of fluid may be required to achieve hemodynamic stability. Short-term morbidity and mortality are increased in patients with RV MI compared with those with IMI alone. Several studies have suggested that primary PCI, rather than thrombolytic therapy, should be the preferred reperfusion method in these high-risk individuals. In patients who stabilize, the prognosis for full recovery of RV function is very good.

## Free Wall Rupture

Rupture of the free wall of the LV is the most catastrophic mechanical complication of acute MI, with a mortality rate in excess of 90%. The presentation is one of pericardial tamponade and hemodynamic collapse, often culminating in pulseless electrical activity. Survival is dependent on prompt recognition, emergent pericardiocentesis, and surgical repair.

The interaction of rupture and thrombolytic therapy is complex. Although early thrombolytic therapy lowers the risk for rupture, late thrombolytic therapy, when given in the setting of a completed infarct with softened necrotic tissue, may actually increase the incidence of rupture. In addition, in the thrombolytic era, rupture appears to be occurring earlier after presentation; although the most common time frame is 1 to 4 days after MI, it may occur within the first 24 hours. Rupture is associated with large transmural infarctions and is more common in the elderly, women, and patients *without* prior MI. Controversy exists about an association with glucocorticoids and nonsteroidal antiinflammatory drugs. The most common location of rupture is in the anterior and lateral distributions of the left anterior descending artery.

Incomplete free wall rupture can lead to formation of a pseudoaneurysm. In this situation, the rupture site is sealed by a hematoma and the pericardium itself, and when the thrombus organizes, a pseudoaneurysm cavity is formed. The pseudoaneurysm is often large and typically remains filled with some degree of thrombus. In distinction to a true aneurysm, in which the wall is composed of myocardial tissue, a pseudoaneurysm communicates with the LV cavity via a narrow neck of myocardial tissue; the wall of the pseudoaneurysm is composed of thrombus and pericardium but no myocardial tissue. Early elective repair is indicated for all suitable patients.

## Septal Rupture

Rupture of the intraventricular septum typically does not present in as catastrophic a manner as does free wall rupture. Septal rupture causes an acute ventricular septal defect, with left-to-right flow across the lesion. The presentation is usually one of CHF that develops over hours to days (depending on the size of the defect), associated with a harsh holosystolic murmur, which may be difficult to distinguish from mitral regurgitation. Either Doppler echocardiography or insertion of a pulmonary artery catheter can be used to confirm the diagnosis. If a step-up in oxygen saturation is noted at the level of the RV when the pulmonary artery catheter is placed, it is diagnostic of a ventricular septal defect in this setting. Septal rupture is more common after anterior infarction, where the apical regions of the septum are involved. With inferior infarction, the basal portions of the septum are involved, and the prognosis is somewhat worse. Patients should be stabilized with pressors, usually an IABP, and vasodilators (if tolerated), followed by surgical repair and revascularization.

## Acute Mitral Regurgitation

Acute mitral regurgitation following acute MI is caused by ischemic dysfunction or frank rupture of a papillary muscle. This complication is more common after IMI, because the posteromedial papillary muscle typically has a single blood supply from the right coronary artery whereas the anterolateral papillary muscle has dual supply from the left anterior descending and circumflex arteries. As opposed to rupture, this complication can occur with relatively small but well localized infarctions. As with septal rupture, a new holosystolic murmur is classically present in the setting of acute pulmonary edema, and cardiogenic shock may even ensue. As blood pressure falls, the murmur may disappear entirely. Doppler echocardiography is particularly helpful in distinguishing acute mitral rupture from septal rupture. Treatment for this complication requires initial stabilization, usually with an IABP, pressors, and vasodilators (if tolerated), followed by prompt surgical correction.

## Ventricular Tachycardia and Ventricular Fibrillation
(See Chapters 16 and 17)

Ventricular tachycardia (VT) is common in patients during the first hours and days after MI and does not appear to be associated with an increased risk for subsequent mortality if the arrhythmia is rapidly terminated. VT occurring after 24 to 48 hours, however, is associated with a marked increase in mortality. *Monomorphic* VT is usually due to a reentrant focus around a scar, whereas *polymorphic* VT is more commonly a function of underlying ischemia, electrolyte abnormalities, or drug effects.

Ventricular fibrillation (VF) is believed to be the primary mechanism of arrythmic sudden death. The incidence of primary VF appears to have declined substantially. In patients with acute MI, the vast majority of the episodes of VF occur early (< 4 to 12 hours) after infarction. As with sustained VT, *late* VF occurs more frequently in patients with severe LV dysfunction or CHF and is associated with a poor prognosis. Patients with VF or with sustained VT associated with symptoms or hemodynamic compromise should undergo cardioversion immediately. Underlying metabolic and electrolyte abnormalities must be corrected, and ongoing ischemia should be addressed. Lidocaine remains an effective agent for the treatment of symptomatic VT or VF but should rarely be used as a prophylactic measure. It should be noted that IV amiodarone may be a particularly effective antiarrhythmic agent in the setting of acute MI owing to its heart rate lowering properties.

### Bradyarrhythmias (See Chapters 16 and 17)

Bradyarrhythmias are common in the setting of acute MI and may be due to either increased vagal tone or ischemia/infarction of conduction tissue. Sinus bradycardia is usually a result of stimulation of cardiac vagal receptors, which are located most prominently on the inferoposterior surface of the LV. If the heart rate is extremely low (< 40 to 50) or if hypotension is present, IV atropine should be given.

Mobitz type I (Wenkebach) second-degree AV block is also very common in patients with IMI and may be a function of either ischemia or infarction of the AV node or increased vagal tone. The level of conduction block is usually within the AV node; therefore, the QRS complex is narrow and the risk for progression to complete heart block is minimal. Again, atropine can be used for patients with significant bradycardia, hypotension, or symptoms. Temporary pacing is rarely required unless there is hemodynamic or electrical instability. Mobitz type II block is much less common than Mobitz type I block in the setting of MI. As opposed to Mobitz type I block, Mobitz type II block is more frequently associated with anterior MI, an infranodal lesion, and a wide QRS complex. Because Mobitz type II block can suddenly progress to complete heart block, a temporary pacemaker is indicated.

Although compete heart block may occur with either inferior or anterior MI, the implications differ considerably depending on the location of the infarct. With IMI, heart block often progresses from first-degree or Wenckebach to third-degree AV block. The level of block is usually within or above the level of the AV node, the escape rate is often stable, and the effect transient. Although temporary pacing is indicated for hemodynamic or electrical instability, a permanent pacemaker is rarely required. With anterior MI, complete heart block is usually a result of extensive infarction that involves the bundle branches. The escape rhythm is usually unstable, and the AV block permanent. Mortality is extremely high, and permanent pacing is performed unless there are contraindications.

### Supraventricular Arrhythmias (See Chapters 16 and 17)

Atrial fibrillation occurs in up to 15% of patients early after MI, with atrial flutter and paroxysmal supraventricular tachycardia occurring much less frequently. Ischemia itself is rarely a cause of atrial fibrillation, except in rare cases of atrial infarction. Precipitants of atrial fibrillation after MI include RV or LV failure and pericarditis. Although the arrhythmia itself is usually transient, it is a marker for increased morbidity and mortality, probably because of the conditions associated with its development. Management of supraventricular arrhythmias in the setting of acute MI is similar to management in other settings (see Chapter 17); however, in the setting of acute MI, the threshold for cardioversion should be lower and the urgency with which the ventricular response is controlled should be greater. Because of their beneficial effects in acute MI, beta blockers should be the first agents used to control rate. Diltiazem and verapamil are appropriate alternatives in patients without heart failure or significant LV dysfunction, and digoxin is indicated for patients with concomitant LV dysfunction. Of the antiarrhythmic agents available, amidarone is probably the safest in the periinfarct setting.

## Left Ventricular Aneurysm

A true LV aneurysm is a discreet outpouching of a thinned, dyskinetic myocardial segment. As opposed to the wall of a pseudoaneurysm, the wall of a true aneurysm contains cardiac and fibrous tissues, and the neck is broad based. The most common site of aneurysm formation is the LV apex, owing to distal occlusion of a noncollateralized left anterior descending artery. As opposed to pseudoaneurysms, true LV aneurysms pose a small risk of rupture. Aneurysms are, however, associated with increased morbidity and mortality. The dyskinetic aneurysmal segment may alter overall LV geometry and impair contractile performance; thrombus frequently lines the thinned wall and may be a source for arterial embolus; and most importantly, the scarred aneurysmal tissue may be a source of malignant ventricular arrhythmias. Surgical aneurysmectomy is rarely indicated, except to control malignant arrhythmias and, rarely, in an attempt to improve LV function. Anticoagulation with long-term warfarin therapy may be indicated to prevent the development of mural thrombus and embolization.

## Left Ventricular Mural Thrombus

LV mural thrombus occurs in approximately 40% of patients with transmural anterior MI. The incidence is lower in patients who receive thrombolytic or anticoagulant therapy. The risk for subsequent arterial embolization is approximately 10% and is higher in patients with mobile thrombus detected by echocardiography. Although echocardiography can detect mural thrombus in many cases, patients with large anterior MI remain at risk for systemic embolization even if no thrombus is seen. IV heparin, followed by warfarin for 3 to 6 months, is indicated as preventive therapy in patients who are candidates for long-term anticoagulation.

## Pericarditis

Asymptomatic pericardial effusion occurs in as many as 25% of patients following transmural MI; these effusions are rarely associated with symptoms or hemodynamic compromise. Fibrinous pericarditis may also occur in the days to weeks following transmural infarction and may be confused with postinfarction angina or recurrent MI. The pain of pericarditis is usually pleuritic and positional, and it often radiates to the trapezius ridge. A pericardial friction rub may be noted. Treatment generally consists of aspirin; nonsteroidal antiinflammatory agents should be avoided because they may inhibit healing of the infarct. If an effusion is seen on echocardiography in a patient with symptomatic pericarditis, anticoagulants should be withheld unless absolutely necessary. Dressler syndrome is an immunologic phenomenon that is characterized by pericardial pain, generalized malaise, fever, elevated white blood cell count, elevated erythrocyte sedimentation rate, and pericardial effusion. It occurs several weeks to several months after MI and is believed to be immunologically mediated. Again, higher aspirin doses should be used as primary therapy, and steroids and nonsteroidal antiinflammatory drugs should be avoided until at least 1 month has elapsed since MI.

## ■ SUMMARY

Dramatic advances have been made in the diagnosis and management of acute MI. The use of newer, more sensitive serum markers of myocardial necrosis and progress in noninvasive imaging modalities have improved the early detection of ischemia and infarction. In ST-elevation MI, early reperfusion with thrombolytic therapy or primary PCI has significantly reduced mortality. Current research is focusing on combining reperfusion regimens to improve efficacy and reduce bleeding risk. For example, combinations of reduced-dose bolus thrombolytic agents, together with GP IIb/IIIa receptor blockers and low-dose unfractionated (or low-molecular-weight) heparin may well improve outcomes. In non–ST-elevation MI, two important advances are GP IIb/IIIa inhibition and LMWH. Finally, as our understanding of the pathobiologic processes underlying the acute coronary syndromes continues to grow, newer therapies will be developed to address the root problems of atherosclerosis and plaque rupture.

## ■ REFERENCES

1. Cannon CP, Braunwald E: GUSTO, TIMI and the case for rapid reperfusion. Acta Cardiol 1994;49:1–8.
2. Fibrinolytic Therapy Trialists' (FTT) Collaborative Group: Indications for fibrinolytic therapy in suspected acute myocardial infarction: Collaborative overview of early mortality and major morbidity results from all randomised trials of more than 1000 patients. Lancet 1994;343:311–322.
3. TIMI IIIB Investigators: Effects of tissue plasminogen activator and a comparison of early invasive and conservative strategies in unstable angina and non–Q-wave myocardial infarction: Results of the TIMI IIIB trial. Circulation 1994;89:1545–1556.
4. TIMI Study Group: The Thrombolysis in Myocardial Infarction (TIMI) trial; Phase I findings. N Engl J Med 1985;312:932–936.
5. The Gusto Investigators: An international randomized trial comparing four thrombolytic strategies for acute myocardial infarction. N Engl J Med 1993;329:673–682.
6. Global Use of Strategies to Open Occluded Coronary Arteries (GUSTO III) Investigators: A comparison of reteplase with alteplase for acute myocardial infarction. N Engl J Med 1997;337:1118–1123.
7. Van de Werf F: Preliminary Results of the ASSENT II trial. 48th Annual Scientific Sessions of the American College of Cardiology, New Orleans, 1999.
8. Neuhaus K-L: Preliminary results of the InTIME II Trial. 48th Annual Scientific Sessions of the American College of Cardiology, New Orleans, 1999.
9. Ohman EM, Califf RM, Topol EJ, et al: Consequences of reocclusion after successful reperfusion therapy in acute myocardial infarction. Circulation 1990;82:781–791.
10. Ellis S, da Silva ER, Heyndrickx G, et al: Randomized comparison of rescue angioplasty with conservative management of patients with early failure of thrombolysis for acute anterior myocardial infarction. Circulation 1994;90:2280–2284.
11. Weaver WD, Simes RJ, Betriu A, et al: Comparison of primary coronary angioplasty and intravenous thrombolytic therapy of acute myocardial infarction. A quantitative review. JAMA 1997;278:2093–2098.
12. Lefkovits J, Ivanhoe RJ, Califf RM, et al: Effects of platelet glycoprotein IIb/IIIa receptor blockade by a chimeric monoclonal antibody (abciximab) on acute and six-month outcomes after percutaneous transluminal coronary angioplasty for acute myocardial infarction. Am J Cardiol 1996;77:1045–1051.
13. Brener SJ, Barr LA, Burchenal JEB, et al: Randomized, placebo-controlled trial of platelet glycoprotein IIb/IIIa blockade with primary angioplasty for acute myocardial infarction. Circulation 1998;98:734–741.
14. Miller J, Ohman E, Schildcrout J, et al: Survival benefit of abciximab administration during early rescue angioplasty: Analysis of 387 patients from the GUSTO-III trial. J Am Coll Cardiol 1998;31 (Suppl A):191A.
15. Antman EM, Giugliano RP, Gibson CM, et al: Abciximab facilitates the rate and extent of thrombolysis: Results of TIMI 14 trial. Circulation (in press).

16. Roux S, Christeller S, Ludin E: Effects of aspirin on coronary reocclusion and recurrent ischemia after thrombolysis: A meta-analysis. J Am Coll Cardiol 1992;19:671–677.
17. Antiplatelet Trialists' Collaboration: Collaborative overview of randomised trials of antiplatelet therapy—I: prevention of death, myocardial infarction and stroke by prolonged antiplatelet therapy in various categories of patients. BMJ 1994;308:81–106.
18. The Platelet Receptor Inhibition For Ischemic Syndrome Management (PRISM) Study Investigators: A comparison of aspirin plus tirofiban with aspirin plus heparin for unstable angina. N Engl J Med 1998;338:1498–1505.
19. The Platelet Glycoprotein IIb/IIIa in Unstable Angina: Receptor Suppression Using Integrilin Therapy (PURSUIT) Trial Investigators: Inhibition of platelet glycoprotein IIb/IIIa with eptifibate in patients with acute coronary syndromes. N Engl J Med 1998;339:436–443.
20. The GUSTO Angiographic Investigators: The comparative effects of tissue plasminogen activator, streptokinase, or both on coronary artery patency, ventricular function and survival after acute myocardial infarction. N Engl J Med 1993;329:1615–1622.
21. Oler A, Whooley MA, Oler J, Grady D: Adding heparin to aspirin reduces the incidence of myocardial infarction and death in patients with unstable angina. A meta-analysis. JAMA 1996;276:811–815.
22. Cohen M, Demers C, Gurfinkel EP, et al: A comparison of low-molecular-weight heparin with unfractionated heparin for unstable coronary artery disease. N Engl J Med 1997;337:447–452.
23. Antman EM, for the TIMI 9B Investigators: Hirudin in acute myocardial infarction: Thrombolysis and Thrombin Inhibition in Myocardial Infarction (TIMI) 9B trial. Circulation 1996;94:911–921.
24. The Global Use of Strategies to Open Occluded Coronary Arteries (GUSTO) IIb Investigators: A comparison of recombinant hirudin with heparin for the treatment of acute coronary syndromes. N Engl J Med 1996;335:775–782.
25. Coumadin Aspirin Reinfarction Study (CARS) Investigators: Randomised double-blind trial of fixed low-dose warfarin with aspirin after myocardial infarction. Lancet 1997;350:389–396.
26. CAPRIE Steering Committee: A randomised, blinded, trial of clopidogrel versus aspirin in patients at risk of ischaemic events (CAPRIE). Lancet 1996;348:1329–1339.
27. The TIMI Study Group: Comparison of invasive and conservative strategies after treatment with intravenous tissue plasminogen activator in acute myocardial infarction: Results of the Thrombolysis in Myocardial Infarction (TIMI) Phase II trial. N Engl J Med 1989;320:618–627.
28. Yusuf S, Peto R, Lewis J, et al: Beta-blockade during and after myocardial infarction: An overview of the randomized trials. Prog Cardiovasc Dis 1985;27:335–371.
29. Furberg CD, Hawkins CM, Lichstein E, for the Beta-Blocker Heart Attack Trial Study Group: Effects of long-term prophylactic treatment on survival after acute myocardial infarction. Circulation 1984;69:761–765.
30. Ryan TJ, Anderson JL, Antman EM, et al: ACC/AHA guidelines for the management of patients with acute myocardial infarction: A report of the American College of Cardiology/American Heart Association Task Force on Practice Guidelines (Committee on Management of Acute Myocardial Infarction). J Am Coll Cardiol 1996;28:1328–1428.
31. Yusuf S, Collins R, MacMahon S, Peto R: Effect of intravenous nitrates on mortality in acute myocardial infarction: An overview of the randomized trials. Lancet 1988;i:1088–1092.
32. Gruppo Italiano per lo Studio della Sopravvivenza nell'Infarto Miocardico: GISSI-3: effect of lisinopril and trasdermal glyceryl trinitrate singly and together on 6-week mortality and ventricular function after acute myocardial infarction. Lancet 1994;343:1115–1122.
33. ISIS-4 Collaborative Group. ISIS-4: Randomized factorial trial assessing early oral captopril, oral mononitrate, and intravenous magnesium sulphate in 58,050 patients with suspected acute myocardial infarction. Lancet 1995;345:669–685.
34. Yusuf S, Held P, Furburg C: Update of effects of calcium antagonists in myocardial infarction or angina in light of the second Danish Verapamil Infarction Trial (DAVIT-II) and other recent studies. Am J Cardiol 1991;67:1295–1297.
35. Multicenter Diltiazem Postinfarction Trial Research Group: The effect of diltiazem on mortality and reinfarction after myocardial infarction. N Engl J Med 1988;319:385–392.
36. Gibson RS, Boden WE, Theroux P, et al: Diltiazem and reinfarction in patients with non–Q wave myocardial infarction. Results of a double-blind, randomized, multicenter trial. N Engl J Med 1986;315:423–429.
37. ACE Inhibitor Myocardial Infarction Collaborative Group: Indications for ACE inhibitors in the early treatment of acute myocardial infarction: Systematic overview of individual data from 100,000 patients in randomized trials. Circulation 1998;97:2202–2212.
38. Woods KL, Fletcher S, Roffe C, Haider Y: Intravenous magnesium sulfate in suspected acute myocardial infarction: Results of the second Leicester Intravenous Magnesium Intervention Trial (LIMIT-2). Lancet 1992;339:1553–1558.
39. Teo KK, Yusuf S, Collins R, et al: Effects of intravenous magnesium in suspected acute myocardial infarction: Overview of randomized trials. BMJ 1991;303:1499–1503.
40. TIMI Research Group: Immediate vs delayed catheterization and angioplasty following thrombolytic therapy for acute myocardial infarction. TIMI II A results. JAMA 1988;260:2849–2858.
41. TIMI Study Group: Comparison of invasive and conservative strategies after treatment with intravenous tissue plasminogen activator in acute myocardial infarction. Results of the Thrombolysis in Myocardial Infarction (TIMI) Phase II Trial. N Engl J Med 1989;320:618–627.

42. Ross AM: Preliminary results from the PACT trial. Presented at a satellite symposium to the 47th Scientific Sessions of the American College of Cardiology, Atlanta, Georgia, March 1998.
43. Boden WE, O'Rourke RA, Crawford MH, et al: Outcomes in patients with acute non–Q-wave myocardial infarction randomly assigned to an invasive as compared with a conservative strategy. N Engl J Med 1998;338:1785–1792.
44. Stone PH, Thompson B, Zaret BL, et al: Factors associated with failure of medical therapy in patients with unstable angina and non–Q-wave MI: A TIMI-IIIB database study. Eur Heart J 1999;15:1084–1093.

## ■ RECOMMENDED READING

Antman EM, Braunwald E: Acute myocardial infarction. *In* Braunwald E (ed): Heart Disease. A Textbook of Cardiovascular Medicine, Vol. 1. Philadelphia: WB Saunders, 1997:1184–1288.
Braunwald E: Evolution of the management of acute myocardial infarction: A 20th century saga. Lancet 1998;352:1771–1774.
Libby P: Molecular bases of the acute coronary syndromes. Circulation 1995;91:2844–2850.
Opie LH: Pharmacologic Options for Treatment of Ischemic Disease. *In* Smith TW (ed): Cardiovascular Therapeutics. Philadelphia: WB Saunders, 1996:22–56.
Topol EJ, Serruys PW: Frontiers in interventional cardiology. Circulation 1998;98:1802–1820.
Wu A. Cardiac Markers. Clifton, NJ: Humana Press, 1998.

# Chapter 26

# Chronic Coronary Artery Disease: Stable and Unstable Angina

*Michael H. Gollob* ■ *Neal S. Kleiman*

As we enter the 21st century, the prevalence of coronary artery disease (CAD) is reaching nearly epidemic proportions in the Western world. In the United States alone, it is estimated that in excess of 11 million people have CAD.[1] As our population ages, these numbers are expected to accelerate exponentially. The associated morbidity and costs exceed those of any other chronic disease in modern society. Although tremendous progress in diagnostic modalities as well as medical and interventional management has occurred in recent decades, the impetus for more novel strategies remains.

This chapter reviews the current approach to the two most common clinical presentations of CAD, stable and unstable angina. Although angina pectoris has various causes (Table 26–1), the discussion here assumes the most common pathology manifesting these entities, coronary artery atherosclerosis.

## ■ STABLE ANGINA

### Clinical History

As with other diseases, a carefully taken history is essential in accurately diagnosing angina pectoris. Attention to specific details allows the clinician to discern between other potential causes of chest discomfort and thus offset the expense and risk of unnecessary testing. Exploring the quality, location, duration, and relieving and exacerbating features of the symptoms often permits a correct diagnosis. Angina pectoris is typically manifested as a heavy, squeezing chest discomfort brought on by exertional stress. The discomfort generally has a retrosternal component, often described as bandlike in nature. Radiation to the throat, jaw, and left shoulder are common. Relief usually occurs within minutes of cessation of the precipitating stress. Sublingual nitroglycerin also succeeds under most circumstances in providing rapid relief. Anginal symptoms are considered stable if the pattern of intensity, frequency, or duration has not changed for several weeks. Grading of the severity of angina pectoris is useful in monitoring progression of symptoms, conveying information to other clinicians, and assessing treatment strategies (Table 26–2). Symptoms that are described as fleeting, sharp, or pinpoint in location are not suggestive of angina pectoris. Similarly, the absence of characteristic precipitating and relieving features should lead the clinician to suspect other diagnoses.

Symptoms of myocardial ischemia may not always present with classic angina pectoris. Particularly in elderly and diabetic patients, symptoms of recurrent nausea

Table 26–1

**Causes of Angina Pectoris**

| Pathology | Disease |
|---|---|
| Coronary artery obstruction | Atherosclerosis |
| | Vasospasm |
| | Vasculitis |
| | Dissection |
| | Myocardial bridge |
| | Anomalous coronary origin |
| | Kawasaki disease |
| Left ventricular hypertrophy | Hypertension |
| | Aortic valvular / subvalvular stenosis |
| | Idiopathic / familial hypertrophic cardiomyopathy |
| Right ventricular hypertrophy | Pulmonary hypertension |
| | Pulmonary stenosis |

or unexplained vomiting may be the first clinical clues. Shortness of breath on minimal exertion may be due to ischemia-induced left ventricular dysfunction or mitral regurgitation. Rarely, syncope due to ischemia-mediated ventricular arrhythmia may be the first presenting symptom.

Independent risk factors for CAD must also be kept in mind during history taking. These include hypertension, diabetes mellitus, hyperlipidemia, smoking, and a family history of ischemic heart disease ($\leq$60 years old). In women older than 50 years, early menopause or a prolonged estrogen-deficient state without hormone replacement should also be considered a possible risk factor, although the role of estrogen replacement therapy is uncertain.

## Physical Examination

No clinical findings are specific to CAD. However, because CAD is the most common heart disease of Western society, any abnormal cardiac findings should be viewed as possibly related to chronic ischemic disease. The physical examination should focus on the detection of general findings that may be relevant to diagnostic and management strategies. For example, hyperlipidemic syndromes may first be discovered on viewing the skin lesions of xanthelasma or tendinous xanthomata. Diabetic patients may show signs of microvascular disease, such as retinopathy,

Table 26–2

**Canadian Cardiovascular Society Classification of Angina Pectoris**

| | |
|---|---|
| Class I | Ordinary physical activity does not cause angina—such as walking or climbing stairs. Angina with strenuous or rapid or prolonged exertion at work or recreation |
| Class II | Slight limitation of ordinary activity—walking or climbing stairs rapidly, walking uphill, walking or stair climbing after meals, in cold or in wind, or when under emotional stress, or only during the few hours after awakening. Walking more than two blocks (100–200 m) on the level and climbing more than one flight of stairs at a normal pace and in normal conditions |
| Class III | Marked limitation of ordinary physical activity—walking one or two blocks on the level and climbing one flight of stairs in normal conditions and at normal pace |
| Class IV | Inability to carry on any physical activity without discomfort—anginal syndrome may be present at rest |

Campeau L: Grading of angina pectoris. Circulation 1976;54:522–523.

before large vessel atherosclerosis. Evidence of peripheral vascular disease may be detected by the presence of carotid or femoral bruits and diminished peripheral pulses. Palpation of the precordium may provide evidence of left ventricular dysfunction by noting a laterally displaced and sustained apical impulse. Auscultation of the chest may reveal a fourth heart sound ($S_4$) gallop, indicating long-standing hypertension with left ventricular hypertrophy.

During an acute anginal attack, the presence of a fourth heart sound may be secondary to ischemic, noncompliant myocardium. Careful examination of the venous system gives an indication of the volume status of a patient as well as ventricular compliance. Elevated jugular venous pressure, peripheral edema, or both may be findings of right heart failure, with or without concomitant left ventricular dysfunction.

Certain physical findings may lead to alternative diagnoses of angina. Palpation of a right ventricular heave at the left sternal border with a prominent pulmonic component of the second heart sound suggests right ventricular hypertrophy secondary to pulmonary hypertension. Characteristic murmurs of hypertrophic obstructive cardiomyopathy or aortic stenosis would implicate these as causes of angina.

Although clinical findings are nonspecific, careful physical examination may influence the direction of diagnostic workup and management focus.

## Diagnostic Testing

### Resting Electrocardiography and Ambulatory Monitoring

A resting 12-lead electrocardiogram (ECG) should be obtained in all patients undergoing evaluation for symptoms of stable angina pectoris. However, with the exception of abnormal Q waves in contiguous leads suggesting prior myocardial infarction, no findings on the resting 12-lead ECG are diagnostic of CAD. In fact, many patients with normal resting ECG results may subsequently be found to have severe coronary atherosclerosis. Conversely, repolarization abnormalities such as T wave inversions or ST-segment sloping are not uncommon in the general population found to have no evidence of CAD. Certain ECG abnormalities—namely, left anterior fascicular block or left bundle branch block—occurring in patients with classic angina pectoris may identify a subset of patients at higher risk of death or myocardial infarction. It is important to remember, however, that the various abnormal ECG findings have a low sensitivity and specificity for reaching diagnostic conclusions.

The principle of ambulatory ECG (Holter) monitoring is to detect symptomatic or asymptomatic evidence of myocardial ischemia by evaluation of ST-segment changes during routine daily activities. Although this test may be useful in some individuals, ambulatory monitoring rarely provides any additional useful information in the diagnosis of angina pectoris beyond that revealed by standard exercise stress testing.

### Exercise Treadmill Electrocardiography

Exercise treadmill ECG is a frequently used test in the diagnostic workup for symptoms of stable angina. The test is readily available, easily performed, and low in cost. The goal is to correlate subjective symptoms of angina with ECG ST-segment changes consistent with myocardial ischemia. Objective parameters assessed during testing include maximal heart rate achieved, blood pressure response, ST-segment shifts, and workload capacity attained. Adequate sensitivity of the test is accomplished with target heart rates 85% of the age-predicted maximum

(220 − age). Inability to reach this target while remaining symptom free is considered submaximal exercise and has a very low negative predictive value, as adequate stress conditions may not have been met to produce myocardial ischemia. Blood pressure measurements at increasing workloads are expected to show incremental increases in systolic blood pressure. Failure to do so suggests left ventricular dysfunction secondary to ischemia. ST-segment depression of 1 mm or greater with a horizontal or downsloping appearance is interpreted as consistent with myocardial ischemia. Workload capacity or metabolic equivalents (METs) achieved is best viewed as a prognostic marker. Treating patients empirically with antianginal medications before testing lowers the sensitivity of the procedure. Therefore, clinicians should use their discretion in opting to discontinue medical therapy a few days before evaluation.

Exercise ECG has an overall sensitivity of 68% and specificity of 77%. Sensitivity is greatest in patients with multivessel disease, noted to be 81% in an overview of 24,000 patients who eventually underwent coronary angiography.[2] Indicators of severity of disease include onset of symptoms or positive ST-segment changes at low workload capacity (≤5 METs), a sustained drop of 10 mm Hg or greater in systolic blood pressure, or prolonged recovery of ST segments after ceasing exercise. In contrast, patients capable of achieving a workload capacity of 10 METs have an excellent prognosis, regardless of the extent of CAD.[3] Clearly, information such as this derived from the exercise study will guide further diagnostic and management decisions, as discussed in a later section.

## Myocardial Perfusion Imaging

Myocardial perfusion or single-photon emission computed tomography (SPECT) imaging by use of low-dose radioactive-labeled perfusion agents is a valuable test in the evaluation of CAD. This technique is most often used in conjunction with exercise ECG. At peak exercise, when myocardial oxygen consumption and coronary blood flow are at their maximum, the perfusion tracer is injected (thallium-201 or technetium-99m). If no obstructive coronary lesions are present, the tracer is taken up equally in all territories of the myocardium. In areas of myocardium that are underperfused owing to significant obstructive coronary lesions, impaired extraction of the tracer demonstrates a less intense radioactive signal or defect on imaging. These stress images may then be compared with images at rest, when the defect may either fill in with signal, reflecting ischemia in the territory, or remain unchanged, indicating a myocardial scar.

The sensitivity and specificity of SPECT imaging are in the range of 80% and 90%, respectively. Sensitivity is highest for single-vessel disease and falls to approximately 70% for multivessel disease.[4] Additional information obtained from SPECT imaging includes identifying involved coronary arteries and the ischemic burden. As well, with the advent of ECG-gated SPECT technology, assessment of stress and resting left ventricular ejection fraction may be acquired.

In patients unable to exercise, pharmacologic stress modalities are available. Dipyridamole and adenosine are vasodilators that enhance blood flow to normally perfused myocardium, thus allowing differential tracer uptake to be visualized in underperfused areas. These agents are safe and provide results with high sensitivity and specificity. They are contraindicated in patients with a history of reactive airway disease, since they may precipitate acute bronchospasm. In this setting, dobutamine stress is a reasonable alternative.

## Exercise Radionuclide Angiography

The value of radionuclide angiography in the detection of CAD is diminished in light of more advanced techniques now used. It had been proposed that failure to increase ejection fraction more than 5% during peak exercise was diagnostic of CAD; however, this finding has poor specificity.[5] Perhaps the best use of this test is in deciding which patients may benefit from revascularization. Observation of wall motion abnormalities that occur at high stress levels but that recover at rest indicates myocardium that may be protected by a revascularization procedure.

## Rest and Stress Echocardiography

Rest echocardiography alone is not sensitive for the detection of CAD, as many patients with disease exhibit normal left ventricular ejection fraction and wall motion at rest. However, other pathologies responsible for nonspecific symptoms may be recognized—for example, hypertrophic cardiomyopathy or valvular disease.

Stress echocardiography used in combination with rest imaging offers the opportunity to observe visual signs of myocardial ischemia. Stress may be performed with exercise or more commonly with dobutamine, adenosine, or dipyridamole administration. The preferred agent is dobutamine, and at high infusion doses, compromised myocardium may reveal localized hypokinesis or impaired systolic wall thickening relative to rest images. Transient left ventricular dilatation and impaired diastolic function as assessed by transmitral Doppler inflows may be other clues to ischemia. Additional benefits of this technique include accurate assessment of ejection fraction and estimates of right and left heart filling pressures using Doppler techniques. Limitations include the inability to achieve adequate two-dimensional views in 5% to 15% of studies. Overall, relative to myocardial perfusion imaging, dobutamine stress echocardiography has been found to detect CAD with a comparable sensitivity and specificity in the hands of experienced operators.[6]

## Coronary Angiography

Although coronary angiography is the best test for defining the anatomic severity of CAD, it is usually not required as the first choice for establishing the diagnosis of angina pectoris in patients with stable symptoms. Exceptions to this include patients presenting with a history of angina associated with malignant ventricular arrhythmias and patients for whom definitive diagnosis is required for occupational reasons, such as aviators. The optimal use of coronary angiography is for patients with highly positive noninvasive test results, for whom knowledge of the degree of CAD may lead to decisions about appropriate revascularization procedures. Such patients include those with myocardial ischemia at low exercise thresholds (≤5 METs) or a myocardial perfusion scan indicating moderate to severe (>15%) defect size. Angiographic lesions reducing the lumen by 70% are thought to be consistent with symptoms and signs of myocardial ischemia. After evaluation of the coronary arteries, left ventriculography is usually performed for assessment of ejection fraction and wall motion abnormalities.

Although coronary angiography remains the gold standard in defining the anatomic appearance of CAD, visual interpretation of the severity of lesions may vary between observers.[7] Furthermore, major discrepancies between angiographic and postmortem findings have been found to exist, usually showing underestimation of lesion severity by angiography.[8] These difficulties arise as a result of the limitations of angiographic imaging. A contrast-filled vessel lumen provides only a planar two-dimensional cross-sectional view of a lesion, the severity of which may be misrepresented by the cineographic viewing angle. Orthogonal views may help resolve this issue; however, optimal imaging is not uncommonly limited by radiographic foreshortening or overlapping vessels obscuring the lesion in question. These limitations may be overcome by the use of intravascular ultrasound examination. This technique allows visualization of the entire circumference of the vessel wall in addition to deeper intramural structures. Tomographic views may demonstrate eccentricity of lesions, diffusely diseased segments, and ostial disease, all of which may be underestimated by conventional angiography. Finally, by virtue of the ability of intravascular ultrasound examination to characterize intramural anatomy, insight into the pathophysiology of coronary lesions is often gained.

It is essential to keep in mind the imperfect sensitivity of noninvasive testing in diagnosing CAD. Therefore, for any patient in whom clinical suspicion is high despite a nondiagnostic noninvasive test, coronary angiography should be performed.

## Diagnostic Strategy

A thoughtful and systematic diagnostic approach is necessary to ensure cost-effective and accurate diagnoses. The value of a diagnostic test is related to the difference between the pretest probability of the diagnosis in question and the posttest probability using information derived from the diagnostic procedure. This concept is the foundation of bayesian theory, which uses a patient's clinical information to arrive at pretest and posttest probabilities for CAD. For example, the use of exercise ECG alone as a diagnostic tool has various degrees of diagnostic power depending on the prevalence of CAD in selected patient populations (Fig. 26–1). Thus, in patients with low pretest probability of CAD, positive results of the test minimally increase the posttest probability, primarily because of high false-positive rates. Conversely, in patients with a high pretest probability, minimal additional information is learned about the likelihood of CAD. It is apparent from Figure 26–1 that the exercise treadmill test is most powerful for predicting CAD in patients with an intermediate probability (30% to 70%) of CAD (Table 26–3). However, clinicians are nevertheless faced with various patients for whom they feel compelled to address the issue of chest pain. Figure 26–2 illustrates an algorithmic approach to diagnostic testing. Patients with a higher likelihood of CAD should receive adjunctive imaging that can provide prognostic information and guide further management decisions. Although myocardial perfusion imaging and stress echocardiography may be comparable in detecting CAD, a great deal more data on prognostic information are available when perfusion defect size is quantified.[9, 10] Thus, it is our opinion that myocardial perfusion imaging is the test of choice when further stratification is needed to influence treatment strategy.

Patients unable to exercise or those with left bundle branch block or hypertrophic or infiltrative cardiomyopathies should undergo pharmacologic stress owing to the poor specificity of stress ECG in these conditions.

## Medical Therapy

### Antiplatelet Agents

Aspirin, used since the 19th century for its pain-relieving effects, was not recognized as an antiplatelet drug until the 1970s. It has now become the mainstay of treatment for both chronic and acute coronary syndromes. The antiplatelet effect of aspirin arises predominantly from its ability to diminish platelet production of thromboxane $A_2$ ($TXA_2$), a vasoconstrictor and proaggregant. In an overview of more than 300 studies involving 140,000 patients with stable angina pectoris, previous myocardial infarction, prior stroke, and coronary bypass, aspirin was shown to significantly reduce the secondary events of myocardial infarction and vascular death.[11] Dose ranges of 81 to 325 mg have been proved effective in smaller studies, and higher doses appear to have no additional benefit.

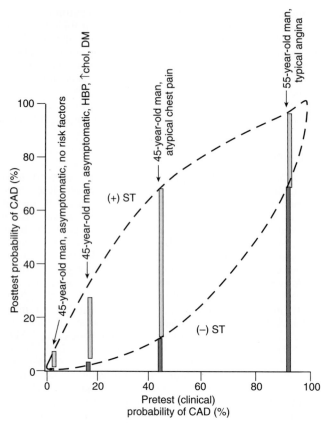

**Figure 26–1** ■ Illustration of Bayes theorem in ascertaining the probability of coronary artery disease (CAD) by exercise electrocardiography. Four specific patient examples are shown, along with pretest and posttest probabilities based on negative (− ST) or positive (+ ST) test results. The value of the test is most useful for patients with intermediate pretest probability for CAD. HBP, hypertension; chol, cholesterol level; DM, diabetes mellitus.

Aspirin is a weak inhibitor of platelet aggregation in the presence of other proaggregate factors. Ticlopidine, a thienopyridine, belongs to a unique class of antiplatelet agents that interfere with adenosine diphosphate (ADP)-mediated platelet activation. Although this class of agents has not been studied specifically in patients with stable angina, evidence from trials enrolling patients with vascular disease has demonstrated a decreased incidence of myocardial infarction and vascular death.[12] Clopidogrel, a newer generation drug lacking the risk of transient neutropenia presented by ticlopidine, may also be an effective secondary prevention agent.[13] For these reasons, ticlopidine or clopidogrel may be an acceptable substitute for aspirin in the rare instances of aspirin intolerance. The effect of aspirin in combination with a thienopyridine on secondary prevention in the setting of CAD seems promising in light of their differing and likely additive actions on platelet activity. These data should be forthcoming in the near future.

## Nitrates

Sublingual nitroglycerin administered during an anginal attack is an effective means of aborting the episode within minutes. Smooth muscle relaxation in vascu-

Table 26-3

**Profiles of Low, Intermediate, and High Probability Coronary Artery Disease**

| | Low Probability (<30%) | | | Intermediate Probability (30%–70%) | | | High Probability (>70%) | | |
|---|---|---|---|---|---|---|---|---|---|
| Age | Any age* | <40 | >45 | A. <40 | >40 | B. >40† | >40 | >40 | >55 |
| Symptoms | Asymptomatic | Atypical | Asymptomatic | Typical | Atypical | Asymptomatic | Typical | Typical | Typical |
| Risk factors‡ | 0 | ≤2 | ≤2 | 0 | ≥2 | ≥2 | ≥2 | ≥2 | 0–5 |
| ECG | Normal | Normal | Normal | Abnormal§ | Abnormal | Normal or abnormal | Normal | Abnormal | Normal |

*Diagnostic testing not indicated.
†Patients considering onset of new vigorous exercise regimen or those with high-risk occupation (aviators, firemen).
‡Risk factors include smoking, family history of coronary artery disease, diabetes mellitus, elevated cholesterol, and hypertension.
§"Abnormal ECG" refers to nonspecific electrocardiographic abnormalities.

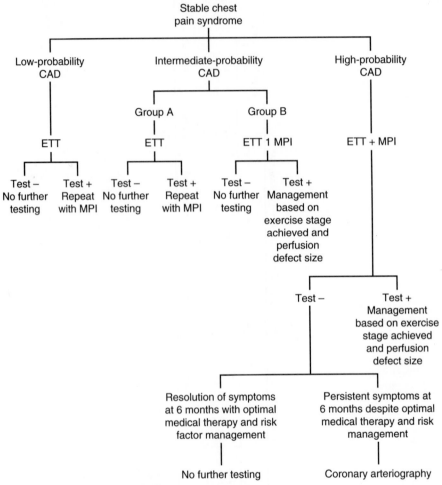

**Figure 26–2** ■ Algorithmic approach to diagnostic testing for coronary artery disease. MPI, myocardial perfusion imaging; ETT, exercise treadmill testing; CAD, coronary artery disease. Refer to Table 26–3 for examples of group A/group B patients.

lar tissue mediated by nitric oxide (NO) and cyclic guanasine monophosphate (cGMP) results in venodilatation, as well as peripheral artery and coronary artery dilatation.[14] Respectively, myocardial oxygen demand is reduced, resulting from decreased preload and afterload, while myocardial oxygen supply is improved. These effects may persist for up to 30 minutes.

Various nitrate formulations exist, extending from short-acting to long-acting preparations (Table 26–4). Owing to the phenomenon of nitrate tolerance, longer-acting derivatives are best suited for patients with more frequent and severe symptoms. To avoid the development of tolerance, an 8 to 10-hour nitrate-free interval is needed. Hence, patients should take nitrates during periods when episodes most commonly occur.

Although nitrates are clearly efficacious in relieving anginal symptoms, no

Table 26–4

**Drugs Commonly Used in Stable Coronary Artery Disease**

| Drug | Dose Range |
|---|---|
| **Antiplatelets** | |
| Aspirin | 75 mg–325 mg qd |
| **Nitrates** | |
| Sublingual NTG tablets | 0.3–0.6 mg prn, maximum three doses in 15 min |
| Sublingual NTG spray | 0.4 mg prn, maximum three doses in 15 min |
| NTG paste / ointment | ½–2″ 2% NTG q 8 hr / off 8 hr–10 hr daily |
| NTG patch | 0.1–0.8 mg / hr, on 12 hr / off 12 hr |
| Isosorbide dinitrate | 10–60 mg (7 AM, noon, 5 PM) |
| Isosorbide mononitrate | 20 mg (8 AM and 3 PM) |
| **Beta blockers** | |
| Cardioselective | |
| Metoprolol | 25–150 mg bid |
| Atenolol | 25–100 mg qd |
| Bisoprolol | 5–10 mg bid |
| Noncardioselective | |
| Propranolol | 20–80 mg qid |
| Nadolol | 40–80 qd |
| **Calcium channel blockers** | |
| Nondihydropyridines | |
| Diltiazem | 30–90 mg qid |
| Verapamil | 80–120 mg tid |
| Dihydropyridines | |
| Nifedipine | 30–60 mg qd |
| Amlodipine | 5–10 mg qd |
| Felodipine | 5–20 mg qd |
| **HMG CoA reductase inhibitors** | |
| Atorvastatin | 10–80 mg qhs |
| Simvastatin | 5–40 mg qhs |
| Pravastatin | 10–40 mg qhs |
| Lovastatin | 20–80 mg qhs |
| Fluvastatin | 20–40 mg qhs |

NTG, nitroglycerin; HMG CoA, hydroxymethylglutaryl coenzyme A.

trials have demonstrated their effect on cardiovascular morbidity or mortality in stable angina pectoris. Nitrates are contraindicated in patients treated with sildenafil (Viagra).

## β-Adrenergic Blockers

β-Adrenergic blocking agents are an essential component in the successful management of stable angina pectoris. Well recognized for their antihypertensive and antiarrhythmic properties, beta blockers exert a powerful antiischemic effect in CAD. $\beta_1$-Receptor blockade in the heart reduces myocardial oxygen demand by reducing heart rate and myocardial contractility. As a result, increased diastolic perfusion time and reduced wall stress improve myocardial oxygen supply. Therapy is usually titrated to achieve a heart rate in the range of 50 to 60 bpm.

Beta blockers are generally well tolerated. Serious side effects include excessive bradycardia, heart block, hypotension, and bronchospasm. More common side effects are fatigue and impotence. Despite the availability of cardioselective $\beta_1$-blocking agents, overlap of $\beta_2$ blockade remains, making beta blockers contraindicated in patients with severe asthma or chronic obstructive pulmonary disease. Patients with remote or mild reactive airway disease generally tolerate cardioselective agents, although dose titration should be implemented cautiously.

Although clinical trials have not evaluated clinical outcomes following beta-blocker therapy in patients with chronic stable angina, abundant data indicate prolonged survival of patients who have suffered myocardial infarction, as well as patients with hypertension, for which beta blockade is a first-line therapy.[15–17] The favorable effects of these agents on ischemia and sudden death in these patient populations can probably be extrapolated to individuals with stable angina pectoris. For this reason, beta blockers are a first-line agent in the management of chronic stable angina, unless absolutely contraindicated.

## Calcium Channel Antagonists

The calcium channel antagonists are a heterogeneous group of compounds that act through the common mechanism of decreasing calcium entry into smooth muscle cells and myocytes. The net effect is both coronary and peripheral vasodilation, improving myocardial oxygen supply and minimizing oxygen consumption through afterload reduction. The nondihydropyridine classes, verapamil (a phenylalklyamine) and diltiazem (a benzothiazepine), have the additional effect of decreasing heart rate. Conversely, dihydropyridines such as nifedipine may produce a reflex tachycardia, although this unwanted effect is less an issue with the predominant availability of longer-acting formulations. Clinically relevant side effects of these agents are few, including ankle edema, headache, flushing, and hypotension. Profound bradycardia may occur with high doses of verapamil owing to its atrioventricular (AV) node blocking ability. In addition, owing to the potent negative inotropic effect of verapamil and to a lesser degree diltiazem, caution should be used in patients with a history of depressed left ventricular function.

All classes of calcium channel antagonists are efficacious antianginal agents, comparable in effect to beta blockers. However, unlike beta blockers, these agents have not been shown to improve survival in patients with known CAD. Evidence does show that verapamil and diltiazem can reduce reinfarction rates when used for secondary prevention after myocardial infarction, provided that there is no evidence of left ventricular dysfunction.[18, 19] Therefore, they may be considered a reasonable alternative when beta-blocker therapy is contraindicated, as in cases of severe reactive airway disease. Beta blockers and calcium channel antagonists may be used in combination for patients requiring a more intensified medical regimen.

## Lipid-Lowering Therapy

Numerous randomized studies of hydroxymethylglutaryl coenzyme A (HMG CoA) reductase inhibitors ("statins") support their routine use in CAD. Lowering total cholesterol and low-density lipoprotein (LDL) levels in patients with hypercholesterolemia reduced the incidence of death and myocardial infarction in the primary prevention West of Scotland Trial.[20] The Air Force/Texas Coronary Atherosclerosis Prevention Trial evaluated men and women with average cholesterol levels and without CAD. This study was terminated prematurely owing to the superior benefit of the treatment arm in preventing the onset of any acute coronary presentations.[21] The Scandinavian Simvastatin Survival Study (4S trial) of hypercholesterolemic patients with stable angina or previous myocardial infarction clearly established the secondary prevention benefit of cholesterol reduction in patients with known CAD.[22] The Cholesterol and Recurrent Events (CARE) trial provided strong evidence that in patients who had suffered myocardial infarction and who had average cholesterol levels, active treatment prolonged survival and reduced recurrent cardiac events.[23] On the basis of these overwhelming data, the National Cholesterol and Education Program (NCEP) recommends lowering cholesterol levels in all patients with CAD or extracardiac atherosclerosis to LDL levels below 100 mg/dl. Although diet therapy has an integral role, it is often difficult to achieve such levels in the absence of HMG CoA reductase inhibitors.

An often forgotten risk factor in CAD is elevated serum triglyceride values. Although most epidemiologic studies have demonstrated an association between triclyceride level and heart disease, the strength of the association often weakens when controlled for high-density lipoprotein (HDL) levels. An 8-year follow-up study of asymptomatic men with elevated triglyceride levels found an increased rate of cardiac events and all-cause mortality, independent of HDL levels.[24] Thus, it seems reasonable that patients with apparent CAD receive strict surveillance of not only LDL cholesterol but also triglyceride levels. Effective treatments include the use of fibric acid derivatives, such as gemfibrozil or clofibrate. Niacin is also an efficacious triglyceride-lowering agent; however, it is intolerable to a substantial number of patients and may worsen glucose intolerance in diabetic patients.

The use of combined therapies for mixed hyperlipidemia disorders raises concerns over increased risk of hepatic toxicity and skeletal myopathy. Combination therapy is not absolutely contraindicated, although patients should be closely monitored for laboratory indicators of these complications. Newer generation HMG CoA reductase inhibitors have been shown to be useful in reducing borderline increases in triglyceride level and may obviate the need for combined therapies in some circumstances.[25]

## Hormone Replacement Therapy

The value of hormone replacement therapy for primary and secondary prevention in CAD is controversial.[26] Although lack of estrogen has been implicated as a risk factor for CAD for more than three decades, only in recent years have well-designed trials been initiated to assess the efficacy of estrogen replacement. The beneficial effect of hormone replacement therapy on the lipid profile is less of an issue. Many studies have demonstrated the lowering of LDL and lipoprotein(a) levels while elevating HDL.[27] The proposed efficacy of hormone replacement therapy is believed to arise from this enhanced lipid profile and from positive effects of estrogen-mediated endothelial vasomotor function.

The data suggesting the benefit of hormone replacement therapy in CAD have come from observational studies.[28, 29] The Nurses Health Study found that a large cohort of women currently using hormone replacement therapy had a 50% reduction of myocardial infarction or all-cause mortality as compared with nonusers.[30] Observational studies such as these may be criticized for inherent selection biases. For example, individuals choosing to use hormone replacement therapy typically lead a healthier lifestyle, seek regular medical care, and follow exercise regimens. The Heart and Estrogen/Progestin Replacement Study (HERS) is a double-blind, randomized secondary prevention trial with hormone replacement therapy. Despite improved lipid profiles in the treatment arm, no significant benefit was found in preventing recurrent myocardial infarction or cardiac death during an average 4-year follow-up. Thromboembolic events, including pulmonary embolism, occurred more frequently in the treated arm, particularly in the first year after beginning therapy.[31] The upcoming results of the ongoing Women's Health Initiative will provide information about the primary prevention benefits of hormone replacement therapy.

Unopposed estrogen therapy increases the risk of endometrial cancer, an effect negated by the addition of progestin. The use of both agents may increase the risk of breast cancer, particularly in women with a strong family history. The current recommendations of the American College of Physicians state that women who are at high risk of developing CAD and who are not at high risk for breast cancer will likely benefit from estrogen/progestin therapy.[32]

## Antioxidant Therapy

It is hypothesized that oxidation of LDL cholesterol particles may have a pivotal role in the initiation and progression of atherosclerosis. Thus, investigators have compiled ample observational data suggesting that naturally occurring antioxidants may slow this process. As previously mentioned, incumbent selection biases of epidemiologic studies render these data inconclusive.

To date, three randomized, double-blind, placebo-controlled trials have examined the effects of antioxidants on cardiovascular events. The Physicians Health Study was a primary prevention trial of 22,000 physicians over a 12-year period. Supplemental betacarotene offered no reduction in cardiovascular morbidity or mortality.[33] Conflicting evidence exists in secondary prevention. A Finnish study failed to detect any benefit of vitamin E or betacarotene in limiting progression to severe symptomatic angina or myocardial infarction among men with established CAD.[34] In contrast, the Cambridge Heart Anti-Oxidant Study (CHAOS), using a higher dose of vitamin E (400 to 800 IU), demonstrated a 47% risk reduction in cardiovascular death and nonfatal myocardial infarction.[35]

Based on the current data, firm recommendations for empiric use of antioxidant therapy cannot be made. Further data are expected to clarify their role in the years to come.

## Revascularization: Catheter-Based Methods

### Percutaneous Transluminal Coronary Angioplasty

The concept of therapeutic percutaneous angioplasty was first introduced in 1964 by Dotter and Judkins.[36] However, widespread acceptance of their technique in the treatment of peripheral vascular stenosis was not realized owing to the frequent occurrence of local trauma and hemorrhage. The subsequent development by Andreas Gruentzig of a double-lumen balloon catheter pioneered the modern era of interventional cardiology. In September 1977 in Zurich, Gruentzig performed the first percutaneous transluminal coronary angioplasty (PTCA) procedure in humans, successfully dilating the proximal left anterior descending (LAD) coronary artery of a 37-year-old man with angina pectoris.[37] Repeat catheterization on the 10th anniversary of the procedure revealed continued vessel patency. This patient has remained symptom free for 20 years.

Since this initial introduction in 1977, operator experience has expanded the selection of patients for whom PTCA may be appropriate to include those with stable multivessel disease and acute coronary syndromes. The ideal candidates for PTCA are patients with stable angina pectoris as a result of single-vessel CAD without complex angiographic characteristics. In such patients, procedural success rates exceed 97% and are associated with a low risk of early complications such as myocardial infarction or death. Clinical variables such as advanced age, history of congestive heart failure or left ventricular dysfunction, and complex lesion features including calcification, presence of thrombus, eccentric morphology, and ostial location increase the periprocedural risk of PTCA.[38] Experienced operators in high-volume catheterization laboratories have lower complication rates when compared with low-volume medical centers.[39]

Early complications of PTCA are most often the result of abrupt vessel closure, defined as sudden occlusion of the target vessel during or shortly after the revascularization procedure. The incidence of this complication is in the range of 5%.[40] The pathophysiology typically involves local vessel dissection with obstructive dissection flaps, often accompanied by development of thrombus secondary to platelet activation from exposed subendothelial vascular wall components. The clinical consequences of such an event may lead to acute myocardial infarction, the need for urgent surgical revascularization, or death. The use of platelet glycoprotein (GP) IIb/IIIa antagonists and intacoronary stenting has successfully reduced the incidence and adverse outcomes of acute vessel closure[41] and has added the ability to approach patients with more complex lesions and multivessel disease. Placement of a coronary stent mandates a 2- to 4-week course of ticlopidine and continued aspirin administration to prevent subacute stent thrombosis. Clopidigrel may ultimately replace ticlopidine because of its better side effect profile.

The principal limitation of PTCA is restenosis, which has been reported in 30% to 40% of patients within 6 months of the procedure.[42] The clinical presentation of restenosis most commonly is recurrence of stable anginal symptoms. Myocardial infarction as the initial presentation of restenosis is a rare occurrence. The pathogenesis of restenosis in response to mechanical injury induced by angioplasty is incompletely understood and likely multifactorial. A number of pharmacologic agents of various classes have been evaluated for the prevention of restenosis, including antiplatelets, anticoagulants, calcium channel blockers, and antiproliferative agents. To date, only coronary stenting has been shown to significantly decrease 6-month restenosis rates to the range of 20%, although in selected cases modern stent implantation techniques may reduce this rate even further.[43, 44]

Over the years, methods adjunctive to angioplasty have been developed to assist with lesions exhibiting complex characteristics. As a result of the increasing frequency with which newer techniques are used, the term *percutaneous transluminal coronary angioplasty* is gradually being replaced by the more accurate term *percutaneous coronary intervention* (PCI). Directional coronary atherectomy uses a blade housed within a balloon catheter. Inflation of the balloon forces the blade's housing against the protruding portion of the plaque, at which time the blade trims away the plaque and forces the debris into the housing, opening the lumen of the artery more widely. Evaluation of this technique versus balloon angioplasty has not shown conclusive improvement in 6-month restenosis rates. Moreover, the use of directional atherectomy is associated with an increased rate of periprocedural non–Q wave infarction.[45, 46] Rotational atherectomy (Rotablator) uses a rotary cone containing diamond chips at the end of a catheter that is capable of abrading rigid or calcified lesions. Observational data suggest rotational atherectomy is useful in managing complex lesion subsets not suitable for balloon angioplasty alone. A direct comparison in a randomized fashion to standard balloon angioplasty has shown superior procedural success rates for complex lesions without an excess of periprocedural complications. However, restenosis rates at 6 months were significantly higher after rotational atherectomy than after balloon angioplasty.[47]

## Angiogenesis

### Percutaneous Transmyocardial Revascularization

A significant number of patients with chronic CAD and severe angina pectoris despite maximal medical therapy are not candidates for revascularization strategies because of their coronary anatomy. Until recently, no alternative therapy has been available for palliation in these patients.

Transmyocardial revascularization is an innovative procedure in which numerous channels 1 mm in width are created in ischemic myocardium. In the surgical approach, channels are generated via a high-powered carbon dioxide laser from the epicardial surface inward. Nonrandomized studies indicate improved exercise treadmill time, and subjective surveys have reported anginal relief.[48] A catheter-based approach creates conduits from the left ventricular cavity into the myocardium and is currently undergoing clinical evaluation. This approach obviates the need for general anesthesia and thoracotomy.

The mechanism by which these myocardial channels lead to neovascularization has remained controversial. Initial conceptions of this technique suggested that the new channels would provide myocardial perfusion directly from the left ventricular cavity, as occurs in the reptilian heart. Perspectives on the mechanism have been elucidated in animal models in which channels using laser were compared with channels created by a hardware store power drill. After several weeks of follow-up, the histologic appearances of the channels were identical and none were patent. However, all previous channels were surrounded by some degree of fibrosis and neovascularization.[49] Thus, the laser channels are not the new vessels, but their creation stimulates chemical signals that lead to new vessel growth. Furthermore, the neovascularization seems not to be dependent on laser therapy but rather on a nonspecific healing response to injury. Complications of these techniques are rare though may have serious consequences. These include ventricular fibrillation, pericardial tamponade, perforation of large arteries, and damage to chordae tendineae or the Pukinje network.

At present, these techniques are reserved for patients with class IV angina that has not responded to traditional therapies. It is conceivable that one day this procedure may become an adjunct to standard revascularization techniques.

## Gene-Related Therapy

Progress in the field of molecular biology and recombinant genetic technology has paved the way for novel strategies in the treatment of chronic ischemic disease. The aim of gene therapy for vascular ischemia is to stimulate the growth of new blood vessels for individuals with advanced, nonreconstructable arterial disease. The development of high-yield gene transfer techniques has allowed for introduction of known angiogenic factors to ischemic tissues. Modes of delivery have used various molecular packages or "vectors." Examples range from simple naked plasmid DNA encoding the desired protein to complex viral particles containing nucleic acid cores.

The two most extensively studied angiogenic growth factors in the context of tissue ischemia are vascular endothelial growth factor (VEGF) and fibroblast growth factor (FGF). VEGF is present in four subtypes, alternative splicing products produced from the same gene. These proteins are secreted by smooth muscle cells and have high-affinity binding sites on the surface of endothelial cells. VEGF stimulates endothelial cell migration and accelerates the process of endothelialization.[50] FGFs are a family of nearly 20 proteins. FGF-1 and FGF-2 are known to stimulate the proliferation of three principal vascular cell types: fibroblasts, endothelial cells, and smooth muscle cells.[51]

Evidence now shows that intramuscular VEGF gene transfer in humans not only achieves expression of VEGF protein but also leads to angiogenesis. Naked plasmid DNA encoding a VEGF isoform was administered into muscle of 10 ischemic limbs of 9 patients. Newly developed collateral vessels were demonstrated angiographically in seven limbs. Ischemic ulcers were markedly improved in four of seven limbs, with salvage of limbs in three patients recommended for below-knee amputation.[52] Further promising data come from a randomized, controlled study of genetically engineered FGF-1 in CAD. Patients received injection of active or denatured FGF-1 protein in close proximity to the LAD artery distal anastomoses after revascularization. At 3 months, coronary angiography revealed the presence of a capillary network sprouting from the LAD in all 20 patients receiving the active agent, as opposed to no angiogenesis in controls.[53]

Trials using catheter-based intramyocardial gene transfer are now under way. This exciting and revolutionary technology shows great hope for improving the future of cardiovascular treatment in the new millennium.

## Coronary Artery Bypass Surgery

Coronary artery bypass grafting (CABG) has remained a very effective procedure for relief of angina pectoris since first used in 1964 as a "bailout" technique by Dr. Michael DeBakey.[54] Success in alleviating symptoms occurs in more than 85% of patients.[55] Although initial costs are high in relation to other strategies, particularly PCI, in selected patients the expenditure is comparable when repeated PCI and intensive medical therapy may be needed long term.

Modifications of the procedure during the past 30 years have continued to lead to high success rates in more complicated cases and in sicker patients. Choice of graft conduit has shown arterial conduits to be superior to saphenous venous grafts. Specifically, the left internal thoracic (mammary) artery is most often reserved for the left coronary system. Patency rates for this graft are approximately 90% at 10 years, compared with 30% for saphenous vein grafts.[56] Evidence suggests that the use of two arterial grafts rather than one may lead to improved long-term symptomatic relief in selected patients.[57] However, a beneficial effect on reoperation or mortality rates remains unclear. The current practice of long-term aspirin and aggressive lipid-lowering therapy in post-CABG patients may make the choice of a second conduit (in addition to an internal thoracic artery) less of an issue, particularly in elderly patients.

Complication rates are related to the extent of CAD, left ventricular dysfunction, and comorbid illnesses. Overall, the perioperative composite rates of mortality and myocardial infarction approximate 5%. Repeat operations are always associated with higher complication rates.

## Management Decision Making

The goals of effective management of stable angina pectoris are to achieve symptom relief and improve long-term survival. Management decisions should be based on prognostic information derived from an appropriately chosen diagnostic test. An approach of medical therapy or revascularization or both should be made after consideration of the known comparative efficacies of the strategy options. However, it must be emphasized that all patients should be encouraged to adopt lifestyle changes known to improve prognosis, such as smoking cessation and following a low-cholesterol diet.

A management algorithm based on current available data is presented in Figure 26–3. As mentioned previously, the diagnostic test shown to provide the most objective prognostic value for risk of cardiac death or myocardial infarction is myocardial perfusion imaging (MPI).[9, 10] The predictive value is enhanced by computer-generated measurement of ischemic defect size. Patients with stable angina and mild perfusion defects (<15%) have been shown to be at low risk (<1% per year) for cardiac death or myocardial infarction.[9, 10] Similarly, patients capable of achieving 10 METS or greater (stage III, Bruce protocol) on exercise treadmill testing have a prognosis with medical therapy as good as with revascularization and are considered to be at low risk for cardiac events.[3] Thus, in such patients, an initial approach of standard medical therapy is reasonable. Standard medical therapy consists of aspirin, beta blockers, short-acting nitrates, and antilipid therapy if LDL levels exceed 100 mg/dl after diet modification. Randomized trial data support such an approach. The Angioplasty Compared to Medicine trial (ACME) for stable angina pectoris demonstrated that 48% of medically treated patients with stable angina may be rendered symptom free by 6 months.[58] The Second Randomized Intervention Treatment of Angina trial (RITA-II) randomized more than 1000 patients with stable angina pectoris to medical therapy or coronary angioplasty. After a median 2.7-year follow-up, interventional management conferred no benefit in terms of death or myocardial infarction.[59] Similarly, data from the Coronary Artery Surgery Study (CASS) registry showed no mortality difference over 10 years when medical therapy was compared with CABG for single-vessel or two-vessel disease

**Management Strategy Based on Diagnostic Test Results**

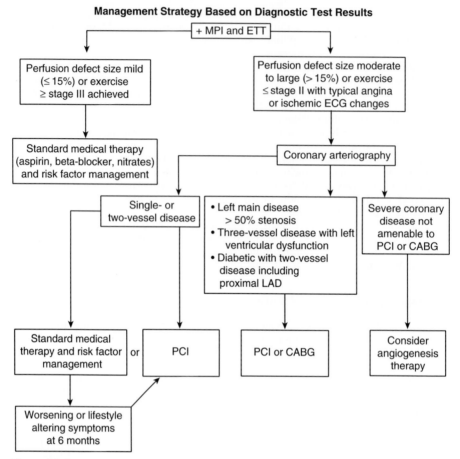

**Figure 26–3** ■ Management strategy based on diagnostic test results. MPI, myocardial perfusion imaging; ETT, exercise treadmill testing; ECG, electrocardiographic; LAD, left anterior descending; PCI, percutaneous coronary intervention; CABG, coronary artery bypass grafting.

excluding the proximal LAD artery in patients with normal left ventricular function.[60]

Although low-risk test results suggest medical therapy is the preferred management approach, there is no dispute that PCI and CABG are efficacious in relieving persistent symptoms of angina despite adequate medical regimens. Therefore, patients with lifestyle-altering stable angina after 6 months of initiation of medical therapy should proceed to undergo coronary angiography with the intent of revascularization.

Coronary angiography should be pursued in patients with moderate to severe perfusion defect size (>15%) or poor treadmill exercise tolerance ($\geq$ 5 METS). Cardiac event rates in these groups are in the range of 3% to 4% per year.[10] After determination of the extent of CAD and the need for revascularization, the decision about PCI versus CABG arises. The CASS registry has clearly shown survival benefit in patients with three-vessel or left main disease in excess of 50% stenosis.[60]

There is little dispute that symptomatic patients with significant disease in the left main coronary artery should proceed directly to CABG. In contrast, PCI has proved to be successful in relieving anginal symptoms in the vast majority of patients who have single-vessel disease and therefore obviates the need for major surgery. The gray zone occurs for patients with two- or three-vessel disease and with anatomy that appears amenable to either surgical or percutaneous revascularization.

To date, five major trials have compared percutaneous revascularization with CABG in patients with stable angina pectoris.[61–65] The results of these trials are uniform and consistent in showing a similar risk of death and nonfatal myocardial infarction in long-term follow-up for as long as 5 years. However, a dramatic increase in the need for repeated revascularization procedures has been seen in percutaneous-treatment arms. In the Bypass Angioplasty Revascularization Investigation trial (BARI), the largest of the studies, an 8% repeat revascularization rate for CABG versus 54% for coronary angioplasty was found.[65] It was also clear from this trial that the subgroup of patients with diabetes mellitus requiring treatment benefited significantly from CABG compared with angioplasty. Although these data may provide general guidelines, decisions about revascularization must still be individualized, with consideration of comorbidities and patients' preference. It should also be kept in mind that percutaneous revascularization techniques have advanced dramatically since these studies were performed. Intracoronary stents have reduced the rate of restenosis from 40% to approximately 20%[43, 44] and permitted much more aggressive use of multivessel angioplasty. The use of adjunctive platelet GP IIb/IIIa antagonists during PCI has reduced the periprocedure infarction rate and is associated with long-term reduction in mortality compared with balloon angioplasty alone.[66] Patients with severe disease not suitable for revascularization should be considered for one of the novel strategies now available, including gene-related therapy or transmyocardial revascularization.

## ■ UNSTABLE ANGINA

Approximately 8 million patients present annually to the emergency room with symptoms of acute chest pain. Of these, 2 million presentations are cardiac in cause, resulting in hospitalization. More than 90% of these patients do not have ST-segment elevation on the ECG.[67] Because the diagnostic sensitivity and specificity of an ECG are poor in this setting, the impetus for effective emergency room stratification is strong. The spectrum of acute coronary syndromes includes unstable angina and non–Q wave myocardial infarction as the predominant clinical presentations. The distinction between these is made retrospectively on the basis of biochemical markers, and hence, initial treatment strategies are identical. The diagnosis of primary unstable angina precludes the presence of factors extrinsic to the coronary bed known to exacerbate the symptoms of coronary ischemia. Such entities include severe anemia, thyrotoxicosis, and tachyarrhythmias.

Four clinical scenarios are consistent with a presentation of unstable angina (Table 26–5). Patients with acute chest pain represent a heterogeneous population. An approach to management must take into account the severity of symptoms, the circumstances in which they are occurring, and associated clinical findings. The Braunwald Classification of Unstable Angina summarizes these important issues and assists in early stratification of patients at higher risk for adverse clinical outcomes (Table 26–6). Clinical features to consider immediately in the emergency room include history of CAD, the presence or absence of ST-segment depression, hemodynamic status, and signs of congestive heart failure. The chosen therapeutic approach reflects the clinical estimation of short-term risk for death or nonfatal myocardial infarction.

Table 26–5

**Unstable Angina Presentations**

Rest angina
New onset angina of CCSC class III or IV within 4 weeks of presentation
Increasing frequency and intensity of previously stable angina to CCSC class III or IV
Angina within 6 wk of myocardial infarction

CCSC, Canadian Cardiovascular Society Classification.

The majority of patients presenting with unstable angina have obstructive CAD. In most studies, however, approximately 20% of patients with suspected acute coronary syndromes are found to have minimally obstructed or normal coronary arteries. The precipitating event of myocardial ischemia is most commonly coronary plaque rupture. Plaques vulnerable to this process tend to be relatively soft and lipid rich, and they display abundant extracellular matrix and smooth muscle cells. After rupture and exposure to local thrombogenic factors such as lipid, and the release of systemic inflammatory mediators from plaque-laden macrophages, platelet activation and development of plaque thrombus ensues. The final component of arterial damage involves local vasoconstriction most likely in response to platelet-derived serotonin and $TXA_2$.

Thrombolytic therapy has been shown to be ineffective in reducing mortality in non–ST-segment-elevation acute coronary syndromes,[68, 69] and treatment is based primarily on antithrombotic and antiplatelet agents. This section reviews the role

Table 26–6

**Classification of Unstable Angina**

| Severity | |
|---|---|
| Class I | New onset, severe, or accelerated angina. |
| | Patients with angina of <2 mo duration, severe or occurring three or more times per day, or angina that is distinctly more frequent and precipitated by distinctly less exertion. No rest pain in the past 2 mo. |
| Class II | Angina at rest. Subacute. |
| | Patients with one or more episodes of angina at rest during the preceding month but not within the preceding 48 hr. |
| Class III | Angina at rest. Acute. |
| | Patients with one or more episodes at rest within the preceding 48 hr. |

| Clinical Circumstances | |
|---|---|
| Class A | Secondary unstable angina. |
| | A clearly identified condition extrinsic to the coronary vascular bed that has intensified myocardial ischemia, e.g., anemia, infection, fever, hypotension, tachyarrhythmia, thyrotoxicosis, hypoxemia secondary to respiratory failure. |
| Class B | Primary unstable angina. |
| Class C | Postinfarction unstable angina (within 2 weeks of documented myocardial infarction). |

| Intensity of Treatment | |
|---|---|
| | Absence of treatment or minimal treatment. |
| | Occurring in the presence of standard therapy for chronic stable angina (conventional doses of oral beta blockers, nitrates, and calcium antagonists). |
| | Occurring despite maximally tolerated doses of all three categories of oral therapy, including nitroglycerin. |

CCSC, Canadian Cardiovascular Society Classification.
Braunwald E: Unstable angina: A classification. Circulation 1989;80:410.

of traditional agents in the initial management of unstable angina as well as more novel antithrombotic and antiplatelet drugs. A discussion of the use of biochemical markers in the setting of unstable angina is included.

## Biochemical Markers and Unstable Angina

The identification of patients who present to the emergency room with acute chest pain and who are at high risk for subsequent cardiac events remains a challenge. New and more sensitive biochemical markers of myocardial injury have been investigated in the hope of providing early risk stratification.

Cardiac troponin T and cardiac troponin I are structural sarcomeric proteins that regulate the calcium-mediated contractile process in striated muscle. A small quantity of cardiac troponins remains free in the cytosol of cardiac myocytes. It has been proposed that the detection of troponin T or I in serum may represent early signs of myocardial damage owing to their absence in the circulation under normal circumstances. Thus, in contrast to the MB fraction of creatine kinase (CK-MB), for which basal levels can be detected in the plasma of normal individuals, the detection of troponins may reveal early minor degrees of myocardial necrosis or severe ischemia due to leakage of cytosolic forms. Elevated blood levels have been found as early as 3 hours after onset of symptoms and may persist beyond 10 days.[70] The envisioned goal of measuring cardiac troponins in the emergency room is to assist in early identification of patients who present with acute chest pain without ST elevation and who may harbor more severe coronary ischemia and may therefore be at increased risk of adverse clinical outcomes. Serial cardiac troponin determinations have not replaced creatine kinase measurement in the diagnosis of myocardial infarction, but rather the two are measured concomitantly in some medical centers.

Numerous studies have indeed demonstrated that early elevation of troponin levels in the emergency room does provide independent prognostic value for adverse outcomes, such as death, recurrent myocardial infarction, and the need for revascularization in patients presenting with and without ST-elevation ischemic chest pain.[71–74] However, these studies were performed in high-risk patients in whom the majority had documented coronary disease and abnormal ECGs on admission. Furthermore, elevation of CK-MB values subsequently occurred in more than 95% of patients developing myocardial infarction.[72] Therefore, although early positive troponin levels may be markers for adverse cardiac events, the positive predictive value of elevated troponin values above and beyond traditional features of risk, such as clinical history, abnormal ECG findings, and serial CK-MB, remains in question. Indeed, in a study assessing more than 10,000 patients admitted for acute chest pain, patients with a less than 1% likelihood of cardiac complications could be predicted using the clinical features of admission ECG, description of chest discomfort, and hemodynamic status.[75]

The largest trial prospectively assessing the value of cardiac troponin I has been completed.[76] In more than 1200 patients presenting to an emergency department with acute chest pain, initial cardiac troponin I and CK-MB levels were measured. This patient population represented the "real-life" situation of a heterogeneous group of patients, without regard to admission ECG or CAD history. The positive predictive value for cardiac events at 72 hours for patients with early positive cardiac troponin I (>0.4 ng/ml) was 19%, versus 22% for those with a positive CK-MB. In patients ruled out for acute myocardial infarction, cardiac troponin I had a positive predictive value for cardiac events of ventricular arrhythmia, hemodynamic collapse, or the need for semiurgent revascularization of only 8%. A similar study assessing initial emergency room troponin levels, CK-MB values, and admission ECG has shown that only ST-segment depression in the baseline ECG carried independent prognostic value of cardiac events at 30 days in patients with acute chest pain without ST elevation.[77]

Although the positive predictive value of troponin determinations is poor, the negative predictive value appears powerful. In patients with negative test results, the risk of major cardiac events appears very low. In a study by Hamm and colleagues, negative troponin T or I results within 12 hours of chest pain and without ST-segment elevation was associated with a 1.1% and 0.03% risk of myocardial infarction or death over 30 days, respectively.[78]

The poor positive predictive value of troponins suggests that their routine use may only confuse the scenario when a well-taken clinical history and benign ECG suggest a presentation not consistent with an acute coronary syndrome. Abnormal levels of troponins may occur in renal insufficiency, cancer, rhabdomyolysis, pulmonary embolism, and accelerated hypertension[79] (personal experience). Perhaps the best use of troponin determinations is in patients with moderate probabilities of having an acute coronary syndrome and minimal ECG abnormalities. In patients in whom cardiac troponin results are negative, triage may be handled in a more cost-effective manner, given the low likelihood of a cardiac event. Consideration of discharge home, admission to a ward other than the intensive care unit, or early stress testing may be warranted.

Other blood serum markers are currently being evaluated for their prognostic value. These include C-reactive protein (CRP) and interleukin-6. These proteins are acute-phase reactants associated with the presence of ongoing inflammation. Elevated levels of CRP have been shown to correlate with adverse clinical outcomes at 14 days in patients presenting with acute coronary syndromes.[80] Further data show the rapid decline of CRP levels paralleling resolution of clinical symptoms but persisting elevation for up to 15 days in patients with unfavorable outcome.[81] These studies strongly implicate inflammation as a key factor in the pathophysiology of the unstable phase of angina.

## Medical Therapy

### Antiischemic Therapy

Unstable angina is often associated with inappropriate vasoconstriction and heart rate elevation due to excessive catecholamine drive. The aim of antiischemic therapy is to alter hemodynamics in order to optimize the balance of myocardial oxygen supply and demand. Nitrates, beta blockers, and calcium channel blockers all are known to improve this ratio.

The recommendation for nitrate therapy is based more on observational evidence and knowledge of its physiologic effect than on availability of clinical trial data. After administration of nitroglycerin, vascular smooth muscle cells convert nitrates to the NO radical. This in turn activates intracellular guanylate cyclase to produce cGMP, triggering smooth muscle relaxation and antiplatelet aggregatory effects. Nitroglycerin decreases preload and afterload and produces coronary vasodilatation.[14]

Similarly, the routine use of beta blockade stems from extrapolation of myocardial infarction data, in which a beneficial effect is clearly evident.[15–17] The heart rate should be targeted to less than 60 bpm. In the event beta blockers cannot be used, calcium channel blockers are also effective in relieving chest pain. The combination of beta blockers and calcium channel blockers is usually reserved for patients with refractory symptoms.

### Antiplatelet Agents

#### Aspirin

Administration of aspirin is a standard therapy in unstable angina. The efficacy of aspirin in reducing early and long-term cardiac events has been well established in randomized trials.[13] Early event rates have been reduced up to 50% with a dose of 81 or 325 mg.[82] Long-term benefits extending to 2 years are noted when daily administration is continued.[83]

Side effects with aspirin are relatively rare and dose dependent, and they usually present after long-term use. A contraindication to immediate aspirin administration in the emergency room is essentially nonexistent. It is recommended that a bolus of 160 mg to 325 mg in chewable form be given to rapidly achieve full inhibition of $TXA_2$-induced platelet aggregation. Maintenance therapy may range from 81 mg to 325 mg daily.

### Thienopyridines

Ticlopidine and clopidogrel are acceptable alternatives when aspirin cannot be tolerated. These agents exert their antiplatelet activity predominantly by interfering with ADP-mediated platelet activation and aggregation.[84] Ticlopidine has been assessed in a randomized trial of patients with unstable angina in the absence of aspirin therapy. Fatal and nonfatal myocardial infarction was 5.1% in the ticlopidine group and 10.9% in the control group, a risk reduction of 53.2%.[85] Clopidogrel, a new-generation thienopyridine derivative, has a longer half-life and a much improved side effect profile. The efficacy of this agent for secondary prevention of recurrent ischemic events in patients with previous stroke, myocardial infarction, or peripheral vascular disease has been shown.[13] No excess neutropenia or gastrointestinal side effects were observed. This agent has not yet been evaluated in acute coronary syndromes.

The beneficial effect of aspirin combined with a thienopyridine may prove useful, although data are not available. This combination is useful, however, in patients undergoing intracoronary stent placement.[86]

### Glycoprotein IIb/IIIa Antagonists

Awareness of the role of the GP IIb/IIIa receptor in platelet aggregation has evolved into a major pharmacologic breakthrough in antiplatelet therapy. Perhaps not since the advent of thrombolytic agents has a new class of drugs received such attention for their potential benefits in acute coronary syndromes. The value of GP IIb/IIIa blockade arises from the fact that binding of this receptor represents the final pathway of platelet aggregation in response to all agonists. Potent inhibition of fibrinogen and von Willebrand factor binding profoundly impairs platelet aggregation.[87]

The prototype agent is c7E3 Fab, or abciximab, a chimeric fragment of a monoclonal antibody, which binds avidly to GP IIb/IIIa. Since development of this drug, many synthetic peptidic and nonpeptidic intravenous and oral formulations have been studied, each mimicking the fibrinogen binding site and allowing for highly specific and reversible inhibition of GP IIb/IIIa (Table 26–7). The clinical use of abciximab is in both elective and urgent PCI, for which its protective effects have been clearly documented. Used concomitantly with aspirin and heparin, abciximab results in significant reduction in periprocedural myocardial infarction.[41, 88] A long-term reduction in mortality has been observed compared with balloon angioplasty alone, particularly in patients receiving intracoronary stents.[66]

The efficacy of GP IIb/IIIa inhibitors in acute coronary syndromes has now been evaluated in four large trials.[89–92] The Platelet Receptor Inhibition for Ischemic Syndrome Management (PRISM) trial investigators randomized patients to receive intravenous tirofiban or heparin for 48 hours in non–ST-elevation ischemic chest pain. Tirofiban significantly reduced the composite endpoint of death, new myocardial infarction, and refractory ischemia; however, this benefit was not evident at 30 days.[89] The PRISM-PLUS investigators evaluated tirofiban in a higher risk population with documented ECG abnormalities or non–Q wave myocardial infarction. In

Table 26–7

**Currently Available Platelet Glycoprotein IIb/IIIa Receptor Antagonists**

| Drug | Indication | Dose |
|------|-----------|------|
| Abciximab (antibody) | Elective PTCA<br>Urgent PTCA<br>Refractory unstable angina<br>  pending PCI | Bolus: 0.25 mg/kg<br>Maintenance: 0.125 μg/kg/min |
| Tirofiban (nonpeptide) | USA/non–Q MI | Bolus: 0.4 μg/kg/min × 30 min<br>Maintenance: 0.1 μg/kg/min × 48–96 hr |
| Eptifibatide (cyclic peptide) | Elective PTCA | Bolus: 135 μg/kg<br>Maintenance: 0.50 μg/kg/min × 24 hr |
| | USA/non–Q MI | Bolus: 180 μg/kg<br>Maintenance: 2 μg/kg/min |
| | Urgent PTCA | |

PTCA, percutaneous transluminal coronary angioplasty; PCI, percutaneous coronary intervention; MI, myocardial infarction.

contrast to PRISM, all patients received heparin and were randomized to tirofiban or placebo. The primary composite endpoint at 7 days revealed a 34% event risk reduction in favor of combined therapy, 12.9% versus 17.9%. A tirofiban-only arm in this study was terminated prematurely owing to an observed excess mortality. The continued advantage of combination therapy persisted to 6 months, although most benefit was in the refractory ischemia component of the composite endpoint.[90] It is relevant to note that all patients received mandatory angiography at 48 hours, and if indicated, angioplasty was performed. The Platelet IIb/IIIa Antagonism for the Reduction of Acute Coronary Syndrome Events in a Global Organization Network (PARAGON) trial assessed the efficacy of lamifiban at high (5 μg/min) and low (1 μg/min) doses, with or without heparin. No benefit was observed at 30 days, and high-dose lamifiban was associated with an excess rate of bleeding. At 6 months, however, the lowest rates of death and myocardial infarction were noted in patients receiving low-dose lamifiban with heparin. When plasma levels were investigated, the lowest cardiac event rate occurred in patients with an intermediate dose of lamifiban, suggesting that the dose-response effect for platelet GP IIb/IIIa antagonists may be J shaped rather than linear.[91]

The largest of the trials, the Platelet Glycoprotein IIb/IIIa in Unstable Angina: Receptor Suppression Using Integrilin (PURSUIT) study, evaluated eptifibatide or placebo with heparin in more than 10,948 patients. In this trial, all management decisions were left to the discretion of the physician in an attempt to mimic "real life." A significant reduction in the rate of death or myocardial infarction was present at 96 hours, 7 days, and 30 days. The effect at 30 days was attenuated to a 10% relative reduction, although the absolute reduction in the number of events was maintained at 15/1000 treated. Rates of transfusion were 11.8% and 9.3% in the eptifibatide and placebo groups, respectively.[92] Considered together, the foregoing trials make a strong case for the use of GP IIb/IIIa antagonists in combination with heparin and aspirin, at least in patients with high-risk features.

The observation that benefit seems to persist long after early administration of these agents is interesting. Perhaps their effect on plaque healing and remodeling are a key feature to their efficacy. Oral GP IIb/IIIa antagonists have been shown to be safe and well tolerated in pilot clinical studies.[93] Initial clinical results from the Orofiban in Patients with Unstable Coronary Syndromes (OPUS) trial have been disappointing (OPUS-TIMI 16).[94] Further trials of oral GP IIb/IIIa antagonists in acute coronary syndromes are continuing.

## Antithrombotic Agents

### Standard Heparin

Heparin consists of an unfractionated mixture of glycosaminoglycans with molecular weights from 5000 to more than 30,000. Various sizes of these molecules bind the serpin antithrombin III. Subsequent binding of this complex to the thrombin enzyme prevents the catalytic cleavage of fibrinogen to fibrin.

The efficacy of intravenous heparin in unstable angina has been suggested by many moderate-sized trials and supported by meta-analyses.[95] A phenomenon of reactivation angina with risk of cardiac events following cessation of heparin has also been observed.[96] This phenomenon is more likely to occur after prolonged administration of heparin exceeding 72 hours. Concomitant use of aspirin may attenuate this effect. Data suggest that prolonged unfractionated heparin infusion decreases antithrombin III levels and that a notable increase in thrombin activity and generation ensues when heparin is abruptly stopped.[97] Therefore, it may be prudent to wean patients off heparin after long-term therapy and to continue close observation for up to 12 hours after cessation of unfractionated heparin infusion.

The therapeutic effect of unfractionated heparin does not constitute a linear dose-effect response. Clinical trial observations of patients presenting with unstable angina or non–Q wave myocardial infarction have shown no additional benefit to activated partial thromboplastin times (aPTTs) in excess of 2.0 times baseline aPTT. In fact, sustained anticoagulation beyond this value is associated with a tendency toward increased adverse outcomes.[98] The mechanism of this paradoxic effect remains uncertain. In vivo and ex vivo studies have demonstrated platelet activation in the presence of unfractionated heparin in normal volunteers.[99] This effect may be more prone to occur at higher heparin blood levels. Thus, therapeutic dosing of unfractionated heparin should target an aPTT 1.5 to 2.0 times baseline value. In most laboratories, this range corresponds to an aPTT in the range of 45 to 60 seconds. Dose titration is easier to achieve by the use of weight-based dosing nomograms. Use of a bedside PTT monitor also facilitates the monitoring of heparin infusions and reduces the time required to obtain a PTT from approximately 90 minutes to less than 5 minutes. In one study, bedside aPTT monitoring was associated with reduced rates of hemorrhage compared with standard laboratory monitoring.[100]

The most common complication of continuous unfractionated heparin administration is bleeding. This occurs in roughly 6% of patients. Heparin-induced thrombocytopenia has been reported in 1% to 2.4% of patients receiving therapeutic doses of unfractionated heparin and most commonly occurs with prolonged dosing. More rare complications include alopecia, skin necrosis, urticaria, and transient transaminase elevations.[101]

### Low-Molecular-Weight Heparins

The low-molecular-weight heparin (LMWH) agents are derived by fractionation of standard heparin and retrieving molecules with a molecular weight less than 8000. Compared with unfractionated heparin, these products bind less avidly to plasma proteins, thereby allowing more predictable anticoagulation dosing. They may be administered subcutaneously and show high bioavailability. These agents have a much more pronounced effect on coagulation factor Xa than on thrombin. Therefore, the total antithrombotic action is not reflected by the aPTT. This anti–factor Xa effect impairs thrombin generation from prothrombin.[102] Because anti–Xa activity is mainly in the lower-molecular-weight fractions, the anti–Xa activity is greater compared with unfractionated heparin and varies among the various LMWH agents.

Four large clinical trials evaluating LMWH in acute coronary syndromes without ST elevation have been completed.[103–105] The Fragmin During Instability in Coronary Artery Disease (FRISC) trial randomized patients to subcutaneous dalteparin (Fragmin) or placebo. Although significant reduction of death and myocardial infarction was present at 6 days, this effect disappeared at 5 months despite continued once daily administration for up to 45 days. This study did not incorporate standard heparin in the control group.[103] The related FRIC study used identical dosing and duration of dalteparin in comparison with standard heparin. No benefit of dalteparin was observed. A negative feature of this trial was the slightly higher mortality observed in the dalteparin-treated patients, 1.5% versus 0.4%.[104] The Efficacy and Safety of Subcutaneous Enoxaperin in Non–Q-wave Coronary Events (ESSENCE) trial compared enoxaparin versus standard heparin and showed a statistical benefit of enoxaparin. At 14 days, the composite endpoint of death, myocardial infarction, or recurrent ischemia occurred in 16.6% of patients randomized to enoxaparin versus 19.9% for the standard heparin group. A nonstatistically significant trend persisted to 30 days. However, recurrent angina, the softest of the three composite endpoints, made up 75% of all events in the trial and most strongly affected outcome.[105]

The TIMI 11 trial investigators evaluated an alternative dosing regimen of enoxaparin versus unfractionated heparin in 3910 patients presenting with non–ST-segment elevation acute coronary syndromes. Enoxaparin was initially administered as an intravenous bolus of 30 mg/kg, followed by 1 mg/kg subcutaneous injections twice daily. The primary composite endpoint of death, myocardial infarction, or refractory ischemia at 8 days noted a statistically significant benefit of enoxaparin. The event rates were 12.4% versus 14.5% for enoxaparin and unfractionated heparin, respectively (TIMI 11B).[106] Long-term follow-up of this patient population is needed to determine whether this apparent benefit extends beyond the early management phase.

Strong evidence suggesting the superiority of LMWH for the prevention of acute myocardial infarction over standard heparin in acute coronary syndromes is lacking. These agents appear safe, however, and may exert efficacy similar to that of unfractionated heparin, although a trial design testing equivalency has not been completed.

### Direct Thrombin Inhibitors

The direct thrombin inhibitors act independently of antithrombin III and are unaffected by heparin-inactivating proteins. They are capable of inhibiting clot-bound thrombin and therefore can theoretically more aggressively prevent the perpetuation of local coagulation.[107] These agents are administered intravenously. Prolongation of the aPTT occurs as a result of their direct effect on thrombin.

The prototype agent is hirudin, a naturally occurring anticoagulant found in the saliva of the medicinal leech. It is now produced through recombinant DNA technology. The clinical value of hirudin has been assessed in the GUSTO-II trial. Patients with acute chest pain with or without ST elevation were randomized to receive intravenous hirudin (0.6 mg/kg bolus and 0.2 mg/kg/hr infusion) or standard heparin. This trial was halted early owing to the observed excess of intracranial bleeding in the hirudin group, particularly in combination with thrombolytics.[108] The GUSTO-IIB trial used a significantly lower dose of hirudin (0.1 mg/kg bolus and 0.1 mg/kg/hr infusion). The primary endpoint of death, nonfatal myocardial infarction, or reinfarction at 30 days was reached in 9.8% of the heparin group as compared with 8.9% of the hirudin group, not reaching statistical significance.[109] The Canadian Organization to Assess Strategies for Ischemic Syndromes (OASIS-2) study evaluated a more intermediate hirudin dose (0.4 mg/kg bolus and 0.15 mg/kg/hr infusion) in patients with acute coronary syndromes without ST elevation. The primary endpoint, a composite of cardiovascular death or myocardial

## Table 26-8

### Early Stratification for Risk of Adverse Outcome in Patients Presenting with Unstable Angina

| | Low Risk | Intermediate Risk | High Risk |
|---|---|---|---|
| Clinical history | Effort angina with little progression <br><br> <Two cardiac risk factors* <br> Negative troponin T or I | Gradual evolution of anginal symptoms to CCSC class III or IV (>4 weeks) <br> Two cardiac risk factors | Rapid evolution of anginal symptoms to CCSC class III or II (<4 weeks) <br> Advanced age (>60 yr) <br> Known CAD <br> Postmyocardial infarction (<6 weeks) <br> Hemodynamic instability <br> Signs of CHF: <br> "+" $S_3$ <br> Lung rales |
| Physical examination | No abnormal cardiovascular findings | Signs of peripheral vascular disease: <br> Carotid/femoral bruits <br> Diminished pulses | ST-segment depression ≥1 mm |
| ECG | Normal or minimal abnormality | Minimal ST- or T-wave abnormalities | |

CCSC, Canadian Cardiovascular Society Classification; CAD, coronary artery disease; CHF, congestive heart failure; ECG, electrocardiogram.
*Risk factors include smoking, elevated cholesterol, hypertension, diabetes mellitus, and family history of coronary artery disease.

infarction at 7 days, occurred in 3.6% of hirudin-treated patients and 4.2% of heparin-treated patients. These results fell just short of statistic significance. Once again, however, major bleeding occurred more frequently with hirudin, 1.2% versus 0.7% for standard heparin.[110]

Hirulog, a synthetic analogue of hirudin, is proposed to inhibit clot-bound thrombin more effectively owing to its smaller size. It is currently being evaluated in large trials for its role as an adjunct to thrombolysis and as an anticoagulant during angioplasty.

The present data suggest that more potent thrombin inhibition is not necessarily beneficial, especially in conjunction with thrombolytics. Perhaps a factor negating the efficacy of direct thrombin inhibitors is their inability to prevent thrombin generation, in contrast to heparin.

## Management Approach

Because clinical presentations of acute chest pain vary, the intensity of the management strategy must vary as well. The clinician must first assess the patient's risk for suffering further cardiac events on the basis of a thorough clinical history, physical examination, and evaluation of the ECG results. Features consistent with a low-, intermediate-, or high-risk presentation are shown in Table 26–8.

Controversy exists about whether and when a more aggressive approach with

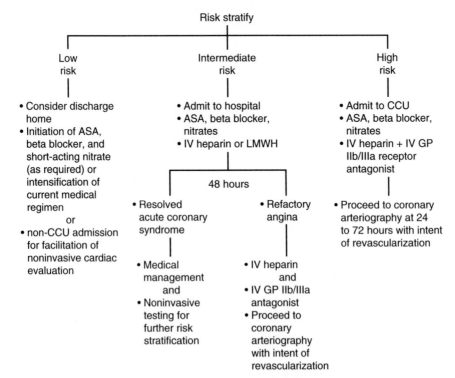

**Figure 26–4** ■ Algorithm for the early management of acute coronary syndromes without ST-segment elevation. ASA, aspirin; CCU, coronary care unit; IV, intravenous; LMWH, low-molecular-weight heparin.

early coronary angiography should be pursued. Based on the results of the TIMI 3B[69] and VANQWISH[111] studies, a *routine* early invasive strategy for all patients with non–ST-elevation acute coronary syndromes confers no benefit in terms of preventing death or myocardial infarction. Similarly, the OASIS registry of more than 7900 consecutive patients with unstable angina or suspected myocardial infarction without ST-segment elevation noted no difference in the rate of cardiovascular death or myocardial infarction in countries with the highest rate of invasive procedures (59%) versus the lowest (21%). As in TIMI 3B, higher rates of invasive and revascularization procedures were associated with lower rates of refractory angina or readmission for unstable angina. This benefit was, however, at the expense of excessive myocardial infarctions and strokes.[112] Nevertheless, early angiography does hasten the triage process. By doing so, it may obviate the waiting period required until noninvasive testing can be performed safely, and it may also aid in identification of the 20% of patients without significant coronary arterial narrowing, for whom alternative diagnostic procedures may be needed.[113]

It is likely that early angiography and revascularization are beneficial in patients presenting with high-risk features and therefore should be performed, although no data support this position. For patients with persisting symptoms after 48 hours of intensive medical therapy, the likelihood of a catastrophic event increases and coronary angiography should be undertaken with a view toward revascularization. Tailoring decision making to the dynamics of the individual clinical scenario is essential. The algorithm presented in Figure 26–4 provides a decision-making guideline for patients presenting to the emergency room with non–ST-elevation acute coronary syndromes.

## ■ REFERENCES

1. Centers for Disease Control and Prevention: National Center for Health Statistics, National Vital Statistics and The United States Bureau of the Census. Health, United States 1993:31.
2. Gianrossi R, Detrano R, Mulvihill D, et al: Exercise-induced ST depression in the diagnosis of coronary artery disease: A meta-analysis. Circulation 1989;80:87.
3. Fletcher, GF, Balady G, Froelicher VF, et al: Exercise standards: A statement for health professionals from the American Heart Association Writing Group. Circulation 1995;91:580.
4. Kaul S, Boucher CA, Newell JB, et al: Determination of the quantitative thallium imaging variables that optimize detection of coronary artery disease. J Am Coll Cardiol 1986;7:527.
5. Gibbons RJ, Fyke FE, Clements IP, et al: Noninvasive identification of severe coronary artery disease using exercise radionuclide angiography. J Am Coll Cardiol 1988;11:28.
6. Quinones MA, Verani MS, Haichin RM, et al: Exercise echocardiography versus T1-201 single photon emission computerized tomography in evaluation of coronary artery disease: Analysis of 292 patients. Circulation 1992;85:1026–1031.
7. Galbraith JE, Murphy ML, Desoyza N: Coronary angiogram interpretation: Interobserver variability. JAMA 1981;240:2053–2059.
8. Grodin CM, Dydra I, Pastgernac A, et al: Discrepancies between cineangiographic and post-mortem findings in patients with coronary artery disease and recent myocardial revascularization. Circulation 1974;49:703–709.
9. Iskandrian AS, Chae SC, Heo J, et al: Independent and incremental prognostic value of exercise single-photon emission computed tomographic (SPECT) thallium imaging in coronary artery disease. J Am Coll Cardiol 1993;22:665–670.
10. Hachamovitch R, Berman DS, Shaw LJ, et al: Incremental prognostic value of myocardial perfusion single photon emission computed tomography for the prediction of cardiac death. Circulation 1998;97:535–543.
11. Antiplatelet Trialists' Collaboration: Collaborative overview of randomized trials of antiplatelet therapy. I: Prevention of death, myocardial infarction, and stroke by prolonged antiplatelet therapy in various categories of patients. BMJ 1994;308:81–98.
12. Gent M, Blakely JA, Easton JD, et al: The Canadian American Ticlopidine Study (CATS) in thromboembolic stroke. Lancet 1989;1:1215–1220.
13. Gent M, Beaumont D, Blanchard J, et al: A randomized, blinded, trial of Clopidogrel versus aspirin in patients at risk of Ischaemic Events (CAPRIE). Lancet 1996;348:1329–1339.
14. Abrams J (ed): Third North American conference on nitroglycerine therapy. Am J Cardiol 1992;70:1B–103B.

15. The BHAT Research Group: A randomized trial of propranolol in patients with acute myocardial infarction. The Beta-blocker Heart Attack Trial. JAMA 1982;247:1707–1714.
16. The MIAMI trial research group: Metoprolol in acute myocardial infarction (MIAMI). A randomized placebo-controlled international trial. Eur Heart J 1985;6:199–211.
17. The ISIS-1 Collaborative Group: Randomized trial of intravenous atenolol among 16027 cases of suspected acute myocardial infarction: ISIS-1. Lancet 1986;ii:57–66.
18. The MDPIT research group: The effect of diltiazem on mortality and reinfarction after myocardial infarction. N Engl J Med 1988;319:385–392.
19. The Danish study group on verapamil in myocardial infarction. Effect of verapamil on mortality and major events after acute myocardial infarction (The Danish Verapamil Infarction Trial II-DAVIT II). Am J Cardiol 1990;66:779–785.
20. The West of Scotland Coronary Prevention Study Group: Prevention of coronary heart disease with pravastatin in men with hypercholesterolemia. N Engl J Med 1995;333:1301–1307.
21. The Air Force/Texas Coronary Atherosclerosis Prevention Research Study Group: Primary prevention of acute coronary events with lovastatin in men and women with average cholesterol levels. JAMA 1998;279:1615–1622.
22. Scandinavian Simvastatin Survival Study Group: Randomized trial of cholesterol lowering in 4444 patients with coronary heart disease: The Scandinavian Simvastatin Survival Study (4S). Lancet 1994;344:1383–1389.
23. The Cholesterol and Recurrent Events Trial Investigators: The effect of pravastatin on coronary events after myocardial infarction in patients with average cholesterol levels. N Engl J Med 1996;335:1001–1009.
24. Jeppesen J, Hein HO, Suadicani P, et al: Triglyceride concentration and ischemic heart disease: An eight-year follow-up in the Copenhagen male study. Circulation 1998;97:1029–1036.
25. McKenney JM, McCormick LS, Weiss S, et al: A randomized trial of the effects of atorvastatin and niacin in patients with combined hyperlipidemia or isolated hypertriglyceridemia. Am J Med 1998;104:137–143.
26. Hemminki E, McPherson K: Impact of post-menopausal hormone therapy on cardiovascular events and cancer: Pooled data from clinical trials. BMJ 1997;315:149–153.
27. The Writing Group for the PEPI Trial: Effects of estrogen or estrogen/progestin regimens on heart disease risk factors in postmenopausal women: The postmenopausal estrogen/progestin interventions (PEPI) trial. JAMA 1995;273:199–208.
28. Belchetz PE: Hormonal treatment of postmenopausal women. N Engl J Med 1994;330:1062–1071.
29. Grady D, Rubin SM, Petitti DB, et al: Hormone therapy to prevent disease and prolong life in postmenopausal women. Ann Intern Med 1992;117:1016.
30. Stampfer MJ, Colditz GA, Willett WC, et al: Postmenopausal estrogen therapy and cardiovascular disease. Ten-year follow-up from the Nurses' Health Study. N Engl J Med 1991;325:756.
31. The Heart and Estrogen/progestin Replacement Study (HERS) Group: Randomized trial of estrogen plus progestin for secondary prevention of coronary heart disease in postmenopausal women. JAMA 1998;280:605–613.
32. American College of Physicians: Guidelines for counseling postmenopausal women about preventive hormone therapy. Ann Intern Med 1992;117:1038.
33. Hennekens CH, Buring JE, Manson JE, et al: Lack of effect of long-term supplementation with beta-carotene on the incidence of malignant neoplasms and cardiovascular disease. N Engl J Med 1996;334:1145–1149.
34. Rapola JM, Virtamo J, Ripatti S, et al: Effects of alpha-tocopherol and beta-carotene supplements on symptoms, progression, and prognosis in angina pectoris. Heart 1998;79:454–458.
35. Stephens NG, Parsons A, Schofiled PM, et al: Randomized controlled trial of vitamin E in patients with coronary disease: Cambridge Heart Antioxidant Study (CHAOS). Lancet 1996;347:781–786.
36. Dotter CT, Judkins MP: Transluminal treatment of arteriosclerotic obstruction: Description of a new technique and a preliminary report of its application. Circulation 1964;30:654–670.
37. King SB III. Angioplasty from bench to bedside to bench. Circulation 1996;93:1621–1629.
38. Kimmel SC, Berlin JA, Strom BL, et al: Development and validation of a simplified predictive index for major complications in contemporary percutaneous transluminal coronary angioplasty practice. J Am Coll Cardiol 1995;26:931.
39. Jollis JG, Peterson ED, DeLong ER, et al: The relation between the volume of coronary angioplasty procedures in hospitals treating Medicare beneficiaries and short-term mortality. N Engl J Med 1994;331:1625.
40. DeFeyter PJ, deJaigere PP, Serruys PW: Incidence, predictors and management of acute coronary occlusion after coronary angioplasty. Am Heart J 1994;19:926.
41. The EPILOG Investigators: Platelet glycoprotein IIb/IIIa blockade and low-dose heparin during percutaneous coronary revascularization. N Engl J Med 1997;336:1689–1696.
42. Kuntz RE, Baim DS: Defining coronary restenosis. Circulation 1993;88:1310.
43. Surruys PW, deJaegere P, Kiemeneij F, et al: A comparison of balloon expandable-stent implantation with balloon angioplasty in patients with coronary artery disease. N Engl J Med 1994;331:489–495.
44. Fischman DL, Leon MB, Baim DS, et al: A randomized comparison of coronary stent placement and balloon angioplasty in the treatment of coronary artery disease. N Engl J Med 1994;331:496–501.

45. Elliott JM, Berdan LG, Holmes DR, et al: One-year follow-up in the coronary angioplasty versus excisional atherectomy trial (CAVEAT I). Circulation 1995;91:2158.
46. Baim DS, Cutlip DE, Sharma SK, et al: Final results of the balloon versus optimal atherectomy trial. Circulation 1998;97:322–331.
47. Reifart N, Vandormael M, Krajcar M, et al: Randomized comparison of angioplasty of complex coronary lesions at a single center. Excimer Laser, Rotational Atherectomy, and Balloon Angioplasty Comparison (ERBAC) Study. Circulation 1997;96:91–98.
48. Horvath KA, Cohn LH, Cooley DA, et al: Transmyocardial laser revascularization: Results of a multicenter trial with transmyocardial laser revascularization used as sole therapy for end-stage coronary artery disease. J Thorac Cardiovasc Surg 1997;113:645–654.
49. Malekan R, Reynolds C, Narula N, et al: Angiogenesis in transmyocardial laser revascularization: A nonspecific response to injury. Circulation 1998;98:II-62–II-66.
50. Isner JM: Vascular endothelial growth factor: Gene therapy and therapeutic angiogenesis. Am J Cardiol 1998;10A:63S–64S.
51. Goncalves LM: Fibroblast growth factor-mediated angiogenesis for the treatment of ischemia. Lessons learned from experimental models and early human experience. Rev Port Cardiol 1998;2S:11–20.
52. Baumgartner I, Pieczek A, Manor O, et al: Constitutive expression of phVEGF after intramuscular gene transfer promotes collateral vessel development in patients with critical limb ischemia. Circulation 1998;97:1114–1123.
53. Schumacher B, Pecher P, von Specht, et al: Induction of neoangiogenesis in ischemic myocardium by human growth factors. Circulation 1998;97:645–650.
54. Garrett HE, Dennis EW, DeBakey ME, et al: Aortocoronary bypass with saphenous vein graft: Seven-year follow-up. JAMA 1973;223:792.
55. Cameron AAC, Davis KB, Rogers WJ, et al: Recurrence of angina after coronary bypass surgery. Predictors and prognosis (CASS Registry). J Am Coll Cardiol 1995;26:895.
56. Goldman S, Copeland J, Moritz T, et al: Internal mammary artery and saphenous vein graft patency. Effects of aspirin. Circulation 1990;82(Suppl IV):237–242.
57. Borger MA, Cohen G, Buth KJ, et al: Multiple arterial grafts. Radial versus right internal thoracic arteries. Circulation 1998;98:II-7–II-14.
58. Parisi AF, Folland ED, Hartigan P: Angioplasty compared to medicine. N Engl J Med 1992;326:10–16.
59. RITA-2 Trial Participants: Coronary angioplasty versus medical therapy for angina: The second Randomized Intervention Treatment of Angina (RITA-2) trial. Lancet 1997;350:461–468.
60. Yusuf S, Zucker D, Pedruzzi P, et al: Effect of coronary artery bypass graft surgery on survival: Overview of 10-year results from randomized trials by the Coronary Artery Bypass Graft Surgery Trialists Collaboration. Lancet 1994;344:563–570.
61. RITA Trialists: Coronary angioplasty versus coronary artery bypass surgery: The Randomized Intervention Treatment of Angina (RITA) trial. Lancet 1993;341:573–580.
62. Hamm CW, Reimers J, Ischinger T, et al: A randomized study of coronary angioplasty compared with bypass surgery in patients with symptomatic multivessel coronary disease. German Angioplasty Bypass Surgery Investigation (GABI). N Engl J Med 1994;331:1037–1043.
63. CABRI Trial Participants: First-year results of CABRI (Coronary Angioplasty versus Bypass Revascularization Investigation). Lancet 1995;346:1178–1184.
64. King SB, Lembo NJ, Weintraub WS, et al: A randomized trial comparing coronary angioplasty with coronary bypass surgery. Emory Angioplasty versus Surgery Trial (EAST). N Engl J Med 1994;331:1044–1050.
65. The BARI (Bypass Angioplasty Revascularization Investigation) Investigators: Comparison of coronary bypass surgery with angioplasty in patients with multivessel disease. N Engl J Med 1996;335:217–225.
66. The EPISTENT Investigators: Randomized placebo-controlled and balloon-angioplasty-controlled trial to assess safety of coronary stenting with use of platelet glycoprotein-IIb/IIIa blockade. Lancet 1998;352:87–92.
67. Rogers WJ, Bowbey L: Treatment of myocardial infarction in the United States: 1990–1993 observations. Circulation 1994;90:2103.
68. Bar FW, Verheugt FW, Col J, et al: Thrombolysis in patients with unstable angina improves the angiographic but not the clinical outcome. Results of UNASEM, a multicenter, randomized, placebo-controlled clinical trial with anistreplase. Circulation 1992;86:131–137.
69. TIMI IIIB Investigators: Effects of tissue plasminogen activator and a comparison of early invasive and conservative strategies in unstable angina and non–Q-wave myocardial infarction: Results of the TIMI IIIB trial. Circulation 1994;89:1545–1556.
70. DeWinter RJ, Koster RW, Sturk A, et al: Value of myoglobin, troponin T, and CK-MB mass in ruling out an acute myocardial infarction in the emergency room. Circulation 1995;92:3401–3407.
71. Lindahl B, Venge P, Wallentin L: Relation between troponin T and the risk of subsequent cardiac events in unstable coronary artery disease. Circulation 1996;93:1651–1657.
72. Ohman EM, Armstrong PW, Christenson RH, et al: Cardiac troponin T levels for risk stratification in acute myocardial ischemia. N Engl J Med 1996;335:1333–1341.
73. Antman EM, Tanasijevic MJ, Thompson B, et al: Cardiac-specific troponin I levels to predict the risk of mortality in patients with acute coronary syndromes. N Engl J Med 1996;335:1342–1349.
74. Newby LK, Christenson RH, Ohman EM, et al: Value of serial troponin T measures for early and late risk stratification in patients with acute coronary syndromes. Circulation 1998;98:1853–1859.

75. Goldman L, Cook EF, Johnson PA, et al: Prediction of the need for intensive care in patients who come to emergency departments with acute chest pain. N Engl J Med 1996;334:1498–1504.
76. Polanczyk CA, Lee TH, Cook EF, et al: Cardiac troponin I as predictor of major cardiac events in emergency department patients with acute chest pain. J Am Coll Cardiol 1998;32:8–14.
77. Holmvang L, Lusher MS, Clemmensen P, et al: Very early risk stratification using combined ECG and biochemical assessment in patients with unstable coronary artery disease (A Thrombin Inhibition in Myocardial Ischemia [TRIM] Substudy). Circulation 1998;98:2004–2009.
78. Hamm CW, Goldman BU, Heeschen C, et al: Emergency room triage of patients with acute chest pain by means of rapid testing for cardiac troponin T or Troponin I. N Engl J Med 1997;337:1648–1653.
79. Bodor GS, Porter S, Landt Y, et al: Development of monoclonal antibodies for an assay of cardiac troponin I and preliminary results in suspected cases of myocardial infarction. Clin Chem 1992;38:2203.
80. Morrow DA, Rifai N, Antman EM, et al: C-reactive protein is a potent predictor of mortality independently of and in combination with troponin T in acute coronary syndromes: A TIMI IIA Substudy. J Am Coll Cardiol 1998;31:1460–1465.
81. Caligiuri G, Liuzzo G, Biasucci LM, et al: Immune system activation follows inflammation in unstable angina: Pathogenetic implications. J Am Coll Cardiol 1998;32:1295–1304.
82. Lewis HD, Davis JW, Archibald DG, et al: Protective effects of aspirin against myocardial infarction and death in patients with unstable angina. N Engl J Med 1983;309:396–403.
83. Cairns JA, Gent M, Singer J, et al: Aspirin, sulfinpyrazone, or both in unstable angina: Results of a Canadian multicenter trial. N Engl J Med 1985;313:1369–1375.
84. Defreyn G, Bernat A, Delebassee D, et al: Pharmacology of ticlopidine: A review. Semin Thromb Hemost 1989;15:159–166.
85. Balsano F, Rizzon P, Violi F, et al: Antiplatelet treatment with ticlopidine in unstable angina. A controlled multicenter clinical trial. Circulation 1990;82:17–26.
86. Leon MB, Baim DS, Popma PC, et al: A clinical trial comparing three antithrombotic-drug regimens after coronary-artery stenting. N Engl J Med 1998;339:1665–1671.
87. Coller BS, Anderson K, Weisman HF: New antiplatelet agents: Platelet GPIIb/IIIa antagonists. Thromb Haemost 1995;74:302–308.
88. The CAPTURE Investigators: Randomized placebo-controlled trial of abciximab before and during coronary intervention in refractory unstable angina. Lancet 1997;349:1429–1435.
89. The PRISM Study Group: A comparison of aspirin plus tirofiban with aspirin plus heparin for unstable angina. N Engl J Med 1998;338:1498–1505.
90. The PRISM PLUS Study Group: Inhibition of the platelet glycoprotein IIb/IIIa receptor in unstable angina and non–Q-wave myocardial infarction. N Engl J Med 1998;338:1488–1497.
91. The PARAGON Investigators: International, randomized, controlled trial of lamifiban (a platelet glycoprotein IIb/IIIa inhibitor), heparin, or both in unstable angina. Circulation 1998;97:2386–2395.
92. The PURSUIT Trial Investigators: Inhibition of platelet glycoprotein IIb/IIIa with eptifibatide in patients with acute coronary syndromes. N Engl J Med 1998;339:436–443.
93. The TIMI Investigators: Randomized trial of an oral platelet glycoprotein IIb-IIIa antagonist, sibrafiban, in patients after an acute coronary syndrome: Results of the TIMI 12 trial. Thrombolysis in Myocardial Infarction. Circulation 1998;97:340–349.
94. Cannon CP. OPUS TIMI-16 Study. Presented at the 48th Annual Scientific Session, American College of Cardiology, New Orleans, March, 1999.
95. Theroux P, Ouimet H, McCans J, et al: Aspirin, heparin, or both to treat unstable angina. N Engl J Med 1988;319:1105–1111.
96. Theroux P, Waters D, Lam J, et al: Reactivation of unstable angina after the discontinuation of heparin. N Engl J Med 1992;327:141–145.
97. Granger CB, Miller JM, Bovill EG, et al: Rebound increase in thrombin generation and activity after cessation of intravenous heparin in patients with acute coronary syndromes. Circulation 1995;91:1929–1935.
98. TIMI IIIB Investigators. Relation between systemic anticoagulation as determined by activated partial thromboploastin time and heparin measurements and in-hospital clinical events in unstable angina and non–Q-wave myocardial infarction. Am Heart J 1996;131:421–433.
99. Xiao Z, Theroux P: Platelet activation with unfractionated heparin at therapeutic concentrations and comparisons with a low-molecular-weight heparin and with a direct thrombin inhibitor. Circulation 1998;97:251–256.
100. The GUSTO Investigators: Use of bedside activated partial thromboplastin time monitor to adjust heparin dosing after thrombolysis for acute myocardial infarction: Results of GUSTO-1. Global Utilization of Streptokinase and TPA for Occluded Coronary Arteries. Am Heart J 1998;136:868–876.
101. Hirsh J, Fuster V: Guide to anticoagulant therapy. Part 1: Heparin. Circulation 1994;89:1449.
102. Boneau B: Low molecular weight heparin therapy: Is monitoring needed? Thromb Haemost 1994;72:330–334.
103. The FRISC Study Group: Low-molecular-weight heparin during instability in coronary artery disease. Lancet 1996;347:561–568.
104. The FRIC Study Group: Comparison of low-molecular-weight heparin with unfractionated heparin acutely and with placebo for 6 weeks in the management of unstable coronary artery disease. Circulation 1997;96:61–68.

105. The ESSENCE Study Group: A comparison of low-molecular-weight heparin with unfractionated heparin for unstable coronary artery disease. N Engl J Med 1997;337:447–452.
106. Antman EM, McCabe CH, Gurfinkel EP, et al: Enoxaparin prevents death and cardiac ischemic events in unstable non-Q-wave myocardial infarction. Results of the thrombolysis in myocardial infarction (TIMI) 11B trial. Circulation 1999;100(15):1593–1601.
107. Johnson PH: Hirudin. Clinic potential of a thrombin inhibitor. Annu Rev Med 1994;45:165–177.
108. GUSTO IIa Investigators. Randomized trial of intravenous heparin versus recombinant hirudin for acute coronary syndromes. The Global Use of Strategies to Open Occluded Coronary Arteries (GUSTO) IIa. Circulation 1994;90:1631–1637.
109. GUSTO IIb Investigators: A comparison of recombinant hirudin with heparin for the treatment of acute coronary syndromes. The Global Use of Strategies to Open Occluded Coronary Arteries (GUSTO) IIb. N Engl J Med 1996;335:775–782.
110. Organization to Assess Strategies for Ischemic Syndromes (OASIS-2) Investigators: Effects of recombinant hirudin (lepirudin) compared with heparin on death, myocardial infarction, refractory angina, and revascularization procedures in patients with acute myocardial ischemia without ST elevation: A randomized trial. Lancet 1999;353:429–438.
111. Boden WE, O'Rourke RA, Crawford MH, et al: Early and late clinical outcomes in acute non–Q-wave myocardial infarction patients randomized to an "invasive" versus "conservative" strategy: Results of the multicentre VA Non–Q-Wave Infarction Strategies in Hospital (VANQWISH) Trial. N Engl J Med 1998;338:1785–1792.
112. OASIS (Organization to Assess Strategies for Ischemic Syndromes) Registry Investigators: Variations between countries in invasive cardiac procedures and outcomes in patients with suspected unstable angina or myocardial infarction without initial ST elevation. Lancet 1998;352:507–514.
113. Braunwald E, Mark DB, Jones RH, et al: Unstable Angina: Diagnosis and management: Clinical Practice Guideline. Rockville, MD: Agency for Healthcare Policy and Research and the National Heart, Lung and Blood Institute. Public Health Service, U.S. Department of Health and Human Services. AHCPR Publication No. 94-0602:154, 1994:28, 92.

## ■ RECOMMENDED READING

Khan MM, Kleiman NS: Novel antiplatelet and antithrombotic agents in the treatment of non–ST-segment elevation coronary ischemia. *In* Cannon CP (ed): Contemporary Cardiology: Management of acute coronary syndromes. Clifton, NJ: Humana Press, 1999:425–461.

Management of stable angina pectoris. Task force of the European Society of Cardiology. Eur Heart J 1997;18:394–413.

Rita-2 Trial Participants: Coronary angioplasty versus medical therapy for angina: Second Randomized Intervention Treatment of Angina (RITA-2). Lancet 1997;350:461–468.

The Bypass Angioplasty Revascularization Investigation (BARI) Investigators: Comparison of coronary bypass surgery with angioplasty in patients with multivessel disease. N Engl J Med 1996;335:217–225.

Theroux P, Fuster V: Acute coronary syndromes: Unstable angina and non–Q-wave myocardial infarction. Circulation 1998;97:1195–1206.

Chapter 27

# Cardiopulmonary Resuscitation

*Joseph P. Ornato*

## ■ SUDDEN CARDIAC DEATH

Sudden cardiac death (SCD) due to unexpected cardiac arrest in adults claims the lives of an estimated 250,000 adult Americans each year. Most episodes of unexpected SCD in adults occur in the home.[1] The typical victim is a man aged 50 to 75 years. The majority of SCD victims have underlying structural heart disease, usually coronary atherosclerosis or cardiomegaly. Although 75% of SCD victims have significant atherosclerotic narrowing (>75%) in at least one major coronary artery, fewer than half of all sudden deaths occur *during* an acute myocardial infarction (AMI).

SCD is usually caused by a chance arrhythmic event that is triggered by an interaction between structural heart abnormalities and transient, functional electrophysiologic disturbances. In the majority of cases, the initiating event is a ventricular tachyarrhythmia, either pulseless ventricular tachycardia (VT) that degenerates rapidly to ventricular fibrillation (VF) or "primary" VF.[2] The majority of neurologically intact survivors of sudden, unexpected cardiac arrest come from a subset of patients whose event is initiated by a ventricular tachyarrhythmia. In such cases, the single most important determinant of survival is the interval from initiation of the cardiac arrest until defibrillation can be provided to terminate the ventricular tachyarrhythmia and restore a more normal rhythm accompanied by effective perfusion of vital organs.

## ■ PRINCIPLES OF RESUSCITATION

The American Heart Association (AHA) has introduced the "chain of survival" metaphor to represent the sequence of events that, ideally, should occur to maximize the odds of successful resuscitation from cardiac arrest in adults.[3] Only about 3% of all out-of-hospital cardiac arrest victims survive to leave the hospital with their neurologic functioning intact.[3] Survival from in-hospital cardiac arrest is not much better (averaging 10% to 20%).[4] There is substantial variability in the odds for survival from one geographic locale to another.[5–7]

For example, it is known that the outcome of resuscitation is strongly influenced by the patient's initial cardiac rhythm. The likelihood of survival is relatively high when the initial rhythm is VT or VF (particularly when the VF is "coarse," the arrest is witnessed, and prompt cardiopulmonary resuscitation [CPR] and defibrillation are provided). The best outcomes from VT/VF in adults occur regularly in the electrophysiology laboratory, where prompt defibrillation (within 20 to 30 seconds) results in virtually 100% survival. The next best reported outcomes are for persons in cardiac rehabilitation programs, where defibrillation occurs within 1 to 2 minutes, and survival is approximately 85% to 90%. Survival from out-of-hospital VT/VF treated by police officers equipped with automated external defibrillators (AED) in Rochester, Minnesota has averaged 50% with a median time from collapse to defibrillation of about 5 minutes.[8] Outcomes in many locations with emergency medical services that cannot provide defibrillation until 10 minutes or more after the patient collapses typically yield survival rates below 10%.[5, 6] Thus, survival from cardiac arrest due to ventricular tachyarrhythmias is highly dependent on the interval from collapse to defibrillation. For every minute's delay from the patient's collapse to defibrillation, the chance for survival diminishes by approximately 7% to 10%.[3]

If the initial rhythm is not VT or VF, survival is typically less than 5% in most reported series. Asystolic patients whose cardiac arrest was not witnessed rarely survive neurologically intact to hospital discharge, even when they are treated promptly with atropine, epinephrine, or an artificial pacemaker. The only common exceptions are those whose cardiac arrest was witnessed and whose initial brady-cardia or asystole (bradyasystole) is due to increased vagal tone or another rela-tively easily correctible factor (e.g., hypoxia of brief duration).

Pulseless electrical activity (PEA) is, by definition, an organized rhythm not accompanied by a detectable pulse in a person whose clinical status is cardiac arrest. The latter part of the definition is important for excluding conditions in which there is unmistakable evidence of blood pressure and cardiac output ade-quate to maintain vital organ perfusion but no detectable pulse (e.g., a conscious patient with profound vasoconstriction due to hypothermia). The underlying physi-ologic cause of PEA in most cases is a marked reduction in cardiac output that is due to either profound myocardial depression or mechanical factors that reduce venous return or otherwise impede the flow of blood through the cardiovascular system. Management of patients with PEA is directed at identifying and treating the underlying cause(s).

There are two fundamental goals in resuscitating an adult from cardiac arrest. First, a rhythm must be restored with a rate that is potentially capable of generating an adequate cardiac output and perfusion pressure. To accomplish this may involve defibrillating a patient out of VF or speeding up a bradyasystolic rhythm with atropine or an artificial pacemaker. Once an acceptable rhythm has been restored, attention should be focused on optimizing cardiac output and perfusion pressure.

# ■ BASIC CARDIAC LIFE SUPPORT

The technique and quality of CPR can dramatically affect critical organ perfu-sion pressure and blood flow. Maintenance of both the systolic and diastolic arterial pressure is even more vital for optimizing critical organ perfusion during CPR than in non-arrest conditions. Since flow to most vital organs (except the heart) occurs during the downstroke of closed chest compression ("systole"), a systolic arterial pressure of at least 50 to 60 mm Hg is usually required to resist arteriolar collapse. Diastolic pressure is particularly important during CPR, because it is a critical determinant of the coronary perfusion pressure (CPP = aortic diastolic − right atrial pressure). CPP is one of the best hemodynamic predictors of return of spontaneous circulation (ROSC) in both animal models and humans. A minimal threshold CPP gradient of approximately 15 mm Hg (usually corresponding to an aortic diastolic pressure of 30 to 40 mm Hg) provides enough myocardial blood flow to meet minimum metabolic needs of the arrested myocardium and to achieve ROSC.[9]

Understanding the mechanisms of blood flow during closed chest CPR and real-time monitoring of hemodynamic parameters allow rescuers to modify chest compression techniques (the force of compression and the downstroke-upstroke ratio), when appropriate, to optimize perfusion pressure and blood flow.[10] There are at least two major mechanisms of blood flow during closed chest CPR: the cardiac pump and the thoracic pump.[11]

It was initially believed that blood flow during CPR was caused by direct compression of the heart between the sternum and the spine (cardiac pump). In the mid-1970s, the cardiac pump theory began to be challenged by investigators who observed that increased intrathoracic pressure alone (without precordial compression) is capable of generating blood flow.[12, 13] Sudden increase in the intrathoracic pressure traps air in the alveoli and small bronchioles during chest compression, creating a pressure gradient between the intrathoracic and extrathoracic cavities.[12] In the thoracic pump theory, the heart functions as a passive conduit.[14] Pressurization of the thorax collapses veins at the thoracic inlet, preventing venous backflow. Forward flow occurs because the more muscular arteries remain open, particularly when epinephrine is administered.

Transesophageal echocardiography studies demonstrate that both mechanisms operate during CPR.[15] Physiologic studies in experimental models and humans suggest a strong, probably dominant, role for the thoracic pump during closed chest compression in adults. In addition, active decompression of the chest by applying negative pressure or suction to the sternum may further enhance cardiac output by improving venous inflow or by increasing the intrathoracic pressure difference between the upstroke and downstroke phases of chest compression (active compression-decompression CPR [ACD-CPR]).[16] Unfortunately, ACD-CPR did not improve survival as compared with standard CPR in a recent large, well-controlled, randomized clinical trial.[17] Other experimental techniques, such as interposing an abdominal compression between chest compressions (IAC-CPR)[18] or phased chest and abdominal compression,[19, 20] are designed to simulate the physiologic effects of intraaortic balloon counterpulsation. Whether any of these techniques is clinically superior to properly performed standard CPR has yet to be determined.

## ■ CARDIOVASCULAR ASSESSMENT DURING RESUSCITATION

### Echocardiography

Conventional transthoracic echocardiography is useful during CPR, but a limitation is the difficulty of imaging the heart when the chest wall is in motion. Transesophageal echocardiography provides high-resolution, real-time images during CPR and can be used to (1) better define the mechanism of blood flow during chest compression; (2) determine the presence of pericardial effusion, intracardiac tumor or clot, chamber enlargement or hypertrophy, severe volume depletion, pneumothorax, or thoracic aortic dissection; (3) better define the cause of PEA; (4) evaluate global and regional wall motion after ROSC; and (5) provide a visual guide for positioning intracardiac catheters and pacemaker wires.[15]

### Capnography

The percentage of carbon dioxide ($CO_2$) contained in the last few milliliters of gas exhaled from the lungs with each breath is termed the end-tidal $CO_2$ concentration ($P_{ETCO_2}$). During normal respiration and circulation, the $P_{ETCO_2}$ averages 4% to 5%. Two units of measure are popularly used in reporting the $P_{ETCO_2}$: % and mm Hg (1% is approximately 7 mm Hg). The $P_{ETCO_2}$ can be used to confirm endotracheal (ET) tube airway placement, particularly in patients who are not in cardiac arrest and who have a pulse and an adequate blood pressure (i.e., sensitivity and specificity of the $PETCO_2$ for detecting correct ET tube placement approach 100% and 90%, respectively).[21] Ventilation through an ET tube that has been properly inserted into the trachea yields a $PETCO_2$ of 4% to 5% in a patient with normal cardiac output and no significant ventilation-perfusion gradient. Ventilation through an ET tube that has been inadvertently inserted into the esophagus results in a $PETCO_2$ of less than 0.5%.

There is a logarithmic relationship between $PETCO_2$ and cardiac output.[22] At normal or elevated cardiac output, ventilation is the rate-limiting factor responsible for eliminating the large volume of $CO_2$ that passes through the pulmonary circuit (e.g., hyperventilation lowers, and hypoventilation raises, $PETCO_2$). In this range, the $PETCO_2$ closely approximates arterial $CO_2$ tension ($PaCO_2$) and can be used as a real-time measure of the adequacy of ventilation. At low levels of cardiac output (below approximately 50% of normal in animal models), ventilation has much less effect on the $PETCO_2$. If ventilation is kept relatively constant in this range, an increase or a decrease in cardiac output is usually reflected by a rise or fall, respectively, in the $PETCO_2$. During CPR the $PETCO_2$ typically decreases to a quarter to a third of normal, paralleling the decrease in cardiac output and pulmonary blood flow.[22, 23] As $CO_2$ builds up in venous blood, hyperventilation cleanses $CO_2$ from the reduced quantity of venous blood traversing the lungs. The result is a low $PaCO_2$ and a high central venous $CO_2$ ($PCVCO_2$) concentration (a venoarterial $CO_2$ and pH gradient). Within seconds after ROSC, the improved cardiac output delivers large quantities of $CO_2$-rich venous blood to the lungs and the $PETCO_2$ climbs suddenly to normal or above normal levels.[23-25] The dramatic change from a low to a high $PETCO_2$ due to venous $CO_2$ washout is often the first clinical indicator of ROSC.

Monitoring the $PETCO_2$ during CPR can be used as a guide to the patient's hemodynamic status. Inadequate chest compression is usually accompanied by a very low (<1%) $PETCO_2$, which increases linearly with increasing sternal compression depth and force.[26] Intravenous (IV) administration of sodium bicarbonate causes a transient rise in $PETCO_2$ as the drug dissociates into water and $CO_2$. Disorders that cause significant ventilation-perfusion mismatch (e.g., pulmonary embolization) or a reduction in production of $CO_2$ (e.g., hypothermia) are accompanied by low $PETCO_2$. The initial $PETCO_2$ also has prognostic value. An end-tidal $CO_2$ level of not more than 10 mm Hg measured 20 minutes after the initiation of advanced cardiac life support (ACLS) accurately predicts death from cardiac arrest associated with electrical activity but no pulse. CPR may be terminated in such cases.[27]

## ▪ ADVANCED AIRWAY MANAGEMENT

### Endotracheal Intubation

One of the most important goals early in resuscitation is to establish an airway that will allow delivery of oxygen in high concentrations, protect the airway from aspiration, and permit administration of aerosolized medications. An ET tube serves all of these purposes and is generally considered the airway of choice during CPR. Medications that are commonly administered via the ET tube during resuscitation include epinephrine, lidocaine, atropine, and naloxone. Endotracheal doses of epinephrine should be at least double IV doses.

### Laryngeal Mask Airway

In the last several years, the laryngeal mask airway (LMA) has become a very well-accepted alternative to ET intubation for many elective operative procedures as well as for resuscitation.[28] The device is easy to use, even for nurses and paramedics, and generally can be inserted much more quickly than an endotracheal tube can. It is inserted "blindly," without a laryngoscope.

## Confirmation of Correct Airway Placement

The $P_{ETCO_2}$ can be used to confirm whether an ET tube or LMA has been positioned in the trachea or the esophagus of a cardiac arrest patient. If the $P_{ETCO_2}$ during CPR is very low (below 0.5%) on at least the seventh breath after intubation, it is very likely that the ET tube has been mistakenly placed in the esophagus. Conversely, a moderately low (>0.5% but <2.0%) $P_{ETCO_2}$ does not necessarily indicate esophageal placement of the ET tube, since there are many other causes for this finding during CPR (Table 27–1). An alternative to the measurement of $P_{ETCO_2}$ for confirming airway placement is an aspiration syringe or bulb device attached to the ET tube immediately after it is inserted. If the tip of the ET tube is in the trachea when suction is applied, air is aspirated readily, since the cartilage of the trachea prevents its collapsing. If the tip is in the esophagus, applying suction causes the esophagus to collapse and obstructs the flow of air during aspiration.

## ■ USE OF VASOPRESSORS AND INOTROPIC AGENTS

### Epinephrine

Epinephrine is the vasopressor of choice for use during CPR. It improves coronary and cerebral blood flow by increasing peripheral vasoconstriction. By enhancing coronary perfusion pressure, it facilitates resynthesis of high-energy phosphates in myocardial mitochondria and enhances cellular viability and contractile force.

What is the optimal dose of epinephrine to augment aortic diastolic blood pressure in humans during CPR has been debated. However, recent prospective, randomized clinical trials have not shown better outcomes with "high doses" (e.g., >1 mg in adults) of epinephrine than with standard doses (0.5 to 1 mg).[29–32] The AHA currently recommends an adult IV dose of 0.5 to 1.0 mg at intervals that do not exceed 3 to 5 minutes. Giving higher doses of epinephrine after the initial 1-mg dose during resuscitation is neither recommended nor discouraged. If the dose is given by peripheral injection, it should be followed by a 20-ml flush of IV fluid to ensure delivery of the drug into the central compartment.

During cardiac arrest, epinephrine also may be given by continuous IV infusion

Table 27–1

**Common Causes of Low\* $P_{ETCO_2}$ During Cardiopulmonary Resuscitation**

| | |
|---|---|
| **Inadequate ventilation** | **Ventilation-perfusion mismatch** |
| Unrecognized esophageal intubation | Pulmonary embolism |
| Airway obstruction | **Decreased metabolic production of carbon** |
| **Inadequate blood flow** | **dioxide** |
| Inadequate chest compression | Hypothermia |
| Hypovolemia | |
| Tension pneumothorax | |
| Pericardial tamponade | |

\* <2%.

(30 ml of a 1:1000 solution added to 250 ml of normal saline or 5% dextrose in water [D5W] and infused at 100 ml/hr and titrated to the desired hemodynamic endpoint). Continuous infusions of epinephrine should be administered centrally to reduce the risk of extravasation. Epinephrine should not be added to infusion bags or bottles that contain alkaline solutions.

## Dopamine

Dopamine is less effective than epinephrine at improving blood flow to vital organs during CPR. During resuscitation, treatment with dopamine is usually reserved for patients with hypotension and shock that develops after return of spontaneous circulation. When dopamine is used to treat shock, norepinephrine should be added when more than 20 μg/kg/min is needed to maintain adequate blood pressure.

## Dobutamine

Dobutamine may be the ideal agent to use after return of spontaneous circulation, particularly if congestive heart failure rather than hypotension is present. In animal models, dobutamine that is given within 15 minutes of successful resuscitation can successfully overcome the global systolic and diastolic left ventricular dysfunction that result from prolonged cardiac arrest and CPR.[33] At present, the AHA recommends giving 2.0 to 20 μg/kg/min of dobutamine (500 mg mixed in 250 ml of D5W or normal saline), using the smallest effective dose that improves hemodynamics. The maximum dose is 40 μg/kg/min.

## Vasopressin

Vasopressin produces significantly higher coronary perfusion pressure and myocardial blood flow than epinephrine during closed chest CPR in a pig model of VF.[34] Both vasopressin and adrenocorticotropin concentrations are higher during CPR when resuscitation is successful than when it fails.[35] Because of these observations, there has been considerable interest in the use of vasopressin for supporting coronary perfusion pressure during CPR in humans.

In a small, blinded, randomized clinical study, 20 patients with out-of-hospital VF resistant to electrical defibrillation were treated during resuscitation with epinephrine (1 mg IV) and another 20 with vasopressin (40 U IV).[36] Seven (35%) patients in the epinephrine group and 14 (70%) in the vasopressin group survived to hospital admission (p = .06). At 24 hours, four (20%) epinephrine-treated patients and 12 (60%) vasopressin-treated ones were alive (p = .02). Three (15%) patients in the epinephrine group and eight (40%) in the vasopressin group survived to hospital discharge (p = .16). Neurologic outcomes were similar in both groups.

## ■ ACID-BASE MANAGEMENT

The marked fall in cardiac output during CPR reduces tissue oxygen delivery to critically low levels. Cells shift to anaerobic metabolism, causing gradual buildup of lactic acid. The $P_{CO_2}$ level begins to increase inside cells, including heart muscle cells, in which the $CO_2$ concentration may become very high. PEA develops when the $P_{CO_2}$ in cells exceeds 400 mm Hg.[37]

A dynamic equilibrium is maintained between intracellular $CO_2$ and the blood traversing each capillary bed in the body. As $CO_2$ diffuses into capillary blood in exchange for oxygen, the $CO_2$ is transported to the heart and lungs in venous blood. Because of this, central (mixed) venous blood during closed chest compression is acidotic (pH approximately 7.15) and hypercarbic ($Pv_{CO_2} \sim 74$ mm Hg). During ventilation, $CO_2$ is removed from the lungs. When closed chest compression is performed capably, usually arterial blood pH is normal, slightly acidotic, or mildly alkalotic. Early in resuscitation, arterial blood can be slightly alkalotic while the venous blood is acidotic. Severe arterial acidosis early during closed chest compression is usually due to inadequate ventilation or other forms of acidosis (e.g., lactic acidosis). The best solution is usually to improve the technique of closed chest compression and to increase ventilation, if possible. When, despite confirmed proper endotracheal intubation, hyperventilation, and proper external chest compression, acidosis persists, an alternate method for providing assisted circulation (e.g., open chest compressions or venoarterial bypass) should be considered.

In the past, the recommended early adjunct to closed chest compression was sodium bicarbonate, because it was believed that bicarbonate would buffer the hydrogen ions produced during anaerobic metabolism. Sodium bicarbonate itself contains a large amount of $CO_2$ (260 to 280 mm Hg). In plasma, the $CO_2$ is released and diffuses into cells more rapidly than $HCO_3^-$, causing a paradoxical rise in intracellular $P_{CO_2}$ and a fall in intracellular pH. The increases in intracellular $P_{CO_2}$ in heart muscle cells decrease cardiac contractility, cardiac output, and blood pressure. Sodium bicarbonate causes other potentially harmful effects, including paradoxical acidosis of cerebrospinal fluid, hyperosmolality, alkalemia, and sodium overload.

At present, there are no convincing data to indicate that treatment with sodium bicarbonate is of benefit during closed chest compression, and it does not improve survival in experimental animals. The AHA no longer recommends routine administration of sodium bicarbonate during resuscitation, because it provides minimal benefit, if any, and adds significant risk. If used at all, bicarbonate should not be given until proven interventions such as defibrillation, cardiac compression, support of ventilation (including intubation), and drug therapies such as epinephrine and antiarrhythmic agents have been employed. The recommended initial dose of sodium bicarbonate is 1 mEq/kg. No more than half of the original dose should be given every 10 minutes thereafter. For a small number of "special situations," sodium bicarbonate is indicated for use early, and in some cases repeatedly, during resuscitation. Such circumstances include severe hyperkalemia, known severe metabolic acidosis, and certain toxic conditions (e.g., tricyclic antidepressant or barbiturate overdose). Alternative buffer agents do not appear to improve survival during cardiac resuscitation.[38]

## ■ MANAGEMENT OF VENTRICULAR TACHYARRHYTHMIAS

Electrical countershock is the treatment of choice for VF and pulseless VT. If three initial countershocks at increasing energies (200, 200 to 300, and 360 J), intubation, epinephrine, and a fourth countershock (360 J) fail to terminate the arrhythmia (refractory VF or VT), or if, as in many cases, the arrhythmia rapidly recurs, antiarrhythmic drug therapy is usually recommended. Until recently, the agents most often used for this purpose included lidocaine, bretylium tosylate, procainamide, beta blockers, and magnesium sulfate. Unfortunately, there are no randomized, placebo-controlled clinical trials that investigated whether any of these agents is any better than just repeating electrical countershocks, continuing CPR, and intermittently administering epinephrine.

## Lidocaine Hydrochloride

For refractory VF and pulseless VT, the AHA guidelines suggest an initial lidocaine dose of 1.5 mg/kg for all adults. After spontaneous circulation has been restored, an IV infusion of lidocaine is continued at a rate of 30 to 50 μg/kg/min (2 to 4 mg/min). The need for additional bolus doses of lidocaine is usually guided by clinical response or by plasma lidocaine concentrations.

## Bretylium Tosylate

Bretylium increases myocardial electrical stability by elevating the VF threshold and by reducing the disparity in action potential duration and refractory periods between ischemic and nonischemic myocardium. No difference in clinical outcome (rate of conversion from VT or VF to a more organized rhythm, or survival) has been observed in small, prospective, randomized studies comparing bretylium and lidocaine for the treatment of prehospital VF.[39, 40]

## Procainamide

Procainamide is a type 1 antiarrhythmic agent with presynaptic ganglionic blocking, vasodilating, and modest negative inotropic properties. During resuscitation, procainamide is usually given in a dose of 1 g administered at a rate of 20 to 30 mg/min, followed by a maintenance infusion of 1 to 4 mg/min. An alternative regimen that achieves therapeutic levels faster (in some patients in only 15 minutes) is a loading dose of 17 mg/kg given over 1 hour followed by a maintenance infusion of 2.8 mg/kg/hr. For patients who might "clear" the agent slowly, the loading dose is reduced to 12 mg/kg and the infusion rate is reduced to 1.4 mg/kg/hr. The rate should be reduced or drug administration stopped temporarily if hypotension or prolongation of the QT interval or QRS complex by 50% or more occurs.

## Other Antiarrhythmic Agents and Treatments

Other conventional antiarrhythmic agents that may be tried in patients with recurrent or refractory VT or VF include IV beta blockers and magnesium sulfate. Unfortunately, beta blockers have not been formally studied during cardiac arrest, and recent randomized, placebo-controlled clinical trials have not shown benefit from IV magnesium sulfate.[41, 42]

Recently, there has been considerable interest in the use of IV amiodarone to treat patients with recurrent, life-threatening ventricular arrhythmias. Studies on hospitalized patients have confirmed that this agent is active within minutes after IV administration.[43, 44] It is at least as effective as bretylium in terminating refractory or recurrent, life-threatening ventricular tachyarrhythmias but causes fewer side effects.

In a recent randomized, controlled clinical prehospital trial conducted on 504 cardiac arrest patients with recurrent or refractory ventricular tachyarrhythmias, rapid IV infusion over 1 to 2 minutes of 300 mg of amiodarone at the time of first IV epinephrine dosing resulted in 26% greater survival to hospital admission as compared with standard ACLS therapy.[45] The study was inadequately powered to determine whether IV amiodarone increases survival to hospital discharge. The principal side effects of IV amiodarone are hypotension and bradycardia, which usually respond readily to therapy (volume infusion and vasopressors; atropine and/or electrical pacing).

Other treatment strategies and troubleshooting checklists should be considered when the patient develops refractory or recurrent VT or VF. Underlying metabolic derangements such as hypokalemia and hypomagnesemia should be sought and corrected. Arterial hypoxemia and acidosis should be reversed or minimized by ET intubation, ventilation with 100% oxygen, and proper CPR technique. Proarrhythmic drug effects, hypokalemia, or hypomagnesemia can induce ventricular arrhythmias such as torsades de pointes. Although magnesium sulfate can be tried, torsades de pointes is best managed with electrical pacing (or another form of overdrive suppression such as isoproterenol until pacing is available).

## ▪ MANAGEMENT OF BRADYASYSTOLIC CARDIAC ARREST

Survival is poor, regardless of therapy, for cardiac arrest patients who present with bradyasystole. It is always important to make sure that a lead or monitor electrode has not been disconnected before concluding that a "flat line" is the patient's rhythm, since some patients with such a tracing may have VF (a rhythm more amenable to treatment) masquerading as asystole. Whenever there is any doubt, the monitor lead should be switched quickly to another lead to confirm the diagnosis before treatment is instituted. Atropine sulfate may improve outcome in patients with bradyasystolic cardiac arrest due to excessive vagal stimulation, but it is less effective when asystole or pulseless idioventricular rhythms are the result of prolonged ischemia or mechanical injury in the myocardium.[46]

For patients with bradyasystolic cardiac arrest, a 1-mg IV dose of atropine is administered and is repeated every 3 to 5 minutes if asystole persists. Three milligrams (0.04 mg/kg) given IV is a fully vagolytic dose for most adult patients. A total vagolytic dose of atropine should be reserved for patients with bradyasystolic cardiac arrest. ET atropine dosing (1 to 2 mg diluted in 10 ml of sterile water or normal saline) produces a rapid onset of action similar to that observed with IV injection.

Pacing (transvenous, transthoracic, or transcutaneous) rarely influences survival in "unwitnessed cardiac arrest patients" who, when first found, have asystole or bradycardia without a pulse.[47, 48] However, pacing is extremely useful for bradycardia patients who have a pulse and for certain patients when a pacemaker can be placed immediately after the conduction disturbance develops. In such cases, a precordial thump can also stimulate ventricular complexes and a pulse ("fist pacing").[49]

Endogenous adenosine released during myocardial hypoxia and ischemia relaxes vascular smooth muscle, decreases atrial and ventricular contractility, depresses pacemaker automaticity, and impairs AV conduction. The cellular electrophysiologic effects of adenosine can be competitively antagonized by methylxanthines but not by atropine. Aminophylline, a competitive, nonspecific adenosine antagonist, has been shown to restore cardiac electrical activity within 30 seconds in 12 of 15 in-hospital, bradyasystolic cardiac arrest patients whose condition was refractory to atropine and epinephrine.[50] Another small randomized clinical pilot study found that adenosine blockade restores normal sinus rhythm in some patients whose bradyasystole does not respond to conventional therapy.[51] Although further clinical research will be necessary to determine the potential value of adenosine blockade for bradyasystolic cardiac arrest, adenosine blockade should not be used when VF is present, as it may make it more difficult to terminate the arrhythmia.[52]

## ▪ MANAGEMENT OF PULSELESS ELECTRICAL ACTIVITY

PEA is present when there is organized electrical activity on the electrocardiogram but no effective circulation, as manifested by absence of a detectable pulse.[53] There are many underlying potential causes, but the most common one may be myocardial ischemia and dysfunction due to intramyocardial increases in $CO_2$. Prognosis is generally poor unless a discrete and treatable cause for PEA can be discerned and corrected. Efforts should be directed toward detecting causes such as hypovolemia, hypoxemia, acidosis, tension pneumothorax, and pericardial tamponade.

## ▪ REFERENCES

1. Becker L, et al: Public locations of cardiac arrest. Implications for public access defibrillation. Circulation 1998;97(21):2106–2109.
2. Bayes de Luna A, Coumel P, Leclercq JF: Ambulatory sudden cardiac death: Mechanisms of production of fatal arrhythmia on the basis of data from 157 cases. Am Heart J 1989;117:151–159.
3. Cummins RO, et al: Improving survival from sudden cardiac arrest: The "chain of survival" concept. A statement for health professionals from the Advanced Cardiac Life Support Subcommittee and the Emergency Cardiac Care Committee, American Heart Association. Circulation 1991;83(5):1832–1847.
4. Saklayen M, Liss H, Markert R: In-hospital cardiopulmonary resuscitation. Survival in 1 hospital and literature review. Medicine 1995;74(4):163–175.
5. Lombardi G, Gallagher J, Gennis P: Outcome of out of hospital cardiac arrest in New York City. The Pre Hospital Arrest Survival Evaluation (PHASE) Study. JAMA 1994;271(9):678–683.
6. Becker LB, et al: Outcome of CPR in a large metropolitan area—Where are the survivors? Ann Emerg Med 1991;20(4):355–361.
7. Eisenberg MS, et al: Cardiac arrest and resuscitation: A tale of 29 cities. Ann Emerg Med 1990;19(2):179–186.
8. White RD, et al: High discharge survival rate after out-of-hospital ventricular fibrillation with rapid defibrillation by police and paramedics. Ann Emerg Med 1996;28(5):480–485.
9. Paradis NA, et al: Coronary perfusion pressure and the return of spontaneous circulation in human cardiopulmonary resuscitation. JAMA 1990;263(8):1106–1113.
10. Ornato JP: Hemodynamic monitoring during CPR. Ann Emerg Med 1993;22(2 Pt 2):289–295.
11. Montgomery WH: Mechanisms and methods of cardiopulmonary resuscitation. Anesthesiol Clin North Am 1995;13(4):767–783.
12. Chandra NC: Mechanisms of blood flow during CPR. Ann Emerg Med 1993;22(2 Pt 2):281–288.
13. Criley JM, Blaufuss AH, Kissel GL: Self-administered cardiopulmonary resuscitation by cough-induced cardiac compression. Trans Am Clin Climatol Assoc 1976;87:138–146.
14. Criley JM, et al: The heart is a conduit in CPR. Crit Care Med 1981;9(5):373–374.
15. Porter TR, et al: Transesophageal echocardiography to assess mitral valve function and flow during cardiopulmonary resuscitation. Am J Cardiol 1992;70(11):1056–1060.
16. Sack JB, Gerber RS, Kesselbrenner MB: Active compression-decompression cardiopulmonary resuscitation. JAMA 1992;268(22):3200–3201.
17. Stiell IG, et al: The Ontario trial of active compression-decompression cardiopulmonary resuscitation for in-hospital and prehospital cardiac arrest. JAMA 1996;275(18):1417–1423.
18. Sack JB, Kesselbrenner MB, Jarrad A: Interposed abdominal compression-cardiopulmonary resuscitation and resuscitation outcome during asystole and electromechanical dissociation. Circulation 1992;86(6):1692–1700.
19. Halle AA 3rd: Alternatives to conventional chest compression. New Horiz 1997;5(2):112–119.
20. Tang W, et al: Phased chest and abdominal compression-decompression. A new option for cardiopulmonary resuscitation. Circulation 1997;95(5):1335–1340.
21. Ornato JP, et al: Multicenter study of a portable, hand-size, colorimetric end-tidal carbon dioxide detection device. Ann Emerg Med 1992;21(5):518–523.
22. Ornato JP, Garnett AR, Glauser FL: Relationship between cardiac output and the end-tidal carbon dioxide tension. Ann Emerg Med 1990;19(10):1104–1106.
23. Garnett AR, et al: End-tidal carbon dioxide monitoring during cardiopulmonary resuscitation. JAMA 1987;257(4):512–515.
24. Weil MH, et al: Cardiac output and end-tidal carbon dioxide. Crit Care Med 1985;13(11):907–909.
25. Falk JL, Rackow EC, Weil MH: End-tidal carbon dioxide concentration during cardiopulmonary resuscitation. N Engl J Med 1988;318(10):607–611.
26. Ornato JP, et al: The effect of applied chest compression force on systemic arterial pressure and end-tidal carbon dioxide concentration during CPR in human beings. Ann Emerg Med 1989;18(7):732–737.
27. Levine RL, Wayne MA, Miller CC: End-tidal carbon dioxide and outcome of out-of-hospital cardiac arrest. N Engl J Med 1997;337(5):301–306.

28. Bryden DC, Gwinnutt CL: Tracheal intubation via the laryngeal mask airway: A viable alternative to direct laryngoscopy for nursing staff during cardiopulmonary resuscitation. Resuscitation 1998;36(1):19–22.

29. Gueugniaud PY, et al: A comparison of repeated high doses and repeated standard doses of epinephrine for cardiac arrest outside the hospital. N Engl J Med 1998;339(22):1595–1601.

30. Callaham M, et al: A randomized clinical trial of high-dose epinephrine and norepinephrine vs standard-dose epinephrine in prehospital cardiac arrest. JAMA 1992;268(19):2667–2672.

31. Brown CG, Martin DR, Pepe PE: A comparison of standard dose epinephrine and high dose epinephrine in cardiac arrest outside the hospital. N Engl J Med 1992;327:1051–1055.

32. Stiell IG, Hebert PC, Weitzman BN: A study of high-dose epinephrine in human CPR. N Engl J Med 1992;327:1047–1050.

33. Kern KB, et al: Postresuscitation left ventricular systolic and diastolic dysfunction. Treatment with dobutamine. Circulation 1997;95(12):2610–2613.

34. Lindner KH, et al: Vasopressin improves vital organ blood flow during closed-chest cardiopulmonary resuscitation in pigs. Circulation 1995;91(1):215–221.

35. Lindner KH, et al: Release of endogenous vasopressors during and after cardiopulmonary resuscitation. Heart 1996;75(2):145–150.

36. Lindner KH, et al: Randomised comparison of epinephrine and vasopressin in patients with out-of-hospital ventricular fibrillation. Lancet 1997;349(9051):535–537.

37. Johnson BA, et al: Mechanisms of myocardial hypercarbic acidosis during cardiac arrest. J Appl Physiol 1995;78(4):1579–1584.

38. Dybvik T, Strand T, Steen PA: Buffer therapy during out-of-hospital cardiopulmonary resuscitation. Resuscitation 1995;29(2):89–95.

39. Haynes RE, Chinn TL, Copass MK: Comparison of bretylium tosylate and lidocaine in management of out-of-hospital ventricular fibrillation: A randomized clinical trial. Am J Cardiol 1981;48:353–356.

40. Olson DW, Thompson BM, Darin JC: A randomized comparison study of bretylium tosylate and lidocaine in resuscitation of patients from out-of-hospital ventricular fibrillation in a paramedic system. Ann Emerg Med 1984;13:807–810.

41. Thel MC, et al: Randomised trial of magnesium in in-hospital cardiac arrest. Duke Internal Medicine Housestaff. Lancet 1997;350(9087):1272–1276.

42. Miller B, et al: Pilot study of intravenous magnesium sulfate in refractory cardiac arrest: Safety data and recommendations for future studies. Resuscitation 1995;30(1):3–14.

43. Scheinman MM, et al: Dose-ranging study of intravenous amiodarone in patients with life-threatening ventricular tachyarrhythmias. The Intravenous Amiodarone Multicenter Investigators Group. Circulation 1995;92(11):3264–3272.

44. Kowey PR, et al: Randomized, double-blind comparison of intravenous amiodarone and bretylium in the treatment of patients with recurrent, hemodynamically destabilizing ventricular tachycardia or fibrillation. The Intravenous Amiodarone Multicenter Investigators Group. Circulation 1995;92(11):3255–3263.

45. Kudenchuk P: Amiodarone in out-of-hospital Resuscitation of Refractory Sustained Ventricular Tachyarrhythmias (ARREST) study. American Heart Association Scientific Sessions Late-Breaking Clinical Trials Presentation, Orlando, FL, 1997.

46. Herlitz J, et al: Predictors of early and late survival after out-of-hospital cardiac arrest in which asystole was the first recorded arrhythmia on scene. Resuscitation 1994;28(1):27–36.

47. Ornato JP, Carveth WL, Windle JR: Pacemaker insertion for prehospital bradyasystolic cardiac arrest. Ann Emerg Med 1984;13(2):101–103.

48. White JD, Brown CG: Immediate transthoracic pacing for cardiac asystole in an emergency department setting. Am J Emerg Med 1985;3(2):125–128.

49. Tucker KJ, Shaburihvili TS, Gedevanishvili AT: Manual external (fist) pacing during high-degree atrioventricular block: A lifesaving intervention. Am J Emerg Med 1995;13(1):53–54.

50. Viskin S, et al: Aminophylline for bradyasystolic cardiac arrest refractory to atropine and epinephrine. Ann Intern Med 1993;118:279–281.

51. Mader TJ, Gibson P: Adenosine receptor antagonism in refractory asystolic cardiac arrest: Results of a human pilot study. Resuscitation 1997;35(1):3–7.

52. Littmann L, et al: Aminophylline fails to improve the outcome of cardiopulmonary resuscitation from prolonged ventricular fibrillation: A placebo-controlled, randomized, blinded experimental study. J Am Coll Cardiol 1994;23(7):1708–1714.

53. Paradis NA, et al: Aortic pressure during human cardiac arrest. Identification of pseudo-electromechanical dissociation. Chest 1992;101(1):123–128.

# ■ RECOMMENDED READING

Becker L, et al: Public locations of cardiac arrest. Implications for pubic access defibrillation. Circulation 198;97(21):2106–2109.

Cummins RO, et al: Improving survival from sudden cardiac arrest: The "chain of survival" concept. A statement for health professionals from the Advanced Cardiac Life Support Subcommittee and the Emergency Cardiac Care Committee, American Heart Association. Circulation 1991;83(5):1832–1847.

Kowey PR, et al: Randomized, double-blind comparison of intravenous amiodarone and bretylium in the treatment of patients with recurrent, hemodynamically destabilizing ventricular tachycardia or fibrillation. The Intravenous Amiodarone Multicenter Investigators Group. Circulation 1995;92(11):3255–3263.

Lindner KH, et al: Randomised comparison of epinephrine and vasopressin in patients with out-of-hospital ventricular fibrillation. Lancet 1997;349(9051):535–539.

White RD, et al: High discharge survival rate after out-of-hospital ventricular fibrillation with rapid defibrillation by police and paramedics. Ann Emerg Med 1996;28(5):480–485.

Chapter 28

# Rehabilitation After Acute Myocardial Infarction

*Fredric J. Pashkow*

Cardiac rehabilitation as practiced today is a synthesis of exercise training, risk factor modification, psychosocial support, and education for the purpose of facilitating readaptation to normal life by means of improved functional performance and coronary artery disease (CAD) risk factors (Fig. 28–1).

Randomized studies performed mainly between 1975 and 1985 typically suggested a 20% to 30% reduction in cardiovascular mortality and sudden cardiac death but generally failed to achieve individual statistical significance largely because of insufficient sample size (Table 28–1). Beyond traditional cardiac endpoints, improved quality of life and cost utility have also become important contemporary outcome goals.

Cardiac rehabilitation is rapidly changing with the dynamics of shortened length of hospital stays, a changing patient population, and the impact of large clinical trials of cholesterol-lowering drugs. It is provided now by many models: institution or center based, community based, or at home. Our observation is that those patients stratified at low risk benefit most by the modification of coronary risk factors and that patients previously thought to be poor candidates for rehabilitation (such as the elderly or those with significant left ventricular [LV] dysfunction and low work capacity) may experience substantial relative functional benefits.

Beyond exercise, the role of risk factor modification for patients with known CAD has become even more established. In addition to the reduction of future acute coronary events and the need for subsequent revascularization, newer data suggest the potential to arrest and in some cases actually effect regression of coronary atherosclerosis.

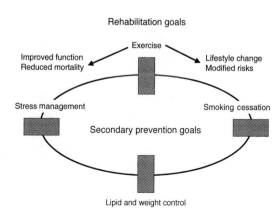

**Figure 28–1** ▪ Components of cardiac rehabilitation. Relative contribution of exercise to rehabilitation versus secondary prevention. (Adapted from Pashkow FJ, Dafoe WA: Cardiac rehabilitation as a model for integrated cardiovascular care. *In* Pashkow FJ, Dafoe WA [eds]: Clinical Cardiac Rehabilitation: A Cardiologist's Guide, 2nd ed. Baltimore: Williams & Wilkins, 1999:7.)

## Table 28-1
### Outcomes of Selected Prospective Cardiac Rehabilitation Trials

| Investigators | Year | Subjects (no.) | Follow-up (mo) | Cardiovascular Deaths | | | Nonfatal MIs | | |
|---|---|---|---|---|---|---|---|---|---|
| | | | | Treatment % | Control % | p | Treatment % | Control % | p |
| Kentala | 1972 | 158 | 24 | 10.39 | 12.35 | NS | 7.79 | 4.94 | NS |
| Wilhelmsen | 1975 | 315 | 48 | 17.72 | 21.02 | NS | 15.82 | 17.83 | NS |
| Palatsi | 1976 | 380 | 29 | 4.20 | 5.80 | NS | 4.90 | 6.00 | NS |
| Hakkila* | 1977 | 350 | 23 | 10.40 | 12.30 | NS | | | |
| Kallio* | 1979 | 375 | 36 | 18.62 | 29.41 | 0.02 | 18.09 | 11.23 | <0.10 |
| Shaw | 1981 | 651 | 36 | 4.33 | 6.10 | 0.4 | 4.64 | 3.35 | NS |
| Carson | 1982 | 303 | 24 | 7.95 | 13.82 | NS(1) | 7.80 | 6.58 | NS |
| Vermeulen | 1983 | 98 | 60 | 4.26 | 9.80 | NS | 8.51 | 17.65 | 0.05 |
| Rechnitzer | 1983 | 733 | 48 | 3.96 | 3.67 | NS | 10.29 | 9.32 | NS |
| Román | 1983 | 193 | 108 | 13.98 | 24.00 | NS(2) | 9.68 | 8.00 | NS(2) |
| WHO | 1984 | 1360 | 36 | 11.91 | 13.44 | NS | 10.64 | 9.16 | NS |
| Froelicher | 1984 | 146 | 12 | 0.00 | 1.35 | NS | 1.39 | 2.70 | NS |
| Marra | 1985 | 167 | 55 | 5.95 | 4.82 | NS | 5.95 | 10.84 | NS |
| Hedbäck† | 1987 | 305 | 60 | 27.21 | 30.38 | NS | 17.30 | 33.30 | 0.02 |
| Hämäläinen* | 1989 | 375 | 120 | 35.10 | 47.10 | 0.02 | 25.60 | 19.30 | NS |
| Hedbäck† | 1993 | 305 | 120 | 36.70 | 48.10 | <0.001 | 28.60 | 39.90 | <0.001 |
| Debusk | 1994 | 585 | 12 | 3.80 | 3.10 | NS | | | |
| Haskell | 1994 | 300 | 48 | 1.38 | 1.94 | NS | 4.14 | 7.10 | 0.23 |

*, †Same study populations.

NS(1) Significant for those with inferior wall MI. p < 0.01.

NS(2) Using life-table analysis. p < 0.05 using crude death rate.

MI, myocardial infarction; WHO, World Health Organization.

Adapted from Pashkow FJ, Pasternak R: Cardiac rehabilitation and risk factor modification. *In* Fuster V, Ross R, Topol EJ (eds): Atherosclerosis and Coronary Artery Disease. Philadelphia / New York: Lippincott-Raven, 1996:1267–1282.

Kentala E: Physical fitness and feasibility of physical rehabilitation after myocardial infarction in men of working age. Ann Clin Res 1972;9(suppl):1–84.

Wilhelmsen L, Sanne H, Elmfeldt D, et al: A controlled trial of physical training after myocardial infarction: Effects on risk factors, nonfatal reinfarction, and death. Prev Med 1975;4:491–508.

Palatsi I: Feasibility of physical training after myocardial infarction and its effect on return to work, morbidity and mortality. Acta Medica Scand 1976;599(suppl):1–84.

Hakkila J: Morbidity and mortality after myocardial infarction. Bib Cardiol 1977;36:159.

Kallio V, Hämäläinen H, Hakkila J, et al: Reduction of sudden deaths by a multifactorial intervention program after acute myocardial infarction. Lancet 1979;2:1091–1094.

Shaw LW: Effects of a prescribed supervised exercise program on mortality and cardiovascular morbidity in patients after myocardial infarction. The National Exercise and Heart Disease Project. Am J Cardiol 1981;48:39–46.

Carson P, Phillips R, Lloyd M, et al: Exercise after myocardial infarction: A controlled trial. J R Coll Physicians Lond 1982;16:147–151.

Vermeulen A, Lie KI, Durrer D: Effects of cardiac rehabilitation after myocardial infarction: changes in coronary risk factors and long-term prognosis. Am Heart J 1983;105:798–801.

Rechnitzer PA, Cunningham DA, Donner AP, et al: Characteristics that predicted recurrence of infarction within 3 years in the Ontario Exercise-Heart Collaborative Study. Can Med Assoc J 1983;1:1.

Román O, Gutierrez M, Luksic I, et al: Cardiac rehabilitation after acute myocardial infarction: 9-year controlled follow-up study. Cardiology 1983;70:223–231.

WHO: Rehabilitation and comprehensive secondary prevention after acute myocardial infarction. Euro Rep Stud 1983;84:1–99.

Froelicher V, Jensen D, Genter F, et al: A randomized trial of exercise training in patients with coronary heart disease. JAMA 1984;252:1291–1297.

Marra S, Paolillo V, Spadaccini F, et al: Long-term follow-up after a controlled randomized post-myocardial infarction rehabilitation programme: Effects on morbidity and mortality. Eur Heart J 1985;6:656–663.

Hedbäck B, Perk J: 5-year results of a comprehensive rehabilitation programme after myocardial infarction. Eur Heart J 1987;8:234–242.

Hämäläinen H, Luurila OJ, Kallio V, et al: Long-term reduction in sudden deaths after multifactorial intervention programme in patients with myocardial infarction: 10-year results of a controlled investigation. Eur Heart J 1989;10:55–62.

Hedbäck B, Perk J, Wodlin P: Long-term reduction of cardiac mortality after myocardial infarction: 10-year results of a comprehensive rehabilitation programme. Eur Heart J 1993;14:831–853.

DeBusk RF, Miller NH, Superko HR, et al: A case-management system for coronary risk factor modification after acute myocardial infarction. Ann Intern Med 1994;120:721–729.

Haskell WL, Alderman EL, Fair JM, et al: Effects of intensive multiple risk factor reduction on coronary atherosclerosis and clinical cardiac events in men and women with coronary artery disease. The Stanford Coronary Risk Intervention Project (SCRIP). Circulation 1994;89:975–990.

## ■ EVOLUTION OF CARDIAC REHABILITATION FROM PROGRESSIVE ACTIVITY

Cardiac rehabilitation had its beginnings as a formalization of escalating physical activity after acute myocardial infarction (MI).[1] Until the early 1950s, exercise following acute MI was thought to be ill advised and patients were prescribed extended periods of bed rest. Levine and Lown experimented with earlier activities such as chair sitting and progressive ambulating.[2] By the late 1960s, 3 weeks' hospitalization after MI was still routine in the United States. Research related to early mobilization burgeoned in the 1970s, particularly in the United Kingdom and in countries where the cost of hospitalization had already become a major social welfare issue. It evolved into structured exercise training before or after hospital discharge, but in the past decade it has matured into a multidisciplinary effort serving as a comprehensive preventive cardiac practice encompassing risk stratification, exercise training, secondary risk factor modification, and personal/vocational adjustment.[3]

## ■ PHYSIOLOGY OF EXERCISE RELEVANT TO CONDITIONING IN PATIENTS WITH CORONARY ARTERY DISEASE

Peripheral adaptations, mainly consisting of more efficient oxygen extraction and use of oxygen by skeletal muscle, account for much of the improvement in functional capacity associated with exercise training. The reduction in activity-related symptoms experienced by many patients with CAD who have received moderate-intensity exercise training is, in large part, a result of the diminished coronary blood supply required to meet the reduced myocardial oxygen demand needed to perform a given amount of physical work. This is especially evident at submaximal workloads, below the anaerobic threshold. Anaerobic threshold is the highest oxygen uptake that can be maintained without an increase in lactate levels.[4] It effectively delineates routine daily activities from athletic endeavors. Exercise training results in a lowering of peripheral vascular resistance, heart rate, and intramyocardial wall tension during exercise, generally producing an improvement in exercise duration.

Exercise alone has not been studied in coronary angiographic regression trials. However, an intensive physical training program in association with moderate diet intervention has been shown to have a favorable effect on the progression of coronary atherosclerotic lesions and stress-induced myocardial ischemia in patients with stable angina pectoris.[5] Furthermore, this same group of trials has shown that the extent of improvement (progression, stabilization, regression) was associated with the weekly amount of physical exercise. Regression was noted only in patients expending an average of 2200 kcal/week, whereas angiographically determined slowing of coronary lesion progression was observed in patients averaging approximately 1500 kcal/week. The salutary effect of exercise training on peripheral vascular resistance, autonomic nervous system adaptations, blood coagulation, and platelet function will likely be linked to both the process of primary atherogenesis and the role of plaque rupture leading to initiation of acute coronary events.

Consistent evidence that exercise stimulates development of coronary collateralization in humans has been lacking,[6] but studies published in the past several years suggest that adaptations can occur and that they may improve coronary blood flow[7] and collateralization.[8] Studies suggest that regression is significantly related to a decrease in collateralization.[9] Improvement in ventricular systolic function as a result of exercise training has been reported in elderly normal persons[10] but generally not in those with CAD.[11]

Ejection fraction is a poor predictor of endurance functional capacity. This appears to be related primarily to the intrinsic capacity of a patient's heart rate to increase appropriately and secondarily to the capability to improve stroke volume by changes in load or contractility. A patient with an extremely large heart and an adequate heart rate reserve (via a normal chronotropic response) may have adequate cardiac output to perform moderate endurance exercise despite a very low ejection fraction.[12]

## ■ COMPONENTS OF PROGRAM DESIGN

Cardiac rehabilitation programs have traditionally been designated by phases according to a patient's temporal and functional status relative to an index coronary event. Although falling out of favor in some institutions, this designative system remains useful for classification purposes. Phase I rehabilitation is an inpatient therapy. The major goal for the physical activity portion of the phase I program is to condition patients for the exertional demands required after discharge. This has been a reasonably straightforward task because most activities of daily living in the home are below the 3 to 4 MET level (1 MET = *met*abolic oxygen requirement for resting conditions). However, shorter hospital stays have reduced the time available for inpatient exercise training. The time available is not adequate to acquire the skills required for self-monitoring of exercise activity or for adequately achieving an understanding of the disease process. With patients often overwhelmed by the chaos of the acute coronary event, it is difficult to do more than begin the process of identifying risk factors and changing lifestyles. Thus, an appropriate trend in phase I programs is to focus more on evaluation of risks and needs and to motivate patients to participate in the appropriate outpatient (phase II or III) rehabilitation program. Phase II programs are both electrocardiogram (ECG) monitored and supervised; phase III programs are supervised only. Current outpatient programs, whether phase II or III, are generally center-based group experiences offering ECG monitoring, exercise supervision, education, and risk factor management. The exercise component occurs concurrently with education and group psychosocial support for modification of CAD-prone behavior and for satisfactory return to a suitable and active lifestyle.[13]

Using a multifactorial approach, all potential risk factors should be addressed.[3] Patients of working age usually have vocational and job-specific issues as well.[14] With an increasing emphasis on quality survival and economic valuation of the service,[15] the major focus of many programs has gone well beyond the presumed impact of exercise training on mortality. Today, cardiac rehabilitation is being refashioned as a "soft technology" with great potential to influence outcomes including, but not limited to, long-term postinfarction survival. It is likely that in the future, the emphasis will be on phase III outpatient programs that can provide supervision and guidance to large numbers of patients in relatively low-cost community-based[16] or at-home programs.[17]

## ■ RISK STRATIFICATION

Cardiac rehabilitation has been the wellspring of several important concepts in contemporary cardiology, including progressive activity after MI, perceived exertion measurement, and risk stratification. The process of risk stratification has become an integral part of the treatment of patients during and after any acute myocardial event.[18] Three factors determine the prognosis for any patient who has had an MI: the amount of myocardium currently ischemic, the extent of LV dysfunction, and the patient's myocardial arrhythmic potential (Fig. 28–2). The results of the risk

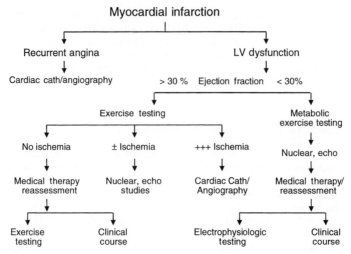

**Figure 28–2** ■ Risk stratification of patients after myocardial infarction. (Adapted from Pashkow FJ, Dafoe WA: Cardiac rehabilitation as a model for integrated cardiovascular care. *In* Pashkow FJ, Dafoe WA [eds]: Clinical Cardiac Rehabilitation: A Cardiologist's Guide, 2nd ed. Baltimore: Williams & Wilkins, 1999:10.)

stratification process thus serve as mileposts for patient care (Table 28–2). In addition, the results of risk stratification define a patient's treatment throughout the rehabilitative process. The designations of low, intermediate, or high risk are then applied for purposes of guidelines and standards used for program planning and operations, for example, staffing and allocation of resources such as ECG telemetry, and for reimbursement of program services.[19, 20]

## ■ TRIALS OF EXERCISE ALONE OR EXERCISE PLUS ADDITIONAL INTERVENTIONS

Individual prospective studies performed mainly from the 1970s into the 1980s (see Table 28–1) showed a trend toward reduced mortality in those participating after an acute MI. Insufficient sample size, limited follow-up duration, and dropout rates as high as 50% resulted in insufficient statistical power for any single random-

Table 28–2

**Characteristics of Low-, Intermediate-, and High-Risk Disease as Defined During Exercise Testing**

| Low Risk | High Risk |
|---|---|
| ≥8 METs 3 wk after cardiac event | ≤5 METs 3 wk after cardiac event |
| No symptoms | Exercise-induced hypotension |
| **Intermediate Risk** | Ischemia induced at low levels of exercise |
| ≤8 METs 3 wk after cardiac event | Persistence of ischemia after exercise |
| Angina with moderate or intense exercise | Sustained arrhythmia |
| History of congestive heart failure | |

METs, metabolic equivalents.
From Pashkow FJ, Dafoe WA: Cardiac rehabilitation as a model for integrated cardiovascular care. *In* Pashkow FJ, Dafoe WA (eds): Clinical Cardiac Rehabilitation: A Cardiologist's Guide, 2nd ed. Baltimore: Williams & Wilkins, 1999:11.

ized trial of exercise training to prove its efficacy.[21, 22] In 1988, Oldridge and colleagues published a meta-analysis of 10 randomized clinical trials that included 4347 patients. It suggested a reduction in the incidence of overall and cardiovascular mortality of about 25% in those participating in exercise rehabilitation.[21] Exercise training started between 8 and 36 weeks after MI, and duration varied between 6 and 48 months. These pooled data showed a significant reduction in both all-cause and cardiovascular mortality with an odds ratio (OR) of 0.76 (95% confidence interval [CI] 0.63 to 0.92, p = 0.004). The reduction in mortality was more marked in those exercising for 52 weeks or more and was only marginally significant among those exercising 12 to 52 weeks. No statistically significant effect on mortality was observed for those exercising 12 weeks or less. This is especially noteworthy because most contemporary programs deliver (and are only maximally reimbursed for) 8 to 12 weeks of program participation, with variable (and largely unknown) participation thereafter.

O'Connor and colleagues published a similar analysis the following year and came to a similar conclusion—namely, that cardiac rehabilitation reduced overall and cardiovascular mortality by 20%. They further noted a 37% reduction in the incidence of sudden cardiac death (OR 0.63; 95% CIs 0.41, 0.97) within the first year after exercise training. The ORs and 95% CIs at 2 and 3 years were 0.76 (0.54, 1.06) and 0.92 (0.69, 1.23), respectively, which suggest a benefit, but they are not statistically significant.[22]

Other studies report that the incidence of sudden death is favorably affected by exercise training. Exercise may contribute to improved electrical stability of the myocardium by virtue of a number of different mechanisms: decreased regional ischemia at submaximal exercise, decreased ambient catecholamines in myocardial substrate at rest and submaximal exercise, and increased ventricular fibrillation threshold due to reduction of cyclic adenosine monophosphate.

Other explanations for the impact on mortality have been postulated. An alteration of the balance between sympathetic and parasympathetic activity occurs in those undergoing endurance exercise training. This has been noted in the modification of heart rate variability observed by spectral analysis indicating an increase in vagal tone with physical training.[23]

Increased surveillance in the rehabilitation environment may in part explain the one-third reduction in the incidence of sudden death.[16] Frequent, regular contact with knowledgeable and experienced staff provides an opportunity for earlier discovery of potentially destabilizing factors such as decompensating ischemia or heart failure. The fact that patients fare well when exercising under direct observation in the rehabilitation environment is further suggested by VanCamp and Peterson's 1986 survey that revealed only 3 deaths among 21 cardiac arrests occurring during more than 2,000,000 patient-hours of exercise training.[24] Cardiac rehabilitation thus may influence both the incidence of sudden death and survival from sudden death.

Both the Oldridge and O'Connor meta-analyses failed to show any decrease in nonfatal reinfarction with exercise-based cardiac rehabilitation programs. In addition to the possibility that this lack of effect is real, other factors may explain this observation, including inadequate attention to other risk factors, selection bias leading to lower participation in rehabilitation programs for patients with ongoing symptoms and risk of reinfarction, and finally, inadequate follow-up.

## ■ MODIFICATIONS OF OTHER RISK FACTORS FOR CORONARY ARTERY DISEASE

Because of the manifold causes of CAD and the multidisciplinary interventions used by contemporary cardiac rehabilitation programs, it is difficult to determine the benefits of individual interventions targeted to specific risk factors. Clearly, the trend toward a more aggressive secondary preventive approach has had an impact on both the design and, in all likelihood, the effects of cardiac rehabilitation programs. Several lines of evidence point to the benefits of the multifactorial approach. In addition to exercise, attention is appropriately directed to psychological factors, diabetes and smoking cessation (see Chapters 22 and 42), and control of lipid abnormalities (see Chapter 24) and hypertension (see Chapter 32).

Advances in our understanding of the pathogenesis of acute coronary syndromes has led to an evolution of secondary preventive approaches that rationally combine multiple risk factor interventions targeted to an individual's unique combination of risk factors. Understanding of patient-based lifestyle and behaviors relevant to modification of appropriate risk factors is ideally managed through the multidisciplinary individualized approach available in comprehensive post-MI cardiac rehabilitation programs.

## ■ PSYCHOLOGICAL STRESS AND DEPRESSION, THEIR IMPACT ON CARDIAC EVENTS AND SURVIVAL, AND THE BENEFITS OF EXERCISE TRAINING

The relationship between the heart and the brain has been the subject of speculation for ages, but an understanding of the details of this association and its impact on the prognosis and treatment of CAD is only relatively recent. A relationship between neural activity and ventricular fibrillation has been observed, and that psychological stress can predispose humans to sudden cardiac death has been documented.[25]

The existence and association of certain specific personality characteristics with CAD has been controversial for many years, since first being reported by Rosenman and Friedman. The type A personality profile includes such behavioral characteristics as aggressiveness/competitiveness, time urgency, and labile hostility. It has been linked to mortality due to CAD as well as to the extent and progression of coronary atherosclerosis. Studies over time have failed to consistently confirm this relationship, however, and the current thought is that some element of the classic personality profile such as anger/hostility constitutes the potentially destructive component.[26]

Depression is common in the post-MI period.[27] Frasure-Smith and colleagues have shown that major depression following MI has a significant *independent* impact on cardiac mortality during the first 6 months after hospital discharge.[28] Depression was the most significant predictor of mortality (hazard ratio, 5.74; 95% CI, 4.61 to 6.87; p = .0006). The impact of depression remained significant even after control for LV dysfunction and previous MI, which were also significant multivariate predictors of mortality (adjusted hazard ratio, 4.29; 95% CI, 3.14 to 5.44; p = .013).

Other manifestations of psychosocial dysfunction are important as well. These include social isolation and degree of life stress. Data also suggest a lack of recognition and treatment of these serious comorbid psychosocial conditions.

Exercise has been popularly described as improving psychological well-being. Anecdotally, patients report significant subjective improvements in mood, anxiety, and self-confidence. The emphasis of studies relevant to this issue has generally been on specific alterations of psychological measures or personality such as positive self-concept and self-esteem. Neurophysiologic improvements have also been observed. For example, in patients with ischemic heart disease, exercise training reduced plasma norepinephrine levels. The addition of psychosocial treatments to standard cardiac rehabilitation regimens reduces mortality and morbidity, psychological distress, and some biologic risk factors.[29]

Thus, cardiac rehabilitation produces measurable worthwhile psychological effects in patients with CAD and provides an alternative or adjunct for improving pathologic psychological conditions. Thus, it appears that affective and stress disorders are potentially important issues to be addressed in patients with CAD, and the cardiac rehabilitation experience provides an excellent opportunity to address psychological issues.

## ■ QUALITY OF LIFE AN ALTERNATIVE ENDPOINT

Quality of life has become an increasingly prominent issue in medicine and cardiology during the past decade.[30] Although interest has been focused on the impact of higher cost modalities of therapy such as coronary bypass surgery on quality of life, many other approaches, regardless of their expense, will now increasingly be analyzed in the same way.[31] Cardiac rehabilitation is no exception, and as measures of quality of life become better understood and more standardized, these subjective outcomes will be more closely and appropriately scrutinized.

Cardiac rehabilitation makes an important difference in perceived quality of life. Many participants enjoy and value their rehabilitation program, but measurable differences attributable to quality have been scarce. In a study in which low-risk patients underwent a brief period of rehabilitation, little difference was observed between those patients who participated in rehabilitation and those who received usual care.[32] Low-risk patients will likely recover normal performance of routine activities of daily living, regardless of whether they participate in an exercise rehabilitation program. Rehabilitation is less likely to affect their perception of quality of life.

The potential impact on quality of life is inherently greater, however, the lower the functional capacity of the patient at the time of program entry. Assuming the absence of other major obstacles to exercise training, conditioning may result in sufficient capacity to perform most activities of daily living—for example, maintaining independence, assisting an invalid spouse, or participating in most socially integrating activities (Fig. 28–3).

## ■ REDUCTION IN CLINICAL EVENTS AS A SURROGATE OF ATHEROSCLEROTIC REGRESSION

During the past decade, the focus on secondary prevention of atherosclerotic CAD within the context of cardiac rehabilitation programs has been heightened.[18] A number of clinically important studies using serial angiography have provided convincing evidence that a slowing of progression or actual regression of coronary atherosclerosis can occur with interventions.[33, 34] Most studies have focused on strategies to improve serum lipid values by lowering serum low-density lipoprotein cholesterol (LDL-C) levels and by raising serum high-density lipoprotein cholesterol

**Figure 28–3** ■ The impact of exercise training on a hypothetical patient with restricted exercise tolerance at the time of entry. Note that the patient, who is essentially sedentary at the time of entry, can achieve a functional capacity that brackets the majority of activities of daily living by the completion of 8 to 12 weeks of exercise training. CO, cardiac output; ADL, activities of daily living; METs, metabolic equivalents, where sitting at rest (1 MET) requires oxygen at a rate of 3.5 ml/kg/min.

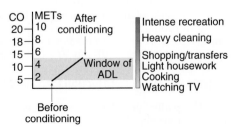

(HDL-C) levels through the use of drugs, diet, exercise, stress reduction, or combinations of these.

Ornish and colleagues published results from a prospective, randomized, controlled trial suggesting that comprehensive lifestyle changes can affect coronary atherosclerosis after only 1 year.[34] In this study, 28 patients were assigned to an experimental group (low-fat vegetarian diet, smoking cessation, stress management training, and moderate exercise) and 20 to a usual-care control group. One hundred ninety-five coronary artery lesions were analyzed by quantitative coronary angiography. The average percentage diameter of stenosis regressed from 40.0% (SD 16.9) to 37.8% (SD 16.5) in the experimental group yet progressed from 42.7% (SD 15.5) to 46.1% (SD 18.5) in the control group. In the experimental group, total cholesterol fell by 24.3% and LDL-C by 37.4%, despite a relatively low fat consumption of about 30% of calories derived from fat before baseline testing.

Significant regression of atherosclerotic lesions after aggressive lipid-lowering treatment without lipid-lowering drugs has also been documented in angiographic studies by Schuler and associates.[5] They tested the appropriateness and effects of intensive physical exercise and low-fat diet on coronary morphology and myocardial perfusion in patients with CAD manifested as active angina. After 12 months of intensive physical exercise and low-fat, low-cholesterol diet (American Heart Association phase 3 diet), total cholesterol decreased by 10% (p < 0.001); triglycerides by 24% (p < .001), and HDL by 3% (p = NS).

Repeat coronary angiography showed relative and minimal diameter reductions using quantitative image processing. Stress-induced myocardial ischemia improved as well. In the intervention group, progression of coronary lesions was noted in nine patients (23%), no change was noted in 18 patients (45%), and regression occurred in 13 patients (32%). These changes were significantly different from those in the intervention group (p < .05).

Haskell and associates found that intensive multiple risk factor reduction delivered via a nurse-mananged, home-based model over an extended period (4 years) can significantly reduce the rate of progression of atherosclerosis in the coronary arteries of men and women with CAD and can decrease hospitalizations for clinical cardiac events.[35] In this study, a multifactorial risk reduction intervention analogous to a comprehensive long-term cardiac rehabilitation program, plus cholesterol-lowering medication when appropriate, resulted in highly significant improvements in several risk factors and a rate of narrowing of diseased coronary artery segments that was 47% less than that for subjects in the usual-care group. Perhaps more importantly, although an equal number of deaths (3) occurred in each group, there were 25 hospitalizations in the risk-reduction group compared with 44 in the usual-care group (rate ratio, 0.61; p = .05; 95% CI, 0.4 to 0.9).

Although evidence of atherosclerotic regression by digital angiography has been the index piece of circumstantial evidence validating the concept of secondary risk factor reduction, the clinical benefit of the intervention (in terms of cardiac event reduction) tends to be of much greater magnitude than expected from the angiographic improvement.[36] Perhaps this is because of a plaque-stabilizing effect of lipid-lowering therapy, with clinical events being prevented by interventions that, through various potential mechanisms (see Chapters 22 and 24), render the atherosclerotic plaque less likely to become disrupted and, if destabilized, less likely to promote local thrombosis. Thus, multifactorial interventions that include cholesterol lowering with medication have resulted in a relative reduction of subsequent events of about 40% to 50% (Table 28–3).

## ▪ IMPACT OF A CHANGING PATIENT POPULATION

The patient population hospitalized for acute coronary syndromes is changing, and as a result, those referred for cardiac rehabilitation are changing as well.

## Table 28-3

### Outcomes of Selected Secondary Prevention Trials

| Study | Year | Follow-up (mo) | CV Events—Experimental | | CV Events—Control | | Rate of Change % | p |
|---|---|---|---|---|---|---|---|---|
| | | | No. of Subjects | % | No. of Subjects | % | | |
| FATS | 1990 | 30 | 10/52 | 19.23 | 05/94 | 5.32 | -0.73 | <0.05 |
| STARS | 1992 | 30 | 10/28 | 35.71 | 01/26 | 3.85 | -0.80 | <0.05 |
| REGRESS | 1992 | 24 | 93/434 | 21.43 | 59/450 | 13.11 | -0.35 | <0.002 |
| PLAC | 1993 | 36 | 13/76 | 17.11 | 05/75 | 6.67 | -0.61 | <0.04 |
| MARS | 1994 | 48 | 31/124 | 25.00 | 22/124 | 17.74 | -0.32 | N/S |
| MAAS | 1994 | 48 | 51/88 | 57.95 | 40/193 | 20.73 | -0.30 | <0.05 |
| SCRIP | 1994 | 48 | 44/155 | 28.39 | 25/145 | 17.24 | -0.40 | <0.05 |

CV, cardiovascular.

FATS, Familial Atherosclerosis Treatment Study[1]; STARS, St. Thomas Atherosclerosis Regression Study[2]; REGRESS, Regression Growth Evaluation Statin Study[3]; PLAC, Pravastatin Limitation of Atherosclerosis in the Coronary Arteries[4]; MARS, Monitored Atherosclerosis Regression Study[5]; MAAS, Multicentre Anti-Atheroma Study[6]; SCRIP, Stanford Coronary Risk Intervention Project.[7]

1. Brown BG, Zhao XQ, Sacco DE, et al: Atherosclerosis regression, plaque disruption, and cardiovascular events: A rationale for lipid lowering in coronary artery disease. Annu Rev Med 1993;44:365–376.

2. Watts GE, Lewis B, Brunt JN, et al: Effects on coronary artery disease of lipid-lowering diet, or diet plus cholestyramine, in the St Thomas' Atherosclerosis Regression Study (STARS). Lancet 1992;339:563–569.

3. Jukema JW, Bruschke AV, van Boven AJ, et al: Effects of lipid lowering by pravastatin on progression and regression of coronary artery disease in symptomatic men with normal to moderately elevated serum cholesterol levels. The Regression Growth Evaluation Statin Study (REGRESS). Circulation 1995;91:2528–2540.

4. Pitt B, Mancini GB, Ellis SG, et al: Pravastatin limitation of atherosclerosis in the coronary ateries (PLAC I): Reduction in atherosclerosis progression and clinical events. PLAC I investigation. J Am Coll Cardiol 1995;26:1133–1139.

5. Blankenhorn DH, Azen SP, Kramsch DM, et al: Coronary angiographic changes with lovastatin therapy. The Monitored Atherosclerosis Regression Study (MARS). The MARS Research Group. Ann Intern Med 1993;119:969–976.

6. Vos J, de Feyter PJ, Kingma JH, et al: Evolution of coronary atherosclerosis in patients with mild coronary artery disease studied by serial quantitative coronary angiography at 2 and 4 years follow-up. The Multicenter Anti-Atheroma Study (MAAS) Investigators. Eur Heart J 1997;18:1081–1089.

7. Haskell WL, Alderman EL, Fair JM, et al: Effects of intensive multiple risk factor reduction on coronary atherosclerosis and clinical cardiac events in men and women with coronary artery disease. The Stanford Coronary Risk Intervention Project (SCRIP). Circulation 1994;89:975–990.

Patients are increasingly older and sicker, and their disease is more complex.[1] These patients were formerly thought to pose increased risk and, because of compromise in their circulatory hemodynamics, to be poor candidates for the exercise portion of the rehabilitation.[37] Ironically, data suggest that formal exercise training may be of significant benefit to patients with medically complex disease, including those with severe LV dysfunction.[38]

## ■ EXERCISE TRAINING IN PATIENTS WITH LEFT VENTRICULAR DYSFUNCTION

Exercise intolerance in patients with significant LV dysfunction appears most consistently related to early onset of anaerobic metabolism in peripheral muscle, leading to the development of leg fatigue.[37] This is thought to result from both reduced muscle perfusion and reduced aerobic enzyme activity. In the majority of patients, it is not related to higher pulmonary capillary wedge pressures or to increased pulmonary dead space and ventilation relation to oxygen uptake. Despite the observation of inconsistent responses to exercise, exercise has theoretic as well as demonstrated benefits in patients with heart failure. Patients with severe LV dysfunction can condition safely by gradually raising their heart rates above resting level. With time, they are able to extract more oxygen from the blood during exercise, thus widening the arterial-venous oxygen difference.

For a person who is severely limited, in distinction to a low-risk patient, even modest improvement is likely to have a noticeable impact on functional capacity.[39] It is ironic that patients with severely reduced exercise tolerance were formerly excluded from exercise rehabilitation on the assumption that they would derive little tangible benefit. Similar reasoning applies to both the elderly and other subsets of patients who with small increments in exercise capacity have the capability of maintaining independence and provision of self-care. Four to five METs, a work capacity achievable by even some of the very elderly,[40] is adequate to perform most activities of daily living, such as light housework, shopping, and other domestic functions (see Fig. 28–3).

## ■ GENDER ISSUES RELEVANT TO CARDIAC REHABILITATION

Women derive comparable benefits from cardiac rehabilitation, but unfortunately, in part because they are usually older and have other concomitant problems, they are not referred as often.[41] There are also more obstacles to their participation. Among these, physician referral appears to be the most frequent. Compared with men, women appear to use cardiac rehabilitation programs less often than men, have higher dropout rates, and return to work less frequently and after a longer period. However, women who complete cardiac rehabilitation can be expected to have similar improvement in risk factors and functional capacity compared with men.[42] Although the risk factors for CAD, other than estrogen or lack of it, are the same for women as for men, the frequency and relative impact of the risk factors differ.[43] These findings have very important implications for the design of rehabilitation programs.

## ■ SUMMARY

Cardiac rehabilitation has evolved from progressive ambulation after MI into a multifactorial therapy of exercise training, psychosocial support, and education, with the twin primary goals of returning patients to normalcy after MI and reducing the chances of subsequent coronary events thereafter. This process appears to succeed especially with patients who are severely deconditioned at the time of program entry. Furthermore, survival itself is likely improved, largely by a decrease in the incidence of sudden cardiac death, but the potential impact of this is hard to assess given the reduction in mortality associated with many other post-MI interventions. Improved quality of life and cost utility have also become important contemporary outcomes. Finally, the impact of risk factor modification on the fundamental pathologic process of coronary atherosclerosis, thereby reducing subsequent coronary events, may be the most exciting and important outcome of cardiac rehabilitation and the one with the most important potential.

## ▪ REFERENCES

1. Pashkow FJ: Issues in contemporary cardiac rehabilitation: A historical perspective. J Am Coll Cardiol 1993;21:822–834.
2. Levine S, Lown B: "Armchair" treatment of acute coronary thrombosis. JAMA 1952;148:1365–1369.
3. Wenger NK, Froelicher ES, Smith LK, et al: Cardiac Rehabilitation. Clinical Practice Guideline No. 17. Rockville, MD: U.S. Department of Health and Human Services, Public Health Service, Agency for Health Care Policy and Research and the National Heart, Lung, and Blood Institute. AHCPR Publication No. 96-0672. October 1995.
4. Wasserman K, Koike A: Is the anaerobic threshold truly anaerobic? Chest 1992;101:211S–218S.
5. Schuler G, Hambrecht R, Schlierf G, et al: Regular physical exercise and low-fat diet. Effects on progression of coronary artery disease. Circulation 1992;86:1–11.
6. Franklin BA: Exercise training and coronary collateral circulation. Med Sci Sports Exerc 1991;23:648–653.
7. McKirnan MD, Bloor CM: Clinical significance of coronary vascular adaptations to exercise training. Med Sci Sports Exerc 1994;26:1262–1268.
8. Senti S, Fleisch M, Billinger M, et al: Long-term physical exercise and quantitatively assessed human coronary collateral circulation. J Am Coll Cardiol 1998;32:49–56.
9. Niebauer J, Hambrecht R, Marburger C, et al: Impact of intensive physical exercise and low-fat diet on collateral vessel formation in stable angina pectoris and angiographically confirmed coronary artery disease. Am J Cardiol 1995;76:771–775.
10. Ehsani AA, Ogawa T, Miller TR, et al: Exercise training improves left ventricular systolic function in older men. Circulation 1991;83:96–103.
11. Jette M, Heller R, Landry F, et al: Randomized 4-week exercise program in patients with impaired left ventricular function [see comments]. Circulation 1991;84:1561–1567.
12. Litchfield RL, Kerber RE, Benge JW, et al: Normal exercise capacity in patients with severe left ventricular dysfunction: Compensatory mechanisms. Circulation 1982;66:129–134.
13. Fletcher GF: Rehabilitative exercise for the cardiac patient. Early phase. Cardiol Clin 1993;11:267–275.
14. Dafoe W, Franklin B, Cupper L: Vocational issues: Maximizing the patient's potential for return to work. In Pashkow F, Dafoe W (eds): Clinical Cardiac Rehabilitation: A Cardiologist's Guide. Baltimore: Williams & Wilkins, 1999:304–323.
15. Oldridge N, Furlong W, Feeny D, et al: Economic evaluation of cardiac rehabilitation soon after acute myocardial infarction. Am J Cardiol 1993;72:154–161.
16. Pashkow FJ, Pashkow PS, Schafer MN: Successful cardiac rehabilitation: The complete guide for building cardiac rehab programs. Loveland, CO: The HeartWatchers Press, 1988.
17. Ades P, Pashkow F, Fletcher G, et al: A controlled trial of cardiac rehabilitation in the home setting: Improvement accessibility. J Am Coll Cardiol 1996; 27(Suppl A): 150A.
18. Pashkow F, Dafoe W: Cardiac rehabilitation as a model of integrated cardiovascular care. In Pashkow F, Dafoe W (eds): Clinical Cardiac Rehabilitation: A Cardiologist's Guide. Baltimore: Williams & Wilkins, 1999:3–25.
19. American Association for Cardiovascular and Pulmonary Rehabilitation: Guidelines for Cardiac Rehabilitation Programs, 2nd ed. Champaign, IL: Human Kinetics Books, 1995.
20. Ryan TJ, Anderson JL, Antman EM, et al: ACC/AHA guidelines for the management of patients with acute myocardial infarction: executive summary. A report of the American College of Cardiology/American Heart Association Task Force on Practice Guidelines (Committee on Management of Acute Myocardial Infarction). Circulation 1996;94:2341–2350.
21. Oldridge NB, Guyatt GH, Fischer ME, et al: Cardiac rehabilitation after myocardial infarction. Combined experience of randomized clinical trials. JAMA 1988;260:945–950.
22. O'Connor GT, Buring JE, Yusuf S, et al: An overview of randomized trials of rehabilitation with exercise after myocardial infarction. Circulation 1989;80:234–244.
23. Seals DR, Chase PB: Influence of physical training on heart rate variability and baroreflex circulatory control. J Appl Physiol 1989;66:1886–1895.

24. VanCamp S, Peterson R: Cardiovascular complications of outpatient cardiac rehabilitation programs. JAMA 1986;256:1160–1163.
25. Leor J, Poole WK, Kloner RA: Sudden cardiac death triggered by an earthquake. N Engl J Med 1996;334:413–419.
26. Mittleman MA, Maclure M, Sherwood JB, et al: Triggering of acute myocardial infarction onset by episodes of anger. Determinants of Myocardial Infarction Onset Study Investigators. Circulation 1995;92:1720–1725.
27. Kavanagh T, Shephard RJ, Tuck JA: Depression after myocardial infarction. Can Med Assoc J 1975;113:23–27.
28. Frasure-Smith N, Lesperance F, Talajic M: Depression following myocardial infarction. Impact on 6-month survival [see comments]. JAMA 1993;270:1819–1825.
29. Linden W, Stossel C, Maurice J: Psychosocial interventions for patients with coronary artery disease: A meta-analysis. Arch Intern Med 1996;156:745–752.
30. Wenger N: Improvement of quality of life in the framework of cardiac rehabilitation. In Pashkow F, Dafoe W (eds): Clinical Cardiac Rehabilitation: A Cardiologist's Guide. Baltimore: Williams & Wilkins, 1999;43–51.
31. Ades PA, Pashkow FJ, Nestor JR: Cost-effectiveness of cardiac rehabilitation after myocardial infarction. J Cardpulm Rehabil 1997;17:222–231.
32. Oldridge N, Guyatt G, Jones N, et al: Effects on quality of life with comprehensive rehabilitation after acute myocardial infarction. Am J Cardiol 1991;67:1084–1089.
33. Brown G, Albers JJ, Fisher LD, et al: Regression of coronary artery disease as a result of intensive lipid-lowering therapy in men with high levels of apolipoprotein B [see comments]. N Engl J Med 1990;323:1289–298.
34. Ornish D, Brown SE, Scherwitz LW, et al: Can lifestyle changes reverse coronary heart disease? The Lifestyle Heart Trial. Lancet 1990;336:129–133.
35. Haskell WL, Alderman EL, Fair JM, et al: Effects of intensive multiple risk factor reduction on coronary atherosclerosis and clinical cardiac events in men and women with coronary artery disease. The Stanford Coronary Risk Intervention Project (SCRIP). Circulation 1994;89:975–990.
36. Brown BG, Zhao, XQ, Sacco DE, et al: Arteriographic view of treatment to achieve regression of coronary atherosclerosis and to prevent plaque disruption and clinical cardiovascular events. Br Heart J 1993;69:S48–S53.
37. Sullivan MJ, Higginbotham MB, Cobb FR: Exercise training in patients with severe left ventricular dysfunction. Hemodynamic and metabolic effects. Circulation 1988;78:506–515.
38. Pashkow FJ: Rehabilitation strategies for the complex cardiac patient. Cleve Clin J Med 1991;58:70–75.
39. Sullivan MJ, Higginbotham MB, Cobb FR: Exercise training in patients with chronic heart failure delays ventilatory anaerobic threshold and improves submaximal exercise performance. Circulation 1989;79:324–329.
40. Lavie CJ, Milani RV, Littman AB: Benefits of cardiac rehabilitation and exercise training in secondary coronary prevention in the elderly. J Am Coll Cardiol 1993;22:678–683.
41. Limacher MC: Exercise and rehabilitation in women. Indications and outcomes. Cardiol Clin 1998;16:27–36.
42. Carhart RL Jr, Ades PA: Gender differences in cardiac rehabilitation. Cardiol Clin 1998;16:37–43.
43. Foody J, Pashkow F: Gender-specific issues related to coronary risk factors in women. In Pashkow F, Dafoe W (eds): Clinical Cardiac Rehabilitation: A Cardiologist's Guide. Baltimore: Williams & Wilkins, 1999:383–402.

# ▪ RECOMMENDED READING

Ades PA, Pashkow FJ, Nestor JR: Cost-effectiveness of cardiac rehabilitation after myocardial infarction. J Cardpulm Rehabil 1997;17:222–231.
Lavie CJ, Milani RV, Littman AB: Benefits of cardiac rehabilitation and exercise training in secondary coronary prevention in the elderly. J Am Coll Cardiol 1993;22:678–683.
Oldridge NB, Guyatt GH, Fischer ME, et al: Cardiac rehabilitation after myocardial infarction. Combined experience of randomized clinical trials. JAMA 1988;260:945–950.
Pashkow F, Dafoe W: Cardiac rehabilitation as a model of integrated cardiovascular care. In Pashkow F, Dafoe W (eds): Clinical Cardiac Rehabilitation: A Cardiologist's Guide. Baltimore: Williams & Wilkins, 1999:3–25.
Pashkow FJ, Pashkow PS, Schafer MN: Successful Cardiac Rehabilitation: The Complete Guide for Building Cardiac Rehab Programs. Loveland, CO: The HeartWatchers Press, 1988.
Wenger NK, Froelicher ES, Smith LK, et al: Cardiac Rehabilitation as Secondary Prevention. Clinical Practice Guideline. Quick Reference Guide for Clinicians, No. 17. Rockville, MD: U.S. Department of Health and Human Services, Public Health Service, Agency for Health Care Policy and Research and National Heart, Lung, and Blood Institute. AHCPR Publication No. 96-0673. October 1995.

*Chapter* 29

# Rheumatic Fever and Valvular Heart Disease

*E. A. W. Brice* ■ *P. J. Commerford*

## ■ ACUTE RHEUMATIC FEVER

Rheumatic fever causes most cases of acquired heart disease in children and young adults worldwide. It is generally classified as a collagen vascular disease whose inflammatory insult is directed mainly against the tissues of the heart, joints, and central nervous system. The inflammatory response, which is characterized by fibrinoid degeneration of collagen fibrils and connective tissue ground substance, is triggered by a throat infection with group A beta-hemolytic streptococci (GAS). The destructive effects on cardiac valve tissue account for most of the morbidity and mortality that the serious hemodynamic disturbances produce.

### Epidemiology

During the 20th century, the two major influences on the reduction of rheumatic fever incidence in many parts of the world were the advent of penicillin and improvements in socioeconomic conditions. At the turn of the 20th century, the reported incidence of rheumatic fever in the United States was 100 per 100,000 population, and by 1960 this had fallen to 45 per 100,000. The most recent U.S. figures show that some regions have rates as low as 2 per 100,000. In stark contrast to these figures are rates as high as a 15 to 21 per 1000 reported in various areas of Africa, Asia, and South America, and in Soweto, South Africa, a prevalence of rheumatic carditis of 19 per 1000 was reported in the early 1970s.[1]

### Pathogenesis

The role of GAS in the genesis of rheumatic fever has been supported by a variety of clinical, epidemiologic, and immunologic observational studies. Pharyngeal infection with this organism is the only known cause of rheumatic fever. In conditions of overcrowding such as schools or military facilities, epidemics of streptococcal throat infection have resulted in approximately 3% of those affected developing rheumatic fever.[2]

GAS have a variety of cell wall antigens, such as the M, T, and R proteins. It

**561**

is the M wall protein that is responsible for type-specific immunity and that is widely regarded as determining streptococcal rheumatogenic potential. Patients with acute rheumatic fever often have high titers of antibody to the M proteins.

The currently accepted mode of development of acute rheumatic fever is that GAS pharyngitis leads to a host response to the GAS antigens and, through cross-reactivity of these with antigens in human tissues such as heart and brain, molecular mimicry.[3] This would explain the frequent observations that (1) after pharyngeal infection, there is a 3-week asymptomatic period and (2) rheumatic fever is rare in very young children (peak incidence is between ages 5 and 18 years).

Host factors such as HLA subtypes have also been cited as possible explanations of variations in susceptibility to disease. Approximately 60% to 70% of patients worldwide are positive for HLA-DR3, DR4, DR7, DRW53, or DQW2.[4]

## Clinical Presentation

No test is specific for rheumatic fever. Therefore, the diagnosis of a patient's first attack of rheumatic fever is usually made by the clinical criteria first formulated by T. Duckett Jones[5] and subsequently modified.[6] These are divided into major and minor criteria. When, after a GAS infection, two major or one major and two minor criteria are found, a diagnosis of rheumatic fever can be made (Table 29–1).

*Carditis* is a pancarditis involving endocardial, myocardial, and pericardial tissues. Valvular involvement is frequent, and, if no evidence of this is found clinically despite myocarditis or pericarditis, rheumatic fever is unlikely. The mitral valve is most often involved, followed by the aortic valve, and this lesion gives rise to the frequent finding of regurgitant murmurs. Mitral systolic murmurs, and occasionally, even mid-diastolic murmurs (Carey-Coombs), detected during the course of an acute attack of rheumatic fever, do not necessarily indicate permanent valvular disease. An aortic early diastolic murmur rarely disappears and is evidence of established valve disease. Echocardiography usually is not required acutely and may give rise to overdiagnosis.[7] As the progression to valvular stenosis through progressive scarring of the valve leaflets is gradual, early routine echocardiography seldom adds any information to clinical findings.

*Arthritis* is symmetric, migratory, and involves the larger joints, such as the wrists, elbows, knees, and ankles. If a patient presents with joint symptoms and evidence of recent GAS pharyngitis but other criteria are insufficient for a diagnosis of rheumatic fever, poststreptococcal reactive arthritis must be considered. This disease may give rise to delayed carditis, and, therefore, patients should be followed closely.

*Sydenham's chorea,* characterized by purposeless, involuntary movements, incoordination, and emotional lability, is seen in about 20% of patients with rheumatic

Table 29–1

**Modified Criteria for Diagnosis of Acute Rheumatic Fever**

| Major | Minor |
|---|---|
| Carditis | Fever |
| Chorea | Arthralgia |
| Polyarthritis | Elevated erythrocyte sedimentation rate |
| Erythema marginatum | Elevated C-reactive protein |
| Subcutaneous nodules | Prolonged PR interval |

fever. It often presents 3 months after the onset of GAS pharyngitis. Even without treatment, symptoms often resolve within 2 weeks.

*Erythema marginatum,* an erythematous macular rash of the trunk and proximal extremities, occurs in approximately 5% of rheumatic fever cases. Lesions have pale centers with rounded or serpiginous, pale pink margins and are not pruritic. They are transient and extremely difficult to detect, particularly in dark-skinned patients.

In 3% of rheumatic fever cases painless, mobile, 0.5- to 2-cm *subcutaneous nodules* develop on the extensor surfaces of joints, the occipital area of the scalp, and over spinous processes.

*Peritoneal* involvement is rare but may simulate acute abdomen, mimicking acute appendicitis in children.

Confirming an antecedent GAS infection is often problematic. Throat swab culture is positive in only about 11% of patients at the time when acute rheumatic fever is identified.[8] A rapid streptococcal antigen test has also been utilized to confirm recent GAS infection. Another confirmatory finding is a rising titer of antistreptococcal antibodies, either antistreptolysin O (ASO) or antideoxyribonuclease B (anti-DNase B).

It is important to maintain a high level of suspicion of rheumatic fever when any patient presents with a pyrexial illness, tachycardia, and progressive symmetric polyarthritis. While most patients are between ages 5 and 15 years at first presentation, much older ones are occasionally diagnosed with an initial attack of acute rheumatic fever. Rheumatic fever can recur at any age and must be distinguished from infective endocarditis.

## Treatment

Once the diagnosis has been made, it is customary for bed rest to be prescribed. Although at the time of presentation for rheumatic fever throat swabs are frequently negative for GAS, a 10-day course of oral penicillin V or a single intramuscular injection of benzathine penicillin is given empirically to eradicate any GAS.

To minimize inflammatory damage to the affected tissues, often joints and the heart, high doses of oral salicylates (100 mg/kg/day in divided doses) is cost-effective therapy. For patients with severe carditis or whose valve lesions require early surgical repair, prednisone (2 mg/kg/day) is often used instead of salicylates. Good evidence for the superiority of prednisone is lacking, but patients with carditis do appear to respond more rapidly to it.[9]

Duration of therapy is determined by clinical and laboratory evidence of resolution of inflammation. This is often achieved in milder cases after a month of salicylate therapy; more severe cases may require 3 months of steroid treatment, and as many as 5% of cases are still active at 6 months.

Heart failure, due to severe valve regurgitation, is the usual cause of death and, when it is resistant to antifailure therapy, may necessitate urgent valve replacement surgery, even in the presence of active carditis.[10]

## Primary Prevention

Prompt recognition and effective treatment of GAS pharyngitis can prevent the development of rheumatic fever, reducing both morbidity and mortality. Penicillin remains the most cost-effective agent in the treatment of GAS pharyngitis. Often, a single intramuscular dose of benzathine penicillin (1.2 MU for patients who weigh at least 27 kg) is effective, and, when compliance is not a concern, an alternative oral regimen such as penicillin V (500 mg three times a day for adults) may be used. Erythromycin estolate (20 to 40 mg/kg/day in two to four doses) can be used in penicillin-allergic persons. True primary prevention of GAS pharyngitis can be achieved only by eliminating conditions of squalor, overcrowding, and socioeconomic deprivation that promote frequent attacks of GAS pharyngitis in communities.

## Secondary Prevention

Recurrent attacks of rheumatic fever are common and can be reduced with prophylactic antibiotics. Duration of secondary prevention must be individualized to each patient and extended for those in poor socioeconomic conditions. Generally, after the first attack of rheumatic fever, patients should receive antibiotics until age 21 years or for at least 5 years. Those with persistent evidence of carditis should receive prolonged therapy. Some authors recommend treatment until age 40 or for at least 10 years after the attack.

Antibiotic regimens whose efficacy is proven include 1.2 MU intramuscular benzathine penicillin every 3 weeks.[11, 12] Oral therapy is often used for patients on warfarin anticoagulation, and penicillin V (250 mg twice daily) is recommended. Penicillin-allergic persons may use erythromycin (250 mg twice daily).

## ■ MITRAL VALVE DISEASE

### Mitral Stenosis

With the rare exception of congenital abnormalities, mitral stenosis (MS) due to abnormalities of the leaflets, commissures, and cusps of the valve is due to rheumatic fever.[13] Some 40% of patients with rheumatic heart disease have combined MS and mitral regurgitation (MR), and a quarter have pure MS. MS is more common in females, but the reason is indeterminate.

### Pathology

The rheumatic process affects the edges of the leaflets. With resolution of the inflammatory process, there is thickening, fibrosis, and fusion of the commissures (Fig. 29–1). Involvement of the chordae tendinae results in thickening, fusion, and contraction with scarring that extends down onto the papillary muscles. Dense fibrosis and calcification may reduce the normal delicate structure of the valve to a rigid, immobile, funnel-shaped orifice.

### Pathophysiology

The normal adult mitral valve orifice area is 4 to 6 $cm^2$. When MS reduces the orifice area to 2 $cm^2$, greater than normal pressure is required to propel blood from the left atrium to the left ventricle. When stenosis is more severe (1 to 1.5 $cm^2$), considerably elevated left atrial pressure is required to maintain normal cardiac output even at rest, the result being a pressure gradient across the valve (Fig. 29–2). The elevated left atrial pressure raises pulmonary capillary pressures, resulting in exertional dyspnea. Dyspnea usually first occurs with exercise, emotional stress, or infection that demands an increased rate of flow across the mitral valve and, thus, higher left atrial pressure. Patients with MS do not tolerate tachycardia. Increased heart rate shortens diastole proportionally more than systole and thus reduces the time available for blood to flow across the mitral valve.[14] Development of atrial fibrillation (AF) with a rapid ventricular rate may precipitate pulmonary edema in previously asymptomatic patients with MS.

Pulmonary hypertension in patients with MS may result from passive backward transmission of the elevated left atrial pressure or organic obliterative changes in the pulmonary vasculature. Reactive pulmonary hypertension due to pulmonary

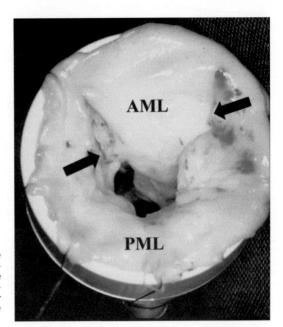

**Figure 29–1** ■ Stenosed mitral valve excised at the time of mitral valve replacement (atrial view). Fusion of the commissures *(arrows)* between the anterior mitral leaflet (AML) and posterior mitral leaflet (PML) is evident. (See Color Figure 29–1.)

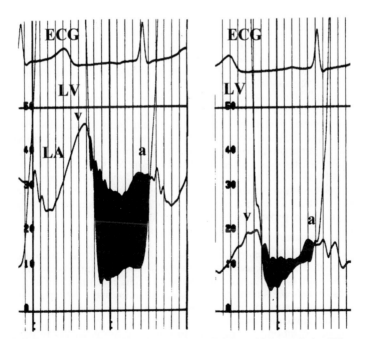

**Figure 29–2** ■ Simultaneous ECG recording of left atrial (LA) and left ventricular (LV) pressure in a patient with severe MS before (left) and immediately after (right) balloon valvuloplasty. Shaded area indicates the gradient. v, v wave; a, a wave.

arteriolar constriction triggered by left atrial and pulmonary venous hypertension may be important in some patients. Prolonged, severe pulmonary hypertension results in dilatation of the right ventricle and secondary tricuspid regurgitation (TR).

## Clinical Features

### History

Subclinical or unrecognized attacks of acute rheumatic fever presumably account for the fact that fewer than half of all patients with MS clearly recall the acute illness. *Dyspnea*, which may be accompanied by cough and wheezing, is the major symptom of MS. This is initially exertional only, but with progression orthopnea and paroxysmal nocturnal dyspnea develop. Patients with severe MS may tolerate modest limitation of ordinary daily activities but are at risk of developing frank pulmonary edema, which can be precipitated by exercise, chest infections, fever, emotional stress, pregnancy, intercourse, or the onset of AF.

Classically, several different kinds of *hemoptysis* have been described as complicating MS:

- Sudden, profuse hemorrhage (pulmonary apoplexy) results from the rupture of thin-walled, dilated bronchial veins.[15] It is more common early in the disease, before bronchial veins thicken and are able to withstand the increased pressure. Often terrifying, it is rarely life threatening.
- Pink, frothy sputum of pulmonary edema
- Blood-stained sputum associated with attacks of paroxysmal nocturnal dyspnea
- Pulmonary infarction, a late complication of long-standing MS associated with heart failure

*Thromboembolism* from left atrial thrombosis is an important and life-threatening complication of MS. Systemic emboli occur at some time in approximately 20% of patients. Emboli are more common in older patients with low cardiac output, a large left atrial appendage, and AF. Embolism may, however, occur with mild MS, and occasionally it is the presenting feature. Cerebral, renal, and coronary emboli may occur, and occasionally a large embolus blocks the aorta at its bifurcation (saddle embolus). Unexpected systemic or cerebral emboli in a young patient should prompt a careful search for MS.

Uncommon manifestations include *chest pain* indistinguishable from angina pectoris, which, in the absence of coronary disease, may be due to right ventricular or left atrial hypertension. Poorly explained, it resolves with successful treatment of the stenosis. *Hoarseness* caused by compression of the left recurrent laryngeal nerve by a dilated left atrium, lymph nodes, and dilated pulmonary artery occurs in isolated cases (Ortner syndrome). Severe untreated MS with pulmonary hypertension and right-sided heart failure produces symptoms due to systemic venous hypertension with hepatomegaly, edema, and ascites.

### Physical Examination

The typical so-called *mitral facies*—pinkish purple patches on the cheeks—is rarely appreciated in dark-skinned patients, in whom the disease is, however, common. The *pulse* is normal in character but of small volume if cardiac output is reduced. The *venous pressure* may be normal if pulmonary hypertension has not developed. When severe pulmonary hypertension is present, a large *a* wave is found. AF and tricuspid incompetence is associated with large *cv* waves and systolic hepatic pulsation. A typical feature on *palpation* is an easily palpable first heart sound (S1). Pulmonary hypertension produces a right ventricular lift and a palpable pulmonic closure sound (P2) in the left parasternal area.

*Auscultation* is best performed with the patient turned into the left lateral position. The first heart sound is typically loud. This accentuation occurs when the anterior leaflet of the mitral valve remains pliable and is due to the abrupt crossover in pressure between left atrium and left ventricle at the onset of systole in mitral stenosis and the rapid acceleration of the closing leaflets.[16] Normally, the leaflets drift closed toward the end of diastole. In MS they are held open by the transmitral pressure gradient. Marked calcification or fibrosis of the leaflets attenuates the accentuation. In patients with pulmonary hypertension, P2 is accentuated. The mitral valve opening snap (OS) is heard only in patients with MS. Caused by sudden tensing of the anterior leaflet, it is best heard in the left parasternal area. The characteristic murmur is a low-pitched diastolic rumble best heard with the bell of the stethoscope and may be limited to the apex. Presystolic accentuation of the murmur is due to atrial contraction, which increases the gradient and flow across the mitral valve just before systole in patients in sinus rhythm. The auscultatory features of MS in obese or emphysematous patients are notoriously difficult to detect. Simple bedside maneuvers (exercise) increase the heart rate and render them easier to hear. Auscultation offers clues to *severity* of stenosis—the longer the murmur and the closer the OS is to the aortic component of the second sound (A2), the more severe is the stenosis—and *mobility* of the valve, a well-heard OS, and loud, easily heard S1 imply that the anterior leaflet is mobile.

The only other important diagnosis to be considered is *left atrial myxoma*, which may produce auscultatory features similar to those of MS. The characteristic inspiratory augmentation of the murmur of *tricuspid stenosis* should readily allow for its differentiation.

### Laboratory Examination

*Electrocardiography* is relatively insensitive but may reveal characteristic changes in patients with moderate or severe MS (Fig. 29–3). The *chest radiograph* usually shows an enlarged atrial appendage, and left atrial enlargement is visible on the left lateral view. *Echocardiography* (Fig. 29–4) both confirms the diagnosis by demonstrating thickening, restricted motion, and doming of the anterior leaflet and provides vital information on the mobility of the anterior leaflet, the presence and severity of valve calcification, and involvement of the subvalvular apparatus, which determines selection of treatment. *Color-flow Doppler* echocardiography demonstrates the high-velocity jet entering the left ventricle (Fig. 29–5) and allows quantitation of severity.

Clinical evaluation and detailed echocardiographic examination, including a Doppler study, usually provide sufficient information to plan management without the need for *cardiac catheterization*, which can be reserved for cases when doubt about severity of associated mitral regurgitation (MR), other valve lesions, or left ventricular function persists. *Coronary angiography* may be indicated for certain patients with chest pain syndromes or those considered at risk for coronary disease before elective valve replacement surgery.

### Treatment

**Medical Treatment.** Medical treatment includes advice on lifestyle and risks of pregnancy, long-term prophylaxis against recurrences of rheumatic fever, when appropriate, antibiotic prophylaxis against infective endocarditis (although the risks are low), and prophylactic anticoagulation with warfarin if AF (sustained or paroxysmal) is present. There is no clear evidence that warfarin anticoagulation benefits patients in sinus rhythm who have not experienced an episode of systemic embolism. Diuretics and dietary sodium restriction reduce pulmonary congestion. Beta-blockers increase exercise capacity by reducing heart rate.[17]

**Surgical Treatment.** Mechanical relief of obstruction may be provided by

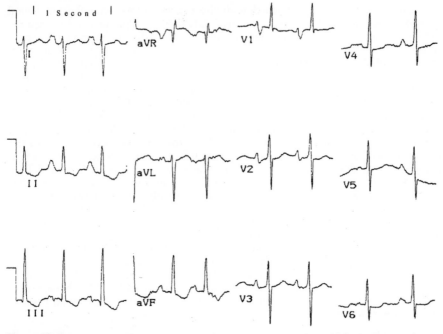

**Figure 29–3** ■ Twelve-lead ECG of a patient with severe isolated mitral stenosis and pulmonary hypertension shows the combination of left atrial enlargement (P wave broadened in lead II, biphasic in lead VI) and right ventricular hypertrophy (right axis deviation, dominant R in lead VI).

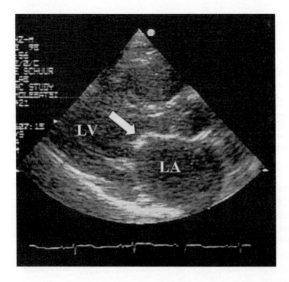

**Figure 29–4** ■ Transthoracic echocardiographic images (parasternal long axis view) reveals left atrial (LA) enlargement and thickened domed anterior leaflet of the mitral valve (*arrow*).

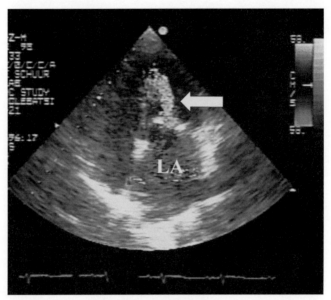

**Figure 29–5** ▪ Color-flow Doppler echocardiography demonstrates the high-velocity jet entering the left ventricle (LV, *arrow*). LA, left atrium. (See Color Figure 29–5.)

closed mitral valvotomy, open mitral valvotomy, percutaneous balloon mitral valvuloplasty (PBMV), or mitral valve replacement. Selection and timing of the procedure require clinical judgment based on the patient's symptoms, the severity of MS, and the risks of the procedure. PBMV has largely superseded surgical valvotomy in suitable patients with pliable leaflets, little or no significant calcification, or MR. A balloon catheter inserted via the femoral vein and a transatrial puncture across a dilated stenotic valve (Fig. 29–6) tears the fused commissures and partially relieves the obstruction. While PBMV is palliative, it preserves the patient's own valvular apparatus and defers mitral valve replacement and its attendant risks. Periprocedural risk is low (1% to 3%), it can be performed as an emergency procedure or in pregnant patients, and it provides excellent relief of symptoms. Severe MR may follow rupture of one of the leaflets. PBMV is usually recommended for patients with significant MS (mitral valve area <0.5 cm$^2$) and symptoms graded New York Heart Association (NYHA) class II or greater. When the valve is badly deformed, heavily calcified, or associated with significant MR, mitral valve replacement surgery is the only option. This is usually recommended for class III or IV disease.

Clinical considerations, including the patient's age, desired level of activity, comorbid conditions, and, for young women, desire for pregnancy, will influence decisions. Each patient with MS requires an individualized assessment recognizing that progression to severe stenosis is almost inevitable, medical treatment can offer only temporary relief, and valvotomy is palliative and restenosis inevitable, although the time to restenosis is unpredictable. Many patients who underwent successful closed mitral valvotomy when the procedure was introduced in the 1950s have had repeat procedures and lead successful and productive lives 40 years later, after inevitable mitral valve replacement.

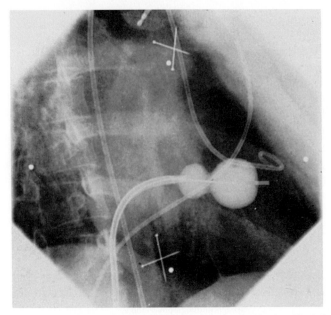

**Figure 29–6** ▪ An Inoue balloon catheter is positioned across the mitral valve. The indentation in the contrast-filled balloon as it ruptures the mitral valve commissures is evident.

# ▪ MITRAL REGURGITATION

## Pathology

A number of pathologic processes may affect components of the mitral valve apparatus and render it incompetent (Table 29–2). The rheumatic disease process leads to fibrosis with resultant scarring and contracture of the valve leaflets, and a similar process affecting the chordae with scarring of the papillary muscles results in mitral regurgitation. The severe MR of acute rheumatic fever in children or adolescents is usually secondary to prolapse of the anterior leaflet, elongation of the chordae, and dilatation of the annulus.[18]

Table 29–2

**Causes of Mitral Regurgitation**

| Chronic | Acute |
| --- | --- |
| Rheumatic heart disease | Infective endocarditis |
| Mitral valve prolapse | Chordal rupture |
| Mitral annular calcification | Trauma (surgery, percutaneous balloon mitral |
| Infective endocarditis | valvuloplasty) |
| Chordal rupture (spontaneous, infective, traumatic) | Ischemic papillary muscle dysfunction, rupture |
| Ischemic papillary muscle dysfunction | Prosthetic valve malfunction |
| Congenital clefts | |
| Systemic lupus erythematosus | |

## Pathophysiology

Isolated or pure MR is uncommon in chronic rheumatic heart disease, and there is almost always some degree of associated stenosis. In chronic MR, the mitral orifice functions in parallel with the aortic valve, and considerable regurgitation into the low-pressure left atrium may occur before the aortic valve opens. This systolic unloading of the ventricle may permit patients with chronic MR many years of relatively symptom-free survival at the risk of developing progressive LV dysfunction. The loading conditions in chronic MR are favorable, the lesion favors LV emptying, and, if myocardial function is normal, the ejection fraction should be supernormal. An understanding of the complex hemodynamic adaptations of chronic MR is important in planning management.[19]

When LV function is impaired, end-diastolic pressure rises, as does left atrial pressure, and pulmonary venous hypertension may increase pulmonary artery pressure. Severe pulmonary hypertension is less common than in patients with isolated mitral stenosis. When MR develops abruptly, the unprepared noncompliant left atrium is unable to accommodate the regurgitant load, and acute heart failure is common.

## Clinical Features

### History

*Dyspnea* is the usual presenting symptom. Most patients tolerate chronic mitral regurgitation very well unless there is a dramatic increase in the degree of MR. The great danger is that, by the time symptoms secondary to reduced cardiac output or pulmonary congestion become apparent, severe and irreversible LV dysfunction may have developed. *Hemoptysis* and *thromboembolism* are less common than in patients with MS. Untreated, severe, chronic MR can result in pulmonary hypertension with secondary TR, hepatomegaly, and ascites with symptoms attributable to these.

### Physical Examination

The *pulse* is usually normal in volume with a brisk upstroke. In the absence of pulmonary hypertension and associated tricuspid valve abnormalities, venous pressure may be normal. On precordial *palpation* the apex beat is volume loaded and displaced to the left. A systolic lift in the left parasternal area due to systolic expansion of the enlarged left atrium may be difficult to differentiate from right ventricular enlargement secondary to pulmonary hypertension.

#### Auscultation

The first heart sound is usually soft, and P2 may be accentuated if pulmonary hypertension has developed. An apical pansystolic murmur commencing immediately after S1 and continuing up to the second sound is characteristic of chronic severe MR. Best heard at the apex, it radiates to the axilla and back. Occasionally, when the regurgitant jet is directed medially, it may be heard maximally parasternally and even in the pulmonary area. The murmur, unlike that of AS, varies little in intensity with alterations in cardiac cycle length. Severity of regurgitation does not correlate with loudness of the murmur. Failure of the murmur to accentuate on inspiration differentiates it from that of TR. An apical third heart sound frequently precedes a short mid-diastolic murmur, the result of the increased forward flow produced by the regurgitant volume and some degree of commissural fusion, which is often present in rheumatic MR.

## Laboratory Examination

*Electrocardiography* may be normal or show left atrial enlargement. A pattern of severe LV hypertrophy with repolarization abnormalities is unusual and, when present, is an indication that the diagnosis may be incorrect and that the MR is secondary to LV dilatation (dilated cardiomyopathy) or that the differential diagnosis of the systolic murmur should be more inclusive (AS, hypertrophic cardiomyopathy). The *chest radiograph* usually reveals cardiomegaly and left atrial enlargement. *Echocardiography* confirms the diagnosis of MR, revealing a high-velocity jet in the left atrium during systole. In addition to its diagnostic value, echocardiography provides vital information on LV function and mitral valve morphology, which, together, determine management and prognosis.

## Treatment

### Medical Treatment

*Medical treatment* for asymptomatic patients must include advice on preventing recurrences of acute rheumatic fever, prophylaxis against infective endocarditis, and advice on lifestyle, pregnancy, and the need for long-term medical supervision. Careful serial evaluations with noninvasive monitoring of LV function are essential. Diuretics relieve symptoms of pulmonary congestion, and digitalis is indicated for patients with severe MR and evidence of heart failure, particularly if AF is present. Chronic afterload reduction with an angiotensin-converting enzyme inhibitor is logical, but unproven, therapy.

### Surgical Treatment

Mitral valve replacement produces symptomatic improvement, but long-term results are far from ideal. Mitral valve annuloplasty or repair is the preferred procedure. The timing of surgery in patients with MR is difficult. Patients with severe symptoms (NYHA class III or IV) should be offered surgery. Asymptomatic patients and those with mild symptoms (NYHA class II) can be observed or treated medically, provided that LV function is monitored meticulously and they are considered for surgery if the ejection fraction falls toward 60% or end-systolic dimension approaches 45 mm.[19] Mitral valve repair is, for technical reasons, often not possible in patients with rheumatic MR, and when it is attempted, results are often unsatisfactory.[20]

## ■ MIXED MITRAL STENOSIS AND REGURGITATION

Rheumatic disease of the mitral valve results in a wide spectrum of clinical presentations, which range from predominant MS to predominant MR. A common and particularly difficult management problem is severe deformity of the valve, which is stenotic during diastole and leaks during systole.

Clinical and laboratory features depend on which pathologic process is dominant, and no brief description can encompass the variety of clinical signs that may be detected. Medical treatment for both asymptomatic and symptomatic patients is the same as that for those with pure MS and pure MR. Surgical treatment by means of valve replacement provides symptomatic relief, and the risks of the procedure need to be weighed against the risks of the underlying disease. Surgery is usually recommended to patients with NYHA class III or IV disability.

## ■ AORTIC VALVE DISEASE

### Aortic Stenosis

#### Pathology

*Congenitally abnormal* valves, which may be bicuspid, may be only mildly obstructive in childhood, but the associated abnormal flow dynamics damage the leaflets, leading to fibrosis, rigidity, and increasing stenosis later in life. Ultimately, the appearance of the congenitally abnormal valve resembles degenerative AS. *Degenerative* or senile calcific disease is the most common cause of AS in older patients. Mechanical stress over many years on a valve originally normal ultimately results in deposition of calcium along the base of the cusps, rendering them immobile and obstructive.

The valvulitis of an attack of acute rheumatic fever results in adhesions along the edges of the cusps and fusion of the commissures. Fibrosis and scarring, which may be associated with calcification, result in thickening and contraction of the cusps so that the normal trileaflet structure becomes fused with a small central orifice. Varying degrees of regurgitation are common. Concentric LV hypertrophy occurs, and evidence of rheumatic mitral valve involvement is common.

## Pathophysiology

Minor commissural fusion produces murmurs due to turbulent blood flow, but significant hemodynamic obstruction occurs only when the cross-sectional area of the valve is reduced to about one fourth the normal size (2.5 to 3.5 $cm^2$). The ventricle adapts to the gradually progressive obstruction by developing concentric LV hypertrophy. Hypertrophy allows for maintenance of cardiac output in the face of a large gradient across the valve for many years without LV dilatation or the development of symptoms. The hypertrophic left ventricle is less distensible than normal, resulting in elevation of the LV end-diastolic pressure.

## Clinical Features

Isolated severe AS without clinically evident aortic regurgitation (AR) or concomitant mitral valve involvement is usually idiopathic and degenerative rather than rheumatic in origin.[21]

### History

A long asymptomatic, latent period is characteristic. *Angina,* which is typical and indistinguishable from that due to atherosclerotic coronary disease, is common, even though the coronary arteries are normal. It is caused by increased myocardial oxygen demand as a result of hypertrophy and reduced coronary flow reserve. *Syncope* is usually exertional and is attributed to failure of an increase in cardiac output to adapt to exercise-associated vasodilatation because of the fixed obstruction at the valve. Alternatively, a vasodepressor mechanism in response to marked elevation of LV systolic pressure is cited. Premonitory symptoms, exertional dizziness, and "grayouts" may predominate and bear the same significance as syncopal episodes. *Dyspnea* on exertion early in the clinical course is due to the elevated LV end-diastolic pressure. Severe manifestations such as orthopnea or paroxysmal nocturnal dyspnea are manifested late in the natural history and, when prominent, suggest that there may be associated mitral valve disease.

### Physical Examination

The *pulse* in mild AS is normal. In advanced AS it is of small volume and sustained (*pulsus parvus et tardus*). The distinctive character is best appreciated by palpating a larger vessel such as the carotid, where the radiation of the basal *systolic thrill* may also be detected. Recognition of the classic features of the pulse is difficult, and they may not be present in older patients with an inelastic arterial bed or in association with aortic regurgitation (AR). The *jugular venous pressure* may be normal unless there is heart failure or associated mitral valve disease. Prominent *a* waves are due to reduced right ventricular compliance secondary to marked septal hypertrophy. Precordial *palpation* reveals a forceful, sustained apical impulse, which may not be greatly displaced in the early stage of the disease.

*Auscultation* typically reveals a normal or soft first heart sound. If it is accentuated, associated MS should be considered. In severe AS, the second sound may be single, owing in part to immobility of the aortic leaflets and inaudibility of A2. A presystolic gallop may be heard that is due to a prominent fourth heart sound reflecting vigorous atrial contraction. An aortic ejection systolic murmur is characteristic. Best heard to the right and left of the sternum and the base of the heart, it radiates to the neck and apex. Usually described as harsh and raspy, its intensity varies markedly. Severity of stenosis usually correlates with the duration of the murmur (long murmur, severe AS) and the timing of the peak intensity (late peak, severe AS). Accentuation of the murmur after a postectopic pause is helpful in differentiating it from that of MR when it is clearly heard at the apex. An early diastolic murmur of associated aortic regurgitation is often detected. Valvar AS must be distinguished from other causes of LV outflow obstruction (Table 29–3).

Clinical determination of the severity of aortic stenosis is notoriously difficult. Even experienced clinicians may fail to evaluate the pulse correctly. When LV failure occurs and cardiac output decreases, the murmur may soften or disappear completely. Operative intervention, even at this late stage, is often successful, and clinical evaluation should be supplemented by echocardiography in any patient with unexplained heart failure. Associated MS may mask manifestations of AS.[22]

### Laboratory Examination

LV hypertrophy with repolarization changes is manifested *electrocardiographically* in the majority of patients with severe AS. In rheumatic heart disease, the pattern may be modified by the effects of concomitant mitral valve disease and pulmonary hypertension. The cardiac silhouette on *chest radiography* may be almost normal in pure AS, some poststenotic dilatation of the ascending aorta or calcification of the aortic valve being the only clue to the diagnosis. This is unusual in rheumatic AS, where associated AR or mitral valve disease often results in LV or left atrial enlargement. *Echocardiography* demonstrates the thickened, poorly mobile leaflets, quantitates severity by the Bernoulli equation, and evaluates LV size and function. Complete "hemodynamic" evaluation of most young patients can now be performed with this technique. *Cardiac catheterization and angiography* is usually indicated only for symptomatic patients being evaluated for valve replacement surgery when there is concern about coronary disease (because of symptoms of angina, age, or risk factor profile) or when doubt remains about the severity of stenosis or the presence or severity of other valve disease after detailed clinical and echocardiographic evaluation.

## Treatment

An understanding of the natural history of the condition aids management. Survival of patients with asymptomatic AS is almost normal until symptoms develop, when the prognosis worsens dramatically.[23]

*Medical treatment* for all patients should include prophylaxis against infective endocarditis and recurrences of rheumatic fever. Asymptomatic patients with severe AS should be advised to avoid vigorous physical activity, particularly competitive contact sports. All patients require education about the natural history of the condition, its gradually progressive nature, the need for regular medical supervision, and the importance of promptly reporting the onset of symptoms.

*Aortic valve replacement surgery* is the only effective treatment for adults with acquired AS. Aortic valve replacement should be recommended for patients with severe AS (aortic valve area 0.8 cm$^2$) and symptoms attributable to it. Although operative mortality is higher in patients with advanced disease, frank heart failure, and apparently impaired systolic function by conventional measures, valve replace-

Table 29-3

**Differential Diagnosis of Aortic Stenosis**

| Type of Stenosis | Maximum Murmur and Thrill | Aortic Ejection Sound | Aortic Component of Second Sound | Regurgitant Diastolic Murmur | Arterial Pulse |
|---|---|---|---|---|---|
| Acquired | Second right sternal border to neck; may be at apex in aged persons | Uncommon | Decreased or absent | Common | Delayed upstroke; anacrotic notch; with or without small amplitude |
| Hypertrophic subaortic | Fourth left sternal border to apex (± regurgitant systolic murmur at apex) | Rare | Normal or decreased | Very rare | Brisk upstroke, sometimes bisferious |
| Congenital valvular | Second right sternal border to neck (along left sternal border in some infants) | Very common in children, disappearing with age | Normal or increased in childhood; decreased with decrease in valve mobility with age | Uncommon in children, not uncommon in adults | Delayed upstroke; anacrotic notch; with or without small amplitude |
| Congenital subvalvular | Discrete: like valvular; tunnel: left sternal border | Rare | Not helpful (normal, increased, decreased, or absent) | Almost all | Delayed upstroke; anacrotic notch; with or without small amplitude |
| Congenital supravalvular | First right sternal border to neck and sometimes to medial aspect of right arm; occasionally greater in neck than in chest | Rare | Normal or decreased | Uncommon | Rapid upstroke in right carotid, delayed in left carotid; right arm pulse pressure greater than left |

From Levinson GE: Aortic stenosis. *In* Dalen JE, Alpert JS (eds): Valvular Heart Disease, 2nd ed. Boston: Little, Brown, 1987:202–203.

ment often results in dramatic improvement in clinical status and LV function. Given the poor prognosis with medical treatment, surgery is usually recommended.

## Aortic Regurgitation

### Pathology

Diseases affecting the aortic valve leaflets, the wall of the aortic root, or both structures may result in incompetence, which develops suddenly or progresses slowly over many years (Table 29–4). The inflammatory process of acute rheumatic valvulitis heals by fibrosis, causing cusp retraction that prevents apposition during diastole and thus allows reflux of blood from the aorta to the left ventricle. Some commissural fusion may produce a degree of stenosis.

### Pathophysiology

Adaptive processes usually account for a long latent period in chronic AR. Diastolic reflux from aorta to left ventricle results in diastolic volume overload, increased end-diastolic volume, and large stroke volume. Increased wall stress leads to eccentric LV hypertrophy and restoration of the ratio of wall thickness to cavity dimension toward normal, and thus tends to normalize end-diastolic wall stress. Despite a very large end-diastolic volume, end-diastolic pressure remains normal or only modestly elevated because of increased diastolic compliance. Ultimately, compensatory mechanisms fail, LV contractile function deteriorates, the ventricle dilates more, and interstitial fibrosis contributes to a decline in compliance. The end-diastolic pressure rises, and symptoms and signs of heart failure develop.

### Clinical Features

#### History

There may be a long latent period in chronic AR (10 to 15 years) before adaptive mechanisms fail. Thus, the disease may first be manifested when the characteristic murmur is recognized at routine examination of an asymptomatic patient. *Dyspnea* on exertion, with orthopnea and nocturnal dyspnea if presentation is delayed, are the most common symptoms. *Angina* is unusual but does occur in young patients with severe AR and normal coronary arteries. Often nocturnal, it is attributed to a slow heart rate, low diastolic blood pressure, and elevated LV end-diastolic pressure resulting in reduced coronary perfusion. Symptoms of apical

Table 29–4

**Causes of Aortic Regurgitation**

| Chronic | Acute |
| --- | --- |
| Rheumatic disease | Infective endocarditis |
| Degenerative disease | Dissecting aortic aneurysm |
| Chronic severe hypertension | Prosthetic valve malfunction |
| Syphilis | Trauma |
| Marfan's syndrome | |
| Infective endocarditis | |
| Discrete subaortic stenosis | |
| Ventricular septal defect with prolapse | |
| Rheumatoid arthritis | |
| Ankylosing spondylitis | |
| Congenital disorder | |

discomfort, awareness of the heart's activity when lying on the left side, and awareness of pulsation in the neck and precordium are manifestations of ventricular dilatation and large stroke volume and may be manifested long before there is evidence of LV dysfunction.

In *acute AR*, however, the situation is very different. The unprepared left ventricle is unable to tolerate the abrupt hemodynamic load. Acute cardiovascular collapse with hypotension and intense dyspnea may occur. The physical signs of acute AR are very different from those of the chronic disorder. Peripheral arterial signs are absent, the apex beat may not be prominent, and the murmur may be short, soft, and difficult to detect.

### Physical Examination

The *pulse* in chronic severe AR is of large volume with a brisk up-stroke and rapid descent (collapsing or water-hammer pulse). Systolic arterial pressure is elevated and diastolic pressure normally low, with Korotkoff sounds persisting until zero. A bisferiens pulse, with both percussion and tidal waves palpable during systole, may be detected in the brachial or carotid arteries. The large pulse volume gives rise to an array of eponymous physical signs (Table 29–5). The *apex beat* is usually markedly displaced and is diffuse and volume overloaded. A systolic thrill at the base may be a manifestation of large stroke volume in pure AR or of a minor degree of commissural fusion in rheumatic disease.

*Auscultation* in chronic severe AR reveals a normal or soft first heart sound, and a third sound may be present. The murmur of AR is an early diastolic decrescendo that commences immediately after the aortic component of the second heart sound. It is best heard with the patient sitting up and leaning forward with breath held in expiration while the diaphragm of the stethoscope is applied firmly between the apex and base. In general, the longer the murmur the more severe is the AR. A rumbling mid-diastolic murmur (Austin-Flint) is common and is attributable to antegrade flow across a normal mitral valve closing early because of the rapidly rising LV end-diastolic pressure. It may be impossible to distinguish this from the murmur of mitral stenosis. A loud first heart sound and an OS suggest associated MS, but their absence does not rule it out.

### Laboratory Examination

The *electrocardiogram* in the early stages shows increased voltage in the precordial leads. With progression of the condition, repolarization abnormalities develop. *The chest radiograph* usually reveals cardiomegaly. Duration and severity of AR determine the degree of cardiac enlargement. In early, mild AR, heart size may be almost normal, whereas in chronic severe AR it is markedly increased with dilatation of the ascending aorta. Doppler *echocardiography* and color-flow imaging readily detect even minor degrees of AR and allow quantification of its severity by measur-

Table 29–5

**Physical Signs of Aortic Regurgitation**

| Sign | Characteristic |
|------|----------------|
| Corrigan pulse | Bounding carotid pulse |
| De Musset sign | Nodding of head with each heartbeat |
| Traube sign | Pistol-shot sound heard over the femoral artery |
| Quincke pulse | Capillary pulsation visible in nailbed with transillumination |
| Duroziez sign | Diastolic murmur over femoral artery when compressed distal to stethoscope (systolic murmur if compressed proximally) |
| Hill sign | Popliteal systolic pressure exceeds brachial by >60 mm Hg |

ing the rate of decline in velocity of the regurgitant jet. Two-dimensional imaging of LV size and function provides information on ventricular adaptation to the regurgitant load. Serial echocardiographic evaluation provides essential information on ventricular response to the regurgitant load and is vital to formulating a management plan for asymptomatic patients. *Cardiac catheterization and angiography* are rarely necessary in young patients with rheumatic AR unless, after careful echocardiographic evaluation, doubt persists about severity of associated mitral valve disease. Coronary angiography is indicated before valve replacement surgery for patients who have angina or are at risk for coronary disease because of age or other risk factors.

### Treatment

Chronic AR may be tolerated well for years. Once symptoms develop, they are usually progressive, and death occurs in 2 to 4 years if aortic valve replacement, the only definitive therapy, is not performed. *Medical treatment* for all patients includes prophylaxis against infective endocarditis and recurrent acute rheumatic fever. Patients with severe AR, even if symptomatic, are conventionally advised to avoid strenuous physical exertion. All asymptomatic patients with severe chronic AR and normal LV function should be informed of the natural history of the disease and advised to have regular evaluations at 6-month intervals with serial measurements of LV size and function.

Vasodilator therapy can logically be expected to reduce the degree of regurgitation and enhance LV performance, delaying the need for valve replacement in *asymptomatic* patients with preserved LV function. While this has been demonstrated with nifedipine,[24] it has not been rigorously tested in young patients with rheumatic AR. Digoxin, diuretics, and vasodilators may temporarily stabilize patients with decompensated AR and heart failure who are awaiting valve replacement surgery. The need to prescribe any such agent, for either symptoms or evidence of LV dysfunction, should prompt consideration of aortic valve replacement.

*Surgical treatment* by aortic valve replacement should be offered to all patients with severe chronic AR as soon as possible after symptoms attributable to the condition develop. Asymptomatic patients with impaired LV function require individualized assessment and evaluation, which must take into account the natural history of the condition and the risk of aortic valve replacement and anticoagulation. Single measures of LV function may be unreliable, and repeated serial observations may be necessary. If these reveal consistent reproducible changes and the LV ejection fraction falls below 50% to 55%, LV end-systolic diameter exceeds 55 mm, or LV end-diastolic diameter exceeds 70 mm, surgery is recommended.[25]

Occasional patients present very late in the course of the disease with severe heart failure, markedly impaired LV function, and severe AR. Aortic valve replacement in this situation carries increased risk of operative mortality, but the long-term outlook for survivors is unpredictable. Most obtain at least temporary relief of symptoms, and, in some, ventricular function improves markedly with removal of the abnormal loading conditions. Short duration of symptoms may help to predict who will obtain maximum benefit.

## ■ TRICUSPID VALVE DISEASE

Rheumatic involvement of the tricuspid valve is reported in autopsy series far more frequently than it is detected clinically, perhaps because of relatively minor involvement or because the physical signs are often evanescent and are rapidly modified by bed rest and diuretic therapy. Severe organic tricuspid valve disease, almost always associated with significant mitral valve disease as part of a syndrome of multiple valve involvement, poses a formidable therapeutic challenge and has a grave prognosis.

## Tricuspid Regurgitation

## Pathology

*Rheumatic* TR is a result of scarring and deformity of the leaflets with fibrosis of chordae impairing mobility and preventing leaflet apposition. A degree of tricuspid stenosis (TS) is common. Infective endocarditis, the carcinoid syndrome, and trauma are other causes. *Functional* TR secondary to tricuspid annular dilatation may occur as a consequence of right ventricular failure secondary to pulmonary hypertension of any cause.

## Clinical Features

### History

Symptoms due to associated involvement of left heart valves usually predominate. Peripheral edema, ascites, and painful hepatomegaly produce prominent symptoms when TR is severe.

### Physical Examination

*Cachexia,* jaundice, ascites, and edema are prominent in untreated patients with severe TR who present late in the course of the disease. The arterial pulse form is determined by associated valve lesions, and AF is common. The *venous pressure* is always elevated with prominent *cv* waves and marked *y* collapse. A degree of associated TS renders the *y* descent less prominent. *Palpation* in severe TR reveals an atrial systolic impulse at the right lower sternal edge that is due to right atrial expansion. *Auscultation* reveals accentuation of P2 and a pansystolic murmur that is best heard in the fourth left intercostal space and typically increases on inspiration. When TR is very severe, this inspiratory accentuation may be very difficult to appreciate, particularly when AF is present. With marked right ventricular dilatation the murmur may be widespread and audible at the apex, and it is easily mistaken for MR. All the clinical features of severe TR, particularly if it is functional in origin, may abate dramatically after a brief period of intensive diuresis.

### Laboratory Examination

*Electrocardiography* is not helpful, usually showing AF and reflecting changes of pulmonary hypertension and the left-sided lesions responsible for its development. *Echocardiography* reveals dilatation of the right atrium and ventricle with paradoxical septal motion. Color Doppler imaging readily demonstrates the regurgitant jet, and evaluation of peak velocity of regurgitant flow allows estimation of pulmonary artery systolic pressure. *Cardiac catheterization* and *angiography,* which may be indicated to assess other valves, LV function, or coronary anatomy, seldom adds any significant information to that obtained by careful clinical and echocardiographic evaluation.

## Tricuspid Stenosis

## Pathology

Fusion of the leaflets at their commissures consequent to rheumatic valvulitis narrows the central orifice. Shortening and fibrosis of chordae limit leaflet motion. The valve is obstructive in diastole, and, almost invariably, there is a degree of systolic regurgitation. Pathologic evidence of TS may be found in 15% of all patients with rheumatic heart disease but is the rarest clinical manifestion (prevalence 5%).

## Clinical Features

The details of history and general physical examination are very similar to those of patients with rheumatic TR. A dominant *a* wave, which is sharp and flicking in the *jugular venous pressure* when sinus rhythm is present, is characteristic and more easily recognized than the slow *y* descent. Presystolic hepatic pulsation may be palpable.

On *auscultation* a diastolic murmur, loudest at the lower left sternal border with pre-systolic accentuation (with sinus rhythm), is heard. The murmur is accentuated on inspiration. A tricuspid OS is frequently recorded, but clinically it is very difficult to distinguish from the OS of associated MS. As MS frequently coexists, only careful attention to respiratory variation allows for differentiation of the two murmurs. A loud early diastolic murmur of AR in patients with multiple valve involvement may further confound clinical detection of the *murmur* of TS.

### Laboratory Examination

Marked right atrial enlargement on *electrocardiography* in the absence of significant right ventricular hypertrophy is suggestive. Cardiomegaly on chest radiography is common, and right atrial enlargement causes prominence of the right heart border. *Echocardiography* reveals thickening and doming, restricted motion, and reduced separation of the leaflets. Doppler echocardiography demonstrates increased antegrade velocity.

## Treatment

Intensive *medical treatment* with bed rest, salt restriction, and diuretic therapy improves the symptoms and physical signs of systemic venous congestion, improves hepatic function, and reduces the risk of valve replacement surgery. *Surgical treatment* of rheumatic tricuspid valve disease is difficult and the results generally unsatisfactory, but it demands careful consideration at the time of correction of mitral and aortic valve abnormalities. Failure to correct significant TR may result in considerable disability over the long term.

The final decision about what procedure is possible or necessary can often be made only after open inspection. Minor degrees of TS and TR that have not caused significant venous pressure elevation are best left alone. Although open commissurotomy may relieve TS, it may also produce severe TR, and tricuspid valve replacement with a bioprosthesis is usually necessary. Minor degrees of functional TR improve dramatically with resolution of pulmonary hypertension after mitral valve surgery. Patients with severe functional or organic TR require repair with a ring annuloplasty. If the immediate result at surgery is unsatisfactory, valve replacement is necessary. Whenever possible, tricuspid valve replacement is avoided, because all prostheses are inherently stenotic in this position and, while the operation relieves symptoms, the additional procedure increases the operative morbidity and mortality of mitral and aortic valve replacement.

## ■ MULTIPLE VALVE DISEASE

It is conventional and convenient to describe the various clinical syndromes of valvular heart disease in isolation. The clinical reality, however, is that a wide variety of combined lesions do occur, particularly in association with rheumatic heart disease. Only some 25% of all patients with rheumatic heart disease have isolated MS. Others have mixed valve disease or a combination of valve lesions that may produce a wide array of clinical syndromes. Correct identification and correction of all lesions is important. Failure to identify and correct an associated *severe* lesion may increase operative risk. Disregard of *mild* or *moderate* associated disease at the time of surgery for the major abnormality may allow it to progress, necessitating reoperation with its attendant risks and thus rendering nil the benefit of the primary procedure.

When several valves are involved, the clinical and hemodynamic manifestations depend on the relative severity of each lesion. Generally, when lesions are of approximately equal extent, clinical manifestations produced by the more proximal (upstream) lesions predominate.[26] Careful clinical evaluation supplemented by two-dimensional and Doppler echocardiography usually serves to estimate the relative contribution of each valve to the clinical syndrome. If doubt remains, catheterization or angiography specifically directed to answer unresolved issues may be necessary. The final decision about the severity of individual lesions, the need for repair, and the method of repair may be possible only at the time of operation.

## ■ SPECIAL CONSIDERATIONS

Acute rheumatic fever is a disease of poverty and overcrowding, and the majority of patients who suffer the sequelae of chronic valvular heart disease live where medical care is far from ideal. Availability of services and patients' access to and compliance with monitoring of anticoagulation, among many other factors, affect decisions on timing and the type of valve replacement surgery. Considerations of this nature, and the hemorrhagic risks attendant on poor supervision of warfarin anticoagulation, may prompt deferral of valve replacement for mildly symptomatic disease even though measures of ventricular function suggest that, under ideal circumstances, it should be performed. Alternatively, despite the known risks of premature degeneration in young patients, bioprostheses may be placed in those who wish to or must return to rural homes remote from medical supervision where warfarin anticoagulation is out of the question. Thromboembolic complications of mechanical prostheses are inevitable when warfarin anticoagulation is not possible.

Pregnancy poses particular problems for young women with valvular heart disease. It often precipitates symptoms in previously asymptomatic patients with MS. If the valve is suitable, then prophylactic PBMV may be possible before the woman conceives or, if necessary, during pregnancy. Asymptomatic or mildly symptomatic patients with other lesions should be advised to complete their families as soon as possible. Then, ideally, an effective form of contraception should be instituted before valve replacement surgery becomes necessary, thus avoiding the risks of warfarin to both mother and fetus.

## ■ REFERENCES

1. McLaren MJ, Hawkins DM, Koornhof HJ, et al: Epidemiology of rheumatic heart disease in black schoolchildren of Soweto, Johannesburg. Br Med J 1975; 3:474–478.
2. Siegel AC, Johnson EE, Stollerman GH: Controlled studies of streptococcal pharyngitis in a pediatric population. 1. Factors related to the attack rate of rheumatic fever. N Engl J Med 1961; 265:559–565.
3. Dale JB, Beachey EH: Sequence of myosin cross-reactive epitopes of streptococcal M protein. J Exp Med 1986; 164:1785–1990.
4. Haffejee I: Rheumatic fever and rheumatic heart disease: The current state of its immunology, diagnostic criteria and prophylaxis. Q J Med 1992; 84:641–658.
5. Jones TD: Diagnosis of rheumatic fever. JAMA 1944; 126:481–484.
6. Dajani AS, Ayoub EM, Bierman FZ, et al: Guidelines for the diagnosis of rheumatic fever: Jones criteria, updated 1992. JAMA 1992; 268:2069–2073.

7. Vasan RS, Shrivastava S, Vijayakumar M, et al: Echocardiographic evaluation of patients with acute rheumatic fever and rheumatic carditis. Circulation 1996; 94:73–82.
8. Dajani AS: Current status of nonsuppurative complications of Group A streptococci. Pediatr Infect Dis J 1991; 10:S25–S27.
9. Albert DA, Harel L, Karrison T: The treatment of rheumatic carditis: A review and meta-analysis. Medicine (Baltimore) 1995; 74:1–12.
10. Lewis BS, Geft IL, Milo S, Gotsman MS: Echocardiography and valve replacement in the critically ill patient with acute rheumatic carditis. Ann Thorac Surg 1979; 27:529–535.
11. Lue HC, Wu MH, Hseih KH, et al: Rheumatic fever recurrences: Controlled study of 3-week versus 4-week benzathine penicillin prevention programs. J Pediatr 1986; 108:299–304.
12. Lue HC, Wu MH, Wang JK, et al: Long-term outcome of patients with rheumatic fever receiving benzathine penicillin G prophylaxis every three weeks versus every four weeks. J Pediatr 1994; 125:812–816.
13. Olson LJ, Subramanian R, Ackermann DM, et al: Surgical pathology of the mitral valve. A study of 712 cases spanning 21 years. Mayo Clin Proc 1987; 62:22–34.
14. Leavitt JI, Coats MH, Falk RH: Effects of exercise on transmitral gradient and pulmonary artery pressure in patients with mitral stenosis or a prosthetic mitral valve. A Doppler echocardiographic study. J Am Coll Cardiol 1991; 17:1520–1526.
15. Ohmichi M, Tagaki S, Nomura N, et al: Endobronchial changes in chronic pulmonary venous hypertension. Chest 1988; 94:1127–1132.
16. Barrington WW, Boudoulas J, Bashore T, et al: Mitral stenosis: Mitral dome excursion at M1 and the mitral opening snap—the concept of reciprocal heart sounds. Am Heart J 1998; 115:1280–1290.
17. Klein HO, Sareli P, Schamroth CL, et al: Effects of atenolol on exercise capacity in patients with mitral stenosis with sinus rhythm. Am J Cardiol 1985; 56:598–601.
18. Marcus RH, Sareli P, Pocock WA, Barlow JB: The spectrum of severe rheumatic mitral valve disease in a developing country: Correlations among clinical presentations, surgical pathologic findings and haemodynamic sequelae. Ann Intern Med 1994; 120:177–183.
19. Carabello BA, Crawford FA: Valvular heart disease. N Engl J Med 1997; 337:32–41.
20. Rahimtoola SH: Valvular heart disease: A perspective. J Am Coll Cardiol 1983;1:199–215.
21. Passik CS, Ackermann DM, Pluth JR, Edwards WP: Temporal changes in the causes of aortic stenosis: A surgical pathologic study of 646 cases. Mayo Clin Proc 1987; 62:119–123.
22. Zitnik RS, Piemme TE, Messer RJ, et al: The masking of aortic stenosis by mitral stenosis. Am Heart J 1965; 69:22–30.
23. Ross J Jr, Braunwald E: Aortic stenosis. Circulation 1968; 38 (Suppl V): V-61–V-67.
24. Scognamiglio R, Rahimtoola SH, Fasoli G, et al: Nifedipine in asymptomatic patients with severe aortic regurgitation and normal left ventricular function. N Engl J Med 1994; 331: 689–694.
25. Rahimtoola SH: Indications for surgery in aortic valve disease. *In* Yusuf S, Cairns JA, Camm AJ (eds): Evidence Based Cardiology. London: BMJ Books, 1998: 811–832.
26. Braunwald EB: Valvular heart disease. *In* Braunwald EB (ed): Heart Disease: A Textbook of Cardiovascular Medicine, 5th ed. Philadelphia: WB Saunders, 1997: 1007–1076.

# ■ RECOMMENDED READING

Bonow RO, Carabello B, de Leon AC Jr, et al: ACC/AHA guidelines for the management of patients with valvular heart disease: A report of the American College of Cardiology/American Heart Association Task Force on Practice Guidelines (Committee on Management of Patients with Valvular Heart Disease). J Am Coll Cardiol 1998; 32:1486–1588.
Carabello BA: Mitral valve disease: Indications for surgery. *In* Yusuf S, Cairns JA, Camm AJ (eds): Evidence Based Cardiology. London: BMJ Books, 1998;798–810.
Dajani A, Taubert K, Ferrieri P, et al: Treatment of acute streptococcal pharyngitis and prevention of rheumatic fever: A statement for health professionals. Paediatrics 1995; 96:758–764.
Otto CM, Burwask IG, Legget ME, et al: Prospective study of asymptomatic valvular aortic stenosis. Clinical, echocardiographic, and exercise predictors of outcome. Circulation 1997; 95: 2262–2270.
Turi ZG: Balloon valvuloplasty: Mitral valve. *In* Yusuf S, Cairns JA, Camm AJ (eds): Evidence Based Cardiology. London: BMJ Books, 1998; 853–870.

# Chapter 30

# Infective Endocarditis

*Adolf W. Karchmer*

Infective endocarditis (IE) results when microbial agents infect the endothelial surface of the heart. Heart valves are the most common site for this process; however, infection occasionally develops on the low-pressure side of a ventricular septal defect, on chordae tendineae, or on mural endocardium that has been damaged by an aberrant jet of blood or an intracardiac foreign device (transvenous pacing lead, pulmonary artery catheter). Very rarely a similar process, infective endarteritis, arises when arteriovenous shunts, arterioarterial shunts (patent ductus arteriosus), or a coarctation of the aorta is involved. The cardinal lesion developing at these sites is the vegetation, a mass of platelets and fibrin, engendered by the procoagulant activity of infecting organisms and injured local tissue, wherein are enmeshed the causative microorganism and scant inflammatory cells.

IE is a relatively infrequent disease. The incidence generally has ranged from 1.5 to 6.2 cases per 100,000 population in developed countries during the past four decades. From 1988 to 1990, in a metropolitan area in the northeastern United States, the incidence was 9.3 cases per 100,000 population; notably, almost half of the cases occurred among injecting drug users (4.3 cases per 100,000 population).[1] The incidence increases progressively with age, reaching rates of 15 to 30 cases per 100,000 among persons in the sixth and later decades of life. In developed countries, prosthetic valve endocarditis (PVE) accounts for 7% to 25% of cases not involving injecting drug users.[1] Based on actuarial estimates, PVE develops in 1.4% to 3.1% of valve recipients within the first year after surgery and in 3.2% to 5.7% after 5 years have elapsed.[2]

## ■ CLINICAL MANIFESTATIONS

Symptomatic IE likely arises within several weeks of the initiating bacteremia, although in some patients with perioperative infection of new implanted prosthetic valves, overt symptoms may be delayed for more than 2 months.[2] The IE syndrome may be acute in onset, with hectic fevers and chills, numerous extracardiac manifestations, and rapid development of intracardiac complications; or it may be a very indolent illness with modest fevers, night sweats, anorexia, weight loss, infrequent extracardiac complications, and little or no progressive intracardiac injury. In fact, the presentations of IE are a continuum between these two extremes, such as between acute and subacute endocarditis. The temporal evolution of IE is in large part a function of the causative microorganism. *Staphylococcus aureus* and β-hemolytic streptococci usually result in acute presentations. In contrast, viridans streptococci, enterococci, coagulase-negative staphylococci, and the fastidious gram-negative coccobacilli, organisms often referred to by the acronym HACEK (*Haemophilus parainfluenzae, Haemophilus aphrophilus, Haemophilus paraphrophilus, Actinobacillus actinomycetemcomitans, Cardiobacterium hominis, Eikenella corrodens,* and *Kingella kingae*) give rise to subacute endocarditis. *Bartonella* species and *Coxiella burnetii* (the rickettsia-like agent that causes Q fever), organisms associated with blood culture–negative IE, also cause indolent IE.

The symptoms and signs of IE are nonspecific (Table 30–1). Nevertheless, the clinical features should suggest the diagnosis in patients with cardiac conditions that are substrates for infection, behavior patterns that predispose to endocarditis (injecting drug use), and bacteremia due to organisms that commonly cause IE. In addition, progressive cardiac valvular dysfunction or arterial emboli in the context of a nonspecific febrile illness should prompt consideration of IE.

Fever, the most common clinical feature of IE, may be absent or minimal in those who are severely debilitated or who have congestive heart failure or chronic renal failure. IE caused by coagulase-negative staphylococci or *Tropheryma whippelii* (the cause of Whipple disease) may present with little or no fever.[3] Some studies of IE among the elderly have suggested an increased frequency of muted presentations with little or no fever, but this has not been confirmed by others.[4, 5]

A heart murmur in a patient with IE involving a native heart valve (NVE) commonly reflects the valve pathology that predisposed the patient to IE. With acute *S. aureus* NVE, a process often engrafted on previously normal heart valves, murmurs are detected in only 30% to 45% of patients on presentation but ultimately develop in 85%. Murmurs are often not heard in tricuspid valve endocarditis or in pacemaker-related IE. Changing murmurs, reflecting new or progressive valve dysfunction rather than alterations in cardiac output, are most commonly encountered in patients with acute IE or PVE and are infrequent in subacute NVE.

The classic noncardiac manifestations of IE—splenomegaly, petechiae, Osler nodes, Janeway lesions, Roth spots, and splinter hemorrhages—are found less frequently today than several decades ago. Because many of these occur as a consequence of long-standing infection, this change likely represents the increasingly prompt diagnosis of endocarditis. None of these is pathognomonic for IE. Splinter hemorrhages, linear or flame-shaped lesions beneath the nails of the fingers or toes, associated with IE are found proximally in the nails. Those seen at the distal nail margin are most likely due to trauma.

Arthralgias, myalgias, true arthritis with nonspecific inflammatory synovial fluid, and localized back pain are common symptoms that remit rapidly with antimicrobial therapy. These focal skeletal symptoms must be distinguished from metastatic infection, which may require additional therapy, including drainage.

Table 30–1

**Signs and Symptoms in Patients with Infective Endocarditis**

| Symptoms | Percent | Signs | Percent |
|---|---|---|---|
| Fever | 80–85 | Fever | 80–90 |
| Chills | 40–75 | Heart murmur | 80–85 |
| Sweats | 25 | Changing or new murmur | 10–40 |
| Anorexia | 25–55 | Systemic emboli | 20–50 |
| Weight loss | 25–35 | Splenomegaly | 15–50 |
| Malaise | 25–40 | Clubbing | 10–20 |
| Cough | 25 | Osler nodes | 7–10 |
| Stroke | 15–20 | Splinter hemorrhage | 5–15 |
| Headache | 15–40 | Janeway lesions | 2–10 |
| Myalgia / arthralgia | 15–30 | Retinal lesions (Roth spots) | 2–10 |
| Back pain | 7–14 | Petechiae | 10–40 |
| Confusion | 10–20 | | |

Adapted from Karchmer AW: Infective endocarditis. *In* Braunwald E (ed): Heart Disease: A Textbook of Cardiovascular Medicine, 5th ed. Philadelphia: WB Saunders, 1996:1084; and Karchmer AW: Approach to the patient with infective endocarditis. *In* Goldman L, Braunwald E (eds): Primary Cardiology. Philadelphia: WB Saunders, 1998:202.

Arterial emboli, which are evident clinically in up to 50% of patients and are also frequently subclinical, discovered only at autopsy, are associated with significant morbidity and mortality in NVE and PVE.[4, 6–8] Systemic emboli are more common in patients with left-sided vegetations that exceed 10 mm in diameter (by echocardiogram) and that are located on the mitral valve, particularly on the anterior leaflet.[9–12] Emboli are often a presenting symptom in patients with IE. After initiation of appropriate therapy, the frequency of emboli decreases rapidly from 13 per 1000 patient-days during the initial treatment week to less than 1.2 per 1000 patient-days during the third week of effective therapy.[13] Emboli that occur late during treatment are not in themselves evidence of failed antimicrobial therapy. Renal emboli may cause gross or microscopic hematuria but rarely result in clinically important renal dysfunction.

Neurologic symptoms and complications occur in as many as 40% of patients and are particularly prominent when infection is due to *S. aureus*.[4, 7, 14–16] Embolic stroke syndromes occur in 10% to 25% of patients and are the most common neurologic consequences of IE; less common complications include mycotic aneurysm, intracranial hemorrhage, meningitis (either aseptic or occasionally purulent), cerebritis with microabscess formation, seizures, and encephalopathy.[14–16] Intracranial hemorrhage, which occurs in 5% of cases, results from hemorrhagic infarction, rupture of an artery due to septic arteritis at a site of embolic occlusion, or rupture of a mycotic aneurysm. Surgically drainable brain abscesses are uncommon in IE, whereas microabscesses of brain and meninges occur in patients with IE due to *S. aureus*.

Disruptions or distortion of left heart valves or chordae tendineae may result in congestive heart failure. Heart failure due to aortic valve insufficiency generally progresses more rapidly than that due to mitral valve regurgitation. Similar hemodynamic consequences occur with mechanical and bioprosthetic PVE due to valve dehiscence with paravalvular leakage or to destruction or disruption of valve parts. Bulky vegetations may obstruct the orifice of a mitral prosthesis, resulting in functional stenosis.[2]

Renal dysfunction in patients with IE most commonly results from reduced cardiac output or antimicrobial toxicity. Glomerulonephritis due to deposition of circulating immune complexes on the glomerular basement membrane results in renal dysfunction, which may progress during initial therapy but then gradually improves with continued antimicrobial treatment.

## ■ DIAGNOSIS

To avoid overlooking the diagnosis of IE, a high index of suspicion must be maintained. A sensitive and specific diagnostic schema, the Duke criteria, has been developed using predispositions plus the clinical, laboratory, and echocardiographic features of IE (Tables 30–2 and 30–3).[17] Using these clinical criteria, 74% and 26% of more than 300 pathologically proven IE cases were classified as definite and possible IE, respectively, and none were rejected.[7, 18] Similarly, among 1395 clinically diagnosed cases, 55% and 35% were classified by the Duke criteria as definite or possible, respectively; the 10% rejection rate often resulted from a suboptimal echocardiographic evaluation at the time of initial diagnosis.[5, 18] Study of rejected cases suggested that the negative predictive value and specificity were high.[18] Among 410 patients with potential endocarditis, IE diagnoses determined by an expert review panel correlated well with those established by the Duke criteria. However, the Duke criteria accepted as possible IE some cases considered by the experts not to be IE—that is, the criteria made a false-positive diagnosis by comparison with experts.[19]

Table 30–2

## Criteria for Diagnosis of Infective Endocarditis

**Definitive Infective Endocarditis**

*Pathologic criteria*

Microorganisms: demonstrated by culture or histology in a vegetation, *or* in a vegetation that has embolized, *or* in an intracardiac abscess, *or*

Pathologic lesions: vegetation or intracardiac abscess present, confirmed by histology showing active endocarditis

*Clinical criteria,* using specific definitions listed in Table 30–3

Two major criteria, *or*

One major and three minor criteria, *or*

Five minor criteria

**Possible Infective Endocarditis**

Findings consistent with infective endocarditis that fall short of definite endocarditis but are not rejected

**Rejected**

Firm alternative diagnosis for manifestations of endocarditis, *or*

Sustained resolution of manifestations of endocarditis, with antibiotic therapy for 4 days or less, *or*

No pathologic evidence of infective endocarditis at surgery or autopsy, after antibiotic therapy for 4 days or less

Adapted from Durack DT, Lukes AS, Bright DK: New criteria for diagnosis of infective endocarditis: Utilization of specific echocardiographic findings. Am J Med 1994;96:200–209.

Table 30–3

## Terminology Used in Criteria for the Diagnosis of Infective Endocarditis*

**Major Criteria**

*Positive results of blood culture*

Typical microorganism for infective endocarditis from two separate blood cultures

Viridans streptococci, *Streptococcus bovis,* HACEK group, *or* community-acquired *Staphylococcus aureus* or enterococci, in the absence of a primary focus, *or*

Persistently positive blood culture, defined as recovery of a microorganism consistent with infective endocarditis from

Blood cultures drawn more than 12 hr apart, *or*

All of three or a majority of four or more separate blood cultures, with first and last drawn at least 1 hr apart

*Evidence of endocardial involvement*

Positive echocardiogram

Oscillating intracardiac mass, on valve or supporting structures, or in the path of regurgitant jets, or on implanted material, in the absence of an alternative anatomic explanation, *or*

Abscess, *or*

New partial dehiscence of prosthetic valve, *or*

New valvular regurgitation (increase or change in preexisting murmur not sufficient)

**Minor Criteria**

Predisposition: predisposing heart condition *or* intravenous drug use

Fever ≥38.0°C (100.4°F)

Vascular phenomena: major arterial emboli, septic pulmonary infarcts, mycotic aneurysm, intracranial hemorrhage, conjunctival hemorrhages, Janeway lesions

Immunologic phenomena: glomerulonephritis, Osler nodes, Roth spots, rheumatoid factor

Microbiologic evidence: positive blood culture but not meeting major criterion as noted previously† *or* serologic evidence of active infection with organism consistent with infective endocarditis

Echocardiogram: consistent with infective endocarditis but not meeting major criterion

*See Table 30–2 for the criteria.

†Excluding single positive cultures for coagulase-negative staphylococci and organisms that do not cause endocarditis.

HACEK, *Haemophilus* species, *Actinobacillus actinomycetemcomitans, Cardiobacterium hominis, Eikenella* species, *Kingella kingae.*

Adapted from Durack DT, Lukes AS, Bright DK: New criteria for diagnosis of infective endocarditis: Utilization of specific echocardiographic findings. Am J Med 1994;96:200–209.

Several modifications of the Duke criteria have been suggested.[18] Inclusion of serologic results for organisms that are either slow growing or not readily isolated from blood cultures (e.g., *Brucella, C. burnetii,* or *Bartonella* sp.) as a major criterion would aid in the diagnosis of culture-negative IE. Expanding the minor criteria could increase the percent of definite cases without loss of specificity. The current major deficiency in the clinical application of the Duke criteria is the somewhat reduced specificity that results from limited capability to reject cases and the resulting expanded possible category. Although this is a conservative position avoiding missed diagnoses, it can result in overtreatment of some patients. This deficiency could be addressed by requiring that at least one major or three minor criteria be present before cases are accepted as possible IE and treated.[18]

The Duke diagnostic schema appropriately emphasizes the role of bacteremia (blood cultures) and echocardiography in the evaluation of patients with potential IE. Endocarditis is characterized by sustained low-density (<100 organisms/ml) bacteremia. Among patients who have IE but no prior antimicrobial therapy and who ultimately will have positive results of blood cultures, at least 95% of all blood cultures will be positive, and in 98% of cases one of the first two sets will yield the causative organism. In addition, organisms isolated from blood cultures can be classified as rarely encountered in blood except as causes of IE, as rare causes of IE, as common contaminants of blood cultures, and as organisms that often cause endocarditis but are frequently isolated from blood cultures as a consequence of infection other than IE. The diagnostic criteria give weight to both the persistence of bacteremia as well as the specific organism isolated. Bacteremia with organisms rarely encountered in the absence of IE (viridans streptococci, HACEK group) are thus highly suggestive, whereas organisms associated with endocarditis as well as other infections (*S. aureus,* enterococci) must be encountered in the absence of another site of infection in order to rank as a major criterion. Organisms that commonly contaminate blood cultures (i.e., coagulase-negative staphylococci or diphtheroids) or that rarely cause IE (i.e., Enterobacteriaceae) must be isolated from blood repetitively or from several cultures as a single molecular clone (coagulase-negative staphylococci) and in the absence of an alternative infection in order to be used as a criterion.[17, 18]

Incorporation of specifically defined echocardiographic findings characteristic of IE as a criterion markedly enhances the clinical utility of the schema. Including echocardiography recognizes the high sensitivity and specificity of two-dimensional echocardiography with color Doppler, especially if a transesophageal study with biplane or multiplane images is performed.[20–24] Echocardiography is not recommended as a screening test for febrile or bacteremic patients when endocarditis is unlikely; however, all patients suspected of having IE should be studied by echocardiogram (Fig. 30–1).[18]

# ■ DIAGNOSTIC TESTING

## Blood Cultures

In patients who are suspected of having endocarditis and who have not received an antibiotic recently, three blood cultures, obtained from separate venipuncture sites and spaced over 24 hours independently of temperature elevations, are sufficient to isolate the causative organism and to demonstrate the persistence of bacteremia characteristic of IE (Table 30–4 and Fig. 30–2). If blood cultures remain negative after 48 to 72 hours and fungi or fastidious organisms are suspected, additional cultures should be obtained, possibly using special techniques such as the lysis centrifugation system or a biphasic system.[18, 25] The microbiology

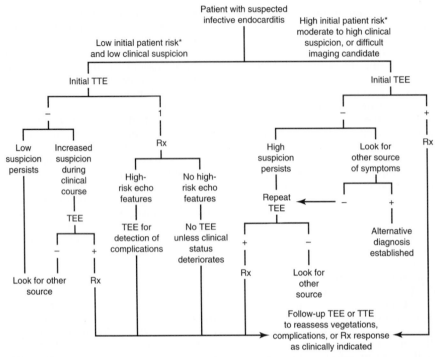

**Figure 30–1** ■ An algorithmic approach to the diagnostic use of echocardiography. High-risk echocardiographic features include large or mobile vegetation, valvular insufficiency, suggestion of perivalvular infection, and prosthetic valve. *See Table 30–9. TTE, transthoracic echocardiography; TEE, transesophageal echocardiography; Rx, drug therapy. (Adapted from Bayer AS, Bolger AF, Taubert KA, et al: Diagnosis and management of endocarditis and its complications. Circulation 1998;98:2936–2948.)

laboratory should be advised that IE is suspected so that it can prolong the incubation of the cultures and perform special subcultures to isolate unusual organisms when appropriate.[18, 25] From 5% to 15% of patients with IE diagnosed clinically have negative blood cultures. Prior receipt of antimicrobials accounts for 35% to 50% of these blood culture–negative cases.[18, 26] In hemodynamically stable patients who have subacute presentations of suspected IE and who have received antibiotics within the previous 2 weeks, empirical antibiotic therapy should be delayed to allow time for additional blood cultures to be obtained without the confounding effects of further antibiotic therapy.[18] This delay, although potentially enhancing culture yields, is unlikely to allow otherwise preventable complications. In contrast, among patients with acute presentations or with deteriorating hemodynamics, empirical therapy should be initiated immediately after the initial cultures have been obtained.

If after 5 days initial blood cultures remain negative (not attributable to confounding antimicrobial therapy), serologic testing to identify infection caused by pathogens that are difficult or unlikely to be recovered from blood (*Brucella, Bartonella, Legionella, C. burnetii,* and some fungi) should be considered[18, 25] (see Table 30–4 and Fig. 30–2). If valve tissue or embolized vegetations become available from these patients, not only should the material be cultured and examined by special microscopic techniques, but also the organism's identity should be sought by using the polymerase chain reaction to recover specific microbial DNA or 16S rRNA.[3, 27]

Table 30–4

## Evaluation of Patients with Suspected Endocarditis*

| Timing | Test or Procedure | Comment |
|---|---|---|
| **Admission** (prior to admission if stable) | CBC, differential, three blood cultures,† urinalysis, ECG, creatinine, bilirubin, AST, alkaline phosphatase, prothrombin time, chest roentgenogram | Tests, other than blood cultures, do not aid with diagnosis but establish baseline for assessing the complications of IE or treatment |
| **After Admission** | | |
| 24 to 48 hours | | |
|   Blood culture results positive | TTE | TEE is the initial study of choice with suspected prosthetic valve IE |
| 48 to 72 hours | | |
|   Blood culture results positive but TTE negative or blood culture results and TTE negative | TEE | See Figure 30–2 and text regarding initiation of therapy |
| 72 to 96 hours | | |
|   Blood culture results negative | Two blood cultures daily for 2 days,† ESR, rheumatoid factor, circulating immune complex titer | ESR, circulating immune complex titer, and rheumatoid factor add little value if results of blood cultures and echocardiogram are positive. May contribute to minor diagnostic criterion |
| Days 5 to 10 | | |
|   Blood culture results remain negative (no antibiotics given) | Serologic testing and special blood cultures for fastidious organisms | See text: Diagnosis of IE and Microbiology of IE. Obtain infectious disease consultation and advice of microbiology laboratory director. Consider empirical therapy (see Fig. 30–2 and text) |
| | Retrieve material embolic to a peripheral artery for culture histologic examination, molecular testing | |
| | Repeat TEE if initially negative | Increases the yield for vegetations |
| **Any Time** | | |
| Focal central nervous system symptoms or finding suggesting localized event | Computed tomography (with enhancement). If evidence of hemorrhage without mass effect, consider magnetic resonance angiogram or formal angiogram. If no mass effect, consider lumbar puncture | Consider mycotic aneurysm; with acute *S. aureus* IE or new focal symptoms without infarct, consider angiography |
| Left upper quadrant pain (with/without left shoulder pain) | Image spleen (and kidney) for abscess or infarct | |
| Intracardiac complication: hemodynamic deterioration, suspected paravalvular infection | ECG, echocardiogram | ECG conduction change insensitive indicator of paravalvular abscess. TEE optimal technique |

*For patients who are hemodynamically stable and have a subacute presentation.
†Request that laboratory incubate blood cultures for 3 wk (indicate diagnosis of infective endocarditis).
CBC, complete blood count; AST, aspartate aminotransferase; ESR, erythrocyte sedimentation rate; TEE, transesophageal echocardiography; TTE, transthoracic echocardiography; IE, infective endocarditis; ECG, electrocardiogram.
Adapted from Karchmer AW: Approach to the patient with infective endocarditis. *In* Goldman L, Braunwald E (eds): Primary Cardiology. Philadelphia: WB Saunders, 1998:204.

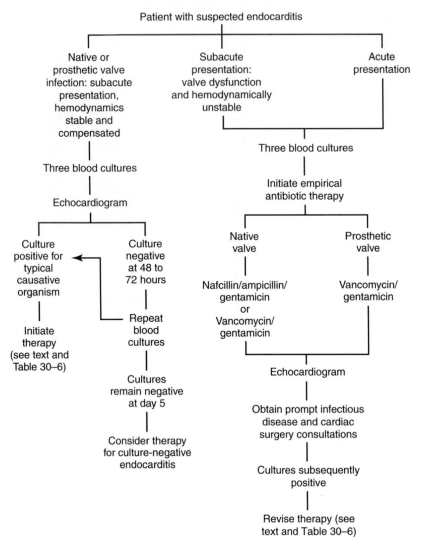

**Figure 30–2** ▪ An algorithmic approach to the initiation of therapy in patients with suspected infective endocarditis. Echocardiogram can initially be performed by the transthoracic approach; however, transesophageal views are required for maximal evaluation and are essential in patients with prosthetic valves.

## Echocardiography

Echocardiographic evaluation with color flow and continuous as well as pulsed Doppler allows anatomic confirmation of IE, identifies intracardiac complications, and allows functional assessment of the heart. Transthoracic echocardiography (TTE), although noninvasive and 98% specific for vegetations, detects vegetations in about 65% of clinical or anatomically established IE.[9, 22] TTE is limited by vegetation size (≤2 mm in diameter) and in 20% of adults by body habitus, chest wall configuration, or lung disease. Furthermore, TTE is not adequate for assessing prosthetic valves (especially in the mitral position) or for detecting perivalvular abscess, leaflet perforations, or intracardiac fistulas.[20, 24, 28–30] In contrast, transesophageal echocardiography (TEE), which though invasive is extremely safe in the hands of experienced operators, detects vegetations in more than 90% of patients with proven NVE and 82% to 94% of patients with clinically diagnosed IE.[9, 22, 23] In patients with PVE, the sensitivity for detecting vegetations by TEE ranged from 74% to 96% whereas the sensitivity with TTE was 13% to 36%.[29, 30] TEE is clearly the optimal technique for diagnosis of PVE and identification of complications that affect management.[28–30] TEE is more sensitive than TTE (78% to 87% vs 28%) in detecting paravalvular abscesses and subaortic invasive infection, without loss of specificity.[20, 31] Although the sensitivity of TEE for detecting abnormalities indicative of NVE and PVE is very high, false-negative results occur in 6% to 18% of patients.[22, 23, 30] The rate of false-negative results can be reduced (4% to 13%) by repeat TEE and multiplane examinations.[23, 24] In patients at low risk of NVE, a nondiagnostic high-quality TTE or TEE is generally sufficient to rule out endocarditis (see Fig. 30–1).[18] In moderate-risk patients, TEE may be required. For example, although earlier studies had suggested that the incidence of IE in patients with catheter-associated *S. aureus* bacteremia averaged 6%, IE was confirmed in 23% when patients were studied with TEE.[32] Still, in patients at high risk of IE, a nondiagnostic TEE is not sufficient to override clinical evidence and exclude the diagnosis.[18, 23] Cardiac catheterization, magnetic resonance imaging, and scintigraphy with various isotopes offer little beyond echocardiography in the anatomic assessment of IE.

## Other Studies

Results of complete blood counts and differential, creatinine determinations, selected liver function tests, prothrombin time, urinalysis, chest radiography, and electrocardiogram are often serially monitored and may be important in patient management (see Table 30–4). Measurements of erythrocyte sedimentation rate, C-reactive protein, quantitative circulating immune complexes, immunoglobulin or cryoglobulin, and rheumatoid factor are commonly abnormal in subacute IE but do not yield significant value beyond clinical observations when monitoring response to therapy. They may be useful if incorporated into a minor criterion in the Duke schema.

## ■ CAUSATIVE MICROORGANISMS

Although almost any bacterial or fungal species can cause IE, in fact, a relative small number of bacterial species cause the majority of cases of IE. Even those species are encountered with different frequencies in various clinical settings (Table 30–5). *S. aureus* is the major organism causing acute NVE, whereas streptococci, enterococci, coagulase-negative staphylococci, and the HACEK group are the major causes of subacute NVE. β-Hemolytic streptococci and *Staphylococcus lugdenensis*, a coagulase-negative *Staphylococcus* species, are associated with valve destruction and acute presentation. Nosocomial NVE occurs as a complication of bacteremia associated with intravascular devices and genitourinary tract manipulations and is caused primarily by staphylococci and enterococci. In two series of *S. aureus* IE, 35% to 46% had nosocomial infection.[33, 34]

Patients with PVE can be divided into three groups: those with infection developing from perioperative events and having onset within 60 days of surgery (early PVE), those with onset a year or more after surgery and arising primarily from community-acquired transient bacteremia (late PVE), and those with onset between 2 and 12 months after valve surgery and largely related to perioperative

Table 30-5

## Microbiology of Infective Endocarditis in Specific Clinical Settings

| | Native Valve Endocarditis‡ | | Prosthetic Valve Endocarditis§ Time of Onset After Valve Surgery | | | Endocarditis in Drug Addicts | | |
|---|---|---|---|---|---|---|---|---|
| | | | | | | | | |
| | | | Number of Cases (%) | | | | | |
| Organism | Community Acquired N = 683 | Nosocomial N = 82 | <2 mo N = 144 | 2–12 mo N = 31 | >12 mo N = 194 | Right Sided‖ N = 346 | Left Sided‖ N = 204 | Total¶ N = 675 |
| Streptococci* | 220 (32) | 6 (7) | 2 (1) | 3 (9) | 61 (31) | 17 (5) | 31 (15) | 80 (12) |
| Pneumococci | 8 (1) | — | — | — | — | — | — | — |
| Enterococci | 57 (8) | 13 (16) | 12 (8) | 4 (12) | 22 (11) | 7 (2) | 49 (24) | 59 (9) |
| Staphylococcus aureus | 241 (35) | 45 (55) | 32 (22) | 4 (12) | 34 (18) | 267 (77) | 47 (23) | 396 (57) |
| Coagulase-negative staphylococci | 29 (4) | 8 (10) | 47 (33) | — | 22 (11) | — | — | — |
| Fastidious gram-negative coccobacilli (HACEK group)† | 22 (3) | — | — | — | 11 (6) | — | — | — |
| Gram-negative bacilli | 22 (3) | 4 (5) | 19 (13) | 1 (3) | 11 (6) | 17 (5) | 26 (13) | 45 (7) |
| Fungi, Candida sp. | 5 (1) | 3 (4) | 12 (8) | 2 (6) | 3 (1) | — | 25 (12) | 26 (4) |
| Polymicrobial / miscellaneous | 41 (6) | 1 (1) | 4 (3) | 2 (6) | 9 (5) | 28 (8) | 20 (10) | 48 (7) |
| Diphtheroids | — | — | 9 (6) | — | 5 (3) | — | — | 1 (0.1) |
| Culture negative | 38 (5) | 2 (2) | 7 (5) | 4 (12) | 16 (8) | 10 (3) | 6 (3) | 20 (3) |

*Includes viridans streptococci; Streptococcus bovis; other non-group A, groupable streptococci; and Abiotrophia species (nutritionally variant streptococci).

†Includes Haemophilus sp., Actinobacillus actinomycetemcomitans, Cardiobacterium hominis, Eikenella sp., and Kingella kingae.

‡Data from Sandre RM, Shafran SD: Infective endocarditis: Review of 135 cases over 9 years. Clin Infect Dis 1996;22:276–286; and Karchmer AW: Treatment of infective endocarditis. In Smith TW (ed): Cardiovascular Therapeutics. Philadelphia: WB Saunders, 1996:718–730.

§Data from Sandre RM, Shafran SD: Infective endocarditis: Review of 135 cases over 9 years. Clin Infect Dis 1996;22:276–286; and Karchmer AW: Infections of prosthetic valves and intravascular devices. In Mandell GL, Bennett JE, Dolin R (eds): Principles and Practice of Infectious Diseases, 5th ed. Philadelphia: Churchill Livingstone, 2000.

‖Data from Sandre RM, Shafran SD: Infective endocarditis: Review of 135 cases over 9 years. Clin Infect Dis 1996;22:276–286.

¶Data from Sandre RM, Shafran SD: Infective endocarditis: Review of 135 cases over 9 years. Clin Infect Dis 1996;22:276–286; and Mathew J, Addai T, Anand A, et al: Clinical features, site of involvement, bacteriologic findings, and outcome of infective endocarditis in intravenous drug users. Arch Intern Med 1995;155:1641–1648.

Adapted from Karchmer AW: Approach to the patient with infective endocarditis. In Goldman L, Braunwald E (eds): Primary Cardiology. Philadelphia: WB Saunders, 1998:205.

events. The causes of early PVE are largely coagulase-negative staphylococci, S. *aureus*, gram-negative bacilli, and fungi (primarily *Candida* sp.). The frequencies of organisms causing late-onset PVE are similar to those noted in community-acquired NVE, except that there is an increased frequency of coagulase-negative staphylococci. Coagulase-negative staphylococci causing PVE within 12 months of valve surgery are predominantly *Staphylococcus epidermidis,* and 85% are methicillin resistant, whereas 50% of those causing PVE a year or more after surgery are nonepidermidis species and only 30% are methicillin resistant.[2]

S. *aureus* causes more than 50% of all IE and 70% of tricuspid valve IE among injecting drug users (see Table 30–5). Streptococci and enterococci infect previously abnormal left heart valves in this population. IE due to gram-negative bacilli, particularly *Pseudomonas aeruginosa,* and fungi occur with increased frequency among drug users. Unusual organisms (e.g., *Corynebacterium, Lactobacillus, Bacillus cereus*) and polymicrobial infections, possibly related to injection of contaminated materials, are occasionally found in drug users with IE. IE in patients with underlying human immunodeficiency virus infection occurs primarily among injecting drug abusers, and its microbiology is very similar to IE in drug abusers in general.[35]

Many unusual and fastidious organisms cause IE.[25] Some cause IE in unique epidemiologic settings (e.g., *C. burnetii* in Europe, *Brucella* in the Middle East and Mediterranean basin), others are associated with unique clinical situations (e.g., *Legionella* and *Mycobacterium chelonei,* and *Mycoplasma hominis* on prosthetic valves), and some appear to be sporadic events. *Bartonella* species have been increasingly implicated as a cause of IE, often with negative results of blood cultures, and may account for as many as 3% of cases of IE overall.[36] *Tropheryma whippelii* has been identified as a cause of very indolent, afebrile IE.[3]

## ■ ANTIMICROBIAL THERAPY

Antimicrobial therapy capable of killing (as opposed to only inhibiting growth) the organism causing IE is required for optimal treatment. The recommended therapies are based on the precise susceptibility of the etiologic agent, combined with prior clinical experience with that species, but must be adjusted in consideration of circumstances unique to the patient—that is, allergies, end organ dysfunction, interactions with other required medications, or other perceived risks of adverse events. Accordingly, it is crucial that efforts to identify the agent be optimal (see Diagnostic Testing, Blood Cultures). The impact of beginning empirical antimicrobial therapy immediately after blood cultures have been obtained must be carefully considered (see Fig. 30–2). In patients who have acute endocarditis or severely compromised hemodynamics and who will require urgent valve surgery, rapid initiation of therapy may prevent further cardiac structural damage or reduce the risk of recrudescent infection after valve surgery. However, among hemodynamically stable patients with subacute IE, especially if antibiotics have been given during the prior 2 weeks, therapy should be delayed for 2 to 5 days while awaiting blood culture results. If initial cultures remain negative, blood cultures should be repeated (see Table 30–4 and Fig. 30–2).

### Organism-Specific Regimens

Expert committees have developed regimens for the treatment of IE caused by the more commonly encountered causative microorganisms (Table 30–6).[37] Choices are provided to address variations in antimicrobial susceptibility within species as well as to avoid anticipated adverse reactions. Regimens for treatment of NVE and PVE are usually qualitatively similar (except for staphylococcal infection), but

## Table 30–6

### Recommended Therapy for Infective Endocarditis Caused by Specific Organisms

| Infecting Organism | Antibiotic | Dose and Route* | Duration (wk)† | Comments |
|---|---|---|---|---|
| 1. Penicillin-susceptible viridans streptococci, *Streptococcus bovis*, and other streptococci, penicillin MIC ≤ 0.1 µg/ml | A. Penicillin G | 12–18 million units IV daily in divided doses q 4 hr | 4 | |
| | B. Penicillin G plus gentamicin‡ | 12–18 million units IV daily in divided doses q 4 hr 1 mg/kg IM or IV q 8 hr | 4 | Avoid aminoglycoside-containing regimens when potential for nephrotoxicity or ototoxicity is increased.‡ See text. |
| | C. Penicillin G plus gentamicin‡ | Same doses as noted previously | 2 2 | |
| | D. Ceftriaxone | 2 g IV or IM daily as single dose | 2 4 | Can be used in patients with nonimmediate penicillin allergy. IM administration of ceftriaxone is painful. |
| | E. Vancomycin§ | 30 mg/kg IV daily in divided doses q 12 hr | 4 | Use for patients with immediate or severe penicillin or cephalosporin allergy. Infuse doses over 1 hr to avoid histamine release (red man syndrome). |
| 2. Relatively penicillin-resistant streptococci Penicillin MIC 0.2–0.5 µg/ml | A. Penicillin G plus gentamicin‡ | 18–24 million units IV daily in divided doses q 4 hr 1 mg/kg IM or IV q 8 hr | 4 2 | Preferred for nutritionally variant (pyridoxal- or cysteine-requiring) streptococci. |
| Penicillin MIC >0.5 µm/ml | B. Penicillin G plus gentamicin‡ | See regimens recommended for enterococcal endocarditis | 4 | |
| 3. Enterococci (in vitro evaluation for MIC to penicillin and vancomycin, β-lactamase production, and high-level resistance to gentamicin and streptomycin required) | A. Penicillin G plus gentamicin‡ | 18–30 million units IV daily in divided doses q 4 hr 1 mg/kg IM or IV q 8 hr | 4–6 | See text for use of streptomycin instead of gentamicin in these regimens. Four weeks of therapy recommended for patients with shorter history of illness (<3 mo) who respond promptly to treatment. |
| | B. Ampicillin plus gentamicin‡ | 12 g IV daily in divided doses q 4 hr Same dose as noted previously | 4–6 4–6 | |
| | C. Vancomycin§ plus gentamicin‡ | 30 mg/kg IV daily in divided doses q 12 hr Same dose as noted previously | 4–6 4–6 | Use for patients with penicillin allergy. Do not use cephalosporins. |

| | | Dose | Duration (wk)* | Comments |
|---|---|---|---|---|
| 4. Staphylococci infecting native valves (assume penicillin resistance), methicillin susceptible | A. Nafcillin or oxacillin plus optional addition of gentamicin‡ | 12 g IV daily in divided doses q 4 hr<br>1 mg/kg IM or IV q 8 hr | 4–6<br>3–5 days | Penicillin—18–24 million units daily in divided doses q 4 hr can be used instead of nafcillin, oxacillin, or cefazolin if strains do not produce β-lactamase. |
| | B. Cefazolin plus optional addition of gentamicin‡ | 2 g IV q 8 hr<br>Same dose as previously | 6<br>3–5 days | Cephalothin or other first-generation cephalosporin in equivalent doses can be used. |
| | C. Vancomycin§ | 30 mg/kg IV daily in divided doses q 12 hr | 6 | Use for patients with immediate penicillin allergy. |
| 5. Staphylococci infecting native valves, methicillin resistant | A. Vancomycin§ | 30 mg/kg IV daily in divided doses q 12 hr | 6 | Use for patients with immediate penicillin allergy. |
| 6. Staphylococci infecting prosthetic valves, methicillin susceptible (assume penicillin resistance) | A. Nafcillin or oxacillin plus gentamicin‡ plus rifampin§ | 12 g IV daily in divided doses q 4 hr<br>1 mg/kg IV or IM q 8 hr<br>300 mg orally q 8 hr | 6<br>2<br>6 | First-generation cephalosporin or vancomycin could be used in penicillin-allergic patients. Use gentamicin during initial 2 wk. See text for alternatives to gentamicin. For patients with immediate penicillin allergy, use regimen 7. |
| 7. Staphylococci infecting prosthetic valves, methicillin resistant | A. Vancomycin§ plus gentamicin‡ plus rifampin‖ | 30 mg/kg IV daily in divided doses q 12 hr<br>1 mg/kg IV or IM q 8 hr<br>300 mg orally q 8 hr | 6<br>2<br>6 | Use gentamicin during the initial 2 wk of therapy. See text for alternatives to gentamicin. Do not substitute a cephalosporin or imipenem for vancomycin. |
| 8. HACEK organisms¶ | A. Ceftriaxone | 2 g IV or IM daily as a single dose | 4 | Cefotaxime or other third-generation cephalosporin in comparable doses may be used. |
| | B. Ampicillin plus gentamicin‡ | 12 g IV daily in divided doses q 4 hr<br>1 mg/kg IV or IM q 8 hr | 4<br>4 | Test organism for β-lactamase production. Do not use this regimen if β-lactamase is produced. |

IE, infective endocarditis; MIC, minimal inhibitory concentration; IV, intravenous; IM, intramuscular.

*Recommended doses are for adults with normal renal and hepatic function. Doses of gentamicin, streptomycin, and vancomycin must be adjusted in patients with renal dysfunction. Use ideal body weight to calculate doses (men = 50 kg + 2.3 kg per inch over 5 ft; women = 45.5 kg + 2.3 kg per inch over 5 ft).

†All durations in weeks except where specifically noted (4.A and B with gentamicin).

‡Aminoglycosides should not be administered as a single daily dose in patients with normal renal function.

§Peak levels obtained 1 hr after completion of the infusion should be 30–45 μg/ml.

‖Rifampin increases the dose of warfarin or dicumarol required for effective anticoagulation.

¶HACEK organisms include *Haemophilus* sp., *Actinobacillus actinomycetemcomitans*, *Cardiobacterium hominis*, *Eikenella corrodens*, and *Kingella kingae*.

From Karchmer AW: Treatment of infective endocarditis. *In* Smith TW (ed): Cardiovascular Therapeutics. Philadelphia: WB Saunders, 1996:722–723.

treatment for PVE is given for several weeks longer than that for NVE. In general, compromises in recommended dosing, duration, and route of administration should be avoided unless supported by medical literature and required by untoward events.

**Streptococcal Infective Endocarditis.** Most viridans streptococci and *Streptococcus bovis* that cause IE are susceptible to penicillin (minimum inhibitory concentration [MIC] ≤ 0.1 μg/ml). IE caused by these organisms can be treated with any of the recommended regimens (see Table 30–6, 1A–E). IE caused by nutritionally deficient streptococci (previously called *Streptococcus adjacens* or *Streptococcus defectivus* but now assigned to the genus *Abiotrophia*), PVE, or complicated streptococcal NVE should not be treated with the 2-week regimen (see Table 30–6, 1C). The ceftriaxone regimen (see Table 30–6, 1D) can be used in patients with a history of an allergy to penicillin that does not result in urticaria or anaphylaxis-like symptoms (immediate-type allergy). In patients who have had an immediate-type allergy reaction to penicillin or a cephalosporin, treatment with vancomycin is recommended (see Table 30–6, 1E). In patients with normal renal function, uncomplicated NVE caused by penicillin-susceptible viridans streptococci has been effectively treated with a 2-week regimen using ceftriaxone 2 g intravenously plus an aminoglycoside (netilmicin 4 mg/kg/day or gentamicin 3 mg/kg/day), each given as a single daily dose.[38, 39] Because experience with short-course therapy using aminoglycosides in single daily doses is very limited, this approach has not been incorporated into recommendations. Combination therapy with penicillin or ceftriaxone for 6 weeks plus gentamicin (1 mg/kg ideal body weight every 8 hours) during the first 2 weeks is advocated for treatment of PVE caused by penicillin-susceptible streptococci.

Endocarditis caused by streptococci that are relatively resistant to penicillin (MIC ≥0.2 μg/ml but <0.5 μg/ml) and IE caused by group B streptococci (*Streptococcus agalactiae*) is treated with combination therapy (see Table 30–6, 2A). If these patients report an immediate-type β-lactam allergy, vancomycin therapy is recommended (see Table 30–6, 1E), whereas for those with milder penicillin allergies, ceftriaxone can be substituted for penicillin. IE caused by even more resistant streptococci (penicillin MIC >0.5 μg/ml) is treated with a regimen used for enterococcal IE (see Table 30–6, 3A). IE caused by nutritionally deficient streptococci (*Abiotrophia* sp.) is treated with penicillin plus gentamicin or streptomycin (see Table 30–6, 3A or B) or by vancomycin alone for 6 weeks.

**Enterococcal Infective Endocarditis.** The enterococci as a genus are more antibiotic resistant than streptococci. They are inhibited but not killed by penicillin, ampicillin, or vancomycin and are resistant to cephalosporins and antistaphylococcal penicillinase-resistant penicillins such as nafcillin, oxacillin, and cloxacillin. Optimal antimicrobial therapy for enterococcal IE requires a bactericidal synergistic interaction between a cell wall–active antibiotic (penicillin, ampicillin, vancomycin, or teicoplanin [not available in the United States]) that at clinically achievable concentrations inhibits the organism and an aminoglycoside (gentamicin or streptomycin) for which the organism does not have high-level resistance.[40] If high concentrations of streptomycin (2000 μg/ml) or gentamicin (500 to 2000 μg/ml) fail to inhibit the growth of an enterococcus (e.g., there is high-level resistance), the aminoglycoside cannot exert a lethal effect or contribute to bactericidal synergism. High-level resistance to gentamicin predicts the inefficacy of kanamycin, amikacin, tobramycin, and netilmicin as well. Additionally, the ability of aminoglycosides other than streptomycin or gentamicin to contribute to synergy, even against organisms not highly resistant to gentamicin, is unpredictable; thus, they should not be used to treat enterococcal IE.

Each of the standard regimens recommended for the treatment of enterococcal IE combines a cell wall–active agent and gentamicin and anticipates that the organism will be inhibited at clinically achievable serum concentrations of the cell wall–active agent and will not exhibit high-level resistance to gentamicin (see Table 30–6, 3A–C). If the causative enterococcus does not exhibit high-level resistance to streptomycin, this aminoglycoside (9.5 mg/kg ideal body weight given intramuscularly or intravenously every 12 hours to achieve peak serum concentrations of 20 µg/ml) can be used in lieu of gentamicin. Patients with a history of an allergic reaction to a penicillin and with enterococcal IE must be treated with vancomycin plus an aminoglycoside (see Table 30–6, 3C) or undergo desensitization and subsequent treatment with a penicillin or ampicillin regimen (see Table 30–6, 3A or B). Cephalosporins are ineffective. Aminoglycosides are not administered in single daily doses. A bacteriologic cure can be achieved in 85% of patients with enterococcal NVE or PVE treated with a synergistic combination regimen.

Enterococci have become increasingly resistant, and regimens that previously were predictably effective now require careful assessment. To structure an effective regimen, the enterococcus must be tested for its susceptibility to ampicillin and vancomycin, for β-lactamase production, and for high-level resistance to gentamicin and streptomycin. With this information, a synergistic bactericidal regimen can be designed, if possible, or alternative nonbactericidal single-drug therapy can be considered (Table 30–7). Treatment with an aminoglycoside if synergy cannot be effected (e.g., high-level resistance is present to both streptomycin and gentamicin) is inappropriate; it offers no benefit and may result in significant toxicity.

**Staphylococcal Infective Endocarditis.** More than 95% of *S. aureus* and coagulase-negative staphylococci produce a β-lactamase and thus are resistant to penicillin. Some *S. aureus* and many coagulase-negative staphylococci are resistant to methicillin also (which implies resistance to all available β-lactam antibiotics);

---

Table 30–7

**Strategy for Selecting Therapy for Enterococcal Endocarditis Caused by Strains Resistant to Components of the Standard Regimen**

1. Ideal therapy includes a cell wall–active agent plus an effective aminoglycoside to achieve bactericidal synergy
2. Cell wall–active antimicrobial
   A. Determine MIC for ampicillin and vancomycin; test for β-lactamase production (nitrocefin test)
   B. If ampicillin and vancomycin susceptible, use ampicillin
   C. If ampicillin resistant (MIC ≥ 16 µg/ml), use vancomycin
   D. If β-lactamase produced, use vancomycin or consider ampicillin-sulbactam
   E. If ampicillin resistant and vancomycin resistant (MIC ≥ 16 µg/ml), consider teicoplanin
   F. If ampicillin-resistant and highly resistant to vancomycin and teicoplanin (MIC ≥ 256 µg/ml), see 4 A–D
3. Aminoglycoside to be used with cell wall–active antimicrobial
   A. If no high-level resistance to streptomycin (MIC < 2000 µg/ml) or gentamicin (MIC < 500–2000 µg/ml), use gentamicin or streptomycin
   B. If high-level resistance to gentamicin (MIC > 500–2000 µg/ml), test streptomycin. If no high-level resistance to streptomycin, use streptomycin
   C. If high-level resistance to gentamicin and streptomycin, omit aminoglycoside therapy; use prolonged therapy with cell wall–active antimicrobial (8–12 wk), see 2 B–E
4. Alternative regimens and approaches
   A. Consider ampicillin, vancomycin (or teicoplanin), and gentamicin (or streptomycin based on absence of high-level resistance)
   B. Treatment with fluoroquinolones, rifampin, or trimethoprim-sulfamethoxazole of questionable efficacy
   C. Consider suppressive therapy with chloramphenicol or tetracycline and surgical intervention
   D. Consider quinupristin/dalfopristin therapy for IE due to susceptible *Enterococcus faecium*

---

MIC, minimal inhibitory concentration; IE, infective endocarditis.
Adapted from Karchmer AW: Infective endocarditis. *In* Braunwald E (ed): Heart Disease, 5th ed. Philadelphia: WB Saunders, 1997.

however, these organisms remain susceptible to vancomycin. Although IE caused by a *Staphylococcus* susceptible to penicillin could be effectively treated by that drug, such strains are so infrequent that the regimens recommended for the treatment of staphylococcal IE are organized around susceptibility or resistance to methicillin (the penicillinase-resistant penicillins) and the valve(s) involved, and infection of a prosthetic valve (see Table 30–6, 4A–C, 5, 6, 7 and Fig. 30–3). Whether strains are coagulase positive (*S. aureus*) or negative does not affect antimicrobial selection beyond susceptibility data.

Methicillin-susceptible staphylococcal infection of a native aortic or mitral valve should be treated with a parenteral penicillinase-resistant penicillin (e.g., nafcillin or oxacillin) plus gentamicin during the initial 3 to 5 days of treatment (see Table 30–6, 4A). The addition of gentamicin seeks to achieve more rapid control of infection through the synergistic interaction of combination therapy. Longer courses of gentamicin are not recommended because nephrotoxicity is increased. Combination therapy has reduced the duration of bacteremia in these patients but has not been shown to reduce the mortality rates. Patients with a history of penicillin allergy can be treated with cefazolin or vancomycin, based on the nature

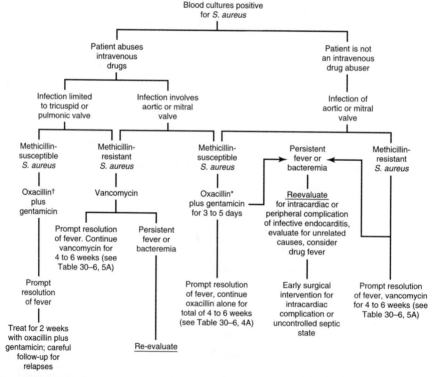

**Figure 30–3** ■ Treatment of native valve endocarditis caused by *Staphylococcus aureus*. *Can use nafcillin; for persons with penicillin allergy that is not anaphylactic/urticarial type, a first-generation cephalosporin may be used instead of oxacillin (see Table 30–6, 4B). If patients have anaphylactic or immediate (urticarial) penicillin allergy, use vancomycin (see Table 30–6, 4C).† Do not use vancomycin instead of oxacillin or nafcillin; patients with penicillin allergy are treated with cefazolin or vancomycin (see Table 30–6, 4B or 5A). (Adapted from Karchmer AW: Approach to the patient with infective endocarditis. *In* Goldman L, Braunwald E [eds]: Primary Cardiology. Philadelphia: WB Saunders, 1998:212).

of the allergic reaction (see Table 30–6, 4B–C). Infection caused by methicillin-resistant staphylococci is treated with vancomycin (see Table 30–6, 4C). In general, rifampin is not used to treat NVE due to staphylococci.

Isolated tricuspid valve endocarditis caused by methicillin-susceptible *S. aureus* that is not complicated by paravalvular extension or metastatic extracardiac focal infection can often be treated with a penicillinase-resistant penicillin plus gentamicin (1 mg/kg ideal body weight every 8 hours) administered for only 2 weeks.[41] A significant percentage of these patients may have prolonged fevers and require longer courses of treatment. Vancomycin does not appear to be a suitable alternative to the penicillinase-resistant penicillin in this short-course regimen, which effectively excludes highly penicillin-allergic patients and infection with methicillin-resistant *S. aureus* from this treatment.

A multidrug regimen administered for 6 to 8 weeks is recommended for the treatment of staphylococcal PVE (see Table 30–6, 6A, 7A).[2] Rifampin, because of its unique ability to kill staphylococci that are adherent to foreign materials or that are not replicating, is an essential component of optimal therapy. Rifampin resistance frequently emerges in this setting, however, despite its being administered in combination with a β-lactam antibiotic or vancomycin. Accordingly, a third antibiotic, preferably gentamicin if the *Staphylococcus* is susceptible to achievable serum concentrations, is included in the initial 2 weeks of treatment. If the *Staphylococcus* is resistant to gentamicin, another aminoglycoside or a fluoroquinolone to which the organism is susceptible should be used.[2] Treatment for staphylococcal PVE should be initiated with a penicillinase-resistant penicillin or vancomycin plus gentamicin; rifampin should be added only after the susceptibility of the *Staphylococcus* to gentamicin has been confirmed or an effective alternative to gentamicin has been initiated.

**HACEK Endocarditis.** β-Lactamase production has been confirmed in some isolates, resulting in resistance to ampicillin. Because the susceptibility of HACEK organisms is difficult to assess, third-generation cephalosporins, which are not inactivated by this β-lactamase, are recommended for the treatment of IE caused by these bacteria (see Table 30–6, 8A).

**Other Organisms Causing Endocarditis.** Limited clinical experience with other causes of IE does not allow consensus therapeutic recommendations.[25] IE caused by *Streptococcus pneumoniae* occurs infrequently but is highly destructive and fatal in more than 63% of patients. Because of the exceptional morbidity of this infection and the increasingly widespread resistance to penicillin among pneumococci, initial therapy with ceftriaxone plus vancomycin (see Table 30–6, 1D and E) is recommended. If the susceptibility of the pneumococcus to penicillin is confirmed, treatment can be continued with penicillin.[37, 42] Penicillin or, in allergic patients, cefazolin or ceftriaxone is recommended for initial therapy for the treatment of IE caused by *Streptococcus pyogenes* (group A).[37]

The preferred treatment for IE caused by *P. aeruginosa* combines an antipseudomonal penicillin (ticarcillin or piperacillin) and high doses of tobramycin (8 mg/kg ideal body weight daily in divided doses every 8 hours to yield peak serum concentrations of 15 μg/ml). Patients with this form of endocarditis often experience intracardiac complications and persistent infection and require valve replacement surgery. The treatment of IE caused by Enterobacteriaceae should be based on reported experience with the specific genus. Treatment often combines a third-generation cephalosporin or a carbapenem (imipenem or meropenem) and an aminoglycoside.

Corynebacterial IE involving prosthetic valves is most commonly caused by *Corynebacterium jeikeium* and that on native valves by *Corynebacterium diphtheriae* (nontoxigenic). The corynebacteria usually are susceptible to penicillin, aminoglycosides, and vancomycin. Aminoglycoside-susceptible strains are killed synergistically by these agents in combination with penicillin. Corynebacterial IE is generally treated with penicillin plus an aminoglycoside or with vancomycin.[43]

Penicillin or ampicillin plus an aminoglycoside has been effectively used to treat many of the reported cases of *Bartonella* IE.[36] Because aminoglycosides have bactericidal activity against *Bartonella,* these regimens may be curative; however, the majority of aminoglycoside-treated patients have also undergone valve replacement surgery. Some authorities suggest that doxycycline or a macrolide be given concurrently with this therapy and for several months thereafter. Treatment of IE caused by *C. burnetii* with doxycycline plus a fluoroquinolone for periods ranging from 4 years to indefinitely, with valve surgery as indicated, yields survival rates exceeding 90%.[44] Shorter courses (18 months to 4 years) of doxycycline 100 mg orally twice daily plus hydroxychloroquine 200 mg orally three times daily (150 to 800 mg daily to maintain a serum concentration of 0.8 to 1.2 μg/ml) was as effective as doxycycline plus a quinolone.[44] Phototoxicity is a consequence of both regimens. Amphotericin B, often in combination with flucytosine, remains the antimicrobial of choice for treating fungal endocarditis, the majority of which is caused by *Candida* sp. and involves prosthetic valves.[45, 46] Limited experience has suggested treatment of *Candida* PVE with amphotericin B should be followed by long-term, if not indefinite, suppression with fluconazole orally.[45, 47]

**Culture-Negative Endocarditis.** In the absence of clinical or epidemiologic information that suggests a specific cause, culture-negative NVE is treated with ceftriaxone (or ampicillin) plus an aminoglycoside. Culture-negative PVE is treated with this regimen plus vancomycin. These recommendations are in part predicted on the unlikely possibility that in the absence of confounding prior antimicrobial therapy, blood culture results would be negative if IE was caused by enterococci or *S. aureus* and that fastidious causes have been sought through serologic tests.

## Monitoring Antimicrobial Therapy

Clinical and laboratory monitoring to assess the response to therapy and to allow prompt detection of complications of IE itself or of therapy is essential to allow timely revision of treatment and to ensure an optimal outcome. Persistent fever beyond 7 to 10 days of presumably effective therapy can indicate treatment failure, paravalvular infection, or an extracardiac focal infection. Recrudescence of fever that had previously resolved suggests systemic emboli, processes unrelated or indirectly related to IE (catheter-related infection, deep vein thrombophlebitis, and others) or drug fever, the latter particularly if fever recurs during the third or fourth week of β-lactam treatment.[48] Monitoring the serum bactericidal titer, the highest dilution of a patient's serum that kills 99.9% of a standard inoculum of the infecting organism, is no longer recommended when patients are treated with a consensus recommendation. Vancomycin and aminoglycoside serum concentrations should be monitored to ensure appropriate dosing. Renal and hepatic function as well as complete blood counts should be monitored regularly when the treatment has the potential to affect these areas adversely. Repeat blood cultures should be obtained to assess persistent or recrudescent fever, to document cure 2 to 8 weeks after completing therapy, and to assess relapse if fever recurs during the 2 to 3 months after treatment. Electrocardiograms, echocardiograms, and special radiologic imaging studies should be obtained or repeated if intracardiac or focal extracardiac complications are suspected (see Table 30–4).

## Outpatient Antimicrobial Therapy

Those patients who have responded to antimicrobial therapy and whose fever has resolved, who have no symptoms or signs suggesting threatening intracardiac or extracardiac complications, who are fully compliant, who have a suitable stable home situation, and who can be carefully monitored can be considered candidates for outpatient therapy. Before beginning home therapy, patients must be fully apprised of the potential complications of IE and instructed to seek medical care immediately if complications or unanticipated symptoms develop. Although outpatient therapy may reduce the cost of treatment, shifting therapy to the outpatient setting must not compromise antimicrobial therapy or the required clinical and laboratory monitoring.

## ■ SURGICAL TREATMENT

Although the mortality associated with IE can be attributed in part to the increased age of patients and comorbidities, intracardiac and central nervous system complications contribute significantly to mortality. Some life-threatening intracardiac complications, as well as instances when antimicrobial therapy fails, can be effectively treated surgically and thus constitute indications for cardiac surgery (Table 30–8). The clinical circumstances in which surgical intervention is considered can be divided into relative indications and more absolute indications; however, even the latter circumstances are to some degree relative. Treatment of each patient requires that the risk-benefit ratio and the timing of surgery be carefully evaluated and the decisions individualized. It is often a combination of findings, rather than a single observation, that indicates the need for surgery.[49]

### Specific Indications

**Congestive Heart Failure Due to Valve Dysfunction.** Severe heart failure due to valve dysfunction regardless of the site portends a very poor prognosis. Mortality rates of 60% to 90% are common within 6 months when IE complicated by new-onset valve dysfunction and moderate to severe heart failure (New York Heart

Table 30–8

**Clinical Circumstances Suggesting Cardiac Surgical Intervention in Patients with Endocarditis**

Indications*
    Moderate to severe congestive heart failure due to valve dysfunction
    Partially dehisced unstable prosthetic valve
    Persistent bacteremia in the presence of optimal antimicrobial therapy
    Absence of effective bactericidal therapy
    Fungal endocarditis, *Brucella* endocarditis
    *Staphylococcus aureus* prosthetic valve endocarditis with an intracardiac complication
    Relapse of prosthetic valve endocarditis after optimal antimicrobial therapy
    Persistent unexplained fever (≥10 days) in culture-negative prosthetic valve endocarditis

Relative indications†
    **Perivalvular extension of infection (myocardial, septal, or annulus abscess, intracardiac fistula)**
    **Poorly responsive** *S. aureus* endocarditis involving the aortic or mitral valve
    Relapse of native valve infective endocarditis after optimal antimicrobial therapy
    Large (>10 mm diameter) hypermobile vegetations
    Persistent unexplained fever (≥10 days) in culture-negative native valve endocarditis
    Endocarditis due to highly antibiotic-resistant enterococci or gram-negative bacilli

*Cardiac surgery required for optimal outcome.
†Surgery, though not always required, must be carefully considered.
Adapted from Karchmer AW: Approach to the patient with infective endocarditis. *In* Goldman L, Braunwald E (eds): *Primary Cardiology.* Philadelphia: WB Saunders, 1998:213.

Association class III or IV) is treated medically. Among patients with comparable hemodynamic dysfunction treated surgically, mortality rates are reduced to 20% to 40% in NVE and 35% to 55% in PVE.[2, 50] Functional stenosis due to a vegetation that obstructs the valve orifice may also cause congestive heart failure and necessitate surgery. Repair of mitral valve fenestrations and ruptured chordae tendineae allows correction of valve dysfunction in the setting of either active or healed IE without the enduring burden of a prosthetic valve.

**Perivalvular Infection.** In 10% to 15% of patients with NVE and 45% to 60% of those with PVE, perivalvular infection complicates endocarditis.[2, 7, 31, 51] In NVE, this complication occurs primarily with aortic valve infection. In patients with PVE or endocarditis involving native aortic valves, clinical findings may suggest perivalvular infection: persistent unexplained fever after 10 days of appropriate antibiotic therapy, pericarditis, and new onset of persistent electrocardiographic conduction disturbance.[2, 31, 48, 51] As an indicator of perivalvular abscess, the specificity of conduction disturbances is high, but sensitivity is low (28% to 41%).[31, 51] The most sensitive method for detection of this abnormality has used multiplane TEE with color Doppler.[20, 24, 31] Among the clinical findings that suggest cardiac surgery, a partially dehisced unstable prosthetic valve and relapse of PVE after optimal therapy are often manifestations of invasive infection. Occasional patients with perivalvular infection are cured with medical treatment alone; the majority, however, require surgical intervention.

**Uncontrolled Infection.** The major manifestations of uncontrolled infection are continued positive blood culture results during therapy and persistent fever. Other causes of continued fever must be precluded before fever can be judged to be due to failure of antimicrobial therapy. Undrained perivalvular abscess may result in failure of antimicrobial therapy. For some organisms, predictable effective bactericidal therapy is not available and surgical excision of infected valves is necessary to cure IE. These include fungi, *P. aeruginosa,* other highly resistant gram-negative bacilli, enterococci for which synergistic killing cannot be effected, *Brucella* sp., and possibly *C. burnetii* (see Specific Therapy).

**S. aureus Infective Endocarditis.** Mortality rates of 22% to 46% have been associated with *S. aureus* infection of native aortic or mitral valves and prosthetic valves.[33, 34, 52] Although not established, the outcome of *S. aureus* left-sided NVE in patients who appear to have perivalvular infection, who remain septic during the initial week of treatment (with or without bacteremia), or who have TTE demonstrable vegetations may be improved by early aggressive surgical intervention.[33, 53] Mortality in patients with *S. aureus* PVE is significantly increased among those with intracardiac complications and is significantly reduced by surgical intervention during active disease.[52] Endocarditis due to *S. aureus* that is restricted to the tricuspid valve, in the vast majority of patients, can be cured without surgical intervention despite persistent fever and pulmonary emboli.

**Unresponsive Culture-Negative Infective Endocarditis.** Patients with echocardiographically confirmed but blood culture–negative IE who fail to become afebrile during empirical antibiotic therapy should be considered for valve replacement. This clinical scenario suggests that empirical therapy is either not effective (wrong organism targeted) or that there is invasive infection. Before proceeding with surgery, especially when valve function is intact, it is important to rule out other causes of persistent fever, including drug reaction, focal undrained metastatic infection, intercurrent complications, and noninfectious endocardial involvement (atrial myxoma, marantic endocarditis, antiphospholipid antibody syndrome, lupus erythematosus with valvular disease).

**Prevention of Systemic Emboli (Vegetations > 10 mm in Diameter).** Vegetations on the aortic or mitral valve greater than 10 mm in diameter are associated with a higher frequency of systemic emboli than are smaller vegetations (33% vs

19%).[12] Furthermore, systemic emboli occurring after initial echocardiography are significantly associated with larger vegetations (>10 mm diameter), mitral valve location, and anterior leaflet of the mitral valve.[9, 11] The risk of embolization, however, is markedly reduced after 2 weeks of effective antimicrobial therapy. Additionally, the mortality and residual morbidity associated with embolic events are largely confined to those emboli that lodge in the central nervous system or the coronary arteries. It is not possible to predict on the basis of echocardiographic findings which patients would experience enhanced survival and reduced morbidity from surgical intervention, particularly when the hazards of surgery and the burden of a prosthetic valve are considered. Consequently, the role of surgery to prevent emboli remains controversial. Rarely is vegetation size alone an indication for surgery (perhaps only with exceptionally large hypermobile vegetations). Benefit from surgery in terms of reduced embolic events is most likely when surgery is undertaken early in therapy, the vegetation has characteristics associated with increased embolic risk, and other clinical features suggest that surgery may be beneficial (e.g., valve dysfunction with moderate congestive heart failure, an antibiotic-resistant organism, suspected paravalvular infection). Vegetectomy and repair of the mitral valve, particularly in younger patients, may reduce the risk of postoperative morbidity and enhance the benefit of surgery in this circumstance.

## Timing of Cardiac Surgery

Surgery to correct valvular dysfunction that has resulted in congestive heart failure must be performed before intractable hemodynamic deterioration results. Delaying surgery under these circumstances risks additional hemodynamic deterioration and a consequent dramatic increase in perioperative mortality. Thus, the timing of surgical intervention to correct valvular dysfunction should be based on hemodynamic status and should be independent of the duration of prior antimicrobial therapy. Similarly, surgery should not be delayed when the indication is uncontrolled infection.[54] Additional antibiotic therapy in this setting does not improve outcome. In fact, only 2% of patients develop recrudescent endocarditis when a prosthetic valve is inserted in patients with active NVE—that is, when blood culture results have been positive during the 48 hours before surgery or when organisms are recovered from the excised valve. Although the presence of perivalvular infection increases the risk of surgical failure and recrudescent infection, approximately 85% of patients survive after surgery for perivalvular abscess, and relapse of IE is rare.[55] Even with surgical treatment of PVE, in which the new valve is typically inserted into an infected annulus that has been debrided and reconstructed, survival approaches 85% and only 15% to 25% of patients develop recurrent endocarditis or require additional cardiac surgery.[56–58] Among patients who have valve dysfunction that will warrant surgery but who are hemodynamically stable and have controlled infection, surgery can often be safely delayed, but other considerations may affect timing. For example, in this circumstance, a large anterior mitral leaflet vegetation that threatened to embolize could justify early surgery.

Patients who have experienced a neurologic complication of IE and who undergo cardiac surgery may experience further neurologic deterioration as a consequence of hypotension, cerebral hemorrhage due to anticoagulation, or cerebral edema due to cardiopulmonary bypass. Morbidity and mortality can be reduced by adjusting the interval between the neurologic complication and surgery or by treating the neurologic complication (e.g., clipping a ruptured mycotic aneurysm) before surgery. Among patients with IE and an embolic cerebral infarction, the frequency of neurologic deterioration postoperatively decreases as the interval between the infarct and surgery increases: within 0 to 7 days, 45% deterioration; from 8 to 14 days, 15%; 15 to 28 days, 10%; greater than 29 days, 2%. Cardiac surgery performed 4 weeks after intracerebral hemorrhage complicating IE is associated with neurologic deterioration in 20% of patients.[59] Depending on the urgency of cardiac surgery, among patients who have had an embolic stroke without hemorrhage, surgery should be delayed for 2 to 3 weeks; among those with a hemorrhagic embolic stroke (no aneurysm), an interval of 4 weeks between the neurologic event and surgery is advised; and with hemorrhage due to rupture of a mycotic aneurysm, the aneurysm should be clipped and cerebral edema allowed to resolve (usually 2 to 3 weeks after neurosurgery) before cardiac surgery.[59, 60]

## ■ EXTRACARDIAC COMPLICATIONS

From 3% to 5% of patients with IE develop a splenic abscess. Although a splenic defect is easily identified with ultrasonography or computed tomography (CT), the distinction between abscess and infarct is difficult. Progressive enlargement of a lesion suggests an abscess, which can be confirmed by guided percutaneous needle aspiration. Successful therapy of splenic abscess requires percutaneous drainage or splenectomy.

Approximately 2% to 12% of patients with IE develop mycotic aneurysm, and half of the aneurysms involve cerebral arteries. In 0.5% to 2% of patients with IE, cerebral mycotic aneurysms rupture.[15, 16] Focal neurologic symptoms and persistent headache may be premonitory symptoms. Based on serial angiograms, 50% of mycotic aneurysms resolve with effective antimicrobial treatment of IE.[61] The risk that an asymptomatic cerebral aneurysm will rupture after completion of effective antimicrobial therapy is estimated to be low.[62] Cerebral angiography is not recommended for all patients with IE and a neurologic deficit; however, head CT with enhancement is advised if there are neurologic symptoms. If intracerebral hemorrhage is detected, angiography is recommended. Ruptured cerebral mycotic aneurysms should be resected. Unruptured cerebral aneurysms should be monitored by angiography, and those that persist or enlarge during therapy should be resected if feasible. Extracranial mycotic aneurysms are managed in an analogous fashion; persistent aneurysms involving intraabdominal arteries should be resected.

## ■ PREVENTION OF ENDOCARDITIS

Although the benefit of periprocedure antibiotic use to prevent IE has not been proved and can be debated, an expert committee of the American Heart Association has identified patients who are at risk for IE, procedures that might increase the risk of IE among endocarditis-prone patients, and regimens that might be used before selected procedures to prevent endocarditis (Tables 30–9 to 30–13).[63] Similar recommendations have been developed by expert committees in other countries. Patients with cardiac abnormalities can be divided into groups with high, moderate, or low to negligible risk for developing IE (see Table 30–9). Prophylaxis is not recommended for those at low to negligible risk. Patients with a secundum atrial septal defect or those lacking other endocarditis-vulnerable defects or having undergone successful repair of an atrial septal defect, patent ductus arteriosus, or ventricular septal defect are at negligible risk for IE.[64] Despite corrective surgery, patients with all other forms of congenital heart disease or coarctation of the aorta remained at high risk for IE; this was in large part the result of coincident unrepaired abnormalities, failed repairs, or placement of prosthetic valves during the repair.[64] Prophylaxis in patients with mitral valve prolapse (MVP) is controversial. The risk is increased relative to the general population but is still significantly less

Table 30–9

**Risk of Infective Endocarditis Associated with Cardiac Abnormalities**

| High Risk | Moderate Risk | Low or Negligible Risk |
|---|---|---|
| Prosthetic heart valves | Congenital cardiac malformations (other than high / low-risk lesions) | Isolated secundum atrial septic defect |
| Prior bacterial endocarditis | Acquired valvular dysfunction | Surgical repair of atrial or ventricular septal defect or patent ductus arteriosus |
| Complex cyanotic congenital heart disease | Hypertrophic cardiomyopathy | Prior coronary artery bypass surgery |
| Surgically constructed systemic-pulmonary shunts | Mitral valve prolapse with valvular regurgitation and / or thickened leaflets | Mitral valve prolapse without valvular regurgitation |
| | | Physiologic, functional, or innocent heart murmurs |
| | | Prior Kawasaki disease or rheumatic fever without valvular dysfunction |
| | | Cardiac pacemakers and implanted defibrillators |

Adapted from Dajani AS, Taubert KA, Wilson W, et al: Prevention of bacterial endocarditis: Recommendations by the American Heart Association from the Committee on Rheumatic Fever, Endocarditis and Kawasaki Disease, Council on Cardiovascular Disease in the Young. JAMA 1997;277:1794–1801.

than that among patients with rheumatic heart disease. Prophylaxis is recommended for patients with MVP and a murmur of mitral regurgitation and for those older than 45 years and who on echocardiography have MVP and thickened valve leaflets even in the absence of mitral regurgitation at rest.

Prophylaxis has been advised for those procedures likely to induce bacteremia with bacteria causally associated with IE (see Tables 30–10 and 30–11). Maintenance of good dental health reduces the risk of IE. Similarly, patients should have dental disease treated before they undergo cardiac valve surgery. Among endocarditis-prone patients with infection in the genitourinary tract, the infection should be eradicated before proceeding with genitourinary manipulation.

Table 30–10

**Dental Procedures for Which Endocarditis Prophylaxis Is Considered**

| Prophylaxis Recommended | Prophylaxis not Recommended |
|---|---|
| Dental extractions | Restorative dentistry (operative and prosthodontic) with / without retraction cord |
| Periodontal procedures (surgery, scaling, root planing, probing) | Local anesthetic injection (not intraligamentary) |
| Dental implant placement, reimplantation of avulsed teeth | Intracanal endodontic treatment (after placement and buildup) |
| Endodontic instrumentation (root canal) or surgery beyond the apex | Placement of rubber dams |
| Subgingival placement of antibiotic fibers / strips | Suture removal |
| Initial placement of orthodontic bands (not brackets) | Placement of removable prosthodontic / orthodontic appliances |
| Intraligamentary local anesthetic injections | Taking oral impressions or radiographs |
| Prophylactic cleaning of teeth or implants when bleeding is anticipated | Orthodontic appliance adjustment |
| | Shedding primary teeth |

Adapted from Dajani AS, Taubert KA, Wilson W, et al: Prevention of bacterial endocarditis: Recommendations by the American Heart Association from the Committee on Rheumatic Fever, Endocarditis and Kawasaki Disease, Council on Cardiovascular Disease in the Young. JAMA 1997;277:1794–1801.

Table 30–11

**Procedures for Which Endocarditis Prophylaxis Is Considered**

| Prophylaxis Recommended | Prophylaxis Not Recommended |
|---|---|
| **Respiratory tract** | **Respiratory tract** |
| Surgical operation involving mucosa | Endotracheal intubation |
| Bronchoscopy with rigid bronchoscope | Bronchoscopy with flexible bronchoscope with or without biopsy* |
| | Tympanostomy tube insertion |
| **Gastrointestinal tract†** | **Gastrointestinal tract** |
| Sclerotherapy for esophageal varices | Transesophageal echocardiography |
| Dilation of esophageal stricture | Endoscopy with or without biopsy* |
| Endoscopic retrograde cholangiography with biliary obstruction | |
| Biliary tract surgery | |
| Surgery involving intestinal mucosa | |
| **Genitourinary tract** | **Genitourinary tract** |
| Prostate surgery | Vaginal hysterectomy* |
| Cytoscopy | Vaginal delivery* |
| Urethral dilatation | Cesarean section |
| | In the absence of infection: |
| | Ureteral catheterization, ureteral dilatation and curettage, therapeutic abortion, sterilization, insertion / removal of intrauterine device |
| | **Other** |
| | Cardiac catheterization, coronary angioplasty |
| | Implantation of pacemakers, defibrillators, coronary stents |
| | Clean surgery |
| | Circumcision |

*Prophylaxis is optional for high-risk patients.
†Recommended for high-risk patients; optional for moderate-risk group.
Adapted from Dajani AS, Taubert KA, Wilson W, et al: Prevention of bacterial endocarditis: Recommendations by the American Heart Association from the Committee on Rheumatic Fever, Endocarditis and Kawasaki Disease, Council on Cardiovascular Disease in the Young. JAMA 1997;277:1794–1801.

Table 30–12

**Regimens for Endocarditis Prophylaxis in Adults: Oral, Respiratory Tract, or Esophageal Procedures**

| Setting | Antibiotic | Regimen* |
|---|---|---|
| Standard | Amoxicillin | 2.0 g PO 1 hr before procedure |
| Unable to take oral medication | Ampicillin | 2.0 g IM or IV within 30 min of procedure |
| Penicillin allergic | Clindamycin | 600 mg PO 1 hr before procedure or IV 30 min before procedure |
| | Cephalexin† | 2.0 g PO 1 hr before procedure |
| | Cefazolin† | 1.0 g IV or IM 30 min before procedure |
| | Cefadroxil† | 2.0 g PO 1 hr before procedure |
| | Clarithromycin | 500 mg PO 1 hr before procedure |

*For patients in high-risk group, administer half the dose 6 hr after the initial dose. Dosing for children: amoxicillin, ampicillin, cephalexin, or cefadroxil 50 mg / kg PO; cefazolin 25 mg / kg IV; clindamycin 20 mg / kg PO, 25 mg / kg IV; clarithromycin 15 mg / kg PO.
†Do not use cephalosporins in patients with immediate hypersensitivity (urticaria, angioedema, anaphylaxis) to penicillin.
PO, orally; IV, intravenously; IM, intramuscularly.
Adapted from Dajani AS, Taubert KA, Wilson W, et al. Prevention of bacterial endocarditis: Recommendations by the American Heart Association from the Committee on Rheumatic Fever, Endocarditis and Kawasaki Disease, Council on Cardiovascular Disease in the Young. JAMA 1997;277:1794–1801.

Table 30–13

**Regimens for Endocarditis Prophylaxis in Adults: Genitourinary and Gastrointestinal\* Tract Procedures**

| Setting | Antibiotic | Regimen† |
|---|---|---|
| High-risk patients | Ampicillin plus gentamicin | Ampicillin 2.0 g IV / IM plus gentamicin 1.5 mg / kg within 30 min of procedure, repeat ampicillin 1.0 g IV / IM or amoxicillin 1.0 g PO 6 hr later |
| High-risk, penicillin-allergic patients | Vancomycin plus gentamicin | Vancomycin 1.0 g IV infused over 1–2 hr plus gentamicin 1.5 mg / kg IM / IV infused or injected 30 min before procedure. No second dose recommended |
| Moderate-risk patients | Amoxicillin or ampicillin | Amoxicillin 2.0 g PO 1 hr before procedure or ampicillin 2.0 g IM / IV 30 min before procedure |
| Moderate-risk, penicillin-allergic patients | Vancomycin | Vancomycin 1.0 g IV infused over 1–2 hr and completed within 30 min of procedure |

\*Excludes esophageal procedures (see Table 30–12).
†Dosing for children: Ampicillin 50 mg / kg IV / IM, vancomycin 20 mg / kg IV, gentamicin 1.5 mg / kg IV / IM (children's doses should not exceed adult doses).
PO, orally; IM, intramuscularly; IV, intravenously.
Adapted from Dajani AS, Taubert KA, Wilson W, et al. Prevention of bacterial endocarditis: Recommendations by the American Heart Association from the Committee on Rheumatic Fever, Endocarditis and Kawasaki Disease, Council on Cardiovascular Disease in the Young. JAMA 1997;277:1794–1801.

The regimens recommended for use in the prophylaxis of IE have been selected because they kill or inhibit the endocarditis-causing bacteria present at the site to be manipulated (see Tables 30–12 and 30–13). Penicillin regimens used to prevent acute rheumatic fever are not suitable for IE prophylaxis, and patients receiving them may have oral and gingival flora that is resistant to penicillins. Accordingly, clindamycin or clarithromycin should be used for prophylaxis in patients repetitively receiving penicillin. Surgical procedures on infected tissues and skin infections may be associated with bacteremia and an increased risk for IE. Antibiotic prophylaxis for IE is recommended for selected surgical procedures. Similarly, skin and wound infections caused by *S. aureus* should be treated vigorously when they occur in IE-prone patients.

# ■ REFERENCES

1. Berlin JA, Abrutyn E, Strom BL, et al: Incidence of infective endocarditis in the Delaware Valley, 1988–1990. Am J Cardiol 1995;76:933–936.
2. Karchmer AW, Gibbons GW: Infections of prosthetic heart valves and vascular grafts. *In* Bisno AL, Waldvogel FA (eds): Infections Associated with Indwelling Devices. Washington, DC: American Society for Microbiology, 1994:213–249.
3. Gubler JGH, Kuster M, Dutly F, et al: Whipple endocarditis without overt gastrointestinal disease: Report of four cases. Ann Intern Med 1999;131:112–116.
4. Gagliardi JP, Nettles RE, McCarty DE, et al: Native valve infective endocarditis in elderly and younger adult patients: Comparison of clinical features and outcomes with use of the Duke criteria and the Duke endocarditis data base. Clin Infect Dis 1998;26:1165–1168.
5. Werner GS, Schulz R, Fuchs JB, et al: Infective endocarditis in the elderly in the era of transesophageal echocardiography: Clinical features and prognosis compared with younger patients. Am J Med 1996;100:90–97.
6. Tornos MP, Permanyer-Miralda G, Olona M, et al: Long-term complications of native valve infective endocarditis in non-addicts: A 15-year follow-up study. Ann Intern Med 1992;117:567–572.
7. Sandre RM, Shafran SD: Infective endocarditis: Review of 135 cases over 9 years. Clin Infect Dis 1996;22:276–286.

8. Tornos P, Almirante B, Olona M, et al: Clinical outcome and long-term prognosis of late prosthetic valve endocarditis: A 20-year experience. Clin Infect Dis 1997;24:381–386.

9. Mugge A, Daniel WC, Frank G, Lichtlen PR: Echocardiography in infective endocarditis: Reassessment of prognostic implications of vegetation size determined by the transthoracic and transesophageal approach. J Am Coll Cardiol 1989;14:631–638.

10. Rohman S, Erbel R, Darius H: Prediction of rapid versus prolonged healing of infective endocarditis by monitoring vegetation size. J Am Soc Echocardiogr 1991;4:465–474.

11. Rohman S, Erbel R, George G, et al: Clinical relevance of vegetation localization by transesophageal echocardiography in infective endocarditis. Eur Heart J 1992;13:446–452.

12. Aragam JR, Weyman AE: Echocardiographic findings in infective endocarditis. *In* Weyman AE (ed): Principles and Practice of Echocardiography. Philadelphia: Lea & Febiger, 1994:1178–1197.

13. Steckelberg JM, Murphy JG, Ballard D, et al: Emboli in infective endocarditis: The prognostic value of echocardiography. Ann Intern Med 1991;114:635–640.

14. Pruitt AA, Rubin RH, Karchmer AW, Duncan GW: Neurologic complications of bacterial endocarditis. Medicine 1978;57:329–343.

15. Salgado AV, Furlan AJ, Keys TF, et al: Neurologic complications of endocarditis: A 12-year experience. Neurology 1989;39:173–178.

16. Kanter MC, Hart RG: Neurologic complications of infective endocarditis. Neurology 1991;41:1015–1020.

17. Durack DT, Lukes AS, Bright DK: New criteria for diagnosis of infective endocarditis: Utilization of specific echocardiographic findings. Am J Med 1994;96:200–209.

18. Bayer AS, Bolger AF, Taubert KA, et al: Diagnosis and management of infective endocarditis and its complications. Circulation 1998;98:2936–2948.

19. Sekeres MA, Abrutyn E, Berlin JA, et al: An assessment of the usefulness of the Duke criteria for diagnosis of active infective endocarditis. Clin Infect Dis 1997;24:1185–1190.

20. Daniel WG, Mugge A, Martin RP, et al: Improvement in the diagnosis of abscesses associated with endocarditis by transesophageal echocardiography. N Engl J Med 1991;324:795–800.

21. Mugge A: Echocardiographic detection of cardiac valve vegetations and prognostic implications. Infect Dis Clin North Am 1993;7:877–898.

22. Shively BK, Gurule FT, Roldan CA, et al: Diagnostic value of transesophageal compared with transthoracic echocardiography in infective endocarditis. J Am Coll Cardiol 1991;18:391–397.

23. Sochowski RA, Chan KL: Implication of negative results on a monoplane transesophageal echocardiographic study in patients with suspected infective endocarditis. J Am Coll Cardiol 1993;21:216–221.

24. Job FP, Franke S, Lethen H, et al: Incremental value of biplane and multiplane transesophageal echocardiography for the assessment of active infective endocarditis. Am J Cardiol 1995;75:1033–1037.

25. Berbari EF, Cockerill FR III, Steckelberg J: Infective endocarditis due to unusual or fastidious microorganisms. Mayo Clin Proc 1997;72:532–542.

26. Hoen B, Selton-Suty C, Lacassin F, et al: Infective endocarditis in patients with negative blood cultures: Analysis of 88 cases from a one-year nationwide survey in France. Clin Infect Dis 1995;20:501–506.

27. Goldenberger D, Kunzli A, Vogt P, et al: Molecular diagnosis of bacterial endocarditis by broad-range PCR amplification and direct sequencing. J Clin Microbiol 1992;35:2733–2739.

28. Khandheria BK: Transesophageal echocardiography in the evaluation of prosthetic valves. Am J Card Imaging 1995;9:106–114.

29. Daniel WG, Mugge A, Grote J, et al: Comparison of transthoracic and transesophageal echocardiography for detection of abnormalities of prosthetic and bioprosthetic valves in the mitral and aortic positions. Am J Cardiol 1993;71:210–215.

30. Morguet AJ, Werner GS, Andreas S, Kreuzer H: Diagnostic value of transesophageal compared with transthoracic echocardiography in suspected prosthetic valve endocarditis. Herz 1995;20:390–398.

31. Blumberg EA, Karalis DA, Chandrasekaran K, et al: Endocarditis-associated paravalvular abscess. Do clinical parameters predict the presence of abscess? Chest 1995;107:898–903.

32. Fowler VG Jr, Li J, Corey GR, et al: Role of echocardiography in evaluation of patients with *Staphylococcus aureus* bacteremia: Experience in 103 patients. J Am Coll Cardiol 1997;30:1072–1078.

33. Fowler VG Jr, Sanders LL, Kong LK, et al: Infective endocarditis due to *Staphylococcus aureus:* 59 prospectively identified cases with follow-up. Clin Infect Dis 1999;28:106–114.

34. Roder BL, Wandall DA, Frimodt-Moller N, et al: Clinical features of *Staphylococcus aureus* endocarditis: A 10-year experience in Denmark. Arch Intern Med 1999;159:462–469.

35. Ribera E, Miro JM, Cortes E, et al: Influence of human immunodeficiency virus 1 infection and degree of immunosuppression in the clinical characteristics and outcome of infective endocarditis in intravenous drug users. Arch Intern Med 1998;158:2043–2050.

36. Raoult D, Fournier PE, Drancourt M, et al: Diagnosis of 22 new cases of *Bartonella* endocarditis. Ann Intern Med 1996;125:646–652.

37. Wilson WR, Karchmer AW, Bisno AL, et al: Antibiotic treatment of adults with infective endocarditis due to viridans streptococci, enterococci, other streptococci, staphylococci, and HACEK microorganisms. JAMA 1995;274:1706–1713.

38. Francioli P, Ruch W, Stamboulian D, The International Infective Endocarditis Study Group: Treatment of streptococcal endocarditis with a single daily dose of ceftriaxone and netilmicin for 14 days: A prospective multicenter study. Clin Infect Dis 1995;21:1406–1410.

39. Sexton DJ, Tenenbaum MJ, Wilson WR, et al: Ceftriaxone once daily for four weeks compared with

ceftriaxone plus gentamicin once daily for two weeks for treatment of endocarditis due to penicillin-susceptible streptococci. Clin Infect Dis 1998;27:1470–1474.

40. Eliopoulos GM: Aminoglycoside resistant enterococcal endocarditis. Infect Dis Clin North Am 1993;7:117–133.

41. Torres-Tortosa M, de Cueto M, Vergara A, et al: Prospective evaluation of a two-week course of intravenous antibiotics in intravenous drug addicts with infective endocarditis. Eur J Clin Microbiol Infect Dis 1994;13:559–564.

42. Aronin SI, Mukherjee SK, West JC, Cooney EL: Review of pneumococcocal endocarditis in adults in the penicillin era. Clin Infect Dis 1998;26:165–171.

43. Petit AIC, Bok JW, Thompson J, et al: Native-valve endocarditis due to CDC coryneform group ANF-3: Report of a case and review of corynebacterial endocarditis. Clin Infect Dis 1994;19:897–901.

44. Raoult D, Houpikian P, Tissot Dupont H, et al: Treatment of Q fever endocarditis: Comparison of 2 regimens containing doxycycline and ofloxacin or hydroxychloroquine. Arch Intern Med 1999;159:167–173.

45. Melgar GR, Nasser RM, Gordon SM, et al: Fungal prosthetic valve endocarditis in 16 patients. An 11 year experience in a tertiary care hospital. Medicine 1997;76:94–103.

46. Gilbert HM, Peters ED, Lang SJ, Hartman BJ: Successful treatment of fungal prosthetic valve endocarditis: Case report and review. Clin Infect Dis 1996;22:348–354.

47. Nguyen MH, Nguyen ML, Yu VL, et al: Candida prosthetic valve endocarditis: Prospective study of six cases and review of the literature. Clin Infect Dis 1996;22:262–267.

48. Douglas A, Moore-Gillon J, Eykyn S: Fever during treatment of infective endocarditis. Lancet 1986;i:1341–1343.

49. Alsip SG, Blackstone EH, Kirklin JW, Cobbs CG: Indications for cardiac surgery in patients with active infective endocarditis. Am J Med 1985;78(Suppl 6B):138–148.

50. Croft CH, Woodward W, Elliott A, et al: Analysis of surgical versus medical therapy in active complicated native valve infective endocarditis. Am J Cardiol 1983;51:1650–1655.

51. DiNubile MJ, Calderwood SB, Steinhaus DM, Karchmer AW: Cardiac conduction abnormalities complicating native valve active infective endocarditis. Am J Cardiol 1986;58:1213–1217.

52. John MVD, Hibberd PL, Karchmer AW, et al: *Staphylococcus aureus* prosthetic valve endocarditis: Optimal management and risk factors for death. Clin Infect Dis 1998;26:1302–1309.

53. Richardson JV, Karp RB, Kirklin JW, Dismukes WE: Treatment of infective endocarditis: A 10-year comparative analysis. Circulation 1978;58:589–597.

54. Baumgartner WA, Miller DC, Reitz BA, et al: Surgical treatment of prosthetic valve endocarditis. Ann Thorac Surg 1983;35:87–102.

55. d'Udekem Y, David TE, Feindel CM, et al: Long-term results of operation for paravalvular abscess. Ann Thorac Surg 1996;62:48–53.

56. Jault F, Gandjbakheh I, Chastre JC, et al: Prosthetic valve endocarditis with ring abscesses: Surgical management and long-term results. J Thorac Cardiovasc Surg 1993;105:1106–1113.

57. Lytle BW, Priest BP, Taylor PC, et al: Surgery for acquired heart disease: Surgical treatment of prosthetic valve endocarditis. J Thorac Cardiovasc Surg 1996;111:198–210.

58. Pansini S, di Summa M, Patane F, et al: Risk of recurrence after reoperation for prosthetic valve endocarditis. J Heart Valve Dis 1997;6:84–87.

59. Eishi K, Kawazoe K, Kuriyama Y, et al: Surgical management of infective endocarditis associated with cerebral complications: Multicenter retrospective study in Japan. J Thorac Cardiovasc Surg 1995;110:1745–1755.

60. Gillinov AM, Shah RV, Curtis WE, et al: Valve replacement in patients with endocarditis and acute neurologic deficit. Ann Thorac Surg 1996;61:1125–1130.

61. Brust JCM, Dickinson PCT, Hughes JEO, Holtzman RNN: The diagnosis and treatment of cerebral mycotic aneurysms. Ann Neurol 1990;27:238–246.

62. Salgado AV, Furlan AJ, Keys TF: Mycotic aneurysm, subarachnoid hemorrhage, and indications for cerebral angiography in infective endocarditis. Stroke 1987;18:1057–1060.

63. Dajani AS, Taubert KA, Wilson W, et al: Prevention of bacterial endocarditis: Recommendations by the American Heart Association, from the Committee on Rheumatic Fever, Endocarditis, and Kawasaki Disease, Council on Cardiovascular Diseases in the Young. JAMA 1997;277:1794–1801.

64. Morris CD, Reller MD, Menashe VD: Thirty-year incidence of infective endocarditis after surgery for congenital heart defect. JAMA 1998;279:599–603.

*Chapter* **31**

# Mechanisms and Diagnosis

*Clive Rosendorff*

Cardiovascular disease is by far the leading cause of death, in males and females, in industrialized nations. In the United States this year, about a million deaths will be due to diseases of the heart and circulation, more than twice the number for the next most frequent cause of death, cancer. The commonest fatal cardiovascular diseases are coronary artery disease, congestive heart failure, and stroke, and these, together with renovascular disease, all have hypertension as a major risk factor. High blood pressure is therefore a highly lethal disease.

The relationship between blood pressure and the relative risks of stroke and coronary heart disease is direct, continuous, and independent, and no evidence has been put forward of any "threshold" level of blood pressure below which humans are entirely safe.[1] In general, men are at greater risk for hypertension-related death than women; black persons than white; and older ones than younger ones. With increasing age, the prevalence of isolated systolic hypertension with a normal diastolic pressure increases considerably, and it is now generally accepted that in adults systolic blood pressure may be a more accurate predictor of cardiovascular risk than diastolic pressure.

An enormous amount of data, experimental, epidemiologic, and clinical, now indicates that reducing elevated blood pressure is beneficial. The first definitive proof of this came from the Veterans Administration (VA) Cooperative Study begun in 1963, and it has been confirmed in a host of studies since, most of which utilized diuretics or beta blockers as antihypertensive agents. More recently, other classes of antihypertensive drugs have been studied—with positive results, at least for cardiovascular morbidity. A very large prospective, randomized study with 40,000 patients is currently under way to assess the efficacy in reducing mortality in hypertension of a calcium channel blocker, an angiotensin-converting enzyme (ACE) inhibitor, an α-adrenergic blocker recently withdrawn from the study, and a diuretic (see Chapter 32).

In spite of the demonstrated benefits of blood pressure reduction, physicians and other health care professionals who are responsible for identifying and treating patients with hypertension are not doing a great job. From 1976 to 1980 and 1988 to 1989, the percentages of Americans who were aware that they had high blood pressure increased from 51% to 73%, but since 1991 that figure has dropped back to 68%. The proportion who were treated at all increased from 31% from 1976 to 1980 to 55% from 1988 to 1991, but it declined to 54% in 1991 to 1994. Most depressing of all were the data for patients whose blood pressure was controlled to normal values: 10% in 1976 to 1980, up to 29% in 1988 to 1991, but back to 27%

since then. So, of every 100 patients with hypertension, 68 are aware of the fact, 54 are receiving treatment, and only 27 are "controlled."[2] This may explain why the dramatic reductions in age-adjusted stroke and coronary heart disease mortality since the 1970s seem to be faltering; the stroke rate has risen slightly since 1993, and the slope of the decline in coronary heart disease appears to be leveling off.[3] Furthermore, rates have increased for end-stage renal disease, for which high blood pressure is the second most common antecedent, and for heart failure, which in a large majority of patients is associated with hypertension.[4, 5]

## ▪ DEFINITION AND CLASSIFICATION

Blood pressure is a continuous variable in any population, with a distribution along a bell-shaped curve. The difference between "normotensive" and "hypertensive" blood pressure values is, therefore, somewhat arbitrary, but, since cardiovascular risk increases with blood pressure, various operational definitions of hypertension have been developed.

The Sixth Joint National Committee on Detection, Evaluation and Treatment of High Blood Pressure (JNC VI)[2] defined hypertension as a systolic blood pressure (SBP) of 140 mm Hg or greater, diastolic blood pressure (DBP) of 90 mm Hg or greater, or taking antihypertensive medication. Another category, "high-normal," was proposed with an SBP of 130 to 139 mm Hg or a DBP of 85 to 89 mm Hg, which, the JNC VI felt, requires advising the patient about lifestyle modifications and rechecking blood pressure in 1 year. It is good clinical policy, however, to check everyone's pressure at least once a year. Another, and simpler, classification of hypertension was developed by the New York Heart Association (NYHA, Table 31–1).[6] The utility of such a classification is, first, to provide an appropriate basis for comparing patients in epidemiologic and clinical studies, and, second, as an indicator of the urgency of starting therapy. For example, a patient with a blood pressure of 142/92 mm Hg (stage 1) need not be treated with antihypertensive therapy right away; repeat visits to the office or clinic should be arranged to confirm the hypertension, and possibly to establish the antihypertensive efficacy of nonpharmacologic interventions (see Chapter 32). On the other hand, a patient with a blood pressure of 220/118 mm Hg (stage 4) usually requires antihypertensive therapy without delay.

## ▪ MEASUREMENT OF BLOOD PRESSURE[7, 8]

Blood pressure is usually measured with a mercury sphygmomanometer, an aneroid manometer, or an electronic manometer with a 12 by 26-cm cuff. For

Table 31–1

**Modified New York Heart Association Classification of Hypertension[6]**

| | Blood Pressure (mm Hg) | | |
|---|---|---|---|
| **Class** | Systolic | | Diastolic |
| Optimal | <120 | and | <80 |
| Normal | ≤130 | and | ≤85 |
| High-normal | 131–140 | or | 86–90 |
| Hypertension | | | |
| Stage 1 | 141–160 | or | 91–100 |
| Stage 2 | 161–180 | or | 101–110 |
| Stage 3 | 181–200 | or | 111–120 |
| Stage 4 | >200 | or | >120 |

patients with arms of greater than 33 cm circumference, pressure should be measured with a large cuff (12 by 40 cm). If an aneroid or electronic manometer is used, it should be calibrated against a mercury manometer at regular intervals. Blood pressures should be measured with subjects both lying and standing, or sitting and standing and repeated 5 minutes later when possible. The cuff should be placed over the brachial artery and the bell of the stethoscope over the artery distal to the cuff; the environment should be quiet and the patient relaxed. Serial measurements should be taken at the same time of day, preferably in the morning, before the patient has taken any antihypertensive medication (i.e., at the trough of the plasma concentration).

The cuff is pumped up to about 20 mm Hg above the systolic level, which point is signaled by the disappearance of the radial pulse, and then the pressure lowered by about 2 mm Hg per second. The systolic blood pressure is the pressure at which the first faint, consistent, tapping sounds are heard (Korotkoff sounds, phase I). The diastolic pressure is the level at which the last regular blood pressure sound is heard and after which all sound disappears (Korotkoff sound, phase V). Below Korotkoff phase I there is sometimes a period of silence referred to as the *auscultatory gap*; otherwise there is a continuum of sound, including swishing beats (Korotkoff II), crisper and louder sounds (Korotkoff III), and muffling of the sound (Korotkoff IV). If the sounds continue down to zero, Korotkoff IV is recorded as the diastolic pressure.

Since blood pressure can vary by as much as 10 mm Hg between arms (and more in conditions such as coarctation of the aorta), it should be measured in both arms, at least at the initial visit. The higher pressure is recorded. All blood pressures should be read to the nearest 2 mm Hg, not rounded off to the nearest 5 or 10 mm Hg, as is done so often.

There are many sources of variability of blood pressure. These include poor technique, faulty equipment, a stressful setting or an anxious patient, and a patient who has been smoking or has had caffeine or alcohol. A common error is the failure to remove patients' garments with tight sleeves. The considerable interobserver variability in blood pressure measurements can be minimized by meticulous attention to correct technique.

Among the biologic variations are short-term ones driven by changes in the autonomic nervous system and a slower, circadian, variability. Blood pressure usually falls about 15% at night, during sleep, to rise to daytime levels an hour or two before awakening. Pressure usually peaks in the late afternoon and evening. Some patients (so-called nondippers) have a smaller fall of BP during sleep, sometimes none; these patients seem to be at greater risk for cardiovascular disease (especially women), ventricular arrhythmias, cerebrovascular disease, and more rapid progression of hypertensive renal disease, ventricular arrhythmias, and cerebrovascular disease.

The *white coat effect* refers to the higher pressures seen in the clinic or the doctor's office as compared with those measured at home, whether by the patient or by 24-hour ambulatory monitoring, and it is quite usual. *White coat hypertension* is an entity in which clinic or office blood pressure is in the hypertensive range but at home is normal. The best current evidence indicates that white coat hypertension is a low-risk, but not entirely harmless, clinical entity, and these patients should be monitored closely for the appearance of (1) features that would require antihypertensive therapy, especially daytime ambulatory blood pressure or home self-measured pressure greater than 130/85 mm Hg, or (2) target organ damage.

## ■ INITIAL WORKUP OF THE HYPERTENSIVE PATIENT

The initial evaluation of patients with hypertension has three objectives: (1) to find clues to secondary causes of hypertension; (2) to assess target organ damage;

and (3) to determine whether there are other risk factors for cardiovascular disease. This requires careful history taking, a complete physical examination, some basic laboratory tests, and electrocardiography (ECG).

The first step is to establish the diagnosis of sustained hypertension. Blood pressure should be measured on at least two occasions. If the hypertension is stage 1 or 2, measurements should be made within 1 month of each other; if stage 3, within a week; and if stage 4, immediate action is necessary to complete the workup and treat the hypertension.

## Secondary Hypertension

Table 31–2 lists the common causes of secondary hypertension. If none of these causes is present, the hypertension is primary. The term *primary hypertension* is preferred to *essential hypertension*, because the latter refers to an obsolete and incorrect concept—that the hypertension is essential to achieving perfusion of organs through arteries narrowed by arteriosclerotic disease.

Of the secondary causes of hypertension, some are often fairly easy to recognize. For example, by the time Cushing syndrome is severe enough to cause hypertension, the clinical features are usually obvious on physical examination. The same is true of acromegaly. Many cases of coarctation of the aorta are detected in infancy or childhood. However, most of the causes of secondary hypertension need to be carefully excluded in the history, the physical examination, and the laboratory workup. Tables 31–3 and 31–4 propose a simple and general approach to this process. Some of the commonest causes of secondary hypertension are described in more detail later in this chapter.

## Target Organ Damage

### Vascular Hypertrophy[9, 10]

*Hypertrophy* refers to growth brought about by an increase in cell *size* rather than *number*. (An increase in cell number is hyperplasia.) In adults, the vascular

---

Table 31–2

**Classification of Hypertension by Etiology**

---

**Secondary Hypertension**
  Renal parenchymal hypertension
  Renovascular disease
  Coarctation of the aorta
  Adrenal disorders
    Adrenal cortical hypertension
    Mineralocorticoid hypertension (e.g., Conn syndrome)
    Glucocorticoid hypertension (e.g., Cushing syndrome)
  Other hormonal disorders
    Hypothyroidism
    Hyperthyroidism
    Hyperparathyroidism
    Acromegaly
  Neurologic disorders: increased intracranial pressure
  Drugs, especially oral contraceptives, erythropoietin, cyclosporin, licorice, sympathomimetic drugs, cocaine, tricyclic antidepressants, prostaglandin synthesis inhibitors (e.g., nonsteroidal antiinflammatory drugs interfere with the effects of many antihypertensive drugs), anabolic steroids

**Primary Hypertension**

---

Table 31–3

**Hypertension Workup: History and Physical Examination**

| Symptoms and Signs | Diagnosis |
|---|---|
| **Secondary Hypertension** | |
| Abdominal or flank masses | Polycystic kidneys |
| Abdominal bruit | Renovascular hypertension |
| Delayed/absent femoral pulses, blood pressure gradient between arm and leg | Aortic coarctation |
| Truncal obesity, moon face, purple striae, buffalo hump | Cushing syndrome |
| Tachycardia, tremor, pallor, sweating | Pheochromocytoma |
| Flank pain, frequency, dysuria, hematuria, prostatism, edema | Renal parenchymal disease |
| **Target Organ Damage** | |
| Vision, fundoscopy | Retinopathy |
| Dyspnea, fatigue, signs of left ventricular failure | Left ventricular failure |
| Angina, previous myocardial infarction | Coronary artery disease |
| Focal neurologic symptoms and signs | Cerebrovascular disease |
| Symptoms and signs of renal failure | Hypertensive renal disease |

smooth muscle cells (VSMC) are relatively quiescent, having an extremely low (<5 %) mitotic index. In persons with hypertension and atherosclerosis, however, VSMC undergo phenotypic modulation with hypertrophy and/or hyperplasia, altered receptor expression, altered lipid handling, and migration from the vascular media to the subintimal portion of the vessel, and the vessel shows enhanced extracellular matrix deposition. All of these result in an increase in stiffness (lower compliance) of the arteries of hypertensive patients. This diffuse arteriosclerosis of hypertension increases with age. Superimposed on this may be accelerated development of atherosclerotic lesions.

Factors that stimulate vascular smooth muscle hypertrophy or hyperplasia in hypertension include endothelin, which activates the $ET_A$ subtype of the endothelin receptor to activate an intracellular transduction pathway involving phospholipase

Table 31–4

**Hypertension Workup: Screening Laboratory Tests**

| Test | Rationale |
|---|---|
| **Blood Chemistry** | |
| Blood urea nitrogen | Impaired renal function |
| Creatinine | Impaired renal function |
| Potassium | Primary aldosteronism |
| | Cushing syndrome |
| | Renal failure |
| Calcium/phosphate | Hyperparathyroidism |
| Cholesterol | |
| Triglycerides | Risk factors for cardiovascular disease |
| Glucose | |
| Uric acid | |
| **Thyroid-stimulating hormone assay** | Hyperthyroidism |
| | Hypothyroidism |
| **Urinalysis** | Renal disease |
| **Electrocardiography** | LVH |
| **Complete blood count** | All new patients should have one |

C (PLC), inositol 1,4,5-trisphosphate ($IP_3$), and 1,2-diacylglycerol (DAG); release of cytosolic calcium from the endoplasmic reticulum; and, possibly, the mitogen-activated protein (MAP) kinase system. Angiotensin II, acting via the $AT_1$ receptor subtype, has a similar intracellular transduction pathway. Other hormones or autocrine or paracrine factors that affect VSMC growth are vasopressin, catecholamines, insulin-like growth factor 1 (IGF-1), platelet-derived growth factor (PDGF), fibroblast growth factor (FGF), and transforming growth factor beta (TGF-β), which all stimulate growth, and nitric oxide, atrial natriuretic peptide, estrogens, and prostacyclin, which are inhibitory. This inhibition is thought to be due to an increase in apoptosis, reversing VSMC proliferation. Many studies have shown improvement in VSMC hypertrophy and hyperplasia in hypertensive patients who take drugs that inhibit the action of angiotensin II (ACE inhibitors or $AT_1$ receptor blockers) or calcium (calcium channel blockers), and it could be predicted that the same effects would occur with agents that enhance inhibitory factors, such as those neutral endopeptidase inhibitors that reduce the breakdown of atrial natriuretic peptide.

## Left Ventricular Hypertrophy[11]

Left ventricular hypertrophy (LVH) is a consequence of mechanical forces such as chronic increased systolic afterloading of the cardiac myofibrils in hypertension. As they do to VSMC hypertrophy, important neurohormonal stimuli contribute to LVH, particularly the renin-angiotensin system (angiotensin II), the sympathetic nervous system, and the other growth factors listed earlier for VSMC. The clinical significance of the prohypertrophic actions of angiotensin II, for instance, is that ACE inhibitors or $AT_1$ receptor blockers could be expected to prevent, or even reverse, LVH more than antihypertensive drugs that reduce blood pressure by the same amount but have no direct action on myocardial cells.[12] This is important, because of the very adverse effect of LVH on the prognosis for patients with hypertension.

Patients with LVH (and many hypertensive patients without LVH) usually have diastolic dysfunction: their left ventricle is stiffer (i.e., less compliant) and thus requires greater distending pressure during diastole. These patients may have dyspnea (secondary to raised pulmonary venous filling pressure), left atrial hypertrophy, a fourth heart sound, and late diastolic flow across the mitral valve (A wave) that is larger than early diastolic flow (E wave). LVH may progress toward the syndrome of systolic dysfunction and dilated cardiomyopathy with congestive heart failure.

## Heart Attack and Brain Attack[13]

Hypertension is a significant risk factor for both acute myocardial infarction and stroke. Both situations are marked by hypertension-induced vascular hypertrophy and/or hyperplasia, endothelial dysfunction, and accelerated atherosclerosis, caused by migration of VSMC into the subintima, subendothelial infiltration of monocytes, cholesterol deposition and oxidation, and calcification. Additional elements in acute myocardial infarction are plaque disruption, platelet adhesion and aggregation, and thrombosis. Strokes, however, are more varied in their pathogenesis. Stroke may be caused by thrombosis, but also by hemorrhage secondary to rupture of cerebral arteries or by embolism from the heart or from aortic or carotid atherosclerotic plaques. Contrary to previous assumptions, stroke is not an all-or-none phenomenon. Reduction of cerebral blood flow due to arterial stenosis or thrombosis may produce any degree of tissue injury from asymptomatic and isolated neuronal dropout to huge infarction and cavitary necrosis. The extent of the ischemic injury depends on the duration and the intensity of the ischemia, and these, in turn, depend on the efficiency of the collateral circulation and the cardiac output. Hemorrhagic stroke in hypertension is probably due to rupture of microaneurysms of the small intracerebral arteries. Hypertensive cerebrovascular disease may also cause white matter ischemic rarefaction (or subcortical arteriosclerotic encephalopathy), which can give rise to a dementia syndrome called *Binswanger's disease*. Hypertension can also cause focal damage to small intracerebral arteries (lipohyalinosis) marked by occlusion of the vessels and the production of small ischemic cavities in the brain known as *lacunar infarcts*. Last, hypertension is a risk factor for berry aneurysms and subarachnoid hemorrhage.

## Acute Hypertensive Encephalopathy[14]

Acute hypertensive encephalopathy is a syndrome of severe hypertension, cerebrovascular dysfunction, and neurologic impairment that resolves rapidly with treatment. The pathophysiologic mechanism is segmental dilatation along the cerebral arterioles (sausage-string appearance); when in severe hypertension the autoregulatory capacity of vessels is exceeded, segments of the vessel dilate. Clinical features are those of encephalopathy (headache, nausea, projectile vomiting, visual blurring, drowsiness, confusion, seizures, coma) in association with severe hypertension. Papilledema, usually with retinal hemorrhages and exudates, may be present, and the sausage-string arteries may be seen in the retina. The differential diagnosis includes intracerebral hemorrhage, subarachnoid hemorrhage, brain tumor, subdural hematoma, cerebral infarction, and epilepsy. These lesions are usually identified by their distinctive clinical features and by computed tomography (CT). Drugs, such as intravenous amphetamines and cocaine, and ingestion of tyramine by patients taking monoamine oxidase inhibitors can produce a similar clinical picture, as can lupus vasculitis, polyarteritis, or uremic encephalopathy.

## Hypertension-Related Renal Damage[15, 16]

Hypertension is both a cause and a consequence of glomerulosclerosis, the hallmark lesion of progressive renal disease (see Chapter 39). It is a frequent cause of end-stage renal disease, second only to diabetes, and is particularly common in black patients. About 15% of patients with primary hypertension have microalbuminuria, and this finding in any patient is predictive of increased cardiovascular risk, but whether hypertensive nephropathy will develop in these patients is not known. The pathologic processes of hypertensive renal injury consist of vascular intimal thickening and fibrosis and hyalinization of arterioles (arteriosclerosis). There may be focal glomerulosclerosis with atrophic tubules. Mechanisms of the hypertensive renal injury include ischemia and increased glomerular capillary pressure. Other mechanisms whose roles are not clearly understood involve free oxygen radicals, glomerular capillary endothelial cell dysfunction, and proteinuria induced by the increased glomerular capillary pressure.

## Hypertensive Retinopathy[17]

Table 31–5 summarizes the features of hypertensive retinopathy, using the Keith and Wagener classification first proposed in 1939. More useful, however, is a careful description of the lesions in any particular patient. In addition to retinopathy, hypertensive choroidopathy occurs, but rarely. In addition to the lesions listed in Table 31–5, hypertension is associated with an increased incidence of central retinal vein occlusion, cotton-wool spots or cytoid bodies (areas of infarction in the retina), capillary microaneurysms (more common in diabetes), arteriolar macroaneurysms, and large, flame-shaped hemorrhages.

Table 31–5

**Keith-Wagener Classification of Hypertensive Retinopathy**

| Degree | A-V Ratio | Hemorrhages | Exudates | Papilledema | Other Findings |
|--------|-----------|-------------|----------|-------------|----------------|
| Normal | 3:4 | 0 | 0 | 0 | |
| Grade I | 1:2 | 0 | 0 | 0 | |
| Grade II | 1:3 | 0 | 0 | 0 | "Copper wire" arterioles, |
| Grade III | 1:4 | + | + | 0 | arteriovenous nipping |
| Grade IV | 1:4 | + | + | + | "Silver wire" arterioles |

0, none; +, at least one.

## ■ HYPERTENSIVE EMERGENCIES AND URGENCIES

*Hypertensive emergencies* are situations in which severe hypertension is associated with acute or rapidly progressive target organ damage. This condition is sometimes referred to as *malignant hypertension* or *accelerated malignant hypertension*, and a frequent, but not universal feature is papilledema (grade IV retinopathy). The mechanism of the often extremely high blood pressure with rapid deterioration of target organ function is not known; hypotheses include vascular endothelial damage with myointimal proliferation, and pressure natriuresis producing hypovolemia with activation of vasoconstrictor hormones such as catecholamines and the renin-angiotensin system. Plasma renin activity is usually very high. Usually, but not always, the diastolic blood pressure is over 120 mm Hg and at least one of the features of rapid target organ damage is evident, such as cerebrovasular (hypertensive encephalopathy, stroke) or cardiac (acute left ventricular failure, myocardial infarction, aortic dissection) lesions or acute renal failure. Obviously, these patients require urgent therapy with parenteral antihypertensive agents (see Chapter 32), although care should be taken not to drop mean arterial pressure too suddenly or below the lower limit of cerebrovascular autoregulation, which could induce an ischemic stroke. *Hypertensive urgencies* describes situations of very high blood pressure (stage 4, New York Heart Association) not related to severe symptoms or acute progressive target organ damage. For this condition the blood pressure should be reduced by oral agents and without delay (i.e., within hours, rather than days or weeks).

## ■ PATHOGENESIS OF PRIMARY HYPERTENSION

Most of the causes of secondary hypertension (see later) have been well-characterized, and their pathophysiologic mechanisms are reasonably well-understood. These causes, however, account for only 5% to 10% of all hypertension cases seen by physicians, and the remaining 90% to 95% of patients with primary hypertension have a disease that is as poorly understood as it is common. Consequently, enormous research efforts have been mobilized to study the pathogenesis of primary hypertension, using animal models, human patients, and, more recently, the powerful tools of cell and molecular biology. The result has been a plethora of mechanisms and theories, not all mutually exclusive, that support the concept devised by Irvine Page of a "mosaic" of mechanisms, each operating in different organs and at different levels of organization. What follows is a brief and selective survey of this topic.

## Genetic Predisposition

Monogenic syndromes are covered in the section on Secondary Hypertension. Primary hypertension also tends to cluster in families, but a specific genotype has not been identified. A number of associations have been suggested, but none has been confirmed. These include mutations in the gene for angiotensinogen, renin, and the $\beta_2$ and $\alpha_2$ receptors, a negative association with transforming growth factor beta$_1$, the adducin protein which affects the assembly of the actin-based cytoskeleton, and polymorphisms of the ACE gene.

## Increased Cardiac Output (Fig. 31–1)

Blood pressure is proportional to cardiac output and total peripheral resistance. Some young "borderline hypertensives" have a hyperkinetic circulation with increased cardiac output. This, in turn, may be due to increased preload associated with increased blood volume or to increased myocardial contractility. Also, LVH has been described in the still normotensive children of hypertensive parents, an observation that suggests that the LVH is not only a consequence of increased arterial pressure but that it may itself reflect some mechanism, such as hyperactivity of the sympathetic nervous system or the renin-angiotensin system, that causes both LVH and hypertension. Plasma volume is usually normal or slightly decreased in primary hypertension; however, some investigators have suggested that the volumes are still higher than they should be, given the elevated blood pressure, which should produce substantial pressure natriuresis and diuresis.

## Excessive Dietary Sodium

We ingest many times more sodium than we need; there is much epidemiologic and experimental evidence to show an association between salt intake and hyper-

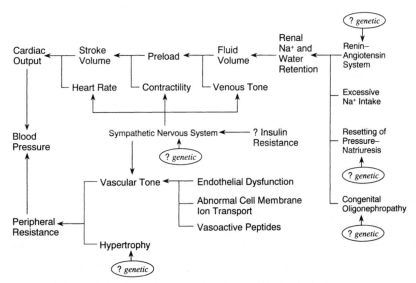

**Figure 31–1** ■ Hemodynamic and renal control of arterial blood pressure.

tension. Sodium excess activates some pressor mechanisms (such as increases of intracellular calcium and plasma catecholamines), and it increases insulin resistance. About half of hypertensive patients are particularly salt sensitive (as defined by the blood pressure rise induced by sodium loading), as compared with about a quarter of normotensive controls. Sodium sensitivity becomes greater with age and has a strong genetic component. The mechanism of sodium sensitivity may be renal sodium retention (see later).

## Renal Sodium Retention

Abnormal renal sodium handling may be due to a rightward shift of the pressure-natriuresis curve of the kidney (Fig. 31–2).[18] When the arterial pressure is raised, the normal kidney excretes more salt and water; balance normally occurs at a mean perfusion pressure of around 100 mm Hg, producing sodium excretion of about 150 mEq/day. Increased salt intake transiently raises blood pressure, and the pressure-natriuresis effectively restores total body sodium to normal. In patients with primary hypertension, this pressure-natriuresis curve is reset to a higher blood pressure, preventing return of the blood pressure to normal, because, at all pressures below the patient's hypertensive level, sodium retention occurs. There is some evidence in certain animal models and in humans that the rightward shift in the pressure-natriuresis curve is inherited.

A variation on this theme is a hormonal mediator of salt sensitivity, a sodium pump inhibitor, endogenous ouabain, which is secreted by the adrenal cortex and is natriuretic in sodium-loaded animals.[19] Renal sodium retention stimulates ouabain

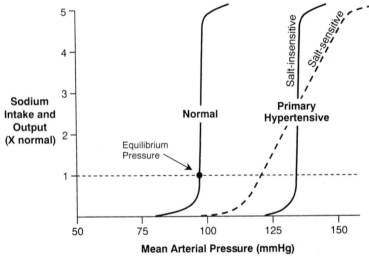

**Figure 31–2** ■ Steady state relations between blood pressure and sodium intake and output in normotensive subjects and in patients with salt-sensitive or salt-insensitive hypertension. Normally, an increase in sodium intake will result in a small increase in mean arterial pressure that is sufficient to increase sodium output by pressure natriuresis, so that the "equilibrium pressure" is restored. In salt-insensitive hypertension, the steep curve is retained but is shifted to the right (i.e., reset at a higher mean arterial pressure). In salt-sensitive hypertension, there is a shift to the right and flattening of the curve so that sodium loading increases blood pressure by a greater amount. (Modified from Hall JE, Brands MW, Shek EW: Central role of the kidney and abnormal fluid volume control in hypertension. J Hum Hypertens 1996;10:633–639.)

release, which, by its inhibition of the sodium pump, increases intracellular sodium. In turn, sodium-calcium exchange is inhibited, and the rise in intracellular calcium causes increased vascular tone and vascular hypertrophy. This is discussed further under Abnormal Cell Membrane Ion Transport, below.

Some investigators believe that a more important role for the kidney is the generation of more renin from nephrons that are ischemic owing to afferent arteriolar vasoconstriction or structural narrowing of the lumen.[20] Some patients with primary hypertension have elevated plasma renin activity, but, even in those with normal levels, it may be inappropriately high, since we would expect the hypertension to suppress renin.[21] Others have developed the idea that hypertension may arise from a congenital reduction in the number of nephrons or in the filtration surface area per glomerulus that limits the ability of the kidney to excrete sodium, raising blood pressure, which destroys more glomeruli, thus setting up a vicious circle of hypertension and renal glomerular dysfunction. This idea has support from the observation that low–birth weight babies are more likely to become hypertensive later in life.

## Increased Activity of the Renin-Angiotensin System

The components of the renin-angiotensin system, the biosynthesis and actions of angiotensin II, and angiotensin II signal transduction in VSMC are all described in Chapter 4. Plasma renin activity is nearly always low in association with primary aldosteronism, high with renovascular or accelerated-malignant hypertension, and low, normal, or high with primary hypertension. Primary hypertension with sodium retention would be expected to depress plasma renin levels; under these circumstances "normal" values are inappropriately high. Three explanations for this have been developed. The first, cited earlier, is that a population of ischemic nephrons contributes excess renin. The second is that the sympathetic hyperactivity associated with primary hypertension stimulates β-adrenergic receptors in the juxtaglomerular apparatus of the nephron to activate renin release. The third proposes that many of the patients with inappropriately normal or even high renin levels have defective regulation of the relationship of sodium and the renin-angiotensin system—that they are "nonmodulators." This results in abnormal adrenal and renal responses to salt loads; in particular, salt loading does not reduce angiotensin II.[22]

## Increased Sympathetic Activity

There is much evidence of sympathetic hyperactivity in patients with primary hypertension. Heart rate and stroke volume are increased, at least in the early, labile phase of blood pressure elevation, and at least part of the increased vascular resistance of the established phase of hypertension may be due to the increased sympathetic tone. Baroreceptor sensitivity is reduced, so that a given increase in blood pressure decreases heart rate less than it normally would. It is not surprising that psychogenic stress seems to predispose to high blood pressure, tension causing hypertension.

## Increased Peripheral Resistance

Small arteries and arterioles are responsible for most of the peripheral resistance, but the microvasculature is difficult to study in humans. It is much easier to study larger arteries, especially by noninvasive methods such as ultrasonography.

We can make measurements of morphology, such as wall thickness and wall:lumen ratio, and of physiologic processes, such as compliance or distensibility (lumen cross-sectional diameter or area change per unit pressure change). Patients with hypertension very frequently have large arteries (e.g., brachial, carotid, femoral) that are thick (owing to hypertrophy, increased wall:lumen ratio) and stiff (owing to decreased compliance). These effects are due to VSMC hypertrophy in the media. Smaller arteries probably undergo either hyperplasia or remodeling, which is a rearrangement of existing cells around a smaller lumen. The growth factors responsible for these changes are summarized in Figure 31–3 and are discussed in more detail in Chapter 4.

## Abnormal Cell Membrane Ion Transport[23]

Because it is so easy to measure red cell cation concentrations, and therefore the kinetics of transmembrane cation flux, the literature on abnormalities of these in primary hypertension is voluminous. There seems to be general agreement that there is decreased activity of the $Na^+$-$K^+$-ATPase pump (which pumps $Na^+$ *out* of the cell), possibly the result of an excess of the endogenous inhibitor ouabain (see earlier in the section on Renal Sodium Retention). There may also be increased activity of the $Na^+$-$H^+$ exchange antiporter (which pumps $Na^+$ *into* the cell). Both mechanisms increase intracellular sodium. This high intracellular sodium concentration (and low intracellular pH) inhibits $Na^+$-$Ca^{2+}$ exchange (normally $Na^+$ *in* and $Ca^{2+}$ *out*) to increase intracellular $Ca^{2+}$, which increases vascular tone and stimulates hypertrophy. Hyperactivity of the $Na^+$-$H^+$ exchanger in renal proximal tubule cells may also cause increased sodium reabsorption and vascular volume expansion.

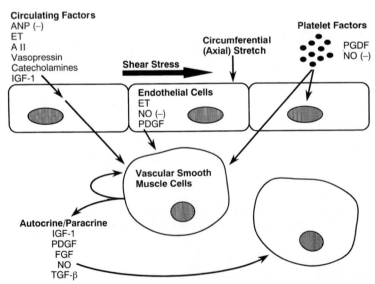

**Figure 31–3** ■ Stimuli to vascular smooth muscle growth. ANP, atrial natriuretic peptide; ET, endothelin; AII, angiotensin II; PDGF, platelet-derived growth factor; NO, nitric oxide (endothelin-derived relaxing factor); IGF-1, insulin-like growth factor-1; FGF, fibroblast growth factor; TGF-β, transforming growth factor beta; ( − ), inhibitory to hypertrophy/hyperplasia.

## Endothelial Dysfunction[10]

Impaired biosynthesis or release of nitric oxide, the vascular endothelium–derived relaxing factor, has been described in animal models of hypertension and in human hypertension. Endothelin, a 21–amino acid vasoconstrictor made by endothelial cells, may or may not be present in increased amounts in the plasma of hypertensives. This uncertainty does not rule out a role for endothelin in hypertension, since there may be paracrine release of endothelin from the endothelial cells, where it is made, toward the VSMC, where it acts. The animal data are also somewhat preliminary; in rats, endothelin production is increased in sodium volume overload forms of hypertension but not in genetic hypertension. Prostaglandin $H_2$ and thromboxane $A_2$ are other vasoconstrictors made by endothelial cells (see Chapter 4).

## Insulin Resistance and Hyperinsulinemia[24]

Hypertension is more common in obese persons, possibly because of insulin resistance and the resulting hyperinsulinemia. The mechanism by which insulin resistance or hyperinsulinemia increases blood pressure is obscure; possibilities include enhanced renal sodium and water reabsorption, increased sympathetic nervous system activity, and vascular hypertrophy, all firmly established actions of insulin. While the physiologic role of insulin resistance and hyperinsulinemia has been studied most intensively in the syndrome of obesity, hypertension, and diabetes, similar abnormalities of insulin action have been described in lean hypertensives who are not diabetic.

## Other Possible Mechanisms

The many other possible mechanisms that have been investigated are supported by more or less solid evidence. Notable ones are abnormal patterns of biosynthesis or secretion of adrenocortical hormones in response to various stimuli, adrenomedullin (an adrenomedullary vasodilator peptide), the kallikrein-kinin system, including bradykinin, other vasoactive peptides (calcitonin gene–related peptide, neuropeptide Y, opioid peptides, vasopressin), dopamine, serotonin, prostaglandins, and medullipin (a renomedullary vasodepressor lipid). In addition to all of the postulated mechanisms for primary hypertension, many other factors may contribute to high blood pressure in susceptible persons. Examples are increased urinary calcium with a low plasma calcium concentration, potassium and magnesium deficiency, smoking, excessive consumption of caffeine or alcohol, physical inactivity, and hyperuricemia.

## ■ COMMON CAUSES OF SECONDARY HYPERTENSION

*Common* is an overstatement. As a rough estimate, only about 5% of all patients who present with hypertension have a demonstrable cause that therefore may qualify the condition as *secondary*. It is, however, critically important to recognize these conditions when they occur, as many are curable—by surgery or some other means.

## Renovascular Hypertension[25-27]

Renal hypoperfusion as a result of renovascular disease accounts for about 1% of all cases of hypertension, but it is much more likely to be the cause when hypertension is rapidly progressive, accelerated or malignant, or is associated with coronary, carotid, or peripheral vascular disease. The mechanism of renovascular hypertension has been firmly established in animal models (based on those developed by Harry Goldblatt in the 1930s). When both renal arteries in the dog are partially occluded by clamps, or when one artery is clamped and the other kidney removed, sustained hypertension develops. The two-clip–two-kidney model resembles bilateral renovascular hypertension, and the one-clip–one-kidney animal is a model for renovascular hypertension plus chronic renal parenchymal disease. A more useful model for the common form of renovascular hypertension, unilateral renal artery stenosis, is the one-clip–two-kidney model.

*Bilateral renovascular hypertension* and *renovascular hypertension (unilateral or bilateral) with chronic renal parenchymal disease* have similar mechanisms. The decreased intrarenal vascular pressure results in increased secretion of renin from the juxtaglomerular apparatus, and, consequently, increased activity of angiotensin II and aldosterone. The systemic vasoconstriction produced by angiotensin II raises the blood pressure (renin-dependent hypertension). With time, however, the renin-angiotensin dependency of the systemic hypertension wanes because of progressive retention of sodium and water, which leads to increases in extracellular fluid volume, blood volume, and blood pressure. Sodium and water retention are consequences of a reduction in the functional renal mass subjected to reduced perfusion pressure, with the associated rightward shift of the pressure-natriuresis curve (see Fig. 31–2), and are secondary to the effects of the angiotensin II, namely intrarenal vasoconstriction, increased net tubular sodium reabsorption, and increased aldosterone levels. At this stage, the hypertension is mainly volume dependent. With progressive diminution in renin release and in circulating angiotensin II levels, salt and water balance is restored, but at the expense of high arterial blood pressure.

This dual mechanism has important therapeutic implications. Therapy with vasodilators reduces the renal perfusion pressure even further and exacerbates volume retention. Diuretics reduce the extracellular fluid volume and enhance the activity of the renin-angiotensin system. Vasodilator drugs in combination with volume depletion can decrease the glomerular filtration rate and can even cause acute renal failure. ACE inhibitors or angiotensin II receptor blockers may also be dangerous because they remove the selective vasoconstrictor action of angiotensin II on efferent arterioles to maintain glomerular filtration pressure.

*Unilateral renovascular hypertension* is much more common than bilateral stenosis in humans. Here, the stenotic kidney releases renin, elevating circulating levels of angiotensin II to increase blood pressure. This hypertension should increase sodium excretion in the nonstenotic kidney to restore blood pressure to normal; however, this pressure-natriuresis effect (see Fig. 31–2) is blunted by the increased angiotensin II levels, because of angiotensin II– and aldosterone-mediated sodium reabsorption, and because of angiotensin II renal vasoconstriction with reduction in renal plasma flow and glomerular filtration rate (GFR). Since the pressure distal to the stenosis is never completely restored to normal, even with high systemic blood pressure, the levels of renin and angiotensin II remain high and the hypertension is "renin dependent."

Treatment of unilateral renovascular hypertension with ACE inhibitors or angiotensin II receptor blockers reduces glomerular filtration pressure and GFR in stenotic kidneys but increases renal blood flow and GFR in nonstenotic kidneys. In some patients, the sustained hypertension of unilateral renovascular disease can cause hypertensive glomerular injury in the nonstenotic kidney, which further compromises renal function and exacerbates the hypertension. In these patients, ACE inhibitors and angiotensin II receptor blockers may further impair renal function—for the reasons described earlier.

## Pathology

The most common cause of renovascular hypertension is atherosclerotic stenosis of a main renal artery. Affected patients are relatively older and usually have vascular disease elsewhere. The second condition is fibromuscular dysplasia, which can be subdivided into intimal fibroplasia, medial fibromuscular dysplasia, and periadventitial fibrosis. Of these, the most common is medial fibromuscular dysplasia (or medial fibroplasia), usually a condition of young women. Other, rare, causes are renal artery aneurysms, emboli, and Takayasu's arteritis and other vasculitides.

## Clinical Features

The only unique clinical finding, an abdominal bruit, is heard in about half of those who have renal artery stenosis. In general, renal artery stenosis should be suspected in severe hypertension associated with any one of the following: progressive renal insufficiency, refractoriness to aggressive treatment, evidence of occlusive vascular disease, in young women, or in patients whose serum creatinine value rises quickly after they start taking an ACE inhibitor. Laboratory findings often include proteinuria, elevated renin and aldosterone levels, and a low serum potassium value.

## Diagnosis

The most cost-effective screening test is the captopril renal scan. Reduced renal uptake of $^{99m}$Tc-diethylenetriamine pentaacetic acid (DTPA) or reduced renal excretion of iodine 121 ($^{121}$I) hippurate or technetium 99m ($^{99m}$Tc) mercaptoacetyltriglycine (MAG) is a measure of renal function in stenotic kidneys. Renal function can be reduced further after a single dose of the ACE inhibitor captopril. If the captopril scan is positive, then magnetic resonance angiography (MRA) should be done. Other useful imaging tests include ultrasonography, spiral CT with contrast, digital subtraction intravenous angiography, and renal arteriography. Various tests detect hypersecretion of renin from the hypoperfused kidney: these are peripherial blood plasma renin activity (PRA), captopril-augmented peripheral blood PRA, and the renal vein renin ratio (ratio of PRA between the two renal veins; a ratio $> 1.5:1$ is diagnostic).

## Therapy

For most patients, renal angioplasty (with or without stenting) or surgery is the treatment of choice. If, however, the hypertension is very well-controlled and renal function does not decline under close monitoring, antihypertensive drug therapy may be appropriate. ACE inhibitors or angiotensin II receptor antagonists should not be used.

## ■ RENAL PARENCHYMAL HYPERTENSION[28]

Renal parenchymal hypertension is discussed in more detail in Chapter 39. Renal disease, the commonest cause of secondary hypertension, is present in about 80% of patients with chronic renal failure (CRF). Primary hypertension also damages the kidneys; in the United States, hypertension ranks just below diabetes among causes of end-stage renal disease. Hypertension is, therefore, both a cause and a consequence of renal disease, and often there is a vicious circle: hypertension causes renal damage, which exacerbates hypertension.

## Pathophysiologic Mechanisms

The following mechanisms have been identified:

### Sodium and Volume Status

A severely reduced GFR (<50 ml/min) causes sodium retention and volume expansion and, therefore, increased cardiac output. The disorder of sodium homeostasis may also be due to increased amounts of an endogenous ouabain-like natriuretic factor that inhibits the $Na^+$-$K^+$-ATPase pump.

### The Renin-Angiotensin-Aldosterone System

The renin-angiotensin-aldosterone system is activated in CRF because of diffuse intrarenal ischemia. The aldosterone contributes to sodium retention. Eventually, however, the expanded fluid volume inhibits renin release, and plasma renin activity may become normal. Even "normal" plasma concentrations of renin are, however, inappropriately high in relation to the state of sodium and water balance, and the hypertension remains partly due to an angiotensin-dependent increase in peripheral vascular resistance.

### The Autonomic Nervous System

CRF activates renal baroreceptors, which effect increases sympathetic nervous system activity and elevates plasma norepinephrine levels (as does reduced catecholamine clearance).

### Other Mechanisms

In uremic patients increased plasma levels of an endogenous compound, asymmetrical dimethylarginine (ADMA), a nitric oxide synthase inhibitor, contribute to the hypertension. Recombinant human erythropoietin (rHu-EPO), used extensively to treat the anemia of CRF, exacerbates hypertension, though how it does so is not known. The secondary hyperparathyroidism of CRF makes the hypertension worse. The mechanism, as yet undefined, is somehow related to the increase in intracellular calcium concentration.

## Management

The problem in treating hypertension in patients with CRF is that diuretics and other antihypertensive agents often produce a transient drop in renal blood flow and GFR and an increase in serum creatinine; so, management is often a delicate balancing act between achieving blood pressure control and maintaining whatever renal function is left. In general, diuretics and ACE inhibitors are the antihypertensive drugs of choice (see Chapter 32).

## ■ PHEOCHROMOCYTOMA[29]

Pheochromocytomas develop in about 0.5% of hypertensives. They can occur at any age, and they arise from neuroectodermal chromaffin cells, mostly in the adrenal medulla (85%) but sometimes elsewhere, usually in the abdomen or pelvis (15%). About 10% of adrenal and about 30% to 40% of extraadrenal tumors are malignant. Ten percent are familial and autosomal dominant. The familial form seems to be due to mutations of the RET protooncogene on chromosome 10 and may be intercurrent with other tumors as a syndrome of multiple endocrine neoplasia (MEN). In MEN 2, pheochromocytoma is associated with medullary thyroid carcinoma (MTC) and parathyroid adenoma or hyperplasia, whereas in MEN 3 there is no parathyroid disease but there is a characteristic phenotype (marfanoid appearance, neuromas of the lips and tongue, thickened corneal nerves, intestinal ganglioneuromatosis).

Pheochromocytomas secrete norepinephrine (NE) mainly and less epinephrine, plus a variety of peptide hormones, adrenocorticotropin (ACTH), erythropoietin, parathyroid hormone, calcitonin gene–related protein, atrial natriuretric peptide, vasoactive intestinal peptide, and others. Most patients have hypertension; in about half it is sustained, with or without paroxysms, and in the other half blood pressure is normal between paroxysms. Paroxysms of hypertension may be signaled by severe headaches, sweating, palpitations with tachycardia, pallor, anxiety, and tremor. Also described are orthostatic hypotension, nausea and vomiting, and weight loss. Any patient with this symptom complex should be screened for pheochromocytoma with measurement of 24-hour urinary catecholamine metabolites (especially metanephrine) and plasma catecholamines. There are some problems with these tests. Results can be normal in patients with paroxysmal hypertension if the test is done during a normotensive interval. Urinary metabolites of an antihypertensive drug, labetalol, may cause a false-positive result. If plasma catecholamines are moderately elevated (600 to 2000 pg/ml), the differential diagnosis includes neurogenic hypertension and hypertension associated with increased sympathetic activity. Here, the clonidine suppression test is useful; clonidine decreases plasma catecholamine levels to normal in neurogenic hypertension, but not in pheochromocytoma. If blood or urine test findings are positive, the next step is to localize the tumor using CT or magnetic resonance imaging. Scintigraphy using [131]I-metaiodobenzylguanidine ([131]I-MIBG) is also useful. Definitive treatment is surgery, but great care must be taken to prevent severe hypertension or hypotension during the operation or in the immediate postoperative period, utilizing sympathetic blocking drugs and careful management of fluid balance.

## ▪ ADRENAL CORTICAL HYPERTENSION[30]

### Mineralocorticoid Hypertension

Aldosterone, the most abundant mineralocorticoid hormone, is synthesized by aldosterone synthase in the outer zone of the adrenal cortex (zona glomerulosa). Its synthesis and release are controlled by adrenocorticotropic hormone (ACTH) and blood levels peak in the early morning, but angiotensin II and the serum concentration of potassium also affect it. Aldosterone increases distal tubular reabsorption of sodium and chloride and secretion of potassium and hydrogen ions. Another mineralocorticoid hormone, deoxycorticosterone, produced by the inner zone of the adrenal cortex (zona fasciculata), is a much weaker mineralocorticoid than aldosterone, but it can cause hypertension when produced in large quantities.

The hypertension produced by mineralocorticoid excess is due to the increase in total exchangeable sodium, but most patients with chronic mineralocorticoid excess have normal plasma volume, because the initial increase in extracellular fluid volume is restored to normal by an increased natriuresis and diuresis due to decreased sodium reabsorption in segments of the nephron other than the distal tubule (mineralocorticoid escape). The hypertension is sustained by increased vascular resistance (possibly due to augmented vascular sensitivity to catecholamines) or by central nervous system mineralocorticoid receptors, which activate the sympathetic nervous system.

Primary hyperaldosteronism (Conn's syndrome) is due either to a benign aldosterone-producing adenoma (APA) or, more rarely, to idiopathic hyperaldosteronism (IHA), in which the adrenal glands are normal or hyperplastic. The classic clinical features of primary hyperaldosteronism are hypertension, excessive urinary potassium excretion, hypokalemia, hypernatremia, and metabolic alkalosis. A hypertensive patient who is treated with diuretics or who has diarrhea may also have a low serum potassium concentration. In this situation, the serum potassium value returns to normal after recovery from the diarrhea or a few weeks after the diuretic is discontinued. Also useful in this situation is measurement of 24-hour urinary potassium excretion; if it is more than 30 mEq/day, then primary hyperaldosteronism should be suspected and plasma renin and aldosterone levels measured. If the plasma renin activity is low and the plasma aldosterone level is high (aldosterone:renin ratio > 20 using traditional units of concentration or > 900 using SI units), primary hyperaldosteronism is confirmed. Diuretics raise both PRA and aldosterone levels. Another test sometimes done to confirm the diagnosis is based on the failure of volume expansion to suppress aldosterone. Serum 18-hydroxycorticosterone, the precursor of aldosterone, should also be measured; serum 18-hydroxycorticosterone levels are higher than 100 ng/dl with APA and lower than 100 ng/dl with IHA. CT or magnetic resonance imaging of the adrenal glands completes the workup.

## Glucocorticoid Hypertension

The principal glucocorticoid in humans, cortisol, is synthesized in the zona fasciculata under the control of ACTH. While cortisol has only a weak mineralocorticoid effect, the circulating levels of the hormone in Cushing's syndrome are usually hundreds of times the normal value. Since most patients with Cushing's syndrome, however, do not have other findings of hypermineralocorticoidism, particularly hypokalemia and hyperreninemia, and since spironolactone, a mineralocorticoid antagonist, does not blunt the hypertensive effect of cortisol, other mechanisms must be operating. Possibilities include glucocorticoids activating gene transcription of angiotensinogen in the liver, increasing vascular reactivity to vasoconstrictor amines, inhibition of the extraneuronal uptake and degradation of norepinephrine, inhibition of vasodilators like kinins and some prostaglandins, and a shift of sodium from cells to the extracellular compartment with an increase in plasma volume and, thus, in cardiac output. Also, in Cushing's syndrome, the ACTH excess may stimulate production and release of endogenous mineralocorticoids, especially deoxycorticosterone.

## Other Clinical Syndromes of Adrenocortical Hypertension

### Glucocorticoid-Remediable Hyperaldosteronism (GRA)

GRA is an autosomal-dominant disorder in which the classic features of primary hyperaldosteronism are completely relieved by glucocorticoids such as dexamethasone. Because dexamethasone suppresses ACTH, the concept was developed of increased adrenal sensitivity to the aldosterone-stimulating effects of ACTH. Recently, it has been shown that this syndrome is due to a chimeric gene produced by unequal crossing over of the 5' regulatory region of 11β-hydroxylase and the coding sequence of aldosterone synthase. As a result, aldosterone synthase, normally found in the zona glomerulosa, is expressed in the zona fasciculata under the control of the ACTH-sensitive 11β-hydroxylase regulatory sequence, which accounts for the aldosterone elevation and the excess formation of products of 11β-hydroxylase activity, such as 18-hydroxycortisol and 18-oxocortisol. This is the first description of a gene mutation as a cause of hypertension in humans.

## Pseudohyperaldosteronism (Liddle's Syndrome)

In 1963, Liddle described members of a family with hypertension and hypokalemic alkalosis who had low levels of aldosterone and no elevations of other mineralocorticoids. Treatment with the mineralocorticoid antagonist spironolactone or with other inhibitors of mineralocorticoid biosynthesis had no effect, but amiloride and triamterene, both inhibitors of distal nephron sodium reabsorption, improved hypertension and hypokalemia. Affected patients have a mutation of the β- or γ-subunit of the renal epithelial sodium channel that increases sodium reabsorption in the distal nephron.

## Enzyme Deficiencies

(1) 11β-Hydroxylase converts 11-deoxycortisol to cortisol. Deficiency of this enzyme leads to reduced cortisol levels, increased ACTH secretion, and increased production of 11-deoxycorticosterone in the zona fasciculata. The 11-deoxycorticosterone induces volume expansion, hypertension, and suppression of aldosterone secretion. These patients also have virilization. (2) 17α-Hydroxylase converts progesterone to 17-hydroxyprogesterone; deficiency of 17-hydroxylase reduces cortisol levels, causing increased ACTH and increased deoxycorticosterone levels. (3) 11-β-Hydroxysteroid dehydrogenase metabolizes cortisol to its metabolites. A deficiency of this enzyme in the kidney produces high renal levels of cortisol, producing all of the features of the hypermineralocorticoid state but with low mineralocorticoid levels (the syndrome of apparent mineralocorticoid excess). An acquired form of this syndrome develops in adults who eat large quantities of licorice. The active alkaloid in licorice, glycyrrhetenic acid, is an inhibitor of 11β-hydroxysteroid dehydrogenase.

## ■ REFERENCES

1. MacMahon S, Peto R, Cutler J, et al: Blood pressure, stroke, and coronary heart disease. Part I. Prolonged differences in blood pressure: Prospective observational studies corrected for the regression dilution bias. Lancet 1990;335:765–773.
2. The Sixth Report of the Joint National Committee on Prevention, Detection, Evaluation, and Treatment of High Blood Pressure. Bethesda: National Institutes of Health, 98-4080, 1997.
3. National Institutes of Health; National Heart, Lung, and Blood Institute: Fact Book, Fiscal Year 1996. Bethesda: National Institutes of Health, 1997.
4. National Institute of Diabetes and Digestive and Kidney Disease: U.S. Renal Data System Annual Report. Bethesda: U.S. Department of Health and Human Services, 1997.
5. Levy D, Larson MG, Vasan RS, et al: The progression from hypertension to congestive heart failure. JAMA 1996;275:1557–1562.
6. The Criteria Committee of the New York Heart Association: Nomenclature and Criteria for Diagnosis of Diseases of the Heart and Great Vessels, 9th ed. Boston: Little, Brown, 1994.
7. American Society of Hypertension: Recommendations for routine blood pressure measurement by indirect cuff sphygmomanometry. Am J Hypertens 1992;5:207–209.
8. Peloff D, Grim C, Flack J, et al: Human blood pressure determination by sphygmomanometry. Circulation 1993;88:2460–2470.
9. Rosendorff C: The renin-angiotensin system and vascular hypertrophy. J Am Coll Cardiol 1996;28:803–812.
10. Rosendorff C: Endothelin, vascular hypertrophy and hypertension. Cardiovasc Drugs Ther 1996;10:795–802.
11. Koren MJ, Devereux RB, Casale PN, et al: Relation of left ventricular mass and geometry to morbidity and mortality in uncomplicated essential hypertension. Ann Intern Med 1991;114:345–352.
12. Schmieder RE, Martus P, Klingbeil A: Reversal of left ventricular hypertrophy in essential hypertension: A meta-analysis of randomized double-blind studies. JAMA 1996;275:1507–1513.
13. Rosendorff C: Stroke in the elderly—risk factors and some projections. Cardiovasc Rev Reports 1999;20(4):244–248.
14. Healton EB, Brust JC, Feinfeld DA, Thomson GE: Hypertensive encephalopathy and the neurological manifestations of malignant hypertension. Neurology 1982;32:127–132.
15. Mountokalakis TD: The renal consequences of arterial hypertension. Kidney Int 1997;51:1639–1653.

16. Rennke HG, Anderson S, Brenner BM: Structural and functional correlations in the progression of renal disease. *In* Tisher CC, Brenner BM (eds): Renal Pathology, 2nd ed. Philadelphia: JB Lippincott, 1994:116–142.
17. Frank RN: The eye in hypertension. *In* Izzo JL Jr, Black HR (eds): Hypertension Primer: The Essentials of High Blood Pressure, 2nd ed. Dallas, TX: Council for High Blood Pressure Research, American Heart Association, 1999:194–196.
18. Guyton AC: Kidneys and fluids in pressure regulation. Small volume but large pressure changes. Hypertension 1992;19(suppl I):I2–I8.
19. de Wardener HE: Sodium transport inhibitors and hypertension. J Hypertens 1996;14(suppl 5):S9–S18.
20. Laragh JH: Renin-angiotensin-aldosterone system for blood pressure and electrolyte homeostasis and its involvement in hypertension, in congestive heart failure and in associated cardiovascular damage (myocardial infarction and stroke). J Hum Hypertens 1995;9:385–390.
21. Brenner BM, Chertow GM: Congenital oligonephropathy and the etiology of adult hypertension and progressive renal injury. Am J Kidney Dis 1994;23:171–175.
22. Williams GH, Hollenberg NK: Non-modulating hypertension. A subset of sodium-sensitive hypertension. Hypertension 1991;17(suppl I):I81–I85.
23. Swales JD: Functional disturbance of ions in hypertension. Cardiovasc Drug Ther 1990;4:367–372.
24. Reaven GM, Lithell H, Landsberg L: Hypertension and associated abnormalities—The role of insulin resistance and the sympathoadrenal system. N Engl J Med 1996;334:374–381.
25. Martinez-Maldonado M: Pathophysiology of renovascular hypertension. Hypertension 1991;17:707–719.
26. Ploth DW: Renovascular hypertension. *In* Jacobson HR, Striker GE, Klahr S (eds): The Principles and Practice of Nephrology, 2nd ed. St. Louis: Mosby–Year Book, 1995:379–386.
27. Pohl MA: Renal artery stenosis, renal vascular hypertension and ischemic nephropathy. *In* Schrier RW, Gottschalk CW (eds): Diseases of the Kidney, 6th ed. Boston: Little, Brown, 1997:1367–1423.
28. Working Group: 1995 Update of the Working Group Reports on Chronic Renal Failure and Renovascular Hypertension. NIH Publication No. 95-3791. Washington: National Heart, Lung and Blood Institute, 1995.
29. Manger WM, Gifford RW Jr: Clinical and Experimental Pheochromocytoma, 2nd ed. Cambridge, MA: Blackwell Scientific, 1996.
30. Ganguly A: Primary aldosteronism. N Engl J Med 1998;339:1828–1834.

## ▪ RECOMMENDED READING

Izzo JL Jr, Black HR (eds): Hypertension Primer. The Essentials of High Blood Pressure, 2nd ed. Dallas, TX: Council on High Blood Pressure Research, American Heart Association, 1999.
Kaplan NK: Clinical Hypertension, 7th ed. Baltimore: Williams & Wilkins, 1998.
Laragh JH, Brenner BM (eds): Hypertension: Pathophysiology, Diagnosis, and Management, 2nd ed. New York: Raven, 1995.

*Chapter* <u>32</u>

# Hypertension Therapy

*Norman M. Kaplan*

Hypertension is almost always easy to treat but often exceedingly difficult to keep under control. The latest survey of a representative sample of the U.S. population reports that more than half of hypertensives are being treated but only 27% have their blood pressure under control (i.e., <140/90 mm Hg on three measurements at two different times).[1] These figures point to a number of problems: many cases of hypertension have not been diagnosed or treated, and many physicians have not provided adequate amounts of medication. The most likely problem, however, is inherent to hypertension: It is a lifelong condition that for many years is usually asymptomatic but that requires daily therapy, which can, of itself, induce symptoms.

Most hypertension is of unknown cause and, therefore, cannot with certainty be prevented (see Chapter 31). Nonetheless, in view of the inherent difficulty of treating the condition after it has developed, here, attention will first be given to lifestyle modifications that may help to delay, if not to prevent, its onset. All are also of value in treating established hypertension; if offered to prehypertensive persons, they may be preventive as well. In the absence of a genetic or physiologic marker, there is no way to identify with certainty the "prehypertensive." Only those with a hypertensive parent could be chosen, but, since more than half of all of us will be hypertensive before we die, the more rational approach is to educate everyone in low-cost, minimally intrusive lifestyle changes. Although as many as half will not derive any protection from hypertension (since they are not destined to develop the condition), they will still derive benefits, including better quality of life and protection from other risk factors for premature cardiovascular morbidity and mortality.

## ■ LIFESTYLE MODIFICATIONS

As the sixth report of the Joint National Committee (JNC-6) states,[1] lifestyle modifications are often the only therapy indicated for patients with relatively mild hypertension and little overall cardiovascular risk, and they are always indicated, along with drug therapy, for the others.

The tendency, for most patients and physicians, is to proceed immediately to drug therapy for hypertension of any degree. For the patient, drug therapy offers almost universal and instantaneous reduction of blood pressure; with current drugs, this benefit comes at little cost in the way of side effects, although the financial cost can be considerable. Moreover, bad habits are hard to break, and, as long as the blood pressure can be controlled with a few pills, patients seem to see little reason not to be what most other people are: overweight, physically inactive consumers of high-calorie, high-sodium fast foods, chased down by a six-pack.

For the physician, drugs are a known quantity: they are easy to prescribe and likely to be effective. Instructing, motivating, and following patients, compliance with lifestyle modifications, on the other hand, is costly in time and energy, costs that are not compensated by the medical insurors.

But the effort is worthwhile. Even when the weight loss and sodium restriction are relatively small, marked benefits have been shown, as among the elderly hypertensives enrolled in the TONE study.[2] Moreover, other cardiovascular risk factors—dyslipidemia, glucose intolerance and diabetes, physical inactivity, cigarette smoking—may incidentally be relieved, an outcome that multiplies the benefits far beyond those of the reduction in blood pressure. The lifestyle modification prescription recommended in JNC-6 for treatment is also applicable to prevention (Table 32–1).

## Prevention of Intrauterine Growth Retardation

Though it is not included in the list of lifestyle modifications, perhaps the most effective preventive measure is the prevention of intrauterine growth retardation. A number of epidemiologic surveys have documented an increased prevalence of hypertension in adults whose birth weight was low for their gestational age (Fig. 32–1).[3] For every kilogram increase in birth weight, on average, systolic blood pressure is 4 mm Hg lower when those infants become adults. Low birth weight, as a reflection of intrauterine growth retardation, is clearly a contributor to adult hypertension.

The mechanism is indeterminate; the most attractive hypothesis is congenital oligonephropathy—fewer than usual nephrons at birth, a condition that leads to both systemic and glomerular hypertension.[4] Regardless of how low birth weight eventuates in hypertension (or diabetes or coronary heart disease), preventing low birth weight may very well be the most effective and achievable way to prevent these diseases in adults.

Low birth weight is more common in disadvantaged populations, in particular among blacks (who have much higher prevalences of both hypertension and renal insufficiency). Associations have been noted between low birth weight and teenage pregnancy, shorter intervals between pregnancies, inadequate nutrition, familial aggregation, and other (unknown) factors linked to the black population. Moreover, low birth weight is part of the inherited predisposition to hypertension, likely because it is also associated with higher maternal blood pressure during pregnancy. All in all, it's a vicious circle, hypertension begetting small babies begetting hypertension.

As I have noted, the opportunity—and the measures—for overcoming most of these contributing factors are obvious. However, recent cutbacks in support for teenage contraception, maternal nutrition, and prenatal care in the United States suggest that we will eventually pay billions for the care of hypertension-related

Table 32–1

**Lifestyle Modifications for Prevention and Management of Hypertension**

Lose weight if necessary
Limit alcohol intake to 1 oz (30 ml) of ethanol (i.e., 24 oz [720 ml] beer, 10 oz [300 ml] wine, or 2 oz [60 ml] 100-proof whiskey per day) or 0.5 oz (15 ml) per day for women and lighter-weight persons
Increase aerobic physical activity (30–45 min most days of the week)
Reduce sodium intake to 100 mmol/day (2.4 g sodium or 6 g sodium chloride)
Maintain adequate dietary intake of potassium (approximately 90 mmol/day)
Maintain adequate dietary intake of calcium and magnesium for general health
Stop smoking and reduce intake of dietary saturated fat and cholesterol for overall cardiovascular health

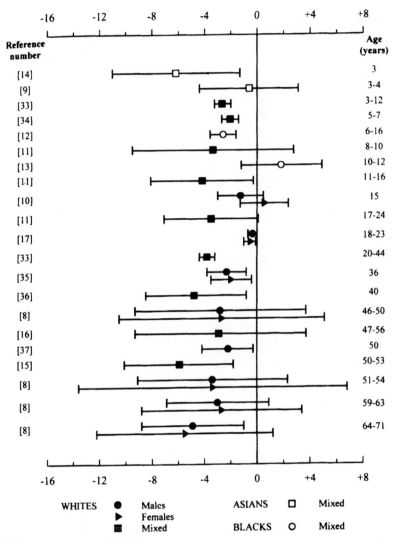

**Figure 32–1** ▪ Difference in systolic blood pressure (mm Hg) per kilogram increase in birth weight according to age, sex, and race in 21 studies arranged in descending order of current age. Symbols show the regression coefficient for birth weight, from the regression of systolic blood pressure on birth weight and current size (weight in children, body mass index in adults). Horizontal bars show the 95% confidence intervals. *Solid circles,* white males; *solid triangles,* white females; *solid squares,* white males and females; *open squares,* Asian males and females, *open circles,* black males and females. (From Law CM, Sheill AW: Is blood pressure inversely related to birth weight? The strength of evidence from a systematic review of the literature. J Hypertens 1996;14:935–941.)

end-stage renal disease, strokes, and heart attacks, instead of the millions required for the preventive care of the disadvantaged among us.

## Prevention of Obesity

As difficult as it may be to prevent low birth weight, it likely will be even harder to correct the three major environmental contributors to the pathogenesis of hypertension: obesity, sodium excess, and stress. Of these three, obesity is growing fastest: more than half of all adult Americans are now overweight (i.e., have a body mass index [BMI]>27) and more than a fourth are now obese (BMI>30). In the Framingham Heart Study, 70% of hypertension in men and 61% in women was directly attributable to obesity; for every 10-lb weight gain, the average increase in systolic blood pressure was 4.5 mm Hg. The association was clearly demonstrated among the 82,500 female nurses aged 30 to 55 years who were followed every 2 years from 1976 to 1992.[5] A weight gain of only 5 kg (11 lb) from weight at age 18 years was responsible for almost doubling the incidence of hypertension; a 10-kg gain tripled the incidence (Fig. 32–2).

When obesity is predominately upper body or visceral in distribution, the dangers for hypertension, diabetes, and dyslipidemia are even greater, and a marked increase in coronary disease is a consequence. The problem is obvious; the solution, perhaps unattainable. As children and their parents become couch potatoes, arising only begrudgingly to change the TV channel or computer game, and as they eat more and more "empty-calorie" fast food and junk food, the prospect of their becoming clinically obese looks ever worse. Nonetheless, even a small weight loss can protect against a rise in blood pressure.[2] In this study, the Nonpharmacologic Interventions in the Elderly (TONE) trial, almost 1000 elderly patients with hypertension that was well controlled with one or two drugs voluntarily discontinued their drug therapy and were randomly assigned to one of four regimens: weight loss by calorie restriction and physical activity; sodium restriction, both weight loss and sodium restriction, or nothing (i.e., usual care). After 30 months, those who had lost an average of only 4.7 kg (10 lb) on the weight

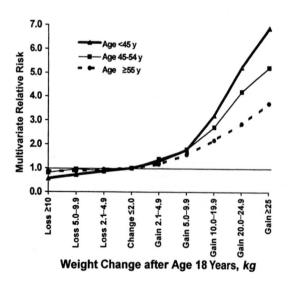

**Figure 32–2** ■ Multivariate relative risk for hypertension according to weight change after age 18 years within strata of age. Adjusted for age, body mass index at age 18 years, height, family history of myocardial infarction, parity, oral contraceptive use, menopausal status, postmenopausal use of hormones, and smoking status (Huang Z, Willett WC, Manson JAE, et al: Body weight, weight change and risk for hypertension in women. Ann Intern Med 1998;128:81–88.)

loss regimen had a 50% greater likelihood of staying normotensive and free of cardiovascular complications than did those who had lost no weight (Fig. 32–3).

This study looked at elderly hypertensives, but equally small weight losses have been shown to decrease the incidence of hypertension in young subjects. Therefore, the effort is worthwhile and is best directed at young people, to prevent them from becoming obese, but also at adults, to help them lose even a little weight.

## Reduction of Sodium Intake

The next target should be easier to accomplish: universal reduction in sodium intake by lowering the amount of sodium added to processed foods, the source of about 80% of all sodium we consume. As many controlled trials amply document, a reduction of 40 to 50 mmol/day, about 25% to 33% of the usual intake, will produce a 4- to 6-mm Hg drop in systolic blood pressure among hypertensives and a 1- to 2-mm Hg drop among normotensives. The TONE trial provides further evidence: Those who reduced daily sodium intake, on average, by 40 mmol had a 50% greater chance of remaining normotensive and free of cardiovascular events than did those who attempted no sodium restriction (see Fig. 32–3).[2]

The small blood pressure reduction that normotensives would realize by such moderate sodium restriction could have a very considerable impact on the incidence of hypertension and the development of cardiovascular disease. As Rose noted,[6] "All the life-saving benefits achieved by current antihypertensive treatment might be equaled by a downward shift of the whole blood pressure distributed by a mere 2 to 3 mm Hg. The benefits from a mass approach in which everybody received a small benefit may be unexpectedly large."

Confirmation of Rose's prediction has come from Law and coworkers,[7] who

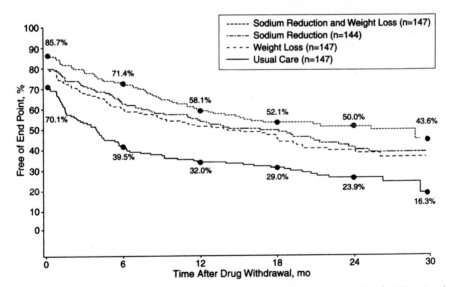

**Figure 32–3** ■ Percentages of the 144 participants assigned to reduced sodium intake, the 147 assigned to weight loss, the 147 assigned to reduced sodium intake and weight loss combined, and the 147 assigned to usual care (i.e., no lifestyle intervention) who remained free of cardiovascular events and high blood pressure and did not have an antihypertensive agent prescribed during follow-up. CI, confidence interval. (Whelton PK, Appel LJ, Espeland MA, et al: Sodium reduction and weight loss in the treatment of hypertension in older persons. JAMA 1998;279:839–846. Copyright 1998, American Medical Association.)

analyzed all of the crossover and randomized controlled trials of dietary sodium restriction published through 1989—78 in total and 18 in normotensive subjects. Although most of these trials were of short duration and studied small numbers of subjects, Law and coworkers found that in 50- to 59-year-old people, a decrease in daily sodium intake of 50 mmol for 4 weeks or longer would lower blood pressure by an average of about 5/2 mm Hg. They then estimated the effect on mortality from stroke and coronary disease of universal reduction of dietary sodium intake by 50 mmol/24 hr. The result was a decrease of 22% in the incidence of stroke and a 16% decrease in ischemic heart disease, effects almost as impressive as those found in some trials of drug therapy for hypertensive patients.

## Doubts About Universal Sodium Restriction

A few hypertension experts question both the role of sodium excess in the pathogenesis of hypertension and the wisdom of advocating a strategy of population-wide moderate sodium restriction. The evidence, although only circumstantial, for a causal role for high dietary sodium (only recently introduced into the food supply of industrialized societies) is so extensive that most investigators are convinced that excessive sodium intake is a necessary, though not sufficient, contributor to the pathogenesis of hypertension. The role of high sodium may never be proved beyond question, since it is not possible to monitor the sodium intake of thousands of people almost from birth through midlife and to observe the effects, particularly since there is considerable individual variability in the pressor sensitivity of humans to sodium. Convincing evidence for a direct and specific hypertensive effect of the amounts of sodium typically consumed by humans has been obtained in studies of chimpanzees, the species closest to us humans.

Those who object to the recommendations for universal sodium restriction point to studies in which short-term, profound reductions in sodium intake induced hormonal and lipid perturbations. Such perturbations do not occur with the moderate sodium restrictions that most experts promote and most patients practice. Therefore, a modest population-wide reduction in sodium will almost certainly be beneficial. It can be easily achieved while, as we wait for food processors to reduce the amount of salt they add, simply reading the labels and rejecting any that contain more than 300 mg of sodium per portion.

## Sodium Potassium Imbalance

Rather than placing the blame on excessive dietary sodium, some investigators point to an imbalance between (too much) sodium and (too little) potassium. For example, surveys have noted lower than recommended potassium intake—but no greater intake of sodium—in poor blacks (particularly those in the southern United States), who, overall, have a higher prevalence of hypertension. Presumably, this reflects the fact that the diets of poor persons contain less meat, fresh fruit, and vegetables.

Potassium supplements will lower blood pressure in those who follow a low-potassium diet, and the salutary effects on blood pressure of a diet rich in fruits and vegetables may be the result of the increased potassium intake.[8] Potassium supplements cannot be recommended for prevention, but more fresh fruits and vegetables likely will be beneficial.

## Relief from Stress

Stress-induced activation of the sympathetic nervous system likely contributes to the development of hypertension. "Job stress," quantitated and used as a measure of what is for most people a major source of stress, has been found to be tightly correlated with hypertension.[9] The investigators found that hypertensives were more likely to be employed in high-stress jobs: the odds ratio was 3.1 after adjusting for other possible confounding variables, including age, race, obesity, alcohol and sodium intake, education, and type A behavior pattern. Moreover, in those aged 30 to 40 years with higher levels of job strain, echocardiographically measured left ventricular mass averaged 10 g/m² more than in those without job strain.

These data, along with much more from both humans and animals, support a role in the pathogenesis of hypertension for stress, which likely interacts with several other factors to increase vascular resistance. Nonetheless, it has not been possible to show that relief of stress, like that provided by various relaxation methods, prevents hypertension; nor does it provide anything more than a placebo effect in lowering the pressure of persons with established hypertension (with rare exceptions).

## Increased Physical Activity

One way to help overcome stress may be physical activity. Regardless of whether that is how physical activity lowers blood pressure, most well-controlled studies do show that regular aerobic exercise reduces blood pressure in hypertensive persons, and numerous surveys show a reduced incidence of hypertension in those who are physically fit. This protection likely involves damping sympathetic nervous system activity.

## Moderation of Alcohol

Beyond the three major factors, many others involved in raising the blood pressure of at least some people may be alterable so that primary prevention of hypertension may be possible.

Excessive alcohol consumption is certainly a pressor mechanism, one responsible for 5% to 10% of hypertension among men. About half of all published data show the pressor effect only when average daily consumption is greater than two drinks, a drink being the equivalent of 1 ounce of ethanol. Some even show lower pressure among those who consumed one or two drinks per day than in those who drank more (Fig. 32–4).[10] The J-shaped pattern of blood pressure noted in this study of 7735 middle-aged men randomly drawn from general practices in 24 British towns closely fits the pattern of coronary morbidity and mortality related to alcohol consumption in multiple populations.

## Cessation of Smoking

Although it appears at the bottom of the list in Table 32–1, cessation of smoking should be addressed first. Quitting smoking reduces overall cardiovascular risk beyond any other maneuver, including normalization of blood pressure. Moreover, each cigarette raises blood pressure acutely and 20 or more cigarettes a day keeps the blood pressure higher throughout the patient's waking hours. Unfortunately, the pressor effect of smoking usually is not recognized. Since smoking is not allowed in clinics and physician's offices, the pressor effect of the last cigarette is almost always gone by the time blood pressure is measured. Therefore, it is essential that smokers take their blood pressure while smoking and that the physician use that blood pressure value as the criterion for therapy. If the recognition of this additional insult does not help to motivate smokers to quit, the physician should

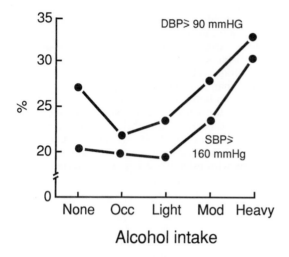

**Figure 32–4** ■ Age-adjusted prevalence rates (in percentages) of measured systolic (SBP) and diastolic (DBP) hypertension by levels of alcohol intake in drinks: Occ, occasional; light, one to two daily; Mod, moderate, three to six daily; heavy, more than six daily. (Shaper AG, Wannamethee G, Whincup P: Alcohol and blood pressure in middle-aged British men. J Hum Hypertens 1988;2:71–78S.).

consider pharmacologic aids. Those that include small amounts of nicotine rarely raise the blood pressure.

### Reduction of Dietary Saturated Fat and Cholesterol

These days, dyslipidemia is being much more effectively treated with statins, but a prudent diet helps to lower high low-density lipoprotein (LDL) cholesterol. However it is accomplished, correction of dyslipidemia may provide a small but significant reduction of elevated blood pressure, likely by producing a virtually immediate improvement in endothelial function that promotes vasodilatation.

### Maintenance of Adequate Intake of Calcium and Magnesium

Although calcium and magnesium supplements continue to be advocated by a few enthusiasts, multiple controlled trials have shown little if any associated reduction of blood pressure.[11] Adequate intake of both can be provided by a balanced diet that includes low-fat dairy products.

### Caffeine

Although the first cup of coffee raises the blood pressure by 5 to 20 mm Hg, tolerance to this pressor effect develops rapidly, and most surveys do not demonstrate a relationship between hypertension and caffeine intake.[12]

A host of other lifestyle modifications, mostly of diet, have been advocated to both prevent and control hypertension. None of these has been documented to be effective in large-scale, randomized, controlled trials, so we are left with resort to the maneuvers previously described. Although the evidence that they will prevent hypertension is not conclusive, in controlled trials that combined sodium restriction, weight loss, exercise, and moderation of alcohol in subjects with "high-normal" blood pressure, a uniform decrease in the incidence of overt hypertension has been reported (Table 32–2). The potential shown in these trials for prevention (at best) or delay of the onset (at least) of hypertension supports vigorous pursuit of these

Table 32–2

**Trials of Lifestyle Modifications and Their Effects on the Incidence of Hypertension**

| Trial (Reference) | Number | Duration (yr) | Reduction of Incidence (%) |
|---|---|---|---|
| Primary prevention (Stamler et al, 1989) | 201 | 5 | 54 |
| Hypertension prevention (HPTR, 1990) | 252 | 3 | 23 |
| Trials of Hypertension Prevention | | | |
|   I (TOHP, 1992) | 564 | 1.5 | 51 |
|   II (TOHP, 1997) | 595 | 4 | 21 |

preventive measures against the disease. Even if they are not preventive, these lifestyle modifications serve as the basis for therapy of established hypertension.

## ■ ANTIHYPERTENSIVE DRUG THERAPY

Drug therapy should begin if blood pressure remains above the goal of therapy after diligent application of lifestyle modifications or if, initially, the patient's blood pressure is so high or cardiovascular risk so great as to mandate immediate treatment with antihypertensive drugs (Table 32–3).

### The Goal of Therapy

It is critically important to recognize a goal for therapy at the outset and to define that goal for the patient. Otherwise, simply taking a medication may be misconstrued as fulfilling the need for treatment. In the JNC-6 treatment algorithm (Fig. 32–5), the goal of therapy is 140/90 mm Hg except for patients known to require further reductions, including those with diabetes or renal insufficiency. Until recently, that goal was based on conjecture. Fortunately, the level of blood pressure that provides the best protection against cardiovascular morbidity and mortality has now been ascertained in a properly designed prospective trial involving more than 19,000 patients whose diastolic blood pressure was between 100 and 115 mm Hg, the Hypertension Optimal Treatment (HOT) Trial,[13] in which patients were randomly assigned to achieve one of three levels of diastolic blood pressure—80, 85, or 90 mm Hg.

In this trial, the lowest rate of major cardiovascular events and mortality

Table 32–3

**Risk Stratification and Treatment**

| Blood Pressure Stages (mm Hg) | Risk Group A (No Risk Factors; No TOD/CCD) | Risk Group B (≥1 Risk Factor, not Including Diabetes; No TOD/CCD) | Risk Group C (TOD/CCD and/or Diabetes, With or Without Other Risk Factors) |
|---|---|---|---|
| High-normal (130–139/85–89) | Lifestyle modification | Lifestyle modification | Drug therapy |
| Stage 1 (140–159/90–99) | Lifestyle modification (up to 12 mo) | Lifestyle modification (up to 6 mo) | Drug therapy |
| Stages 2 and 3 (≥160/≥100) | Drug therapy | Drug therapy | Drug therapy |

TOD, target organ damage; CCD, clinical cardiovascular disease.

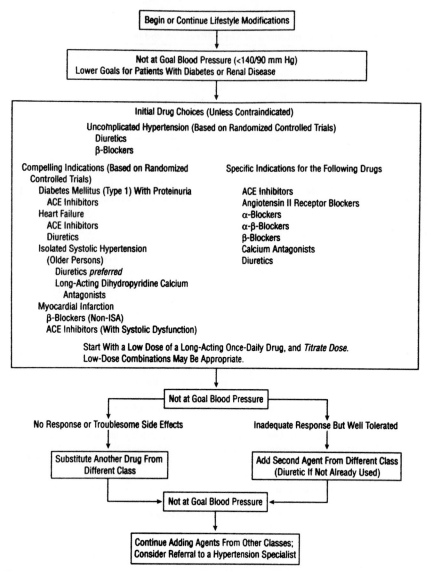

**Figure 32–5** ■ Simplified algorithm for treatment of hypertension. ISA, intrinsic sympathomimetic activity. (Joint National Committee on Detection, Evaluation, and Treatment of High Blood Pressure: The Sixth report to the Joint National Committee on Detection, Evaluation, and Treatment of High Blood Pressure [JNC VI]. Arch Intern Med 1997;157:2413–2446. Copyright 1997, American Medical Association.)

overall was around 139/84 mm Hg (Fig. 32–6). Therefore, the appropriate goal for most, relatively uncomplicated hypertension should be 140/85 rather than 140/90 mm Hg (as given in the JNC-6). Diastolic pressures below 80 mm Hg were more protective in the 1500 diabetics enrolled in the HOT trial, in keeping with the JNC-6 recommendations for lower goals for diabetics and other high-risk patients.

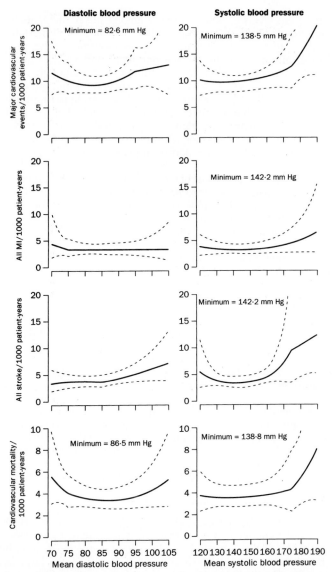

**Figure 32–6** ▪ Estimated incidence (95% CI) of cardiovascular events in relation to achieved mean diastolic and systolic blood pressures. (Hansson L, Zanchetti A, Carruthers SG, et al: Effects of intensive blood-pressure lowering and low-dose aspirin in patients with hypertension: Principal results of the hypertension optimal treatment [HOT] randomised trial. Lancet 1998;351:1755–1762.)

## The J Curve

The HOT trial was originally designed to prospectively ascertain the presence or absence of a J curve (i.e., an increase in coronary ischemic events when diastolic pressure is reduced much below 85 mm Hg, an effect seen in multiple small, and mainly retrospective, studies). Although the HOT trial was not able to obtain significantly different levels of blood pressure among the participants to settle the issue, there does appear to be an upswing in both morbidity and mortality at levels of diastolic blood pressure below 80 mm Hg. Therefore, a J curve may exist for coronary disease, although neither stroke nor renal damage has been found to increase with lower pressures. The myocardium may be uniquely susceptible to reduced perfusion from lower diastolic levels for several reasons: all coronary flow occurs during diastole; the myocardium usually becomes hypertrophic and needs more blood whereas the brain and kidneys often shrink. Unlike the brain and kidneys, the heart cannot extract any more oxygen in response to increased demand than under basal conditions; the atherosclerotic coronary vessels may not be able to dilate to increase blood flow when perfusion pressure falls (i.e., poor autoregulation).

Therefore, caution remains advisable in reducing diastolic blood pressure much below 85 mm Hg in persons known to have coronary heart disease (CHD) or very likely to have unrecognized CHD. In the elderly with isolated systolic hypertension and "natural" low diastolic pressure, no J curve has been recognized with antihypertensive therapy, even though the diastolic pressure has been further reduced. Perhaps, over long periods, adjustments are made in those with naturally low diastolic pressures that cannot be made quickly in patients when high diastolic pressures are abruptly lowered.

## Initial Choice of Therapy

The first choice is likely to be the most critical one. If it is correct, not only will the blood pressure be well-controlled but concomitant conditions will also improve, and the patient will remain asymptomatic and therefore more likely to stick with therapy. If it is incorrect, the blood pressure will be poorly controlled, other conditions exacerbated, and the patient will have symptoms and, perhaps, be lost to therapy.

JNC-6 recommends a diuretic or beta blocker as the initial choice for uncomplicated hypertension or, for compelling indications, a variety of agents (see Fig. 32–5). These choices are mandated by the results of multiple randomized controlled trials (RCT), the evidence behind "evidence-based medicine," which is increasingly the mantra of correct medical practice. Less convincing clinical evidence supports specific choices wherein comorbid conditions may be favorably affected.

### Patients with Uncomplicated Hypertension

Such paragons may be hard to find: in the Framingham cohort, only about 10% of all cases of hypertension were truly uncomplicated. For persons younger than 65 without any of the compelling indications for another choice, however, a diuretic or beta-blocker should be chosen, since their benefits have been documented in 18 RCT (Fig. 32–7).[14] As of this time, no RCT of any other type of drug using mortality as an end point have been published for such patients.

Note, in particular the greater protection against the most common and deadly cardiovascular catastrophe, coronary heart disease, afforded by low doses of diuretics (12.5 to 25 mg per day of hydrochlorothiazide (HCTZ) or its equivalent), as compared with high doses (>25 mg/day). Although higher doses were commonly used from the time that diuretics became available in the late 1950s until the 1990s, more recent experiences have documented the usually equal efficacy of low doses and fewer, if any, of the biochemical perturbations seen with higher doses (Table 32–4).[15] The relative potency of bendrofluazide is 10 times that of HCTZ, so that the 1.25-mg dose would be equivalent to 12.5 mg.

Even lower doses of HCTZ (6.25 mg/day) have been shown to improve the

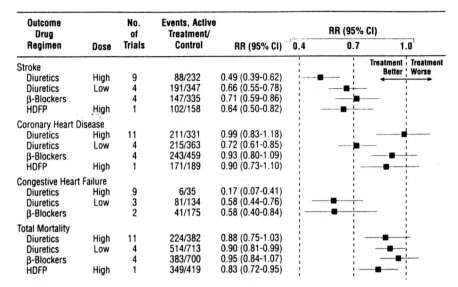

| Outcome Drug Regimen | Dose | No. of Trials | Events, Active Treatment/ Control | RR (95% CI) |
|---|---|---|---|---|
| **Stroke** | | | | |
| Diuretics | High | 9 | 88/232 | 0.49 (0.39-0.62) |
| Diuretics | Low | 4 | 191/347 | 0.66 (0.55-0.78) |
| β-Blockers | | 4 | 147/335 | 0.71 (0.59-0.86) |
| HDFP | High | 1 | 102/158 | 0.64 (0.50-0.82) |
| **Coronary Heart Disease** | | | | |
| Diuretics | High | 11 | 211/331 | 0.99 (0.83-1.18) |
| Diuretics | Low | 4 | 215/363 | 0.72 (0.61-0.85) |
| β-Blockers | | 4 | 243/459 | 0.93 (0.80-1.09) |
| HDFP | High | 1 | 171/189 | 0.90 (0.73-1.10) |
| **Congestive Heart Failure** | | | | |
| Diuretics | High | 9 | 6/35 | 0.17 (0.07-0.41) |
| Diuretics | Low | 3 | 81/134 | 0.58 (0.44-0.76) |
| β-Blockers | | 2 | 41/175 | 0.58 (0.40-0.84) |
| **Total Mortality** | | | | |
| Diuretics | High | 11 | 224/382 | 0.88 (0.75-1.03) |
| Diuretics | Low | 4 | 514/713 | 0.90 (0.81-0.99) |
| β-Blockers | | 4 | 383/700 | 0.95 (0.84-1.07) |
| HDFP | High | 1 | 349/419 | 0.83 (0.72-0.95) |

**Figure 32–7** ▪ Meta-analysis of randomized, placebo-controlled clinical trials in hypertension according to first-line treatment strategy. For these comparisons, the numbers of participants randomized to activate therapy and placebo were 7758 and 12,075 for high-dose diuretic therapy; 4305 and 5116 for low-dose diuretic therapy; and 6736 and 12,147 for β-blocker therapy. RR, relative risk; CI, confidence interval; HDFP, Hypertension Detection and Followup Program. (Psaty BM, Smith NL, Siscovick DS, et al: Health outcomes associated with antihypertensive therapies used as first-line agents. JAMA 1997;277:739–745. Copyright 1997, American Medical Association.)

efficacy of other drugs when given in combination. For most patients, when HCTZ is given alone, 12.5 mg is an appropriate starting dose. Even though there was only a minimal fall in serum potassium in the study of Carlsen and coworkers[15] with a dose equivalent to 12.5 mg, the combination of HCTZ and a potassium-sparing agent, usually triamterene, blunts the fall in potassium at little extra cost. In practice, half of a tablet with 25 mg HCTZ plus 37.5 mg triamterene every morning works very well. Low doses of other long-acting diuretics such as indapamide do as well as HCTZ, possibly with even fewer biochemical changes and additional antihypertensive effects. For uncomplicated hypertension, loop diuretics are not needed and a single daily dose of furosemide is almost totally ineffective. For those with renal insufficiency, loop diuretics are needed, but either metolazone or

Table 32–4

**Efficacy and Safety of Low Doses of Thiazides**

| | Dose of Bendrofluazide (mg/day) | | | | |
|---|---|---|---|---|---|
| Change from 0 to 10 weeks | 0 | 1.25 | 2.5 | 5 | 10 |
| Blood pressure (mm Hg) | −3/3 | −13/10 | −14/11 | −13/10 | −17/11 |
| Potassium (mmol/l) | +.09 | −0.16 | −0.2 | −0.33 | −0.45 |
| Glucose (mg/dl) | −1.4 | −3.4 | +2.5 | +0.7 | +4.9 |
| Cholesterol (mg/dl) | −2.2 | −1.1 | 0 | +4.6 | +9.5 |

From Carlsen JE, Kober L, Torp-Pedersen C, Johansen P: Relation between dose of bendrofluazide, antihypertensive effect, and adverse biochemical effects. Br Med J 1990; 300:974–978.

torsemide will provide efficacy with one dose a day, whereas two or three doses of short-acting furosemide will be needed.

The antihypertensive effect of low doses of diuretic may be overcome by very high dietary intake of sodium and blunted by nephrosclerosis that has not yet induced renal insufficiency. For most uncomplicated hypertensives, a single morning dose of HCTZ works well.

A beta-blocker along is not recommended for those older than 65 (see section on Treatment of the Elderly Hypertensive). If there are reasons to use a beta-blocker in an elderly hypertensive, it should be given with a diuretic.

## Compelling Indications

Four conditions are listed in Figure 32–5 as compelling indications for specific drugs. The need for three of the four has long been recognized: angiotensin-converting enzyme (ACE) inhibitors for diabetic nephropathy; ACE inhibitors and diuretics for heart failure, beta-blockers without intrinsic sympathomimetic activity (ISA) and ACE inhibitors for systolic dysfunction after myocardial infarction. Despite their long-known value, surveys indicate that fewer than half of the patients in each category are currently receiving the appropriate drugs.

The fourth compelling indication involves isolated systolic hypertension in elderly persons, the largest single group of hypertensive patients. Diuretics are the preferred choice, again in low doses. In addition, long-acting dihydropyridine (DHP) calcium antagonists are recommended on the basis of findings of the only RCT in such patients that used any drug other than a low dose of diuretic (Table 32–5). The first three trials, the U.S. Systolic Hypertension in the Elderly Program (SHEP), the Swedish STOP-HTN trial, and the English MRC trial, started with a diuretic. The fourth, the Syst-Eur trial performed throughout Europe[16] started with the long-acting DHP calcium antagonist, nitrendipine, adding an ACE inhibitor to about half and a diuretic to about a fourth to achieve adequate control. Protection against stroke, the primary end point, and all cardiovascular events was significant and as good as that seen in the other trials. Two additional trials performed in China, the Shanghai Trial of Nifedipine in the Elderly (STONE) and the Syst-China trial, also reported excellent protection in elderly patients with long-acting DHP calcium antagonists—nifedipine in the first, nitrendipine in the second.

## Favorable Effects on Comorbid Conditions

The third path for initial choice of therapy described in JNC-6 is a variety of drugs known to favorably affect one of the many comorbid conditions that often

### Table 32–5

### Effects of Therapy on Elderly Hypertensive Patients

| | SHEP (1991)[38] | STOP-HTN (Dahlof, 1991)[39] | MRC (1992)[40] | SYST-EUR (Staessen, 1997)[41] |
|---|---|---|---|---|
| Mean blood pressure at entry | 170/77 | 195/102 | 185/91 | 174/85 |
| *Relative difference in rate between treated and placebo groups* | | | | |
| Stroke | −33* | −47* | −25* | −42* |
| CAD | −27* | −13† | −19 | −30 |
| CHF | −55* | −51* | | −29 |
| All CVD | −32* | −40* | −17* | −31* |

*Statistically significant.
†Myocardial infarction only; sudden deaths reduced from 13 to 4.
BP, blood pressure; SHEP, Systolic Hypertension in the Elderly Program; STOP-HTN, Swedish Trial in Old Persons with Hypertension; MRC, Medical Research Council Trial in Older Adults; SYST-EUR, Systolic Hypertension–Europe Trial; CAD, coronary artery disease; CHF, congestive heart failure; CVD, cardiovascular disease.

accompany hypertension (Table 32–6). These recommendations do not have the force of RCT behind them, but they are well-supported by extensive clinical experience. As one example, alpha-blockers are now the first choice for relief of the obstructive symptoms of benign prostatic hypertrophy. Therefore, it seems appropriate to use an alpha-blocker to treat an elderly man who also has benign prostatic hyperplasia. One could argue that a low dose of,* a diuretic should also be given to provide its proven protection against cardiovascular death.

Table 32–6

**Considerations for Individualizing Antihypertensive Drug Therapy**

| Indication | Drug Therapy |
|---|---|
| **Compelling Indications Unless Contraindicated** | |
| Diabetes mellitus (type 1) with proteinuria | ACE I |
| Heart failure | ACE I, diuretics |
| Isolated systolic hypertension (older patients) | Diuretics (preferred), CA (long-acting DHP) |
| Myocardial infarction | β-Blockers (non-ISA), ACE I (with systolic dysfunction) |
| **May Have Favorable Effects on Comorbid Conditions** | |
| Angina | β-Blockers, CA |
| Atrial tachycardia and fibrillation | β-Blockers, CA (non-DHP) |
| Cyclosporine-induced hypertension (caution with dose of cyclosporine) | CA |
| Diabetes mellitus (types 1 and 2) with proteinuria | ACE I (preferred, CA) |
| Diabetes mellitus (type 2) | Low-dose diuretics |
| Dyslipidemia | α-Blockers |
| Essential tremor | β-Blockers (non-CS) |
| Heart failure | Carvedilol, losartan potassium |
| Hyperthyroidism | β-Blockers |
| Migraine | β-Blockers (non-CS), CA (non-DHP) |
| Myocardial infarction | Dilitiazem hydrocholoride, verapamil hydrochloride |
| Osteoporosis | Thiazides |
| Preoperative hypertension | β-Blockers |
| Prostatism (BPH) | α-Blockers |
| Renal insufficiency (caution in renovascular hypertension and creatinine level ≥265.2 μmol/l [≥3 mg/dl]) | ACE I |
| **May Have Unfavorable Effects on Comorbid Conditions** | |
| Bronchospastic disease | β-Blockers |
| Depression | β-Blockers, central α-agonists, reserpine‡ |
| Diabetes mellitus (type 1 or 2) | β-Blockers, high dose diuretics |
| Dyslipidemia | β-Blockers (non-ISA), diuretics (high dose) |
| Gout | Diuretics |
| Second- or third-degree heart block | β-Blockers,* CA (non DHP)* |
| Heart failure | β-Blockers (except carvedilol), CA (except amlodipine besylate; felodipine) |
| Liver disease | Labetalol hydrochloride, methyldopa* |
| Peripheral vascular disease | β-Blockers |
| Pregnancy | ACE I,* angiotensin II receptor blockers* |
| Renal insufficiency | Potassium-sparing agents |
| Renovascular disease | ACE I, angiotensin II receptor blockers |

ACE I, angiotensin-converting enzyme inhibitors; BPH, benign prostatic hyperplasia; CA, calcium antagonists; DHP, dihydropyridine; ISA, intrinsic sympathomimetic activity; MI, myocardial infarction; non-CS, noncardioselective.
*Contraindicated.

## The Safety of Calcium Antagonists

In addition to the compelling indication, after diuretics, for long-acting DHP calcium antagonists for elderly persons with isolated systolic hypertension, members of the calcium antagonist family are recommended for a number of the comorbid conditions listed in Table 32–6. The various indications for members of this family are partly responsible for their current position as the drugs most often prescribed for the treatment of hypertension in the United States, one, amlodipine, now being the most popular antihypertensive worldwide.

In addition, effective marketing has almost certainly played a major role in the popularity of these drugs. Marketing would not translate into use, however, if they were not both effective and well tolerated. Nonetheless, a series of reports over the past few years have implicated various calcium antagonists in increasing the incidence of coronary disease, cancer, gastrointestinal bleeding, and suicide. At the same time, the evidence, known since 1982, that large doses of short-acting nifedipine increase mortality when given in the immediate post–myocardial infarction period has been published again.

The majority of these reports were uncontrolled, retrospective case-control studies comparing the frequency of the use of various of calcium antagonists against other drugs in patients who had coronary disease, cancer, or gastrointestinal bleeding or who had attempted suicide. Almost all of these reports involved short-acting formulations of verapamil, diltiazem, or nifedipine, but the long-acting formulations were also faulted in the manner of guilt by association. Whereas large doses of such short-acting agents may aggravate coronary disease by the sympathetic activation induced by abrupt drops in blood pressure, long-acting agents do not induce such reactions, and they clearly should not have been incriminated.

The same conclusions have now been reached in regard to long-acting formulations of calcium antagonists.[17] As noted, the incidence of coronary disease has been shown in large-scale, prospective, nonrandomized controlled trials to be lower in persons who take long-acting DHP calcium antagonists. No increase in the incidence of cancer was noted, either in those RCT or in multiple case-controlled studies involving much larger numbers of patients than in the original studies purporting to show an association.

Of all the claims of serious adverse effects, an increase in the risk of gastrointestinal bleeding may be the only one that has any validity, since calcium antagonists do inhibit platelet aggregation, though to a lesser degree than does aspirin. In addition, there is convincing evidence that calcium antagonists do not protect against coronary events in diabetic hypertensives, in contrast to the excellent protection provided by ACE inhibitors. The evidence supports, not a deleterious effect but rather a lack of protective action and, if additional antihypertensive effect is needed, calcium antagonists can safely be used in such patients (see section on Treatment of Diabetic Hypertensives).

We have witnessed a concerted campaign to blame the entire family of calcium antagonists for one sin of a distant relative; that is, increased coronary risk from large doses of short-acting nifedipine given in the immediate post–myocardial infarction period. This campaign has caused considerable discomfort to patients and physicians. It is certainly true that the pharmaceutical marketers of these agents were at fault for not having documented their long-term safety and efficacy in large RCT that should have been started as soon as the drugs were approved for use. The lesson has been learned, as witnessed by the prompt performance of such RCT with various statin agents. These RCT have clearly documented the ability of statin drugs to reduce mortality, effectively countering earlier claims that they increased deaths from noncardiovascular causes.

Perhaps the only other positive outcome of this misguided campaign is the recognition that sublingual nifedipine was being greatly overused for hypertensive "pseudocrises." In truth, the dangers of sublingual nifedipine may be no greater than those of other drugs that rapidly lower blood pressure, and the larger number of reports of adverse effects may simply reflect its much wider use. Nonetheless, sublingual nifedipine should be used only when life-threatening hypertension cannot be properly managed with a parenteral agent (see later). Other than in this situation there is no reason to use short-acting nifedipine for hypertension. For the majority of patients with nonthreatening but severe hypertension that needs to be reduced in a matter of hours, one or more rapidly acting oral agents should be used.

## General Recommendations

Whatever drug is chosen for initial therapy, three additional general recommendations are appropriate:
- Start with a low dose and gradually titrate upward.
- Use a long-acting formulation once a day.
- When appropriate to the needs of the patient, use low-dose combinations.

### Low Starting Doses

Many patients—and most physicians—are in a hurry to bring hypertension under control. The motives are usually good: reduce the time and money needed to control the disease, thereby more quickly protecting the patient from the dangers of untreated hypertension. (Limitations imposed by managed care may further the push toward "quick and easy" control.)

Unfortunately, the consequences are often bad: fast and marked falls in blood pressure often provoke symptoms of fatigue and dizziness, likely consequences of reduced perfusion to the brain when systemic pressure is lowered even to levels that are not "hypotensive" and that normotensive people tolerate well (Fig. 32–8). Autoregulation maintains normal cerebral blood flow over a range of arterial blood pressure from as low as 90/50 to 180/120 mm Hg in normotensives. In hypertensives, the autoregulatory curve is shifted to the right as thickened vessels are able to maintain perfusion despite pressures that could not be tolerated in normotensives. On the other hand, if blood pressure is lowered below a mean of 100 to 110 mm Hg (i.e., 140/90 mm Hg), cerebral blood flow is reduced. Fortunately, over time treated patients do "shift their curve" toward the left so that lower pressures can be tolerated.

Other organs may also be underperfused if blood pressure is abruptly lowered. These include the heart and kidneys and, perhaps most bothersome to many men, the penis. Penile blood flow must increase almost 10-fold to achieve and maintain an erection. Particularly when blood flow to the genitals is already compromised by arteriosclerotic narrowing, an abrupt drop in systemic pressure may induce impotence, whereas a slower and smaller fall in pressure may be tolerated.

By "starting low and going slow," good control should be achieved within a few months and symptoms related to tissue hypoperfusion should be few, if they occur at all. If patients monitor their own blood pressure with home devices, manipulations of therapy can easily be made without the need for office visits. For most patients in no distress, increments should be made only after 4 to 6 weeks, to enable the full effectiveness of the previous dose to be expressed.

### Low-Dose Combinations

Two drugs in low doses sometimes achieve better control with fewer adverse effects than do larger doses of a single drug. The concept was portrayed by Fagan[18] in an idealized manner (Fig. 32–9). If a submaximal dose of one drug is started, the

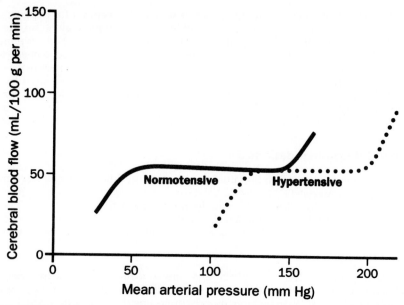

**Figure 32–8** ▪ Idealized curves of cerebral blood flow at varying levels of systemic blood pressure in normotensive and hypertensive subjects. Rightward shift is shown in autoregulation with chronic hypertension. (Adapted from Strandgaard S, Olesen J, Skinhoj E, Lassen NA: Autoregulation of brain circulation in severe arterial hypertension. Br Med J 1973;1:507–510.)

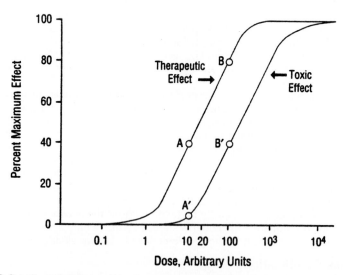

**Figure 32–9** ▪ Theoretical therapeutic and toxic logarithmic-linear dose-response curves. The horizontal axis is a logarithmic scale with arbitrary dose units. The vertical axis is a linear scale showing percent of maximum possible response. (Fagan TC: Remembering the lessons of basic pharmacology. Arch Intern Med 1994;154:1430–1431. Copyright 1994, American Medical Association.)

effect on blood pressure will be partial (point A) but the dose-dependent side effects will be minimal (point A'). If the dose of the first drug is raised to achieve better antihypertensive efficacy (point B), side effects will then become obvious (point B').

Rather than doubling the dose of the first drug, a second drug from a different class may be added, again in a dose so low that no side effects will be noted but the two in combination will provide additional efficacy. This concept has been nicely documented, perhaps best with truly low doses of a diuretic (6.25 mg of HCTZ) and a beta blocker (2.5 mg of bisoprolol).[19] Each drug alone had only a small antihypertensive effect but minimal adverse effects; in combination, fully additive efficacy was achieved with no increase in adverse effects (Table 32–7).

Availability of low-dose combinations is increasing. Those with a low-dose diuretic component are most attractive for initial therapy. Others may find their major place as second-line therapy when the first choice is only partially effective.

## Once-a-Day Dosing

As stated in the JNC-6, "Long-acting formulations that provide 24-hour efficacy are preferred over short-acting agents for many reasons: (1) compliance is better with once-daily dosing; (2) for some agents, fewer tablets cost less; (3) control of hypertension is persistent and smooth rather than intermittent; and (4) protection is provided against whatever risk for sudden death, heart attack, and stroke that is due to the abrupt increase of blood pressure after arising from overnight sleep. Agents with a duration of action beyond 24 hours are attractive because many patients inadvertently miss at least one dose of medication each week." The first three reasons are obvious. The fourth deserves additional comment, since all cardiovascular catastrophes occur at a greater frequency in the first few hours after arising from sleep (Fig. 32–10). If drugs with less than full 24-hour efficacy are taken only once a day in the morning, the patient's blood pressure will be poorly controlled in the hours just before and after arising from sleep, when the need for control is most critical. Therefore, drugs with full 24-hour effectiveness should be chosen, in the hope that they will provide full protection from early morning catastrophes.

As noted in the JNC-6 statement, "Many patients inadvertently miss at least one dose of medication each week," which gives additional reason for the use of "agents with a duration of action beyond 24 hours." Two such agents that have been shown to provide continued significant antihypertensive efficacy for a full 48 hours are the calcium antagonist amlodipine and the ACE inhibitor trandolapril (Fig. 32–11). In this study,[20] patients on a once-a-day regimen of enalapril or trandolapril purposely missed a dose. Whereas the enalapril did not provide even

Table 32–7

**Mean Changes in Seated Blood Pressure (4 Weeks), Serum Potassium, and Uric Acid (12 Weeks)**

| HCTZ (mg) | Bisoprolol (mg) | Decrease (Syst/Diast) (mmHg) | Potassium (mmol/l) | Uric Acid (mg/dl) |
| --- | --- | --- | --- | --- |
| 0 | 0 | 2.5 / 3.8 | −0.04 | +0.2 |
| 0 | 2.5 | 9.0 / 8.4 | +0.17 | +0.2 |
| 0 | 10.0 | 12.6 / 10.9 | +0.07 | +0.4 |
| 6.25 | 0 | 6.2 / 6.4 | −0.05 | +0.2 |
| 6.25 | 2.5 | 12.8 / 10.8 | +0.03 | +0.1 |
| 6.25 | 10.0 | 16.4 / 13.4 | −0.01 | +0.6 |

Frishman WH, Bryzinski BS, Coulson LR, et al: A multifactorial trial design to assess combination therapy in hypertension. Arch Intern Med 1994; 154:1461–1468. Copyright 1994, American Medical Association.

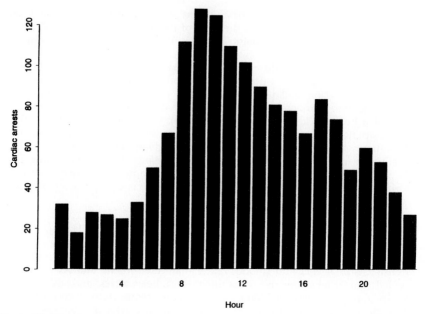

**Figure 32–10** ■ Distribution of time of dispatch for 1558 unwitnessed, untreated cardiac-etiology epi-sodes of cardiac arrests. (Peckova M, Fahrenbruch CE, Cobb LA, Hallstrom AP: Circadian variations in the occurrence of cardiac arrests. Circulation 1998;98:31–39.)

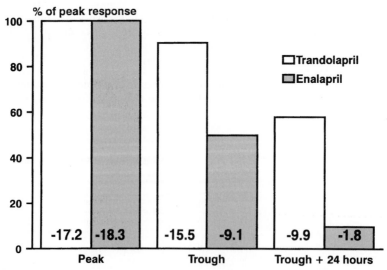

**Figure 32–11** ■ Systolic BP responses to enalapril *(shaded bars)* and trandolapril *(open bars)* at steady state and 24 hours after a missed dose. (Meredith PA: Implications of the links between hypertension and myocardial infarction for choice of drug therapy in patients with hypertension. Am Heart J 1996;132:222–228.)

full 24-hour efficacy, trandolapril maintained considerable effectiveness for the entire 48 hours. We can hope that more such inherently long-acting formulations will be marketed so that patients will be protected even if they occasionally miss a daily dose.

A special formulation of the calcium antagonist verapamil has been marketed that does not release the drug for 4 to 6 hours (i.e., Covera HS). It is to be taken at bedtime, thus ensuring early morning efficacy. Although this "chronobiologic approach" is rational, equal efficacy can be provided by 24-hour effective formulations that can be taken literally at any time of the day. If, as is true of many formulations, the maximal effect occurs within 2 to 6 hours, bedtime dosing could induce nocturnal tissue hypoperfusion, since blood pressure usually falls spontaneously during sleep. The author's preference is to give all antihypertensives drugs with 24-hour efficacy as early in the morning as possible. If because of nocturia the patient awakens some 2 to 3 hours before arising for the day, the medications can be taken at that time.

## The Second Step in Therapy

Even if all of the cautions about the initial choice of drug are observed, as many as 40% to 50% of patients who faithfully take the medication for 6 weeks or longer will not reach the goal of therapy with the first drug alone. One of two paths may then be followed: if little or no response has been achieved or bothersome side effects develop, a drug from another class should be substituted for the first one; if a definite but only partial response has been produced by a well-tolerated drug in a moderate dose, a second drug should be added.

Note the parentheses in the JNC-6 algorithm under the addition path: "Diuretic if not already used." Some practitioners have literally quit using diuretics because of concerns about the real biochemical aberrations induced by high doses, which likely blunted their cardioprotective effectiveness. Low doses that provide adequate efficacy induce few if any of these aberrations, and such small doses should always be used.

The need for some diuretic is based on the principles of pressure-natriuresis that were clearly elucidated by Arthur Guyton in describing the usual relationship between systemic blood pressure and renal sodium excretion that must be reset in order for hypertension to develop and persist. If this resetting did not occur, the higher pressure would effect natriuresis and the shrinkage in fluid volume would return the pressure to normal. Only with a rightward shift of the relation would hypertension persist. As a corollary to this rightward shift, when the blood pressure is lowered by a nondiuretic agent, the kidney perceives the pressure to be so low as to interfere with its normal functions and responds by retaining extra sodium and water. Consequently, circulating fluid volume is expanded and the blood pressure rises (Fig. 32–12). The problem is even worse with direct vasodilators such as minoxidil, which stimulate renin secretion.

Such reactive fluid retention was recognized soon after the introduction of nondiuretic antihypertensive agents, which were found to lose their effectiveness over time when used alone only to regain full efficacy after addition of a diuretic. The problem may be less with newer agents such as calcium antagonists, which have some intrinsic natriuretic action, or with ACE inhibitors, which blunt the renin-angiotensin-aldosterone mechanism. Nonetheless, such reactive sodium retention may still blunt full expression of the efficacy of those agents, and their efficacy is clearly increased by the addition of a diuretic.[21]

## The Third Step in Therapy

If the goal still has not been reached, agents from other classes should be added sequentially, even if four or five are needed. Fortunately, only about 5% of

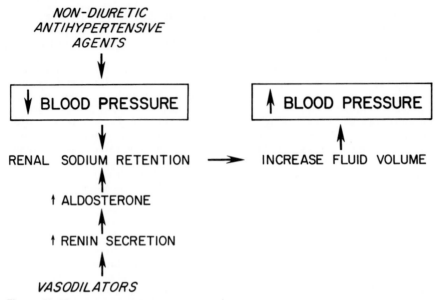

**Figure 32–12** ■ Manner by which nondiuretic antihypertensive agents may lose their effectiveness by reactive renal sodium retention. (Kaplan NM: Treatment of hypertension: Drug therapy. *In* Clinical Hypertension, 7th ed. Baltimore: Williams & Wilkins, 1998.)

patients do not respond to moderate doses of three drugs, one of them a diuretic. As will be described in the next section, resistance to therapy is usually defined as persistence of blood pressure above 140/90 mm Hg despite the use of three drugs.

If resistance persists and cannot be overcome by the steps described in the next section, referral to a hypertension specialist should be considered. Such specialists are being identified by the American Society of Hypertension, which is certifying those whose expertise in dealing with complicated hypertensives has been identified either by community recognition or by a qualifying examination.

## ■ MANAGEMENT OF REFRACTORY HYPERTENSION

If office blood pressure readings are persistently elevated despite increasing therapy, the possibility of pseudoresistance from the white-coat effect should be considered. If significant target organ damage is present, the assumption must be that resistance is genuine and additional therapy is needed (Fig. 32–13). But in the absence of progressing target organ damage, home blood pressure readings and, if available, ambulatory monitoring should be obtained before proceeding with more therapy.

Of all the causes for true resistance to therapy shown in Table 32–8, likely the most common one is failure of compliance with therapy. If the patient is taking the prescribed medications, drug interactions, one or another associated conditions, or identifiable (secondary) forms of hypertension should be sought.

In a number of studies of such groups of patients, the most common cause for resistance has turned out to be volume overload from multiple causes, most likely inadequate diuretic therapy. In turn, this is often attributable to once-a-day dosing with the short-acting loop diuretic furosemide. Used once a day, the short duration

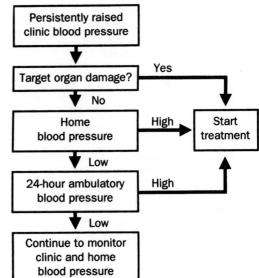

**Figure 32–13** ■ Proposed schema of blood pressure measurement for patients with apparently resistant hypertension. (Pickering TG: Blood pressure monitoring outside the office for the evaluation of patients with resistant hypertension. Hypertension 1998;11(Suppl II):II96–II100.)

of action provides only transient natriuresis and contraction of effective blood volume. When lunch or dinner is eaten, all of the sodium initially excreted is retained, so, at the end of the day, the patient is no different than before, except for the discomfort of having to empty a full bladder for the first 2 or 3 hours after taking the diuretic.

For those patients with intact renal function, a single morning dose of a thiazide usually provides the continued shrinkage of fluid volume that is needed to reduce blood pressure. In persons with markedly high blood pressure who are taking one or more other drugs, the tendency for reactive sodium retention (see Fig. 32–12) may require larger doses than most patients need.

For those with renal insufficiency, two or three doses of a short-acting loop diuretic may work, but better control will likely be achieved with one dose a day of such long-acting and potent agents as metolazone or torsemide.

# ■ THERAPY OF HYPERTENSIVE EMERGENCIES

The small number of patients who present with a hypertensive emergency (Table 32–9) almost always should receive parenteral therapy (Table 32–10) in an intensive care facility, where careful monitoring is feasible. The choice of drug is usually based on the experience of the caregiver, although emergencies of certain types are best treated with specific parenteral agents (see Table 32–10).

Many patients with markedly elevated blood pressure but no advancing target organ damage or other features of a true hypertensive emergency have been deemed to have a hypertensive "urgency" (i.e., need for immediate reduction in blood pressure but not for parenteral therapy). By far the most common therapy for such patients has been sublingual nifedipine.

In late 1996, a paper was published that described the use of sublingual nifedipine as a "pernicious and widespread practice [that] was repeatedly deplored in influential journals."[22] The authors presented 16 cases marked by serious adverse, mostly ischemic, events related to precipitous falls in blood pressure after they took

Table 32–8

### Causes of Inadequate Responsiveness to Therapy

**Pseudoresistance**
  White coat or office elevations
  Pseudohypertension in the elderly
**Nonadherence to therapy**
  Side effects or costs of medication
  Lack of consistent and continuous primary care
  Inconvenient and chaotic dosing schedules
  Instructions not understood
  Organic brain syndrome (e.g., memory deficit)
**Drug-related causes**
  Doses too low
  Inappropriate combinations
  Rapid inactivation (e.g., hydralazine)
  Drug actions and interactions
    Sympathomimetics
    Nasal decongestants
    Appetite suppressants
    Cocaine and other street drugs
    Caffeine
  Oral contraceptives
  Adrenal steroids
  Licorice (as may be found in chewing tobacco)
  Cyclosporine, tacrolimus
  Erythropoietin
  NSAIDS
**Associated conditions**
  Smoking
  Increasing obesity
  Sleep apnea
  Insulin resistance or hyperinsulinemia
  Ethanol intake more than 1 ounce a day
  Anxiety-induced hyperventilation or panic attacks
  Chronic pain
  Intense vasoconstriction (Raynaud phenomenon, arthritis)
**Identifiable causes of hypertension**
**Volume overload**
  Excess sodium intake
  Progressive renal damage (nephrosclerosis)
  Fluid retention from reduction of blood pressure
  Inadequate diuretic therapy

Reprinted with permission from the Joint National Committee on Detection, Evaluation and Treatment of High Blood Pressure: The sixth report of the Joint National Committee on Detection, Evaluation and Treatment of High Blood Pressure (JNC-VI). Arch Intern Med 1997;157:2413–2446.

10 to 30 mg of nifedipine sublingually. Liquid nifedipine is actually absorbed move slowly from the small area under the tongue than when the capsule is swallowed whole or is chewed and the contents swallowed (the fastest absorption of all). Nonetheless, these hypotensive sequelae are neither unexpected nor unique to sublingual nifedipine. They have been observed with almost every fast-acting antihypertensive agent given to patients with markedly high blood pressure. It is almost certain that the apparently larger number of adverse effects reported with sublingual nifedipine reflects the fact that a much larger number of patients take it. It is likely that, in fact, the incidence of serious adverse effects is quite low, perhaps lower than those associated with other fast-acting agents, but there is no way to know.

It is likely that the relative danger of sublingual nifidipine has been exaggerated, since many millions of hypertensive patients swallowed the capsules for

Table 32–9

**Causes of Hypertensive Emergencies (Usually Diastolic Pressure >120 mm Hg)**

| | |
|---|---|
| **Accelerated-malignant hypertension** | **Excess of circulating catecholamines** |
| Papilledema | Pheochromocytoma crisis |
| **Cerebrovascular** | Food or drug interactions with monoamine |
| Hypertensive encephalopathy | oxidase inhibitors |
| Atherothrombotic brain infarction with severe | Sympathomimetic drug (e.g., cocaine) |
| hypertension | Rebound hypertension after sudden cessation of |
| Intracerebral hemorrhage | antihypertensive drugs |
| Subarachnoid hemorrhage | Autonomic hyperreflexia after spinal cord injury |
| Head trauma | Eclampsia |
| **Cardiac** | **Surgical** |
| Acute aortic dissection | Severe hypertension in patients requiring |
| Acute left ventricular failure | immediate surgery |
| Acute or impending myocardial infarction | Postoperative hypertension |
| After coronary bypass surgery | Postoperative bleeding from vascular suture |
| **Renal** | lines |
| Acute glomerulonephritis | **Severe body burns** |
| Renal crises from collagen vascular diseases | **Severe epistaxis** |
| Severe hypertension after kidney transplantation | |

decades, before long-acting calcium antagonists became available, without inciting acute ischemic events. Nonetheless, Grossman and colleagues are certainly correct in describing gross overuse of this agent in patients with a "pseudoemergency" (i.e., high blood pressure but no other indications for rapid reduction of the pressure).

A sizable number of patients, however, need fairly fast treatment, including most whose sustained blood pressure is above 210/120 mm Hg. The prudent physician treats such patients until their blood pressure is at a safer level, likely below 180/110 mm Hg. A variety of oral agents are available that begin working within 30 to 60 minutes and bring blood pressure down in 2 to 6 hours, not so fast as to induce ischemia but fast enough to allow the patient to be sent home on a regimen of long-acting medications—with close follow-up to ensure that control is achieved and necessary evaluation is performed. The fast-acting agents include oral furosemide, propranolol, captopril, nicardipine, felodipine, and nifedipine.

## ■ SPECIAL PATIENT POPULATIONS

The limitations of space preclude coverage of all of the special populations that clinicians may encounter—from neonates to children to pregnant women to patients with a variety of comorbid conditions. Additional attention will be given to three groups of hypertensives, because they both are common and need special considerations: the elderly, those with diabetes, and those who have coexisting cardiac diseases.

Pregnant women with preexisting hypertension can continue taking the drugs they used before pregnancy, with the exception of ACE inhibitors and angiotensin II receptor blockers, which must be stopped as soon as the pregnancy is recognized. Since few trials have documented the safety of newer drugs for the fetus as they have for methyldopa, this drug is still chosen by most U.S. obstetricians, along with parenteral hydralazine if needed.

### The Elderly Hypertensive

The largest portion of the hypertensive population, and the portion that is growing most rapidly, are those older than 65 years. More than half are hyperten-

## Table 32–10

### Parenteral Drugs for Hypertensive Emergency

| Drug* | Dose | Onset of Action | Duration of Action | Adverse Effects† | Special Indications |
|---|---|---|---|---|---|
| **Vasodilators** | | | | | |
| Nitroprusside (Nipride, Nitropress) | 0.25–10 µg/kg/min as IV infusion (10 µg/kg dose‡ <10 min) | Immediate | 1–2 min | Nausea, vomiting, muscle twitching, sweating, thiocyanate and cyanide intoxication | Most hypertensive emergencies; caution with high intracranial pressure or azotemia |
| Glyceryl trinitrate | 5–100 µg/min as IV infusion‡ | 2–5 min | 3–5 min | Headache, vomiting, methemoglobinemia, tolerance with prolonged use | Coronary ischemia |
| Diazoxide (Hyperstat) | 50–100 mg IV bolus repeated, or 15–30 mg/min infusion | 2–4 min | 6–12 hr | Nausea, flushing, tachycardia, chest pain | None (now obsolete) |
| Nicardipine§ (Cardene) | 5–15 mg/hr IV | 5–10 min | 1–4 hr | Headache, nausea, flushing, tachycardia, local phlebitis | Most hypertensive emergencies; caution with acute heart failure |
| Hydralazine (Apresoline) | 10–20 mg IV | 10–20 min | 3–8 hr | Tachycardia, flushing, headache, vomiting aggravation of angina | Eclampsia |
| Enalaprilat (Vasotec IV) | 1.25–5 mg q 6 hr | 15 min | 6 hr | Precipitous fall in pressure in high-renin states; response varies | Acute left ventricular failure |
| **Adrenergic inhibitors** | | | | | |
| Phentolamine | 5–15 mg IV | 1–2 min | 3–10 min | Tachycardia, flushing, headache | Catecholamine excess |
| Trimethaphan‖ (Arfonad) | 0.5 mg/min as IV infusion | 1–5 min | 10 min | Paresis of bowel and bladder, blurred vision, dry mouth, apnea | Aortic dissection (no longer available in the United States) |
| Esmolol (Brevibloc) | 200–500 µg/kg/min for 4 min, then 50–300 µg/kg/min IV | 1–2 min | 10–20 min | Hypotension, nausea | Aortic dissection, postoperative hypertension |
| Labetalol (Normodyne, Trandate) | 20–80 mg in IV bolus q 10 min | 5–10 min | 3–6 hr | Vomiting, scalp tingling, burning in throat, dizziness, nausea, heart block, orthostatic hypotension | Most hypertensive emergencies except acute heart failure |

*In order of rapidity of action.
†Hypotension can occur with any agent.
‡Requires special delivery system.
§Intravenous formulations of other calcium channel blockers are also available.
‖No longer available in the United States.

sive, and almost two thirds have isolated systolic hypertension (ISH).[23] As the Framingham Study has clearly shown, ISH is a serious risk factor for all cardiovascular complications, including myocardial infarction. Fortunately, treatment of elderly persons with either ISH or combined systolic and diastolic hypertension provides excellent protection against all of these morbidities (see Table 32–5). Over the short time of these RCT, even greater protection was noted among elderly patients than younger ones,[24] likely because the elderly start at so much greater immediate risk. Therapy in three of these four large recent RCT began with a low dose of diuretic and in the fourth (the Syst-Eur trial[16]) with a long-acting dihydropyridine calcium antagonist. These drugs are given preference in JNC-6 for treatment of elders with ISH (i.e., a compelling indication). Other drugs work well in the elderly, and, if comorbid conditions recommend one or another, they may logically be used alone or probably best with a small dose of diuretic (see Table 32–6). This is particularly true of a beta-blocker: in the two RCT involving elderly hypertensives, beta-blockers given alone did not reduce coronary or overall mortality.[25] Therefore, if an elderly hypertensive is deemed in need of a beta-blocker, as after an acute myocardial infarction, it should be given with a small dose of a diuretic.

## Avoid Risks of Therapy

Elders are more susceptible to a variety of potential risks from antihypertensive drug therapy (Table 32–11). In particular, they frequently have postural and postprandial hypotension,[26] which may be converted from an occassional but tolerable nuisance to a frequent and intolerable danger by the addition of antihypertensive therapy. Often, their supine and seated hypertension can be treated only after their postural and postprandial hypotension is managed by a variety of helpful maneuvers, including slow rising, elevation of the head of the bed, isometric exercises, support hose, and small meals. A few require additional drugs, including the alpha-antagonist midodrine and octreotide.[27]

Since the only medical condition more common than hypertension in the elderly is osteoarthritis, many use nonsteroidal antiinflammatory drugs (NSAID). Any NSAID may interfere with the antihypertensive efficacy of any antihypertensive with the probable exception of calcium antagonists. Therefore, whenever possible, other analgesics, including acetaminophen, should be used instead of NSAID.

Since the elderly are susceptible to both overtreatment and undertreatment, home blood pressure self-monitoring is particularly useful for them. Thereby, the white-coat effect, which is quantitatively greater in elderly persons, can be recognized and assurance provided that therapy is sufficient but not excessive.

Table 32–11

**Possible Contributors to Increased Risk from Drug Treatment
of Hypertension in Elderly Persons**

| Factor | Potential Complications |
| --- | --- |
| Diminished baroreceptor activity | Orthostatic hypotension |
| Impaired cerebral autoregulation | Cerebral ischemia with small falls in systemic pressure |
| Decreased intravascular volume | Orthostatic hypotension |
| | Volume depletion, hyponatremia |
| Sensitivity to hypokalemia | Arrhythmia, muscle weakness |
| Decreased renal and hepatic function | Drug accumulation |
| Polypharmacy | Drug interaction |
| Central nervous system changes | Depression, confusion |

## Diabetic Hypertensives

Diabetes patients are more likely to have hypertension than nondiabetics, and more hypertensives than normotensives have diabetes. The combination is deadly: all diabetic microvascular and macrovascular complications are accelerated by the presence of hypertension. As diabetics survive longer, they are prone to develop cardiomyopathy and nephropathy, both worsened by hypertension and now the leading causes of their premature death. Antihypertensive therapy should be started at lower levels of blood pressure in diabetics, likely at a level above 130/ 85 mm Hg, and the goal of therapy may be even lower.[13] Since most diabetics are obese, weight reduction must be vigorously pursued by calorie restriction and physical activity. If drugs are needed, ACE inhibitors or, if trials now in progress document their equal or greater efficacy, angiotensin II receptor blockers should be the first drug, combined with a low dose of diuretic. ACE inhibitors appear to protect diabetic hypertensives better than do calcium antagonists both from coronary disease[28] and likely from progressive proteinuric nephropathy.[29] If calcium antagonists are needed to control the hypertension, however, they should not be avoided, since the combination of an ACE inhibitor and a calcium antagonist was even more protective than either drug alone.[28]

## Hypertensives with Cardiac Diseases

Since these various diseases are extensively covered elsewhere in this book, only a few specific issues relative to the coexistence of hypertension will be highlighted here.

### Left-Ventricular Hypertrophy (LVH)

LVH is recognizable by electrocardiography in perhaps 25% of hypertensives and by echocardiography in more than half. As an independent risk factor for coronary mortality in hypertensives, LVH is being more diligently sought and its regression is being used as a surrogate endpoint for effective therapy. Data still do not document that knowledge of either the presence or the regression of LVH adds enough useful information to make routine echocardiography worthwhile.

Nonetheless, numerous studies have examined the relative ability of various antihypertensive drugs to regress LVH with the assumption that regression in itself is beneficial beyond its value in simply lowering the blood pressure. All lifestyle modifications and antihypertensive drugs except direct vasodilators will cause regression of LVH.[30] ACE inhibitors likely cause LVH to regress somewhat better than do drugs of other classes that provide equal antihypertensive efficacy.[31]

### Heart Failure

LVH is often the progenitor of heart failure, particularly when it is primarily the result of diastolic dysfunction. In the Framingham study population, hypertension was a factor in more than 90% of patients with heart failure. The role of hypertension may not be recognized because, as cardiac output falls, systemic blood pressure may drop despite the neurohumoral activation that attempts to maintain tissue perfusion.

Therapy usually includes a diuretic and an ACE inhibitor with angiotensin II receptor blockers a possible alternative. Beta-blockers, or the alpha-beta-blocker carvedilol, may also be useful. If needed to treat angina or hypertension in patients with heart failure, the long-acting dihydropyridine calcium antagonists amlodipine and felodipine have been found to be safe.

## Coronary Heart Disease

Beyond the particular ability of beta-blockers and long-acting calcium antagonists to treat both angina and hypertension, non-ISA beta-blockers and, in the presence of systolic dysfunction, ACE inhibitors have clearly been shown to be protective for patients who have survived an acute myocardial infarction.

Two caveats apply to hypertensives with CHD: first, the diastolic blood pressure likely should not be lowered below 80 to 85 mm Hg because of the likely presence of a J curve (see Fig. 32–6); second, short-acting calcium antagonists should be avoided, since they may abruptly lower blood pressure and thereby stir up the sympathetic nervous system, further stressing the already compromised mycocardium.

## ■ THE NEED TO IMPROVE COMPLIANCE

As noted at the beginning of this chapter, most hypertensives, in the United States and elsewhere, are not being adequate treated. A good deal of the blame can be laid onto physicians who are noncompliant in pushing therapy to the goal. Even more is due to patient noncompliance with therapy.

Only a few interventions have been proven effective in improving patient adherence to therapy[32]: more convenient care; special pill containers that monitor removal of the contents; home self-monitoring of blood pressure; and special staff that provide remainders, support, feedback, and reinforcement. These maneuvers may cost a bit more and require greater involvement of physician and staff, but the benefits outweigh the costs.[32]

Easier-to-use medications should help. The quality of life has been shown to be improved by effective, once-a-day drug therapy as well as by weight loss and increasing physical activity.[33] On the other hand, male sexual potency may be diminished by the use of the type of drug that is most frequently recommended, small doses of diuretic.[34] Obviously, care should be taken to recognize any sexual dysfunction related to the treatment of hypertension. Fortunately, the most widely used treatment for impotence, sildenafil, does not interact adversely with any oral antihypertensive drug, but it should be used with caution in patients with coronary artery disease, and not at all if the patient is taking nitrates.

## ■ THE PAST AND THE FUTURE

Obviously, the treatment of hypertension has improved greatly over the past 30 years. Despite the evidence that only 53% of current U.S. hypertensives are being treated and only 27% are well-controlled,[1] recognition should be given to the fact that these figures are much improved over those from 1980. The improvements have clearly played a significant role in the marked decreases in mortality from CHD and stroke in the U.S. population.

Just as clearly, more needs to be done. Even among presumably well-treated hypertensives, long-term rates of cardiovascular disease remain higher than among normotensives.[35] In particular, hypertensives with high levels of overall cardiovascular risk from other known risk factors have not been well-protected from morbidity and mortality despite successful antihypertensive therapy.[36]

More intensive antihypertensive therapy, always pushed to the appropriate goal of therapy, is one likely solution. New and, we hope, better antihypertensive drugs are being developed,[37] so that it may be easier to achieve good blood pressure control. Beyond that, greater attention must be given to other cardiovascular risk factors so that the full benefits of health care can be provided to all hypertensive patients.

# ■ REFERENCES

1. The Sixth Report of the Joint National Committee on Prevention, Detection, Evaluation and Treatment of High Blood Pressure. Arch Intern Med 1997;157:2413–2446.
2. Whelton PK, Appel LJ, Espeland MA, et al: Sodium reduction and weight loss in the treatment of hypertension in older persons. JAMA 1998;279:839–846.
3. Law CM, Sheill AW: Is blood pressure inversely related to birth weight? The strength of evidence from a systematic review of the literature. J Hypertens 1996;14:935–941.
4. Kaplan NM. Primary hypertension: Pathogenesis. In Clinical Hypertension, 7th ed. Baltimore: Williams & Wilkins, 1998.
5. Huang Z, Willett WC, Manson JE, et al: Body weight, weight change and risk for hypertension in women. Ann Intern Med 1998;128:81–88.
6. Rose G: Strategy of prevention. Br Med J 1981;282:1847–1849.
7. Law MR, Frost CD, Wald NJ: Analysis of data from trials of salt reduction. Br Med J 1991;302:819–824.
8. Appel LJ, Moore TJ, Obarzanek E, et al: A clinical trial of the effects of dietary patterns on blood pressure. N Engl J Med 1997;336:1117–1124.
9. Schnall PL, Pieper C, Schwartz JE, et al: The relationship between "job strain," workplace diastolic blood pressure and left ventricular mass index. Results of a case-control study. JAMA 1990;263:1929–1935.
10. Shaper AG, Wannamethee G, Whincup P: Alcohol and blood pressure in middle-aged British men. J Hum Hypertens 1988;2:71–78.
11. Sacks FM, Willett WC, Smith A, et al: Effect on blood pressure of potassium, calcium, and magnesium in women with low habitual intake. Hypertension 1998;31:131–138.
12. James JE: Is habitual caffeine use a preventable cardiovascular risk factor? Lancet 1997;349:279–281.
13. Hansson L, Zanchetti A, Carruthers SG, et al: Effects of intensive blood-pressure lowering and low-dose aspirin in patients with hypertension: Principal results of the hypertension optimal treatment (HOT) randomised trial. Lancet 1998;351;1755–1762.
14. Psaty BM, Smith NL, Siscovick DS, et al: Health outcomes associated with antihypertensive therapies used as first-line agents: A systematic review and meta-analysis. JAMA 1997;277:739–745.
15. Carlsen JE, Kober L, Torp-Pedersen C, Johansen P: Relation between dose of bendrofluazide, antihypertensive effect, and adverse biochemical effects. Br Med J 1990;300:974–978.
16. Staessen JA, Fagard R, Thijs L, et al: Randomised double-blind comparison of placebo and active treatment for older patients with isolated systolic hypertension. Lancet 1997;350:757–764.
17. Ad Hoc Subcommittee of the Liaison Committee of the World Health Organization and the International Society of Hypertension: Effects of calcium antagonists on the risks of coronary heart disease, cancer and bleeding. J Hypertens 1997;15:104–115.
18. Fagan TC: Remembering the lessons of basic pharmacology. Arch Intern Med 1994;154:1430–1431.
19. Frishman WH, Bryzinski BS, Coulson LR, et al: A multifactorial trial design to assess combination therapy in hypertension. Arch Intern Med 1994;154:1461–1468.
20. Meredith PA: Implications of the links between hypertension and myocardial infarction for choice of drug therapy in patients with hypertension. Am Heart J 1996;132:222–228.
21. Manning G, Miller-Craig MW: Calcium antagonists and diuretics: A useful combination in the management of hypertension? J Hum Hypertens 1996;10:441–442.
22. Grossman E, Messerli FH, Grodzicki T, Kowey P: Should a moratorium be placed on sublingual nifedipine capsules given for hypertensive emergencies and pseudoemergencies? JAMA 1996;276:1328–1331.
23. Kannel WB: Prospects for prevention of cardiovascular disease in the elderly. Prev Cardiol 1998;1:32–39.
24. Mulrow CD, Cornell JA, Herrera CR, et al: Hypertension in the elderly. JAMA 1994;272:1932–1938.
25. Messerli FH, Grossman E, Goldbout U: Are β-blockers efficacious as first-line therapy for hypertension in the elderly? JAMA 1998;279:1903–1908.
26. Imai C, Muratani H, Kimura Y, et al: Effects of meal ingestion and active standing on blood pressure in patients ≥60 years of age. Am J Cardiol 1998;81:1310–1314.
27. Hoeldtke RD, Horvath GG, Bryner KD, Hobbs GR: Treatment of orthostatic hypotension with midodrine and octreotide. J Clin Endocrinol Metab 1998;83:339–343.
28. Tatti P, Pahor M, Byington RP, et al: Outcome results of the Fosinopril Versus Amlodipine Cardiovascular Events Randomized Trial (FACET) in patients with hypertension and NIDDM. Diabetic Care 1998;21:597–603.
29. Klock HJ, Branten AJ, Huysmans T, Wetzels JF: Antihypertensive treatment of patients with proteinuric renal diseases? Risks or benefits of calcium channel blockers? Kidney Int 1998;53:1559–1573.
30. Ofili EO, Cohen JD, St Vrian JA, et al: Effect of treatment of isolated systolic hypertension on left ventricular mass. JAMA 1998;279:778–780.
31. Roman MJ, Alderman MH, Pickering TG, et al: Differential effects of angiotensin converting enzyme

inhibition and diuretic therapy on reductions in ambulatory blood pressure, left ventricular mass and vascular hypertrophy. Am J Hypertens 1998;11:387–396.

32. Haynes RB, McKibbon KA, Kannai R: Systematic review of randomised trials of interventions to assist patients to follow prescriptions for medications. Lancet 1996;348:383–386.

33. Grimm RH Jr, Grandits GA, Cutler JA, et al: Relationships of quality-of-life measures to long-term lifestyle and drug treatment in the treatment of mild hypertension study. Arch Intern Med 1997;157:638–648.

34. Grimm RH Jr, Grandits GA, Prineas RJ, et al: Long-term effects on sexual function of five antihypertensive drugs and nutritional hygienic treatment in hypertensive men and women. Hypertension 1997;29:8–14.

35. Anderson OK, Almgren T, Persson B, et al: Survival in treated hypertension: Follow up study after two decades. Br Med J 1998;317:167–171.

36. Alderman MH, Cohen H, Madhavan S: Distribution and determinants of cardiovascular events during 20 years of successful antihypertensive treatment. J Hypertens 1998;16:761–769.

37. Krum H, Viskoper RJ, Lacourciere Y, et al: The effect of an endothelin-receptor antagonist, bosentan, on blood pressure in patients with essential hypertension. N Engl J Med 1998;338:784–790.

38. SHEP Cooperative Research Group: Prevention of stroke by antihypertensive drug treatment in older persons with isolated systolic hypertension: Final results of the Systolic Hypertension in the Elderly Program (SHEP). JAMA 1991;265:3255–3264.

39. Dahlöf B, Lindholm LH, Hansson L, et al: Morbidity and mortality in the Swedish Trial in Old Patients With Hypertension (STOP-Hypertension). Lancet 1991;338:1281–1285.

40. MRC Working Party: Medical Research Council trial of treatment of hypertension in older adults: Principal results. BMJ 1992;304:405–412.

41. Staeseen JA, Fagard R, Thijs L, et al, for the Systolic Hypertension—Europe (Syst-Eur) Trial Investigators: Morbidity and mortality in the placebo-controlled European Trial on Isolated Systolic Hypertension in the Elderly. Lancet 1997;360:757–764.

# ■ RECOMMENDED READING

Cohn JN: Arteries. myocardium, blood pressure and cardiovascular risk: Towards a revised definition of hypertension. J Hypertens 1998;16:2117–2124.

Gueyffier F, Boutitie F, Boissel J-P, et al: Effect of antihypertensive drug treatment on cardiovascular outcomes in women and men. Ann Intern Med 1997;126:761–767.

Jennings G, Wong J: Regression of left ventricular hypertrophy in hypertension. J Hypertens 1998;16(S6):S29–S34.

Kaplan NM: Clinical Hypertension, 7th ed. Baltimore: Williams & Wilkins, 1998.

The Sixth Report of the Joint National Committee on Detection, Evaluation, and Treatment of Blood Pressure (JNC-VI). Arch Intern Med 1997;157:2413–2446.

# OTHER CONDITIONS THAT AFFECT THE HEART

*Chapter* 33

# Myocarditis and Cardiomyopathies

*Kenneth L. Baughman*

## ▪ MYOCARDITIS

Myocarditis is one of the most challenging diseases in medicine today. Myocarditis is rarely recognized; its pathophysiology is ill-understood; there is no diagnostic gold standard; and all current treatments are controversial. Myocarditis may have secondary causes: drugs, other chemicals, physical agents, rickettsiae, bacteria, spirochetes, fungi, protozoa, and systemic illnesses such as lupus erythematosus and Kawasaki disease, among others. In this section I concentrate on primary myocarditis, which most believe is a viral or "postviral" autoimmune disease. This analysis will include pathophysiology, signs and symptoms, methods of diagnosis, and classification schemes and will briefly mention treatment.

As early as the 1800s, it was recognized that cardiac symptoms could be associated with mumps. Sometime about 1929, the influenza epidemic produced autopsy evidence of associated myocarditis. By 1942, other enteral viruses, particularly the poliomyelitis virus, were associated with post-mortem evidence of myocarditis. By the 1950s, a number of other viruses, including 70 enterovirus subtypes, had been "identified" as being associated with myocardial inflammation. Viruses that can cause myocarditis may be either RNA core or DNA core viruses (Table 33–1).[1] The most common pathogens of myocarditis are the picornoviruses (Coxsackie type B). That a virus is the agent of myocarditis is proven by one of the following mechanisms: direct isolation from the myocardium, polymerase chain reaction identification of a viral pathogen associated with biopsy-proven myocarditis, isolation of a virus from an extracardiac source at the time when cardiac inflammation is documented, or a fourfold or greater rise in convalescent titer of antibody to a viral pathogen associated with new cardiac systolic dysfunction.

The pathophysiologic course of viral myocarditis begins with systemic viremia of 1 to 3 days' duration after a viral infection. This disorder often produces a vasoactive response that is usually characterized by hypotension. By day 3 or 4, the virus is replicating in myocardial tissue and causing myocytolysis (cell death) and dysfunction. By days 5 to 10, there is a nonspecific inflammatory infiltrate produced by macrophage and immunoglobulin M (IgM) antibody response. By day

Table 33–1

**Viruses That Cause Myocarditis**

| RNA Core | DNA Core |
|---|---|
| **Picornavirus** | **Poxvirus** |
| Coxsackie A and B viruses | Variola |
| Echovirus | Vaccinia |
| Poliovirus | **Herpesvirus** |
| **Orthomyxovirus** | Varicella-zoster virus |
| Influenza A and B | Cytomegalovirus |
| | Epstein-Barr |
| | **Adenovirus** |

14, there is an IgG antibody response associated with a myofiber dropout pattern and variable interstitial fibrosis. In most humans, viral myocarditis clears without producing clinical evidence of cardiac dysfunction. Perhaps 10% of those with viremia have active myocarditis. Animal models have demonstrated that the manifestations of myocardial inflammation due to a virus are dependent on the viral pathogen and the host response.

In humans, however, after the onset of the viral illness comes some delay before symptoms appear.[2] The symptoms may be the onset of congestive heart failure, arrhythmia (including sudden death), or an embolic event. Unfortunately, the clinical manifestations of myocarditis are subtle and not unique to this entity. They include fatigue, dyspnea, chest pain, and palpitations. Signs include heart rate excessive for the level of activity, a decreased first heart sound due to diminished contractility, gallop rhythms, murmurs, and/or a pericardial friction rub associated with pericarditis. Laboratory manifestations include a nonspecific change in the electrocardiogram (ECG), including ST-T wave changes, atrial or ventricular arrhythmias, and atrioventricular or intraventricular block. The chest radiograph may be normal or may demonstrate an increased cardiothoracic ratio and pulmonary congestion. Laboratory study results are also nonspecific. Cardiac enzymes are not usually very helpful. In 88 patients with histologically demonstrated myocarditis, creatine phosphokinase elevation was demonstrated in only 6%, and cardiac troponin I elevation in only 34%.[3] Noninvasive scintigraphic techniques are not universally reliable in establishing a definitive diagnosis. Gallium scanning has sensitivity of 36% and specificity of 98%; antimyosin antibody scanning has sensitivity of 83% and specificity of only 53%.[4, 5]

Currently, the diagnosis of myocarditis is based on histologic criteria. In 1986, a group of pathologists met in Dallas, Texas, and proposed histologic criteria that have since been termed *the Dallas criteria*.[6] The diagnosis of myocarditis demands an inflammatory infiltrate that is lymphocytic and either focal or diffuse. The patient must also exhibit myocyte degeneration, either necrosis or myocyte damage. The diagnosis of borderline myocarditis requires a less severe inflammatory infiltrate and no light microscopic evidence of myocyte destruction. These changes must be separate and distinct from those usually identified with inflammation due to coronary atherosclerosis and myocardial infarction.

The histologic diagnosis requires endomyocardial biopsy. Biopsies may be associated with significant complications. In more than 546 consecutive biopsies in cardiomyopathy patients performed at The Johns Hopkins Hospital, complication rates were 2.7% during introduction (inadvertent carotid artery puncture with the anesthetic needle, bleeding, local nerve infiltration) and 3.3% during biopsy. These include arrhythmias (1.1%), transient conduction abnormalities (1%), and myocardial perforation (0.5%).[7] Myocardial perforation can result in cardiac tamponade and death. The risks associated with the performance of endomyocardial biopsy are directly associated with the experience and skill of those who perform the procedure. Although endomyocardial biopsy is the "gold standard," concern persists about its specificity and sensitivity. In two different studies,[8, 9] repeated biopsies were acquired post mortem from the hearts of patients who succumbed to autopsy-proven myocarditis. With a single biopsy, there is a 17% to 28% chance of diagnosing myocarditis in a patient who died from it, and, even with more than five biopsies, there is only a 64% chance of making the histologic diagnosis. Adding borderline myocarditis to the true histologic diagnosis would increase the positivity of five specimens to approximately 75%.

The diagnosis of myocarditis can be enhanced by utilizing certain techniques, including mononuclear cell typing and staining for upregulation of major histocompatibility complex (MHC) class I and class II antigens. The polymerase chain reaction and other molecular biologic techniques may increase our ability to identify viral pathogens as agents of myocardial failure. Recent studies[10] have demonstrated, first, that, in children, as many as two thirds of endomyocardial biopsy samples may demonstrate polymerase chain reaction evidence of a previous viral infection. Second, the pathogen is often an adenovirus, as opposed to an enterovirus, and, third, as many as two thirds of the adenovirus-infected myocardial specimens display no evidence of an inflammatory infiltrate. Therefore, patients with biopsy-negative myocarditis may have myocardial destruction that is not associated with an active inflammatory infiltrate.

Fenoglio[11] proposed a classification for human myocarditis based on duration of illness, degree of cellular inflammation, amount of healing as determined by biopsy, and mortality rate. We have proposed an alternative classification. At The Johns Hopkins Hospital, more than 750 consecutive patients with left ventricular dysfunction of new onset had endomyocardial biopsies.[12] Of these, 147 had myocarditis; 11 were negative by immunopathologic studies, and six had incompatible histologic findings. Of the 130 remaining cases, 58 were due to secondary myocarditis and 72 were primary. The secondary causes included peripartum cardiomyopathy, HIV-related left ventricular dysfunction, sarcoidosis, lupus erythematosus, cocaine, and other less common ones. Utilizing only data from patients with primary myocarditis, we suggested four different clinical pathologic categories of myocardial inflammation, which were similar to the categories of acute hepatic inflammation. These categories of myocarditis include fulminant myocarditis, acute myocarditis, chronic active myocarditis, and chronic persistent myocarditis (Table 33–2). In our experience, 17% of patients have fulminant myocarditis, 65% acute, 11% chronic active, and 7% chronic persistent disease.

The specific features of these forms of myocarditis that differentiate them are

Table 33–2

## Clinicopathologic Forms of Myocarditis

|  | Fulminant | Acute | Chronic Active | Chronic Persistent |
|---|---|---|---|---|
| Onset | Distinct | Indistinct | Indistinct | Indistinct |
| Heart dysfunction | Severe | Moderate | Moderate | None |
| Biopsy | Multiple foci active | Active or borderline | Active or borderline | Active or borderline |
| Clinical history | Complete recovery or death | Incomplete recovery | Restrictive cardiomyopathy | Normal |
| Histologic findings | Complete resolution | Complete resolution | Ongoing fibrosis and inflammation | Ongoing myocarditis |

of great interest. Patients with fulminant myocarditis have a distinct onset, usually within 2 weeks of a systemic viral illness. They present abruptly with profound left ventricular compromise. Their echocardiograms often show normal-sized hearts but with thickened walls owing to myocardial inflammation and swelling. Their biopsies show multiple foci of myocyte necrosis and an extensive inflammatory infiltrate. Patients either die or recover entirely within 2 weeks. Patients are treated with supportive therapy only. We do not believe that immunosuppressive agents have a role in the management of this population of patients. Chronic active myocarditis is characterized by indistinct onset and progressive left ventricular compromise that, ultimately, results in a restrictive, minimally dilated heart with profoundly elevated filling pressures. Biopsy demonstrates ongoing inflammation and severe fibrosis, and this process appears not to be interrupted by immunosuppressive therapy. Patients with chronic persistent myocarditis have ongoing histologic evidence of inflammation but not evidence of left ventricular compromise. These patients have other cardiac signs or symptoms, including atypical chest pain or ventricular premature contractions. Immunosuppressive therapy appears to be of no benefit to these patients.

The vast majority of patients have acute myocarditis. This entity has an indistinct onset, and affected persons present with a mildly dilated heart and reduced ventricular function. Limited focal myocarditis is usually found after an extensive search of their biopsy specimens. Although the inflammatory infiltrate resolves, these patients usually have persistent mild to severe left ventricular compromise. It is for this population that treatment with immunosuppressive or immunomodulating agents remains controversial.

Treatment options include immune regulation (suppression, absorption, or stimulation), cytokine alteration, interferon, immunoglobulin, antiviral agents, and calcium channel blockade. The largest trial to date in patients with acute myocarditis was concluded in 1996.[13] More than 2200 patients with recent (≤2 years) onset of heart failure but no coronary disease were included. Only 214 were judged to have histologic myocarditis. Of those with myocarditis, patients were excluded because of an ejection fraction of greater than 45%, refusal to participate in the trial, or some other study criterion. Ultimately, only 110 patients were entered in the study. Of these patients, only 64% actually had histologic myocarditis as determined by review by an expert panel of pathologists. Treatment with placebo was compared with treatment with prednisone and cyclosporine. Treatment produced no change in 1-year survival and no alteration in the ejection fraction at the completion of week 28. It was noted that prognosis was better for patients who initially had a higher ejection fraction and whose illness was of shorter duration. Drucker and colleagues[14] completed a nonrandomized trial of gammaglobulin infusion in 21 consecutive children presumed to have acute myocarditis. They demonstrated improved recovery of left ventricular function and a tendency toward better survival during the first year after presentation. Parrillo[15] evaluated by endomyocardial biopsy patients with chronic myocardial dysfunction and inflammatory markers in a prospective, randomized, controlled trial using corticosteroids. While a transient improvement was reported in those with an inflammatory infiltrate, the improvement was not persistent after 12 months. Jones[16] has demonstrated in an observational study that patients with borderline myocarditis may respond as well or better to immunosuppressive agents than do patients with active "histologic" myocarditis, a phenomenon presumably related to the greater autoimmune activity associated with the borderline myocarditis.

Currently, we recommend that patients whose history is compatible with fulminant myocarditis be submitted to endomyocardial biopsy to establish the diagnosis and create an expectation of outcome. The patient should then be supported for at least 2 weeks to determine whether or not myocardial function will improve. This support includes the use of a left ventricular assist device and intraaortic balloon counterpulsation, as necessary. Patients with chronic persistent and chronic active myocarditis do not appear to benefit from currently available immunosuppressive therapies. Most practicing physicians will have to diagnose patients with acute myocarditis. These patients are difficult to distinguish from those who present with cardiomyopathy of new onset from another cause. Currently, we manage patients who present with new systolic dysfunction with standard heart failure treatment. Patients who fail to improve after approximately 2 weeks of appropriate heart failure treatment are submitted to endomyocardial biopsy to determine whether or not they have myocarditis. If the patient is found to have myocarditis but continues to show lack of improvement or deterioration, immunosuppressive therapy is probably justified. Immunosuppressive agents that have been tested include prednisone, azathioprine, and cyclosporine. Other immunomodulating agents include intravenous gamma globulin. The treatment options must be followed closely because of the potential for side effects, and therapy should be discontinued if, after 4 weeks, noninvasive studies demonstrate no improvement in overall contractility.[17]

Myocarditis remains a challenging and ill-understood disease. It is our hope that, with additional molecular biologic approaches and their application to myocardial samples, significant progress will be made in understanding and treating it.

## ■ CARDIOMYOPATHIES

Cardiomyopathies are defined by abnormalities in heart muscle function. These disorders are either primary (indicating an abnormality of the myocardium itself) or secondary to causes such as coronary artery disease or valvular dysfunction, which may cause left ventricular compromise. Cardiomyopathies are categorized by histopathologic types (Table 33–3): dilated, hypertrophic, and restrictive cardiomyopathy.

Approximately 90% of cardiomyopathies are of the dilated histopathologic form. These are typified by hearts that are large, thin-walled, and have decreased contractility. On histologic examination, they demonstrate individual muscle fiber hypertrophy and interstitial fibrosis. Patients with hypertrophic cardiomyopathy (prevalence 5% to 10%) are, "histopathologically," the antithesis of those with dilated cardiomyopathy. Hypertrophic cardiomyopathy is characterized by thick walls, increased contractility, and a small left ventricular cavity. Histologically, specimens reveal marked fiber hypertrophy and fiber disarray. Interstitial fibrosis increases with the duration and severity of the hypertrophy. Patients with restrictive cardiomyopathy (fewer than 5%) have normal wall thickness and normal cavity size. Their contractility is normal until late in the course of the illness that has caused the restrictive cardiomyopathy. Diastolic compliance abnormalities appear

Table 33–3

**Characteristics of the Cardiomyopathies**

| Types | Wall Thickness | Left Ventricular Cavity | Systolic Function | Diastolic Compliance | Histology |
|---|---|---|---|---|---|
| Dilated | Thin | Large | Decreased | Altered late | Hypertrophy and interstitial scar |
| Hypertrophic | Thick | Small | Increased | Altered early | Hypertrophy and myocyte disarray |
| Restrictive | Normal | Normal | Normal | Altered early | Varies with cause |

early in the course of restrictive cardiomyopathy, in the middle phase of hypertrophic cardiomyopathy, and not until the advanced stage of dilated cardiomyopathy. Alternatively, systolic dysfunction appears at the time of presentation of persons with dilated cardiomyopathy and late in those with restrictive cardiomyopathy, and, usually, it does not appear at all in those with hypertrophic cardiomyopathy.

The symptoms of all three types of cardiomyopathy are the same and are attributable to congestion and low cardiac output. Symptoms of low output reflect a small stroke volume caused by decreased contractility in a patient with a large heart or by a left ventricular cavity of small size. Low-output symptoms include fatiguability, weakness, malaise, and, ultimately, decreased cerebral and renal perfusion.

Low cardiac output stimulates a neurohormonal response that results in elevated levels of norepinephrine, renin, angiotensin, atrial naturetic factor, cytokine stimulation, and a host of other factors.[18–21] Initially, these neurohormonal responses are compensatory. The increased sympathetic drive enhances contractility and diastolic relaxation (lusitropy). Increases in renin and angiotensin are associated with salt and water retention, which increases left ventricular volume and improves cardiac output (at the expense of increased filling pressures). Atrial naturetic factor elevation secondary to atrial stretch may result in increased diuresis. Ultimately, the increase in neurohormonal stimulation exceeds compensatory benefit and is associated with signs and symptoms of excessive sympathetic drive, including tachycardia, diaphoresis, and elevated diastolic blood pressure. Elevation of angiotensin II and sympathetic stimulation result in an increase in systemic resistance owing to their vasoconstrictive properties. Persistent elevations of cytokines such as tumor necrosis factor are associated with wasting and, ultimately, with the cachexia seen with advanced cardiac dysfunction. These changes cause cell death (apoptosis)[22] and are associated with a poor prognosis.

Low cardiac output stimulates the kidney to produce renin and angiotensin, which in turn results in salt and water retention. The additional volume enhances cardiac output by increasing diastolic filling. As the ventricular compliance is altered, the increased volume causes high end-diastolic pressures, which cause symptoms of congestive heart failure. Congestive symptoms reflect increased blood and water in the lungs or systemic veins and liver, depending on whether or not left- or right-sided congestive symptoms are displayed. Fluid retention in these areas is due to altered left ventricular compliance and an elevation of the left and/or right ventricular end-diastolic pressure. Increase ventricular diastolic pressures increase left and right atrial pressures and transmit increased pressures in the pulmonary and/or hepatic and systemic venous systems. These pressure elevations can result in retention or exudation of fluid by the affected organs. The end-diastolic pressures may be elevated in any of the three forms of cardiomyopathy owing to altered compliance. Even in a normal heart, pressures can be elevated if an abrupt increase in volume expands the myocardium to the limits of a noncompliant pericardium or cardiac fibrous tissue network. Therefore, patients who have any form of cardiomyopathy present with symptoms of shortness of breath, dyspnea on exertion, orthopnea, paroxysms of nocturnal dyspnea, and lower extremity and abdominal/hepatic distension.

## ■ EVALUATION

The patient who presents with congestive heart failure or low-output symptoms should have a thorough evaluation to determine the type of myopathic abnormality and its cause. All patients should have a very thorough history and examination. The jugular venous pressure may be markedly elevated in each of the three forms of cardiomyopathy; however, those with restrictive cardiomyopathy often have a dramatic elevation of the jugular venous pressure and display prominent *a* and *v* waves. Patients with hypertrophic cardiomyopathy frequently display a large jugular venous *a* wave; whereas those with dilated cardiomyopathy often display a giant *v* (or S) wave due to tricuspid regurgitation. Patients with dilated cardiomyopathy have decreased carotid pulsations (volume and rate of rise), those with restrictive cardiomyopathy have normal to decreased pulsations, and those with hypertrophic cardiomyopathy display dynamic (and often bifid) pulsations. The point of maximum impulse in persons with dilated cardiomyopathy is displaced and large; in those with hypertrophic cardiomyopathy, it is usually minimally displaced, active, and muscular; and those who have restrictive cardiomyopathy have a barely discernible point of maximum pulse with weakened dynamics. A dilated heart is often associated with mitral and tricuspid regurgitant murmurs, restrictive cardiomyopathy with no murmur, and hypertrophic cardiomyopathy with harsh outflow and mitral murmurs that sometimes increase with the Valsalva maneuver or another mechanism that decreases left ventricular filling. Patients with dilated cardiomyopathy often have $S_3$ gallops; those with hypertrophic cardiomyopathy $S_4$ gallops; and those with restrictive cardiomyopathy often have no gallops at all. Peripheral edema is much more marked in persons with dilated cardiomyopathy; those with restrictive cardiomyopathies have ascites and hepatic congestion; and those with hypertrophic cardiomyopathy usually have little or no edema.

The ECG pattern is abnormal in each entity. Dilated cardiomyopathy produces variable voltage and nonspecific ST-T wave changes. Hypertrophic cardiomyopathy is associated with large increases in left ventricular voltage and, often, a "strain" pattern of ST segment depression. Restrictive cardiomyopathy often produces low voltage and a pseudoinfarct pattern. A chest film usually shows a very large heart in humans with dilated cardiomyopathy. The hearts of those with hypertrophic cardiomyopathy are usually normal to slightly increased in size and those of persons with restrictive cardiomyopathy may be of normal size.

The most discriminating noninvasive test is the echocardiogram. It clearly determines whether the patient has dilated or hypertrophic cardiomyopathy. Restrictive cardiomyopathy is usually less evident on noninvasive echocardiographic studies. The myocardium of restrictive cardiomyopathy occasionally has a ground-glass appearance, which is compatible with fibrosis or amyloidosis. Abnormalities of mitral valve inflow suggest decreased compliance.

Persons who have dilated cardiomyopathy of indeterminate cause after history taking, physical examination, or echocardiography should have thyroid-stimulating hormone, serum or urinary catecholamines, and antinuclear antibodies measured to rule out "reversible" conditions (e.g., hyper- or hypothyroidism, pheochromocytoma, and connective tissue disease). Those who have significant risk factors for coronary atherosclerosis—male gender, age greater than 45 years, hypertension, hypercholesterolemia, diabetes, and/or a family history of early atherosclerosis—should be studied with coronary angiography to rule out coronary atherosclerosis. Alternatively, noninvasive techniques such as ultrafast computed tomography (CT) or magnetic resonance imaging (MRI) may demonstrate coronary calcification severe enough to suggest atherosclerosis as the cause. If atherosclerosis is suspected, investigation of areas of myocardium "in jeopardy" owing to severe coronary artery disease but free of "completed" myocardial damage, should be undertaken with positron emission tomography, dobutamine echocardiography, or MRI. Patients with hypertrophic cardiomyopathy should undergo catheterization only as a guide to invasive interventions such as myectomy or alcohol injection of the first septal perforating artery of the left anterior descending coronary artery. Similarly, for patients with hypertrophic cardiomyopathy who might have intercurrent ischemic heart disease, angiography may be of benefit. Coronary angiography is of little benefit to those with restrictive cardiomyopathy.

Endomyocardial biopsy may be helpful in those with dilated cardiomyopathy, is of no benefit to those with hypertrophic cardiomyopathy, and is usually diagnostic in those with restrictive cardiomyopathies. Patient with dilated cardiomyopathies should have an endomyocardial biopsy if they are young, have had their illness for less than 6 months, and have no other cause suggested by history, examination, or other laboratory values.

The diagnosis of hypertrophic cardiomyopathy can be confirmed by finding evidence of a similar myopathic state in first-degree relatives. Looking back, patients with hypertrophic cardiomyopathy often notice that symptoms have been present throughout their life, and, typically, they include light-headedness, presyncope, and fatiguability as well as atypical chest pain and exercise limitation. If the transthoracic echocardiogram is not diagnostic, dobutamine echocardiography may show the left ventricular outflow obstruction.

Restrictive cardiomyopathy must be differentiated from constrictive pericarditis. Constrictive pericarditis is curable; restrictive cardiomyopathy is usually rapidly fatal. If the chest radiograph does not show features of pericardial calcification, MRI or CT may show marked pericardial thickening suggestive of constrictive pericarditis. The greatest challenge in patients with restrictive features is to differentiate them from constrictive pericarditis and to define their cause.

## ■ CAUSES

### Dilated Cardiomyopathies

The causes of dilated cardiomyopathy are many. Most patients with dilated cardiomyopathy have idiopathic cardiomyopathy, ischemic cardiomyopathy, inflammatory left ventricular compromise, or a metabolic abnormality or suffer the effects of a toxic agent. Drugs may more frequently be the cause of cardiomyopathy than we once thought. Examples of drugs with potential direct cardiotoxicity are doxorubicin, cyclophosphamide, chloroquine, emetine, and the phenothiazines. Left ventricular dysfunction may also be associated with drug hypersensitivity and eosinophilic myocarditis due to agents such as penicillin, sulfonamides, and methyldopa. Familial dilated cardiomyopathy may account for 10% to 15% of all patients with dilated cardiomyopathy. Therefore, searching the family history will become as important with patients who have dilated cardiomyopathy as it is with those with hypertrophic features.

In evaluating the causes of dilated cardiomyopathy, it is important to concentrate on causes that may be treatable or reversible. These include, but are not limited to, hyper- or hypothyroidism, pheochromocytoma, myocarditis, tachycardia-induced cardiomyopathy, peripartum cardiomyopathy, drug hypersensitivity, carnitine deficiency, and some ischemic cardiomyopathies. Among investigators, some confusion persists concerning the response of the heart to exercise. "Aerobic athletes" may display diastolic left ventricular dimensions at the upper limit of normal, whereas "anaerobic athletes" (e.g., weight lifters) may display increased wall thickening. These physiologic responses virtually never exceed the upper limits of normal.

The physician must also be certain that a patient is not presenting with a dilated cardiomyopathy "look-alike." Patients with end-stage aortic stenosis or mitral regurgitation may appear to have primary cardiomyopathy, their murmurs having decreased intensity because of very low cardiac output and blood flow through the affected valve. The patient with left ventricular aneurysm or left ventricular pseudo-aneurysm may appear to have dilated cardiomyopathy if the functional walls (usually the lateral and posterointerior walls) are not visualized well during the noninvasive study. Patients with pericardial effusions may appear to have a dilated cardiomyopathy by chest radiography and examination, whereas the echocardiogram clearly demonstrates the potential for pericardial compression or tamponade.

## Hypertrophic Cardiomyopathy

Patients with hypertrophic cardiomyopathy are usually easily identified by noninvasive transthoracic echocardiography. Patients with hypertrophic cardiomyopathy display increased left ventricular wall thickness by echocardiographic analysis (>1.5 cm). One of three patterns is usually displayed: diffuse hypertrophy, apical hypertrophy, or asymmetric septal hypertrophy, distinguished by the diffuse apical or proximal septal location of the hypertrophy. The inherited form of hypertrophic cardiomyopathy is confirmed by echocardiographic or autopsy evidence of the disorder in other family members. Although hypertrophic cardiomyopathy has an autosomal-dominant pattern of inheritance, sometimes it appears "spontaneously." Some patients develop hypertensive hypertrophic cardiomyopathy, a pattern of diffuse increased wall thickness usually observed in elderly women with a long history of significant hypertension and evidence of diffuse hypertrophy (as opposed to asymmetric left ventricular growth) on noninvasive studies. All patients with familial inherited hypertrophic cardiomyopathy have a genetic basis for the cardiac abnormality. Those with hypertensive hypertrophic cardiomyopathy are likely to have an abnormal response to left ventricular growth factors associated with pressure overload.

## Restrictive Cardiomyopathy

Patients with restrictive cardiomyopathy have a limited number of diagnoses. They may have profound left ventricular hypertrophy, interstitial fibrosis (familial or independent), amyloidosis, sarcoidosis, or hemochromatosis. The endomyocardial biopsy tissue provides the diagnosis for each of these ("tissue is the issue"). Biopsy tissue from patients with suspected amyloidosis should be stained with Congo red and studied by electron microscopy. The patients should then be evaluated to determine whether their amyloidosis is primary or secondary to an associated protein abnormality (multiple myeloma, familial). Patients with amyloidosis often have associated periorbital purpura, submandibular nodal enlargement and macroglossia, and they bruise easily. Hepatic and abdominal engorgement are other features. Patients with sarcoidosis may have x-ray evidence of mediastinal adenopathy, retinitis, or oligoarticular arthritis. Patients with fibrosis may have a familial disorder, primary fibrosis, or fibrosis associated with chronic active myocarditis or giant cell myocarditis. Obviously, the noncaseating granuloma diagnostic of sarcoidosis or giant cell myocarditis may be missed because of the focal nature of these findings. Persons with hemochromatosis often have more features of dilated than of restrictive cardiomyopathy; however, on endomyocardial biopsy, their iron study findings are definitive. These often subtle histologic disorders will not be found unless the pathologist examining appropriate biopsy samples is looking for them.

## ▪ PROGNOSIS

Patients with restrictive cardiomyopathy often have the worst prognosis owing to the advanced state of their primary abnormality at the time of presentation.

Patients with dilated cardiomyopathy have an intermediate prognosis, which depends in part on the identification of treatable or reversible disorders. The prognosis of patients with hypertrophic cardiomyopathy depends on the genetic form of the disease. Some genetic inheritance patterns are associated with early and sudden death, others with features of outflow obstruction.

In general, patients with dilated cardiomyopathy have a worse prognosis when there is advanced heart failure (NYHA class IV symptoms), age greater than 55 years, male gender, $S_3$ on examination, intraventricular conduction delay on ECG, cardiothoracic ratio greater than 0.55 on chest films, ejection fraction below 10%, wall thickness by echocardiogram less than 0.9 cm, metabolic exercise stress test maximal oxygen consumption below 12 ml/kg/min, Holter monitor evidence of increased ventricular ectopy or ventricular tachycardia, elevated plasma norepinephrine levels, elevated neurohormonal stimulation (plasma renin activity), or elevated filling pressures, particularly a pulmonary capillary wedge pressure above 20 mm Hg. Even patients who present with many of these adverse features often respond to treatment (i.e., the features just listed improve) and, thus, their potential for survival is enhanced. Increasingly, agents that interrupt the neurohormonal cycle of stimulation and decline (angiotensin-converting enzyme inhibitors and beta-blockers) appear to improve prognosis.[23–26]

Patients with hypertrophic cardiomyopathy have a worse prognosis if there is a family history of sudden death, a personal history of cardiac arrest, or symptoms of congestive heart failure. Prognosis is not determined by the degree of outflow obstruction or wall thickness as demonstrated by echocardiography. The prognosis for patients with restrictive cardiomyopathy is determined not just by the findings of heart failure when they come to diagnosis but also by the prognosis of the underlying illness.

Patients with dilated or hypertrophic cardiomyopathy who have ventricular tachycardia that is prolonged (more than 10 bpm) or is associated with symptoms, should undergo electrophysiologic study to determine their potential for sudden cardiac death and receive an automatic implantable cardiac defibrillator (AICD) or be treated with amiodarone.

## ■ TREATMENT

The treatment of heart failure has been discussed in other sections of this book. Special features that deserve mention in dealing with patients with cardiomyopathies are noted below.

Patients with dilated cardiomyopathy should be treated for any reversible causes that have been identified. Angiotensin-converting enzyme inhibitors and beta-blockers appear to improve symptoms and prognosis. Although diuretics have not been demonstrated to improve prognosis, they remain the mainstay for treatment of symptoms of congestion. Inotropic agents have been uniformly disappointing, and with the exception of digoxin have not been better than placebo in clinical trials.[27–29] Patients with dilated cardiomyopathy due to ischemia and ventricular tachycardia should have an AICD implanted. Those with idiopathic dilated cardiomyopathy and symptomatic ventricular tachycardia should have an electrophysiology study and be treated with either an AICD or amiodarone. Other cardiomyopathy patients who frequently experience ventricular tachycardia may be candidates for amiodarone.

Patients with dilated cardiomyopathy may be treated with digoxin, the only inotrope that appears not to increase mortality and ameliorates symptoms and decreases the frequency of hospitalizations.

Patients with hypertrophic cardiomyopathy are initially treated with negative inotropic agents to improve left ventricular filling time (rate effect) or compliance. If these agents are ineffective, patients may be considered for atrioventricular sequential pacemaker therapy. This form of treatment has been championed by the National Institutes of Health, and ongoing studies will determine whether atrioventricular sequential pacing improves symptoms and allows ventricular remodeling over time. Patients may also undergo left ventricular myectomy if they have asymmetric septal hypertrophy and the proximal septum interferes with left ventricular outflow. Such patients should undergo definitive catheterization studies to determine their eligibility. Recently, some investigators have been injecting alcohol into the proximal septal branch of the left anterior descending coronary artery to induce a limited myocardial infarction—a "chemical myectomy." Data are too preliminary to recommend this broadly.

The cause of restrictive cardiomyopathy must be treated. Patients with amyloidosis, whether primary or secondary, often have disappointing results of treatment. Hemochromatosis, sarcoidosis, and other causes of restrictive cardiomyopathy are usually more responsive.

When these therapies fail, the patient may be considered for experimental surgical intervention. In the case of dilated cardiomyopathy, this might include myoplasty or left ventricular reduction surgery. Today, mitral valve reconstruction is also being performed in patients with dilated cardiomyopathy and significant mitral regurgitation.

Patients with dilated or hypertrophic cardiomyopathy and some forms of restrictive cardiomyopathy (those that would not recur in a transplanted organ) may be candidates for cardiac transplantation. The criteria for transplantation remain stringent, and only a limited number of transplants can be performed due to a shortage of donors.

Treatment of the cardiomyopathies remains one of the most challenging and poorly understood areas of cardiology today. We are in a period of rapid advancement, and can anticipate that significant strides will be made over the next 10 years.

## ■ REFERENCES

1. Brown CA, O'Connell JB: Myocarditis and idiopathic dilated cardiomyopathy. Am J Med 1995;99:309–314.
2. Lange LG, Schreiner GF: Immune mechanisms of cardiac disease. N Engl J Med 1994;330:1129–1135.
3. Smith SC, Ladenson JH, Mason JW, Jaffe AS: Elevations of cardiac troponin I associated with myocarditis: Experimental and clinical correlates. Circulation 1997;95:163–168.
4. O'Connell JB, Henkin RE, Robinson JA, et al: Gallium-67 imaging in patients with dilated cardiomyopathy and biopsy-proven myocarditis. Circulation 1984;70:58–62.
5. Dec GW, Palacios I, Yasuda T, et al: Antimyosin antibody cardiac imaging: Its role in the diagnosis of myocarditis. J Am Coll Cardiol 1990;16:97–104.
6. Aretz HT, Billingham ME, Edwards WD, et al: Myocarditis: A histopathologic definition and classification. Am J Cardiol Pathol 1986;1:3–14.
7. Deckers JW, Jare JM, Baughman KL, et al: Complications of transvenous right ventricular endomyocardial biopsy in adult patients with cardiomyopathy: A seven-year survey of 546 consecutive diagnostic procedures in a tertiary referral center. J Am Coll Cardiol 1992;19:43–47.
8. Hauck AJ, Kearney DL, Edwards WD: Evaluation of postmortem endomyocardial biopsy specimens from 38 patients with lymphocytic myocarditis: Implications for role of sampling error. Mayo Clinical Proc 1989;64:1235–1245.
9. Chow LH, Radio SJ, Sears TD, Mc Manus BM: Insensitivity of right ventricular endomyocardial biopsy in the diagnosis of myocarditis. J Am Coll Cardiol 1989;14:915–920.
10. Bowles NE, Towbin JA: Molecular aspects of myocarditis. Curr Opin Cardiol 1998;13:179–184.
11. Fenoglio JJ Jr, Ursell PC, Kellogg CF, et al: Diagnosis and classification of myocarditis by endomyocardial biopsy. N Engl J Med 1983;308:12–18.
12. Lieberman EB, Herskowitz A, Rose NR, Baughman KL: A clinicopathologic description of myocarditis. Clin Immunol Immunopathol 1993;68:191–196.
13. Mason JW, O'Connell JB, Herskowitz A, et al: A clinical trial of immunosuppressive therapy for myocarditis. N Engl J Med 1995;333:269–275.

14. Drucker NA, Colan SD, Lewis AB, et al: γ-Globulin treatment of acute myocarditis in the pediatric population. Circulation 1994;89:252–257.
15. Parrillo JE, Cunnion RE, Epstein SE, et al: A prospective, randomized, controlled trial of prednisone for dilated cardiomyopathy. N Engl J Med 1989;321:1061–1068.
16. Jones SR, Herskowitz A, Hutchins GM, Baughman KL: Effects of immunosuppressive therapy in biopsy-proved myocarditis and borderline myocarditis on left ventricular function. Am J Cardiol 1991;68:370–376.
17. Caforio AL, McKenna WJ: Recognition and optimum management of myocarditis. Drugs 1996;52:515–525.
18. Cohn JN, Levine TB, Olivari MT, et al: Plasma norepinephrine as a guide to prognosis in patients with chronic congestive heart failure. N Engl J Med 1984;311:819–823.
19. Bristow MR, Ginsburg R, Minobe W, et al: Decreased catecholamine sensitivity and β-adrenergic–receptor density in failing human hearts. N Engl J Med 1982;307:205–211.
20. Margulies KB, Hildebrand FL, Lerman A, et al: Increased endothelin in experimental heart failure. Circulation 1990;82:2226–2230.
21. Haber HL, Leavy JA, Kessler PD, et al: The erythrocyte sedimentation rate in congestive heart failure. N Engl J Med 1991;324:353–358.
22. Narula J, Haider N, Virmani R, et al: Apoptosis in myocytes in end-stage heart failure. N Engl J Med 1996;335:1182–1189.
23. Pfeffer MA, Braunwald E, Moyé LA, et al: Effect of captopril on mortality and morbidity in patients with left ventricular dysfunction after myocardial infarction. N Engl J Med 1992;327:669–677.
24. Yusuf S, et al: Effect of enalapril on survival in patients with reduced left ventricular ejection fractions and congestive heart failure. N Engl J Med 1991;325:293–302.
25. Waagstein F, Hjalmarson A, Varnuskas E, Wallentin I: Effect of chronic beta-adrenergic receptor blockade in congestive cardiomyopathy. Br Heart J 1975;37:1022–1036.
26. Swedberg K, Hjalmarson A, Waagstein F, Wallentin I: Prolongation of survival in congestive cardiomyopathy by beta-receptor blockade. Lancet 1979;1:1374–1376.
27. Massie B, Baurassa M, DiBianco R, et al: Long-term oral administration of amrinone for congestive heart failure: Lack of efficacy in a multicenter controlled trial. Circulation 1985;71:963–971.
28. Krell MJ, Kline EM, Bates ER, et al: Intermittent, ambulatory dobutamine infusions in patients with severe congestive heart failure. Am Heart J 1986;112:787–791.
29. Lee DC, Johnson RA, Bingham JB, et al: Heart failure in outpatients: A randomized trial of digoxin versus placebo. N Engl J Med 1982;306:699–705.

# ■ RECOMMENDED READING

Baughman KL: Hypertrophic cardiomyopathy (clinical conference). JAMA 1992;267(6):846–849.
Kasper EK, Agema WR, Hutchins GM, et al: The causes of dilated cardiomyopathy: A clinicopathologic review of 673 consecutive patients. J Am Coll Cardiol 1994;23:586–590.
Manolio TA, Baughman KL, Rodeheffer R, et al: Prevalence and etiology of idiopathic dilated cardiomyopathy (summary of a National Heart, Lung and Blood Institute workshop). Am J Cardiol 1992;69:1458–1466.
McKee PA, Castelli WP, McNamara PM: The natural history of congestive heart failure: The Framingham Study. N Engl J Med 1971;285:1441–1446.
Rose NR, Herskowitz A, Neumann DA: Autoimmunity in myocarditis: Models and mechanisms. Clin Immunol Immunopathol 1993;68:95–99.
Towbin JA: Molecular genetic aspects of cardiomyopathy (review). Biochem Med Metab Biol 1993;49(3):285–320.

# Chapter 34

# Pericardial Disease

*David H. Spodick*

The pericardium is a complex, mesothelium-lined serous sac surrounding the heart and clasped externally by a fibrous sac so that the layer on the heart (visceral pericardium) is mesothelium while the external portion (parietal pericardium) is composed of mesothelium internally and fibrosa externally. Normally, 15 to 35 ml of serous fluid surrounds the heart. The normal microphysiology of the visceral and parietal pericardia is complex and is discussed in detail elsewhere.[1] The pericardium is involved in every known kind of disease, and abnormal fluid accumulation in it frequently seriously compromises cardiac function (tamponade) and raises important questions in differential diagnosis and treatment.

Table 34–1 lists the nine major categories of pericardial disease, each of which must be considered in any new case. A vast array of individual conditions under each of these categories is described in detail elsewhere.[2]

## ■ CONGENITAL PERICARDIAL DEFECTS AND CYSTS

Gaps in the pericardium, although usually left sided, may occur anywhere and have the potential to compress herniating cardiac structures, including parts of chambers and coronary vessels. Predictable syndromes, however, may be difficult to identify, although imaging is usually successful, especially magnetic resonance imaging (MRI). Congenital cysts, the majority occurring in the right cardiophrenic angle, usually require imaging to distinguish them from solid tumor or cardiac aneurysm.

## ■ PERICARDIAL INFLAMMATIONS: ACUTE PERICARDITIS

Acute pericarditis is the most common—and therefore the most important—of all pericardial disorders, although subclinical cases may be missed. Every category of inflammatory, including infectious, agent has been identified. Most patients, particularly younger ones, present the "idiopathic pericarditis syndrome." There is no proved cause, but it is most likely viral. This syndrome is typically the epitome of acute pericarditis, because it includes all the classic manifestations: pain, pericardial rubs, and electrocardiographic (ECG) changes (usually classic).[3] Coxsackie virus and other enteroviruses are the most common agents in the United States. Effusion is frequent, usually without tamponade. Adhesions are indetectable except by imaging, but constrictive scarring occurs occasionally. The differential diagnosis includes systemic diseases like lupus and other vasculitides that frequently involve the pericardium.

## ■ CLINICALLY DRY ACUTE PERICARDITIS

*Clinically dry* indicates either that the condition is without effusion or that any effusion has no clinical significance; it is the most common presentation of acute

Table 34–1

**Causes and Pathogenesis of Acquired Diseases of the Pericardium***

I. Idiopathic pericarditis (syndromes)
II. Living agents, infections, parasitic
III. Vasculitis, connective tissue disease
IV. Immunopathies/hypersensitivity states
V. Disease of contiguous structures
VI. Disorders of metabolism
VII. Trauma, direct or indirect
VIII. Neoplasms, primary, metastatic, or multicentric
IX. Of uncertain pathogenesis or in association with various syndromes

*Considerable overlap (e.g., categories III and IV; V and VII).
Modified from Spodick DH: The Pericardium: A Comprehensive Textbook. New York: Marcel Dekker, 1997.

pericarditis. Onset may be gradual or sudden with central chest pain, usually pleuritic, that is exacerbated by body movements and by breathing. Occasionally it mimics ischemic forms of chest pain, including substernal pressure sensations. The pain is simultaneously (or occasionally only) perceived in one or both trapezius ridges, a finding *virtually pathognomonic for acute pericarditis*. Frequently, the onset follows an upper respiratory tract infection. Fever varies according to the cause but is usually between 37° and 38.8° C. A pericardial friction sound (rub) is usual[4]: it has a high frequency, is often loud, is nearly always strongest at the left middle to lower sternal edge, and has a peculiar shuffling, grating, scratching, or creaking quality. Usually, three components are distinguishable by careful auscultation: presystolic, systolic, and early diastolic (Fig. 34–1). Biphasic—and even monophasic—rubs are relatively common. When all three components are distinguishable, this rules out similar-sounding murmurs. Rubs are supposedly due to friction between pericardial surfaces, yet effusions, including large effusions, often occur with rubs. Moderate leukocytosis is common, but the infective agent or any systemic disorder causing the pericarditis dictates the variation in cell count, sedimen-

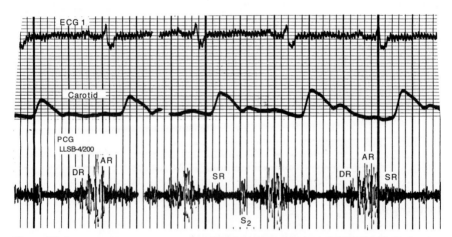

**Figure 34–1** ▪ Electrocardiogram (ECG 1), carotid displacement pulse (carotid), and phonocardiogram (PCG) show a quasidiagnostic, three-part pericardial rub. DR, late diastolic component; AR, atrial component; SR, ventricular systolic component. In this example, the AR is the most intense. (Spodick DH: The Pericardium: A Comprehensive Textbook. New York: Marcel Dekker, 1997, with permission.)

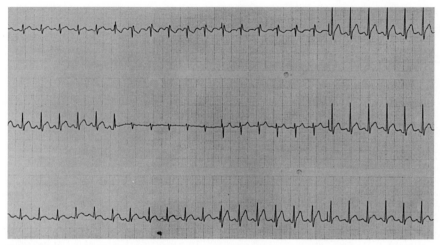

**Figure 34–2** ▪ A 12-lead ECG shows typical, quasidiagnostic stage 1 changes of acute pericarditis. The J points (ST segments) are elevated in most leads. (aVR is always an exception, and V1 nearly always; aVL is almost algebraically zero.) PR segments are oppositely deviated, reflecting the atrial T waves due to atrial pericarditis. (Spodick DH: The Pericardium: A Comprehensive Textbook. New York: Marcel Dekker, 1997, with permission.)

tation rate, and other acute phase reactants. Cardiac enzyme studies vary much, from normal to small increases depending directly on the extent of any accompanying myocarditis. Indeed, some degree of myocarditis is entirely responsible for electrocardiographic (ECG) PR segment and ST-T changes. When typical, ECG changes are quasidiagnostic, particularly stage 1 (Fig. 34–2) of four sequential stages. J-point (ST) elevations with normal-looking T waves in all leads except aVR and occasionally $V_1$ and $V_2$ characterize stage 1.[5] Atypical ECG variants are described in detail elsewhere.[6] In stage 2, all J points return to the baseline together with little change in the T waves until later. In stage 3, T waves progressively flatten and invert. Stage 4 is a recovery stage. A typical transition from stage 1 to 2 to 3 is diagnostic; however, in modern times, many patients stop at stage 2, which is virtually a return to normal, probably because of early diagnosis and antiinflammatory treatment. Equally characteristic are PR segment deviations, mostly depression, occurring in most leads. These tend to appear earlier than ST elevations and may be the only ECG abnormality. Heart rate is quite variable and is proportional to the systemic reaction. Usually, it is relatively rapid (>90 bpm), but it can be slow, especially in uremic patients. Rhythm abnormalities are not due to pericarditis but to an accompanying heart disorder such as severe myocarditis.

A similar ECG pattern, "early repolarization," must be distinguished, particularly in males younger than 40 years. Here, PR segment deviations are uncommon and never generalized, while the J-point elevation is usually less than 25% of the T wave height in lead $V_6$.

## ▪ PERICARDIAL EFFUSION

Inflammation of the pericardium or a fluid-retaining state (e.g., congestive heart failure) can cause pericardial effusion if fluid is produced too fast to be reabsorbed. There may be one of four general consequences: clinically insignificant amounts; a larger effusion without apparent physiologic effects; a relatively large

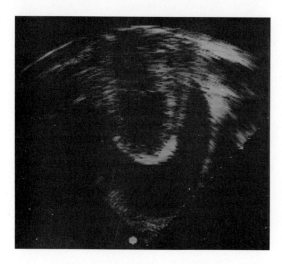

**Figure 34–3** ▪ Large circumcardiac pericardial effusion is compressing the heart. Apical 4-chamber echocardiogram. (Spodick DH: The Pericardium: A Comprehensive Textbook. New York: Marcel Dekker, 1997, with permission.)

effusion compressing the heart but checked by compensatory mechanisms; and frank cardiac tamponade with cardiac compression limiting cardiac output with life-threatening consequences. Heart sounds may be distant, especially with tamponade. The effusion may be asymptomatic but can compress adjacent organs, causing dyspnea, cough, hoarseness, abdominal fullness, hiccups, and nausea.

Ordinary x-ray films show cardiomegaly with a "water bottle" outline and clear lung fields in the absence of independent pulmonary disease. Echocardiography (Fig. 34–3) is the standard for identifying and following the course of pericardial effusion. Other imaging modalities may be required. Pleural effusions, especially on the left, are common. Larger effusions, particularly with tamponade, permit "swinging" of the heart, with electric alternation on the ECG.

## ▪ ACUTE CARDIAC TAMPONADE

Tamponade is the decompensated phase of cardiac compression resulting from an unchecked increase in pericardial fluid pressure. Tamponade may be slow to develop, owing to slow effusion, or sudden, usually owing to hemorrhage. In either case, compression of the heart must be relieved by drainage. Clinically, patients have signs of low-output state, including air hunger, which often resembles congestive heart failure, but without pulmonary edema. There is equalization of diastolic pressures throughout the heart. Pulsus paradoxus, a drop in systolic blood pressure greater than 10 mm Hg during inspiration, is usual. Imaging, particularly Doppler echocardiography, usually shows right ventricular and/or atrial diastolic collapse, and occasionally left atrial collapse. In volume-expanded patients, however, signs of tamponade may not be present.

## ▪ PERICARDIAL CONSTRICTION

Pericardial inflammation may heal with tight or thick scar tissue, sometimes compressing the heart much as tamponade does but more slowly. Some degree of pericardial bleeding has been necessary to produce experimental constrictive scarring. Constrictive pericarditis was formerly regarded as a chronic disease, but earlier diagnosis by better-trained physicians and a shift in its major causes now make most cases subacute or even relatively acute. Any pericardial inflammation (except rheumatic) can cause constriction. Tuberculosis was the major detectable cause but is no longer so in developed countries, where constriction after cardiac surgery is an increasingly important factor. The acute pericardial inflammation may be manifest or totally silent so that the patient presents with constrictive pericarditis de novo.

The pathophysiology of constrictive pericarditis is distinct from that of tamponade. Catheterization traces usually show a diastolic "dip" and plateau (the square root sign). As a rule, atrial $x$ and $y$ descents are deep. Chest films are of no use unless there is pericardial calcification, which is best seen in lateral views. Doppler echocardiography and other imaging modalities usually give the diagnosis, although it is sometimes difficult to distinguish constriction from its mimic, restrictive cardiomyopathy.

Pedal edema is common. Symptoms correspond to those of congestive heart failure without pulmonary edema. There is frequently a loud early third heart sound, which is sometimes palpable and may have a "knocking" quality. ECG changes are nonspecific, although they may resemble stage 3 of the acute pericarditis ECG, with frequent interatrial block (notched, wide P waves).

In effusive-constrictive pericarditis, intercurrent effusion produces acute and subacute clinical pictures. The clinical and physiologic signs depend on whether tamponade or constriction predominates. The treatment for all forms of constriction is surgical removal.

## ▪ IDIOPATHIC PERICARDITIS

Cases in which the cause cannot be established can be considered "idiopathic," although, in this case most patients have a viral pericardial syndrome and the designation of *idiopathic* persists because it is usually not productive to search for a particular virus. As in acute viral pericarditis, tamponade and constriction occur occasionally.

## ▪ INFECTIOUS ACUTE PERICARDITIS

Viruses are perhaps the most common cause of infectious acute pericarditis in the United States, especially coxsackievirus and enterovirus. Other viral etiologies include the agents for hepatitis, mumps, and other childhood diseases. Elements of myopericarditis or perimyocarditis are common, especially in children. Although the pericardial syndrome dominates, patients may have dyspnea, cough, and pulmonary infiltrates. Viral pericarditis is much more common in men, usually in young, healthy male patients. Patients less likely to have a viral infection always raise questions of acute myocardial infarction, tuberculosis, and vasculitis. Patients may have recurrent attacks within the first few months, but others have attacks for years owing to a persistent immunopathy in the absence of living organisms.

## ▪ BACTERIAL PERICARDITIS

Bacterial infection is the most serious of the common infectious forms of pericarditis. The control of bacteria, except in compromised hosts, has reduced its incidence; but serious tamponade and constriction are much more likely with aggressive bacterial infections, which are more destructive of tissues than most viral ones. These appear to be increasingly evident in hospitalized patients and may be dramatic, with septic manifestations, though in many elderly patients with severe systemic disease they are silent. Tachycardia is the rule, and about half the patients have a very high fever. Leukocytosis with a marked leftward shift is characteristic. Blood culture may help, but pericardial fluid culture is more specific. Pericardial drainage with resection for any signs of constriction of the pericardium or loculation is virtually mandatory.

Tuberculosis, although its prevalence is decreasing, is still a significant cause, particularly in immunocompromised hosts, who may also have atypical organisms. There is a broad spectrum of tuberculous pericarditis from painful acute pericarditis with minimal to large effusions, to tamponade. Others may lack acute symptoms, except fever. Some patients have chronic pericardial effusion and pericardial calcification with or without hemodynamic impairment. Tuberculin testing is of little help for the diagnosis. Treatment is drainage for tamponade and surgical resection for any suggestion of pericardial constriction, under triple antituberculous drug therapy.

## ▪ FUNGAL PERICARDITIS

Fungal pericarditis is seen increasingly in immunocompromised patients. Organisms include fungi like *Histoplasma* and *Coccidiodes,* each with a geographic distribution that makes consideration of these diagnoses important in edemic areas. Many other fungi also attack the pericardium. Treatment is with an agent specific for a particular fungus, as well as amphotericin, as indicated.

## ▪ PARASITIC PERICARDIAL DISEASE

Parasitic infestations are mainly endemic, particularly echinococcosis, amebiasis, and toxoplasmosis. Indeed, any parasite may attack the pericardium. Patients returning from endemic areas should always raise the question of parasitosis.

## ▪ PERICARDITIS IN DISEASES OF CONTIGUOUS STRUCTURES

Pericarditis is common in anatomically *transmural myocardial infarction* and usually has no clinical importance. Occasionally, rubs and pleuritic pain are associated. Most cases are self-limited. Fluid retention may cause hydropericardium. Tamponade is usually due to hemorrhagic effusion but is rare unless there is antithrombotic therapy or cardiac rupture. The ECG does not change unless there is a postinfarction (Dressler) syndrome, which can occur after (and sometimes with) the acute infarct.

*Type 1 aortic dissections* commonly rupture into the pericardium with rapid hemopericardium and tamponade. Although the pericardium may be irritated if blood leaks beneath the epicardium producing signs and symptoms of acute pericarditis, a compressed coronary vessel may cause infarction. Emergency surgical management is virtually mandatory.

*Pulmonary diseases,* including pulmonary embolism, can involve the pericardium. *Esophageal disorders,* including inflammation, ulcers, and malignancies, can extend to the pericardium, usually with tamponade and a stormy clinical picture, although, rarely, they are relatively silent.

*Postmyocardial and pericardial injury syndromes* are considered to be immunopathic with common features, including response to corticosteroids, latent period, recurrences, fever with pulmonary infiltrates and pleuritis, and sterile blood and pericardial fluid cultures. Immunopathies also include the postmyocardial infarction syndrome and related ones. *Traumatic pericarditis* due to penetrating wounds or nonpenetrating chest injuries (including radiation) produces the signs typical of acute pericarditis or pericardial effusion, with or without tamponade or constriction.

## ▪ VASCULITIS–CONNECTIVE TISSUE DISEASE GROUP

Every member of this group, notably *rheumatoid arthritis,* produces pericardial lesions of every description, except acute rheumatic fever, which scars the pericardium but does not provoke constriction. The differential diagnosis includes idiopathic (presumably viral) pericarditis, which in itself can present with arthropathy. *Systemic lupus erythematosus* is particularly important in this group and must be ruled out in women with the "idiopathic" viral pericardial syndrome, since the latter is so common in men and lupus so frequent in women. Antiinflammatory agents suppress most attacks unless there are complications.

## ▪ DISORDERS OF METABOLISM

In *renal failure,* especially when chronic, pericarditis is quite common, though it occasionally accompanies uncomplicated acute renal failure. Bacterial or viral infection can occur, although bacteria are much less common in the antibiotic era. ECG usually is not helpful. A stubborn form in patients on dialysis, *dialysis pericarditis,* is difficult to treat and sometimes causes huge effusions with variable symptoms. Resection of the pericardium is often necessary. *Myxedema,* increasingly rare, produces large pericardial effusions that are often asymptomatic, often with small electrocardiographic voltage. Tamponade is rare.

## ▪ NEOPLASTIC PERICARDIAL DISEASES

Primary malignant tumors are rare, and benign tumors (like fibromas and lipomas) are uncommon. More important are metastases, particularly from the lungs and breasts, which are relatively common and can present as anything from apparent acute pericarditis to florid tamponade. Hodgkin's disease is the most important of the lymphomas.

## ▪ RECURRENT AND INCESSANT PERICARDITIS

Patients with acute pericarditis, particularly those receiving corticosteroid therapy may have frequently recurring pericarditis requiring new therapy. The term "incessant pericarditis" applies to patients who are asymptomatic only when taking medication. This difficult problem is discussed in detail elsewhere.[7]

## ▪ REFERENCES

1. Spodick DH: Macro- and microphysiology and anatomy of the pericardium. Am Heart J 1992;124:1046–1051.
2. Spodick DH: The Pericardium: A Comprehensive Textbook. New York, Marcel Dekker, 1997, 98–100.
3. Spodick DH: Idiopathic pericarditis: Pericarditis of unknown origin. *In* Spodick DH: The Pericardium: A Comprehensive Textbook. New York, Marcel Dekker, 1997, 417–421.
4. Spodick DH: The pericardial rub: A prospective, multiple observer investigation of pericardial friction in 100 patients. Am J Cardiol 1975;35:357–362.
5. Spodick DH: Diagnostic electrocardiographic sequences in acute pericarditis: Significance of PR segment and PR vector changes. Circulation 1973;48:575–580.

6. Spodick DH: Pathogenesis and clinical correlations of the electrocardiographic abnormalities of pericardial disease. *In* Rios G (ed): Clinico-Electrocardiographic Correlations. Philadelphia: FA Davis, 1977:201–214.
7. Spodick DH: Recurrent and incessant pericarditis. *In* Spodick DH: The Pericardium: A Comprehensive Textbook. New York, Marcel Dekker, 1997, 422–431.

## ▪ RECOMMENDED READING

Fowler NO: The Pericardium in Health and Disease. Mt. Kisco, NY: Futura, 1985.
Reddy PS, Leon DF, Shaver JA (eds): Pericardial Disease. New York: Raven, 1982.
Shabetai R: The Pericardium. New York: Grune & Stratton, 1981.
Spodick DH: The Pericardium: A Comprehensive Textbook. New York: Marcel Dekker, 1997.

*Chapter* 35

# Disorders of the Pulmonary Circulation

*Sean P. Gaine*

Disorders of the pulmonary circulation constitute a diverse group of conditions that arise as a consequence of lung or left-sided heart disease (e.g., emphysema or mitral valve disease), from the pulmonary arteries (e.g., primary pulmonary hypertension [PPH]), or as a consequence of diseases that originate outside of the lungs (e.g., pulmonary embolism, [PE]). This chapter outlines the major causes of pulmonary vascular disease and describes the chief complications of these disorders, pulmonary hypertension and cor pulmonale.

## ■ PULMONARY HYPERTENSION

### Classification of Disorders of the Pulmonary Circulation

Because of the heterogeneity of causes of pulmonary hypertension, no thoroughly satisfactory classification system has been devised. Perhaps the most clinically useful method is to group disorders into three broad groups, intrinsic pulmonary vascular diseases, parenchymal lung disease, and diseases of the left side of the heart.

*Intrinsic pulmonary vascular diseases* include diseases that result from a precapillary increase in pulmonary vascular resistance. These disorders include PPH, Eisenmenger syndrome due to chronic left-to-right intracardiac shunts, and connective tissue diseases such as scleroderma and systemic lupus erythematosus. These diverse conditions result in indistinguishable pathologic findings on lung biopsy. The characteristic findings of smooth muscle hypertrophy, intimal proliferation, and in situ thrombosis are found to various degrees in each of these conditions (Fig. 35–1), so that the pathologic injury pattern is similar, as are the approaches to treatment. Venous thromboembolism can also lead to precapillary or intrinsic pulmonary vascular hypertension either as a result of acute obstruction of a significant portion of the pulmonary vascular bed or as a result of chronic recurring obstruction.

*Parenchymal lung disease* can cause pulmonary hypertension. Chronic bronchitis and emphysema result in a mixture of hypoxic pulmonary vasoconstriction and obliteration of the pulmonary vascular bed. Similarly, individuals with interstitial pulmonary fibrosis (IPF) can develop pulmonary hypertension.

*Diseases of the left side of the heart* can result in postcapillary pulmonary hypertension. Once again, it appears that the degree of pulmonary hypertension may be related to the susceptibility of the host; for example, not all individuals with severe mitral stenosis develop significant pulmonary hypertension. Postcapillary causes of pulmonary hypertension can be identified by elevated pulmonary capillary wedge pressure or left ventricular end-diastolic pressure.

**683**

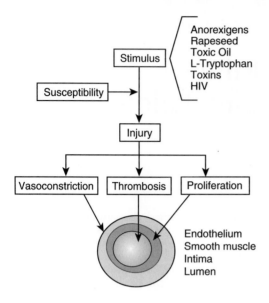

**Figure 35–1** ▪ The development of intrinsic pulmonary vascular disease. An insult or stimulus, in a susceptible individual, results in a characteristic injury pattern (smooth muscle hypertrophy and vasoconstriction, intimal proliferation, and in situ thrombosis).

## Clinical Findings

### Signs and Symptoms

The earliest symptom of pulmonary hypertension is exertional shortness of breath, the gradual onset of which can result in a considerable delay in diagnosis. Other common symptoms include angina (related to right ventricular ischemia), lightheadedness or frank syncope, undue fatigue, and peripheral edema. The degree of symptomatic involvement can be assessed by using the New York Heart Association (NYHA) classification system, grading symptoms I through IV.

Physical examination may suggest the presence of a systemic disease associated with the pulmonary hypertension. Scleroderma may be identified by cutaneous telangiectases and sclerodactyly, and the presence of significant systemic hypertension may suggest underlying obstructive sleep apnea or left ventricular diastolic dysfunction. Clubbing is not seen in PPH; therefore, its presence suggests alternative diagnoses such as congenital heart disease, lung disease, or liver disease.

The findings on physical examination in pulmonary hypertension depend on the severity of disease. The most common findings are an accentuated pulmonic component of the second heart sound in the pulmonic region and a right ventricular S₄ gallop. These may be difficult to appreciate in patients with hyperinflation secondary to emphysema. Patients with severe right ventricular hypertrophy may have a heave palpable along the left sternal border or in the epigastrium. Examination of the neck veins may reveal a prominent "a" wave indicating a noncompliant right ventricle, and as the right ventricle enlarges, "v" waves indicative of tricuspid regurgitation may be seen. When right ventricular decompensation and right-sided heart failure finally develop, the jugular venous pressure increases. Dilatation of the pulmonic valve annulus or right ventricular outflow tract can produce a soft-blowing early diastolic murmur along the upper left sternal border, the Graham Steell murmur of pulmonary regurgitation. The presence of a right ventricular S₃ gallop signifies advanced right heart failure.

## Diagnostic Testing

An extensive battery of diagnostic tests is required in evaluating patients with pulmonary hypertension to define the cause of the condition. If all test results are negative, a diagnosis of PPH can be made (Fig. 35–2). Screening blood tests should include an evaluation of liver function, antibodies to human immunodeficiency virus, and an antinuclear antibody (ANA) and rheumatoid factor to preclude occult collagen-vascular disease. The ANA result may be positive in PPH, usually in a low titer and without other evidence of connective tissue disease. The chest radiograph demonstrates prominence of the central pulmonary arteries and clear lung fields in individuals with intrinsic pulmonary vascular disease but reveals evidence of IPF

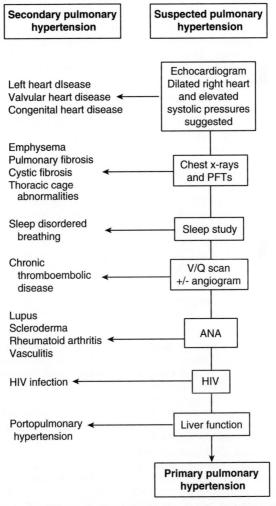

**Figure 35–2** ■ Algorithm for the evaluation of suspected pulmonary hypertension. V/Q, ventilation-perfusion scan; ANA, antinuclear antibody; PFTs, pulmonary function tests; HIV, human immunodeficiency virus. (Gaine SP, Rubin LJ: Primary pulmonary hypertension. Lancet. 1998;352:9124.)

or emphysema in pulmonary hypertension secondary to parenchymal lung disease. The presence of Kerley B lines and pulmonary edema suggests left heart or postcapillary causes of the pulmonary hypertension. An electrocardiogram (ECG) usually demonstrates right-axis deviation, right ventricular hypertrophy, and T-wave changes suggesting strain. Echocardiography is helpful in precluding congenital heart disease or postcapillary causes of pulmonary hypertension such as mitral valve disease or left ventricular dysfunction, and it may be useful in monitoring the response to therapy.[1] The echocardiographic findings of pulmonary hypertension include right heart chamber dilatation, right ventricular hypertrophy, and paradoxic movement of the septum toward the left ventricle during systole. Left ventricular filling may be impaired when there is severe dilatation of the right heart chambers. Doppler studies can estimate the pulmonary artery systolic pressure by measuring either systolic flow velocity across the pulmonic valve or the regurgitant flow across the tricuspid valve. Transesophageal is more sensitive than transthoracic echocardiography in evaluating intracardiac defects such as a patent foramen ovale.

Pulmonary function tests are used to detect the presence of significant parenchymal or airways disease. The 6-minute walk test has also been demonstrated to correlate with both resting hemodynamics and survival in patients with PPH.[2] Arterial blood gas determinations frequently show a chronic respiratory alkalosis, perhaps due to increased activity of intrapulmonary stretch receptors or intravascular baroreceptors causing hyperventilation. An increased carbon dioxide tension may be noted in individuals with underlying obstructive lung disease or hypoventilation due to obesity. Mild hypoxemia is frequently secondary to ventilation-perfusion (V/Q) mismatching; however, more severe hypoxia, when present, may be due to either decreased cardiac output or intracardiac shunting through a patent foramen ovale. Right heart catheterization has a central role in the evaluation of pulmonary hypertension (discussed later).

A V/Q lung scan is essential for precluding chronic thromboembolic disease, and pulmonary angiography is indicated only when segmental or subsegmental perfusion defects are present and suggestive of large-vessel, unresolved chronic thromboembolic disease. Polysomnography is recommended in patients with daytime hypersomnolence, because sleep apnea is associated with the development of pulmonary hypertension.[3] Lung biopsy is rarely necessary in pulmonary hypertension and is reserved for cases in which the clinical diagnosis is unclear.

## Management (Figs. 35–3 and 35–4)

### General Approach

The first step in the management of pulmonary hypertension is to identify and treat the underlying cause (Fig. 35–3). Therefore, in pulmonary hypertension secondary to parenchymal lung disease, improving gas exchange with bronchodilators and reversing hypoxia with oxygen therapy may significantly improve the pulmonary hypertension. Similarly, patients with IPF may experience improvement in their pulmonary hypertension in response to oxygen, high-dose steroids, and immunosuppression. Individuals with obstructive sleep apnea may benefit from nocturnal continuous positive airway pressure (CPAP).[3] Surgical intervention with a pulmonary thromboendarterectomy may be warranted in selected patients with chronic thromboembolic disease involving the more proximal pulmonary arteries.

In all patients with significant pulmonary hypertension, general measures recommended include limiting physical activity to tolerance, avoidance of concomitant medications that can aggravate pulmonary hypertension such as vasoactive decongestants, cardiodepressant antihypertensives such as β-adrenergic blockers, and agents that interfere with warfarin. Environments with reduced oxygen levels

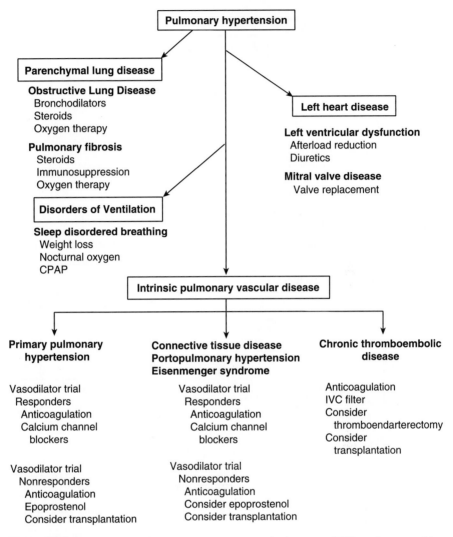

**Figure 35–3** ■ Algorithm for the treatment of pulmonary hypertension. CPAP, continuous positive airway pressure; IVC, inferior vena cava.

such as unpressurized aircraft or high altitude can worsen the condition, and supplemental oxygen may be needed by individuals with borderline oxygenation. The hemodynamic stresses of pregnancy are poorly tolerated. Women with pulmonary hypertension should be counseled on effective nonpharmacologic contraception, because oral contraceptives may increase the risk of venous thrombosis and may directly exacerbate the underlying pulmonary hypertension. Hormone replacement therapy appears to be without significant adverse hemodynamic effects in the postmenopausal population.

## An Approach to Vasodilator Therapy

Smooth muscle hypertrophy and vasoconstriction are present to various degrees in both PPH and secondary pulmonary hypertension. Although vasodilators

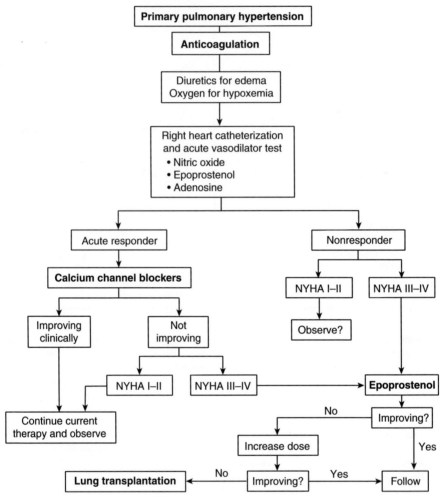

**Figure 35–4** ■ Algorithm for the management of primary pulmonary hypertension. NYHA, New York Heart Association.

may be beneficial in many types of intrinsic pulmonary vascular disease such as PPH, they do not have a significant role in pulmonary hypertension secondary to parenchymal lung disease or disorders of left heart filling. Treatment with vasodilators in pulmonary hypertension can be unpredictable and hazardous, and great care must be exercised to decrease the risk of serious adverse events such as systemic hypotension, syncope, and sudden death.

Patients with intrinsic pulmonary vascular disease should undergo right heart catheterization and a vasodilator trial before empirical vasodilator therapy is begun. Hemodynamic assessment at catheterization can determine the degree of pulmonary hypertension, preclude left heart filling problems, and allow prediction of survival. A vasodilator trial using short-acting agents such as inhaled nitric oxide, epoprostenol, or adenosine (Table 35–1) at the time of catheterization can also

Table 35–1

**Short-Acting Pulmonary Vasodilators**

Nitric oxide (10–80 ppm inhaled)
Adenosine (50–200 ng/kg/min IV)
Prostacyclin (2–12 ng/kg/min IV)

IV, intravenously.

provide a guide to therapy. A decrease in mean pulmonary artery pressure of at least 10 mm Hg and an increase in cardiac output identifies patients with PPH who tend to have sustained hemodynamic improvement and prolonged survival on oral vasodilators.[4] Although approximately 20% to 30% of patients with PPH demonstrate an acute response to vasodilators, the number is even smaller in secondary causes of intrinsic pulmonary vascular disease such as scleroderma. Oral vasodilators are contraindicated in patients who have an adverse hemodynamic response such as a decline in systemic pressure, a reduction in oxygen saturation, or a decrease in cardiac output during the vasodilator trial.

### Calcium Channel Blockers

Patients with PPH and a favorable response to an acute vasodilator trial during right-sided heart catheterization demonstrate improved survival and regression of right ventricular hypertrophy with calcium channel blockers. Indiscriminate use of a calcium channel blocker without first determining the response during a vasodilator trial may result in worsening gas exchange, depressed systolic function, and right heart failure, hypotension, or death.[5] Calcium channel blockers should be started at a low dose, but the final dose required to achieve benefit is generally higher than that used in systemic hypertension. The most commonly used agents are amlodipine (2.5 to 20 mg/day), nifedipine (30 to 240 mg/day), and diltiazem (90 to 900 mg/day). Abrupt discontinuation of these drugs can lead to fatal rebound pulmonary hypertension.

### Epoprostenol (Prostacyclin, PGI₂, Flolan).

Epoprostenol, a potent vasodilator, has been approved in the United States for treatment of PPH. Because of its short half-life (3 to 5 minutes), epoprostenol is delivered intravenously through a permanent indwelling catheter by a continuous-infusion pump. Individuals who have severe PPH and who do not demonstrate a favorable response during acute vasodilator testing are treated with continuous intravenous epoprostenol. In a randomized trial, epoprostenol improved hemodynamics and exercise tolerance and prolonged survival in severe PPH (NYHA III–IV).[2] Epoprostenol may be a bridge to transplantation in patients with PPH, or it may function to defer or avoid lung transplantation. Although epoprostenol is currently approved only for treatment in PPH, the results of a completed randomized trial of epoprostenol in the treatment of secondary pulmonary hypertension in scleroderma also suggest benefit at least in the short term.

Minor side effects of epoprostenol include jaw pain, headache, rash, diarrhea, and joint pain. More serious side effects are related predominantly to the drug delivery system and include life-threatening line sepsis or accidental discontinuation of drug delivery. Dose increments are frequently required during the first year of therapy. The reason for the increased dose requirement over time is unknown but may be related either to increased drug degradation or to increased vasoconstrictive mediators such as thromboxane. Epoprostenol should be avoided in postcapillary pulmonary hypertension because of the risk of acute pulmonary edema.[6] Furthermore, the pulmonary hypertension of parenchymal lung disease is also a relative contraindication to epoprostenol therapy, because nonspecific pulmonary vasodilatation can lead to worsening shunt and hypoxemia.

Inhaled therapy with aerosolized iloprost, a stable prostacyclin analogue, and a long-acting stable prostacyclin analogue, UT15, which is biologically active when delivered subcutaneously, is currently undergoing large-scale prospective study in Europe, North America, and Australia.

## Long-Term Oxygen Therapy

Long-term oxygen therapy is indicated in patients with pulmonary hypertension and documented hypoxemia, either at rest or with exercise. Patients with intrinsic vascular disease such as PPH usually do not have significant hypoxemia, and when it is present, it is usually as a result of right-to-left intracardiac shunting or reduced cardiac output. However, hypoxemia is frequently observed in parenchymal lung disease such as chronic obstructive pulmonary disease (COPD) and IPF. In these patients, survival is improved when hypoxemia is corrected by long-term oxygen therapy.[7] The mechanisms responsible for the beneficial effects of oxygen therapy are likely to be multifactorial, as the improvements in pulmonary hemodymamics in COPD are variable and slow to develop.[8] Continuous positive airway pressure (CPAP) or bilevel positive airway pressure (BiPAP) is used to treat obstructive sleep apnea or chronic alveolar hypoventilation and the hypercarbia that can exacerbate the pulmonary hypertension.

## Anticoagulation

Local thrombus formation on dysfunctional pulmonary vascular endothelium and the development of venous thrombosis secondary to right-sided heart failure, diminished cardiac output, and impaired mobility all are potential risks in all forms of pulmonary hypertension. Two nonrandomized studies have suggested a benefit of anticoagulation in prolonging life in PPH.[9, 10] Recommendations for anticoagulation have been extrapolated to include secondary pulmonary hypertension. Particular care should be taken when initiating warfarin therapy in patients with a history of hemoptysis or with right-sided heart failure and liver dysfunction.

## Diuretics, Inotropes, and Glycosides

Diuretic therapy is frequently required to control edema and reduce right ventricular end-diastolic volume in advancing right-sided heart failure. Patients receiving high-dose calcium channel blocker therapy may also require diuretic therapy for drug-induced edema formation. Patients with ascites require an aldosterone antagonist such as spironolactone. In patients with severe right-sided heart failure, long-term low-dose dopamine may improve right ventricular contractility and enhance diuresis. In parenchymal lung disease, ankle edema may occur as a result of salt retention secondary to hypoxia or steroid use and may not denote a deterioration in right-sided heart function.

Digoxin has been shown to be of benefit in patients with hypoxemic pulmonary hypertension and concomitant left-sided heart dysfunction.[11] The role of digoxin in other forms of pulmonary hypertension is controversial, however. Digoxin may also have a role in counteracting the negative inotropic effect of calcium channel blockers and in antagonizing the neurohumoral activation of right-sided heart failure.[12]

## Nonpharmacologic Therapy

The right ventricular dysfunction in pulmonary hypertension is reversible on restoration of normal pulmonary artery pressures; therefore, double lung transplantation has become the treatment of choice for patients with severe and refractory pulmonary hypertension, reserving heart-lung transplantation for patients with left-sided heart disease or congenital structural abnormalities. Single lung transplantation has also been successfully used as an alternative for patients with pulmonary hypertension. Atrial septostomy, the controlled opening of a right-to-left shunt at the atrial level, is reserved for patients with severe right-sided heart failure or recurrent syncope. The procedure, by decompressing the right ventricle and improving cardiac output, may provide palliation and improved survival. It is hoped that the impact of oxygen desaturation that results is offset by the overall increase in cardiac output and systemic oxygen delivery.

## ▪ VENOUS THROMBOEMBOLISM

Venous thromboembolism has two common clinical manifestations. First, venous thromboembolism may occur as deep venous thrombosis (DVT), most usually in the deep veins of the calf, and then propagate proximally. Second, it is estimated that more than half of all patients with DVT will develop PE. PE is estimated to cause 50,000 deaths per year in the United States.[13] Death due to PE generally occurs rapidly before the diagnosis can be established and treatment implemented. As a result, management of venous thromboembolism focuses primarily on prevention in patients at risk. Indeed, if PE is diagnosed and the patient survives more than 1 hour, mortality is less than 10%; however, if the diagnosis is missed, mortality is sixfold greater.[14, 15] In a study in which PE was found at autopsy to be the cause of death, 24% of cases had undergone surgery a mean period of 7 days before the fatal embolic event.[16]

### Deep Venous Thrombosis

### Risk Factors

DVT usually develops in the deep veins of the calf muscle. Clinical conditions and diseases associated with venostasis, vascular injury, or enhanced blood viscosity increase the risk for DVT. Therefore, the major factors predisposing to DVT include venous stasis due to any cause, trauma, childbirth, malignancy, and increasing age.[13] Other conditions predisposing to DVT include hyperhomocysteinemia, elevated levels of antiphospholipid antibodies, and polycythemia. Activated protein C resistance, an inherited abnormality that involves substitution of glutamine for arginine at position 506 on factor V, renders the factor, termed *factor V Leiden*, more resistant to degradation.[17] The heterozygote state, present in 5% of whites in North America and Europe, carries as great as a fivefold increased lifetime risk for DVT, and homozygotes have an even higher risk. The combination of inheritance of this mutation and oral contraceptive therapy increases the risk of thrombosis some 30-fold. Other less common abnormalities that predispose an individual to venous thromboembolism include deficiencies of antithrombin or of proteins C or S. These risk factors for thrombosis are considered cumulative when more than one is present in an individual.

### Prevention

Anticoagulants are used in those at risk for the development of venous thromboembolism. Low-dose subcutaneous heparin administered at doses of 10,000 to 15,000 units/day in two divided doses is the most frequent form of prophylaxis in both medical and surgical patients. The newer low-molecular-weight heparins have some advantages over the unfractionated heparins, however, and are more effective than warfarin after hip or knee replacement surgery. Mechanical prophylactic methods, such as graded elastic compression stockings and pneumatic compression devices, are also effective. A meta-analysis has shown that elastic stockings, when worn by moderate-risk surgical patients, can reduce the incidence of postoperative DVT by 68%.[18] A combination of anticoagulants and mechanical methods has additive benefits in individuals undergoing abdominal or cardiac surgery or neurosurgery.[19] Vena caval filters are reserved for those patients who have not responded to anticoagulants or for whom anticoagulants are contraindicated.[20] Furthermore, it is recommended that filters be considered in those who would not tolerate a further embolism, such as in those with chronic thromboembolic pulmonary hypertension or poor cardiopulmonary reserve.

## Diagnosis

The differential diagnosis for a suspected DVT includes cellulitis, ruptured Baker cyst, and chronic venous insufficiency. The clinical diagnosis of acute DVT of the lower extremities is insensitive and nonspecific. Duplex ultrasound examination has emerged as the most common technique for diagnosing DVT. The noncompressibility of a venous segment is good indirect evidence of venous thrombosis.[21] Contrast venography is reserved for situations in which ultrasound findings are equivocal, when a false-negative ultrasound result is strongly suspected, or in patients with recurrent DVT. Serial noninvasive evaluations can also be helpful in equivocal cases.[22] Magnetic resonance imaging (MRI) has emerged as a promising tool in the diagnosis of DVT, particularly when ultrasound examination is less helpful, such as for lesions in the calf and pelvis and with recurrent DVT.

Considerable attention has been directed at developing a blood test to aid in the diagnosis of venous thrombosis. The D-dimer, a fibrin degradation product, has utility as a screening agent when used in combination with a noninvasive technique such as ultrasonography, but it is not yet diagnostic when used alone.[23]

## Pulmonary Embolism

### Epidemiology

Like DVT, the diagnosis of PE is often difficult because the presenting symptoms may be nonspecific. A PE is present in only one in four patients in whom it is clinically suspected.[24] Less than 1% of individuals who survive a PE go on to develop chronic thromboembolic pulmonary hypertension (CTPH).[25] Most patients who develop CTPH have no definable abnormality in the clotting cascade, although of all the known abnormalities, the presence of lupus anticoagulant confers the highest risk for developing this condition.

### Clinical Presentation

The PIOPED study identified a triad of dyspnea, tachypnea, and chest pain in 97% of those with a confirmed PE.[24] Patients most commonly present with dyspnea with or without pleuritic chest pain (Table 35–2). Patients with larger emboli may present with hemodynamic instability and syncope. Less common is a chronic nonspecific course mimicking chronic pneumonia or congestive heart failure, particularly in elderly patients. Although numerous signs of PE have been described, tachypnea is the only consistent clinical finding (Table 35–3). Tachycardia is present only 40% of the time, and heart rate rarely exceeds 120 bpm. On auscultation, rales may be heard in 50% of patients, and wheezing is distinctly uncommon. Transient low-grade fevers are not uncommon.[26] In patients with more severe embolic events, the signs of right ventricular dysfunction may be prominent. An increased pul-

Table 35–2

**Symptoms in Patients with Pulmonary Embolism**

| Symptoms | % |
|---|---|
| Dyspnea | 81 |
| Pleuritic chest pain | 72 |
| Apprehension | 59 |
| Cough | 54 |
| Hemoptysis | 34 |
| Syncope | <5 |
| Substernal chest pain | <5 |

Moser KM: Pulmonary embolism: State of the art. Am Rev Respir Dis 115:829, 1977.

monic component of the second heart sound, a right ventricular diastolic gallop, and prominent jugular venous pulse indicate significant right ventricular strain. Hypotension and shock indicate the presence of a massive PE.

## Pathophysiology

### Respiratory Consequences

The degree of cardiopulmonary compromise following an acute PE correlates with the extent of occlusion and the degree of underlying cardiopulmonary disease. Almost every form of abnormal gas exchange has been described in PE. The hypoxia and hypocarbia that generally occur are perhaps best explained by the presence of V/Q inequality and low mixed venous oxygen saturation. Lung units with low V/Q ratios predominate for a number of reasons, resulting in physiologic shunt. Overperfusion of unembolized regions of the lung, atelectasis in lung tissue beyond the embolic obstruction as a result of the loss of surfactant and splinting secondary to pleuritic chest pain, and regional pulmonary hypoperfusion all may lead to alveolar hypocapnia, which can produce localized bronchconstriction and further atelectasis. Bronchoconstriction may also occur as a result of the local release from the clot of factors such as serotonin, which further promote atelectasis. Furthermore, once perfusion resumes and reperfusion occurs, the lung units are further compromised by hemorrhage and edema. The development of an intracardiac shunt secondary to the opening of a patent foramen ovale in the setting of increased right-sided heart pressures can further worsen hypoxemia and shunt.

Table 35–3

**Physical Findings in Patients with Pulmonary Embolism**

| Physical Findings | % |
|---|---|
| Tachypnea | 88 |
| Rales | 54 |
| Increased pulmonic $P_2$ | 54 |
| Pulse >100 bpm | 43 |
| Temperature >37.8°C | 42 |
| $S_3$ or $S_4$ heart sound | 34 |
| Thrombophlebitis | 34 |
| Diaphoresis | 33 |
| Arrhythmias | 15 |
| Blood pressure <100 mm Hg | 3 |

Reproduced with permission from Moser KM: Pulmonary embolism: State of the art. Am Rev Respir Dis 115:829, 1977.

Right ventricular dysfunction and a decrease in cardiac output reduce mixed venous oxygen saturation and exacerbate the hypoxia.

Lung infarction is uncommon because the lungs have a number of possible sources of oxygen, including the pulmonary artery, the bronchial circulation, alveolar oxygen, and back-perfusion from the venous side of the pulmonary circulation. Infarction, when present, is most likely to occur in the periphery, where the bronchial circulation is minimal, and particularly in patients with antecedent cardiopulmonary disease, in whom oxygen supply to the lungs is already compromised.

### Hemodynamic Consequences

The hemodynamic effects of a PE correlate with loss of vascular surface area. In previously normal individuals, the pulmonary artery pressure does not rise until at least 50% of the pulmonary vascular bed is compromised.[27] The right ventricle is poorly equipped to deal with increased afterload. In patients without previous disease, the maximal mean arterial pressure that can be developed and maintained is estimated to be 40 mm Hg. If this load is exceeded, acute cor pulmonale and shock develop. As the right ventricle fails and dilates, left ventricular filling is impeded by a shift in the interventricular septum. Moreover, a decline in systemic pressure may produce right ventricular ischemia due to decreased coronary perfusion during diastole. As the right ventricle fails, the flow through the pulmonary vascular bed decreases and the pulmonary artery pressure may decrease. Therefore, the central venous pressure or right atrial pressure is more reliable than the actual pulmonary artery pressure as a measure of the hemodynamic sequelae of the embolism under these circumstances.

In nonfatal PE, the process of vascular restoration and healing begins, with the objective of restoring vascular luminal patency. In general, both the V/Q scan and the pulmonary angiogram results remain positive for weeks to months after the acute event.[15] Less than 1% of patients have persistent unresolved thrombus and go on to develop CTPH.[25]

## Laboratory Diagnostic Aids

The standard laboratory tests should enhance a clinician's suspicion that an acute PE has occurred. The ECG and chest radiographic findings in acute PE are nonspecific and difficult to distinguish from the abnormalities of preexisting cardiopulmonary disease. The ECG is perhaps most useful in ruling out other acute cardiopulmonary disorders such as acute myocardial infarction or pericarditis. The most frequent ECG finding of PE is tachycardia and non–ST-T wave changes. In the setting of a massive PE, the classic S1-Q3-T3 pattern, right-axis deviation, and P-pulmonale are described.[28] The findings on a chest radiograph can be normal in an acute PE, although nonspecific abnormalities are frequently found, such as focal atelectasis, small pleural effusions, elevation of a hemidiaphragm, or subtle pleural based infiltrates. In more severe cases, engorgement of the central pulmonary arteries or an absence of peripheral vessels (Westermark sign) may be seen.

Arterial blood gas determinations may be useful in the diagnosis of PE. However, arterial blood gas values can be normal in previously healthy young patients. When they are abnormal, the most common finding is a low oxygen tension and widened alveolar-arterial oxygen difference. A normal alveolar-arterial oxygen gradient may be helpful in reducing the need for V/Q scanning. The carbon dioxide tension is usually low but can be elevated in the setting of a massive PE.

V/Q lung scanning remains central to the evaluation of suspected PE. Two or more moderate to large perfusion defects with intact ventilation and normal chest radiographic finding in the involved area represent a high probability of PE. Bronchospasm and pleural effusions can, however, result in an indeterminate scan by altering the ventilation component. The final arbitrator remains the pulmonary angiogram, which, despite its expense and invasiveness, is relatively safe in experienced hands.[24] An intravascular filling defect, when seen on two or more projections, defines the presence of a PE. Newer imaging studies include spiral computed tomography (CT) and MRI. Spiral CT has a sensitivity of greater than 80% and specificity of greater than 90% when compared with pulmonary angiography and is reported to be particularly useful with larger, more proximal PE.[29] Whether the smaller, more distal emboli missed by CT or MRI have any impact on outcome is not yet known.

## Approach to Diagnosis

Clinical diagnosis in PE is unreliable, V/Q scanning is most often nondiagnostic, and angiography is not readily available. Clinical decision making in PE requires integration of both clinical and laboratory data. Clinical suspicion can be expressed by the use of a clinical probability scale divided into three groups: high, intermediate, and low probability[30] (Table 35–4). By viewing DVT and PE as part of a continuum in the disease of venous thromboembolism, we can integrate the information from tests for lower extremity DVT and noninvasive screening for PE to narrow the indications for angiography. Individuals with a nondiagnostic V/Q scan, or either a low- or high-probability scan with discordant clinical probability, should undergo evaluation for DVT. If results of the leg ultrasound study are positive, the patient should be treated for PE. If the ultrasound findings are negative, an angiogram is recommended if there is considerable discrepancy between the V/Q scan findings and the clinical impression (Fig. 35–5).

## Treatment of Venous Thromboembolism

The first step in the management of PE is supportive, including supplemental oxygen and adequate intravenous fluids to maintain right ventricular function. Generally, heparin therapy is initiated on the suspicion of PE before a definitive diagnosis is made. Patients remain on heparin as the evaluation algorithm is pursued. Therapies for PE include pharmacologic, surgical, and combinations of both.

## Heparin

If venous thromboembolism is suspected, intravenous heparin should be administered immediately while the patient is evaluated. Once the diagnosis is confirmed, heparin is either continued intravenously or converted to low-molecular-weight heparin. The intravenous heparin is monitored by measuring the activated partial thromboplastin time (aPTT) and kept 1.5 to 2.3 times control. Because of the obvious difficulties of administering intravenous heparin, attention has focused on alternative anticoagulants with more predictable dose-response characteristics. Low-molecular-weight heparins are the first class of these new agents to enter widespread use and are assuming an increasing role in the everyday management

Table 35–4

### Clinical Probability Scale

| | |
|---|---|
| High probability | Risk factors, unexplained symptoms |
| Intermediate probability | Does not fall neatly into the high or low probability groups |
| Low probability | No risk factors, symptoms can be explained by another condition that is present |

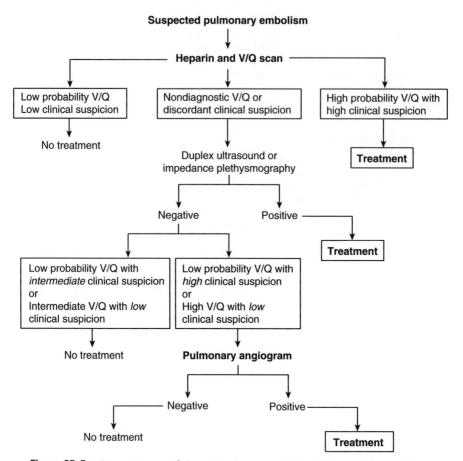

**Figure 35–5** ■ Diagnostic approach for acute pulmonary embolism. V/Q, ventilation-perfusion.

of venous thromboembolism, for both prophylaxis and treatment, facilitating outpatient management of venous thromboembolism. Low-molecular-weight heparins produce less thrombocytopenia and osteopenia than the unfractionated. They are administered subcutaneously in a weight-based dose either once or twice a day. They have a longer effective half-life than unfractionated heparin and interact less with cells and proteins. Because these low-molecular-weight heparins lose their anti-IIa activity, they cannot be monitored using the aPTT, although when indicated, their activity can be followed using an anti-Xa assay.

## Warfarin

Warfarin-based anticoagulants remain the standard of care for long-term outpatient management of venous thromboembolism. Oral anticoagulation is initiated soon after heparin, and the dose adjusted depending on the International Normalized Ratio, which is maintained between 2.0 and 3.0 with a target of 2.5. Numerous drugs, foods, and comorbid conditions can interact with warfarin; thus, careful monitoring is essential. Warfarin has teratogenic side effects and is therefore contraindicated in pregnancy. The length of time that anticoagulation should be continued is controversial and generally tailored to the individual patient, depending on the risk of recurrence. The two greatest risk factors for recurrence are advancing age and a previous episode of thrombosis. Therefore, patients with a first episode before the age of 60 years are generally treated for 3 to 6 months, older individuals for 6 to 12 months, and those with recurrent disease or a nonreversible risk factor, such as cancer or a defined clotting abnormality, are treated for at least a year and probably lifelong.

## Thrombolytics

Urokinase, streptokinase, and tissue plasminogen activator are thrombolytic agents that have been used to treat venous thromboembolism. Thrombolytics are considered for use in those with extensive iliofemoral venous thrombosis because of the high prevalence and morbidity associated with the postthrombotic syndrome after DVT.[31] Thrombolytics should be considered for PE in patients who do not have risk factors for bleeding and who are unstable or have evidence of significant right ventricular dysfunction.[32] The scientific evidence to date has not supported the use of thrombolytics for less extensive PE.[15, 32]

## Nonpharmacologic Interventions

Radiologic intervention using transvenous extraction or fragmentation of pulmonary thromboemoli has been described, although experience with them is limited. Surgical intervention for acute pulmonary embolectomy using cardiopulmonary bypass is available for patients with large, acute, life-threatening clots when standard methods have failed. CTPH develops in less than 1% of patients with PE. These patients may be candidates for pulmonary thromboendarterectomy. This difficult surgery is reserved for centers with considerable expertise. Individuals with proximal accessible pulmonary artery occlusion identified at angiography, spiral CT, or angioscopy are potential candidates. Those with more distal, inaccessible disease should be considered for lung transplantation.

## ■ SUMMARY

Disorders of the pulmonary circulation may result acutely in right ventricular failure; more chronically, the right ventricle adapts and can tolerate considerable pulmonary hypertension. If the afterload is not reduced, however, either with long-term oxygen therapy, with oral or intravenous vasodilators, or by thromboendarterectomy or lung transplantation, the right ventricle inevitably becomes increasingly more dysfunctional, resulting in cor pulmonale and death. Although a significant number of the disorders affecting the pulmonary circulation are idiopathic, many can be prevented either by effective prophylaxis against venous thromboembolism or by rigorous attention to smoking cessation. Although the treatment modalities remain few, significant progress has been made during the past decade, and further advances can be expected in the next few years.

## ■ REFERENCES

1. Hinderliter AL, Willis PW, Barst RJ, et al: Effects of long-term infusion of prostacyclin (epoprostenol) on echocardiographic measures of right ventricular structure and function in primary pulmonary hypertension. Primary Pulmonary Hypertension Study Group. Circulation 1997; 95(6):1479–1486.
2. Barst RJ, Rubin LJ, Long WA, et al: A comparison of continuous intravenous epoprostenol (prostacyclin) with conventional therapy for primary pulmonary hypertension. The Primary Pulmonary Hypertension Study Group. N Engl J Med 1996;334(5):296–302.

3. Weitzenblum E, Krieger J, Apprill M, et al: Daytime pulmonary hypertension in patients with obstructive sleep apnea syndrome. Am Rev Respir Dis 1988;138:345–349.
4. Rich S, Brundage BH: High dose calcium channel blocking therapy for primary pulmonary hypertension: Evidence for long term reduction in pulmonary artery pressure and regression of right ventricular hypertrophy. Circulation 1987;76:135–141.
5. Weir E, Rubin L, Ayres S, et al: The acute administration of vasodilators in primary pulmonary hypertension: Experience from the National Institutes of Health Registry on primary pulmonary hypertension. Am Rev Respir Dis 1989;140:1623–1630.
6. Rubin LJ, Mendoza J, Hood M, et al: Treatment of primary pulmonary hypertension with continuous intravenous prostacyclin (epoprostenol). Results of a randomized trial. Ann Intern Med 1990;112:485–491.
7. Group NOTT: Continuous or nocturnal oxygen therapy in hypoxemic chronic obstructive lung disease. Ann Intern Med 1980;93:391–398.
8. Timms R, Khaja F, Williams GEA: Hemodynamic response to oxygen therapy in chronic obstructive pulmonary disease. Ann Intern Med 1985;102:29–36.
9. Fuster V, Steele PM, Edwards WD, et al: Primary pulmonary hypertension: Natural history and the importance of thrombosis. Circulation 1984;70(4):580–587.
10. Rich S, Kaufmann E, Levy PS: The effect of high doses of calcium-channel blockers on survival in primary pulmonary hypertension. N Engl J Med 1992;327(2):76–81.
11. Mathur P, Powles R, Pugsley S, et al: Effect of digoxin on right ventricular function in severe chronic airflow obstruction. Ann Intern Med 1981;95:283–288.
12. Nootens M, Kaufmann E, Rector T, et al: Neurohumoral activation in patients with right ventricular failure from pulmonary hypertension: Relation to hemodynamics and endothelin levels. J Am Coll Cardiol 1995;26:1581–1585.
13. Clagett G, Anderson F, Heit J, et al: Prevention of venous thromboembolism. Chest 1995;108:312S–334S.
14. Dalen J, Alpert J: Natural history of pulmonary embolism. In Sasahara A, Sonnenblick E, Lesch M (eds): Pulmonary Embolism. New York: Grune & Stratton, 1975:77–88.
15. Urokinase Trial. Urokinase pulmonary embolism trial: A cooperative study. Circulation 1973;47(Suppl II):1–108.
16. Sandler D, Martin J: Autopsy proven pulmonary embolism in hospital patients: Are we detecting enough deep vein thrombosis? J R Soc Med 1989;82:203–205.
17. Price D, Ridker P: Factor V Leiden mutation and the risks of thromboembolic disease: A clinical perspective. Ann Intern Med 1997;127:895–903.
18. Wells P, Lensing A, Hirsh J: Graduated compression stockings in the prevention of postoperative venous thromboembolism: A meta-analysis. Arch Intern Med 1994;154:67–72.
19. Agnelli G, Piovella P, Buoncristiani P, et al: Enoxaparin plus compression stockings alone in the prevention of venous thromboembolism following elective neurosurgery. N Engl J Med 1998;339:80–85.
20. Decousus H, Leizorovicz A, Parent F, et al: A clinical trial of vena cava filters in the prevention of pulmonary embolism in patients with proximal deep-vein thrombosis. N Engl J Med 1998;338:409–415.
21. Heijboer H, Buller H, Lensing A, et al: A comparison of real-time compression ultrasonography with impedence plethysmography for the diagnosis of deep venous thrombosis in symptomatic outpatients. N Engl J Med 1993;329:1365–1369.
22. Huisman M, Buller H, ten Cate J, Vreeken J: Serial impedence plethysmography for suspected deep venous thrombosis in outpatients: The Amsterdam General Practioners Study. N Engl J Med 1986;314:823–828.
23. Ginsberg J, Kearon C, Douketis J, et al: The use of D-dimer testing and impedence plethysmographic examination in patients with clinical indications of deep venous thrombosis. Arch Intern Med 1997;157:1077–1081.
24. PIOPED: Value of the ventilation/perfusion scan in acute pulmonary embolism—results of the prospective investigation of pulmonary embolism diagnosis (PIOPED). JAMA 1990;263:2753–2759.
25. Moser K, Auger W, Fedullo P: Chronic major-vessel thromboembolic pulmonary hypertension. Circulation 1990;81:1735–1743.
26. Bell W, Simon T, De Mets D: The clinical features of submassive and massive pulmonary emboli. Am J Med 1977;62:355–360.
27. Dexter L, Smith G: Quantitative studies of pulmonary embolism. Am J Med Sci 1964;247:641–648.
28. Stein P, Dalen J, McIntyre K, et al: The electrocardiogram in acute pulmonary embolism. Prog Cardiovasc Dis 1975;17:247–257.
29. Reny-Jardin M, Reiny J, Deschildre F, et al: Diagnosis of acute pulmonary embolism with spiral CT: Comparison with pulmonary angiography and scintigraphy. Radiology 1996;200:6998–7006.
30. Stein P, Henry J, Gottschalk A: The addition of clinical assessment to stratification according to prior cardiopulmonary disease further optimizes the interpretation of ventilation/perfusion scans in pulmonary embolism. Chest 1993;104:1472–1476.
31. Pradoni P, Lensing A, Cogo A, et al: The long-term clinical course of acute deep venous thrombosis. Ann Intern Med 1996;125:1–7.
32. Dalen J, Alpert J: Thrombolytic therapy for pulmonary embolism: Is it effective? Is it safe? When is it indicated? Arch Intern Med 1997;157:2550–2556.

# ▪ RECOMMENDED READING

D'Alonzo G, Bower J, et al: The mechanism of abnormal gas exchange in acute massive pulmonary embolism. Am Rev Respir Dis 1983;128:170–172.

D'Alonzo G, Barst RJ, Ayres SM, et al: Survival in patients with primary pulmonary hypertension. Results from a national prospective registry. Ann Intern Med 1991;115(5):343–349.

Fedullo P, Auger W, Channick R, et al: Chronic thromboembolic pulmonary hypertension. Clin Chest Med 1995;16:353–374.

Gaine S, Rubin L: Medical and surgical treatment options for pulmonary hypertension. Am J Med Sci 1998;315(3):179–184.

Gaine S, Rubin L: Primary pulmonary hypertension. Lancet 1998;352:9124.

Hyers T: Venous thromboembolism: State of the art. Am J Respir Crit Care Med 1999;159:1–14.

Rubin LJ: Primary pulmonary hypertension. N Engl J Med 1997;336(2):111–117.

Wagenvoort C, Wagenvoort N: Pathology of pulmonary hypertension. New York: John Wiley & Sons, 1977.

# Chapter 36

# Diseases of the Aorta

Eric M. Isselbacher

The largest artery in the body, the aorta, receives blood pumped from the left ventricle and distributes it distally to the branch arteries. Although it is one continuous vessel, its segments have been distinguished anatomically. The aorta begins in the anterior mediastinum above the aortic valve as the ascending aorta, the most proximal portion of which is also called the *aortic root*. This is followed in the superior mediastinum by the aortic arch, which gives rise to the brachiocephalic arteries. The descending thoracic aorta then courses in the posterior mediastinum to the level of the diaphragm, after which it becomes the abdominal aorta, which then bifurcates distally into the common iliac arteries.

## ■ AORTIC ANEURYSMS

Aortic aneurysm, a pathologic dilatation of the aorta, is one of the most commonly encountered aortic diseases. Aneurysms may involve any part of the aorta, but they are much more common in the abdominal than in the thoracic aorta. Abdominal aortic aneurysms have a prevalence of at least 3% in the population older than 50 years and are four to five times more common in men than in women.[1] The infrarenal aorta is the segment most often involved. Among thoracic aortic aneurysms, aneurysms of the descending aorta are most common. Frequently, such descending thoracic aortic aneurysms extend distally and involve the abdominal aorta as well, producing a *thoracoabdominal aortic aneurysm.*

### Causes

Atherosclerosis is the major underlying cause of abdominal aortic aneurysms. While the mechanism by which atherosclerosis promotes the growth of aneurysms is not known for certain, it appears that the atherosclerotic thickening of the aortic intima reduces diffusion of oxygen and nutrients from the aortic lumen to the media, in turn causing degeneration of the elastic elements of the media and weakening of the aortic wall.[2] As the aorta begins to dilate, tension on the wall increases, thus promoting further expansion of the aneurysm. There also appears to be a genetic predisposition to the development of abdominal aortic aneurysms: as many as 28% of first-degree relatives of persons with abdominal aneurysms may be affected.[3]

Atherosclerosis is also a common cause of aneurysms of the descending thoracic aorta. However, the most important cause of ascending aortic aneurysms is a process known as *cystic medial necrosis* or *degeneration,* which appears histologically as smooth muscle cell necrosis and degeneration of elastic layers within the media. Cystic medial necrosis is found in almost all patients with Marfan syndrome, a group at very high risk for aortic aneurysm formation at relatively young age. Among patients without overt evidence of connective tissue disease, it is unclear what, specifically, predisposes to the development of such medial degeneration, although a history of hypertension is a common risk factor. Syphilis was once a common cause of thoracic aortic aneurysms but today is rare. Less common causes of thoracic aortic aneurysms include great vessel arteritis (aortitis), aortic trauma, and aortic dissection. Often, thoracic aortic aneurysms are idiopathic.

## Clinical Manifestations

The large majority of abdominal and thoracic aortic aneurysms are asymptomatic and are discovered incidentally on a routine physical examination or imaging study. When patients with abdominal aortic aneurysms do experience symptoms, the most frequent complaint is pain in the hypogastrium or lower back. The pain typically has a steady, gnawing quality and may last for hours or days. New or worsening pain may herald aneurysm expansion or impending rupture. Rupture of an abdominal aneurysm is often accompanied by the triad of pain, hypotension, and a pulsatile abdominal mass. Thoracic aortic aneurysms may cause chest or back pain from aneurysm expansion or compression of adjacent structures. Aneurysms of the ascending aorta often produce aortic insufficiency (due to dilatation of the aortic root), so patients may present with congestive heart failure or a diastolic murmur.

## Diagnosis

Abdominal aortic aneurysms may be palpable on physical examination, although even large aneurysms are sometimes obscured by body habitus. Typically, abdominal aortic aneurysms are hard to "size" accurately by physical examination alone, as adjacent structures often make an aneurysm feel larger than it actually is. Thoracic aortic aneurysms, on the other hand, cannot be palpated at all.

The definitive diagnosis of an aortic aneurysm is made by radiographic examination. Abdominal aortic aneurysms can be detected and sized by either abdominal ultrasonography or computed tomography (CT). Ultrasound is extremely sensitive and is the most practical method of screening for abdominal aortic aneurysms. While mass screening is not currently considered cost-effective, screening with ultrasound is generally recommended for patients considered to be at risk for aortic aneurysms.[4] CT is even more accurate and can size aneurysms to within a diameter of $\pm$ 2 mm. Thus, it is the preferred modality for following growth of an aneurysm over time.

Thoracic aortic aneurysms are frequently recognized on chest radiographs, where they often produce widening of the mediastinal silhouette, enlargement of the aortic knob, or displacement of the trachea from the midline. CT is an excellent modality for detecting and sizing thoracic aneurysms and for following growth over time. Transthoracic echocardiography, which generally visualizes the aortic root and ascending aorta well, is useful for screening patients with Marfan syndrome because they are at particular risk for aneurysms in this area.

## Prognosis

Most aneurysms expand over time, and the rate of growth tends to increase with the aneurysm's size. The major risk associated with an aortic aneurysm in any location is rupture. The risk of rupture increases with aneurysm size, because, in accordance with Laplace's law (i.e., wall tension is proportional to the product of pressure and radius), as the diameter of the aorta increases its wall tension rises. Abdominal aortic aneurysms smaller than 4.0 cm have no more than a 2% risk of rupture, whereas those larger than 5.0 cm have a 22% risk of rupture within 2 years.[5] The overall mortality rate associated with rupture of an abdominal aortic aneurysm is 80%; even for those who reach the hospital, it is 50%. Thoracic aneurysms smaller than 5.0 cm typically expand slowly and rarely rupture, but the rate of growth and risk of rupture increase significantly for aneurysms of 6.0 cm or larger. Rupture of thoracic aneurysms carries an early mortality risk of 76% at 24 hours.[6]

## Treatment

Patients whose aneurysms are not at significant risk of rupture should be managed medically. The goal of medical therapy is to reduce the rate of aneurysm expansion and the risk of future rupture. Beta blockers are the mainstay of this approach, but additional antihypertensive agents are often required. Both thoracic and abdominal aortic aneurysms should be followed closely with serial imaging studies (such as CT) to detect progressive enlargement over time that may indicate the need for surgical repair.

Size is the major indicator for repair of aortic aneurysms. Abdominal aortic aneurysms larger than 5.0 cm should be repaired in good operative candidates, and aneurysms larger than 4.0 cm should be monitored every 6 months. Patients with thoracic aortic aneurysms greater than 6.0 cm should undergo surgical repair, while those with Marfan syndrome should have repair when the aneurysm is 5.5 cm or larger.[7] Surgical repair consists of resection of the aneurysmal portion of the aorta and insertion of a synthetic, prosthetic tube graft. When aneurysms involve aortic segments with branch arteries, such branches may need to be reimplanted into the graft. Similarly, when a dilated aortic root must be replaced in the repair of an ascending thoracic aortic aneurysm, the coronary arteries must be reimplanted. A promising alternative approach currently under investigation for repair of abdominal aortic—and some descending thoracic—aneurysms is the placement of an expandable endovascular stent graft inside the aneurysm via a percutaneous catheter.[8]

## ■ AORTIC DISSECTION

Although aortic dissection is far less common than aortic aneurysms, it is a life-threatening condition with an early mortality rate as high as 1% per hour. With prompt early diagnosis and treatment, however, survival can be dramatically improved. The process of aortic dissection begins with a tear in the aortic intima that exposes a diseased medial layer to the systemic pressure of blood in the aortic lumen. The systolic force of aortic blood flow may cleave the media longitudinally into two layers, producing a blood-filled false lumen within the aortic wall that propagates distally (or sometimes retrograde) for some distance. The result is two lumens, a true one and a false lumen, separated by an intimal flap.

Aortic dissections are classified by location, according to one of several systems (Fig. 36–1). Two thirds of aortic dissections are type A, and the remainder are type B. The classification schemes are intended to distinguish dissections that involve the ascending aorta from those that do not. Involvement of the ascending aorta carries a high risk of early aortic rupture and death from cardiac tamponade, whereas lesions that do not involve the ascending aorta carry much lower risk. Therefore, prognosis and management differ according to the extent of aortic involvement.

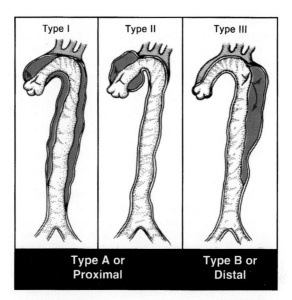

**Figure 36–1** ■ Classification systems for aortic dissection. (From Isselbacher EM, Eagle KA, DeSanctis RW: Diseases of the aorta. *In* Braunwald E (ed): Heart Disease: A Textbook of Cardiovascular Medicine, 5th ed. Philadelphia: WB Saunders, 1997:1555.)

## Causes

Disease of the aortic media, with degeneration of the medial collagen and elastin, is the most common predisposing factor for aortic dissection. Patients with Marfan syndrome have classic cystic medial degeneration and are at particularly high risk for aortic dissection at a relatively young age. The incidence of aortic dissection in patients without Marfan syndrome peaks in the sixth and seventh decades of life, men being affected twice as often as women.[9] A history of hypertension is present in the large majority of cases. A biscupid aortic valve is a less common risk factor. Iatrogenic trauma from catheterization procedures or cardiac surgery may also cause aortic dissection.

## Clinical Manifestations

The most common presenting symptom of aortic dissection is severe pain, which occurs in 74% to 90% of cases. The pain is typically retrosternal or interscapular, but it can appear in the neck or throat or in the lower back, abdomen, or lower extremities, depending on the location of the dissection. In fact, the pain may migrate as the dissection propagates distally. The pain is often of abrupt onset and is most severe at the start. It is sometimes described as *tearing, ripping,* or *stabbing.* Less typical presentations include congestive heart failure (due to acute aortic insufficiency), syncope, stroke, and mesenteric ischemia.

Hypertension on presentation is a common finding, especially among most of those with type B aortic dissection. Hypotension can also occur, particularly among those with type A dissections, and it suggests rupture into the pericardium (causing cardiac tamponade) or severe aortic insufficiency. It is essential to recognize *pseudohypotension,* a falsely low blood pressure that is due to involvement of the affected extremity's subclavian artery by the dissection. Pulse deficits are a common finding on physical examination when there is involvement of any of the subclavian, carotid, or femoral arteries. Acute aortic insufficiency may occur in as many as half of persons with type A dissection. While congestive heart failure or a widened pulse pressure should raise suspicion, the diastolic murmur is often difficult to appreciate.

Involvement of branch arteries by the aortic dissection may produce a variety of vascular complications. Compromise of the ostium of a coronary artery (the right is most often involved) may cause myocardial ischemia or acute infarction.[9] Involvement of the brachiocephalic or left common carotid artery may produce a stroke or coma. A dissection that extends into the abdominal aorta may compromise flow to one or both renal arteries and produce acute renal failure with an exacerbation of hypertension. Another consequence may be mesenteric ischemia presenting as abdominal pain. Finally, an extensive dissection may compromise one of the common iliac arteries, causing femoral pulse deficits or lower extremity ischemia.

The findings on chest radiography typically are nonspecific and rarely diagnostic. An enlarged mediastinal silhouette is present in as many as 90% of cases[9, 10] and is often the factor that first prompts suspicion of aortic dissection in patients with chest pain. A small left pleural effusion (a transudate produced by the inflamed aortic wall) is commonly seen when the descending thoracic aorta is involved. It should be emphasized that a normal chest film *never* rules out the diagnosis of aortic dissection.

## Diagnosis

When the possibility of aortic dissection is being considered, it is essential that the examiner promptly confirm or exclude the diagnosis with an appropriate imaging study. CT, magnetic resonance imaging (MRI), transesophageal echocardiography (TEE), and aortography can accurately demonstrate aortic dissection. In a tertiary care center, when suspicion of aortic dissection is great, TEE (Fig. 36–2) is usually the study of choice, as it provides sufficient detail to enable the surgeon to take the patient directly to the operating room for aortic repair if necessary.[11] When clinical suspicion is lower and the goal is to rule out aortic dissection, contrast-enhanced CT (Fig. 36–3) is generally preferred, since it is entirely noninvasive. In community hospitals where TEE is not readily available, contrast-enhanced CT should be performed in all cases; if findings are positive, the patient can be transferred promptly to a tertiary care center for definitive treatment. When clinically significant branch artery involvement is suspected, aortography may be necessary to adequately define the arterial anatomy.[11]

## Treatment

The goal of medical therapy is to halt further progression of the aortic dissection and to reduce the risk of rupture. Whenever there is a suspicion of aortic dissection, medical therapy should be instituted immediately while imaging studies are ordered, rather than waiting for the diagnosis to be confirmed. The primary goal of therapy is to reduce the systolic force of blood ejected from the heart into the aortic lumen by reducing $dP/dt$. The secondary goal is to reduce systolic blood pressure to 100 to 120 mm Hg, or to the lowest level that sustains cerebral, cardiac, and renal perfusion. Beta-blockers are the first-line therapy to achieve these goals, and intravenous agents such as propranolol, metoprolol, or (ultrashort-acting) esmolol should be administered. Intravenous labetalol, which acts as both an alpha- and a beta-blocker, may be particularly useful in aortic dissection for reducing both

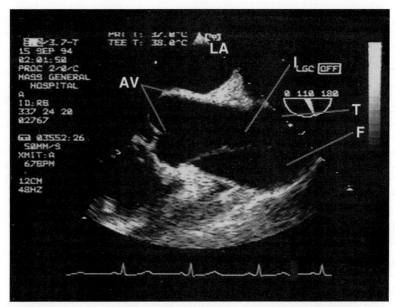

**Figure 36–2** ■ A transesophageal echocardiogram of the ascending aorta in long axis in a patient with a type A aortic dissection. The aortic valve (AV) is on the left, and the ascending aorta extends to the right. Within the aorta is an intimal flap (I) that originates at the level of the sinotubular junction. The true (T) and the false (F) lumens are separated by the intimal flap. LA, left atrium. (Isselbacher EM, Eagle KA, DeSanctis RW: Diseases of the aorta. *In* Braunwald E (ed): Heart Disease: A Textbook of Cardiovascular Medicine, 5th ed. Philadelphia: WB Saunders, 1997.)

dP/dt and hypertension. Finally, after beta-blocker therapy has been instituted, intravenous nitroprusside may be added to control hypertension more precisely minute to minute.

When a patient first presents with aortic dissection the physician must always document which arm has the higher blood pressure and then use only that arm for subsequent hemodynamic monitoring. Moreover, when patients present with

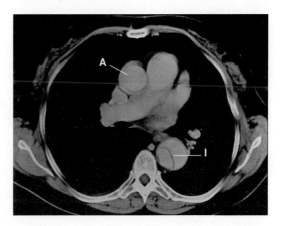

**Figure 36–3** ■ Contrast-enhanced CT of the chest shows an intimal flap (I) separating the two lumens of the descending thoracic aorta in a type B aortic dissection. Note that there is no evidence of a dissection flap in the ascending aorta (A).

significant hypotension, *pseudohypotension* should be conclusively excluded. When true hypotension occurs due to hemopericardium and cardiac tamponade, patients should be treated with volume expansion and taken to surgery without delay, as early mortality in this setting is extremely high. Pericardiocentesis should be performed only as a last resort in this setting as it may precipitate hemodynamic collapse and death.[12]

After the diagnosis of aortic dissection has been confirmed, medical or surgical therapy must be chosen. Whenever an acute dissection involves the ascending aorta, surgical repair is indicated to minimize the risk of life-threatening complications such as rupture, cardiac tamponade, or severe aortic insufficiency. Conversely, if the dissection is confined to the descending aorta, patients have been found to fare as well with medical therapy as with surgical repair.[13] When a type B dissection is associated with a serious complication, such as end-organ ischemia, surgery is indicated.

## Prognosis

Regardless of whether they are treated medically or surgically, patients with acute aortic dissection who survive the initial hospitalization generally do well thereafter. Possible late complications include aneurysm formation (and possible rupture), recurrent dissection, and aortic insufficiency. Medications to reduce dP/dt and control hypertension can dramatically reduce the risk of such late complications and should, therefore, be continued indefinitely.[14] A beta-blocker is the drug of choice in this setting, but, typically, additional medications will be needed to bring systolic blood pressure below 130 mm Hg. Patients are at highest risk of complications during the first 2 years after aortic dissection. Progressive aneurysm expansion typically occurs without symptoms, so patients must be followed closely with serial aortic imaging. This can be done with CT, MRI, or TEE. We prefer MRI, as it is entirely noninvasive and provides superior anatomic detail in multiple imaging planes. All patients should have a baseline imaging study before hospital discharge and follow-up examinations, initially at 6-month intervals and then annually provided that the anatomy is stable.

## ■ INTRAMURAL HEMATOMA OF THE AORTA

Intramural hematoma of the aorta is best defined as an atypical form of classic aortic dissection. It occurs when the vasa vasorum ruptures within the aortic media, producing a contained hemorrhage in the aortic wall.[15] This hematoma may then propagate longitudinally along the aorta, but, since the intimal layer remains intact, the hematoma does not communicate with the aortic lumen. While intramural hematoma of the aorta is clinically indistinguishable from aortic dissection, on cross-sectional imaging it appears as a crescent-shaped thickening around the aortic wall (Fig. 36-4) rather than as true and false lumens separated by an intimal flap.[16] It is important to note that an intramural hematoma may go undetected on aortography. The prognosis and management of intramural hematoma are essentially the same as those for classic aortic dissection.[15]

## ■ TAKAYASU ARTERITIS

### Definition

Takayasu arteritis is a chronic inflammatory disease of unknown cause that involves the aorta and its branches. Typically, it affects young women: mean age of

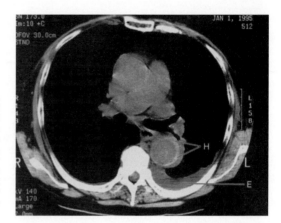

**Figure 36–4** ■ Intramural hematoma of the aorta. CT scan without contrast enhancement demonstrates crescentic thickening (of increased density) of the aortic wall, a finding consistent with an intramural hematoma (H). A left pleural effusion (E) is also present. (Isselbacher EM, Eagle KA, DeSanctis RW: Diseases of the aorta. *In* Braunwald E (ed): Heart Disease: A Textbook of Cardiovascular Medicine, 5th ed. Philadelphia: WB Saunders, 1997:1568.)

onset is 29 years and women are affected eight times as often as men.[17] It occurs more often in Asia and Africa than in Europe or North America and, typically, has two stages. The first is an early stage of active inflammation involving the aorta and its branches. This progresses (at a variable rate) to a sclerotic stage marked by intimal hyperplasia, medial degeneration, and obliterative changes of the aorta and affected arteries. The majority of the resulting arterial lesions are stenotic, but aneurysms can also occur. The aortic arch and brachiocephalic vessels are most often affected, but the abdominal aorta is also commonly involved. The pulmonary artery is occasionally involved. The disease may be diffuse or patchy, affected areas being separated by lengths of normal aorta.

## Clinical Manifestations

Most patients present initially with symptoms of a systemic inflammatory process such as fever, night sweats, arthralgias, and weight loss. There is often a delay of months to years between the onset of symptoms and the time the diagnosis is made. Indeed, at the time of diagnosis, 90% of patients have already entered the sclerotic phase and suffer symptoms of vascular insufficiency, typically with pain in the upper (or, less often, the lower) extremities.[18] Often pulses are absent and blood pressures diminished in the upper extremities, and bruits may be heard over affected arteries. Significant hypertension due to renal artery involvement occurs in more than half of patients, but it may be difficult to recognize because of the diminished pulses. Aortic insufficiency may result from proximal aortic involvement. Congestive heart failure may result from either the hypertension or aortic insufficiency. Involvement of the coronary artery ostia may cause angina or myocardial infarction, and carotid artery involvement may cause cerebral ischemia or stroke. Abdominal angina may result from mesenteric artery compromise. The overall 15-year survival for persons diagnosed with Takayasu arteritis is 83%, the majority of deaths being due to stroke, myocardial infarction, or congestive heart failure.[19] The survival rate for those with major complications of the disease is as low as 66%, whereas it may be as high as 96% for those without a major complication.

## Diagnosis

During the acute phase, laboratory abnormalities include an elevated erythrocyte sedimentation rate, mild leukocytosis, anemia, and elevated immunoglobulin levels. The diagnosis is made most accurately, however, by the angiographic findings of stenosis of the aorta and stenosis or occlusion of its branch vessels, often with poststenotic dilatation or associated aneurysms. Specific clinical criteria have been proposed for making a definitive diagnosis of Takayasu arteritis.[20]

## Treatment

The primary therapy for persons in the acute inflammatory stage of Takayasu arteritis is corticosteroids, which may ameliorate the constitutional symptoms and slow the erythrocyte sedimentation rate and the progression of disease.[21] When steroid therapy is ineffective, cyclophosphamide or methotrexate may be added. Nevertheless, it is not known whether medical therapy actually reduces the risk of major complications or prolongs life. Surgery may be necessary to bypass or reconstruct segments of the aorta or branch arteries. Most often, surgery is performed to bypass the coronary, carotid, or renal arteries or to treat aortic insufficiency. More recently, as an alternative to surgery, balloon angioplasty has been used successfully to dilate stenotic lesions of either the aorta or the renal arteries.

## ▪ REFERENCES

1. Bengtsson H, Bergquist D, Sternby NH: Increasing prevalence of abdominal aortic aneurysms: A necropsy study. Eur J Surg 1992;158:19–23.
2. Holmes DR, Liao S, Parks WC, Thompson RW: Medial neovascularization in abdominal aortic aneurysms: A histopathologic marker of aneurysm degeneration with pathophysiologic implications. J Vasc Surg 1995;21:761–771.
3. Webster MW, Ferrell RF, St Jean PL, et al: Ultrasound screening of first-degree relatives of patients with abdominal aortic aneurysm. J Vasc Surg 1991;13:9–13.
4. Cole CW: Prospects for screening for abdominal aortic aneurysms. Lancet 1997;349:1490–1491.
5. Limet R, Sakalihassan N, Adelin A: Determination of the expansion rate and incidence of rupture of abdominal aortic aneurysms. J Vasc Surg 1991;14:540–548.
6. Johansson G, Markström U, Swedenborg J: Ruptured thoracic aortic aneurysms: A study of incidence and mortality rates. J Vasc Surg 1995;21:985–988.
7. Treasure T: Elective replacement of the aortic root in Marfan's syndrome (Editorial). Br Heart J 1993;69:1013.
8. Katzen BT, Becker GJ, Benenati JF, Zemel G: Stent grafts for aortic aneurysms: The next interventional challenge. Am J Cardiol 1998;81(7A):33E–43E.
9. Spittell PC, Spittell JA, Joyce JW, et al: Clinical features and differential diagnosis of aortic dissection: Experience with 236 cases (1980 through 1990). Mayo Clin Proc 1993;68:642–651.
10. Slater EE, DeSanctis RW: The clinical recognition of dissecting aortic aneurysm. Am J Med 1976;60:625–633.
11. Cigarroa JA, Isselbacher EM, DeSanctis RW, Eagle KA: Diagnostic imaging in the evaluation of suspected aortic dissection: Old standards and new directions. N Engl J Med 1993;328:35–43.
12. Isselbacher EM, Cigarroa JE, Eagle KA: Cardiac tamponade complicating proximal aortic dissection: Is pericardiocentesis harmful? Circulation 1994;90:2375–2378.
13. Glower DD, Fann JI, Speier RH, et al: Comparison of medical and surgical therapy for uncomplicated descending aortic dissection. Circulation 1990;82(Suppl IV):IV–39–46.
14. Neya K, Omoto R, Kyo S, et al: Outcome of Stanford type B acute aortic dissection. Circulation 1992;86(Suppl II):II–1–7.
15. Nienaber CA, von Kodolitsch Y, Petersen B, et al: Intramural hemorrhage of the thoracic aorta. Circulation 1995;92:1465–1472.
16. Lui RC, Menkis AH, McKenzie FN: Aortic dissection without intimal rupture: Diagnosis and management. Ann Thorac Surg 1992;53:886–888.
17. Procter CD, Hollier LH: Takayasu's arteritis and temporal arteritis. Ann Vasc Surg 1992;6:195–198.
18. Lupi-Herrera E, Sanchez-Torres G, Marcushamer J, et al: Takayasu's arteritis. Clinical study of 107 cases. Am Heart J 1977;93:94–103.
19. Ishikawa K, Maetani S: Long term outcome for 120 Japanese patients with Takayasu's disease. Circulation 1994;90:1855–1860.
20. Ishikawa K: Diagnostic approach and proposed criteria for the clinical diagnosis of Takayasu's arteriopathy. J Am Coll Cardiol 1988;12:964–972.
21. Shelhamer JH, Volkman DJ, Parrillo JE, et al: Takayasu's arteritis and its therapy. Ann Intern Med 1985;103:121–126.

# ■ RECOMMENDED READING

Cigarroa JA, Isselbacher EM, DeSanctis RW, Eagle KA: Diagnostic imaging in the evaluation of suspected aortic dissection: Old standards and new directions. N Engl J Med 1993;328:35.

Davies MJ: Aortic aneurysm formation: Lessons from human studies and experimental models. Circulation 1998;98:193–195.

Isselbacher EM, Eagle KA, DeSanctis RW: Diseases of the aorta. *In* Braunwald E (ed): Heart Disease: A Textbook of Cardiovascular Medicine, 5th ed. Philadelphia: WB Saunders, 1997:1546–1581.

Nienaber CA, von Kodolitsch Y, Petersen B, et al: Intramural hemorrhage of the thoracic aorta. Circulation 1995;92:1465.

Shores J, Berger KR, Murphy EA, Pyeritz RE: Progression of aortic dilatation and the benefit of long-term β-adrenergic blockade in Marfan's syndrome. N Engl J Med 1994;330:1335.

Section XI
## MISCELLANEOUS

*Chapter 37*

# Pregnancy and Cardiovascular Disease

*Samuel C. Siu* ▪ *Jack M. Colman*

## ▪ THE CARDIOVASCULAR SYSTEM DURING PREGNANCY

During pregnancy, hormonally mediated changes in blood volume, red cell mass, and heart rate produce a 50% increase in intravascular volume and cardiac output that peaks during the second trimester and remains constant through the remainder of the pregnancy.[1] Gestational hormones, circulating prostaglandins, and the low-resistance vascular bed in the placenta contribute to concomitant decreases in peripheral vascular resistance and blood pressure. During labor and delivery, pain and uterine contractions further increase cardiac output and blood pressure. Immediately after parturition, relief of caval compression and autotransfusion from the emptied and contracted uterus produce yet another increase in cardiac output. The hemodynamic changes of pregnancy persist at least several days post partum and may not fully resolve for 6 months.

As a result of physiologic changes, many pregnant women without cardiac disease may have symptoms that mimic those associated with cardiac disease.[2] Common symptoms experienced by pregnant women without heart disease include fatigue, dyspnea, and light-headedness. A displaced apical impulse, prominent jugular venous pulsations, widely split first and second heart sounds, and soft ejection systolic murmurs are frequent during normal pregnancy. Sinus tachycardia, premature atrial or ventricular ectopic beats, right or left axis deviation, ST segment depression, and T wave changes have also been observed on 12-lead electrocardiograms (ECG) of normal, healthy pregnant women. There may be straightening of the left upper heart border and increased lung markings on the chest radiograph. In the post-partum period, small pleural effusions can be present. Echocardiographic studies of normal pregnant women have described a mild increase in left ventricular (LV) diastolic dimension with preservation of contractility and ejection fraction. Functional tricuspid regurgitation and small pericardial effusion are normal findings.

## ▪ OUTCOMES ASSOCIATED WITH SPECIFIC CARDIAC LESIONS

In the presence of maternal heart disease, the physiologic changes of pregnancy can lead to maternal and fetal deterioration. With the exception of patients with

**711**

Eisenmenger syndrome, pulmonary vascular obstructive disease, or Marfan syndrome with aortopathy, death during pregnancy in women with heart disease is rare.[3-6] Nevertheless, pregnant women with heart disease remain at risk for other complications, including heart failure, arrhythmia, and stroke. With advances in the pediatric treatment of congenital heart disease, women with congenital heart disease now comprise the majority of pregnant women with heart disease seen at referral centers. Rheumatic heart disease is the second most common lesion encountered during pregnancy. Hypertension, whether preexisting or gestational, is common. Peripartum cardiomyopathy is frequent but is mentioned because of its unique relationship to pregnancy. Isolated mitral valve prolapse is probably the most prevalent cardiac lesion of pregnant women; however, patients with this condition may not be referred to a cardiovascular specialist owing to their excellent outcomes during pregnancy.[7]

## Congenital Heart Lesions

### Left-to-Right Cardiac Shunts

The principal lesions in this group are *atrial septal defect (ASD)*, *ventricular septal defect (VSD)*, and *patent ductus arteriosus (PDA)*. The effect of increased cardiac output of pregnancy on the volume-loaded right ventricle in ASD or the left ventricle in VSD and PDA may be counterbalanced by the decrease in peripheral vascular resistance to the extent that the increase in left-to-right shunt is attenuated. In the absence of pulmonary hypertension, pregnancy, labor, and delivery are well tolerated.[4] However arrhythmias, ventricular dysfunction, and progression of pulmonary hypertension can occur, especially when the shunt is large or when pulmonary artery pressure was already elevated. Infrequently, particularly in ASD, paradoxical embolization may be encountered when systemic vasodilatation or elevation of pulmonary resistance promotes transient right-to-left shunting.

### Bicuspid Aortic Valve and Left Ventricular Outflow Tract Obstruction

A bicuspid aortic valve is often functionally normal. Its presence is an indication for prophylaxis against endocarditis and a reminder to exclude its associated lesions, aortic coarctation and ascending aortopathy. When *aortic stenosis (AS)* complicates pregnancy, it is usually due to congenital bicuspid aortic valve; other causes of LV outflow tract obstruction—at, below, and above the valve—have similar hemodynamic consequences. Women with symptomatic AS should defer conception until it has been surgically corrected. However the absence of symptoms ante partum is not sufficient assurance that pregnancy will be well tolerated; patients suspected to have AS should be assessed by transthoracic echocardiography to define the level and severity of the obstruction and the degree of LV dysfunction. In a pregnant woman with severe AS, the limited ability to augment cardiac output may result in abnormal elevation of LV systolic and filling pressures, which in turn lead to precipitation or exacerbation of heart failure or ischemia. In addition, the noncompliant, hypertrophic ventricle is sensitive to reductions in preload like that that may result from inferior vena cava compression late in pregnancy, vasodilator effects of anesthetic agents, peri-partum blood loss, or bearing down. The consequent exaggerated drop in cardiac output may lead to hypotension. In a compilation of many small published series, 106 pregnancies of 65 patients were associated with a maternal mortality rate of 11% and perinatal mortality of 4%.[8] Most of the complications were reported in the earlier studies. Although in 25 pregnancies managed more recently, there were no maternal deaths, deterioration of maternal functional status occurred in 20% of pregnancies.[8] Thus, severe AS imparts a hazard, and can be fatal. Antepartum palliation by balloon valvuloplasty may be helpful in certain cases.

## Coarctation of the Aorta

Coarctation of the aorta often is corrected before the woman becomes pregnant. It is commonly associated with a bicuspid aortic valve; other associations include aneurysm of the circle of Willis, VSD, and Turner syndrome. Maternal mortality with uncorrected coarctation has been reported as 3% to 4% higher in presence of associated cardiac defects, aortopathy, or long-standing hypertension. Aortic rupture is a risk in the third trimester and during labor. The management of hypertension of uncorrected coarctation is particularly problematic in pregnancy, because satisfactory control of upper body hypertension may lead to excessive hypotension below the coarctation site and compromise the fetus. Intrauterine growth retardation and premature labor and delivery are more common. After coarctation repair, the risk of dissection and rupture is reduced but not eliminated. A preliminary report described encouraging maternal and fetal outcomes: no maternal deaths and one early neonatal death among 87 pregnancies.[9]

## Pulmonary Stenosis

Echocardiographic estimation of the pressure gradient allows classification of disease into mild (<49 mm Hg), moderate (50–79 mm Hg), and severe (≥80 mm Hg) pulmonic stenosis (PS). Gradients increase with cardiac output during pregnancy, however, so the severity of the stenosis may be overestimated if no antenatal data are available. Mild PS or PS that has been alleviated by valvuloplasty or surgery is tolerated well during pregnancy. Fetal outcome in pregnancy complicated by PS is favorable. Even though a woman with severe PS may be asymptomatic, the increased hemodynamic load of pregnancy may precipitate right heart failure or atrial arrhythmias. Such a patient should be considered for correction before she conceives. Even during pregnancy, balloon valvuloplasty may be feasible if symptoms of PS progress.

## Cyanotic Heart Disease, Unrepaired and Repaired

Tetralogy of Fallot is the most common form of cyanotic congenital heart disease. Its essential features are right ventricular outflow tract obstruction and a large, nonrestrictive VSD. In uncorrected or palliated pregnant patients with tetralogy, the usual pregnancy-associated fall in systemic vascular resistance and rise in cardiac output exacerbate right-to-left shunting, an effect that leads to increased maternal hypoxemia and cyanosis. Fetal loss may be as high as 30%, and reported maternal mortality is 4% to 15%, fetal risk increasing in proportion to the hematocrit value.[10] A recent report examining the outcomes of 96 pregnancies in 44 women with a variety of cyanotic congenital heart defects also reported high rates of maternal cardiac events (32%, including 1 death) and prematurity (37%), and a low live birth rate (43%).[11] The lowest live birth rate (12%) was observed in mothers whose arterial oxygen saturation was no higher than 85%.

Pregnancy risk is low for women who have had successful correction of tetralogy[4, 6]; however, residua and sequelae such as residual shunt, right ventricular outflow tract obstruction, arrhythmias, pulmonary regurgitation, right ventricular systolic dysfunction, pulmonary hypertension (due to the effects of a previous palliative shunt), or LV dysfunction (due to previous volume overload) increase the likelihood of pregnancy complications and must be considered independently.

An increasing number of women who have undergone atrial repair or the Fontan procedure for complex cyanotic heart defects are undergoing pregnancy.

Atrial repair (Mustard or Senning procedure) was developed for the surgical correction of complete transposition of the great arteries. It redirects systemic venous return to the left ventricle, thence to the pulmonary artery, and pulmonary venous return to the right ventricle and thence the aorta. The anatomic right ventricle supports the systemic circulation. Late adult complications after atrial repair include sinus node dysfunction, atrial arrhythmias, and systolic dysfunction of the systemic ventricle. In 30 pregnancies in 20 women described in recent reports, there were no maternal deaths.[12, 13] There was a 23% prematurity rate and a 17% incidence of maternal heart failure, arrhythmias, or cardiac deterioration. Few recipients of the current repair of choice for complete transposition, the arterial switch procedure, have yet reached reproductive age.

The Fontan operation for patients with univentricular circulation involves diversion of systemic venous return to the pulmonary artery without a functional subpulmonary ventricle. Cyanosis and volume overload of the functioning systemic ventricle are both eliminated, but the ability to increase cardiac output is limited. In a recent review of 33 pregnancies in 21 women who were doing well after the Fontan operation, there were 15 term pregnancies (45%) and no maternal deaths, although two women (14%) had cardiac complications and the incidence of first trimester abortion was high (39%).[14] Since 10-year survival after the Fontan operation is only 60% to 80%, it is important that long-term maternal prognosis be discussed during preconception counseling.

## Marfan Syndrome

Marfan syndrome is a heritable autosomal-dominant connective tissue disorder. Life-threatening aortic complications are due to medial aortopathy that results in dilatation, dissection, and valvular regurgitation. Risk increases during pregnancy owing to hemodynamic stress and perhaps hormonal effects. Although older case reports suggested a very high mortality risk (in the range of 30%), more recent data suggested an overall maternal mortality rate of 1% and fetal mortality of 22%.[15] A prospective evaluation of 45 pregnancies in 21 patients reported no increase in obstetric complications or significant changes in aortic root size in most patients. Importantly, in the eight patients with a dilated aortic root (>40 mm) or a history of aortic root surgery, three of their nine pregnancies were complicated by either aortic dissection (two) or rapid aortic dilatation (one).[16] Thus, patients with aortic root involvement should receive preconception counseling that emphasizes their risk, and early in pregnancy, they should be offered termination. In contrast, women with little cardiovascular involvement and with aortic root diameter (by echocardiography) less than 40 mm may tolerate pregnancy well, though serial echocardiography should be used to identify progressive aortic root dilatation, prophylactic beta-blockers should be administered, and the possibility of dissection, even with a normal aortic root, should be acknowledged.[17]

## Eisenmenger Syndrome and Pulmonary Hypertension

The Eisenmenger syndrome consists of pulmonary vascular obstructive disease that develops as a consequence of a preexisting left-to-right shunt. The results are pulmonary pressures that approach systemic levels and bidirectional or right-to-left shunt flow. Maternal risk of death is approximately 30% in each pregnancy.[18] The preponderance of complications occur at term and during the first week post partum. Preconception counseling should stress the extreme pregnancy-associated risks. Termination of pregnancy should always be offered to such patients, as should sterilization. Fetal outcome is also poor: spontaneous abortion is common, intrauterine growth retardation is seen in 50% of pregnancies, and pre-term labor is common. Perinatal mortality is due mainly to prematurity and is seen in as many as 28% of pregnancies. A recent review of outcome of 52 pregnancies in patients with primary or secondary pulmonary hypertension reported equally poor outcomes.[19] Maternal mortality rates were 36% and 30% in the Eisenmenger and primary pulmonary hypertension groups, respectively. The overall neonatal mortality rate was 12%.

## Rheumatic Heart Disease

Mitral stenosis is the most common rheumatic valvular lesion encountered during pregnancy. The hypervolemia and tachycardia associated with pregnancy exacerbate the impact of mitral valve obstruction. The resultant elevation in left atrial pressure increases the likelihood of atrial fibrillation. Thus, even patients with mild to moderate mitral stenosis who were asymptomatic before they conceived can still develop atrial fibrillation and heart failure during gestation or the puerperium. Atrial fibrillation is a frequent precipitant of heart failure in pregnant women with mitral stenosis (owing, principally, to uncontrolled ventricular rate), and equivalent tachycardia of any cause may produce the same detrimental effect. Earlier studies of a pregnant population composed predominantly of women with rheumatic mitral disease showed that the mortality rate varied directly with antenatal functional class.[5] A more recent study found no deaths but described substantial morbidity from heart failure and arrhythmia.[6] Pregnant women whose predominant lesion is rheumatic AS have outcomes similar to those of women with congenital AS. Severe aortic or mitral regurgitation is generally tolerated well during pregnancy, although deterioration in maternal functional class has been observed.

## Hypertensive Disorders in Pregnancy

Hypertensive disorders are the cause of as many as a third of all maternal deaths, and they predispose women to other complications, such as placental abruption, stroke, disseminated intravascular coagulation, renal and/or hepatic failure, and congestive heart failure.[20] The fetus is at increased risk for intrauterine growth restriction, prematurity, and intrauterine death.

Recently, attempts have been made to standardize definitions and criteria for diagnosis.[20–24] We have adopted the recommendations of the Canadian Hypertension Society and the Society of Obstetricians and Gynaecologists of Canada.[20, 23, 24] Hypertension in pregnancy may be *preexisting hypertension* (elsewhere called *chronic hypertension, renal hypertension, underlying hypertension,* or *essential* or *secondary hypertension*), or it may be *gestational hypertension, without or with proteinuria and other adverse conditions* (elsewhere called *pregnancy-induced hypertension, transient hypertension, preeclampsia, eclampsia, HELLP* [hemolysis, elevated liver enzymes, low platelet count] syndrome, or *gestational proteinuric hypertension*). Hypertension in pregnancy is defined as a seated diastolic blood pressure of at least 90 mm Hg. Proteinuria in pregnancy is defined as at least 0.3 g of protein in a 24-hour urine collection. Severe hypertension is defined by diastolic blood pressure greater than 109 mm Hg and severe proteinuria by 24-hour urine protein excretion of more than 3 g. Gestational hypertension may be *superimposed* on preexisting hypertension.

The pathophysiology of gestational hypertension differs from other forms of hypertension. As a result of placental dysfunction, the normal cardiovascular adaptations to pregnancy (increased plasma volume and decreased peripheral resistance) do not develop. Perfusion to placenta, liver, kidneys, and brain is reduced. It is thought that endothelial dysfunction, perhaps a consequence of the decreased perfusion, results in excessive vasoactive toxins, which produce most (if not all) of the manifestations of gestational hypertension. Thus, hypertension is but one effect—not a cause—of the clinical syndrome.

Certain conditions are associated with worse outcomes. Frontal headache, severe nausea and vomiting, visual disturbances, chest pain and shortness of breath, and right upper quadrant pain are significant symptoms. The components of the HELLP syndrome may occur in isolation or in combination. Other adverse maternal manifestations are severe hypertension, severe proteinuria, hypoalbuminemia (<18 g/l), oliguria, pulmonary edema, and convulsions. Fetoplacental manifestations are suspected placental abruption, intrauterine growth retardation, oligohydramnios, and absent or reversed umbilical artery end-diastolic flow.

## Peripartum Cardiomyopathy

Peripartum cardiomyopathy is an idiopathic form of dilated cardiomyopathy defined by otherwise unexplained myocardial dysfunction that occurs during the last month of gestation or in the first 5 post-partum months.[25] It usually manifests as heart failure, although arrhythmias and embolic events have been described. Most affected women show improvements in functional status and ventricular function post partum, but others have persistent or progressive clinical deterioration. The relapse rate during subsequent pregnancies is substantial in women with evidence of persisting cardiac enlargement or LV dysfunction.[26]

## ■ MANAGEMENT

### Risk Stratification and Counseling

Risk stratification and counseling of women with heart disease is best done before they conceive. The data required for risk stratification can be readily acquired from a thorough cardiovascular history and examination, 12-lead ECG, and transthoracic echocardiogram. In patients with cyanosis, arterial oxygen saturation should be assessed by percutaneous oximetry. In counseling, six areas should be considered: the underlying cardiac lesion, maternal functional status, the possibility of further palliative or corrective surgery, additional associated risk factors, maternal life expectancy and ability to care for a child, and the risk of congenital heart disease in offspring.

Defining the *underlying cardiac lesion* is an important part of stratifying risk and determining management. The nature of residua and sequelae should be clarified, especially ventricular function, pulmonary pressure, severity of obstructive lesions, persistence of shunts, and presence of hypoxemia. Patients at low risk include those with small left-to-right shunts, repaired lesions without residual cardiac dysfunction, isolated mitral valve prolapse without significant regurgitation, bicuspid aortic valve without stenosis, mild to moderate pulmonic stenosis, or valvular regurgitation with normal ventricular systolic function. Intermediate-risk lesions include unrepaired or palliated cyanotic congenital heart disease, large left-to-right shunt, uncorrected coarctation of the aorta, mitral or aortic stenosis, prosthetic valves, severe pulmonic stenosis, and moderate to severe systemic ventricular dysfunction. Those at high risk include patients with New York Heart Association (NYHA) class III or IV symptoms, significant pulmonary hypertension, Marfan syndrome with aortic root or major valvular involvemet, or severe AS.

*Maternal functional status* is widely used as a predictor of outcome and most often is defined by NYHA functional class. In a study of 482 pregnancies in women with congenital heart disease, cardiovascular morbidity was less (8% versus 30%) and live birth rate higher (80% versus 68%) for mothers whose disease was NYHA functional class I, as compared with the others.[3] Recently, we examined 276 pregnancies in 221 women and showed that poor functional status (NYHA >II) or cyanosis, myocardial dysfunction, left heart obstruction, or a history of arrhythmia or cardiac events were independent predictors of maternal cardiac complications.[6] Poor maternal functional class and cyanosis were also predictive of adverse neonatal events.

Both maternal and fetal outcomes are improved by further palliative or corrective surgery to correct cyanosis, when possible, which should be undertaken before the woman conceives. Patients with symptomatic obstructive lesions are also better served by intervention before they become pregnant. Valve replacement requires weighing the need for ongoing anticoagulation with a mechanical valve against the likelihood of early reoperation if a xenograft valve is used. Other alternatives include homografts and, for aortic stenosis, the pulmonary autograft (Ross procedure).

*Additional associated risk factors* that can complicate pregnancy include a history of arrhythmia or heart failure, prosthetic valves and conduits, anticoagulant therapy, and teratogenic drugs such as warfarin or angiotensin-converting enzyme inhibitors.

Maternal life expectancy and ability to care for her child is obviously an important issue. A patient with limited physical capacity or with a condition that may result in her premature death should be advised of her potential inability to look after her child. Women whose condition imparts great likelihood of fetal complications, such as those who have cyanosis or are taking anticoagulants, must be apprised of these added risks.

The *risk of occurrence of congenital heart disease in offspring* should be addressed in the context of a 0.4% to 0.6% risk in the general population. When a first degree relative is affected, the recurrence risk increases about 10-fold. Left heart obstructive lesions have a higher occurrence rate. Certain conditions, such as Marfan syndrome and the 22q11 deletion syndrome, are autosomal dominant, conferring a 50% risk of occurring in an offspring. Patients with congenital heart disease who reach reproductive age should be offered genetic assessment and counseling so that they are fully informed of the mode of inheritance, risk, and available prenatal diagnosis options. Preventive strategies to decrease the incidence of congenital defects, such as preconception use of multivitamins, can be discussed during prepregnancy counseling.[27]

## Antepartum Management

Pregnant women with heart disease may be at particular risk for congestive heart failure, arrhythmias, thrombosis, emboli, and adverse effects from anticoagulants. When ventricular dysfunction is a concern, activity limitation is helpful, and for severely affected women with class III or IV symptoms, hospital admission by the middle of the second trimester may be advisable. Pregnancy-induced hypertension, hyperthyroidism, infection, and anemia should be identified early and treated vigorously. For patients with important MS, beta-adrenergic blockers, or digoxin for control of heart rate should be considered.

Arrhythmias—premature atrial or ventricular beats—are common in uncomplicated pregnancies, although sustained tachyarrhythmias have also been reported. In women with preexisting arrhythmias, pregnancy may exacerbate the frequency or hemodynamic severity of arrhythmic episodes. Pharmacologic treatment of arrhythmias is usually reserved for patients with severe symptoms or when sustained episodes are poorly tolerated in the presence of ventricular hypertrophy, ventricular dysfunction, or valvular obstruction. Sustained tachyarrhythmias such as atrial flutter and atrial fibrillation should be treated promptly, avoiding teratogenic antiarrhythmias. Digoxin and beta-adrenergic blockers are antiarrhythmics of choice in view of their established safety profiles.[28] Quinidine, adenosine, sotalol, and lidocaine are also "safe," but published data on their use during pregnancy is more limited. Electrical cardioversion is safe in pregnancy. A recent report of 44 pregnant women with implantable cardioverter-defibrillators reported favorable maternal and fetal outcomes.[29]

Pregnancy is a hypercoagulable state that may be complicated by thrombosis and thromboembolism. When a pregnant woman requires anticoagulation, heparin and warfarin are used, but controversy persists on the matter of which is better at a given stage of gestation.[30] Anticoagulation with oral warfarin is better accepted by patients and is effective, but teratogenicity during organogenesis produces warfarin embryopathy. Uteroplacental bleeding sometimes associated with warfarin is a cause of increased fetal loss. Fetal intracranial hemorrhage during vaginal delivery is a risk with warfarin unless it is withdrawn at least 2 weeks before labor. Adjusted-dose subcutaneous heparin has no teratogenic effects, as the drug does not cross the placenta. Maternal thrombocytopenia is a risk, and maternal osteoporosis may develop after use for more than 3 months. Low–molecular weight heparin may be equally effective and is easier to administer. Claims of inadequate effectiveness of heparin in patients with mechanical heart valves have been countered by arguments that the doses were inadequate; clinical trials examining the optimal anticoagulation strategy for these patients have not been performed. In North America, heparin is used almost universally, either throughout pregnancy or at least during the first trimester and the last 6 weeks before the anticipated delivery.

If a woman with the Eisenmenger syndrome does not accept advice to terminate or presents late in pregnancy, meticulous ante-partum management is necessary, including early hospitalization, supplemental oxygen, and, possibly, empiric anticoagulation.

## Multidisciplinary Approach and High-Risk Pregnancy Units

Women with heart disease who are at intermediate or high risk for complications should be managed in a high-risk pregnancy unit by a multidisciplinary team from obstetrics, cardiology, anesthesia, and pediatrics. When the problem is complex, the team should meet early in the pregnancy. At this time, the nature of the cardiac lesion, anticipated effects of pregnancy, and potential problems are explored. Since often it is not possible for every member of the team to be at the patient's bedside at a moment of crisis, it is helpful to develop a written management plan for most contingencies. Women with heart disease in the "low-risk" group can be managed in a community hospital, but if the mother's status or risk is in doubt, consultation at a regional referral center should be arranged.

## Labor and Delivery

Vaginal delivery is recommended, with very few exceptions. The only cardiac indications for cesarean section are aortic dissection, Marfan syndrome with dilated aortic root, and a mother who did not stop taking coumadin at least 2 weeks before labor begins. Pre-term induction is uncommon, but once fetal lung maturity is ensured, a planned induction and delivery in high-risk situations will ensure availability of appropriate staff and equipment. Invasive monitoring, including indwelling pulmonary artery catheter, should be considered only when the information sought is not otherwise available and the situation warrants the risk of the procedure, which may be significant, especially in women who have pulmonary hypertension. Although there is no consensus on the use of invasive hemodynamic monitoring during labor and delivery, we commonly utilize intraarterial monitoring (with or without concurrent pulmonary artery catheterization) when we are concerned about the interpretation and deleterious effects of a sudden drop in systemic blood pressure (e.g., in patients with severe aortic stenosis, pulmonary hypertension, or more than moderate systemic ventricular systolic dysfunction).

Heparin anticoagulation is discontinued at least 6 hours before induction or is reversed with protamine if spontaneous labor develops. Dosing can usually be resumed 6 to 12 hours post partum.

Endocarditis prophylaxis is initiated at onset of active labor when indicated. The American Heart Association recommendations state that delivery by cesarean section and vaginal delivery in the absence of infection do not require endocarditis prophylaxis, except, perhaps, for patients at high risk.[31] Many centers with extensive experience in caring for pregnant women with heart disease utilize endocarditis prophylactics routinely, as an uncomplicated delivery cannot always be anticipated.

Epidural anesthesia with adequate volume preloading is the technique of choice. Epidural fentanyl is particularly useful for patients with shunt lesions, because it does not lower peripheral vascular resistance. In the presence of a shunt, air and particulate filters should be placed in all intravenous lines.

Labor is conducted with the parturient in the left lateral decubitus position to attenuate hemodynamic fluctuations associated with contractions in the supine position. The latter part of the second stage of labor is shortened, and delivery is assisted by forceps or vacuum extraction. As hemodynamic values do not return to baseline for many days after delivery, patients at intermediate or high risk may require monitoring for at least 72 hours post partum. Patients with Eisenmenger syndrome require longer close post-partum observation, since mortality risk persists for as long as 7 days.

## Management of Hypertensive Disorders in Pregnancy

In general, preexisting hypertension is managed as it is in nonpregnant persons but using antihypertensive drugs known to be safe for the fetus. There is no evidence of benefit from drug treatment of mild preexisting hypertension without target organ involvement, although such patients should be under close surveillance for possible development of superimposed gestational hypertension.[32] There is some evidence that the incidence or severity of gestational hypertension may be reduced by calcium supplementation, fish oil supplementation, or small doses of aspirin.[23] Mild gestational hypertension, especially at early gestational age, may be managed conservatively by activity limitation—and perhaps modest bed rest. Pharmacologic therapy is generally instituted if the diastolic pressure exceeds 90 mm Hg but may be withheld for diastolic blood pressures between 90 and 94 mm Hg that is first noted after 28 weeks' gestation and in the absence of associated symptoms, proteinuria, pre-existing hypertension, and target organ damage. Although blood pressure control is important to protect the mother from adverse consequences of hypertension, it has no benefit for the fetus and does not reverse the pathophysiologic processes.[33]

Drugs for which evidence of safety and efficacy is best include methyldopa, labetalol, pindolol, oxprenolol, and nifedipine.[24] Other drugs that may be used include hydralazine, clonidine, and other beta-blockers. The drug of choice for convulsions is magnesium sulfate. Diuretics may be useful in the management of preexisting hypertension, but they are contraindicated in gestational hypertension, a volume-contracted state. Angiotensin-converting enzyme inhibitors and angiotensin II–receptor blockers should not be used in pregnancy because they are teratogens.[34]

The only definitive treatment for severe gestational hypertension is delivery of the fetus.[21–23]

## Acknowledgment

This work is supported in part by an operating grant from the Medical Research Council of Canada.

## ▪ REFERENCES

1. Elkayam U, Gleicher N: Hemodynamics and cardiac function during normal pregnancy and the puerperium. *In* Elkayam U, Gleicher N (eds): Cardiac Problems in Pregnancy: Diagnosis and Management of Maternal and Fetal Heart Disease. New York: Wiley-Liss, 1998:3–19.
2. Elkayam U, Gleicher N: Cardiac evaluation during pregnancy. *In* Elkayam U, Gleicher E (eds): Cardiac Problems in Pregnancy: Diagnosis and Management of Maternal and Fetal Heart Disease. New York: Wiley-Liss, 1998:23–32.
3. Whittemore R, Hobbins J, Engle M: Pregnancy and its outcome in women with and without surgical treatment of congenital heart disease. Am J Cardiol 1982;50:641–651.
4. Shime J, Mocarski E, Hastings D, et al: Congenital heart disease in pregnancy: Short- and long-term implications. Am J Obstet Gynecol 1987;156:313–322.
5. McFaul P, Dornan J, Lamki H, et al: Pregnancy complicated by maternal heart disease. A review of 519 women. Br J Obstet Gynaecol 1988;95:861–867.
6. Siu S, Sermer M, Harrison D, et al: Risk and predictors for pregnancy-related complications in women with heart disease. Circulation 1997;96:2789–2794.
7. Rayburn W: Mitral valve prolapse and pregnancy. *In* Elkayam U, Gleicher N (eds): Cardiac Problems in Pregnancy: Diagnosis and Management of Maternal and Fetal Heart Disease. New York: Wiley-Liss, 1998:175–182.
8. Lao T, Sermer M, MaGee L, et al: Congenital aortic stenosis and pregnancy—a reappraisal. Am J Obstet Gynecol 1993;169:540–545.
9. Connolly H, Ammash N, Warnes C: Pregnancy in women with coarctation of the aorta. J Am Coll Cardiol 1996;27:43A.
10. Whittemore R: Congenital heart disease: Its impact on pregnancy. Hosp Pract 1983;18:65–74.
11. Presbitero P, Somerville J, Stone S, et al: Pregnancy in cyanotic congenital heart disease. Outcome of mother and fetus. Circulation 1994;89:2673–2676.
12. Lao T, Sermer M, Colman J: Pregnancy following surgical correction for transposition of the great arteries. Obstet Gynecol 1994;83:665–668.
13. Clarkson P, Wilson N, Neutze J, et al: Outcome of pregnancy after the Mustard operation for transposition of the great arteries with intact ventricular septum. J Am Coll Cardiol 1994;24:190–193.
14. Canobbio M, Mair D, van der Velde M, et al: Pregnancy outcomes after the Fontan repair. J Am Coll Cardiol 1996;28:763–767.
15. Pyeritz R: Maternal and fetal complications of pregnancy in the Marfan syndrome. Am J Med 1981;71:784–790.
16. Rossiter J, Repke J, Morales A, et al: A prospective longitudinal evaluation of pregnancy in the Marfan syndrome. Am J Obstet Gynecol 1995;173:1599–1606.
17. Shores J, Berger K, Murphy E, et al: Progression of aortic dilatation and the benefit of long-term β-adrenergic blockade in Marfan's syndrome. N Engl J Med 1994;330:1335–1341.
18. Gleicher N, Midwall J, Hochberger D, et al: Eisenmenger's syndrome and pregnancy. Obstet Gynecol Surv 1979;34:721–741.
19. Weiss B, Zemp L, Seifert B, et al: Outcome of pulmonary vascular disease in pregnancy: A systematic overview from 1978 through 1996. J Am Coll Cardiol 1998;31:1650–1657.
20. Helewa M, Burrows R, Smith J, et al: Report of the Canadian Hypertension Society Consensus Conference: 1. Definitions, evaluation and classification of hypertensive disorders in pregnancy (see Comments). Canadian Medical Association Journal 1997;157:715–725.
21. National High Blood Pressure Education Program Working Group Report on high blood pressure in pregnancy. Am J Obstet Gynecol 1990;163:1689–1712.
22. Australasian Society for the Study of Hypertension in Pregnancy: Management of hypertension in pregnancy. Consensus Statement, Melbourne: The Society, 1993.
23. Moutquin J, Garner P, Burrows R, et al: Report of the Canadian Hypertension Society Consensus Conference: 2. Nonpharmacologic management and prevention of hypertensive disorders in pregnancy. Canadian Medical Association Journal 1997;157:907–919.
24. Rey E, LeLorier J, Burgess E, et al: Report of the Canadian Hypertension Society Consensus Conference: 3. Pharmacologic treatment of hypertensive disorders in pregnancy. Canadian Medical Association Journal 1997;157:1245–1254.

25. Demakis J, Rahimtoola S, Sutton G, et al: Natural course of peripartum cardiomyopathy. Circulation 1971;44:1053–1061.
26. Witlin A, Mabie W, Sibai B: Peripartum cardiomyopathy: An ominous diagnosis. Am J Obstet Gynecol 1997;176:182–188.
27. Czeizel A: Reduction of urinary tract and cardiovascular defects by periconceptional multivitamin supplementation. Am J Med Genet 1996;62:179–183.
28. Chow T, Galvin J, McGovern B: Antiarrhythmic drug therapy in pregnancy and lactation. Am J Cardiol 1998;82:58I–62I.
29. Natale A, Davidson T, Geiger M, et al: Implantable cardioverter-defibrillators and pregnancy: A safe combination? Circulation 1997;96:2808–2812.
30. Elkayam U: Anticoagulation in pregnant women with prosthetic heart valves: A double jeopardy. J Am Coll Cardiol 1996;27:1704–1706.
31. Dajani A, Taubert K, Wilson W, et al: Prevention of bacterial endocarditis: Recommendations by the American Heart Association. JAMA 1997;277:1794–1801.
32. Sibai B: Drug therapy: Treatment of hypertension in pregnant women. N Engl J Med 1996;335:257–265.
33. Chari R, Frangieh A, Sibai B: Hypertension during pregnancy: Diagnosis, pathophysiology, and management. *In* Elkayam U, Gleicher N (eds): Cardiac Problems in Pregnancy. Diagnosis and Management of Maternal and Fetal Heart Disease. New York: Wiley-Liss, 1998:257–273.
34. Elkayam U, Gleicher N: Cardiac Problems in Pregnancy: Diagnosis and Management of Maternal and Fetal Disease. New York: Wiley-Liss, 1998.

# ■ RECOMMENDED READING

Dajani A, Taubert K, Wilson W, et al: Prevention of bacterial endocarditis: Recommendations by the American Heart Association. JAMA 1997;277:1794–1801.

Helewa M, Burrows R, Smith J, et al: Report of the Canadian Hypertension Society Consensus Conference: 1. Definitions, evaluation and classification of hypertensive disorders in pregnancy (see Comments). Canadian Medical Association Journal 1997;157:715–725.

Lao T, Sermer M, MaGee L, et al: Congenital aortic stenosis and pregnancy—a reappraisal. Am J Obstet Gynecol 1993;169:540–545.

McFaul P, Dornan J, Lamki H, et al: Pregnancy complicated by maternal heart disease. A review of 519 women. Br J Obstet Gynaecol 1988;95:861–867.

Moutquin J, Garner P, Burrows R, et al: Report of the Canadian Hypertension Society Consensus Conference: 2. Nonpharmacologic management and prevention of hypertensive disorders in pregnancy. Canadian Medical Association Journal 1997;157:907–919.

Rey E, LeLorier J, Burgess E, et al: Report of the Canadian Hypertension Society Consensus Conference: 3. Pharmacologic treatment of hypertensive disorders in pregnancy. Canadian Medical Association Journal 1997;157:1245–1254.

Rossiter J, Repke J, Morales A, et al: A prospective longitudinal evaluation of pregnancy in the Marfan syndrome. Am J Obstet Gynecol 1995;173:1599–1606.

Shime J, Mocarski E, Hastings D, et al: Congenital heart disease in pregnancy: Short- and long-term implications. Am J Obstet Gynecol 1987;156:313–322.

Sibai B: Drug therapy: Treatment of hypertension in pregnant women. N Engl J Med 1996;335:257–265.

Siu S, Sermer M, Harrison D, et al: Risk and predictors for pregnancy-related complications in women with heart disease. Circulation 1997;96:2789–2794.

Weiss B, Zemp L, Seifert B, et al: Outcome of pulmonary vascular disease in pregnancy: A systematic overview from 1978 through 1996. J Am Coll Cardiol 1998;31:1650–1657.

Whittemore R, Hobbins J, Engle M: Pregnancy and its outcome in women with and without surgical treatment of congenital heart disease. Am J Cardiol 1982;50:641–651.

*Chapter* 38

# Heart Disease in the Elderly

*Michael W. Rich*

The 20th century saw a dramatic shift in the demographics of the U.S. population, as average life expectancy at birth increased from approximately 49 years in 1900 to almost 80 years at the end of the century. As a result, both the absolute number and the relative proportion of older persons in the population have increased exponentially, and these trends are expected to continue well into the 21st century. Of particular note is the fact that the "oldest old"—those aged 85 years or older—is the fastest-growing segment of the U.S. population.

Cardiovascular disease is the leading cause of death and of major disability in the United States and a disproportionate number of persons with cardiovascular disease are older than 65 years. Indeed, it is estimated that 70% of persons over age 70 have clinically manifested cardiovascular disease (including hypertension). In addition, 84% of all deaths attributable to cardiovascular disease occur in patients older than 65, and 64% in those older than 75. The elderly also account for 65% of all cardiovascular hospitalizations and for an increasing proportion of all cardiovascular procedures (Table 38–1).

For these reasons, it is important for the practitioner to understand the effects of aging on the cardiovascular system, to have a working knowledge of cardiovascular therapeutics in the elderly, and to appreciate the limitations of currently available data on the treatment of older patients with cardiac disease.

## ■ EFFECTS OF AGING ON THE CARDIOVASCULAR SYSTEM

Aging is associated with diffuse changes in cardiovascular structure and function (Table 38–2).[1] From the clinical perspective, the principal effects of aging are as follows:

- Increased vascular stiffness resulting in increased impedance to left ventricular ejection
- Impaired ventricular filling due to altered relaxation and decreased ventricular compliance
- Diminished responsiveness to beta-adrenergic stimulation
- Reduced capacity to augment adenosine triphosphate (ATP) production in response to increased demands
- Progressive decline in sinus node function

These changes affect disease expression, clinical manifestations, and response to therapy in older patients. Thus, increased vascular stiffness contributes to the progressive rise in systolic blood pressure with advancing age. In turn, systolic hypertension is a key risk factor for coronary heart disease, heart failure, and stroke in elderly persons.

Impaired diastolic filling, a hallmark of cardiovascular aging, is caused by increased interstitial collagen deposition, compensatory myocyte hypertrophy, and altered calcium flux leading to impaired relaxation during early diastole. These changes result in decreased filling during early and mid-diastole and are accompanied by increased reliance on atrial contraction to optimize left ventricular end-

Table 38-1

**Rates of Major Cardiovascular Procedures by Age: 1995**

| | Age (yr) | | | | | |
|---|---|---|---|---|---|---|
| | <45 | | 45–64 | | ≥65 | |
| Procedure | (No)* | (%) | (No)* | (%) | (No)* | (%) |
| Cardiac catheterization | 100 | 8.9 | 460 | 41.0 | 561 | 50.0 |
| Percutaneous coronary revascularization | 32 | 7.4 | 193 | 44.5 | 209 | 48.2 |
| Coronary bypass surgery | 17 | 3.0 | 236 | 41.2 | 320 | 55.8 |
| Placement of permanent pacemaker | 9 | 2.9 | 47 | 15.1 | 256 | 82.1 |
| Implantation of cardioverter-defibrillator | 8 | 13.6 | 14 | 23.7 | 37 | 62.7 |
| Carotid endarterectomy | 35 | 5.1 | 270 | 39.6 | 376 | 55.2 |

*In thousands.
Data from American Heart Association, Biostatistical Fact Sheets, 1998, www.americanheart.org

Table 38-2

**Effects of Aging on the Cardiovascular System**

**Gross anatomy**
  Increased left ventricular wall thickness
  Decreased left ventricular cavity size
  Endocardial thickening and sclerosis
  Increased left atrial size
  Valvular fibrosis and sclerosis
  Increased epicardial fat
**Histologic changes**
  Increased lipid and amyloid deposition
  Increased collagen degeneration and fibrosis
  Calcification of fibrous skeleton, valve rings, and coronary arteries
  Shrinkage of myocardial fibers with focal hypertrophy
  Decreased mitochondria, altered mitochondrial membranes
  Decreased nucleus-myofibril size ratio
**Biochemical changes**
  Decreased protein elasticity
  Numerous changes in enzyme content and activity affecting most metabolic pathways, but no change
    in myosin ATPase activity
  Decreased catechol synthesis, especially norepinephrine
  Decreased acetylcholine synthesis
**Conduction system**
  Degeneration of sinus node pacemaker and transition cells
  Decreased number of conducting cells in the atrioventricular node and His-Purkinje system
  Increased connective tissue, fat, and amyloid
  Increased calcification around conduction system
**Vasculature**
  Decreased distensibility of large and medium-sized arteries
  Dilation, elongation, and tortuosity of aorta and muscular arteries
  Increased wall thickness
  Increased connective tissue and calcification
**Autonomic nervous system**
  Decreased responsiveness to β-adrenergic stimulation
  Increased circulating catecholamines, decreased tissue catecholamines
  Decreased α-adrenergic receptors in left ventricle
  Decreased cholinergic responsiveness
  Diminished response to Valsalva and baroreceptor stimulation
  Decreased heart rate variability

Table 38–3

**Effects of Aging on Related Organ Systems**

Kidneys
  Gradual decline in glomerular filtration rate ($\sim$8 ml / min / decade)
  Impaired fluid and electrolyte homeostasis
Lungs
  Reduced ventilatory capacity
  Increased ventilation-perfusion mismatch
Neurohumoral system
  Reduced cerebral perfusion autoregulatory capacity
  Diminished reflex responsiveness
  Impaired thirst mechanism

diastolic volume. Clinical implications of these alterations include progressive increases in the prevalence of both atrial fibrillation and the syndrome of heart failure with normal left ventricular systolic function and a diminished capacity to augment stroke volume via the Frank-Starling mechanism.[2]

The effects of reduced responsiveness to beta-adrenergic stimulation include a linear decline of approximately 10 beats per decade in the maximum attainable heart rate, reduced ability to augment contractility, and impaired $beta_2$-mediated vasodilatation. Taken together, these effects greatly reduce the capacity of the older heart to increase cardiac output in response to increased demands, and this capacity is further diminished by the inability of cardiac mitochondria to maximally upregulate ATP production in response to increased energy requirements.

Finally, degenerative changes in the sinus node and atrial conducting tissues produce a rising prevalence of "sick sinus syndrome" with advancing age and predispose older persons to supraventricular tachyarrhythmias, especially atrial fibrillation. More than 80% of permanent pacemakers are implanted in patients older than 65 years, and sinus node dysfunction is by far the most common indication for pacemaker insertion (see Table 38–1).

In addition to age-related changes in the cardiovascular system, there are also important changes in renal, pulmonary, and neurohumoral function that have implications for older patients with cardiovascular disease (Table 38–3). Older patients are also subject to numerous behavioral, psychosocial, and financial constraints that may have an impact on symptoms, compliance with prescribed therapy, and overall prognosis. Finally, aging is associated with significant changes in the absorption, distribution, metabolism, and elimination of virtually all medications.

## ■ CARDIOVASCULAR RISK FACTORS

In general, the major risk factors for cardiovascular disease are similar in older and younger patients, but the relative importance of some risk factors (e.g., smoking, total cholesterol) declines with age. Since the prevalence of cardiovascular disease increases with age, however, the clinical significance of these risk factors persists (or even increases) with age.

### Relative and Attributable Risk

*Relative risk* refers to the likelihood that a person with a given "risk factor" will develop a specific disease, as compared with someone without that risk factor.

*Attributable risk* is the actual number of cases of a disease than can be attributed to a specific risk factor. Thus, the attributable risk reflects both relative risk and disease prevalence, and it provides a more accurate estimate of the potential impact of risk factor modification (i.e., the number of cases prevented by the eradication of a given risk factor). Stated another way, since older persons are at higher risk for cardiovascular disease, the potential benefit of treating a specific risk factor is often greater in older patients than in younger ones, even though the relative risk may be lower in the elderly.

## Hypertension

Systolic blood pressure increases with age in both men and women, whereas diastolic blood pressure tends to peak and plateau in middle age and then declines slightly in old age (Fig. 38–1). Although systolic and diastolic blood pressure are each independent risk factors for cardiovascular disease in the elderly, systolic hypertension is more common, and it is also a more powerful risk factor.

To date at least nine prospective, randomized clinical trials have evaluated the effects of antihypertensive therapy in the elderly (Table 38–4).[3–12] Six of these studies focused on diastolic hypertension,[3–9] two enrolled patients with isolated systolic hypertension,[10, 11] and one included subjects with either systolic or diastolic hypertension.[12] These studies provide compelling evidence that treatment of systolic and diastolic hypertension substantially reduces the incidence of stroke, coronary heart disease, and cardiac failure in older adults. Moreover, the benefits of treating diastolic hypertension persist at least to age 80, whereas the benefits of treating systolic hypertension are apparent at least up to age 90.

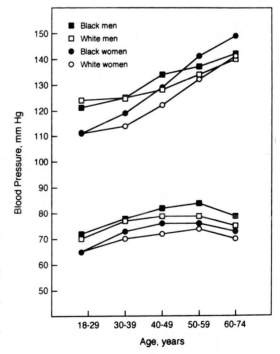

**Figure 38–1** ▪ Average systolic and diastolic blood pressures in the U.S. population as a function of age, sex, and race: NHANES III. (Adapted from Burt VL, Cutler JA, Higgins M, et al: Trends in the prevalence, awareness, treatment, and control of hypertension in the adult U.S. population. Data from the health examination surveys, 1960–1991. Hypertension 1995;26:60–69.)

Table 38–4

## Trials of Antihypertensive Treatment in the Elderly

| Trial | Number of Participants | Age (yr) | Risk Reduction (%) | | | |
|---|---|---|---|---|---|---|
| | | | CVA | CAD | CHF | All CVD |
| Australian[3] | 582 | 60–69 | 33 | 18 | NR | 31 |
| EWPHE[4] | 840 | >60 | 36 | 20 | 22 | 29 |
| Coope[5] | 884 | 60–79 | 42 | −3 | 32 | 24 |
| STOP-HTN[6] | 1627 | 70–84 | 47 | 13 | 51 | 40 |
| MRC[7] | 4396 | 65–74 | 25 | 19 | NR | 17 |
| HDFP[8,9] | 2374 | 60–69 | 44 | 15 | NR | 16 |
| SHEP[10] | 4736 | ≥60 | 33 | 27 | 55 | 32 |
| Syst-Eur[11] | 4695 | ≥60 | 42 | 26 | 36 | 31 |
| STONE[12] | 1632 | 60–79 | 57 | 6 | 68 | 60 |

CAD, coronary artery disease; CHF, congestive heart failure; CVA, cerebrovascular accident; CVD, cardiovascular disease; EWPHE, European Working Party on High Blood Pressure in the Elderly; HDFP, Hypertension Detection and Followup Program; MRC, Medical Research Council; NR, not reported; SHEP, Systolic Hypertension in the Elderly Program; STONE, Shanghai Trial of Nifedipine in the Elderly; STOP-HTN, Swedish Trial in Old Patients with Hypertension; Syst-Eur, Systolic Hypertension in Europe.

Treatment of hypertension is similar in older and younger patients, but older ones are more susceptible to adverse drug reactions, so therapy should generally be initiated with lower drug doses, and close follow-up is essential to assess efficacy and tolerability.

## Hyperlipidemia

In men, total cholesterol levels tend to peak in late middle age then decline modestly thereafter.[13] In the absence of estrogen replacement, women's cholesterol levels rise rapidly after menopause, surpassing men's after age 60. In the Framingham Heart Study, the importance of total cholesterol as a risk factor for coronary heart disease declined with age, but the ratio of total cholesterol to high-density lipoprotein cholesterol (HDL-C) remained a strong independent risk factor in both men and women of older age.[14] Similar findings from other studies confirm the importance of hyperlipidemia as a cardiovascular risk factor in the elderly.

To date, no large-scale randomized trials have evaluated the effects of lipid lowering therapy in the elderly; however, age-specific subgroup analyses from several trials provide strong evidence that treatment with an hydroxymethylglutaryl-coenzyme A (HMG-CoA) reductase inhibitor ("statin") reduces mortality and nonfatal coronary events, at least to age 75 (Table 38–5).[15–18] Based on these trials, it seems reasonable to recommend an HMG-CoA reductase inhibitor, in conjunction with an appropriate low-fat diet, for most older persons known to have coronary heart disease or multiple risk factors in the absence of other major life-limiting illness. The benefits of such treatment in persons older than 75 years are not yet known.

## Smoking

Smoking prevalence declines with age owing to smoking-related deaths and successful smoking cessation. Nonetheless, continued smoking remains an important risk factor for myocardial infarction (MI) and stroke in older persons. Moreover, there is strong evidence that smoking cessation is beneficial at any age.

Table 38–5

**Impact of HMG-CoA Reductase Inhibitors on Coronary Events**

| Study | Patient Age (yr) | Number of Participants | Risk Reduction (%) | |
|---|---|---|---|---|
| | | | Coronary Events | Death |
| 4S[15] | | | | |
| | <65 | 3423 | 34 | 28 |
| | 65–70 | 1021 | 34 | 34 |
| CARE[16] | | | | |
| | <65 | 2876 | 19 | −11 |
| | 65–75 | 1283 | 32 | 45 |
| LIPID[17] | | | | |
| | <65 | 5500 | 23 | NR |
| | 65–75 | 3514 | 21 | NR |
| AFCAPS/TexCAPS[18] | | | | |
| | ≤Median age* | 3425 | 46 | NR |
| | >Median age* | 3180 | 30 | NR |

*57 years for men, 62 years for women.

4S, Scandinavian Simvastatin Survival Study; CARE, Cholesterol and Recurrent Events; LIPID, Long-term Intervention with Pravastitin in Ischemic Disease; AFCAPS/TexCAPS, Air Force/Texas Coronary Atherosclerosis Prevention Study; NR, not reported.

In the Coronary Artery Surgery Study (CASS) Registry, for example, coronary disease patients over 70 years of age who continued to smoke had a 3.3-fold higher risk of death and a 2.9-fold higher risk of death or MI during a 6-year follow-up period as compared with those who stopped smoking.[19]

The efficacy of smoking cessation programs, nicotine replacement therapy, and other medications (e.g., bupropion) for elderly smokers is not known, but older smokers tend to be more receptive to counseling interventions than younger ones. In addition, the motivation to quit smoking often peaks after an index cardiovascular event, and the importance of smoking cessation should be strongly emphasized to persons of all ages who suffer such an event.

## Other Risk Factors

Left ventricular hypertrophy, physical inactivity, elevated fibrinogen levels, and increased homocysteine levels remain important risk factors in older men and women. Diabetes mellitus and hypertriglyceridemia are risk factors for older women but not older men. The impact of treating these risk factors in elderly patients is not yet known.

## ▪ CORONARY ARTERY DISEASE

### Acute Myocardial Infarction

The incidence of acute MI increases with age in both men and women. In 1995, 61.1% of patients hospitalized with acute MI in the United States were older than 65 years and nearly a third older than 75. Case fatality rates increase with age, and 85% of persons who die of acute MI are over age 65 and 60% over 75. In addition, women comprise nearly half of all patients with acute MI older than 65, and MI is the leading cause of death in both men and women of this age group.

## Clinical Manifestations

After age 75, patients with acute MI are less likely to present with typical ischemic chest discomfort, and shortness of breath is the most common initial symptom in those older than 80.[20] Diaphoresis occurs less frequently in older persons, whereas nonspecific neurologic symptoms such as light-headedness, confusion, and syncope are more common in the elderly and may be the presenting manifestations in as many as 20% of MI patients older than 85.

In older MI patients electrocardiograms (ECG) are often nondiagnostic owing to preexisting ECG abnormalities (e.g., paced rhythm, left bundle branch block, or left ventricular hypertrophy) and a high prevalence of non–Q wave MI. The combination of atypical symptoms and a nondiagnostic ECG may confound the diagnosis unless a high index of suspicion is maintained. Lack of diagnostic certainty is also an important contributor to reduced utilization of reperfusion therapy and other interventions in older patients.

In addition to increased mortality, older patients with acute MI are more likely to develop heart failure, hypotension, atrial fibrillation, conduction abnormalities, myocardial rupture, and cardiogenic shock. Although ventricular arrhythmias are also more common in the elderly, older patients are less likely to develop primary ventricular fibrillation.

## Reperfusion Therapy

Pooled data from five large, randomized, placebo-controlled trials indicate that thrombolytic therapy administered within 6 hours of symptom onset in elderly patients with acute MI accompanied by electrocardiographic ST segment elevation is associated with a significant reduction in mortality (Table 38–6).[21] Indeed, the absolute mortality benefit, in terms of the number of lives saved per 100 patients treated, is actually somewhat greater in the elderly than in younger patients (3.5 and 2.2, respectively). Moreover, among 401 patients over age 80 enrolled in the ISIS-2 (Second International Study of Infarct Survival) trial, treatment with streptokinase reduced mortality by 41% as compared with placebo and saved 14.1 lives per 100 treated patients, the largest differential for any age group.[22]

Intracranial hemorrhage occurs in 0.3% to 0.5% of patients who receive thrombolytic therapy for acute MI, but the risk increases with age. Other major bleeding complications occur slightly more frequently in patients receiving thrombolysis, but the risk is not age dependent.[23]

The choice of a thrombolytic agent for patients older than 75 remains controversial. In the GUSTO-I trial, recombinant tissue plasminogen activator (rt-PA) was associated with a somewhat lower mortality rate than streptokinase in patients over 75 (19.3% vs. 20.6%), but the difference was not statistically significant.[24] In

Table 38–6

**Early Mortality in Five Major Placebo-Controlled Thrombolytic Trials: Pooled Results by Age for 36,925 Subjects**

|  | Younger (N = 26,941) | Older (N = 9,984) |
|---|---|---|
| Mortality (%) |  |  |
| Control group | 8.4 | 20.7 |
| Thrombolysis | 6.2 | 17.2 |
| Mortality reduction (%) | 25.7 | 16.9 |
| Lives saved / 100 patients | 2.2 | 3.5 |
| $p$ Value | <.0001 | <.0001 |

addition, rt-PA was associated with more intracranial hemorrhages in this age group (1.2% and 2.1%, P < .05).

Percutaneous transluminal coronary angioplasty (PTCA) is an effective alternative to thrombolytic therapy for patients with acute MI, and it is associated with improved patency rates and fewer intracranial hemorrhages than thrombolysis. Among 300 patients older than 70 enrolled in the GUSTO-IIb trial, which compared PTCA with rt-PA in patients with acute MI, the composite end points of death, reinfarction, or disabling stroke tended to occur less frequently in patients randomized to PTCA, suggesting that PTCA may be the preferred reperfusion strategy for selected elderly patients.[25] Very few patients over age 80 were enrolled in GUSTO-IIb, however, and the value of PTCA in this age group remains undefined.

## Aspirin

Among 3411 patients over 70 years of age enrolled in the ISIS-2 trial, the administration of aspirin, 162.5 mg daily, was associated with 21% mortality reduction at 35 days.[22] Moreover, the *absolute* benefit of aspirin increased with advancing age, from 1.0% in patients younger than 60 years to 4.7% in those 70 or older. Long-term aspirin therapy after MI also reduces the list of death, reinfarction, or stroke by approximately 25% in patients of all ages.

## Other Antiplatelet Agents

The roles of ticlopidine, clopidogrel, and the glycoprotein IIb/IIIa inhibitors in the treatment of elderly patients with acute MI are not currently known.

## Heparin

Although older patients with acute MI often receive intravenous heparin, the value of this treatment is unproven. In a recent study involving 6935 Medicare patients hospitalized with acute MI, heparin therapy was associated with more bleeding complications and increased lengths of hospital stay, but there was no evidence of beneficial effects on mortality or reinfarction.[26]

Low–molecular weight heparins such as enoxaparin and dalteparin offer several advantages over conventional unfractionated heparin, and recent studies indicate that these agents are associated with better clinical outcomes for patients with unstable coronary syndromes, including the elderly. Several ongoing trials should help to clarify the role of these agents in treating patients with acute coronary ischemia.

## Warfarin

Long-term warfarin therapy after acute MI reduces the risk of death, reinfarction, and stroke in elderly patients.[27] It is not clear, however, that warfarin is superior to aspirin, and aspirin is less costly, easier to use, and associated with fewer bleeding complications. For these reasons, warfarin is generally reserved for patients who are intolerant of aspirin and for those who have clear indications for long-term anticoagulation (e.g., chronic atrial fibrillation).

## Beta Blockers

Table 38–7 summarizes data from three large randomized trials of intravenous beta blockers in patients with acute MI.[21] Intravenous beta blockade reduced mortality by 23% in older patients, but there was no significant effect on younger patients. In these trials, beta blockers also reduced the incidence of supraventricular and ventricular arrhythmias and of recurrent ischemic events. Although these studies were conducted before the advent of reperfusion therapy, the results remain appli-

Table 38–7

**Mortality in Three Large Trials of Intravenous Beta Blockers:
Pooled Results by Age for 23,200 Subjects**

|  | Younger (N = 14,687) | Older (N = 8,513) |
|---|---|---|
| Mortality (%) |  |  |
|    Control group | 2.6 | 8.9 |
|    Beta-blocker group | 2.5 | 6.9 |
| Mortality reduction (%) | 5.0 | 23.2 |
| Lives saved / 100 patients | 0.1 | 2.1 |
| p Value | NS | .0005 |

NS, not significant.

cable today, since the majority of older patients with acute MI do not receive thrombolytic therapy or primary PTCA.

Long-term beta-blocker therapy is also associated with greater benefits in older than in younger patients (6.0 and 2.1 lives saved, respectively, per 100 treated patients).[21] In addition, since event rates are higher in the elderly, beta blockade is more cost-effective in older than in younger persons.

## Nitrates

Nitrates can be administered safely to most elderly patients with acute MI, and data from the GISSI-3 trial indicate that early treatment with transdermal nitroglycerin is associated with favorable trends in mortality and in the combined end points of death, heart failure, and severe left ventricular dysfunction in patients older than 70 years.[28] The value of long-term nitroglycerin therapy after MI is currently unknown.

## Calcium Channel Blockers

Calcium channel blockers have not been shown to improve outcomes in elderly patients with acute MI, and routine use of these agents is not recommended.

## Angiotensin-Converting Enzyme (ACE) Inhibitors

In the GISSI-3 trial, treatment with lisinopril within 24 hours of symptom onset reduced the combined end points of death, heart failure, and severe left ventricular dysfunction by 17% in patients older than 70 years.[28] Similarly, in patients with anterior MI who were not receiving a thrombolytic agent, early treatment with zofenopril reduced the incidence of death or severe heart failure by 34%, and the absolute benefit was threefold greater in patients older than 65 years than in younger ones.[29]

In patients with acute MI complicated by heart failure or left ventricular dysfunction (ejection fraction ≤40%), long-term ACE inhibitor therapy reduces mortality, hospitalizations, and heart failure progression, and the benefits of treatment are at least as great in older patients as in younger ones.[30, 31] Indeed, in the Acute Infarction Ramipril Efficacy (AIRE) trial, the mortality benefit of ramipril was limited to older patients.[31] Since the risk for drug-induced hypotension and renal dysfunction is greater in older patients, those using these agents must be carefully monitored.

## Magnesium

Although some older patients with acute MI may benefit from intravenous magnesium, data are insufficient to support widespread use of magnesium at this time.

## Antiarrhythmic Agents

Antiarrhythmic agents have not been shown to reduce mortality or improve clinical outcomes in elderly MI patients, and routine use of these agents is not recommended.

## Non–Q Wave Myocardial Infarction

Non–Q wave MI (NQMI) increases in frequency with advancing age and accounts for more than 50% of all MI in patients older than 70. Although the short-term prognosis after NQMI is more favorable than that after Q wave MI, NQMI patients are at increased risk for reinfarction and death during follow-up.

In general, the treatment of NQMI is similar in younger and older patients (see Chapter 25). The Thrombolysis in Myocardial Infarction IIIB (TIMI-IIIB) study, however, found that compared with conservative management, an initial strategy of early cardiac catheterization and revascularization was associated with a significant reduction in adverse events at 6 weeks' follow-up in older patients (7.9% and 14.8%, respectively, $p = .02$).[32] Moreover, these benefits were sustained for at least 1 year. Unfortunately, the recently completed VANQWISH (Veterans Affairs Non–Q Wave Infarction Strategies in Hospital) trial failed to confirm these findings in older patients with NQMI.[33] Thus, the role of early catheterization and revascularization in elderly patients with NQMI remains undefined.

## Chronic Coronary Artery Disease

Coronary artery disease (CAD) is very prevalent in the elderly, and older patients account for more than half of hospital admissions for angina pectoris. Older CAD patients usually have more diffuse disease than younger ones, and they are more likely to have multivessel and left main coronary disease. Because older patients tend to be more sedentary than their younger counterparts, they are more likely to be asymptomatic or minimally symptomatic despite having more severe CAD. Older patients also have a higher prevalence of silent ischemia and infarction than younger patients.

The treatment of chronic CAD is similar in older and younger patients and will not be reviewed here; however, a brief discussion of revascularization procedures is in order.

## Percutaneous Transluminal Coronary Angioplasty

Almost 50% of PTCA in the United States are performed in patients older than 65 years (see Table 38–1). Compared to younger patients, older ones referred for PTCA are more likely to be women and to have more severe symptoms, more comorbidity, and more complex "target" lesions.[34] These factors, in conjunction with age-related reductions in cardiovascular reserve, increase procedure-related morbidity and mortality rates in older patients, particularly those over 80, and hospital mortality after PTCA in octogenarians ranges from 7% to 10%. In addition, although late survival after successful PTCA in older patients is good, the incidence of recurrent angina is higher than in younger patients, owing principally to incomplete revascularization. Intracoronary stents offer an alternative to conventional

PTCA in older patients, but preliminary studies indicate that technical success rates are lower and complication rates higher in the very elderly.

## Coronary Artery Bypass Surgery

More than 50% of all coronary artery bypass graft (CABG) operations performed in the United States are in patients over age 65, and the proportion continues to rise. Like PTCA candidates, older patients referred for CABG are more likely to be female and have more advanced coronary disease, more symptoms, and more comorbidity. Perioperative mortality rates range from 5% to 10% in patients over age 75 undergoing isolated CABG, as compared with 1% to 2% in patients younger than 65.[35] Older patients also have higher rates of perioperative complications, including atrial fibrillation, heart failure, stroke, bleeding, cognitive dysfunction, respiratory disorders, and renal insufficiency. As a result, postoperative lengths of stay are substantially longer for older patients. Despite these difficulties, the long-term results after CABG in older patients are excellent: as many as 90% of patients experience sustained symptomatic improvement, and the majority report improved functional capacity and quality of life. In addition, although none of the randomized trials comparing CABG to PTCA or medical therapy have included a substantial number of elderly patients, registry data indicate that, in elderly patients with severe symptoms, CABG is associated with better survival than is medical therapy.[36]

## ■ VALVULAR HEART DISEASE

### Aortic Valve

Aortic stenosis severe enough to warrant surgical consideration affects 2% to 3% of persons older than 75, and aortic valve replacement is the second most common major cardiac operation in this age group (after CABG).[37, 38] Age-related degenerative changes occurring on a normal trileaflet aortic valve account for the majority of cases. Other causes include congenital bicuspid aortic valve and rheumatic disease.

Aortic stenosis in the elderly is often occult, because sedentary older persons may experience few symptoms or may attribute their symptoms to old age. Similarly, the physician may ascribe the symptoms of aortic stenosis to other causes. In addition, the murmur of aortic stenosis in older patients may be less prominent owing to changes in chest wall geometry (increased anteroposterior diameter) and reduced stroke volume. An $S_4$ gallop is a nonspecific finding in older persons, but the *absence* of an $S_4$ during sinus rhythm makes the diagnosis of aortic stenosis unlikely. The $A_2$ component of the second heart sound is frequently diminished in older patients with severe aortic stenosis, but this may be difficult to appreciate on routine examination. As a result of decreased vascular compliance, the carotid upstrokes may be well-preserved in older patients with severe aortic stenosis. In addition, although the ECG usually shows left ventricular hypertrophy with ST segment and T wave changes, these findings may be attributed to long-standing hypertension or other causes. For these reasons, echocardiography should be performed whenever an elderly patient has unexplained symptoms that could be due to aortic stenosis. Cardiac catheterization should also be performed in patients with severe aortic stenosis who are suitable candidates for valve replacement.

Aortic valve replacement is the treatment of choice for severe aortic stenosis in adults of all ages; however, some elderly patients, such as those with dementia, advanced frailty, or major comorbidity, may not be suitable candidates for the procedure. The results of aortic valve replacement in the elderly are excellent, even in octogenarians: several series report perioperative mortality rates of 4% to 7% for isolated valve replacement.[38] Death rates are somewhat higher when valve replacement is combined with CABG. The majority of patients experience marked improvement in symptoms and functional capacity after the procedure, and long-term survival is comparable to that of the general population of similar age.

The prevalence of aortic regurgitation increases with age, but most cases are not severe enough to require surgery. Causes of acute aortic regurgitation in the elderly include type A aortic dissection, infective endocarditis, prosthetic valve dysfunction, and sinus of Valsalva rupture. Causes of chronic aortic regurgitation include rheumatic or calcific aortic valve disease, healed endocarditis, and aneurysms of the aortic root due to atherosclerosis, syphilis, or another disorder. Treatment of aortic regurgitation is similar in older and younger adults.

## Mitral Valve

Mitral stenosis in the elderly is usually rheumatic in origin, but severe mitral valve annulus calcification occasionally causes mitral stenosis in patients with a small left ventricular cavity.[37] As in younger patients, the symptoms of mitral stenosis are often insidious, and it is not unusual for the diagnosis to be clinically inapparent until echocardiography is performed. In most elderly patients with mitral stenosis, the valve apparatus is heavily calcified or significant mitral regurgitation is present, conditions that preclude percutaneous valvuloplasty or open commissurotomy. In elderly patients who are suitable candidates for valvuloplasty, however, the procedure can be performed safely, and it produces significant hemodynamic and clinical improvement in the majority of cases. For other patients with severe symptoms, mitral valve replacement offers the only viable therapeutic option.[38] Like aortic valve replacement, mitral valve surgery in elderly patients is associated with increased morbidity and mortality. The perioperative mortality rate for elective mitral valve surgery in elderly patients is 10% to 20%, although some centers are now reporting mortality rates less than 10%.

Mitral regurgitation is the most common valvular lesion in elderly patients, but in most cases it is not severe enough to require surgical intervention. Common causes of mitral regurgitation in the elderly include ischemic mitral valve dysfunction, ischemic or nonischemic dilated cardiomyopathy, mitral valve prolapse, rheumatic heart disease, and mitral valve annulus calcification.[37] Less often, mitral regurgitation is due to infective or noninfective endocarditis, prosthetic valve dysfunction, or hypertrophic cardiomyopathy. In patients with mild to moderate mitral regurgitation, medical management with afterload reduction (e.g., ACE inhibitors, hydralazine) is appropriate. For patients with severe symptomatic mitral regurgitation and satisfactory left ventricular function, surgical treatment should be considered. As in younger patients, mitral valve repair, when feasible, is associated with more favorable outcomes. Long-term results after successful mitral valve repair or replacement in elderly patients are generally favorable, with significant symptomatic improvement occurring in the majority of cases.

## Infective Endocarditis

The incidence of infective endocarditis increases progressively with age, reflecting age-related changes in valve structure, the increasing prevalence of specific valvular lesions in the elderly, and the increased prevalence of potential sources of bacteremia (e.g., poor dentition, respiratory and urinary tract infections, and procedures such as cystoscopy).[39] Detecting endocarditis in the elderly is often difficult, since the clinical manifestations are usually nonspecific and protean. The classic peripheral manifestations of endocarditis, such as Roth spots, Osler nodes, and Janeway lesions, are also uncommon in elderly patients.

In general, the pathogens of endocarditis are similar in older and younger patients, streptococci, staphylococci, and enterococci being the most common, followed by gram-negative bacilli and other less common organisms. In addition, as many as 10% of cases may be culture negative, usually because antibiotic therapy is instituted before an adequate number of blood cultures have been obtained. As in younger patients, vegetations are visualized with transthoracic echocardiography in fewer than 50% of cases, but the yield is substantially higher with the transesophageal approach. The treatment and complications of endocarditis are similar in older and younger patients, although mortality is higher among the elderly.

## ■ HEART FAILURE

The effects of aging on the cardiovascular system markedly reduce cardiovascular reserve and predispose older patients to heart failure (HF). The prevalence of cardiovascular disease, particularly hypertension and coronary artery disease, also increases with age, and these factors combine to produce an exponential rise in HF with increasing age.[40] Indeed, HF is relatively uncommon in younger adults, but the prevalence doubles with each decade after age 45, and HF affects 1 in 10 persons over the age of 80. As a result, HF is the most common indication for hospitalization after age 65 years, and it is the most costly diagnosis-related group (DRG) by a factor of almost 2. HF is also a major cause of long-term disability in the elderly, and mortality rates from HF increase progressively with age (Fig. 38–2).

Hypertension is the most common antecedent illness in elderly patients with HF, and 70% to 80% of cases can be attributed to either hypertension or CAD. Valvular disease is the third most common cause of HF in the elderly, followed by nonischemic cardiomyopathy. Importantly, the prevalence of HF with preserved systolic function (so-called diastolic HF) increases with age and accounts for more than 50% of cases after age 80.

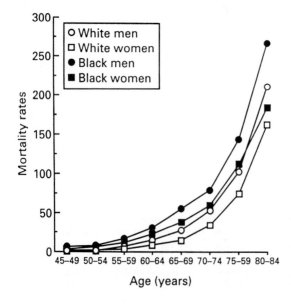

**Figure 38–2** ■ Mortality rates for heart failure in the U.S. by age, sex, and race: 1990. (Adapted from Gillum RF: Epidemiology of heart failure in the United States. Am Heart J 1993; 126:1042–1047.)

HF in the elderly is both overdiagnosed and underdiagnosed. The cardinal symptoms of HF—shortness of breath, edema, fatigue, and exercise intolerance—are common in elders, and these symptoms are often attributed to HF, even when caused by other disorders. Conversely, sedentary elderly persons may not report exertional symptoms, and neurologic symptoms such as altered sensorium or irritability, or gastrointestinal disturbances such as anorexia or bloating may be the only overt manifestations of HF. Similarly, the physical findings are often nonspecific, and the chest radiograph may be difficult to interpret in patients with mild HF. Finally, left ventricular systolic function is often normal in older HF patients.

## Management

The principal goals of HF management in elderly patients are to maximize quality of life, reduce medical resource utilization, and extend functional survival. In the past 20 years, major advances have been made in the treatment of HF, but older patients are much less likely to receive aggressive therapy. In addition, management of older HF patients is often confounded by a variety of behavioral and psychosocial factors, particularly noncompliance, which contribute to the high rate of repetitive hospitalizations.[41] For these reasons, many centers are now utilizing a multidisciplinary disease management strategy to optimize medication prescribing practices, enhance compliance with medications and diet, and provide appropriate follow-up for older HF patients. Several studies have now documented the efficacy of this approach in reducing hospitalizations and costs of care while improving quality of life and overall compliance.[42]

## Medical Therapy

In general, the pharmacologic treatment of patients with systolic HF is similar for older and younger patients (see Chapter 20). Considerations specific to the elderly are discussed briefly in the following paragraphs.

### Angiotensin-Converting Enzyme Inhibitors

Although none of the ACE inhibitor trials has specifically targeted older patients, the average age of patients in CONSENSUS (Cooperative North Scandinavian Enalapril Survival Study) was 71 years,[43] and the beneficial effects of enalapril were also similar in older and younger patients enrolled in the SOLVD (Studies of Left Ventricular Dysfunction) trials.[44, 45] Moreover, in the post-MI ACE inhibitor trials, the benefits of ACE inhibitors were, if anything, greater in older patients,[30, 31] and a metaanalysis of all the ACE inhibitor studies concluded that there is substantial benefit in all age groups, including the elderly.[46] Thus, ACE inhibitors are indicated for all elderly persons with significant left ventricular systolic dysfunction (ejection fraction <40% to 45%), regardless of whether overt HF symptoms are present. As in younger patients, the ACE inhibitor dose should be incrementally increased to achieve a minimum daily dose of captopril 150 mg, enalapril 20 mg, or an equivalent. Older patients usually tolerate ACE inhibitors well, but hyperkalemia and renal dysfunction occur more frequently than in younger patients.

### Other Vasodilators

The angiotensin II receptor blockers (ARB) are a rational alternative to ACE inhibitors for patients unable to tolerate ACE inhibitors because of cough, allergic reactions, or other side effects. In the ELITE (Evaluation of Losartan in the Elderly) trial, losartan was associated with fewer limiting side effects (including cough) than was captopril, and during a 48-week follow-up period, mortality was lower among patients who took losartan.[47] However, in the recently completed ELITE II trial, mortality was similar in patients treated with losartan or captopril, although losartan was better tolerated. Several ongoing studies will help to further clarify the role of ARB in the treatment of HF.

The combination of hydralazine and isosorbide dinitrate increased survival relative to placebo in V-HeFT-I (Veterans Administration Heart Failure Trial)[48] but was less effective than enalapril in V-HeFT-II.[49] Although few elderly patients were enrolled in these trials, this combination is an acceptable alternative to ACE inhibitors in appropriately selected patients.

## Digoxin

The positive inotropic effects of digoxin persist at older age, but the therapeutic range of serum digoxin concentration is lower in older patients (0.5 to 1.3 ng/ml) owing to changes in lean body mass and renal function.[50] Higher serum digoxin levels are associated with greater toxicity but no greater clinical benefit, and should therefore be avoided.

The value of digoxin in patients with symptomatic HF was recently confirmed in the DIG (Digitalis Investigation Group) trial.[51] Although digoxin had no net effect on mortality, HF deaths and hospitalizations were significantly reduced. Moreover, although both mortality and hospital admissions increased sharply with age, the effects of digoxin were similar in all age groups, including octogenarians. Thus, digoxin is a useful adjunct to ACE inhibitors and diuretics in older patients, particularly those with more advanced symptoms and left ventricular dysfunction.

## Diuretics

Although conventional diuretics such as furosemide may not improve long-term outcomes in HF patients, diuretics remain a cornerstone of therapy owing to their efficacy in relieving congestive symptoms and edema. Recently, spironolactone was shown to reduce mortality in patients with advanced HF, and the benefits were similar in older and younger patients. Older patients are more susceptible to dehydration and to diuretic-induced electrolyte disturbances, so older patients receiving chronic diuretic therapy should be monitored closely with daily weights and periodic electrolyte assessments.

## Other Agents

Data from three large trials indicate that beta blockers reduce hospitalizations and mortality in patients with systolic HF of mild to moderate severity. Moreover, the U.S. Carvedilol Study and CIBIS II (Cardiac Insufficiency Bisoprolol Study) found these agents to be equally efficacious in older and younger patients.[52, 53] Unfortunately, few patients over age 75 have been treated with beta blockers, and the value of these agents in the very elderly is unknown. Nonetheless, beta blockers should be considered for older patients with stable HF and no contraindications, especially those with underlying CAD or an elevated resting heart rate.

In the PRAISE (Prospective Randomized Amlodipine Survival Evaluation) study, the calcium channel blocker amlodipine was associated with a favorable trend in mortality as compared with placebo[54]; however, the apparent benefit was limited to patients with nonischemic left ventricular dysfunction, and these findings were not confirmed in the recently completed PRAISE II trial. At the present time, calcium channel blockers are not recommended for older patients with systolic HF.

Aspirin, 75 to 325 mg daily, is recommended for all patients with known CAD, regardless of their age. Warfarin is indicated for those with chronic atrial fibrillation, advanced rheumatic mitral valve disease, a history of thromboembolic events, or mechanical prosthetic valves. The value of antithrombotic therapy in other HF patients is not yet known and is the subject of the ongoing WATCH (Warfarin-Antiplatelet Therapy in Chronic Heart Failure) trial.

## Diastolic Heart Failure

As many as 50% of older HF patients have preserved left ventricular systolic function, and this is a major clinical problem because no large-scale clinical trials have focused on the treatment of this disorder. As a result, the management of diastolic HF remains largely empirical and generally includes some combination of diuretics, nitrates, beta blockers, calcium channel blockers, and ACE inhibitors.

Diuretics are effective in relieving congestion and edema, but they must be used cautiously because patients with diastolic dysfunction are dependent on a sufficient preload to maintain adequate stroke volume. Such patients are often "volume sensitive" and are prone to develop pulmonary edema with modest volume overload, whereas volume contraction and prerenal azotemia may occur in response to overdiuresis.

Limited data suggest that some patients with diastolic HF derive symptomatic benefit from beta blockers, calcium channel blockers, ACE inhibitors, and ARB. Unfortunately, none of these studies has been of sufficient size or duration to provide meaningful data on the effects of these agents on major clinical outcomes. On the other hand, data from the DIG ancillary study, which involved a cohort of 988 HF patients with ejection fractions of 45% or greater, indicate that digoxin may reduce hospitalizations for HF in this population.[51] Thus, digoxin may play a role in the management of patients with diastolic HF that is not responsive to other agents.

## Prevention

Given the high rates of morbidity and mortality among older patients with established HF, preventing this disorder is clearly desirable. At the present time, the best preventive measures include aggressive treatment of hypertension and other known CAD risk factors. Indeed, based on data from the SHEP (Systolic Hypertension in the Elderly) program, treatment of hypertension may reduce the risk of incident HF by as much as 50% during a 5-year follow-up period, and this benefit is most pronounced in patients 80 years of age or older (Fig. 38–3).[55]

## ■ ARRHYTHMIAS AND CONDUCTION DISORDERS

Supraventricular, ventricular, and bradyarrhythmias all increase in frequency with advancing age, as do supranodal, nodal, and infranodal conduction abnormalities. Each of these disorders is discussed briefly in the following paragraphs.

### Supraventricular Arrhythmias

Atrial fibrillation is the most common and clinically important sustained supraventricular arrhythmia in older adults. The prevalence of atrial fibrillation increases from less than 1% in persons younger than 40 to more than 10% in those older than 80, and the median age of patients with atrial fibrillation is 75 years. Atrial fibrillation is more common in men than in women at all ages, but the proportion of women increases with age.

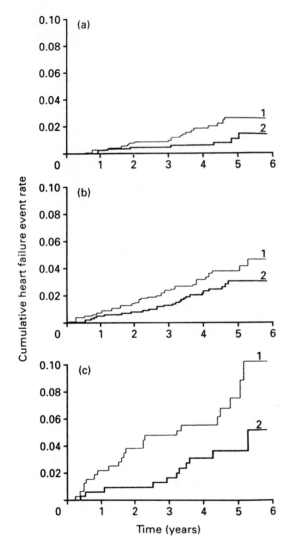

**Figure 38–3** ▪ Effect of antihypertensive drug therapy on the incidence of heart failure in the Systolic Hypertension in the Elderly Program (SHEP): (a) 60–69 years; (b) 70–79 years; (c) 80 years and older. In each panel, line 1 represents placebo and line 2 active treatment. (Kostis JB, Davis BR, Cutler J, et al: Prevention of heart failure by antihypertensive drug treatment in older persons with isolated systolic hypertension. JAMA 1997;278:212–216. Copyright 1997, American Medical Association.)

Atrial fibrillation in the elderly is almost always associated with significant underlying cardiac disease, with hypertension, CAD, valvular heart disease, and sick sinus syndrome being the most common precursors. Hyperthyroidism, alcoholism, nonischemic cardiomyopathies, chronic lung disease, and electrolyte disturbances (especially hypokalemia) are also important causes of atrial fibrillation in the elderly. In addition, atrial fibrillation frequently complicates major cardiac and noncardiac surgery in older patients.

The symptoms of atrial fibrillation in the elderly are highly variable. Many patients are asymptomatic or experience only mild palpitations. Others describe fatigue, shortness of breath, or poor exercise tolerance, and still others present with acute pulmonary edema or stroke. In the Framingham Heart Study, the proportion of strokes attributable to atrial fibrillation increased from 1.5% in patients aged 50 to 59 years to 23.5% after age 80,[56] thus demonstrating the importance of atrial fibrillation as a cause of stroke at older ages.

Although it is clear that the risk of stroke in patients with atrial fibrillation increases with age, particularly after age 75, the management of atrial fibrillation in the very elderly remains somewhat controversial. The greatest effect of warfarin in reducing the absolute risk of thromboembolic stroke occurs in patients over age 75, but the risk of major bleeding complications, including intracranial hemorrhage, is also highest in this age group. Indeed, in the second Stroke Prevention in Atrial Fibrillation (SPAF-II) trial, the net benefits of warfarin and aspirin were similar after age 75.[57] Despite these findings, most experts recommend that patients over age 75 with chronic atrial fibrillation and no major contraindications be treated with warfarin to maintain an international normalized ratio (INR) in the range of 2.0 to 3.0. Aspirin is a less effective alternative in patients with contraindications to warfarin.

In patients with atrial fibrillation of recent onset (i.e., within 6 to 12 months), many clinicians attempt cardioversion at least once and prescribe antiarrhythmic therapy to maintain sinus rhythm after successful cardioversion. However, the value of this approach versus a strategy of rate control with atrioventricular nodal blocking agents in combination with anticoagulation is currently unknown and is the subject of the ongoing AFFIRM (Atrial Fibrillation Followup Investigation of Rhythm Management) trial. In certain elderly patients with chronic atrial fibrillation that does not respond to conventional atrioventricular nodal blocking agents, atrioventricular nodal ablation with placement of a permanent ventricular pacemaker often provides significant symptomatic palliation. Since atrial fibrillation persists in these patients, antithrombotic therapy with warfarin or aspirin is indicated.

The treatment of other supraventricular arrhythmias, including atrial flutter, is generally similar for older and younger patients, but the risk of antiarrhythmic drug toxicity is greater in the elderly.

## Ventricular Arrhythmias

The prevalence and complexity of ventricular ectopic activity increase with age, and men are affected more often than women.[58] As in younger patients, the prognostic significance of ventricular arrhythmias is related principally to the underlying cardiac disease. Therefore, therapy should be directed at the primary disorder (e.g., CAD, hypertension), and the arrhythmias should be treated only if they produce severe symptoms or threaten to be fatal. When indicated, treatment is similar for older and younger patients. In particular, age is not a contraindication to an implanted cardioverter-defibrillator (ICD). Indeed, the majority of ICD recipients are older than 65 (see Table 38–1), and long-term survival is similar for older and younger patients.

## Bradyarrhythmias and Conduction Disturbances

Aging is associated with degenerative changes throughout the conduction system, and the prevalences of virtually all bradyarrhythmias and conduction abnormalities increase with age. From the clinical perspective, "sick sinus syndrome" is the most important disorder of the conduction system in older adults.[59] Increasing age is associated with a decline in the number of functioning pacemaker cells in the sinus node, and, by age 75, only about 10% of the cells remain capable of initiating an impulse. In addition, conduction of the impulse from the sinus node to the atrial tissues may be impaired (sinus exit block), and conduction within the atria and through the atrioventricular node may be delayed. Sick sinus syndrome thus is a generalized disorder of sinoatrial function that is often manifested by both bradyarrhythmias and supraventricular tachyarrhythmias ("tachy-brady syndrome"). Importantly, most medications used to treat the tachyarrhythmias, including beta blockers, diltiazem, verapamil, and antiarrhythmic agents, can exacerbate bradyarrhythmias.

Bradyarrhythmias commonly associated with the sick sinus syndrome include marked sinus bradycardia, sinus pauses and sinus arrest, sinus exit block, advanced atrioventricular nodal block, and atrial fibrillation with slow ventricular response. These arrhythmias can produce a spectrum of symptoms ranging from fatigue, shortness of breath, angina, and reduced exercise tolerance to dizziness, impaired cognition, and syncope. For patients with major symptoms directly attributable to bradycardia, permanent pacemaker implantation is indicated. In the United States, more than 80% of all pacemakers are implanted in older persons (see Table 38–1), and sick sinus syndrome is the most common underlying disorder. For patients in sinus rhythm, dual-chamber pacing is associated with better quality of life as compared with single-chamber ventricular pacing.[60]

## Cardiopulmonary Resuscitation

The value of cardiopulmonary resuscitation (CPR) in elderly patients remains a matter of debate. Fewer than 10% of older patients who suffer cardiac arrest and receive CPR have favorable neurological outcomes and survive longer than 30 days.[61] In addition, there is little difference in outcomes, whether the arrest occurs in a hospital, a nursing home, or a community setting. Despite these grim statistics, a subgroup of older patients can be identified who enjoy substantially better outcomes. For example, previously healthy persons who receive prompt CPR for a witnessed cardiac arrest and who are subsequently found to be in ventricular fibrillation have a 25% to 40% chance of surviving with a good neurologic outcome. Thus, although the decision to initiate CPR must be based on both clinical and psychosocial considerations, the results of CPR can be quite gratifying, even in the very old.

## ▪ EXERCISE AND CARDIAC REHABILITATION

As it is in younger patients, physical inactivity is a risk factor for cardiovascular events in older adults, and regular physical exercise is associated with improved health status and sense of well-being in elderly persons. In addition, the benefits of cardiac rehabilitation after MI or cardiac surgery are comparable for older and younger patients.[62] Despite these considerations, physicians are less likely to recommend regular exercise or cardiac rehabilitation for older patients. Nonetheless, the dictum, *use it or lose it* is most applicable to the elderly, and maintaining a physically, intellectually, and emotionally active lifestyle is perhaps the best way to preserve independence and to ensure optimal quality of life.

## ▪ ETHICAL ISSUES AND END-OF-LIFE CARE

Older patients with cardiovascular disease are at increased risk for a multitude of complications, including death. Elders have widely divergent views about the use of life-sustaining interventions and other invasive medical procedures, and about what constitutes acceptable quality of life in the face of chronic or terminal illness.[63] Moreover, studies have shown that patient surrogates, including spouses and physicians, cannot reliably predict patients' wishes in specific end-of-life scenarios. To ensure that patients' wishes are honored, if and when they are no longer capable of expressing them, the physician should make an effort to address these issues when patients are still competent and lucid. Patients should also be encouraged to develop a living will and appoint durable power of attorney. In addition, for patients with a progressive illness such as HF, it is helpful to discuss where they wish to spend their final days. Potentially suitable environments include the home, a reputable hospice, a chronic care facility, and a hospital.

## ■ SUMMARY AND CONCLUSIONS

Aging is associated with extensive changes in cardiovascular structure and physiology, many of which have a direct impact on the clinical manifestations, response to treatment, and prognosis of cardiovascular disease in older adults. As a general principle, older patients are at increased risk for adverse outcomes, and the potential benefits to be derived from specific therapeutic interventions are therefore greater in older patients than in younger ones. Although additional research is needed to define the precise role of many therapies for older patients, the available evidence strongly suggests that age alone is not sufficient justification for withholding treatment. Similarly, it is quite clear that more effective preventive strategies are needed to reduce the tremendous physical, emotional, and financial burdens imposed on our society by cardiovascular disease in the ever growing elderly population.

## ■ REFERENCES

1. Wei JY: Age and the cardiovascular system. N Engl J Med 1992;327:1735–1739.
2. Kitzman DW, Higginbotham MB, Cobb FR, et al: Exercise intolerance in patients with heart failure and preserved left ventricular systolic function: Failure of the Frank-Starling mechanism. J Am Coll Cardiol 1991;17:1065–1072.
3. Management Committee: Treatment of mild hypertension in the elderly. Med J Aust 1981;II:398–402.
4. Amery A, Birkenhager W, Brixko P, et al: Mortality and morbidity results from the European Working Party on High Blood Pressure in the Elderly Trial. Lancet 1985;I:1349–1354.
5. Coope J, Warrender TS: Randomised trial of treatment of hypertension in elderly patients in primary care. Br Med J 1986;293:1145–1151.
6. Dahlof B, Lindholm LH, Hannson L, et al: Morbidity and mortality in the Swedish Trial in Old Patients with Hypertension (STOP-Hypertension). Lancet 1991;338:1281–1285.
7. MRC Working Party: Medical Research Council Trial of Treatment of Hypertension in Older Adults: Principal results. Br Med J 1992;304:405–412.
8. Hypertension Detection and Follow-up Program Cooperative Group: Five-year findings of the Hypertension Detection and Follow-up Program. I. Reduction in mortality of persons with high blood pressure, including mild hypertension. JAMA 1979;242:2562–2571.
9. Hypertension Detection and Follow-up Program Cooperative Group: Five-year findings of the Hypertension Detection and Follow-up Program. II. Mortality by race, sex and age. JAMA 1979;242:2572–2577.
10. The Systolic Hypertension in the Elderly Program (SHEP) Cooperative Research Group: Prevention of stroke by antihypertensive drug treatment in older persons with isolated systolic hypertension: Final results of SHEP. JAMA 1991;265:3255–3264.
11. Staessen JA, Fagard R, Thijs L, et al: Randomised double-blind comparison of placebo and active treatment for older patients with isolated systolic hypertension. The Systolic Hypertension in Europe (Syst-Eur) Trial Investigators. Lancet 1997;350:757–764.
12. Gong L, Zhang W, Zhu Y, et al: Shanghai Trial of Nifedipine in the Elderly (STONE). J Hypertens 1996;14:1237–1245.
13. Johnson CL, Rifkind BM, Sempos CT, et al: Declining serum total cholesterol levels among U.S. adults. The National Health and Nutrition Examination Surveys. JAMA 1993;269:3002–3008.
14. Kannel WB, Wilson PWF: An update on coronary risk factors. Med Clin North Am 1995;79:951–971.
15. Miettinen TA, Pyorala K, Olsson AG, et al: Cholesterol-lowering therapy in women and elderly patients with myocardial infarction or angina pectoris. Findings from the Scandinavian Simvastatin Survival Study (4S). Circulation 1997;96:4211–4218.
16. Lewis SJ, Moye LA, Sacks FM, et al: Effect of pravastatin on cardiovascular events in older patients

with myocardial infarction and cholesterol levels in the average range. Results of the Cholesterol and Recurrent Events (CARE) Trial. Ann Intern Med 1998;129:681–689.

17. The Long-Term Intervention with Pravastatin in Ischaemic Disease (LIPID) Study Group: Prevention of cardiovascular events and death with pravastatin in patients with coronary heart disease and a broad range of initial cholesterol levels. N Engl J Med 1998;339:1349–1357.

18. Downs JR, Clearfield M, Weis S, et al: Primary prevention of acute coronary events with lovastatin in men and women with average cholesterol levels: Results of AFCAPS/TexCAPS. Air Force/Texas Coronary Atherosclerosis Prevention Study. JAMA 1998;279:1615–1622.

19. Hermanson B, Omenn GS, Kronmal RA, Gersh BJ, and participants in the Coronary Artery Surgery Study: Beneficial six-year outcome of smoking cessation in older men and women with coronary artery disease. N Engl J Med 1988;319:1365–1369.

20. Tresch DD: Management of the older patient with acute myocardial infarction: Difference in clinical presentations between older and younger patients. J Am Geriatr Soc 1998;46:1157–1162.

21. Rich MW: Therapy for acute myocardial infarction in older persons. J Am Geriatr Soc 1998;46:1302–1307.

22. ISIS-2 (Second International Study of Infarct Survival) Collaborative Group: Randomised trial of intravenous streptokinase, oral aspirin, both, or neither among 17187 cases of suspected acute myocardial infarction: ISIS-2. Lancet 1988;II:349–360.

23. Fibrinolytic Therapy Trialists' (FTT) Collaborative Group: Indications for fibrinolytic therapy in suspected acute myocardial infarction: Collaborative overview of early mortality and major morbidity results from all randomised trials of more than 1000 patients. Lancet 1994; 343:311–322.

24. The GUSTO Investigators: An international randomized trial comparing four thrombolytic strategies for acute myocardial infarction. N Engl J Med 1993;329:673–682.

25. The Global Use of Strategies to Open Occluded Coronary Arteries in Acute Coronary Syndromes (GUSTO IIb) Angioplasty Substudy Investigators: A clinical trial comparing primary coronary angioplasty with tissue plasminogen activator for acute myocardial infarction. N Engl J Med 1997;336:1621–1628.

26. Krumholz HM, Hennen J, Ridker PM, et al: Use and effectiveness of intravenous heparin therapy for treatment of acute myocardial infarction in the elderly. J Am Coll Cardiol 1998;31:973–979.

27. Aronow WS: Management of older persons after myocardial infarction. J Am Geriatr Soc 1998;46:1459–1468.

28. Gruppo Italiano per lo Studio della Sopravvivenza nell'Infarto Miocardico: GISSI-3: Effects of lisinopril and transdermal glyceryl trinitrate singly and together on 6-week mortality and ventricular function after acute myocardial infarction. Lancet 1994;343:1115–1122.

29. Ambrosioni E, Borghi C, Magnani B, for the Survival of Myocardial Infarction Long-Term Evaluation (SMILE) Study Investigators: The effect of the angiotensin-converting enzyme inhibitor zofenopril on mortality and morbidity after anterior myocardial infarction. N Engl J Med 1995;332:80–85.

30. Pfeffer MA, Braunwald E, Moye LA, et al: Effect of captopril on mortality and morbidity in patients with left ventricular dysfunction after myocardial infarction. Results of the Survival and Ventricular Enlargement Trial. N Engl J Med 1992;327:669–677.

31. The Acute Infarction Ramipril Efficacy (AIRE) Study Investigators: Effect of ramipril on mortality and morbidity of survivors of acute myocardial infarction with clinical evidence of heart failure. Lancet 1993;342:821–828.

32. The TIMI IIIB Investigators: Effects of tissue plasminogen activator and a comparison of early invasive and conservative strategies in unstable angina and non–Q wave myocardial infarction. Results of the TIMI IIIB Trial. Circulation 1994;89:1545–1556.

33. Boden WE, O'Rourke RA, Crawford MH, et al: Outcomes in patients with acute non–Q wave myocardial infarction randomly assigned to an invasive as compared with a conservative management strategy. N Engl J Med 1998;338:1785–1792.

34. Thompson RC, Holmes DR: Percutaneous transluminal coronary angioplasty in the elderly. Clin Geriatr Med 1996;12:181–194.

35. Alexander KP, Peterson ED: Coronary artery bypass grafting in the elderly. Am Heart J 1997;134:856–864.

36. Gersh BJ, Kronmal RA, Schaff HV, et al: Comparison of coronary artery bypass surgery and medical therapy in patients 65 years of age or older. A nonrandomized study from the Coronary Artery Surgery Study (CASS) registry. N Engl J Med 1985;313:217–224.

37. Cheitlin MD: Valve disease in the octogenarian. In Wenger NK (ed): Cardiovascular Disease in the Octogenarian and Beyond. London: Martin Dunitz, 1999;255–266.

38. Aranki SF, Nathan M, Cohn LH: Surgery for valvular heart disease in the octogenarian. In Wenger NK (ed): Cardiovascular Disease in the Octogenarian and Beyond. London: Martin Dunitz, 1999;267–277.

39. Erbelding EJ, Gerding DN, Chesler E: Infective endocarditis. In Chesler E (ed): Clinical Cardiology in the Elderly. Armonk, NY: Futura, 1994;427–445.

40. Rich MW: Epidemiology, pathophysiology, and etiology of congestive heart failure in older adults. J Am Geriatr Soc 1997;45:968–974.

41. Krumholz HM, Parent EM, Tu N, et al: Readmission after hospitalization for congestive heart failure among Medicare beneficiaries. Arch Intern Med 1997;157:99–104.

42. Rich MW: Heart failure disease management: A critical review. J Cardiac Failure 1999;5:64–75.

43. The CONSENSUS Trial Study Group: Effects of enalapril on mortality in severe congestive heart

failure. Results of the Cooperative North Scandinavian Enalapril Survival Study. N Engl J Med 1987;316:1429–1435.

44. The SOLVD Investigators: Effect of enalapril on mortality and the development of heart failure in asymptomatic patients with reduced left ventricular ejection fractions. N Engl J Med 1992;327:685–691.

45. The SOLVD Investigators: Effect of enalapril on survival in patients with reduced left ventricular ejection fractions and congestive heart failure. N Engl J Med 1991;325:293–302.

46. Garg R, Yusuf S, for the Collaborative Group on ACE Inhibitor Trials: Overview of randomized trials of angiotensin-converting enzyme inhibitors on mortality and morbidity in patients with heart failure. JAMA 1995;273:1450–1456.

47. Pitt B, Segal R, Martinez FA, et al: Randomised trial of losartan versus captopril in patients over 65 with heart failure (Evaluation of Losartan in the Elderly Study, ELITE). Lancet 1997;349:747–752.

48. Cohn JN, Archibald DG, Ziesche S, et al: Effect of vasodilator therapy on mortality in chronic congestive heart failure. Results of a Veterans Administration Cooperative Study. N Engl J Med 1986;314:1547–1552.

49. Cohn JN, Johnson G, Ziesche S, et al: A comparison of enalapril with hydralazine-isosorbide dinitrate in the treatment of chronic congestive heart failure. N Engl J Med 1991;325:303–310.

50. Rich MW: Heart failure: Epidemiology, pathophysiology and management. *In* Wenger NK (ed): Cardiovascular Disease in the Octogenarian and Beyond. London: Martin Dunitz, 1999;73–91.

51. The Digitalis Investigation Group: The effect of digoxin on mortality and morbidity in patients with heart failure. N Engl J Med 1997;336:525–533.

52. Packer M, Bristow MR, Cohn JN, et al: The effect of carvedilol on morbidity and mortality in patients with chronic heart failure. N Engl J Med 1996;334:1349–1355.

53. CIBIS-II Investigators and Committees: The Cardiac Insufficiency Bisoprolol Study II (CIBIS II): A randomized trial. Lancet 1999;353:9–13.

54. Packer M, O'Connor CM, Ghali JK, et al: Effect of amlodipine on morbidity and mortality in severe chronic heart failure. N Engl J Med 1996;335:1107–1114.

55. Kostis JB, Davis BR, Cutler J, et al: Prevention of heart failure by antihypertensive drug treatment in older persons with isolated systolic hypertension. JAMA 1997;278:212–216.

56. Wolf PA, Abbott RD, Kannel WB: Atrial fibrillation as an independent risk factor for stroke: The Framingham Study. Stroke 1991;22:983–988.

57. Halperin JL, Hart RG, Kronmal RA, et al: Warfarin versus aspirin for prevention of thromboembolism in atrial fibrillation: Stroke Prevention in Atrial Fibrillation II Study. Lancet 1994;343:687–691.

58. Fleg JL: Arrhythmias and conduction disturbances in the octogenarian: Epidemiology and progression. *In* Wenger NK (ed): Cardiovascular Disease in the Octogenarian and Beyond. London: Martin Dunitz, 1999;279–290.

59. Rodriguez RD, Schocken DD: Update on sick sinus syndrome, a cardiac disorder of aging. Geriatrics 1990;45(1):26–30, 33–36.

60. Lamas GA, Orav EJ, Stambler BS, et al: Quality of life and clinical outcomes in elderly patients treated with ventricular pacing as compared with dual-chamber pacing. Pacemaker Selection in the Elderly Investigators. N Engl J Med 1998;338:1097–1104.

61. Tresch DD, Amirani H: Cardiopulmonary resuscitation in the elderly: Beneficial or an exercise in futility? *In* Wenger NK (ed): Cardiovascular Disease in the Octogenarian and Beyond. London: Martin Dunitz, 1999;291–304.

62. Lavie CJ, Milani RV: Effects of cardiac rehabilitation programs on exercise capacity, coronary risk factors, behavioral characteristics, and quality of life in a large elderly cohort. Am J Cardiol 1995;76:177–179.

63. Hofmann JC, Wenger NS, Davis RB, et al: Patient preferences for communication with physicians about end-of-life decisions. SUPPORT Investigators. Study to Understand Prognoses and Preference for Outcomes and Risks of Treatment. Ann Intern Med 1997;127:1–12.

## ■ RECOMMENDED READING

Aronow WS, Tresch DD (eds): Coronary artery disease in the elderly. Clin Geriatr Med 1996;12(1):1–236.

Tresch DD, Aronow WS (eds): Cardiovascular Disease in the Elderly Patient, 2nd ed. New York: Marcel Dekker, 1999.

Wenger NK (ed): Cardiovascular Disease in the Octogenarian and Beyond. London: Martin Dunitz, 1999.

# Chapter 39

# Cardiovascular Complications in Patients with Renal Disease

*Richard A. Preston* ■ *Simon Chakko* ■ *Murray Epstein*

The heart and kidneys are invariably intertwined. Heart failure is associated with the important alterations in renal hemodynamics and function that constitute a major problem of clinical management. Conversely, in persons with chronic renal disease, the heart rarely escapes consequences. Cardiovascular complications are the major cause of death in the end-stage renal disease (ESRD) population.[1] The effects of chronic renal failure on the heart are diverse and involve numerous anatomic and functional aspects of the cardiovascular system.

Given the broad scope of this subject, we have elected to focus our review primarily on the more common cardiovascular alterations that complicate the course of progressive renal disease: pericarditis, renal parenchymal hypertension, coronary arteriosclerosis, and left ventricular dysfunction. Finally, we have included a discussion of ischemic renal disease, a common but underdiagnosed disorder that is an important complication of systemic arteriosclerosis.

## ■ PERICARDITIS (See also Chapter 34)

Pericarditis is a common and often severe complication of advanced chronic renal failure. Before emergency dialysis was available, the appearance of a pericardial friction rub in a patient with ESRD was a harbinger of death within the ensuing 2 weeks. Many authorities group pericarditis associated with ESRD into two main categories.[1–3] Early or uremic pericarditis occurs in ESRD patients before chronic dialysis therapy is instituted and is probably secondary to the biochemical perturbations of uremia per se. Early or uremic pericarditis generally responds rapidly to renal replacement therapy in the majority of patients. Late or dialysis-associated pericarditis develops in patients who are already receiving renal replacement therapy. In general, dialysis-associated pericarditis tends to be more severe, has a higher rate of complications, responds less readily to dialysis, and is more likely to result in pericardial tamponade.[1–3]

### Incidence

In 1968, a 41% prevalence of uremic pericarditis was reported in patients beginning dialysis. The incidence of uremic pericarditis has fallen in recent years, probably because of the greater availability and earlier initiation of renal replacement therapy. More recent reports indicate a much lower prevalence, less than 10%. Pericarditis has been found to occur in approximately 10% to 20% of patients receiving regular dialysis therapy, figures that have not changed appreciably over the past decade.

## Pathology

The basic pathologic process of pericarditis associated with ESRD, an aseptic inflammatory reaction with fibrin formation, is similar in both uremic pericarditis and dialysis-associated pericarditis. Both parietal and visceral pericardium are covered with a fibrinous exudate. Fibrinous bands are usually present and form adhesions and areas of loculation between the two layers. The effusion is usually serosanguinous but is uniformly hemorrhagic in cases of tamponade. The white blood cell count in the effusion is variable but usually in the range of 500 to 700 per cubic millimeter with variable proportions of polymorphonuclear and mononuclear leukocytes. Cultures are routinely negative.

## Pathogenesis

Pericarditis in ESRD patients who have not yet begun dialysis is most likely related to the biochemical milieu of untreated uremia as evidenced by the rapid response to the initiation of dialysis and the clinical correlation with biochemical control of uremia in the majority of patients.[1-3] Dialysis-associated pericarditis, on the other hand, is less well-understood. It is not clear why a substantial percentage of patients receiving regular renal replacement should develop pericarditis. Dialysis-associated pericarditis may be related to underdialysis in some patients, but this is not always the case. The cause of dialysis-associated pericarditis is probably multifactorial and is ill-understood.

A number of potential pathogenic factors have been proposed to explain dialysis-associate pericarditis, including inadequate dialysis therapy, hypercatabolic states, poorly controlled hyperparathyroidism, heparin received during dialysis, and an abnormal immune response. Underdialysis has been noted in a significant percentage of patients with dialysis-associated pericarditis, often as a result of vascular access failure or missing dialysis treatments. In addition, pericarditis has been observed to occur during periods of hypercatabolism such as after major surgery or during sepsis.

A possible role for severe secondary hyperparathyroidism in the genesis of dialysis-associated pericarditis has been proposed, but this has not been established. Heparin most likely does not initiate inflammation of the pericardium but can contribute to ongoing inflammation by causing bleeding from the friable membranes. Evidence for an infectious cause (e.g., viral, bacterial, tuberculous) has been demonstrated in a minority of cases. Finally, certain autoantibodies have been demonstrated in patients with dialysis-associated pericarditis, a finding that implies that an immune-mediated mechanism may be responsible in some cases.

## Clinical Features

The presentation of pericarditis in a patient with ESRD may be dramatic, marked by a fulminant course resulting in acute tamponade. On the other hand, a patient may present with only vague chest pain or mild constitutional symptoms. Dialysis-associated pericarditis may occasionally present as recurrent hypotension during hemodialysis. Clinical and laboratory features of the pericarditis of ESRD are summarized in Table 39–1. Pericardial friction rub and chest pain are important in the diagnosis of pericarditis but are not always present. Dialysis-associated pericarditis is a more severe clinical illness marked by more systemic manifestations, a higher likelihood of tamponade, and a less favorable response to dialysis.[1-4]

The majority of patients have chest pain, which may be variable in character and severity. The pain may be located anywhere in the precordium and may

Table 39–1

**Prevalence of Clinical Features of Pericarditis
Associated with End-Stage Renal Disease**

| Finding | Prevalence (%) |
| --- | --- |
| Pericardial rub | 95 |
| Chest pain | 60–70 |
| Hypotension | 13–56 |
| Fever | 63–76 |
| Leukocytosis | 35–71 |
| Classic ECG changes for pericarditis | 2–5 |
| Arrhythmias | 20–28 |
| Pericardial effusion (echocardiogram) | 89 |

antedate the development of a friction rub. There is often a pleuritic component to the pain, and it may be aggravated by lying supine and partially relieved by sitting forward. A pericardial friction rub may be detected in more than 90% of patients. The rub is typically evanescent and may change in quality from moment to moment. Thus, the absence of a rub on any given physical examination does not rule out pericarditis.

Hemodynamic compromise, including hypotension during hemodialysis, may be a presenting clinical feature. Dialysis-associated pericarditis should be sought when any patient suffers repeated episodes of hypotension during dialysis or one with ESRD presents with hypotension despite signs of fluid overload.

Fever and leukocytosis may more often be associated with dialysis-associated pericarditis and, if severe, may predict a less favorable response to intensification of the dialysis regimen. The electrocardiogram (ECG) is of very limited usefulness in the diagnosis of pericarditis in ESRD. ECG abnormalities are common but nonspecific. The classic ST segment elevations described in several types of acute pericarditis are uncommon in this form; the most common findings are nonspecific ST and T wave abnormalities. Atrial arrhythmias, including atrial flutter and fibrillation, have been observed in a significant number of cases.

Echocardiography is the easiest and most accurate method for detecting pericardial effusion. It can be done rapidly and at the bedside, if necessary. The echocardiogram provides useful information on the size of a pericardial effusion and can detect early or impending tamponade. Information on the volume of the effusion and its hemodynamic significance is important when reaching a decision regarding early management of uremic pericarditis. A large effusion or one that causes hemodynamic embarrassment generally does not respond to conservative management with dialysis alone; often surgical drainage is required.

Acute cardiac tamponade is the most serious—and potentially lethal— complication of pericarditis associated with ESRD and is more common in dialysis-associated pericarditis than in uremic pericarditis. It has been reported that as many as 35% of patients with dialysis-associated pericarditis experience tamponade or impending tamponade.[4] Tamponade may occur during or shortly after a dialysis session. It may be difficult to distinguish acute tamponade from hypovolemia-induced hypotension. In patients with unexplained hypotension during or shortly after dialysis, the echocardiogram may be very useful in making this important differential diagnosis. It is important to maintain a high index of suspicion for pericarditis-related tamponade in patients with hypotension during hemodialysis because it is potentially reversible.

## Management

When uremic pericarditis develops in a patient with renal disease approaching ESRD, institution of renal replacement therapy is indicated. Cardiac tamponade is unusual in this form of pericarditis, and most patients respond well to dialysis therapy with resolution of the signs and symptoms of pericarditis.

Management of dialysis-associated pericarditis has been less satisfactory. The initial treatment is determined by the hemodynamic stability of the patient. For a stable patient who does not have evidence of tamponade or impending tamponade, the first line of treatment is generally intensification of dialysis therapy, monitored by repeat echocardiographic evaluations of effusion size. This approach has yielded a response rate of approximately 60% to 70%. In the majority of cases, the response is seen within the first 10 to 14 days after initiating intensive dialysis therapy. If hemodynamic compromise develops or the effusion fails to reduce in size or becomes larger over a course of 10 to 14 days, a drainage procedure should be undertaken.

A positive effect from the use of nonsteroidal antiinflammatory agents in the treatment of pericarditis has been difficult to prove and these drugs are associated with gastrointestinal toxicity and bleeding complications. Similarly, systemic corticosteroids have been reported to improve the clinical course of pericarditis but are associated with side effects and do not seem to prevent the development of constrictive pericarditis. Nonsteroidal antiinflammatory agents and steroids are controversial for pericarditis associated with ESRD.

Several clinical features predict the failure of intensive dialysis intervention and thus the need for early surgical drainage for treatment of pericarditis. A report by De Pace and coworkers[5] suggests that, in the presence of a large pericardial effusion, temperature greater than 102°F, and rales, peritoneal dialysis is required because the patient is too hemodynamically unstable to tolerate hemodialysis. Systolic blood pressure under 100 mm Hg, jugular venous distention, white blood cell count over 15,000 per cubic millimeter, and white blood cell count leftward shift all correlated with poor outcomes with dialysis treatment alone. The simultaneous presence of several of these features describes disease that likely will not respond favorably to intensive dialysis therapy. Thus, the febrile, toxic patient with a large effusion and evidence of hemodynamic compromise is at high risk of failing to respond to dialysis alone, and the need for a drainage procedure should be anticipated.

Pericardiocentesis is associated with a high rate of severe complications, including lacerations of the atrial or ventricular wall or coronary arteries. Most series report high morbidity and mortality rates for pericardiocentesis. In addition, pericardiocentesis has a high rate of reaccumulation of pericardial fluid and thus is not a definitive procedure. Because purulent pericarditis is rare in patients with ESRD, there is little need for diagnostic pericardiocentesis. Therefore, it is generally recommended only for extreme emergency situations as a last resort.

Subxiphoid pericardiotomy is a safe, effective, and relatively easy procedure to achieve pericardial drainage. It is generally tolerated better by uremic patients who are ill and often have hemodynamic compromise in comparison with the more extensive (albeit more definitive) pericardiectomy. Subxiphoid pericardiotomy is associated with a 6% failure rate but a low rate of complications. Experts recommend instillation of intrapericardial steroid (triamcinolone hexacetine, 50 mg every 6 hours) after pericardiotomy.

Pericardiectomy is a definitive surgical procedure almost never associated with fluid reaccumulation. Pericardiectomy also prevents the late complication of constrictive pericarditis. It is, however, an extensive major surgical intervention requiring general anesthesia and either a median sternotomy or anterior thoracotomy. Pericardiectomy remains the treatment of choice for constrictive pericarditis.

## ■ RENAL PARENCHYMAL HYPERTENSION (See also Chapter 31)

Any consideration of cardiovascular complications in persons who have renal disease must, a priori, consider the generation of renal parenchymal hypertension and its effects on cardiac structure and function. Renal parenchymal hypertension[6-11] is hypertension that is caused by kidney disease and is the most common type of secondary hypertension. Chronic renal disease and systemic hypertension may coexist in three very different clinical settings. First, primary hypertension is an important cause of chronic renal disease. Poorly controlled, severe, sustained hypertension over an extended period results in hypertensive nephrosclerosis. In the second situation, renal parenchymal disease is a well-established and important cause of secondary hypertension. Therefore, hypertension is both a cause and a consequence of renal disease. Renal parenchymal hypertension is the most common secondary form of hypertension and accounts for 3% to 5% of all cases of systemic hypertension. The secondary hypertension produced by the diseased kidneys may accelerate the decline in renal function if it is not adequately controlled. Sometimes, it may be difficult to distinguish clinically between primary hypertension causing nephrosclerosis and renal disease causing hypertension. The third clinical setting in which chronic renal disease and hypertension may coexist is ischemic renal disease, which is discussed briefly later in this chapter.

Renal parenchymal hypertension may be caused by almost any disease of the renal parenchyma (Table 39–2). A patient who appears to have primary hypertension may have underlying renal disease that is causing the hypertension. The initial evaluation of all hypertensive patients should include a screen for renal disease. Determination of blood urea nitrogen and serum creatinine values and careful urinalysis with examination of the urinary sediment, often, but not invariably, rules out significant underlying renal disease. Urinary findings that suggest that a renal disease is causing the hypertension are cellular and granular casts, significant hematuria, pyuria, and urine protein excretion greater than 150 mg in 24 hours.

### Pathogenesis

Renal parenchymal hypertension most probably represents the combined interactions of many independent mechanisms: potential factors include sodium retention leading to volume expansion, increases in endogenous pressor activity, and decreases in endogenous vasodepressor compounds. The precise mechanisms that lead to hypertension in chronic renal failure have not been completely defined, but

---

Table 39–2

**Common Causes of Renal Parenchymal Hypertension**

| Glomerular diseases | Interstitial diseases |
|---|---|
| Postinfectious glomerulonephritis | Polycystic kidney disease |
| Focal segmental sclerosis | Chronic interstitial nephritis |
| Renal vasculitis | |
| Diabetic nephropathy | |
| Crescentic glomerulonephritis | |
| Systemic lupus erythematosus nephritis | |

recent investigations have provided exciting new insights. Traditionally, the focus has been on volume-mediated mechanisms, the renin-angiotensin system, and renal prostaglandins; recently, increasing attention has been given to other pressor and vasodilator systems, including endogenous digitalis-like factor (DLF), endothelin, and nitric oxide (NO). The sodium intake and the volume-mediated mechanisms of renal parenchymal hypertension are of central importance to management and will be discussed in more detail.

## Sodium Intake

Impaired renal sodium excretion leads to positive sodium balance and contributes to the development of renal parenchymal hypertension. Abnormal renal sodium excretion is the most important mechanism of renal parenchymal hypertension, from a clinical standpoint. Patients with renal failure have increased total extracellular fluid volume (ECFV) sodium as compared with normal controls and patients with primary hypertension. This increase in ECFV sodium correlates directly with increased ECFV and with hypertension. Changes in sodium intake directly influence blood pressure in patients with chronic renal failure, and this relationship seems stronger at lower levels of renal function. Increasing sodium intake in patients with chronic renal failure increases ECFV and blood pressure. The increment in blood pressure for a given increase in ECFV tends to be greater in the patients with farther advanced renal failure. Reduction of dietary sodium lowers ECFV and blood pressure in many patients with chronic renal insufficiency. This sodium sensitivity of the hypertension caused by renal disease is key to appropriate antihypertensive therapy.

Despite the importance of impaired sodium excretion and ECFV expansion in the genesis of renal parenchymal hypertension, the most consistently observed hemodynamic alteration in established cases is elevation of peripheral vascular resistance rather than increased cardiac output. The mechanism(s) for this elevation in peripheral vascular resistance are not known exactly: the relationship of ECFV expansion to pressure elevation appears to be complex and may involve alterations in autonomic function, in neurohumoral control of blood pressure, and possibly in local vascular factors such as increased cytosolic calcium concentration in vascular smooth muscle. There is a complex connection between volume expansion and peripheral vascular resistance in patients with the sodium-sensitive hypertension of chronic renal disease. Part of this connection may be explained by the existence of an endogenous DLF, believed to be a steroid produced in the adrenal, the hypothalamus, or both. DLF is believed to act by inhibiting cellular Na-K-ATPase activity, resulting in increased smooth muscle calcium. Increased intracellular calcium, in turn, favors increased vascular smooth muscle tone and elevated peripheral vascular resistance. Studies in humans suggest that DLF activity is increased in the hypertension secondary to chronic renal failure and ESRD.

## Nephron Number, Hypertension, and Renal Injury

The number of functioning nephron units present at birth may determine a person's predisposition to the subsequent development of hypertension and renal damage. Low birth weight may impair renal development, reduce the number of glomeruli, or decrease the filtration surface area (FSA).[10] This decrease in FSA could eventually lead to an increase in glomerular capillary hydraulic pressure (glomerular hypertension) with consequent development of glomerular sclerosis. Thus, the "dose" of functioning nephrons present at birth may determine the risk of developing hypertension and renal disease later in life.

There may be a balance between nephron number and metabolic requirements imposed upon the kidney. Consequently, a nephron dose smaller than some critical value (relative to the metabolic demands of the patient) may be inadequate for survival of the kidney. Therefore, the number of functioning nephrons in the kidney may not suffice for the patient and the single-nephron glomerular filtration rate may increase, leading to intraglomerular hypertension, proteinuria, and declining glomerular filtration rate. Although the role of nephron dosing in the pathogenesis of renal parenchymal hypertension has not been established, it has been proposed that the number of nephrons is related to the risk of developing hypertension in association with the progression of chronic renal disease.

## Treatment of Renal Parenchymal Hypertension: Focus on Sodium Balance (See also Chapter 32)

Regardless of what mechanisms lead from ECFV expansion to hypertension, sodium retention with associated ECFV expansion plays a central role in the pathogenesis of renal parenchymal hypertension. Consequently, therapeutic modalities that reduce total body sodium are frequently very effective in lowering blood pressure in patients with renal parenchymal hypertension. Even small net gains in total body sodium can produce significant increases in blood pressure. The first step in managing renal parenchymal hypertension is reduction of ECF sodium.

The management of patients with hypertension secondary to chronic renal insufficiency is a common and often perplexing problem for general internists. Elevated systemic arterial blood pressure indicates a poor prognosis for a number of renal disorders, and there is extensive evidence that hypertension of any cause accelerates the deterioration of renal function. Therefore, preservation of renal function is a compelling reason for early identification and vigorous treatment of hypertension: Regardless of what mechanism(s) are involved, treatment of hypertension has been shown to retard progression of renal impairment in several disease states. Because both the prevalence and the severity of hypertension increase as the glomerular filtration rate declines, it is important to continue close follow-up and frequent reassessment of therapy.

## Sodium Restriction

Renal sodium retention with associated ECFV expansion plays a central role in the genesis of renal parenchymal hypertension, and therapeutic measures that reduce extracellular fluid sodium are frequently very effective in lowering blood pressure. Sodium restriction and diuretics are critical components of effective antihypertensive therapy in patients with renal disease. Controlling blood pressure in patients with chronic renal disease is difficult, if not impossible, without dietary sodium restriction.

Reasonable guidelines for dietary sodium restriction are summarized in Table 39–3. Realistically, 2 g of sodium per day (i.e., 88 mEq) is the minimum sodium intake attainable on an outpatient basis. To maintain this modestly low level of sodium intake requires intensive dietary education and patient compliance. For example, processed foods such as canned vegetables and soups, prepared meat products, and most so-called fast foods contain a very great deal of sodium, as do most seasonings. The preparation of many processed foods adds a great deal of sodium. A variety of educational material listing the sodium contents of different foods for sodium-restricted diets is readily available, and we find repeated counseling and education by clinical dietictians along with diligent follow-up to be quite useful. Patients should be cautioned about the use of salt substitutes: many contain

Table 39–3

**Dietary Sodium Restriction for Chronic Renal Failure**

Restrict sodium to 2 g/day (88 mEq/day)
Measure weight and blood pressure frequently
Measure blood urea nitrogen and creatinine serially
If sodium bicarbonate replacement is required, reevaluate Na intake
Avoid salt substitutes with potassium

potassium and should be avoided altogether by patients with renal impairment and diminished potassium excretory capacity.

Because the chronically diseased kidney may adapt poorly to rapid changes in sodium intake, sodium restriction should be initiated under close observation. When confronted with an abrupt reduction in dietary sodium, some patients may not be able to reduce urinary sodium excretion quickly and a period of negative sodium balance may ensue. This sodium-wasting tendency is generally reversible after several weeks, but early negative sodium balance may decrease ECFV and lead to prerenal azotemia.

Sodium intake must be individualized and carefully monitored. Every renal disease patient should be followed closely for signs of ECFV depletion (i.e., orthostatic blood pressure change or rapid decline in body weight) or worsening azotemia. Serial measurements of body weight and blood chemistries are often useful for identifying an "ideal" weight (ECFV) for optimal blood pressure control.

As renal failure progresses, metabolic acidosis develops in most patients. If sodium bicarbonate is prescribed to counter the metabolic acidosis, the additional sodium must be taken into account when planning total dietary sodium intake or deciding to add loop diuretics to the therapeutic regimen. A typical daily dose of oral sodium citrate solution (1 mEq/ml) is approximately 45 ml. This volume contains 45 mEq of sodium (which is 45 mEq $\times$ 23 mg of sodium per milliequivalent, or 1035 mg per day) fully 50% of the daily sodium allowance! (Citrate is a commonly prescribed bicarbonate precursor that is converted to bicarbonate in the liver.) Although it has been assumed that a patient with advanced renal failure would require more drastic sodium restriction, recent studies demonstrated that the anionic component of an orally administered sodium salt can affect the salt's capacity to increase blood pressure. They reported that replacing supplemental sodium chloride with an equimolar amount of sodium citrate abolished the increase in blood pressure induced by sodium chloride. Consequently, concerns about the pressor effects of sodium citrate solutions may not be warranted.

Because, often, attempts to lower blood pressure by rigid dietary salt restriction are not tolerated by patients, particularly in view of the other dietary restrictions often needed to manage renal failure (i.e., protein restriction), in most cases the next step to control sodium balance is a trial of diuretic therapy.

## Diuretic Therapy

If a trial of sodium restriction is not tolerated or does not produce an adequate reduction of total body sodium, a diuretic should be added to the antihypertensive regimen.[11]

### Thiazide Diuretics

Thiazides alone are not usually effective natriuretics in patients whose serum creatinine value is greater than 2.0 mg/dl or a creatinine clearance rate below 30 ml/min, probably owing to diminished delivery of the sodium load to the distal nephron and of the drug to its site of action. Therefore, the use of thiazide diuretics alone is not recommended for patients with compromised renal function.

## Loop Diuretics

The loop-acting diuretics (furosemide, ethacrynic acid, bumetanide, torasemide) are the agents of choice for the management of ECFV and hypertension when the glomerular filtration rate falls below 30 ml/min. Unlike the thiazides, the loop agents are effective natriuretics at filtration rates well below 30 ml/min, even when used alone, although very high doses may be required as renal failure progresses. The loop diuretics act by inhibiting chloride (and sodium) reabsorption at the medullary thick ascending limb of the loop of Henle, which reabsorbs approximately 25% to 30% of the filtered sodium load. Because so much filtered sodium is reabsorbed in this nephron segment, it is understandable why these agents are such potent natriuretics.

Because loop diuretics act from the luminal side, they must enter the tubular lumen, both by glomerular filtration and by tubular secretion, before they can act. The dose-response curve of the loop diuretics is sigmoid, because the natriuretic response depends on a threshold concentration of drug being delivered to its site of action. One approach to obtaining the optimal diuretic dose is to increase the dose of diuretic carefully until the desired natriuresis occurs. This dose would correspond to some point on the "steep" part of the curve, where a small increase in diuretic delivery results in a large increase in natriuresis.

A common pitfall in the practical use of loop diuretics is increasing dose frequency rather than dose size: when a chosen dose fails to produce sufficient natriuresis, rather than increasing the dose, the clinician administers the *same* dose but more often, mistakenly expecting an additive response. The size of single doses should be increased until satisfactory natriuresis is achieved. If still more natriuresis is desired, either the dose size or the dose frequency can be increased. The dose-response curve flattens above a certain dose. Beyond this point, there is no advantage to increasing single doses. If further sodium excretion is required than is produced with the maximum single effective dose, then additional *effective* doses of the diuretic may be prescribed. In general, furosemide requires twice daily dosing, whereas bumetanide is usually given once daily. If the response is insufficient, single doses can be increased to a maximum of about 480 mg. Larger single doses are unlikely to be more effective, and they increase the risk of ototoxicity.

Dietary sodium restriction is important during diuretic therapy because sodium retention may occur between doses of diuretic. This sodium retention may be sufficient to completely neutralize the natriuretic effects of the loop diuretics if sodium restriction is not imposed.

In our clinical practice, we have found daily weighing to be the most useful indicator of changes in extracellular sodium. Done at the same time each day and on the same scale, the daily weight is quite helpful in determining net changes in sodium balance. An "ideal" weight can often be established at which the blood pressure becomes easier to manage. Measurements of 24-hour urinary excretion of sodium are somewhat time consuming and cumbersome but may be useful to confirm patient compliance with sodium restriction or suspected sodium wasting.

Patients with the nephrotic syndrome may demonstrate diuretic resistance, even with a preserved glomerular filtration rate, possibly owing to intraluminal binding of the diuretic by albumin, which inactivates the diuretic before it reaches its site of action at the loop of Henle. Conclusive human data have been difficult to obtain, but diuretic resistance is a serious clinical problem in nephrotic patients.

The initial dose of furosemide for patients with a 50% or greater reduction in glomerular filtration rate is about 40 mg IV or 80 mg PO. The corresponding dose of bumetanide is about 1 mg IV or PO. Furosemide may be titrated as high as 120 to 160 mg IV or 240 to 320 mg PO and bumetanide as high as 4 to 6 mg IV or PO.

Hypokalemia and glucose intolerance may complicate therapy with the loop diuretics. The risk of ototoxicity is increased by renal insufficiency and by concomitant administration of aminoglycosides. In addition, care must be taken to avoid overdiuresis and consequent intravascular volume depletion and prerenal azotemia.

## ■ CORONARY ATHEROSCLEROSIS

Ischemic heart disease[12–16] is common in patients with ESRD. In the United States Renal Data System, ischemic heart disease was already present in 40.8% of 3399 patients when they began chronic hemodialysis. The incidence of ischemic heart disease is even higher among patients receiving dialysis therapy. In the Canadian Hemodialysis Morbidity Study, the prevalence of myocardial infarction or angina requiring hospitalization was 10% per year. Symptomatic myocardial ischemia is usually caused by atherosclerotic obstructive disease of epicardial coronary arteries; however, small vessel disease has been reported in association with hypertension, left ventricular hypertrophy, and diabetes, all common among patients with ESRD. In hypertensive patients without epicardial coronary disease, angina may be caused by vasoconstriction of the coronary microvasculature, which leads to myocardial ischemia. In patients with left ventricular hypertrophy, angina pectoris may occur in the presence of a normal coronary angiogram. In such patients, fibromuscular hyperplasia leading to narrowing of the small coronary arteries has been demonstrated in histologic studies. A decrease in coronary reserve may occur from the deposition of calcium in the small coronary arteries.

In general, risk factors for epicardial coronary artery disease in the general population apply to patients with ESRD. Advancing age is associated with arteriographic coronary disease in patients with ESRD. Hypertension, a well-known risk factor for coronary artery disease, is common among patients with ESRD. Diabetes mellitus is an independent risk factor for coronary artery disease, although many diabetics have other risk factors such as hypertension and dyslipidemia. Diabetics tend to have more extensive involvement of small and large coronary arteries owing to a variety of factors, including hyperinsulinemia, dyslipidemia, platelet hypercoagulability, and hyperhomocysteinemia. With intercurrent hypertension and diabetes, the development and progression of coronary atherosclerosis is even more pronounced.

Lipid abnormalities have been reported in ESRD. Elevated triglyceride levels and decreased high-density lipoprotein levels are seen in hemodialysis patients and in peritoneal dialysis patients, who may also have high levels of low-density lipoprotein. Hypertriglyceridemia is caused by impaired degradation of very low-density lipoprotein. Lipoprotein (a) levels are increased in hemodialysis patients, and for them lipoprotein (a) is an independent risk factor for cardiovascular disease. Elevated homocysteine, a risk factor for atherosclerosis, is also found in ESRD patients.

Clinical presentation of ischemic heart disease in patients with ESRD may be different from that in patients without renal disease. Myocardial ischemia may be silent owing to autonomic neuropathy induced by diabetes mellitus or another disease. Anemia, left ventricular hypertrophy, and hypertension may cause myocardial ischemia and angina in the absence of significant coronary atherosclerosis. ECG findings such as ST segment and T wave abnormalities, which suggest ischemia, are common in many ESRD patients without coronary disease. The specificity of stress testing with thallium imaging to diagnose coronary disease is poor in these patients.

Dobutamine stress echocardiography may be a better diagnostic test. Coronary angiography may be necessary for definitive diagnosis.

Management of ischemic heart disease is similar to the approach used in patients without kidney disease. Maintaining the hematocrit above 30 using erythropoietin improves exercise capacity. Patients on long-term dialysis have a poor prognosis after acute myocardial infarction. Mortality from cardiac causes was 41% at 1 year, 52% at 2 years, and 70% at 5 years after acute myocardial infarction. Thus, an aggressive approach to the prevention and treatment of acute myocardial infarction is justified. If coronary angiography is performed, nonionic contrast medium is preferred. Coronary angioplasty provides good initial results but the restenosis rate is high. Coronary bypass surgery is a good option for certain patients, but the mortality rate is increased to about 10% and the perioperative morbidity rate is also higher.

## ▪ LEFT VENTRICULAR FUNCTION

Among chronic renal failure patients, alterations in cardiac structure and function[16-20] have been demonstrated with hemodynamic and echocardiographic studies. The causes of these alterations are several (Table 39–4). Knowledge of the pathophysiology of these factors is essential for understanding how renal disease affects cardiac structure and function. They can be divided into four major categories: (1) loading conditions that affect the myocardial function; (2) conditions that impair systolic function directly by their negative inotropic effect or indirectly by causing myocardial damage; (3) impaired diastolic filling of the heart; and (4) alterations in neural control of circulation.

### Loading Conditions

Low cardiac output stimulates the sympathetic nervous system, renin-angiotensin-aldosterone axis, and arginine vasopressin, which results in salt and water retention. In accordance with the Frank-Starling mechanism, the increase in preload (left ventricular end-diastolic volume or pressure) leads to an increase in stroke volume; however, an increase in preload beyond an optimal level causes pulmonary venous congestion. Usually, pulmonary capillary wedge pressure greater than 20 mm Hg leads to pulmonary congestion and pressure above 30 mm Hg leads to pulmonary edema. If the pulmonary capillary permeability is increased or plasma oncotic pressure is low, however, pulmonary congestion and edema may result at lower pressures. Retention of water and sodium may cause pulmonary edema in patients with acute renal failure or with chronic renal failure when fluid intake is excessive. In addition, an increase in pulmonary capillary permeability leading to

Table 39–4

**Factors that Affect Myocardial Function in Chronic Renal Failure**

| Loading conditions | Systolic dysfunction | Diastolic filling |
|---|---|---|
| Anemia | Myocardial ischemia, infarction | Pericardial disease |
| Hypertension | Hyperkalemia | Left ventricular hypertrophy |
| Fluid retention | Hypocalcemia | Myocardial fibrosis |
| Arteriovenous fistula | Metabolic acidosis | **Neural control** |
| Thiamine deficiency | Toxins of uremia (?) | Autonomic neuropathy |
| | Myocardial fibrosis | |
| | Valvular disease | |

pulmonary edema, even in the absence of elevated pulmonary capillary wedge pressure, has been reported in ESRD. The ease with which these patients develop pleural and pericardial effusions supports this possible mechanism. Diluting effect of volume overload on plasma protein concentration, which may already be reduced if significant proteinuria is a feature of the underlying nephropathy, accentuates the tendency for fluid transudation and edema formation. Although increased afterload has little effect on the stroke volume of normal ventricle, it can lead to marked decrease in stroke volume when myocardial dysfunction is present. Most patients with chronic renal failure are hypertensive. With ESRD, and in the dialysis population, severe hypertension is usually secondary to sodium and water retention. Such hypertension is usually present even in anephric patients and is exquisitely sensitive to blood volume.

In some patients, the hypertension is secondary to elevation of peripheral resistance due to increased plasma renin activity; it is not controlled by lowering the blood volume but responds to bilateral nephrectomy. Thus, retention of water and sodium leads to increases in both preload and afterload in chronic renal failure and may precipitate congestive heart failure. Chronic renal failure causes reduced compliance of the aorta and large arteries, thus increasing the afterload. Pressure and volume overload lead to concentric and eccentric left ventricular hypertrophy, respectively. Regression of left ventricular hypertrophy has been demonstrated after renal transplantation.

Heart failure exists when the cardiac output is insufficient to meet the demands of the metabolizing tissue. With anemia and arteriovenous fistula, a high cardiac output state is present; cardiac output and mean arterial pressure are elevated, but the systemic vascular resistance is normal. Using hypertrophy and dilatation as compensatory mechanisms, the normal heart can maintain tissue oxygenation for long periods, but when myocardial function is impaired, these compensatory mechanisms are insufficient and the high–cardiac output state will lead to clinical manifestations of heart failure. An increase in cardiac output occurs when the hematocrit falls below 25%; lowered blood viscosity is the major cause of increased cardiac output. In patients with congestive heart failure who are receiving hemodialysis, use of erythropoietin to raise the hematocrit to 42% did not improve survival over that of patients with a hematocrit of 30%. Many ESRD patients treated with erythropoietin experience an increase in arterial pressure that is due to increased peripheral vascular resistance. It has also been demonstrated that tissue hypoxia resulting from anemia can lead to an autonomic reflex response resulting in reduced arteriolar resistance.

High-output heart failure resulting from the arteriovenous shunts constructed surgically for vascular access for hemodialysis is not uncommon. Mean flow rate through these shunts is 1.5 l/min; however, cardiac outputs as high as 11 l/min per square meter, which decrease substantially during the occlusion of the shunt, have been reported. Although anemia may play a role in such high–cardiac output states, the added hemodynamic burden of the shunt may explain heart failure. Banding or revising the fistula to an appropriate size may relieve heart failure symptoms. Water-soluble vitamins are dialyzable, and it has been suggested that, rarely, loss of thiamine may lead to high-output heart failure secondary to beriberi.

## Systolic Dysfunction

Although cardiomyopathy caused by "uremic toxins" has been suspected for five decades, it has not been clearly demonstrated to be a separate entity. Since uremic patients often have other conditions that may alter myocardial function (e.g., anemia, arteriovenous fistula, hypertension, coronary artery disease), it is difficult to establish the independent contribution of uremia to ventricular dysfunction. In an echocardiographic study, uremic patients had left ventricular dilatation, hypertrophy, and a higher ratio of left ventricular radius to wall thickness, indicating inadequate hypertrophy. Myocardial dysfunction associated with uremia is often multifactorial but is reversible. Left ventricular systolic function has been demonstrated to improve after peritoneal and hemodialysis; however, such improvement may be secondary to reductions in preload and afterload. After renal transplantation, four patients with dilated cardiomyopathy, normal coronary angiograms, and severe left ventricular dysfunction were reported to exhibit resolution of heart failure symptoms and return to normal of left ventricular ejection fraction. Thus, although the existence of uremic cardiomyopathy is controversial, it is important to remember that the idiopathic cardiomyopathy seen in uremia may be reversible.

Calcium is fundamental to the process of myocardial contraction, since its influx through sarcolemmal channels regulates the force of contraction. Chronic hypocalcemia usually does not cause heart failure, however. Severe hypocalcemia (<6 mg/dl) in association with congestive heart failure has been described in dialysis patients after parathyroidectomy, with prompt improvement in cardiac function and resolution of heart failure after intravenous calcium replacement. Parathyroid hormone may be a myocardial depressant, since cardiac function reportedly improves after parathyroidectomy, but the negative inotropic effect of parathyroid hormone has not been established. Dystrophic calcification of the myocardial fibers occurs in secondary hyperparathyroidism of chronic renal failure. Hyperkalemia has a negative inotropic effect, but the principal drawback is its electrical effect on the heart. Severe metabolic acidosis impairs calcium release from sarcoplasmic reticulum and myocardial contractility is impaired at a systemic pH below 7.2. Increased rates of calcific aortic stenosis and mitral annular calcification have been reported in chronic renal failure. When valvular lesions are severe, myocardial dysfunction may result.

## Diastolic Filling

Recently, it has become apparent that diastolic dysfunction may lead to heart failure, even in the presence of normal systolic function, especially in patients with left ventricular hypertrophy and in older persons. Doppler echocardiography is now used to evaluate the diastolic function of the ventricles, and numerous studies have shown that diastolic filling is abnormal in the majority of patients with ventricular hypertrophy. Echocardiographic left ventricular hypertrophy has been noted in 38% of patients with chronic renal failure. Left ventricular hypertrophy develops and progresses with time on dialysis. In a longitudinal study of nondiabetic hemodialysis patients without dilated cardiomyopathy, the prevalence of left ventricular hypertrophy was 71%. After follow-up of 3 to 5 years, the hypertrophy persisted or had even increased in the majority of patients. Progression to severe hypertrophy could not be discriminated on the basis of the degree of hypertension or anemia. Asymmetric septal hypertrophy has also been reported, but this is an unusual manifestation of the hypertrophy resulting from hemodynamic stress and is not associated with left ventricular outflow obstruction.

Hypotension during dialysis that cannot be explained by changes in intravascular volume is a clue to impaired diastolic filling. Effect of hemodialysis on diastolic filling has been evaluated using Doppler echocardiography. Fluid removal during hemodialysis reduces the left ventricular preload to the extent that early diastolic filling becomes impaired if there is no compensatory increase in the atrial phase of filling. Hemodialysis without fluid removal does not alter the left ventricular diastolic filling pattern.

## ■ ISCHEMIC RENAL DISEASE (See also Chapter 31)

To this point, our review has been limited to a discussion of cardiac problems that arise in patients with renal disease. Ischemic renal disease (IRD), however, is a renal disease that occurs in cardiac patients. We include a discussion of this entity because IRD is very common in patients with arteriosclerotic cardiovascular disease, and consequently, the cardiologist may encounter the patient with IRD well in advance of the nephrologist. IRD is now recognized as an important, and *potentially reversible,* cause of ESRD that often goes unrecognized by physicians caring for patients with arteriosclerotic complications.[21-30] In addition, the prevalence of IRD is increasing. For these reasons, we feel that a working knowledge of when to suspect IRD and how to recognize its chief clinical manifestations and an understanding of the potential benefits of intervention before ESRD supervenes can be very valuable to practicing cardiologists.

IRD is defined as a clinically significant reduction in glomerular filtration rate or loss of renal parenchyma caused by hemodynamically significant arteriosclerotic renal artery stenosis. IRD is an important cause of progressive renal disease, and the prevalence of ischemic renal disease is increasing, especially among older patients. IRD is an important and common consequence of arteriosclerotic renal artery stenosis that is separate and distinct from the problem of renovascular hypertension. In the past, the focus of treatment of patients with renal artery stenosis was principally on the goal of lowering blood pressure, but it has been recognized that renal artery stenosis secondary to atherosclerosis may produce progressive loss of renal function due to renal ischemia. Renal ischemia is now understood to be an important and potentially reversible cause of ESRD. Because of increasing recognition of ischemic nephropathy as a common and important clinical entity, there is greater potential for favorably altering the course of this disease. Consequently, recent interest in renovascular disease has been directed at *preservation of renal function* in addition to correction of hypertension.

### Prevalence

Unsuspected renal artery stenosis is common in patients with coronary artery disease. Patients screened for renal artery disease with abdominal aortography while undergoing elective cardiac catheterization have been found to have a high prevalence of renal artery disease: a study of 1302 of 1651 consecutive cardiac catheterizations revealed significant unilateral renal artery stenosis in 11% of the patients and bilateral renal artery stenosis in 4%. Other large studies estimate that some 18% to 30% of patients undergoing cardiac catheterization had significant renal artery stenosis.

A recent review[23] compiled 11 angiographic studies of the prevalence of unsuspected renal artery stenosis in patients with peripheral vascular and cardiac atherosclerosis dating from 1975 to 1995. The 11 studies had a total of 3698 patients. The average prevalence of unsuspected renal artery stenosis (>50%) for the 11 studies was 23%. These reports all suggest that significant unsuspected renovascular disease is very common in patients with extrarenal atherosclerosis, regardless of whether renovascular hypertension is suspected.

### Natural History

Stenosis of the renal arteries, when of high grade, is very likely to progress over a 2-year period, and progression is associated with loss of renal mass and function. Progressive arterial obstruction occurs in 42% to 53% of patients with renal artery stenosis and progression to complete renal artery occlusion in 9% to 16%. Complete occlusion is more likely to develop in patients who have high-grade stenosis on initial examination.

The prevalence of IRD as the cause of ESRD may be between 11% and 14%. Moreover, when IRD is the cause of ESRD, the mortality rate after the initiation of renal replacement therapy is high, possibly because of the severity of the underlying atherosclerotic disease. IRD patients have a median survival of 27 months and 5- and 10-year survival rates of 18% and 5%, respectively. Patients with renal insufficiency secondary to IRD are often considered poor candidates for intervention, but the poor survival of these patients once they have ESRD makes intervention with percutaneous transluminal renal angioplasty (PTRA) or surgical revascularization a reasonable alternative to "conservative" medical therapy.

## Pathophysiology

For a reduction in glomerular filtration rate to be sufficient to cause elevation of the serum creatinine concentration requires that *both* kidneys be injured. Therefore, IRD may arise from one of two principal clinical situations. The first situation is bilateral hemodynamically significant renal artery stenosis leading to bilateral renal ischemia. The second is hemodynamically significant renal artery stenosis in a solitary functioning kidney or in a kidney that is providing the majority of a patient's glomerular filtration. In the second situation, the stenotic kidney suffers from chronic ischemia, whereas the contralateral kidney has been damaged from other causes. Possible causes of impaired function of the contralateral kidney are damage from severe renovascular hypertension induced by the stenotic kidney and renal diseases that typically are unilateral, such as pyelonephritis or trauma.

Chronic reduction of blood flow to the kidney results in decreased renal size: the well-known clinical hallmark of chronic renal ischemia from atherosclerotic renovascular disease is a (unilateral) small kidney.

## Diagnosis

Clinical features that suggest renovascular hypertension point to IRD as the cause of renal insufficiency in a patient with coexisting renal failure and hypertension. In healthy humans, the lengths of the two kidneys normally differ by less than 1 to 1.5 cm. Asymmetry of renal size in a hypertensive patient strongly suggests IRD. Hypertension is often abrupt in onset, severe, and drug resistant, and may first present after age 50 years. An abdominal bruit that is localized over the kidneys, prolonged into diastole, or heard in the flank suggests renovascular disease. In addition, there are six major clinical settings in which the clinician could suspect IRD (Table 39–5).

Table 39–5

**Clinical Findings Suggestive of Ischemic Renal Disease**

Acute renal failure caused by treatment of hypertension, especially with angiotensin-converting enzyme inhibitors
Progressive azotemia in a patient with known renovascular hypertension
Acute pulmonary edema superimposed on poorly controlled hypertension and renal failure
Progressive azotemia in an elderly patient with refractory or severe hypertension
Progressive azotemia in an elderly patient with evidence of atherosclerotic disease
Unexplained progressive azotemia in an elderly patient

A typical clinical presentation of IRD is a patient older than 50 years who has generalized atherosclerosis and refractory hypertension demonstrating progressive azotemia in conjunction with antihypertensive drug therapy. Patients with occult arteriosclerotic IRD may present with acute renal failure (ARF) caused by treatment of hypertension, particularly with angiotensin-converting enzyme inhibitors (ACEI). Reversible worsening of azotemia during ACEI therapy should raise suspicion of IRD. ACEI may acutely alter intrarenal hemodynamics. The stenotic kidney depends on angiotensin II to maintain glomerular filtration rates. Angiotensin II causes vasoconstriction of both afferent and efferent arterioles but has preferential effects on the efferent ones. This differential vasoconstriction increases the glomerular capillary pressure and thus maintains or increases the single-nephron glomerular filtration rate. When the vasoconstrictor effect of angiotensin II on the efferent arteriole is blocked by an ACEI, efferent arteriolar constriction relaxes and glomerular capillary filtration pressures and glomerular filtration rate decrease. Although ACEI-induced ARF is an important clinical marker for IRD, the absence of ARF does not rule out the possibility of significant IRD, because only 6% to 38% of patients with significant renal vascular disease will develop ARF when treated with these agents. The ARF associated with the use of antihypertensive agents in patients with IRD is generally reversible and demands further clinical evaluation.

Recurrent acute pulmonary edema in patients with poorly controlled hypertension and renal insufficiency has also been reported to be a marker of severe bilateral atherosclerotic renal artery disease. Volume-dependent renovascular hypertension caused by bilateral renal artery stenosis appears to be the dominant agent in producing the pulmonary edema. Patients with pulmonary edema, uncontrolled hypertension, and azotemia have not been prospectively evaluated to establish what portion of those with this clinical picture have IRD, but it should alert the clinician to the possibility of IRD. The episodes of pulmonary edema may cease after renal revascularization.

A common presentation of IRD is unexplained progressive azotemia in an elderly patient with evidence of atherosclerotic disease. Angiographic studies have indicated a high prevalence of renal artery stenosis among patients who have atherosclerotic disease in other vessels. Therefore, a history or physical findings of generalized arteriosclerosis are strongly suggestive of ischemic nephropathy.

## Post-ACEI Renography

ACEI renography is the most accurate noninvasive functional test for diagnosing *renovascular hypertension,* but its accuracy is diminished in patients with renal failure. ACEI renography generally has difficulty differentiating ischemic renal disease from intrinsic renal disease.

## Duplex Doppler Sonography

Duplex Doppler sonography (DDS) is useful for diagnosing IRD. DDS combines ultrasound and Doppler techniques to locate the renal artery and assess renal artery blood flow velocity. DDS has several major advantages: it is useful in the presence of azotemia; it is not necessary to discontinue antihypertensive agents as in ACEI renography; there is no risk of contrast nephropathy or cholesterol embolization; and bilateral renal artery stenosis can be assessed. Even total obstruction of a renal artery can be diagnosed by scanning over the kidney. The main limitation of DDS is inadequate imaging because of obesity, bowel gas, or previous abdominal surgery.

Magnetic resonance angiography and spiral computed tomography angiography (spiral CT) are recently developed techniques that have been used to detect renal vascular disease with high sensitivity and specificity, but 100 to 150 ml of contrast medium must be given in the latter procedure.

## Treatment

The prognosis for medically treated IRD is poor: many patients show deterioration of renal function during follow-up. Patients with high-grade (>75%) arterial stenosis bilaterally or in a solitary functioning kidney are at risk for complete renal arterial occlusion. Intervention is indicated to restore renal arterial blood flow to preserve renal function. Total occlusion of the renal artery does not always indicate irreversible ischemic parenchymal damage, because the viability of the kidney can be maintained through development of collateral arterial supply. This occurs when the arterial occlusion develops gradually. Several clinical clues suggest that reestablishment of renal arterial flow can lead to recovery of renal function: (1) kidney size more than 9 cm; (2) evidence of acceptable function of the involved kidney on isotope renography; (3) angiographic filling of the distal renal arterial tree by collateral circulation in patients with total renal arterial occlusion proximally; (4) renal biopsy demonstrating well-preserved glomeruli with minimal arteriolar sclerosis; (5) preoperative serum creatinine levels less than 3.0 mg/dl; and (6) presentation with acute deterioration of renal function after initiation of medical antihypertensive therapy, especially with an ACEI.

The rate of decline in renal function is another important determinant of the outcome after intervention in atherosclerotic ischemic renal disease. Rapid deterioration of renal function in a patient with renal artery stenosis (especially in association with ACEI therapy) suggests a strong possibility of retrieval of function by intervention to restore renal arterial flow. Patients with chronic severe azotemia (serum creatinine >4 mg/dl) are likely to have severe renal parenchymal disease, and, for them, improvement in renal function after revascularization or angioplasty is less likely. Exceptions to this observation are cases of total main renal artery occlusion where kidney viability is maintained via collateral circulation

## Percutaneous Transluminal Renal Angioplasty

PTRA does not require general anesthesia and can be repeated if needed. In patients with nonostial renal artery disease, the success rate of PTRA has been excellent. PTRA is less effective for ostial lesions. Restenosis, the predominant cause of failure in patients with ostial lesions, can be due to elastic recoil of the dilated artery, neointimal hyperplasia, or recurrent atheromatous disease. Technical difficulties and complications of angiographic investigation and PTRA in these patients include contrast media–induced acute renal failure and atheroembolic renal disease. In addition, a recent randomized study of 106 hypertensive patients with atherosclerotic renal artery stenosis reported that angioplasty had little advantage over antihypertensive drug therapy.[31] Clearly, additional studies are required to reconcile these ostensible differences.

Endovascular stents are a newer treatment option for patients who have ostial lesions or are considered poor risks for surgical revascularization. Early recurrent arterial stenosis is a problem. This technique requires further experience and evaluation but offers promise to patients with ostial lesions who are not candidates for surgery.

## ▪ SURGICAL REVASCULARIZATION

The surgical treatment of renovascular disease was recently reviewed by Novick.[30] Surgical revascularization to preserve renal function in patients with high-grade atherosclerotic arterial occlusive disease affecting both kidneys or a solitary kidney may result in improvement or stabilization of renal function postoperatively in 75% to 89% of patients. For example, the Cleveland Clinic performed surgical revascularization for preservation of renal function in 161 patients with critical bilateral stenosis or a solitary kidney and achieved postoperative improvement in renal function in 93 patients (58%), stabilization in 50 patients (31%), and deterioration in only 18 patients (11%).

Recent reports indicate that surgical renal vascular reconstruction can be performed with operative mortality rates in the range of 2.1% to 6.1% and a high technical success rate. Risk of operative mortality has been higher with simultaneous bilateral renal revascularization or when renal revascularization is performed in conjunction with another major vascular operation such as aortic replacement. Most studies have indicated a high technical success rate for surgical vascular reconstruction, with postoperative thrombosis or stenosis rates less than 10%.

# ▪ SUMMARY

It is readily apparent that progressive renal disease is complicated by several common cardiovascular alterations, including pericarditis, renal parenchymal hypertension, primary arteriosclerosis, and left ventricular dysfunction. We have reviewed the pathogenesis, clinical features, and management of the cardiovascular disorders and have included a review of IRD, a common albeit underdiagnosed disorder that cardiologists may encounter frequently well before nephrologists do. Increasing recognition that IRD is a *potentially reversible* cause of ESRD underscores the importance of its inclusion in our review. We are hopeful that the management approaches proposed in this chapter will facilitate optimal care of these difficult patients.

# ▪ REFERENCES

1. Rostand SG, Rutsky EA: Cardiac disease in dialysis patients. *In* Nissenson AR, Fine RN, Gentile DE (eds): Clinical Dialysis, 3rd ed. Norwalk: Appleton and Lange, 1995:652–698.
2. Lundin AP: Cardiovascular system in uremia. Part 1. Pericarditis. *In* Massry SG, Glassock RJ (eds): Textbook of Nephrology, 3rd ed. Baltimore: Williams & Wilkins, 1995:1339–1363.
3. Preston RA, Chakko S, Materson BJ: End-stage renal disease. *In* Rapaport E (ed): Cardiology and Co-existing Disease. New York: Churchill Livingstone, 1994:175–196.
4. Rutsky EA, Rostand SG: Treatment of uremic pericarditis and pericardial effusion. Am J Kidney Dis 1987;10:2–8.
5. De Pace NL, Nestico PF, Schwartz AB, et al: Predicting success of intensive dialysis in the treatment of uremic pericarditis. Am J Med 1984;76:38–46.
6. Preston RA, Epstein M: Hypertension and renal parenchymal disease. Semin Nephrol 1995;15:138–151.
7. Preston RA, Singer I, Epstein M: Renal parenchymal hypertension: Current concepts of pathogenesis and management. Arch Intern Med 1996;154:637–642.
8. Smith, MC, Dunn MJ: Hypertension associated with renal parenchymal disease. *In* Schrier RW, Gottschalk CW (eds): Diseases of the Kidney. Boston: Little, Brown, 1997:1333–1365.
9. Joint National Committee on Detection, Evaluation and Treatment of High Blood Pressure (JNC VI): The sixth report of the Joint National Committee on Detection, Evaluation and Treatment of High Blood Pressure (JNC VI). Arch Intern Med 1997;157:2413–2444.
10. Mackenzie HS, Garcia DL, Anderson S, Brenner BM: The renal abnormality in hypertension: A proposed defect in glomerular filtration surface area. *In* Laragh JH, Brenner BM (eds): Hypertension: Pathophysiology, Diagnosis, and Management. New York: Raven, 1995:1539–1552.
11. Brater DC: Diuretic therapy. N Engl J Med 1998;339:387–395.
12. Foley RN, Harnett JD, Parfrey PS: Cardiovascular complications of end-stage renal disease. *In* Schrier RW, Gottschalk CW (eds): Diseases of the Kidney. Boston: Little, Brown, 1997:2647–2660.
13. Zonszein J, Sonnenblick EH: Endocrine diseases and cardiovascular diseases. *In* Alexander RW, Schlant RC, Fuster V (eds): Hurst's The Heart. New York: McGraw-Hill, 1998:2117.
14. Reis G, Marcovitz PA, Leichtman AB, et al: Usefulness of dobutamine stress echocardiography in detecting coronary artery disease in end-stage renal disease. Am J Cardiol 1995;75:707–710.
15. Herzog CA, Ma JZ, Collins AJ: Poor long-term survival after acute myocardial infarction among patients on long-term dialysis. N Engl J Med 1998;339:799–805.

16. Pastan SO, Mitch WE: The heart and kidney disease. *In* Hurst JW (ed): The Heart. New York: McGraw-Hill, 1998:2413–2424.
17. London GM, Pannier B, Guerin AP, et al: Cardiac hypertrophy, aortic compliance, peripheral resistance and wave reflection in end-stage renal disease: Comparative effects of ACE inhibitors and calcium channel blockade. Circulation 1994;90:2786–2796.
18. Besarab A, Bolton WK, Browne JK, et al: The effects of normal as compared with low hematocrit values in patients with cardiac disease who are receiving hemodialysis and epoetin. N Engl J Med 1998;339:584–590.
19. Chakko S, Girgis I, Contreras G, et al: Effects of hemodialysis on left ventricular diastolic filling. Am J Cardiol 1997;79:106–108.
20. Feldman AM, Fivush B, Zakha KG, et al: Congestive cardiomyopathy in patients on continuous ambulatory peritoneal dialysis. Am J Kidny Dis 1988;11:76–79.
21. Preston RA, Epstein M: Ischemic renal disease: An emerging cause of chronic renal failure and end-stage renal disease. J Hypertens 1997;15:1365–1377.
22. Preston RA, Epstein M: Ischemic renal disease. Am J Therapeutics 1998;5:203–210.
23. Greco BA, Breyer JA: The natural history of renal artery stenosis: Who should be evaluated for ischemic nephropathy? Semin Nephrol 1996;16(1):2–11.
24. Greco BA, Breyer JA: Atherosclerotic ischemic renal disease. Am J Kidney Dis 1997;29(2):167–187.
25. Pohl MA: Renal artery stenosis, renal vascular hypertension, and ischemic nephropathy. *In* Schrier RW, Gottschalk CW (eds): Diseases of the Kidney. Boston: Little, Brown, 1997:1367–1423.
26. Alcazar JM, Caramelo CA, Alegre ER, Abad J: Ischaemic renal injury. Curr Opin Nephrol Hypertens 1997;6:157–165.
27. Harding MB, Smith LR, Himmestein SI, et al: Renal artery stenosis: Prevalence and associated risk factors in patients undergoing routine cardiac catheterization. J Am Soc Nephrol 1992;2:1608–1616.
28. Messina LM, Zelenock GB, Yao KA, Stanley JC: Renal revascularization for recurrent pulmonary edema in patients with poorly controlled hypertension and renal insufficiency: A distinct subgroup of patients with arteriosclerotic renal artery occlusive disease. J Vasc Surg 1992;15:73–82.
29. Dorros G, Jaff M, Jain A, et al: Follow-up of primary Palmaz-Shatz stent placement for atherosclerotic renal artery stenosis. Am J Cardiol 1995;75:1051–1055.
30. Novick AC: Options for therapy in ischemic nephropathy: Role of angioplasty and surgery. Semin Nephrol 1996;16(1):53–60.
31. van Jaarsveld BC, Krijnen P, Pieterman H, et al: The effect of balloon angioplasty on hypertension in atherosclerotic renal artery stenosis. N Engl J Med 2000;342(14):1007–1014.

# ■ RECOMMENDED READING

Kaplan N: Renal parenchymal hypertension. *In* Kaplan N (ed): Clinical Hypertension, 7th ed. Baltimore: Williams & Wilkins, 1998:281–299.
Mandelbaum AP, Ritz E: Cardiac complications of uremia. *In* Glassock RJ (ed): Current Therapy in Nephrology and Hypertension, 4th ed. St. Louis: Mosby–Year Book, 1998:309–316.
Pohl MA: Renal vascular disease. *In* Glassock RJ (ed): Current Therapy in Nephrology and Hypertension, 4th ed. St Louis: Mosby–Year Book, 1998:327–330.
Walls MJ, Breyer JA: Hypertension in chronic renal failure, dialysis and transplantation. *In* Glassock RJ (ed): Current Therapy in Nephrology and Hypertension, 4th ed. St Louis: Mosby–Year Book, 1998:335–352.

# Chapter 40

# Assessment of Patients with Heart Disease for Fitness for Noncardiac Surgery

*Lee A. Fleisher*

The evaluation of the patient scheduled for anesthesia for noncardiac surgery remains a diagnostic dilemma because of competing issues of economics, expediency, and the desire to have complete knowledge of the extent of cardiovascular disease. Additionally, multiple medical specialists are involved in the evaluation of high-risk patients, each of whom may have complementary or divergent needs. In many institutions, anesthesiologists have established preoperative evaluation centers and the surgeon defers to the anesthesiologist's judgment about the need for extensive cardiovascular consultation. Frequently, the staff of these centers communicate directly with the primary caregivers to define the extent of disease. Alternatively, the surgeon may initiate a cardiology consultation or the referring internist or cardiologist may initiate one. The goal of all professionals involved in the care of the surgical patient with heart disease is to ensure that critical information is communicated to the appropriate personnel so that optimal care can be provided. In this chapter I will focus on what information is required and whether preoperative testing has additive value.

## ■ CONCEPTS FOR PREOPERATIVE CARDIAC EVALUATION

The underlying concept, with respect to the need for preoperative evaluation, is that the information will be used to modify perioperative care. In some circumstances, the preoperative evaluation also provides the patient and physicians with information on risks so they can determine if the benefits of the planned surgical procedure outweigh these risks. The benefits of some elective surgeries may be small or may not accrue for several years. For example, radical prostatectomy is indicated only if the patient has at least 10 years' life expectancy because of the slow progression of prostate cancer. In such circumstances, patients with advanced cardiac disease who might not stand to live long would not be candidates for the procedure, and preoperative testing might help to better define life expectancy. Another example is elective repair of abdominal aortic aneurysms or lower extremity bypass procedures, which may not be indicated or performed in patients with the highest perioperative risks.

Information from the preoperative evaluation can be used to direct multiple points of care. The most important application is to evaluate patients with unstable symptoms, since they have been shown to be at prohibitive risk.[1] Medical management of these unstable symptoms is essential before elective or urgent surgery is undertaken. Alternative treatment strategies need to be considered if the procedure is emergent. Particularly with respect to vascular surgery, a great deal of attention has focused on the role of coronary revascularization before the noncardiac procedure. Invasive monitoring is not without cost or risks; therefore, directed utilization is essential. Postoperative intensive care is expensive, and resources are frequently limited, and the preoperative evaluation should be used to identify for whom a benefit can accrue.

## ■ ROLE OF THE CONSULTANT

As outlined in the recent American Heart Association/American College of Cardiology Guidelines on Perioperative Cardiovascular Evaluation for Non-cardiac Surgery, the role of the consultant is to define the extent and stability of a patient's cardiac disease and determine if they are in their optimal medical condition.[2] From the anesthesiologist's perspective, these are the critical factors necessary to modify intraoperative technique and monitoring. Importantly, the guidelines state that the specific choice of anesthesia is best left to the discretion of the anesthesia providers.[2] In fact, choice of anesthesia did not appear to affect cardiovascular outcome in several well-controlled randomized clinical trials. Specifically, there appears to be no difference between regional (epidural and spinal) anesthesia and general anesthesia. Therefore, the preoperative evaluation should depend not on the type of anesthesia but rather on the extent of surgery (outlined later in this chapter). Good communication among all caregivers should ensure optimal outcomes.

## ■ PATHOPHYSIOLOGY OF PERIOPERATIVE CARDIAC EVENTS

The pathophysiology underlying perioperative cardiac events is multifactorial, a fact that influences the potential value of preoperative cardiac testing. A great deal of attention has focused on the association between perioperative myocardial ischemia and cardiac morbidity. In several large-scale studies, postoperative myocardial ischemia had the strongest association with myocardial infarction and cardiac death.[3, 4] Further analysis has suggested that prolonged ischemia is a critical predictor of such events.[5] If mismatches of supply and demand in patients with critical coronary stenoses are the underlying cause of these events, either coronary revascularization or tight hemodynamic management should reduce morbidity (Fig. 40–1). The value of coronary revascularization will be discussed later in the chapter. The use of beta-adrenergic blockade has been associated with a reduction in perioperative myocardial ischemia and significantly improved long-term survival.[6, 7] Maintenance of normothermia was associated with a significantly lower rate of cardiac complications in a randomized clinical trial of intraoperative forced-air warming.[8] Anemia (hematocrit <28%) was associated with an increased incidence of cardiac morbidity in a small cohort study.[9] All of these factors could lead to ischemia, which, if prolonged, can lead to infarction. Yet, symptomatic cardiac events and cardiac death may result from acute coronary thrombosis on noncritical stenoses or areas without significant collaterals.[10] For the former case (noncritical stenoses), preoperative evaluation would not identify the critical lesion and strategies aimed at decreasing the hypercoagulable state observed in the perioperative period would be the optimal strategy.[11]

## ■ CARDIAC RISK INDICES

Many of the studies have adopted the approach of defining a cohort of patients, determining their clinical and laboratory risk factors, and using multivariate modeling to determine which factors are associated with increased risk. A major limitation

## Pathophysiology of Acute Coronary Syndromes During the Perioperative Period

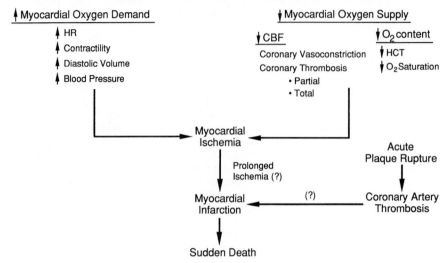

**Figure 40–1 ■** Pathophysiology of acute coronary syndromes during the perioperative period. The perioperative period is associated with acute changes in myocardial oxygen supply and demand, which can lead to myocardial ischemia. If the ischemia is prolonged, there is evidence to suggest that it can lead to MI. Alternatively, acute thrombosis may be the cause of perioperative MI, and ischemia may simply be the manifestation of the underlying disease. (Perioperative myocardial ischemia and infarction. IN: Perioperative myocardial and infarction (Beattie, Fleisher-editors) Int Anesthesiol Clin 1992;30(1):xx.)

in the use of multivariate modeling for this purpose is the assumption that the intraoperative period is a "black box" and that care is not modified when the risk factor is known. However, when a risk factor is known (e.g., uncontrolled hypertension), anesthesiologists frequently modify care and thus reduce risk. Therefore, many of the indices developed previously may no longer be clinically valid if they identify treatable risk factors.

Many particular disease states increase perioperative risk. Cardiovascular disease has been studied most extensively with the goal of identifying patients at greatest risk for fatal and nonfatal myocardial infarctions. One of the earliest attempts to define cardiac risk was performed by Goldman and colleagues at the Massachusetts General Hospital.[12]

Using multivariate logistic regression, they demonstrated nine clinical factors associated with increased morbidity and mortality in a population of 1001 patients older than 45 years (Table 40–1). Each of these risk factors was associated with a given weight in the logistic regression equation, which was converted into points in the index. Greater numbers of points were associated with increasing perioperative cardiac morbidity or mortality.

Several attempts have been made to validate the Goldman Cardiac Risk Index. Zeldin and coworkers prospectively determined the Cardiac Risk Index for 1140 surgical patients.[13] They reported that the overall accuracy of the index was as high as in the original study, although the rate of complications in the highest-risk group was lower than that originally reported.[14, 15] Several other studies failed to demonstrate any relationship between the Cardiac Risk Index and perioperative

Table 40–1

**Computation of the Cardiac Risk Index**

| Criteria | Multivariate Discriminant Function Coefficient | Points |
|---|---|---|
| **I. History:** | | |
| (a) Age >70 yr | 0.191 | 5 |
| (b) MI in previous 6 mo | 0.384 | 10 |
| **II. Physical examination:** | | |
| (a) S₃ gallop or JVD | 0.451 | 11 |
| (b) Important VAS | 0.119 | 3 |
| **III. Electrocardiogram:** | | |
| (a) Rhythm other than sinus or PAC on last preoperative ECG | 0.283 | 7 |
| (b) >5 PVC/min documented at any time before operation | 0.278 | 7 |
| **IV. General status:** | | |
| Po₂ <60 or Pco₂ >50 mm Hg, K <3.0 or HCO₃ <20 mEq/l, BUN >50 or Cr >3.0 mg/dl, abnormal SGOT, signs of chronic liver disease, or patient bedridden from noncardiac causes | 0.132 | 3 |
| **V. Operation:** | | |
| (a) Intraperitoneal, intrathoracic, or aortic operation | 0.123 | 3 |
| (b) Emergency operation | 0.167 | 4 |
| **Total possible points** | | 53 |

MI, myocardial infarction; JVD, jugular vein distention; VAS, valvular aortic stenosis; PAC, premature atrial contractions; ECG, electrocardiogram; PVC, premature ventricular contractions; Po₂, partial pressure of oxygen; Pco₂, partial pressure of carbon dioxide; K, potassium; HCO₃, bicarbonate; BUN, blood urea nitrogen; Cr, creatinine; SGOT, serum glutamic oxaloacetic transaminases.

From Goldman L, Caldera DL, Nussbaum SR, et al: Multifactorial index of cardiac risk in noncardiac surgical procedures. N Engl J Med 1977;297:845–850.

cardiac complications, reporting high incidences of complications in patients with a Cardiac Risk Index of I or II, particularly in a vascular disease population.[16, 17]

Other investigators have attempted to develop risk indices. Detsky studied a cohort of patients who were referred to an internal medicine service for preoperative evaluation, as opposed to an unselected group of surgical patients (Table 40–2).[18] Many of the factors identified by Goldman were confirmed or slightly modified in the Detsky index, although angina was added to the risk factors. Importantly, Detsky advocated calculating a pretest probability of complications based on the type of surgery, after which the Modified Risk Index is applied using a nomogram. In this manner, the overall probability of complications can be determined as a function of both the surgical procedure and the patient's disease. The Detsky index has been advocated as the starting point for risk stratification for the American College of Physicians Guideline on preoperative evaluation.[19] Although risk indices may be extremely helpful in defining the prior probability of disease, they are not sufficient for providing anesthesiologists with information they can use to modify perioperative management. They also appear to be insufficiently sensitive for patients undergoing major vascular surgery.

## ■ CLINICAL RISK FACTORS (Table 40–3)

In virtually all studies, active congestive heart failure (CHF) is associated with the highest perioperative risk.[12, 18] The ACC/AHA Guidelines differentiate active congestive heart failure, which is considered a major risk factor, from compensated CHF, which is considered an intermediate risk factor.

Table 40–2

**Modified Cardiac Risk Index by Detsky et al.**

| Variables | Points |
|---|---|
| Angina | |
|    Class IV | 20 |
|    Class III | 10 |
|    Unstable angina <3 mo | 10 |
| Suspected critical aortic stenosis | 20 |
| Myocardial infarction | |
|    <6 mo | 10 |
|    >6 mo | 5 |
| Alveolar pulmonary edema | |
|    <1 wk | 10 |
|    ever present | 5 |
| Emergency surgery | 10 |
| Sinus plus atrial premature beats or rhythm other than sinus on preoperative ECG | 5 |
| >5 Premature ventricular contractions at any time before surgery | 5 |
| Poor general medical status | 5 |
| Age >70 yr | 5 |

Reproduced with permission from Detsky A, Abrams H, McLaughlin J, et al: Predicting cardiac complications in patients undergoing noncardiac surgery. J Gen Intern Med 1986;1:211–219.

Table 40–3

**Clinical Predictors of Increased Perioperative Cardiovascular Risk (Myocardial Infarction, Congestive Heart Failure, Death)**

**Major**
Unstable coronary syndromes
   Recent myocardial infarction* with evidence of important ischemic risk with clinical symptoms
      or noninvasive study
   Unstable or severe angina (Canadian class III or IV)†
Decompensated congestive heart failure
Significant arrhythmias
   High-grade atrioventricular block
   Symptomatic ventricular arrhythmias in the presence of underlying heart disease
   Supraventricular arrhythmias with uncontrolled ventricular rate
Severe valvular disease
**Intermediate**
Mild angina pectoris (Canadian class I or II)
Prior myocardial infarction by history or pathologic Q waves
Compensated or prior congestive heart failure
Diabetes mellitus
**Minor**
Advanced age
Abnormal ECG (left ventricular hypertrophy, left bundle branch block, ST-T abnormalities)
Rhythm other than sinus (e.g., atrial fibrillation)
Low functional capacity (e.g., inability to climb one flight of stairs with a bag of groceries)
History of stroke
Uncontrolled systemic hypertension

ECG, electrocardiogram.
*The American College of Cardiology National Database Library defines recent myocardial infarction as one that occurred >7 days but ≤1 month (30 days) earlier.
†May include "stable" angina in patients who are unusually sedentary.
Reproduced with permission from Campeau L: Grading of angina pectoris. Circulation 1976;54:522–523.

Time since a previous myocardial infarction (MI) has traditionally been an important predictor of perioperative risk: the more recent the MI, particularly within 3 to 6 months, the greater is the perioperative risk (Table 40–4).[20–22] However, recent advances in the management of acute MI make the older data less valid, and no studies have been performed recently in the perioperative period to confirm these data.[23] The ACC/AHA advocate using 30 days as the acute period (of major clinical risk) and associate high risk with the period of 6 to 8 weeks.[2] After that time, a prior MI places that patient in the intermediate clinical risk category and further evaluation depends on other clinical symptoms.

Angina has not consistently been a risk factor in the various studies, although unstable angina was associated with a 28% incidence of perioperative MI.[1] Such patients would benefit from delay of surgery and more intensive medical therapy. For those with chronic stable angina, exercise tolerance appears to be a good method of assessing risk. The ACC/AHA Guidelines Endorse the Canadian Cardiovascular Society Classification as a means of stratifying risk, disease of class III or IV carrying high risk and class I and II intermediate risk.

## Risk Factors for Coronary Artery Disease

In evaluating patients with hypertension, it is important to determine how the information will affect perioperative management. Hypertension has not been found to be an independent risk factor for perioperative MI in the vast majority of studies, but it was shown to be predictive of perioperative myocardial ischemia. The history of hypertension should be viewed in the context of the general medical condition to determine the need for further evaluation of cardiovascular status.

A second major issue related to hypertension is the need for further preoperative management in a patient who presents with markedly elevated blood pressure (diastolic >110 mm Hg). Traditionally, further treatment for these patients has been deferred. However, when evaluating the original study of Goldman and Caldera, on which this recommendation is partially grounded, it is clear that there are insufficient data to validate such a claim.[24] In fact, none of the patients with "uncontrolled systemic hypertension" sustained a major cardiac event, and the authors simply state that surgery is safe for those with hypertension up to a diastolic of 110 mm Hg. These patients may be at risk for perioperative hemodynamic lability, but not irreversible myocardial necrosis. Left ventricular hypertrophy, particularly with a strain pattern, has been associated with increased risk of perioperative myocardial ischemia.[25]

Diabetes has been associated with a high incidence of perioperative cardiac morbidity in several studies, particularly those involving vascular surgery patients.[26] Diabetics have high rates of both silent ischemia and silent MI.[27] Based on

Table 40–4

**Reinfarction Rates in Different Studies and Number of Patients Studied**

| Interval Between Myocardial Infarction and Operation (mo) | Investigator | | |
| --- | --- | --- | --- |
| | Tarhan (1972) | Rao (1983) | Shah (1990) |
| 0–3 | 37%, N = 18 | 5.8%, N = 52 | 4.3%, N = 23 |
| 4–6 | 16%, N = 19 | 2.3%, N = 86 | 0%, N = 18 |
| >6 | 5.6%, N = 322 | 1.5%, N = 595 | 5.7%, N = 174 |
| Unknown | — | — | 33.3%, N = 60 |

the preponderance of evidence about the high incidence of cardiac morbidity in diabetic patients, particularly those with intercurrent peripheral vascular disease, the ACC/AHA Guidelines consider diabetes a moderate risk.

# ■ IMPORTANCE OF SURGICAL PROCEDURE

It is well recognized that the surgical procedure itself significantly influences perioperative risk. In virtually every study, emergency surgery carries additional risk. In some cases, the risk related to surgery is a function of both the underlying disease processes and the stress related to the surgical procedure. Vascular surgery has the highest risk among noncardiac procedures. Although, traditionally, aortic reconstructive surgery was considered the highest-risk procedure, infrainguinal procedures have had similar rates of cardiac morbidity in several recent studies.[28] In attempting to determine the cause of the high complication rate on a peripheral procedure, L'Italien demonstrated that the extent of coronary artery disease was higher in the "infrainguinal patients," a finding that most likely accounts for the excessive morbidity and mortality.[28]

Many studies have evaluated the perioperative complication rate for superficial procedures. Backer evaluated the rate of perioperative myocardial reinfarction in patients undergoing ophthalmic surgery.[29] They demonstrated that the rate of perioperative cardiac morbidity after ophthalmic surgery was extremely low, even in patients with a history of recent MI. Virtually all studies have confirmed that ophthalmic surgery is very safe under anesthesia. Warner and coworkers studied patients undergoing ambulatory surgery and reported anesthesia-related deaths in more than 45,000 cases.[30]

Eagle and colleagues evaluated the contribution of coronary artery disease and its treatment on perioperative cardiac morbidity and mortality.[31] They evaluated patients enrolled in the Coronary Artery Surgery Study who had documented coronary artery disease and who received either medical therapy or coronary revascularization and then underwent noncardiac surgery sometime during the next 10 years. Their rates of perioperative MI and death were determined, and the surgical procedures were divided into three broad categories. Major vascular surgery was again demonstrated to be associated with the highest risk (combined morbidity and mortality rates >10%). Procedures associated with a combined complication rate of at least 4% included intraabdominal, thoracic, and head and neck operations. In all of these cases, patients who earlier had had coronary artery bypass grafting had significantly lower combined morbidity and mortality rates than did the medically treated group. Low-risk procedures included breast, skin, urologic, and orthopedic surgery. These broad groups of surgical procedures were the basis for defining surgical risk in the AHA/ACC Guidelines on Perioperative Cardiovascular Evaluation for Noncardiac Surgery (Table 40–5).[2]

# ■ IMPORTANCE OF EXERCISE TOLERANCE

There is disagreement on the value of exercise tolerance as a means of determining perioperative risk. Specifically, the AHA/ACC Guidelines advocate using it, whereas the American College of Physicians Guidelines suggest that evidence for its use is insufficient. Importantly, a lack of evidence does not translate into evidence for a lack of effect, and most clinicians have advocated its use. Several studies demonstrate that the ability to raise heart rate on a stress test is the strongest predictor of perioperative outcome.[32] Excellent exercise tolerance, even in patients with stable angina, suggests that the myocardium can tolerate the stress of surgery without becoming dysfunctional. Additionally, these patients are at risk for devel-

Table 40–5

## Cardiac Risk* Stratification for Noncardiac Surgical Procedures

**High** (Reported cardiac risk often >5%)
    Emergent major operations, particularly in the elderly
    Aortic and other major vascular
    Peripheral vascular
    Anticipated prolonged surgical procedures associated with large fluid shifts and / or blood loss
**Intermediate** (Reported cardiac risk generally <5%)
    Carotid endarterectomy
    Head and neck
    Intraperitoneal and intrathoracic
    Orthopedic
    Prostate
**Low†** (Reported cardiac risk generally <1%)
    Endoscopic procedures
    Superficial procedure
    Cataract
    Breast

*Combined incidence of cardiac death and nonfatal myocardial infarction.
†Do not generally require further preoperative cardiac testing.
From Eagle K, Brundage B, Chaitman B, et al: Guidelines for perioperative cardiovascular evaluation for noncardiac surgery. Circulation 1996;93:1278–1317.

oping hypotension with ischemia and, therefore, may benefit from more extensive monitoring or coronary revascularization. Exercise tolerance can be assessed with formal treadmill testing or with a questionnaire that investigates activities of daily living (Table 40–6).[2]

## ▪ APPROACH TO THE PATIENT

The ACC/AHA Task Force has published Guidelines on Perioperative Evaluation of the Cardiac Patient undergoing Noncardiac Surgery that are based on the available evidence and expert opinion. The approach integrates clinical history (see

Table 40–6

## Estimated Energy Requirement for Various Activities

| 1 MET | | 4 METs | |
|---|---|---|---|
| | Can you take care of yourself? Eat, dress, or use the toilet? | | Climb a flight of stairs or walk up a hill? Walk on level ground at 4 mph or 6.4 km / h? |
| | Walk indoors around the house? | | Run a short distance? |
| | Walk a block or two on level ground at 2–3 mph or 3.2–4.8 km / h? | | Do heavy work around the house like scrubbing floors or lifting or moving heavy furniture? |
| | Do light work around the house like dusting or washing dishes? | | Participate in moderate recreational activities like golf, bowling, dancing, doubles tennis, or throwing a baseball or football? |
| | | >10 METs | Participate in strenuous sports like swimming, singles tennis, football, basketball, or skiing? |

MET indicates metabolic equivalent.
Adapted from the Duke Activity Status Index and AHA Exercise Standards.
From Eagle K, Brundage B, Chaitman B, et al: Guidelines for perioperative cardiovascular evaluation for noncardiac surgery. Circulation 1996;93:1278–1317.

Table 40–3), surgery-specific risk, and exercise tolerance (Fig. 40–2).[2] First, the clinican must evaluate the urgency of the surgery and the appropriateness of a formal preoperative assessment. Next he must determine whether the patient has had a previous revascularization procedure or coronary evaluation. Patients with unstable coronary syndromes should be identified and appropriate treatment instituted. Finally, the decision to undergo further testing depends on the interaction among the clinical risk factors, surgery-specific risk, and functional capacity. For patients at intermediate clinical risk, both exercise tolerance and the extent of the surgery are taken into account to determine the need for further testing. The authors of the guidelines suggest that all patients undergoing aortic or infrainguinal bypass surgery be considered at high surgical risk, and, therefore, that further evaluation be considered. In an editorial in *Annals of Internal Medicine,* two of the authors of the guidelines (Fleisher and Eagle) suggest that routine preoperative testing of all major vascular surgery patients would produce a high incidence of false-positive results and advocate a more Bayesian approach.[33]

The American College of Physician Guideline attempts to apply the evidence-based approach (Figs. 40–3, 40–4).[19] The initial decision point is the assessment of risk using the Detsky modification of the Cardiac Risk Index. Patients whose disease is class II or III are considered at high risk. For class I disease, other clinical factor (according to work by Eagle and colleagues[26] or Vanzetto and colleagues[34]) are used to further stratify risk. Those with multiple markers for cardiovascular disease according to these risk indices and those undergoing major vascular surgery are considered appropriate for further diagnostic testing by either dipyridamole imaging or dobutamine stress echocardiography.

## Coronary Revasculariation

Before cardiovascular testing is performed, it is important to determine whether the results will affect perioperative management. Among the various interventions discussed earlier, several investigators have proposed coronary revascularization before noncardiac surgery as a means of reducing perioperative risk. No randomized trials have addressed this issue, and such a trial would require a very large sample and have multiple confounding issues. Several large cohort studies, however, suggest that, for patients who survive coronary artery bypass grafting (CABG), the risk of subsequent noncardiac surgery is low.[31, 35] While there are few data to support the notion of coronary revascularization solely for the purpose of improving perioperative outcome, it is true that, for certain patient subsets, long-term survival may be enhanced by revascularization. Rihal and colleagues utilized the Coronary Artery Surgery Study database and found that CABG significantly improved survival in patients with both peripheral vascular disease

---

**Figure 40–2** ■ The American Heart Association/American College of Cardiology Task Force on Perioperative Evaluation of cardiac patients undergoing noncardiac surgery has proposed an algorithm for decisions on further evaluation. This is one of multiple algorithms proposed in the literature. It is based on expert opinion and incorporates six steps. First, the clinician must evaluate the urgency of the surgery and the appropriateness of a formal preoperative assessment. Next, she must determine whether the patient has had a previous revascularization procedure or coronary evaluation. Patients with unstable coronary syndromes should be identified, and appropriate treatment should be instituted. The decision to have further testing depends on the interaction of the clinical risk factors, surgery-specific risk, and functional capacity. CHF, congestive heart failure; ill, myocardial infarction. (Adapted from Eagle K, Brundage B, Chaitman B, et al: Guidelines for perioperative cardiovascular evaluation for noncardiac surgery. A report of the American Heart Association/American College of Cardiology Task Force on Assessment of Diagnostic and Therapeutic Cardiovascular Procedures. Circulation 1996;93:1278–1317.)

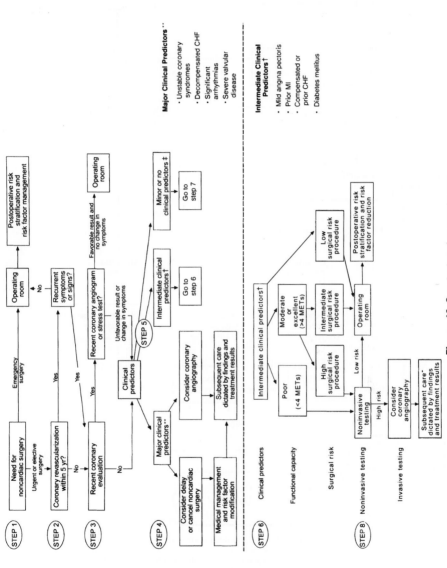

**Figure 40-2** ■ *See legend on opposite page*

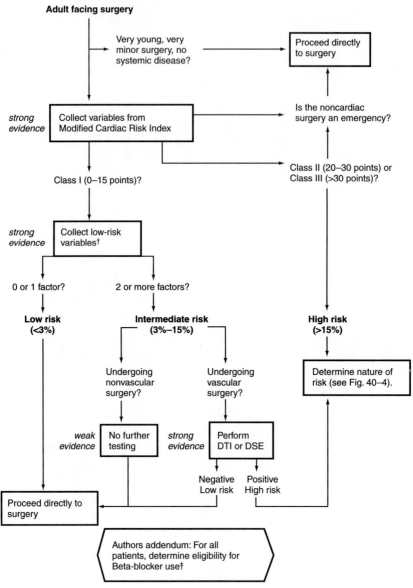

**Figure 40–3** ▪ The American College of Physicians Guidelines for assessing and managing the perioperative risk from coronary artery disease associated with major noncardiac surgery. The commentary in italics represents the strength of evidence to support each decision in the algorithm. An evidence-based analysis of the literature accompanied the algorithm in a paper by Detsky and Palda. Initially, patients are assessed using the Detsky modification of the cardiac risk index to determine if their risk is class I (low) or class II or III (high; see Table 41–2). If class I, clinical predictors such as those identified by Eagle are collected to determine whether they are associated with low or high clinical risk. Only patients with several clinical predictors are then determined to be at intermediate perioperative risk. Those at intermediate risk who are to undergo vascular surgery should be considered for noninvasive imaging with dipyridamole thallium imaging (DTI) or dobutamine stress echocardiography (DSE). No further testing is suggested for patients undergoing nonvascular surgery. (Palda VA, Detsky AS: Perioperative assessment and management of risk from coronary artery disease. Ann Intern Med 1997;127:313–328.)

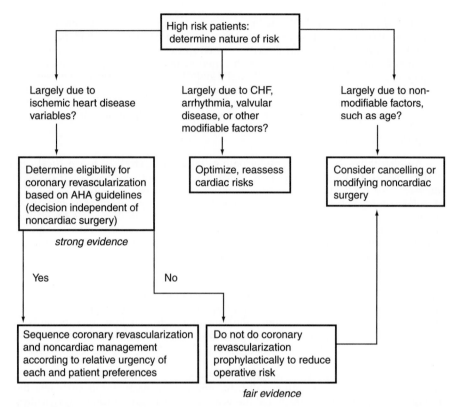

**Figure 40–4** ■ Further defining interventions for the high risk group in the American College of Physicians Guidelines. If the noninvasive testing is positive or the patient is at high clinical Detsky risk, then it is important to determine the nature of the risk. If the risk is largely due to ischemic heart disease, then it is important to determine if the patient would be eligible for coronary revascularization based on AHA Guidelines independent of noncardiac surgery. If the risk is due to nonischemic origins then the ideal choice is to optimize and reassess. Finally, if it is due to largely nonmodifiable factors then either canceling the case or modifying the noncardiac surgery should be considered. (Adapted from Eagle K, Brundage B, Chaitman B, et al: Guidelines for perioperative cardiovascular evaluation for noncardiac surgery. A report of the American Heart Association/American College of Cardiology Task Force on Assessment of Diagnostic and Therapeutic Cardiovascular Procedures. Circulation 1996;93:1278–1317.)

and triple-vessel coronary disease, especially the group with depressed ventricular function.[36]

The value of percutaneous transluminal coronary angioplasty (PTCA) like that of newer techniques such as stenting and rotoblade, is less firmly established. In several series, the incidence of cardiovascular complications was low for patients treated with "prophylactic" PTCA before vascular surgery, but it is difficult to determine the expected complication rate in a comparison group with single- or double-vessel disease.[37, 38] For patients who have perioperative MI as a result of plaque rupture and coronary thrombosis in noncritical lesions, single-vessel PTCA of more critical stenoses, theoretically, produces little benefit. Ellis and coworkers studied 21 patients who had coronary angiography before major vascular surgery and sustained a perioperative cardiac event.[10] None of the MI occurred in areas distal to a critical stenosis, but approximately a third occurred distal to a noncritical stenosis.[10] An administrative dataset from Washington State was analyzed to assess the value of preoperative PTCA using a case-control approach.[39] Patients who had undergone PTCA more than 6 weeks before noncardiac surgery had better outcomes than did matched controls with coronary artery disease, whereas no difference in outcome was observed when the period between PTCA and noncardiac surgery was less than 6 weeks. Although analysis of administrative datasets has some inherent limitations owing to the inability to determine the potential selection bias for those being treated, these data suggest that "prophylactic" PTCA intended simply to get the patient through surgery may confer minimal benefit or none.

### Risks and Benefits

An alternative approach to determining the optimal strategy for medical care in the absence of clinical trials is to construct a decision analysis. Two decision analyses have been published on the issue of cardiovascular testing before major vascular surgery.[40, 41] Both assumed that patients with significant coronary artery disease would undergo CABG before noncardiac surgery. Both models found that the optimal decision was sensitive to local morbidity and mortality rates within the clinically observed range. These models suggest that preoperative testing for the purpose of coronary revascularization is not the optimal strategy if perioperative morbidity and mortality are low.

Importantly, the greatest cost (in both dollars and morbidity) of preoperative testing and revascularization is the revascularization procedure itself. Therefore, the indications for revascularization, and thus the frequency of its use, have significant impact on the model. Second, the fact that potential long-term benefits of coronary revascularization in this population were not included in the analysis might bias against the revascularization arm. If long-term survival is included in the models, coronary revascularization may improve outcomes overall and be a cost-effective intervention, although a patient's age should be included in the equation. For example, an 80-year-old diabetic patient with significant comorbid diseases may gain little in additional life years by undergoing coronary revascularization and may actually have poorer quality of life in their final years than they would have otherwise. In contrast, a 55-year-old man with an abdominal aortic aneurysm who is found to have occult left main coronary artery disease would realize substantial increases in both the length and quality of his life from preoperative cardiovascular testing and coronary revascularization. Therefore, identification of patients with diffuse disease or a significant left main stenosis amenable to surgery should undergo CABG before noncardiac surgery. In this instance, the procedure is justified by long-term benefit, and performing it before noncardiac surgery reduces the risk of a fatal or nonfatal perioperative myocardial infarction.

## ■ CHOICE OF DIAGNOSTIC TEST

Many tests are available to further investigate the presence and extent of coronary artery disease, and are described in greater detail elsewhere in this book. Exercise electrocardiography (ECG) is a useful test to diagnose CAD but is rarely indicated preoperatively since it requires that the patient have good exercise capacity (which would render the test unnecessary). A number of studies have suggested that preoperative ambulatory ECG for silent MI is a sensitive and specific test for perioperative cardiac events, but it has two major problems. The majority of patients at highest risk have an ECG that prevents accurate diagnosis of silent ischemia.[42, 43] Additionally, attempts have been made to quantitate preoperative ischemia as a means of identifying a high-risk cohort. In a study comparing preoperative ambulatory ECG with dipyridamole thallium imaging, those patients who had more prolonged preoperative ischemia had no greater perioperative and long-term risks than those with shorter-lived preoperative ischemia.

For patients who are unable to exercise, particularly candidates for major vascular surgery, pharmacologic stress testing has been advocated. Dipyridamole thallium imaging has been studied extensively as a preoperative diagnostic test since the original report by Boucher and colleagues was published. The negative predictive value of dipyridamole thallium imaging has consistently been high (>90%), although the positive predictive value has decreased over time owing to the overall reduction in cardiac morbidity in these studies. In particular, recent studies of a consecutive cohort of vascular surgery patients have not been able to demonstrate additive value for dipyridamole thallium imaging. Eagle and colleagues studied 200 consecutive vascular surgery patients referred to a preoperative evaluation clinic and defined five risk factors: age older than 70 years, diabetes, ventricular ectopic activity that is being treated, angina, and Q waves on the preoperative ECG. Patients who had no risk factors had only a 3% cardiac complication rate, a finding that suggests that testing would have minimal value. Similarly, those with three or more risk factors have a 50% risk of complications. For patients at moderate clinical risk (i.e., one or two risk factors), the diagnostic test was able to delineate a low-risk and a high-risk group. The test is best utilized and has its best predictive value in persons at moderate clinical risk. Using such an approach, a recent blinded study by Vanzetto and colleagues demonstrated high predictive value when the test was reserved for patients with multiple risk factors who are to undergo major vascular surgery.[34] Second, the patients at greatest risk have larger areas of reversible defect or increased lung uptake on thallium imaging. Fleisher and coworkers found that those with these findings had both increased risk of perioperative cardiac morbidity and decreased survival 2 years after surgery.

Dobutamine stress echocardiography has received a great deal of attention. Its positive and negative predictive values are among the best of any preoperative diagnostic test. This test may most closely mimic the hyperdynamic state associated with the perioperative period. Patients at greatest risk develop new regional wall motion abnormalities at slower heart rates.[44] Like dipyridamole thallium imaging, dobutamine stress echocardiography has the best predictive value in persons at moderate clinical risk. In two recent meta-analyses, dobutamine stress echocardiography had the best predictive value, but there was a great deal of overlap with dipyridamole imaging.[45, 46]

## ■ SUMMARY

Preoperative evaluation should focus on obtaining information on the extent and stability of the cardiovascular system so that perioperative management may be modified, if necessary. The decision to perform further evaluation and diagnostic testing depends on the interactions of patients and surgery-specific factors and on exercise capacity.

## ■ REFERENCES

1. Shah KB, Kleinman BS, Rao T, et al: Angina and other risk factors in patients with cardiac diseases undergoing noncardiac operations. Anesth Analg 1990;70:240–247.
2. Eagle K, Brundage B, Chaitman B, et al: Guidelines for perioperative cardiovascular evaluation for noncardiac surgery. A report of the American Heart Association/American College of Cardiology Task Force on Assessment of Diagnostic and Therapeutic Cardiovascular Procedures. Circulation 1996;93:1278–1317.
3. Mangano DT, Browner WS, Hollenberg M, et al: Association of perioperative myocardial ischemia with

cardiac morbidity and mortality in men undergoing noncardiac surgery. N Engl J Med 1990;323:1781–1788.

4. Raby KE, Barry J, Creager MA, et al: Detection and significance of intraoperative and postoperative myocardial ischemia in peripheral vascular surgery. JAMA 1992;268:222–227.

5. Fleisher LA, Nelson AH, Rosenbaum SH: Postoperative myocardial ischemia: Etiology of cardiac morbidity or manifestation of underlying disease? J Clin Anesth 1995;7:97–102.

6. Mangano DT, Layug EL, Wallace A, Tateo I: Effect of atenolol on mortality and cardiovascular morbidity after noncardiac surgery. Multicenter Study of Perioperative Ischemia Research Group (see Comments). N Engl J Med 1996;335:1713–1720.

7. Wallace A, Layug B, Tateo I, et al: Prophylactic atenolol reduces postoperative myocardial ischemia. McSPI Research Group (see Comments). Anesthesiology 1998;88:7–17.

8. Frank SM, Fleisher LA, Breslow MJ, et al: Perioperative maintenance of normothermia reduces the incidence of morbid cardiac events. A randomized clinical trial (see Comments). JAMA 1997;277:1127–1134.

9. Nelson AH, Fleisher LA, Rosenbaum SH: Relationship between postoperative anemia and cardiac morbidity in high-risk vascular patients in the intensive care unit. Crit Care Med 1993;21:860–866.

10. Ellis SG, Hertzer NR, Young JR, Brener S: Angiographic correlates of cardiac death and myocardial infarction complicating major nonthoracic vascular surgery. Am J Cardiol 1996;77:1126–1128.

11. Rosenfeld BA, Beattie C, Christopherson R, et al: The effects of different anesthetic regimens on fibrinolysis and the development of postoperative arterial thrombosis. Perioperative Ischemia Randomized Anesthesia Trial Study Group (see Comments). Anesthesiology 1993;79:435–443.

12. Goldman L, Caldera DL, Nussbaum SR, et al: Multifactorial index of cardiac risk in noncardiac surgical procedures. N Engl J Med 1977;297:845–850.

13. Zeldin RA: Assessing cardiac risk in patients who undergo noncardiac surgical procedures. Can J Surg 1984;27:402.

14. Larsen SF, Olesen KH, Jacobsen E, et al: Prediction of cardiac risk in non-cardiac surgery. Eur Heart J 1987;8:179–185.

15. Domaingue CM, Davies MJ, Cronin KD: Cardiovascular risk factors in patients for vascular surgery. Anaesth Intensive Care 1982;10:324–327.

16. McEnroe CS, O'Donnell TF, Yeager A, et al: Comparison of ejection fraction and Goldman risk factor analysis to dipyridamole-thallium imaging 201 studies in the evaluation of cardiac morbidity after aortic aneurysm surgery. J Vasc Surg 1990;11:497–504.

17. Lette J, Waters D, Lassonde J, et al: Postoperative myocardial infarction and cardiac death. Predictive value of dipyridamole-thallium imaging and five clinical scoring systems based on multifactorial analysis. Ann Surg 1990;211:84–90.

18. Detsky A, Abrams H, McLaughlin J, et al: Predicting cardiac complications in patients undergoing noncardiac surgery. J Gen Intern Med 1986;1:211–219.

19. Palda VA, Detsky AS: Perioperative assessment and management of risk from coronary artery disease. Ann Intern Med 1997;127:313–328.

20. Tarhan S, Moffitt EA, Taylor WF, Giuliani ER: Myocardial infarction after general anesthesia. JAMA 1972;220:1451–1454.

21. Rao TK, Jacobs KH, El-Etr AA: Reinfarction following anesthesia in patients with myocardial infarction. Anesthesiology 1983;59:499–505.

22. Shah KB, Kleinman BS, Sami H, et al: Reevaluation of perioperative myocardial infarction in patients with prior myocardial infarction undergoing noncardiac operations. Anesth Analg 1990;71:231–235.

23. Ryan TJ, Anderson JL, Antman EM, et al: ACC/AHA guidelines for the management of patients with acute myocardial infarction: Executive summary. A report of the American College of Cardiology/American Heart Association Task Force on Practice Guidelines (Committee on Management of Acute Myocardial Infarction). Circulation 1996;94:2341–2350.

24. Goldman L, Caldera DL: Risks of general anesthesia and elective operation in the hypertensive patient. Anesthesiology 1979;50:285–292.

25. Hollenberg M, Mangano DT, Browner WS, et al: Predictors of postoperative myocardial ischemia in patients undergoing noncardiac surgery. The Study of Perioperative Ischemia Research Group (see Comments). JAMA 1992;268:205–209.

26. Eagle KA, Coley CM, Newell JB, et al: Combining clinical and thallium data optimizes preoperative assessment of cardiac risk before major vascular surgery. Ann Intern Med 1989;110:859–866.

27. Kannel W, Abbott R: Incidence and prognosis of unrecognized myocardial infarction: An update on the Framingham Study. N Engl J Med 1984;311:1144–1147.

28. L'Italien GL, Cambria RP, Cutler BS, et al: Comparative early and late cardiac morbidity among patients requiring different vascular surgery procedures. J Vasc Surg 1995;21:935–944.

29. Backer CL, Tinker JH, Robertson DM, Vlietstra RE: Myocardial reinfarction following local anesthesia for ophthalmic surgery. Anesth Analg 1980;59:257–262.

30. Warner MA, Shields SE, Chute CG: Major morbidity and mortality within 1 month of ambulatory surgery and anesthesia. JAMA 1993;270:1437–1441.

31. Eagle KA, Rihal CS, Mickel MC, et al: Cardiac risk of noncardiac surgery: Influence of coronary disease and type of surgery in 3368 operations. CASS Investigators and University of Michigan Heart Care Program. Coronary Artery Surgery Study. Circulation 1997;96:1882–1887.

32. McPhail N, Calvin JE, Shariatmadar A, et al: The use of preoperative exercise testing to predict cardiac complications after arterial reconstruction. J Vasc Surg 1988;7:60–68.
33. Fleisher LA, Eagle KA: Screening for cardiac disease in patients having noncardiac surgery. Ann Intern Med 1996;124:767–772.
34. Vanzetto G, Machecourt J, Blendea D, et al: Additive value of thallium single-photon emission computed tomography myocardial imaging for prediction of perioperative events in clinically selected high cardiac risk patients having abdominal aortic surgery. Am J Cardiol 1996;77:143–148.
35. Huber KC, Evans MA, Bresnahan JF, et al: Outcome of noncardiac operations in patients with severe coronary artery disease successfully treated preoperatively with coronary angioplasty. Mayo Clin Proc 1992;67:15–21.
36. Rihal CS, Eagle KA, Mickel MC, et al: Surgical therapy for coronary artery disease among patients with combined coronary artery and peripheral vascular disease. Circulation 1995;91:46–53.
37. Elmore J, Hallett J, Gibbons R, et al: Myocardial revascularization before abdominal aortic aneurysmorrhapy: Effect of coronary angioplasty. Mayo Clin Proc 1993;68:637–641.
38. Gottlieb A, Banous M, Sprung J, et al: Perioperative cardiovascular morbidity in patients with coronary artery disease undergoing vascular surgery after percutaneous transluminal coronary angioplasty. J Cardiothorac Vascu Anesth 1998;12:501–506.
39. van Norman GA, Posner KL, Wright IH, Spiess BD: Adverse cardiac outcomes after noncardiac surgery in patients with prior PTCA compared to patients with nonrevascularized CAD and no CAD (Abstract). Circulation 1997;96:I–734.
40. Fleisher LA, Skolnick ED, Holroyd KJ, Lehmann HP: Coronary artery revascularization before abdominal aortic aneurysm surgery: A decision analytic approach. Anesth Analg 1994;79:661–669.
41. Mason JJ, Owens DK, Harris RA, et al: The role of coronary angiography and coronary revascularization before noncardiac surgery. JAMA 1995;273:1919–1925.
42. Raby KE, Goldman L, Creager MA, et al: Correlation between perioperative ischemia and major cardiac events after peripheral vascular surgery. N Engl J Med 1989;321:1296–1300.
43. Fleisher LA, Rosenbaum SH, Nelson AH, et al: Preoperative dipyridamole thallium imaging and Holter monitoring as a predictor of perioperative cardiac events and long term outcome. Anesthesiology 1995;83:906–917.
44. Poldermans D, Arnese M, Fioretti PM, et al: Improved cardiac risk stratification in major vascular surgery with dobutamine-atropine stress echocardiography. J Am Coll Cardiol 1995;26:648–653.
45. Mantha S, Roizen MF, Barnard J, et al: Relative effectiveness of four preoperative tests for predicting adverse cardiac outcomes after vascular surgery: A meta-analysis. Anesth Analg 1994;79:422–433.
46. Shaw LJ, Eagle KA, Gersh BJ, Miller DD: Meta-analysis of intravenous dipyridamole-thallium-201 imaging (1985 to 1994) and dobutamine echocardiography (1991 to 1994) for risk stratification before vascular surgery (see Comments). J Am Coll Cardiol 1996;27:787–798.

# ▪ RECOMMENDED READING

Eagle K, Brundage B, Chaitman B, et al: Guidelines for perioperative cardiovascular evaluation for noncardiac surgery. A report of the American Heart Association/American College of Cardiology Task Force on Assessment of Diagnostic and Therapeutic Cardiovascular Procedures. Circulation 1996;93:1278–1317.
Fleisher LA, Eagle KA: Screening for cardiac disease in patients having noncardiac surgery. Ann Intern Med 1996;124:767–772.
Fleisher LA, Skolnick ED, Holroyd KJ, Lehmann HP: Coronary artery revascularization before abdominal aortic aneurysm surgery: A decision analytic approach. Anesth Analg 1994;79:661–669.
Mangano DT: Perioperative cardiac morbidity. Anesthesiology 1990;72:153–184.
Palda VA, Detsky AS: Perioperative assessment and management of risk from coronary artery disease. Ann Intern Med 1997;127:313–328.

# Chapter 41

# Myocardial and Vascular Gene Therapy

*Afshin Ehsan* ▪ *Michael J. Mann* ▪ *Victor J. Dzau*

The application of gene therapy technology to the treatment of both identifiable single genetic defects and common multifactorial diseases has begun a slow but progressive evolution from the laboratory to the clinic. Recent discoveries about the molecular basis of cardiovascular diseases (such as atherosclerosis and restenosis after balloon angioplasty), have created an opportunity for the application of genetic manipulation as definitive therapy. Increasingly, researchers have been able to identify molecular and cellular abnormalities that form the basis of cardiovascular disease, and these processes can, at times, be linked to the pattern of activity of certain critical genes in vascular cells. The development of tools for the successful manipulation of gene expression in living tissues has been critical to the potential realization of gene therapies. These systems have included recombinant viral vectors that allow relatively efficient insertion of genetic information and oligonucleotides that can be used to alter native gene expression.[1, 2]

A growing body of data afford researchers the ability to target common cardiovascular problems at the level of gene expression. Such intervention can be geared toward the prevention of complications that limit the long-term efficacy of traditional cardiovascular therapies (such as balloon angioplasty, bypass grafting, and cardiac transplantation) and toward the reduction of susceptibility to myocardial infarction or congestive heart failure. Furthermore, as our knowledge of the specific genetic elements involved in determining the risk of cardiovascular disease expands, genetic therapies may evolve as a primary form of cardiovascular disease prevention. In this chapter, we describe the current state of gene therapy in the treatment of cardiovascular disease and vascular grafts, with emphasis on illustrating a variety of methods for genetic intervention and their applicability to the different cellular elements and pathologic processes encountered in this complex system.

## ▪ CARDIOVASCULAR GENE THERAPY STRATEGIES

Gene therapy can be defined as any manipulation of gene activity, or gene "expression," that influences disease. This manipulation is generally achieved by introducing foreign DNA into cells in a process known as *transduction* or *transfection*. Gene therapy can involve either the delivery of whole, active genes (gene transfer) or the blockade of native gene expression by transfection of cells with short chains of nucleic acids known as *oligonucleotides* (Fig. 41–1).

The gene transfer approach allows for replacement of a missing gene product or for "overexpression" of a native or foreign protein that can prevent or reverse a disease process. The transfer of a gene into a target cell where subsequently it is expressed, is known as *transduction*, and the new gene as the *transgene*. Gene *replacement* or *augmentation* involves transfer of a gene that is missing from a cell,

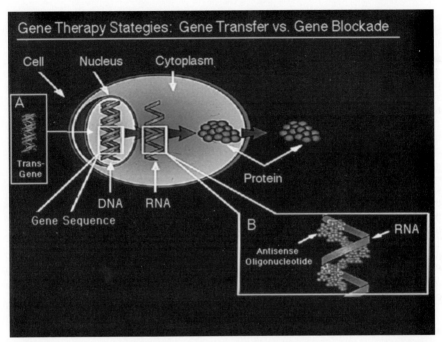

**Figure 41–1** ■ Gene therapy strategies. (*A*) Gene transfer involves delivery of an entire gene, either by viral infection or by nonviral vectors, to the nucleus of a target cell. Expression of the gene via transcription into mRNA and translation into a protein gene product yields a functional protein that either achieves a therapeutic effect within a transduced cell or is secreted to act on other cells. (*B*) Gene blockade involves the introduction into the cell of short sequences of nucleic acids that block gene expression, such as antisense ODN that bind mRNA in a sequence-specific fashion and prevent translation into protein.

is present in a defective form, or is simply underexpressed (relative to the level of protein expression desired by the clinician). The protein expressed may be active only within the cell, in which case very high gene transfer efficiency may be necessary to alter the overall function of an organ or tissue. Alternatively, proteins secreted by target cells may act on other cells in a paracrine or endocrine manner, in which case delivery to a small subpopulation may yield a sufficient therapeutic result.

Gene blockade can be accomplished by transfection of cells with short chains of DNA known as *antisense oligodeoxynucleotides* (ODN).[3] This approach attempts to alter cellular function by inhibiting specific gene expression. Genes are defined by a specific sequence of bases that make up the DNA chain. Antisense ODN are designed to have a base sequence that is complementary in terms of Watson-Crick binding to a segment of the target gene. These 15 to 20 base single-stranded sequences confer specificity to a single site within the genome. This complementary sequence allows the ODN to bind specifically to the corresponding segment of messenger RNA (mRNA) that is transcribed from the gene during expression. This binding of ODN to mRNA prevents the translation of RNA into the protein product of the gene.

Another form of gene blockade is use of "ribozymes," segments of RNA that can act as enzymes do to destroy only certain sequences of target mRNA.[4] Ribozymes contain both a catalytic region that can cleave other RNA molecules in sequence-specific manner and an adjacent sequence that confers the specificity of the target. Because the sequence recognition portion of the ribozymes is generally limited to approximately six bases, these gene-inhibitory agents are generally more susceptible than their antisense counterparts to nonspecific interactions.

A third type of gene inhibition involves the blockade of gene regulatory proteins known as *transcription factors*. Transcription factors regulate gene expression by binding to chromosomal DNA at specific promoter regions, and this binding turns on, or activates, an adjacent gene. Double-stranded ODN can, therefore, be designed to mimic the chromosomal binding sites of these transcription factors and to act as "decoys," binding up the available transcription factor and preventing subsequent activation of target genes.[5]

Transfer of genetic sequences exogenous to the human genome has been envisioned, for example, the gene encoding thymidine kinase [TK] from the herpes simplex virus. This technique has been used to enhance metabolic activation of the cytotoxic prodrug ganciclovir, an effect that may be useful in treating vascular proliferative disorders such as restenosis.[6] Scientists studying gene transfer technology have often relied on a class of genes known as *reporter* or *marker genes*. These genes encode proteins, such as the β-galactosidase found in *Escherichia coli* organisms (known as *lacZ* or *β-gal*), or a small fluorescent molecule known as *green fluorescent protein* (GFP), that can be detected easily via histochemistry, fluorescent microscopy, or other techniques that allow rapid identification and quantification of successful gene transfer.

## ▪ CARDIOVASCULAR GENE THERAPY VECTOR SYSTEMS

Although many cells naturally take up DNA in small amounts from their extracellular environment, this uptake is inefficient and generally unsuitable for exerting a physiologically significant influence on the genetic function of either healthy or diseased tissues. Clinical gene therapies will, therefore, depend on the development of vectors that enhance the efficiency of DNA transfer, both in vitro and in vivo. The "ideal" DNA vector would be capable of safe and highly efficient delivery to all cell types, both proliferating and quiescent, with the opportunity to select either short-term or indefinitely prolonged gene expression. This ideal vector would also have the flexibility to accommodate genes of all sizes, to incorporate control of the temporal pattern and degree of gene expression, and to recognize specific cell types for tailored delivery or expression. While progress is being made on each of these fronts individually, researchers are still far from developing a single vector with all of these characteristics. Instead, a spectrum of vectors has evolved, each of which may find a niche in some early clinical gene therapy strategies.

Viruses are the most common vehicles for exogenous gene delivery into mammalian cells. Although they take on many distinctive forms, all viruses consist of a genetic nucleic acid code encapsulated in a machinery that facilitates gene transfer and, in many cases, gene expression. Recombinant DNA technology has allowed scientists to alter the genetic material contained within viral particles, both to include target genes of interest and to remove viral genes toxic to the host tissue.

Recombinant virus particles employed as gene transfer vectors are distinguished from their naturally occurring derivative viruses by their inability to replicate (Fig. 41–2). This is achieved by deleting structural and functional genes from the native viral genome that, in the normal virus life cycle, provide the blueprint for production of new virus in infected host cells. Instead, these endogenous viral genes are replaced by the gene chosen for transfer, which is coupled to necessary regulatory elements using recombinant technology. To "package" these

# Genetic Organization of MMLV Retrovirus

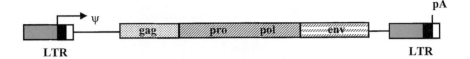

# Recombinant Retroviral Vector for Gene Transfer

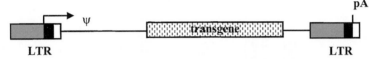

**Figure 41–2** ■ Generation of recombinant retroviral particles for gene transfer. The MMLV genome is depicted schematically. There are four major viral gene products encoded by the genes *gag, pro, pol,* and *env.* At either end of the single-stranded RNA genome are the long-terminal repeat (LTR) sequences, which contain important regulatory elements. The ψ sequence is a packaging signal that must be present for the encapsidation of viral constructs. Gene transfer constructs are made by removing the structural genes and inserting the gene of interest downstream from ψ.

vectors into particles, cell lines are engineered to provide the missing structural viral proteins separately. The final vector particle is assembled to include the transgene construct in the genetic information, which is capable of infecting suitable target cells without producing the complete viral replication life cycle.

Although viral vectors are Nature's solution to the problem of efficient gene transfer, humans' attempts to harness these resources have also been confounded by the biologic barriers that have evolved to protect cells and organisms from viral infection. Immune responses not only limit the efficacy of viral gene transfer, particularly when repeated administration is considered, but the inflammatory response to viral antigens, even those associated with replication-deficient vectors, may impede or nullify the benefits of expression of the transferred gene.[7] Furthermore, engineering of viral genomes does not always preclude residual cytotoxicity in infected cells, and the possibility for regression to replication proficiency or for further mutation and recombination with other virulent viruses in the environment pose biologic hazards that are difficult to quantify or predict.

Scientists have therefore continued to explore nonviral vectors for achieving efficient DNA delivery. One advantage of nonviral delivery systems is that they can be used not only for gene transfer but also for delivery of oligonucleotides and protein–nucleic acid complexes that can be used for alternative forms of genetic manipulation. Whereas *transduction* refers generally to the delivery of an intact gene to a target cell and *infection* is used to describe the process of viral gene delivery, *transfection* is a term used to describe nonviral (i.e., physical or chemical) delivery of genes or oligonucleotides. What follows is a brief description of DNA delivery vectors that have been exploited in the cardiovascular system (Table 41–1).

## Retroviral Vectors

Retroviruses contain RNA genomes and express an enzyme, known as *reverse transcriptase,* that generates double-stranded DNA from the viral RNA template.

Table 41-1

## Comparison of Vectors Used for Cardiovascular Gene Transfer

| | Efficiency in Vivo | DNA Integration | Target Cells | Gene Size (max) | Ease of Preparation | Host Response | Risks |
|---|---|---|---|---|---|---|---|
| **Viral** | | | | | | | |
| Retrovirus | + | Yes | Replicating | ~6 kb | +++ | + | Oncogenesis<br>Viral mutation |
| Adenovirus | ++++ | No | Replicating and nonreplicating | ~7.5 kb | ++ | ++++ | Cytotoxicity<br>Viral mutation |
| Adenoassociated virus | + | Sometimes | Replicating and nonreplicating | ~4 kb | + | + | Oncogenesis<br>Viral mutation<br>Viral contamination |
| **Nonviral** | | | | | | | |
| Liposome | + | No | Replicating and nonreplicating | Unlimited | ++++ | + | Cytotoxicity at high concentrations |
| Fusigenic liposome | ++ | No | Replicating and nonreplicating | Unlimited | + | + | Cytotoxicity at high concentrations |
| Naked plasmid | + | No | Replicating and nonreplicating | Unlimited | +++ | + | Cytotoxicity at high concentrations |

+, lowest, +++, highest.

This DNA is then inserted into the chromosomal genome of the host cell, from which it is expressed. For this insertion to take place, the infected cell must undergo cell division shortly after infection, so a traditional retrovirus can deliver DNA effectively only to actively replicating cells. Once viral gene insertion has taken place, this exogenous genetic material continues to be passed on to subsequent generations of progeny cells, creating the possibility for long-term stable gene expression. Recombinant, replication-deficient retroviral vectors have been used extensively for gene transfer in cultured cells in vitro, where cell proliferation can be manipulated easily. Their use in vivo has been more limited owing to low transduction efficiency, particularly in the vascular system, where most cells remain quiescent. Nabel and coworkers[8] first demonstrated the feasibility of transducing blood vessels with foreign DNA in vivo by infecting porcine iliofemoral arteries with a recombinant retroviral vector containing the β-galactosidase gene. Several cell types in the vessel wall were transduced, including endothelial and vascular smooth muscle cells (VSMC). Using a β-galactosidase retroviral vector to genetically modify endothelial cells in vitro, Wilson and colleagues[9] demonstrated expression as long as 5 weeks after implantation of a prosthetic vascular graft seeded with genetically transformed cells. The random integration of traditional retroviral vectors such as Moloney murine leukemia virus (MMLV) into chromosomal DNA carries the potential hazard of oncogene activation and neoplastic cell growth. Although the risk may be exceedingly low, safety monitoring will be an important aspect of clinical trials using viral vectors. Recent improvements in packaging systems (particularly the development of "pseudotyped" retroviral vectors that incorporate vesicular stomatitis virus G protein) have improved the stability of retroviral particles and facilitated their use in a wider spectrum of target cells.

## Adenoviral Vectors

Recombinant adenoviruses have become the most widely used viral vectors for experimental gene transfer in vivo and have been used extensively in animal models of cardiovascular disease. Adenoviruses can infect nondividing cells and generally are not integrated into the host genome. These vectors can, therefore, achieve relatively efficient gene transfer in quiescent vascular tissue, but transgenes are generally lost when cells are stimulated into rounds of cell division. Expression of DNA in a nonchromosomal (or episomal) state also appears to be less stable, and adenoviral transduction has proved to be transitory in cells, even in the absence of replication. Most experimental adenoviral vectors have undergone deletion of the viral genes known as E1a and E1b (genes that play a critical role in the adenoviral replication cycle) so as to render the vectors incapable of replication. Deletion of the E3 region provides enough space in the recombinant genome for insertion of as much as 7.5 kb of DNA. Researchers are currently exploring removal of nearly all adenoviral genes, both to reduce the immunogenicity of the vector and to increase the size of possible transgene insertions.

Many scientists have concluded that the immune response to adenoviral antigens is the greatest limitation to their use in gene therapy. Conventional vectors have generally achieved gene expression for only 1 to 2 weeks after infection. It is not certain to what extent the destruction of infected cells contributes to the termination of transgene expression, given that episomal transgene promoters appears to be suppressed as well. Longer expression has, however, been documented after injection of tissues in immunodeficient mice. Even in the context of such reactions, some have postulated that the adenoviral vector provides an adjuvant effect that amplifies the immune response. In the vasculature, physical barriers such as the internal elastic lamina apparently limit infection to the endothelium and gene transfer to the media and adventitia occurs only after injury has disrupted the vessel architecture. Although after balloon injury gene delivery to 30% to 60% of cells has been reported with adenoviral vectors carrying reporter genes, the fact that atherosclerotic disease has also been found to limit the efficiency of adenoviral transduction may pose a significant problem for the treatment of human disease.

## Adenoassociated Viral Vectors

Adenoassociated virus (AAV) is a dependent human parvovirus that is not able to replicate unless a helper virus, such as adenovirus or herpesvirus, is present in the same cell. AAV has not been linked to human disease. It can infect a wide range of target cells and can establish a latent infection by integrating into the genome of the cell, thus yielding stable gene transfer, as in the case of retroviral vectors. Although AAV vectors transduce replicating cells more rapidly, they possess the ability to infect nonreplicating cells both in vitro and in vivo. AAV is limited by its small size (transgenes cannot be longer than about 4 kb) and the need to eliminate helper viruses from viral preparations. Early applications of AAV vectors to human gene therapy have included phenotypic correction of Fanconi anemia in hematopoietic cells and stable in vivo expression of the cystic fibrosis transmembrane conductance regulator in airway epithelial cells. The efficiency of AAV-mediated gene transfer to vascular cells, and the potential use of AAV vectors for vascular gene therapy in vivo, remain to be determined; however a number of groups have reported successful transduction of myocardial cells after direct injection of AAV suspensions into the heart tissue, and these infections have yielded relatively stable expression for more than 60 days.[10, 11] It has not yet been clearly established whether long-term recombinant AAV transgenic expression is associated with genomic integration as the wild-type AAV infection is. In general, AAV transgene expression does not occur at significant levels during the first 2 to 4 weeks after infection, although the reason for this delay is a matter of speculation.

## Lipid-Mediated Gene Transfer

Numerous nonviral methods are available for the delivery of DNA into cells in vitro, including calcium phosphate, electroporation, and particle bombardment. The development of similarly effective methods of transfection in vivo, however, has posed a significant challenge to cardiovascular (and other clinical) researchers who hope to avoid the cumbersome and invasive steps of harvesting and culturing tissues or cells from the patient. The encapsulation of DNA in artificial lipid membranes (liposomes) can facilitate its uptake and cellular transport. The principal advantages of lipid-based gene transfer methods are ease of preparation and flexibility in substituting different transgene constructs as compared with the relatively complex process of producing recombinant viral vectors. Cationic liposomes have been used extensively during the last 5 years for cellular delivery of plasmid DNA and antisense oligonucleotides.

A wide variety of cationic lipid preparations are currently available for DNA transfer both in vitro and in vivo. Early clinical trials with cationic:DNA complexes focused principally on direct injection into malignant tumors (such as metastatic melanoma) to induce a heightened antitumor immune response.[12] In addition to cationic lipids, other substances, such as lipopolyamines and cationic polypeptides, are now being investigated as potential vehicles for enhanced DNA delivery, for both gene transfer and gene blockade strategies.

## Fusigenic Liposome–Mediated Gene Transfer (HVJ Liposomes)

Fusigenic liposome–mediated gene transfer utilizes a combination of fusigenic proteins of the Sendai virus (hemagglutinating virus of Japan, HVJ) in conjunction with neutral liposomes.[13] HVJ is an RNA virus and belongs to the paramyxovirus family, which has HN and F glycoproteins on its envelope. HN binds with glycol-type sialic acid groups that act as receptors on the cell surface, and F protein can interact directly with a cellular lipid bilayer and induce fusion. HVJ liposomes consist of neutral liposomes complexed with ultraviolet light–inactivated HVJ. Fusion of HVJ-liposome complexes with the cell membrane may result in the release of DNA directly into the cytosol. Additionally, the viral coat proteins appear to influence the intracellular fate of DNA delivered by this fusion. HVJ-liposome methods have been employed successfully for gene transfer in vivo to many tissues, including liver, kidney, and the vascular wall. A major limitation to current HVJ liposome techniques is the need to perform a multistep liposome preparation procedure immediately before use and the poor long-term stability of the complexes.

## Other in Vivo Gene Transfer Methods

Plasmids are circular chains of DNA that were originally discovered as a natural means of gene transfer between bacteria. Naked plasmids can also be used to transfer DNA into mammalian cells. Direct injection of plasmid DNA into tissues in vivo can result in transgene expression. Plasmid uptake and expression, however, have generally been achieved at reasonable levels only in skeletal and myocardial muscle.[14] The uptake of naked oligonucleotides is also inefficient after either intravascular administration or direct injection. Various catheters that have been designed to enhance local drug delivery to isolated segments of target vessels have been proposed as vehicles for local vascular gene therapy. The controlled application of a pressurized environment to vascular tissue in a nondistended manner was recently been found to enhance oligonucleotide uptake and nuclear localization. This method may be particularly useful for applications ex vivo such as vein grafting or transplantation and may also be a means of enhancing plasmid gene delivery.[15]

## Regulation of Transgene Expression

In addition to effective gene delivery, many therapeutic problems demand some degree of control over the duration, location, and degree of transgene expression. To this end, researchers have developed early gene promoter systems that allow the clinician to regulate the spatial or temporal pattern of gene expression. These systems include tissue-specific promoters that have been isolated from genetic sequences encoding proteins that are naturally restricted to the target tissue, such as the von Willebrand factor promoter in endothelial cells and the α-myosin heavy chain promoter in myocardium. Promoters have also been isolated from nonmammalian systems that can either promote or inhibit downstream gene expression in the presence of a drug, such as tetracycline, zinc, or a steroid. In addition, regulation of transgene expression may even be relegated to physiologic conditions, by incorporating promoters or enhancers that respond to particular conditions such as hypoxia or increased oxidative stress.[16]

# ▪ MYOCARDIAL GENE THERAPY

Failure of the myocardium secondary to insults such as ischemia, infection, metabolic disorders, or substance abuse afflicts millions of Americans each year. Traditional pharmacotherapy and surgical intervention have successfully ameliorated these problems, but the advent of gene transfer technology has heightened interest in correcting, preventing, or limiting the functional deficits sustained by the myocardium. The myocardium has been shown to be receptive to the introduction of foreign genes. As in noncardiac muscle, measurable levels of gene activity have been observed after direct injection of plasmids into myocardial tissue in vivo.[14] Although the effect was limited to a few millimeters surrounding the injection site, these observations have laid the basis for consideration of gene transfer as a therapeutic approach to cardiac disease. The distribution of myocardial expression of genes after direct injection in rats has been enhanced via incorporating the gene into an adenovirus vector.[17] Additionally, both adenovirus and adeno-associated virus vectors may be delivered to the myocardial and coronary vascular cells via intracoronary infusion of highly concentrated preparations.[18] Gene transfer into the myocardium has also been achieved, via direct injection or intracoronary infusion of myoblast cells that have been genetically engineered in cell culture.[19]

## Gene Therapy for Neovascularization

The vascularization observed in neoplastic tissue led researchers, such as Judah Folkman in the 1970s, to investigate the role of molecular factors in the induction of new blood vessel growth.[20] Subsequent identification and characterization of "angiogenic" growth factors created an opportunity not only to target growth of solid tumors but also to attempt therapeutic "neovascularization" of tissue rendered ischemic by occlusive disease in the native arterial bed. *Angiogenesis* has come to refer more strictly to the sprouting of new capillary networks from preexisting vascular structures, whereas *vasculogenesis* is development de novo of both simple and complex vessels during embryonic development. Although it has been clearly established in a number of animal models that angiogenic factors can, in fact, stimulate the growth of capillary networks in vivo, it is less clear that these molecules can induce the development of larger, more complex vessels in adult tissues that would be capable of carrying significantly increased bulk blood flow. Nevertheless, the possibility of an improvement, even of only the microvascular collateralization, as a "biologic" approach to the treatment of tissue ischemia has sparked the beginning of human clinical trials of neovascularization therapy.

After the first description of the angiogenic effect of fibroblast growth factors (FGF), an abundance of "proangiogenic" factors were discovered to stimulate either endothelial cell proliferation or enhanced endothelial cell migration, or both. Many of these factors possess heparin-binding domains, which not only increase their retention in heparin-rich extracellular matrix but also play critical roles in mediating the interaction of the factors with cell surface receptors. Although the list of angiogenic factors includes such diverse molecules as insulin-like growth factor, hepatocyte growth factor, angiopoietin, and platelet-derived endothelial growth factor, the molecules that have received the most attention as potential therapeutic agents for neovascularization are vascular endothelial growth factor (VEGF) and two members of the FGF family, acidic FGF (FGF-1) and basic FGF (FGF-2).

Whereas all angiogenic factors share some ability to stimulate capillary growth in classic models such as the chick allantoic membrane, much debate persists about the optimal agent and the optimal route of delivery for angiogenic therapy in the ischemic human myocardium or lower extremity. VEGF may be the most selective agent for stimulating endothelial cell proliferation, although VEGF receptors are also expressed on a number of inflammatory cells, including members of the monocyte-macrophage lineage.[21] This selectivity has been viewed as an advantage, since the unwanted stimulation of fibroblasts and VSMC in native arteries might exacerbate the growth of neointimal or atherosclerotic lesions. Despite this theoretical selectivity, however, experimental use of VEGF in animal models has been associated not only with capillary growth but also with development of more complex vessels involving these other cell types.[22] The FGF are believed to be even more potent stimulators of endothelial cell proliferation, but, as their name implies, they are much less selective in their "pro-proliferative" action.

Optimizing the route of drug delivery depends much on the pharmacokinetic properties of any agent. Angiogenesis, however, is a very complex biologic process that involves multiple cell types engaged in multiple activities, including extracellular tissue dissolution and remodeling, cell proliferation, cell migration, cell recruitment, and programmed cell death. The role of any single agent must be understood in the context of the complicated orchestration of multiple signaling agents and effectors. Despite the large amount of data that have become available in the past two decades, details of the cellular and molecular mechanisms of angiogenesis remain poorly understood. Nevertheless, it is believed that many of the known angiogenic factors, including VEGF and the FGF, are exquisitely potent and would not, therefore, require large doses or prolonged dosing. These conclusions are based partly on the results of experiments in vivo in which a broad range of dosing strategies, ranging from implantation of sustained-release formulations to single intraarterial boluses, have been reported to induce similarly successful increases in tissue perfusion.[21]

Preclinical studies of angiogenic gene therapy have utilized a number of models of chronic ischemia. An increase in capillary density was reported in an ischemic rabbit hindlimb model after VEGF administration, and these results did not differ significantly, regardless of whether VEGF was delivered as a single intraarterial bolus of protein, plasmid DNA applied to surface of an upstream arterial wall, or direct injection of the plasmid into the ischemic limb.[21] Direct injection of an adenoviral vector encoding VEGF also succeeded in improving regional myocardial perfusion and ventricular fractional wall thickening at stress in a model of chronic myocardial ischemia induced via placement of a slowly occluding Ameroid constrictor around the circumflex coronary artery in pigs.[23]

Unlike VEGF, FGF-1 and -2 do not possess signal sequences that facilitate secretion of the protein, so transfer of these genetic sequences is less likely to yield an adequate supply of growth factor to target endothelial cells. To overcome this limitation, Tabata and associates constructed a plasmid that encodes a modified FGF-1 molecule onto which a hydrophobic leader sequence had been added to enhance secretion.[24] Delivery of this plasmid to the femoral artery wall, even at very low transfection efficiencies, was found to improve capillary density and reduce vascular resistance in ischemic rabbit hindlimb. Applying a similar strategy, Giordano and coworkers employed intracoronary infusion of $10^{11}$ viral particles of an adenoviral vector encoding human FGF-5, which does contain a secretory signal sequence at its amino terminus, to achieve enhanced wall thickening with stress and a larger number of capillary structures per myocardial muscle fiber 2 weeks after gene transfer.[25]

Another novel approach to molecular neovascularization has been the combination of growth factor gene transfer with a potentially synergistic method of angiogenic stimulation, transmyocardial laser therapy. The formation of transmural laser channels, though not yet firmly established as an effective means of generating increased collateral flow, has had documented clinical success in reducing angina scores and improving myocardial perfusion in otherwise untreatable patients. In a porcine Ameroid model, Sayeed-Shah and coworkers found that direct injection of plasmid DNA encoding VEGF in the region surrounding laser channel formation yielded better normalization of myocardial function than either therapy alone,[26] and this plasmid can now be delivered through a minimally invasive thoracotomy or a percutaneous catheter.

A number of phase I safety studies have already been reported in which angiogenic factors or the genes encoding these factors have been administered to small numbers of patients.[27, 28] These studies have involved either the use of angiogenic factors in patients with peripheral vascular or coronary artery disease who were not candidates for conventional revascularization therapies or the application of proangiogenic factors as an adjunct to conventional revascularization. The modest doses of either protein factors or genetic material delivered in these studies were not associated with any acute toxicity. Concerns remain, however, about the safety of potential systemic exposure to molecules known to enhance the growth of possible occult neoplasms or ones that can enhance diabetic retinopathy—and, potentially, even occlusive arterial disease itself. Despite early enthusiasm, the experience with the administration of live viral vectors in extremely large numbers to a large number of patients is extremely limited, and it is not clear whether potential biologic hazards of reversion to replication-competent states or mutation and recombination will eventually be manifested.

In addition to issues of safety, it is also unclear whether the clinical success of conventional revascularization, which has involved the resumption of lost bulk blood flow through larger conduits, will be reproduced via biologic strategies that principally increase microscopic collateral networks. Neovascularization is a natural process, and the addition of a single factor may not overcome an inadequate endogenous neovascularization response in patients suffering from myocardial and lower limb ischemia. Despite these limitations, angiogenic gene therapy may provide an alternative not currently available to a significant number of patients suffering from untreatable disease and may offer an adjunct to traditional therapies that improves their long-term outcomes.

## Gene Therapy to Enhance Contractility

The β-adrenergic receptor (β-AR) is known to be a critical player in mediating the ionotropic state of the heart and has received significant attention as a target for genetic therapeutic intervention in congestive heart failure. Milano and coworkers,[29] using transgenic mice expressing the $β_2$-AR under the control of the cardiac α-myosin heavy chain promoter, demonstrated approximately a 200-fold increase in the level of $β_2$-AR along with much enhanced contractility and increased heart rates in the absence of exogenous β-agonists. This genetic manipulation of the myocardium has generated considerable interest in the transfer of the β-AR gene into the ailing myocardium as a therapeutic intervention. To date, attempts at exploring this exciting possibility have been limited to cell culture systems. Akhter and colleagues[30] demonstrated improved contractility after adenovirus-mediated gene transfer of the human $β_2$-AR into chronically paced rabbit ventricular myocytes. An enhanced chronotropic effect resulting from the injection of a $β_2$-AR plasmid construct into the right atrium of mice was demonstrated by Edelberg and associates,[31] but no evaluation of enhanced contractility by transfer of this gene into the ventricle has been reported. These results demonstrate the feasibility of using the β-adrenergic pathway and its regulators as a treatment for heart failure.

Recently there has also been interest in the enhancement of contractility through the manipulation of intracellular calcium levels. Sarcoplasmic reticulum $Ca^{++}$-ATPase (SERCA2a)–transporting enzyme, which regulates $Ca^{++}$ sequestration into the sarcoplasmic reticulum (SR), has been shown to be decreased in a variety human and experimental cardomyopathies. Using adenoviral-mediated gene transfer, Hajjar and coworkers[32] were able to overexpress the SERCA2a protein in neonatal rat cardiomyocytes. This led to an increase in peak $[Ca^{++}]_i$ release, a decrease in resting $[Ca^{++}]_i$ levels, and, more important, enhanced contraction of the myocardial cells as detected by shortening measurements. The success of this approach to improving myocardial contractility has yet to be documented in vivo, but, once again, it provides a novel and potentially exciting means through which to treat the failed heart.

## Gene Therapy for Myocardial Infarction

Coronary artery atherosclerosis and resulting myocardial ischemia is a leading cause of death in developed countries. Reperfusion injury has been linked to significant cell damage and progression of the ischemic insult. In addition to stimulating therapeutic neovascularization, genetic manipulation may be used to limit the degree of injury to the myocardium after ischemia and reperfusion.

The process of tissue damage secondary to ischemia and reperfusion has been characterized well. Briefly, the period of ischemia leads to accumulation of adenosine monophospate, which then leads to increased levels of hypoxanthine within and around cells in the affected area. Additionally, conversion of xanthine dehydrogenase into xanthine oxidase increases, and on exposure to oxygen during the period of reperfusion, hypoxanthine converts to xanthine, leaving behind the cytotoxic oxygen radical, superoxide anion ($O_2^-$). $O_2^-$ can then go on to form hydrogen peroxide ($H_2O_2$), another oxygen radical species. Ferrous iron ($Fe^{++}$), which accumulates during ischemia, reacts with $H_2O_2$, a reaction that leads to the formation of the most potent oxygen radical, hydroxyl anion ($OH^-$). These oxygen radicals produce cellular injury via lipid peroxidation of the plasma membrane, oxidation of sulfhydryl groups of intracellular and membrane proteins, nucleic acid injury, and breakdown of components of the extracellular matrix, such as collagen and hyaluronic acid. Natural oxygen radical scavengers, such as superoxide dismutase (SOD), catalase, glutathione peroxidase, and hemoxygenase function through various mechanisms to remove oxygen radicals produced in normal and injured tissues.[33]

The degree of oxygen radical formation produced after ischemia and reperfusion in the heart can overwhelm the natural scavenger systems. Overexpression of either extracellular SOD (ecSOD) or manganese SOD (MnSOD) in transgenic mice has produced improved postischemic cardiac function and decreased cardiomyocyte mitochondrial injury in adriamycin-treated mice, respectively.[34, 35] These findings suggest a role for the gene transfer of these natural scavengers as a means of protecting the myocardium in the event of an ischemia-reperfusion event. Li and coworkers[36] demonstrated substantial protection against myocardial stunning using intraarterial injection of an adenovirus that contained the gene for Cu/ZnSOD (the cytoplasmic isoform) into rabbits, although no studies have investigated the direct antioxidant effect and ensuing improvement in myocardial function of this treatment after ischemia and reperfusion. This application of gene therapy technology, if incorporated into a system of long-term, regulatable transgene expression, may offer a novel and exciting approach to prophylaxis against myocardial ischemic injury. In addition to the overexpression of antioxidant genes, some researchers have proposed intervening in the program of gene expression within the myocardium that leads to the deleterious effects of ischemia reperfusion. For example, transfection of rat myocardium with decoy oligonucleotides that block activity of the oxidation-sensitive transcription factor NFk-B (linked to expression of a number of proinflammatory genes), succeeded in reducing infarct size after coronary artery ligation.[37]

At the cellular level, myocardial infarction results in the formation of scar, which is composed of cardiac fibroblasts. Because cardiomyocytes are terminally differentiated, there is no regeneration of myocytes to repopulate the wound after infarction. Researchers have therefore pursued the possibility of genetically converting cardiac fibroblasts into functional cardiomyocytes. The feasibility of this notion gained support from the work of Tam and colleagues,[38] who demonstrated the conversion in vitro of cardiac fibroblasts into cells resembling skeletal myocytes via the forced expression of a skeletal muscle lineage–determining gene, MyoD, using retrovirus-mediated gene transfer. Fibroblasts expressing the MyoD gene were observed to develop multinucleated myotubes similar to those seen in striated muscle, which expressed MHC and myocyte-specific enhancer factor 2. Additionally, Murry and associates,[39] also showed expression of myogenin and embryonic skeletal MHC after transfection of rat hearts injured by freeze-thaw with an adenovirus containing the MyoD gene. At this time, however, functional cardiomyocytes have not yet been identified in regions of myocardial scarring treated with gene transfer in vivo.

## Gene Therapy for Immunomodulation

Genetic manipulation of donor tissues affords the opportunity to design organ-specific immunosuppression during cardiac transplantation. Although transgenic animals are being explored as potential sources for immunologically protected xenografts, the delivery of genes for immunosuppressive proteins or the blockade of certain genes in human donor grafts may allow site-specific, localized immunosuppression and reduction or elimination of the need for toxic systemic immunosuppressive regimens. Gene activity has been documented in transplanted mouse hearts for at least 2 weeks after intraoperative injection of the tissue with plasmid DNA or retroviral or adenoviral vectors.[40] The transfer of a gene for either TGF-β or interleukin 10 in a small area of the heart via direct injection in this model succeeded in inhibiting cell-mediated immunity and delaying acute rejection.[41, 42] In another study, systemic administration of antisense ODN directed against intercellular adhesion molecule 1 (ICAM-1), when combined with a monoclonal antibody against the ligand for ICAM-1, leukocyte function antigen, also prolonged graft survival and induced long-term graft tolerance.[43]

## ▪ VASCULAR GENE THERAPY

### Gene and Oligonucleotide Therapy of Recurrence of Stenosis

Recurrent narrowing of arteries after percutaneous angioplasty, atherectomy, or another disobliterative technique is a common clinical problem that severely limits the durability of these procedures for patients with atherosclerotic occlusive diseases. After balloon angioplasty, restenosis occurs in approximately 30% to 40% of treated coronary lesions and 30% to 50% of superficial femoral artery lesions within the first year. Intravascular stents may reduce the restenosis rates; however, the incidence remains high and long-term data are limited. Despite impressive technologic advances in the development of minimally invasive and endovascular approaches to treating arterial occlusions, the full benefit of these gains awaits the solution of this fundamental biologic problem.

Restenosis is an attractive target for gene therapy, not only because of its prevalence (and, therefore, its economic burden) but also because it is a local tissue reaction that develops precisely at a site of intervention to which access has already been achieved. A potential advantage of the genetic approach over more conventional pharmacotherapies is that a single dose of a gene therapy agent may have a prolonged biologic effect. The appropriate genetic modification, performed locally at the time of angioplasty, could induce a long-term benefit in patency by altering the healing response. The potential role for gene therapy in the prevention of restenosis will depend on identification of an appropriate molecular target, a suitable vector system for efficiently targeting vessel wall cells, and methods of achieving local delivery without producing undue damage or distal tissue ischemia. Today, considerable hurdles remain, even though significant progress has been made in each of these areas.

Restenosis is comprised of contraction and fibrosis of the vessel wall known as *remodeling* and active growth of a fibrocellular lesion composed principally of vascular smooth muscle cells (VSMC) and extracellular matrix. The latter process, known as *neointimal hyperplasia*, involves stimulation of the normally "quiescent" VSMC in the arterial media into the "activated" state characterized by rapid proliferation and migration. A number of growth factors are believed to play roles in the stimulation of VSMC during neointimal hyperplasia, including platelet-derived growth factor (PDGF), basic fibroblast growth factor (bFGF), transforming growth factor beta (TGF-β), and angiotensin II. Activated VSMC have also been found to produce a variety of enzymes, cytokines, adhesion molecules, and other proteins that not only enhance the inflammatory response in the vessel wall but also stimulate further vascular cell abnormality.[44]

Although it is now thought that remodeling may account for the majority of late lumen loss after balloon dilation of atherosclerotic vessels, proliferation has been the principal target of experimental genetic interventions. There have been two general approaches, cytostatic, in which cells are prevented from progressing through the cell cycle to mitosis, and cytotoxic, in which cell death is induced. A group of molecules known as *cell cycle regulatory proteins* act at different points along the cell cycle, mediating progression toward division. It has been hypothesized that, by blocking expression of the genes for one or more of these proteins, one could prevent the progression of VSMC through the cell cycle and inhibit neointimal hyperplasia. Morishita and coworkers demonstrated nearly complete inhibition of neointimal hyperplasia after carotid balloon injury, via HVJ-liposome–mediated transfection of the vessel wall with a combination of antisense ODN against cell cycle regulatory genes.[45] Arrest of the cell cycle via antisense blockade of either of two protooncogenes, *c-myb* or *c-myc*, has been found to inhibit neointimal hyperplasia in models of arterial balloon injury,[46, 47] although the specific antisense mechanism of the ODN used in these studies was subsequently questioned.[48]

In addition to transfection of cells with antisense ODN, cell cycle arrest can also be achieved through manipulation of transcription factor activity. The activity of a number of cell cycle regulatory genes is affected by a single transcription factor known as *E2F*. In quiescent cells, E2F is bound to a complex of other proteins, including a protein known as the *retinoblastoma gene product* (Rb), that prevents its interaction with chromosomal DNA and its stimulation of gene activity. In proliferating cells, E2F is released, resulting in cell cycle gene activation. A transcription factor decoy bearing the consensus binding sequence recognized by E2F can be employed to inhibit cellular proliferation (Fig. 41–3). Morishita and associates demonstrated the use of this strategy to prevent VSMC proliferation and neointimal hyperplasia after rat carotid balloon injury.[49] Alternatively, Chang and colleagues showed that localized arterial infection with a replication-defective adenovirus encoding a nonphosphorylatable, constitutively active form of Rb at the time of balloon angioplasty significantly reduced VSMC proliferation and neointima formation in both rat carotid and porcine femoral artery models of restenosis.[50]

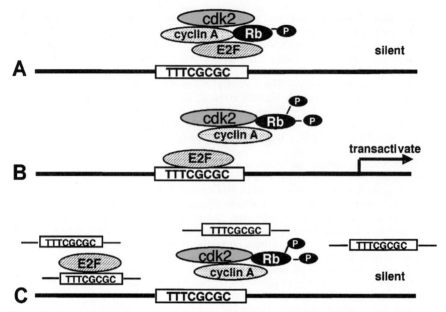

**Figure 41–3** ■ Principle of E2F "decoy" strategy. TTTCGCGC, consensus sequence for the E2F binding site. (*A*) In quiescent cell state, the transcription factor E2F is complexed Rb (retinoblastoma gene product), cyclin A, and cyclin-dependent kinase cdK2. (*B*) Phosphorylation of releases free E2F, which binds to *cis* elements of the cell cycle regulatory genes, resulting in the transactivation of these genes. (*C*) The E2F decoy *cis*-element double-stranded oligonucleotide binds to free E2F, preventing E2F-mediated transactivation of cell cycle–regulatory genes.

Similar results were also obtained by adenovirus-mediated overexpression of a "natural" inhibitor of cell cycle progression, the cyclin-dependent kinase inhibitor p21, which likely prevents hyperphosphorylation of Rb in vivo.[51] In addition to blockade of cell cycle gene expression, interruption of mitogenic signal transduction has been achieved in experimental models. For example, *Ras* proteins are key transducers of mitogenic signals from membrane to nucleus in many cell types. Local delivery of DNA vectors expressing *Ras*-dominant negative mutants, which interfere with *Ras* function, reduced neointimal lesion formation in a rat carotid artery balloon injury model.[52]

Nitric oxide mediates a number of biologic processes that are thought to mitigate neointima formation in the vessel wall, such as inhibition of VSMC proliferation, reduction of platelet adherence, vasorelaxation, promotion of endothelial cell survival, and, possibly, reduction of oxidative stress. Transfer in vivo of plasmid DNA coding for endothelial cell nitric oxide synthase (ecNOS), has been investigated as a potential paracrine strategy to block neointimal disease. EcNOS cDNA driven by a β-actin promoter and CMV enhancer was transfected into the VSMC of rat carotid arteries after balloon injury. This model is known to exhibit no significant regrowth of endothelial cells within 2 to 3 weeks after injury and, therefore, is capable of loss of endogenous ecNOS expression. Results revealed expression of the transgene in the vessel wall, along with improved vasomotor reactivity and 70% inhibition of neointima formation (Fig. 41–4).[53]

An example of a direct cytotoxic approach to the prevention of neointima formation is the transfer of a so-called suicide gene such as the herpes simplex virus-TK (HSV-TK) gene into VSMC. Using an adenoviral vector, HSV-TK was

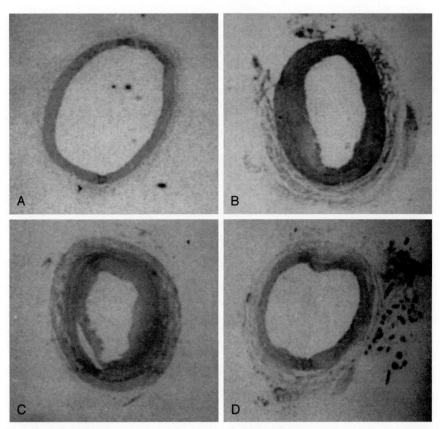

**Figure 41–4** ■ Inhibition of neointimal hyperplasia by gene transfer in vivo of endothelial cell–nitric oxide synthase (ecNOS) in balloon-injured rat carotid arteries. (*A*) Uninjured control artery (CTRL), (*B*) injured, untransfected artery (INJ), (*C*) injured, control vector transfected artery (INJ + CV), (*D*) injured, ecNOS-transfected artery (INJ + NOS).

introduced into the VSMC of porcine arteries, rendering the smooth muscle cells sensitive to the nucleoside analogue gancyclovir given immediately after balloon injury. After one course of gancyclovir treatment, neointimal hyperplasia decreased by about 50%.[6] More recently, Pollman and associates[54] induced endogenous machinery for VSMC suicide, in a strategy designed to inhibit the growth or achieve regression of neointimal lesions. This strategy involved antisense ODN blockade of a "survival" gene known as Bcl-x that helps to protect cells from activation of programmed cell death (apoptosis).

Another potentially relevant biologic strategy for treatment of restenosis is reendothelialization, which might be accelerated by local delivery of a proangiogenic factor (e.g., VEGF) at the angioplasty site. This is the basis for the only current U.S. clinical trial of gene therapy for prevention of restenosis in the peripheral circulation, in which the human VEGF gene is delivered as a "naked" circular DNA plasmid directly to the injured arterial wall on the surface of the angioplasty balloon.[55] The investigators hypothesize that the low efficiency of this delivery method is balanced by the high biologic potency of this secreted angiogenic cytokine, an effect that produces a significant local biologic effect despite poor gene transfer.

Successful and efficient gene transfer to the injured, atherosclerotic arterial wall presents unique mechanical and kinetic challenges. For strategies designed to attenuate or prevent VSMC proliferation, the target cell mass lies within the media of the vessel wall. After balloon angioplasty, mechanical disruption and dissection of plaque may facilitate particle delivery to deeper layers of the vessel wall; however, uniform gene delivery to the bulk of target VSMC has been difficult to achieve, despite the development of a number of specialized local delivery catheters. Experimental models of neointima formation in animals may not be clinically relevant, given their high, uniform cell content and absence of the more predominant noncellular components of complex atherosclerotic plaque in humans.

A gene transfer ex vivo approach involving implantation of genetically modified endothelial cells or VSMC at sites of arterial injury is also being investigated. The need to harvest autologous donor tissue for target cells, coupled with the increased costs and complexity of tissue culture, have greatly damped enthusiasm for this strategy, and more direct methods are favored. Nonetheless, it remains clinically feasible, and, in the case of endothelial cells, the implanted cells alone may confer beneficial properties to the healing arterial wall. Application of these cell transplantation approaches would be greatly facilitated by the development of "universal donor" cell lines from which major histocompatibility antigens have been "knocked out." Such a development, while clearly years or decades away, may no longer be merely science fiction or fantasy.

In summary, it would appear that application of gene therapy for postangioplasty restenosis may be somewhat premature. In addition to major obstacles in delivering gene transfer agents to the atherosclerotic vessel wall, the fundamental biologic process remains incompletely understood. Nonetheless, continued progress on each of these fronts warrants an optimistic view for genetic approaches to control the arterial injury response.

## Vein Graft Engineering with E2F Decoy Oligodeoxynucleotides

The long-term success of surgical revascularization in the lower extremity and coronary circulations has been limited by significant rates of autologous vein graft failure (30% in 5 years and 50% in 10 years for both). No pharmacologic approach has been successful at preventing long-term graft diseases such as neointimal hyperplasia or graft atherosclerosis. Gene therapy offers a new avenue for the modification of vein graft pathobiology that might lead to a reduction in clinical morbidity from graft failures. Intraoperative transfection of the vein graft also offers an opportunity to combine intact tissue DNA-transfer techniques with the increased safety of transfection ex vivo, and a number of studies have documented the feasibility of ex vivo gene transfer into vein grafts using viral vectors.

The vast majority of vein graft failures have been linked to the neointimal disease that is part of graft remodeling after surgery. Although neointimal hyperplasia contributes to the reduction of wall stress in vein grafts after bypass, this process can also lead to luminal narrowing of the graft conduit during the first years after operation. Furthermore, the abnormal neointimal layer, with its production of proinflammatory proteins, is believed to form the basis for an accelerated form of atherosclerosis that causes late graft failure.

As in the arterial balloon injury model, treatment of vein graft with antisense ODN that inhibit expression of at least two cell cycle regulatory genes could significantly block neointimal hyperplasia. Additionally, E2F decoy ODN yielded efficacy in the vein graft similar to that of the arterial injury model. In contrast to arterial balloon injury, however, vein grafts are not only subjected to a single injury at the time of operation but are also exposed to chronic hemodynamic stimuli for remodeling. Despite these chronic stimuli, a single, intraoperative ODN treatment of vein grafts resulted in resistance to neointimal hyperplasia that lasted at least 6 months in the rabbit model. During that time, the grafts treated with antisense ODN were able to adapt appropriately to arterial conditions via hypertrophy of the medial layer. Furthermore, these genetically engineered conduits proved resistant to diet-induced graft atherosclerosis (Fig. 41–5) and were associated with preserved endothelial function.[56, 57]

A large-scale, prospective, randomized double-blind trial of human vein graft

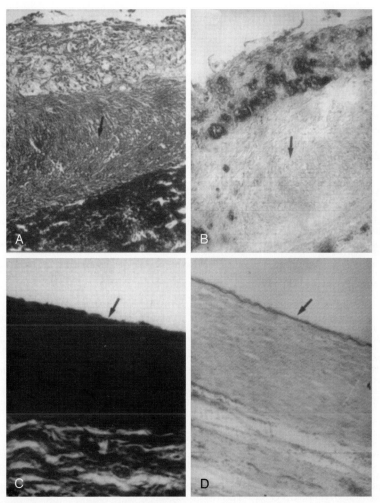

**Figure 41–5** ▪ Control oligonucleotide-treated (*A, B*) and antisense oligonucleotide (against cdc2 kinase/ PCNA)-treated vein grafts (*C, D*) in hypercholesterolemic rabbits, 6 weeks after surgery. (×70). Arrows indicate the location of the internal elastic lamina. (Original magnification × 70; hematoxylin/van Gieson (*A, C*) and monoclonal antibody against rabbit macrophages (*B, D*) stains.)

treatment with E2F decoy ODN has been undertaken.[58] Efficient delivery of the ODN is accomplished within 15 minutes during the operation by placement of the graft after harvest in a device that exposes the vessel to ODN in physiologic solution and allows simultaneous application of pressure of 300 mm Hg to all sides of the vessel, avoiding any potential mechanical injury. Preliminary findings indicated delivery of ODN to more than 80% of graft cells and effective blockade of target gene expression. This study, which will measure the effect of cell cycle gene blockade on primary graft failure rates, represents one of the first attempts to definitively determine the feasibility of clinical gene manipulation in the treatment of a common cardiovascular disorder.

# ■ SUMMARY

Gene therapy for the treatment of cardiovascular diseases may affect the care of a large segment of the population. Although traditional pharmacologic and surgical treatments have significantly improved the lives of patients suffering from cardiovascular disease, significant limitations in their care still exist. The complexity and variety of cardiovascular diseases require the use of more than one gene therapy for any given patient. Furthermore, the systems available today are likely to be combined with or replaced by new methods of gene therapy that will enhance their effectiveness. As this exciting technology evolves, so will the horizons of its application to human disease. Nevertheless, great challenges remain that must be overcome before clinicians routinely look toward the molecular machinery driving pathobiology as a target for intervention.

# ■ REFERENCES

1. Danos O, Mulligan RC: Safe and efficient generation of recombinant retroviruses and amphotrophic and ecotrophic host ranges. Proc Natl Acad Sci USA 1988;85:6460–6464.
2. Berg P, Singer MF: The recombinant DNA controversy twenty years later. Proc Natl Acad Sci USA 1995;92:9011–9013.
3. Colman A: Antisense strategies in cell and developmental biology. J Cell Sci 1990;97:399–409.
4. Zaug A, Been M, Cech T: The Tetrahymena ribozyme acts like an RNA restriction endonuclease. Nature 1986;324:429–433.
5. Bielinska A, Schivdasani RA, Zhang L, et al: Regulation of gene expression with double-stranded phosphorothioate oligonucleotides. Science 1990;250:997–1000.
6. Ohno T, Gordon D, San H, et al: Gene therapy for vascular smooth muscle cell proliferation after arterial injury. Science 1994;265:781–784.
7. Newman KD, Dunn PF, Owens JW, et al: Adenovirus-mediated gene transfer into normal rabbit arteries results in prolonged vascular cell activation, inflammation, and neointimal hyperplasia. J Clin Invest 1995;96:2955–2965.
8. Nabel EG, Plautz G, Nabel GJ: Site-specific gene expression in vivo by direct gene transfer into the arterial wall. Science 1990;249:1285–1288.
9. Wilson JM, Birinyi LK, Salomon RN, et al: Implantation of vascular grafts lined with genetically modified endothelial cells. Science 1989;244:1344–1346.
10. Brody SL, Crystal RG: Adenovirus-mediated in vivo gene transfer. Ann NY Acad Sci 1994;716:90–101.
11. Svensson EC, Marshall DJ, Woodard K, et al: Efficient and stable transduction of cardiomyocytes after intramyocardial injection or intracoronary perfusion with recombinant adeno-associated virus vectors. Circulation 1999;99:201–205.
12. Nabel GJ, Gordon D, Bishop DK, et al: Immune response in human melanoma after transfer of an allogeneic class I major histocompatibility complex gene with DNA-liposome complexes. Proc Natl Acad Sci USA 1996;93:15388–15393.
13. Dzau VJ, Mann MJ, Morishita R, et al: Fusigenic viral liposome for gene therapy in cardiovascular diseases. Proc Natl Acad Sci USA 1996;93:11421–11425.
14. Lin H, Parmacek MS, Morle G, et al: Expression of recombinant gene in myocardium in vivo after direct injection of DNA. Circulation 1990;82:2217–2221.
15. Mann MJ, Whittemore AD, Donaldson MC, et al: Preliminary clinical experience with genetic engineering of human vein grafts: Evidence for target gene inhibition. Circulation 1997;96:I4.

16. Rinsch C, Regulier E, Deglon N, et al: A gene therapy approach to regulated delivery of erythropoietin as a function of oxygen tension. Hum Gene Ther 1997;8:1881–1889.

17. Guzman RJ, Lemarchand P, Crystal RG, et al: Efficient gene transfer into myocardium by direct injection of adenovirus vectors. Circ Res 1993;73:1202–1207.

18. Kaplitt MG, Xiao X, Samulski RJ, et al: Long-term gene transfer in porcine myocardium after coronary infusion of an adeno-associated virus vector. Ann Thorac Surg 1996;62:1669–1676.

19. Blau HM, Springer ML: Muscle-mediated gene therapy. N Engl J Med 1995;333:1554–1556.

20. Folkman J, Merler E, Abernathy C, et al: Isolation of a tumor factor responsible or angiogenesis. J Exp Med 1971;133:275–288.

21. Ware JA, Simons M: Angiogenesis in ischemic heart disease. Nat Med 1997;3:158–164.

22. Banai S, Jaklitsch MT, Shou M, et al: Angiogenic-induced enhancement of collateral blood flow to ischemic myocardium by vascular endothelial growth factor in dogs. Circulation 1994;89:2183–2189.

23. Mack CA, Patel SR, Schwarz EA, et al: Biologic bypass with the use of adenovirus-mediated gene transfer of the complementary deoxyribonucleic acid for vascular endothelial growth factor 121 improves myocardial perfusion and function in the ischemic porcine heart. J Thorac Cardiovasc Surg 1998;115:168–176.

24. Tabata H, Silver M, Isner JM: Arterial gene transfer of acidic fibroblast growth factor for therapeutic angiogenesis in vivo: Critical role of secretion signal in use of naked DNA. Cardiovasc Res 1997;35:470–479.

25. Giordano FJ, Ping P, McKirnan MD, et al: Intracoronary gene transfer of fibroblast growth factor-5 increases blood flow and contractile function in an ischemic region of the heart. Nat Med 1996;2:534–539.

26. Sayeed-Shah U, Mann MJ, Martin J, et al: Complete reversal of ischemic wall motion abnormalities by combined use of gene therapy with transmyocardial laser revascularization. J Thorac Cardiovasc Surg 1998;116:763–769.

27. Schumacher B, Pecher P, von Specht BU, et al: Induction of neoangiogenesis in ischemic myocardium by human growth factors: First clinical results of a new treatment of coronary heart disease. Circulation 1998;97:645–650.

28. Losordo DW, Vale PR, Symes JF, et al: Gene therapy for myocardial angiogenesis: Initial clinical results with direct myocardial injection of phVEGF165 as sole therapy for myocardial ischemia. Circulation 1998;98:2800–2804.

29. Milano CA, Allen LF, Rockman HA, et al: Enhanced myocardial function in transgenic mice overexpressing the beta 2-adrenergic receptor. Science 1994;265:582–586.

30. Akhter SA, Skaer CA, Kypson AP, et al: Restoration of beta-adrenergic signaling in failing cardiac ventricular myocytes via adenoviral-mediated gene transfer. Proc Natl Acad Sci USA 1997;94:12100–12105.

31. Edelberg JM, Aird WC, Rosenberg RD: Enhancement of murine cardiac chronotropy by the molecular transfer of human beta2 adrenergic receptor DNA. J Clin Invest 1998;101:337–343.

32. Hajjar RJ, Kang JX, Gwathmey JK: Physiological effects of adenoviral gene transfer of sarcoplasmic reticulum calcium ATPase in isolated rat myocytes. Circulation 1997;95:423–429.

33. Flaherty JT: Myocardial injury mediated by oxygen free radicals. Am J Med 1991;91(Suppl 3C):79S–85S.

34. Chen EP, Bittner HB, Davis D, et al: Extracellular superoxide dismutase transgene overexpression preserves postischemic myocardial function in isolated murine hearts. Circulation 1996;94(Suppl II):II412–II417.

35. Yen H-C, Oberley TD, Vichitbandha S, et al: The protective role of manganese superoxide dismutase against adriamycin-induced acute cardiac toxicity in transgenic mice. J Clin Invest 1996;98:1253–1260.

36. Li Q, Bolli R, Qiu Y, et al: Gene therapy with extracellular superoxide dismutase attenuates myocardial stunning in conscious rabbits. Circulation 1998;98:1438–1448.

37. Morishita R, Sugimoto T, Aoki M, et al: In vivo transfection of cis element "decoy" against nuclear factor-kappaB binding site prevents myocardial infarction. Nat Med 1997;3:894–899.

38. Tam SK, Gu W, Nadal-Ginard B: Molecular cardiomyoplasty: Potential cardiac gene therapy for chronic heart failure. J Thorac Cardiovasc Surg 1995;109:918–924.

39. Murry CE, Kay MA, Bartosek T, et al: Muscle differentiation during repair of myocardial necrosis in rats via gene transfer with MyoD. J Clin Invest 1996;98:2209–2217.

40. Qin L, Chavin KD, Ding Y, et al: Multiple vectors effectively achieve gene transfer in a murine cardiac transplantation model. Immunosuppression with TGF-beta 1 or vIL-10. Transplantation 1995;59:809–816.

41. Qin L, Ding Y, Bromberg JS: Gene transfer of transforming growth factor-beta 1 prolongs murine cardiac allograft survival by inhibiting cell-mediated immunity. Hum Gene Ther 1996;7:1981–1988.

42. Qin L, Chavin KD, Ding Y, et al: Retrovirus-mediated transfer of viral IL-10 gene prolongs murine cardiac allograft survival. J Immunol 1996;156:2316–2323.

43. Poston RS, Mann MJ, Rode S, et al: Ex vivo gene therapy and LFA-1 monoclonal antibody combine to yield long-term tolerance to cardiac allografts. J Heart Lung Transp 1997;16:41.

44. Tanaka H, Sukhova GK, Swanson SJ, et al: Sustained activation of vascular cells and leukocytes in the rabbit aorta after balloon injury. Circulation 1993;88:1788–1803.

45. Morishita R, Gibbons GH, Ellison KE, et al: Single intraluminal delivery of antisense cdc2 kinase and proliferating-cell nuclear antigen oligonucleotides results in chronic inhibition of neointimal hyperplasia. Proc Natl Acad Sci USA 1993;90:8474–8478.

46. Simons M, Edelman ER, DeKeyser JL, et al: Antisense *c-myb* oligonucleotides inhibit intimal arterial smooth muscle cell accumulation in vivo. Nature 1992;359:67–70.
47. Shi Y, Fard A, Galeo A, et al: Transcatheter delivery of *c-myc* antisense oligomers reduces neointimal formation in a porcine model of coronary artery balloon injury. Circulation 1994;90:944–951.
48. Burgess TL, Fisher EF, Ross SL, et al: The antiproliferative activity of *c-myb* and *c-myc* antisense oligonucleotides in smooth muscle cells is caused by nonantisense mechanism. Proc Natl Acad Sci USA 1995;92:4051–4055.
49. Morishita R, Gibbons GH, Horiuchi M, et al: A novel molecular strategy using *cis* element "decoy" of E2F binding site inhibits smooth muscle proliferation in vivo. Proc Natl Acad Sci USA 1995;92:5855–5859.
50. Chang MW, Barr E, Seltzer J, et al: Cytostatic gene therapy for vascular proliferative disorders with a constitutively active form of the retinoblastoma gene product. Science 1995;267:518–522.
51. Chang MW, Barr E, Lu MM, et al: Adenovirus-mediated over-expression of the cyclin/cyclin dependent kinase inhibitor, p21 inhibits vascular smooth muscle cell proliferation and neointima formation in the rat carotid artery model of balloon angioplasty. J Clin Invest 1995;96:2260–2268.
52. Indolfi C, Avvedimento EV, Rapacciuolo A, et al: Inhibition of cellular ras prevents smooth muscle cell proliferation after vascular injury in vivo. Nat Med 1995;1:541–545.
53. von der Leyen HE, Gibbons GH, Morishita R, et al: Gene therapy inhibiting neointimal vascular lesion: In vivo gene transfer of endothelial-cell nitric oxide synthase gene. Proc Natl Acad Sci USA 1995;92:1137–1141.
54. Pollman MJ, Hall JL, Mann MJ, et al: Inhibition of neointimal cell bcl-x expression induces apoptosis and regression of vascular disease. Nat Med 1998;4:222–227.
55. Isner JM, Walsh K, Rosenfield K, et al: Clinical protocol: Arterial gene therapy for restenosis. Hum Gene Ther 1996;7:989–1011.
56. Mann MJ, Gibbons GH, Kernoff RS, et al: Genetic engineering of vein grafts resistant to atherosclerosis. Proc Natl Acad Sci USA 1995;92:4502–4506.
57. Mann MJ, Gibbons GH, Tsao PS, et al: Cell cycle inhibition preserves endothelial function in genetically engineered rabbit vein grafts. J Clin Invest 1997;99:1295–1301.
58. Mann MJ, Whittemore AD, Donaldson MC, et al: The PREVENT trial of vein graft genetic engineering: Preliminary molecular and clinical findings. Circulation 1998;98:I321.

# ▪ RECOMMENDED READING

Berg P, Singer MF: The recombinant DNA controversy twenty years later. Proc Natl Acad Sci USA 1995;92:9011–9013.
Guzman RJ, Lemarchand P, Crystal RG, et al: Efficient gene transfer into myocardium by direct injection of adenovirus vectors. Circ Res 1993;73:1202–1207.
Nabel EG, Plautz G, Nabel GJ: Site-specific gene expression in vivo by direct gene transfer into the arterial wall. Science 1990;249:1285–1288.
Ohno T, Gordon D, San H, et al: Gene therapy for vascular smooth muscle cell proliferation after arterial injury. Science 1994;265:781–784.
Simons M, Edelman ER, DeKeyser JL, et al: Antisense c-myb oligonucleotides inhibit intimal arterial smooth muscle cell accumulation in vivo. Nature 1992;359:67–70.
von der Leyen HE, Gibbons GH, Morishita R, et al: Gene therapy inhibiting neointimal vascular lesion: In vivo gene transfer of endothelial -cell nitric oxide synthase gene. Proc Natl Acad Sci USA 1995;92:1137–1141.
Ware JA, Simons M: Angiogenesis in ischemic heart disease. Nat Med 1997;3:158–164.

# Chapter 42

# Preventive Cardiology

*Michael Miller*

Preventive cardiology is a relatively new subspecialty of cardiovascular medicine that focuses on a wide variety of factors aimed at reducing the risk of a first cardiovascular event (primary prevention) or subsequent events (secondary prevention). It demands an understanding of initiators and promoters of atherothrombosis (see Chapter 22) and the complex interplay between genetic factors and environmental influences. In this era of managed care and cost containment, selected primary and secondary cardiac interventions have recently been shown to be cost-effective (Table 42–1), and 10 important measures for preventive care were recently endorsed by the American Heart Association (AHA) and American College of Cardiology (ACC; Table 42–2). Yet risk factors among patients who have coronary artery disease (CAD) remain undertreated, in both clinical and academic practice. This is, in part, reflective of underemphasis on cardiovascular prevention in medical school curricula. Similarly, medical house officers receive little formal training in preventive cardiology. Fortunately, the recent endorsement by the ACC of incorporating preventive cardiology in cardiovascular fellowship training programs and the establishment of a task force aimed at broadening the scope of preventive cardiology within cardiovascular medicine will be the first steps in an initiative that asks trainees to consider preventive cardiology as a rewarding career choice for the 21st century. This section complements Chapters 1, 23, 28, 31, and 32.

## ▪ NUTRITIONAL ASPECTS

### Important Lessons from Our Paleolithic Ancestors

The influence of diet on cardiovascular disease prevention cannot be overstated: diet and cigarette smoking are the most important agents of the development

Table 42–1

**Cost per Year of Life Saved with Certain Cardiovascular Treatments**

| Treatment | Cost Saving ($/yr of life) |
|---|---|
| Single vessel percutaneous transcatheter angioplasty | 102,100 |
| Stent | 83,900 |
| Coronary artery bypass | 34,400 |
| Thrombolytic therapy (70-yr-old) | 21,200 |
| Cholesterol reduction in primary prevention (West of Scotland) | 17,600 |
| Exercise | 11,300 |
| Cholesterol reduction in secondary prevention (Scandinavian Simvastatin Survival Study) | 7,100–16,000 |
| Beta-blocker after myocardial infarction | 5,900 |
| Smoking cessation (nurse-based) | 220 |

Data from Krumholz HM, Cohen BJ, Tsevat J, et al: J Am Coll Cardiol 1993; 22:1697–1702; Hatziandreu EI, Kaplan JP, Weinstein MC, et al: Am J Public Health 1988; 78:1417–1421; Johannesson M, Jonsson B, Kjekhus J, et al: N Engl Med 1997; 336:332–336; Hay JW, Yong Y, Ford I, et al: Circulation 1997; 96:S1:184.

Table 42–2

### Key Measures for Quality of Preventive Care

Smoking status should be documented in all patients with vascular disease.
Smoking cessation programs should be available.
Physician advice and self-help materials should be available to smokers.
Fasting lipid profile should be performed in all CAD patients.
Nutrition evaluation and counseling should be provided to all CAD patients.
Lipid-lowering therapies should be prescribed in CAD patients with LDL >130 mg/dl not responsive to
  nutritional measures.
CAD patients should be considered for exercise counseling or cardiac rehabilitation, if appropriate.
Aspirin therapy should be offered to all patients with CAD; if contraindicated, medical record
  documentation should be provided.
Blood pressure measurements should be recorded at each visit.
BP measurements of 140/90 mm Hg (on three occasions) should be treated with lifestyle and
  pharmacologic therapy, if appropriate.

Modified from Pearson TA, McBride PE, Miller NH, Smith SC: 27th Bethesda Conference: Matching the intensity of risk factor management with the hazard for coronary disease events. Task Force 8. Organization of Preventive Cardiology Service. J Am Coll Cardiol 1996; 27:1039–1047.

and acceleration of atherothrombosis. Barring atherogenic genetic abnormalities (e.g., familial hypercholesterolemia), avoidance of cigarette smoking, in concert with a diet low in saturated fat, often translates into low overall risk of CAD. This is exemplified by the lifestyles observed in today's hunter-gatherer societies. A comparison of the dietary composition of the foods consumed by the descendants of modern preliterate societies (e.g., our paleolithic ancestors) with that of present Westernized societies is outlined in Table 42–3. The reduced percentage of fat in the diets of Stone Age societies reflects a predominantly low intake of *saturated* fat. Wild game, the primary source of fat, contains considerably less carcass fat (4%) than domesticated livestock do (30%). Equally important was the absence of dairy products from the diets of our paleolithic ancestors. The processing of milk products was developed during the agricultural revolution within the past 5000 years. Harvesting of tobacco also began during this period. Thus, not only was the relative intake of dietary fat reduced in these preagrarian societies, but the percentage of saturated fat was also low, a fact reflected in the polyunsaturated-saturated fat (P:S) ratio. Moreover, although the relative protein intake was higher by today's standards, comparative increases in protein consumption (in the absence of preexisting hypertension or diabetes mellitus) has not been associated with increased preva-

Table 42–3

### Comparison of Dietary Patterns in the Late Paleolithic Era and Contemporary America

|  | Energy (%) | |
| --- | --- | --- |
|  | **Late Paleolithic** | **Contemporary America** |
| Carbohydrate | 46 | 46 |
| Fat | 21 | 42 |
| Protein | 33 | 12 |
| Polyunsaturated:saturated fat | 1.4:1 | 0.44 |
| Cholesterol (mg) | 520 | 300–500 |
| Fiber (g) | 100–150 | <20 |
| Sodium (mg) | <700 | 2300–6900 |

Data from Eaton SB, Konner M, Shostak M: Stone agers in the fast lane: Chronic degenerative diseases in evolutionary perspective. Am J Med 1988; 84:739–749; J Nutr 1996; 126:1732–1740.

Table 42–4

**Cholesterol and Triglyceride Values in Selected Preliterate Populations**

| Population | Cholesterol (mg/dl) | Triglyceride (mg/dl) |
|---|---|---|
| Tanzanian villagers | 110 | 99 |
| New Guinea Melanesians | 135 | 95 |
| Tarahumara Indians | 121 | 91 |
| Australian aborigines | 139 | 102 |

Data from Eaton SB, Eaton SB 3rd, Konner MJ, Shostak M: Am J Med 1988; 84:739–749; J Nutr 1996; 126:1732–1740; Pauletto P, Puato M, Caroli MG, et al: Lancet 1996; 348:784–788; McMurry MP, Cerqueira MT, Connor SL, Connor WE: N Engl J Med 1991; 325:1704–1708.

lence of renal disease. Although the foragers' dietary cholesterol intake was greater, it likely had little clinical impact (except for persons afflicted with abnormalities of the low-density lipoprotein cholesterol (LDL-C) receptor, owing to the highly regulated homeostatic feedback mechanism that governs cholesterol metabolism. It is noteworthy that fiber intake was considerably higher and sodium intake lower, as compared with those of modern day societies. Taken together, the earlier dietary habits support the notion that atherothrombosis was uncommon. Similar findings extend to present preliterate societies: autopsy reports among these groups confirm the virtual absence of atherothrombotic disease. Levels of cholesterol and triglycerides for some of these societies are listed in Table 42–4.

## The Impact of Dietary Fat in Cardiovascular Disease Prevention

### Saturated Fat

It has been conclusively established that diets high in saturated fat (>40% of calorie intake) are associated with an increased tendency to atherothrombosis. Nearly 35 years ago, Connor demonstrated the impact of saturated fatty acids on coagulation and thrombosis.[1] Saturated fatty acids may also inhibit LDL-C receptor activity, thus raising the level of LDL-C.[2] In general, for each 1% rise in saturated fat there is a 2.7 mg/dl increase in total cholesterol. Of the major saturated fats (Table 42–5), only stearate is believed to have no effect on cholesterol levels.

### *Trans* Fatty Acids

*Trans* fatty acids are present in animal and dairy fats and in polyunsaturated vegetable oils such as soybean oil that are partially hydrogenated to increase the stability and shelf life of a variety of commercially available food products (see

Table 42–5

**Sources of Saturated Fats**

| Carbon | Fatty Acid | Sources | Food Products |
|---|---|---|---|
| C12:0 | Lauric | Coconut, palm kernel oil | Baked goods |
| C14:0 | Myristic | Coconut | Baked goods, butter |
| C16:0 | Palmistic | Palm oil | Beef tallow, butter, lard, shortening |
| C18:0 | Stearic | Cocoa butter | Chocolate |

later). A study by Mensink and Katan revealed that substitution of *trans* fatty acids for *cis* (e.g., oleic acid) raised LDL and triglycerides (TG) and reduced high-density lipoprotein (HDL).[3] *Trans* fatty acids may also be associated with elevated lipoprotein(a) [Lp(a)].[4] It has been estimated that *trans* fatty acids account for as much as 20% of total dietary fat. (The most common sources are listed in Table 42–6.) They include shortening used in baked goods (e.g., doughnuts, cookies), packaged foods (e.g., potato chips, crackers), solid margarine, and cooking oil. While epidemiologic studies have suggested a link between *trans* fatty acid intake and CAD development and progression,[5–6] there are confounding factors related to self-reporting that limit interpretation of the data. In addition, the American Heart Association Nutrition Committee has also determined that measurement of *trans* fatty acids in various foods must be standardized before suitable guidelines on *trans* fatty acid intake and CAD risk are instituted.[7]

## Monounsaturated Fat

The Mediterranean diet gained prominence after publication of the Seven Countries Study, which reported significantly lower incidences of CAD in southern European countries (e.g., Italy, Spain) as compared with North America. The primary fatty acid, oleate, reduces very low-density lipoprotein (VLDL-C) and LDL-C and may reduce macrophage uptake of LDL-C by inhibiting oxidation.[8] In addition to olive oil, the Mediterranean diet also includes a high concentration of fruits and vegetables (excellent sources of antioxidant vitamins and flavanoids), supplemented with fish, poultry, and, occasionally, red meat. Alcoholic beverages (particularly red wine) and nuts, which contain the antioxidant resveratrol (see below), are also permitted (see the Mediterranean diet pyramid in Fig. 42–1). Milk products, when consumed, were often grated cheese added to pasta. Eggs (as many as four a week) were also part of the diet. In addition to its palatability, the Mediterranean diet is also among the most cardioprotective. Countries that have adopted this diet include the island of Crete and Southern Italy, which have the lowest rates of CAD and chronic diseases in the world. The Lyon Diet Heart Study (605 subjects) prospectively evaluated the effect of a Mediterranean Diet on preventing secondary CAD. Subjects randomized to this diet experienced a 73% reduction in CAD deaths and nonfatal myocardial infarction (MI) and a 70% reduction in overall mortality over a 27-month (mean) follow-up period.[9] Extension of the study to 4 years revealed a 78% decline in cardiac death and nonfatal MI (Fig. 42–2). It has also been suggested that, in addition to CAD patients, patients with type II non–insulin-dependent diabetes mellitus (NIDDM) may benefit from eating a Mediterranean—rather than

Table 42–6

**Sources of *Trans* Fatty Acids**

| Sources | Average *Trans* (%) |
|---|---|
| **Vegetable fats** | |
| Shortening | 25.3 |
| Solid margarine | 23.0 |
| Cooking oils | 10.2 |
| **Animal and dairy fats** | |
| Butter | 3.1 |
| Beef fat | 3.0 |
| Beef tallow | 10.2 |

Modified from Enig MG, et al: Isomeric *trans* fatty acids in the U.S. diet. J Am Coll Nutr 1990; 9:471–486.

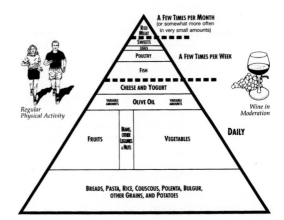

**Figure 42–1** ▪ The Mediterranean diet pyramid. (Willett WC, Sacks F, Trichopoulou A, et al: Mediterranean diet pyramid: A cultural model for healthy eating. Am J Clin Nutr 1995; 61(Suppl):1402S–1406S.)

The Mediterranean diet pyramid: a cultural model for healthy eating. © Copyright 1994 Oldways Preservation & Exchange Trust.

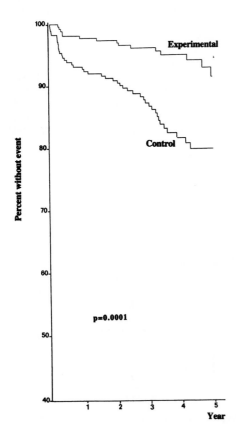

**Figure 42–2** ▪ Survival Curves. De Lorgeril et al: The Mediterranean diet, traditional risk factors, and the rate of cardiovascular complications after myocardial infarction. Final report of the Lyon Diet Heart Study. Circulation 1999;99:779–785.

a high-carbohydrate, low-fat—diet. As carbohydrate intake exceeds 65% of total calorie intake, VLDL-C production is increased, thus raising the plasma TG level. Even 55%-carbohydrate diets have been associated with elevated TG, reduced HDL levels, and potential deterioration of blood glucose control.[10] A randomized trial comparing CAD event rates associated with a Mediterranean diet and a low-fat, high-carbohydrate one in non–insulin dependent diabetics would provide clinically useful information. In addition to olive oil, other important sources of monounsaturated fats are certain nuts.[11–13] Addition of peanuts to a low-fat diet improved serum lipids in hyperlipidemic persons and may retard atherosclerosis.[11, 12] Other nuts that have demonstrated favorable effects on lipids and lipoproteins are almonds and walnuts.[13]

## Diets Rich in Omega-3 Fatty Acids

Omega-3 fatty acids are long-chain polyunsaturated fats that contain the first double bond at the third position adjacent to the methyl terminal of the molecule. As precursors of arachidonic acid, they may be incorporated through the cyclooxygenase or leukotriene pathway (Fig. 42–3), providing both antiplatelet and antiinflammatory effects. The clinical impact of these fatty acids was demonstrated in Greenland Eskimos, whose diet of predominantly fatty fish was enriched with omega-3s (e.g., whale, salmon, herring, and mackerel). Bang and Dyerberg found that these subjects had longer bleeding times and a low incidence of CAD and astutely attributed these effects to the large amounts of omega-3 fatty acids such as eicosapentanoic acid (EPA; C20:5–3) and dicosahexanoic acid (C22:4–3). In addition, significant TG lowering (20% to 50%) was also observed and is attributable to reduced hepatic VLDL-C secretion. Observational studies have disclosed an inverse association between fish consumption and CAD. In the Western Electric Study, middle-aged men who were free of CAD at baseline and who consumed about 2 oz of fish per day had a 38% reduction in CAD deaths as compared with those who did not eat fish. The most impressive finding of the study was a 67% reduction in nonsudden MI deaths during the 30-year follow-up period.[14] The diet and reinfarction trial (DART) assessed the impact of fatty fish intake, fiber intake, and increases in the P:S ratio on CAD events in patients with preexisting disease. Total

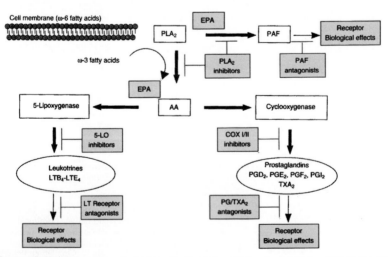

**Figure 42–3** ■ Eicosanoid and platelet activating factor. (Heller A, et al: Drugs 1998;55:487–496.)

mortality was reduced to the greatest extent (29%, $p < .05$) in the group who were advised to eat fatty fish, an effect that was observed early during the first 2 years of the study. After 46 months of follow-up, there were 50% to 70% reductions in cardiac death, MI, stroke, and unstable angina (Fig. 42–4). Recently, consumption of at least one fish meal per week translated into a 52% lower risk of sudden cardiac death; this finding held, no matter what the type of fish.[15] Manufacturers of fish oil capsules have also supported randomized, double-blind, placebo-controlled trials in patients with very high TG (type V phenotype). Because many affected subjects also had elevated total cholesterol, the significant reductions were attributable to the fish oil, and one upshot was the media "hype" of the mid 1980s promoting fish oil as an important cholesterol-lowering agent. In normolipidemic subjects, however, fish oils continue to reduce TG without exerting an appreciable effect on total cholesterol (TC) and LDL-C. In the United States, fish oil preparations are generally sold in health food stores and contain relatively small amounts of active omega-3 compounds (30%) per capsule. As significant TG reduction (e.g., >20%) is observed with daily doses of 2 to 4 g, at least eight to twelve capsules may be required for significant TG lowering. In addition to the added calorie burden, side effects of fish oil capsules may include esophagitis and a fishy body odor that is more noticeable during the summer. Manufacturers produce a more concentrated omega-3 capsules marketed as MaxEPA (France), Omacor (Pronova, Norway), and Epadil (Mochida Pharmaceuticals, Japan). These more concentrated products (65% to 95%) vary in their proportions of EPA and DHA. Alternatively, eating fatty fish remains the best way to consume omega-3 fatty acids. Table 42–7 lists the most important sources and content of these fatty acids.

## Very Low–Fat Diets

Diets low in total and saturated fat were popularized by Pritikin. He reduced his own dietary fat intake after an MI and reportedly had minimal evidence of coronary disease on post-mortem examination.[16] More recently, The Lifestyle Heart Trial evaluated the efficacy of a very low–fat diet (10% of calorie intake) in combination with lifestyle changes (aerobic exercise, stress management training, smoking cessation, and group support) on arteriographic progression of preexisting CAD.

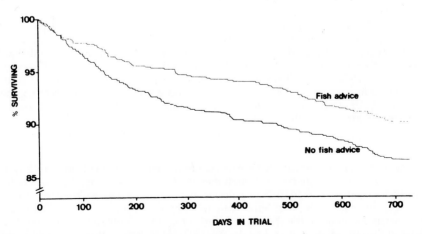

**Figure 42–4** ▪ Survival: fish advice. (Burr ML, Fehily AM, Gilbert JF et al: Effects of changes in fat, fish and fibre intakes on death and myocardial reinfarction: Diet and reinfarction trial (DART). Lancet 1989;334:757–761.)

Table 42–7

**Total Fat and Content of Fish Containing the Most Omega-3**

| Fish | Total Fat | Omega-3 Content (grams per 3.6 oz serving) |
|---|---|---|
| Sardines in sardine oil | 15.5 | 3.3 |
| Atlantic mackerel | 13.9 | 2.5 |
| Pacific herring | 13.9 | 1.7 |
| Atlantic herring | 9.0 | 1.6 |
| Lake trout | 9.7 | 1.6 |
| Anchovy | 4.8 | 1.4 |
| Chinook salmon | 10.4 | 1.4 |
| Sablefish | 15.3 | 1.4 |
| Bluefish | 6.5 | 1.2 |
| Sockeye salmon | 8.6 | 1.2 |
| Atlantic salmon | 5.4 | 1.2 |
| Pink salmon | 8.6 | 1.2 |

Data from Connor SL, Connor WE: Are fish oils beneficial in the prevention and treatment of coronary artery disease? Am J Clin Nutr 1997; 66(Suppl):1020S–1031S. © Am J Clin Nutr. American Society for Clinical Nutrition.

The dietary components of the treated (experimental) group consisted primarily of fruits, vegetables, grains, legumes, and soybean products. Eating red meat, poultry, and fish was not permitted. After 1 year, the experimental group evidenced reduced progression and slight regression of lesions.[17] At the 5-year follow-up, total fat intake represented 8.5% of calories, LDL-C was reduced 20%, and reduced coronary arteriographic progression, as compared with the control group, became more apparent. Nevertheless, there were still 25 cardiac events among the 28 experimental patients during the 5-year follow-up.[18] As TG levels in the experimental group were elevated (mean TG 258 mg/dl), these results suggest that intensive lifestyle measures may not be sufficient for optimal CAD event reduction. Other low-fat, nonpharmacologic trials, including the St. Thomas Arteriographic Regression Study (STARS; 27% fat)[19] and the Heidelberg Exercise/Diet Study (<20% fat),[20] also reduced arteriographic progression of CAD in patients assigned to the intervention group. While evidence supports reduction of total fat intake to less than 40% of total calorie burden, it remains unclear whether very low–fat diets (<10% fat) like the Lifestyle Heart Diet offer any advantages over more palatable diets of the Mediterraneans (25% to 35% fat), our paleolithic ancestors (21% fat, see earlier), or an American Heart Association low-fat (<30% fat) diet supplemented with lipid-lowering therapy. The combination of intensive diet, exercise, and lipid-lowering agents may yield the most favorable effects on TC, LDL, and TG (Fig. 42–5), but the relative impact on CAD event rates has not been established. Whatever regimen is adopted, it is important also to implement other lifestyle modifications, such as quitting smoking and reducing stress.

### The American Heart Association Statement on Very Low–Fat Diets

Recently, the American Heart Association issued a statement on very low–fat (10% of total calories) diets.[21] Although they continue to recommend dietary reduction of total fat to 25% to 30% of calories and saturated fats to less than 10% of calories, there are few long-term data to support extremely low-fat diets like that recommended in the Lifestyle Heart Program. Compared to an olive oil (Mediterranean) diet, a diet low in fat (22% of calories) was associated with reductions in HDL and elevations in TG (Fig. 42–6). In addition, very low–fat diets have not promoted weight loss, as investigators initially theorized (see below).[22]

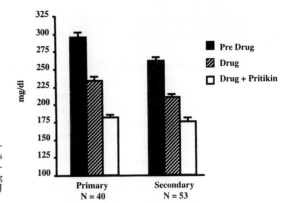

**Figure 42–5** ▪ Total serum cholesterol. (Barnard RJ, DiLauro SC, Inkeles SB: Effects of intensive diet and exercise intervention in patients taking cholesterol lowering drugs. Am J Cardiol 1997;79:1112–1114.)

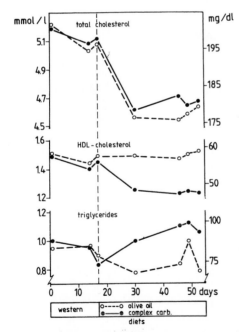

Mean serum total and HDL cholesterol and serum triacylglycerol as a function of fat intake in student volunteers. All 48 participants first received a Western diet that provided 38% of energy as fat, of which 20% was saturated. Over the next 36 d, 12 men and 12 women received a diet high in olive oil providing 41% of energy from fat (O) and another 12 men and 12 women a diet high in complex carbohydrates that provided 22% of energy as fat and 60 g dietary fiber/d (●). Reproduced with permission from The Lancet Ltd (22).

**Figure 42–6** ▪ Effects of blood lipids. (Mensink, Katan: Effect of monounsaturated fatty acids versus complex carbohydrates on high-density lipoproteins in healthy men and women. Lancet 1987: 1:122–125.)

Thus, until clinical outcome data become available, the primary recommendation is to restrict dietary saturated far intake and limit *total* fat intake to no more than 30% of calories.

### Labeling Requirements for Dietary Supplements

In recent years, the FDA has required food manufacturers to provide more accurate descriptions of calories and sources for product labeling. When evaluating a "Nutrition Facts" label (Fig. 42–7), it is important to evaluate the serving size and the total calorie and saturated fat burdens per serving. For example, a food label may list only 120 calories and 2 g of saturated fat per serving, an appropriate amount with a serving size of 3 oz but densely caloric if the serving size were ½ oz. Unfortunately, some densely caloric "low-fat" products may be advertised as being low in total and saturated fat and lead consumers to eat too much simple carbohydrates and promote central adiposity and insulin resistance in susceptible ones. Because the dietary focus often centers on reduction of calories and saturated fat, substitution for saturated fat with mono- and polyunsaturated fats and complex carbohydrates may improve the lipoprotein profile and reduce atherogenic risk, especially when coupled with aerobic activity. In addition to the traditional labeling requirements, the U.S. Food and Drug Administration also recently mandated that labeling requirements include a "Supplement Facts" panel for products that contain amino acids, herbs, minerals, and vitamins.

## Antioxidants in Preventive Cardiology

Important sources of antioxidants include natural substances in selected fruits, vegetables, and beverages. Certain vitamins also possess antioxidant properties when taken as supplements in doses larger than those ordinarily consumed in the diet.

| Nutrition Facts | |
|---|---|
| Serving size 8 wafers (32g) | |
| Servings per Container About 8 | |

| Amount Per Serving | |
|---|---|
| **Calories** 130  Calories from Fat 25 | |

| | % Daily Value |
|---|---|
| **Total Fat** 3g | **4%** |
| Saturated Fat 0.5g | **3%** |
| Polyunsaturated Fat 0g | |
| Monounsaturated Fat 1g | |
| **Cholesterol** 0mg | **0%** |
| **Sodium** 180 mg | **7%** |
| **Total Carbohydrate** 24g | **8%** |
| Dietary Fiber 4g | **17%** |
| Sugars 0g | |
| **Protein** 3g | |

Vitamin A 0% ● Vitamin C 0% ● Calcium 0%
● Iron 10% ● Phosphorous 15%

**Figure 42–7** ■ Nutrition Facts

## Lycopene

Lycopene, a powerful antioxidant, is a carotenoid that imparts the red color to tomatoes. In the European Community Multicenter Study on Antioxidants, Myocardial Infarction and Breast Cancer (EURAMIC), subjects in the upper decile of adipose tissue levels of lycopene had a 40% lower likelihood of an MI as compared with those in the lowest decile.[23] Dietary supplementation with lycopene significantly reduces serum peroxidation and LDL oxidation. The richest sources of lycopene are tomato products (e.g., tomato juice, ketchup, spaghetti sauce), but watermelon, grapefruit, and guava also contain this antioxidant.

## Flavonoids

Flavonoids are nonnutritive, plant-derived, polyphenolic compounds present in fruits, vegetables, and teas, and they have both antioxidant and antiplatelet properties. Flavonoids such as quercetin and myricetin inhibit cyclic adenosine monophosphate (cAMP) and cyclic quanosine monophosphate (cGMP) phosphodiesterases and reduce intraplatelet calcium concentration and activity.[24] Clinically, increased flavonoid intake has been associated with reduced incidence of CAD. Moreover, in the Zutphen Study, drinking approximately 2.5 (8 oz) cups of black tea daily was associated with a 69% reduction in the risk of stroke as compared with drinking less than 1.5 cups daily.[25] In addition to teas, other important sources of flavonoids include red wine, purple grape juice, dark beer, vegetables (e.g., broccoli), fruits (e.g., cranberries, apples), and soybeans. Soybeans were also shown to lower TC, LDL-C, and TG in a recent meta-analysis.[26] Some have proposed that high concentrations of isoflavones or soy estrogens may in part account for the hypolipidemic effects observed.

## Resveratrol

Resveratrol is a naturally occurring phytoestrogen and powerful antioxidant present in nuts (e.g., peanuts), red wine, and grapes. In the Nurses Study of 86,000 women aged 34 to 59 years, frequent consumption of nuts (at least 1 ounce at least five times a week) was associated with a 35% reduction in fatal CAD events and nonfatal MI as compared with eating nuts occasionally or not at all.[27] One ounce of peanuts or 2 pounds of grapes contains approximately 73 μg of resveratrol, whereas red wine contains approximately 160 μg per fluid ounce.

## Vitamins

Inhibition of LDL-C modification is a mechanism proposed to account for the in vitro effect of certain vitamins on CAD risk.[28] While the data for vitamin A (beta carotene) supplementation have been less compelling, observational studies have demonstrated reduced risks of initial MI in men and women who ate products containing vitamin E. Dietary sources of vitamin E, especially nuts and seeds, contain principally γ-tocopherol whereas vitamin E supplements sold in the United States contain α-tocopherol. Although serum levels of γ-tocopherol (but not α-tocopherol) were low in CAD patients, the relative impact of these tocopherol derivatives on the CAD event rate are not known. In one secondary prevention study that demonstrated reduction in cardiovascular events with vitamin E supplementation, natural $d$-α-tocopherol was employed (Fig. 42–8); natural $d$-α-tocopherol has greater antioxidant activity than racemic ($d$ or $l$)-α-tocopherol. Studies in vitro have also reported a synergistic effect for vitamin C and vitamin E on lipid peroxidation.[29] Another antioxidant, Probucol, was shown to impede restenosis after percutaneous transcatheter angioplasty (PTCA).[30] While these studies suggest a favorable effect for antioxidants in preventing CAD, two recent randomized

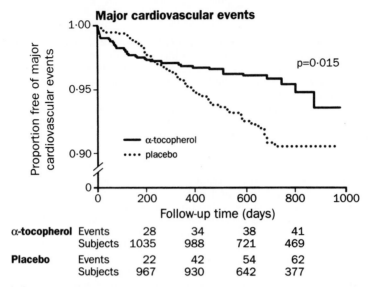

**Figure 42–8** ■ Kaplan-Meier survival analysis (upper graph only). (Stephens NG, Parsons A, Schofield PM, et al: Randomized controlled trial of vitamin E in patients with coronary disease: Cambridge Heart Antioxidant Study (CHAOS). Lancet 1996;347:781–786.)

studies did not show benefit with vitamin E supplementation.[31, 32] At present, therefore, there are no formal recommendations for vitamin supplementation to prevent CAD.

### Folate

Folate is discussed later, in the section on Homocysteine.

## Minerals

Because selenium is a cofactor for the superoxide dismutase metabolic pathway, deficiency has been linked to elevated CAD rates. One study of selenium supplementation observed an associated reduction in recurrent CAD events.[33] The mineral chromium has been shown to elevate levels of HDL-C,[34] which, theoretically, may reduce CAD events. No outcome studies have been performed to evaluate this potential effect, however.

## Neutraceuticals in Preventive Cardiology

The neutraceutical market is a rapidly growing, multibillion-dollar industry in the United States. Because these compounds have much increased in popularity, it is important that physicians familiarize themselves with the industry and recognize its impact on health care because of the growing concern that many patients either are not initiating or are discontinuing conventional therapies in favor of less solidly established holistic ones.

## Selected Herbal Supplements

### Garlic

Even though the oil in garlic contains the potent antiplatelet activator allicin, some have proposed that it may inhibit HMG CoA* reductase and thus lower LDL-

---

*HMG CoA: 3-hydroxy-3 methylglutaryl coenzyme A.

C and TC. Indeed, a meta-analysis of 16 trials detected reductions in TC (12%) in subjects treated with garlic. More recently, no significant changes in lipids or lipoproteins were observed in a multicenter trial of 28 hyperlipidemic subjects (mean TC 274 mg/dl) who received 900 mg of garlic powder tablets (Kwai) daily.[35] Participating subjects also adhered to a low-fat, low-cholesterol diet, an important element that, the authors note, previously published trials did not control rigorously. It is likewise unclear whether allicin processed in garlic tablets loses some of its antithrombotic properties. A crossover trial evaluating effects of garlic clove supplementation on lipoprotein and hemostatic parameters may help to resolve this question.

### Ginkgo Biloba

Reportedly the oldest living tree species, the ginkgo contains flavonoids such as quercetin and terpene lactones, compounds believed to contribute to its antioxidant effects. In candidates for coronary artery bypass grafting (CABG), pretreatment with ginkgo biloba reduced ischemic events, putatively by lowering free radical production.[36] In addition to potentially favorable effects on the cerebral circulation,[37] a study of 60 patients with occlusive peripheral arterial disease assigned to take ginkgo biloba special extract experienced significant improvement in pain-free walking distance during the 6-month trial, even though no changes in the Doppler index were reported.[38] Despite these favorable results, no randomized, placebo-controlled trials have studied the effect of this herb on cardiovascular mortality rates.

### Ginseng

Indigenous principally to China, North Korea, Japan, and Russia, ginseng has only recently been cultivated in the United States. Its principal components, referred to as *ginsenosides*, are steroidlike, saponin-derived, triterpenoid glycosides. Although much of the research on ginseng has centered on its potential impact on enhancing mental concentration and cognition, animal studies have revealed that it may also lower blood pressure and blood glucose and increase insulin release. Ginseng may also stimulate release of nitric oxide.[39] At high doses, however, it has been reported to cause hypertension and other untoward side effects. No randomized clinical trials have been conducted.

## ■ THE IMPACT OF EXERCISE ON CARDIOVASCULAR DISEASE PREVENTION

Humans with high aerobic capacity have a lower incidence of CAD than do sedentary subjects. While it has been widely reported that the best-conditioned athletes have the lowest case fatality rates of MI,[40] moderate physical activity has also been associated with favorably reduced rates. Such activities must be pursued throughout life; a high school athlete who quits exercising later in life is not protected from subsequent development of CAD.[41] Table 42–8 outlines some of the cardioprotective advantages of aerobic conditioning. Exercise is beneficial throughout all age groups. In fact, among elderly persons, regular exercise (walking or cycling for 20 minutes thrice weekly) resulted in a 30% reduction in CAD and in total mortality. In addition to CAD events, moderate physical activity may also reduce stroke rates. In the Harvard Alumni Health Study, approximately a 50% reduction in stroke was observed in men (mean age 58 years) who expended 2000 to 3000 kcal of energy weekly. Interestingly, greater effort (e.g., >3000 kcal/wk) reduced rates only 22%, and low-intensity effort (<1000 kcal/wk or <4.5 METs) was not associated with improvement. These results suggest that there may be diminishing returns, *vis-à-vis* cardiovascular rates, when physical activity is strenu-

Table 42–8

**Ten Cardiovascular Benefits Attributable to Aerobic Conditioning**

| Effect | Consequence |
| --- | --- |
| Enhanced efficiency of tissue $O_2$ extraction | Increased exercise capacity |
| Coronary vasodilatation | Improved myocardial perfusion |
| Increased expression of nitric oxide synthase | Restoration of endothelial function |
| Reduces circulating catecholamines | Decreased platelet aggregation |
| Calorie expenditure | Weight loss |
| Reduction in peripheral vascular resistance | Decreased blood pressure |
| Reduction in oxidative stress | Decreased low-density lipoprotein modification |
| Enhanced activity of lipoprotein lipase | Triglyceride reduction, high-density lipoprotein elevation |
| Enhanced insulin sensitivity | Improved blood glucose control |
| Release of serotonin | Improved sense of well-being |

Modified from Chandrashekhar Y, Anand IS: Exercise as a coronary protective factor. Am Heart J 1991;122:1723–1739.

ous and that moderate-intensity exercise may be the most suitable recommended regimen for lowering CAD risk.

## ■ THE IMPACT OF OBESITY IN CARDIOVASCULAR DISEASE PREVENTION

As exercise reduces CAD event rates in an otherwise active adult, failure to exercise is often accompanied by an increase in body weight. Throughout adult life, every attempt should be made to maintain approximately the body weight at age 21 years. While increases of up to 10 lb do not appear to produce untoward effects, increases greater than 20 lb during adulthood have been associated with higher overall mortality.[42] The body mass index (BMI) is another index used to assess obesity. The formula for BMI is weight (kg) divided by height squared ($m^2$) or weight (lb) divided by height (in) squared multiplied by 704.5. The new Federal Obesity Guidelines define *overweight* as a BMI between 25 and 29.9; *obesity* is defined as BMI greater than 30. The age-adjusted prevalences of overweight and obesity are shown in Figure 42–9. Since 1960, the prevalence of obesity—in men and in women—has nearly doubled. In women, the prevalence rose from 15% to 25% during the 32-year period 1962 to 1994. This is believed to reflect increases in calorie consumption (by 300 calories/day) and reductions in physical activity. Summary recommendations of the recently released obesity guidelines are presented in Table 42–9. Another sensitive index of weight as a marker of enhanced CAD risk is central adiposity (fat distributed in the abdomen is more metabolically active than gluteal fat), a parameter defined by the waist to hip circumference. A normal waist-to-hip circumference ratio is less than 0.8. An elevated ratio (>1) may be a marker of enhanced CAD risk and is common in patients with Reaven's syndrome (syndrome X), which is characterized by a constellation of findings, including hyperinsulinemia, glucose intolerance, hypertension, hypertriglyceridemia, and low HDL-C. Elevated levels of leptin, a protein associated with obesity, has been found in association with syndrome X.[43]

## ■ THE IMPACT OF NONTRADITIONAL CARDIOVASCULAR RISK FACTORS IN PREVENTIVE CARDIOLOGY

Because traditional coronary risk factors (e.g., cigarette smoking, diabetes mellitus, hypertension, hypercholesterolemia) have been reported to explain only 50%

## AGE-ADJUSTED PREVALENCE OF OVERWEIGHT AND OBESITY IN MEN

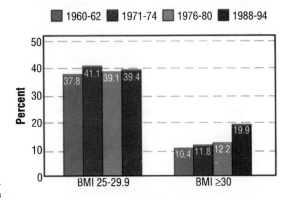

■ 1960-62 ■ 1971-74 ■ 1976-80 ■ 1988-94

**Figure 42–9** ■ Age-adjusted prevalence of overweight and obesity in men. (Clinical guidelines on the identification, evaluation, and treatment of overweight and obesity in adults: Executive summary. Am J Clin Nutr 1998;68:899–917.)

BMI = body mass index
CDC/NCHS, United States, 1960-94 (ages 20-74 years).

of coronary events, additional CAD risk factors have been actively sought. The main nonlipid factors are homocysteine, infectious agents, and mental stress.

## Homocysteine

McCulley's pathologic description of increased intimal thickness and fibrous plaque in the renal and coronary arteries of an infant who succumbed to the complications of homocysteinemia in 1969 anticipated the pyridoxine (vitamin $B_6$)-deficient acceleration of atherosclerosis reported in monkeys 20 years later. These and other early histologic reports in subjects with metabolic alterations in homocysteine regulation suggested a role for this amino acid in the pathogenesis of atherothrombosis. The metabolism of homocysteine begins with its precursor, the essential amino acid methionine. Methionine is converted to homocysteine after intermediary metabolism to S-adenosylmethionine and S-adenosylhomocysteine.

### Table 42–9

#### Summary Recommendations of the Obesity Guidelines

1. Physical activity (30–45 min, 3 × weekly) is recommended as part of a comprehensive weight loss program.
2. Reducing dietary fat alone without reducing calories is not sufficient for weight loss.
3. Initial goal of weight loss therapy is to reduce body weight by approximately 10% from baseline.
4. Weight loss should be about 1–2 lb/wk (or a deficit of 500–1000 kcal/day) for the first 6 mo; additional recommendations are based on the amount of weight loss achieved.
5. Lifestyle therapy should be initiated for 6 months before FDA-approved weight loss drugs are tried.
6. If these therapies fail, patients with BMI >40, or >35 will coexisting risk factors, may be considered for weight loss surgery.

Clinical guidelines on the identification, evaluation, and treatment of overweight and obesity in adults: Executive summary. Am J Clin Nutr 1998;68:899–917.

Cystathione β-synthase initiates a series of reactions that convert homocysteine to cysteine in which vitamin $B_6$ serves as cofactor. Alternatively, homocysteine may be remethylated via transfer of a methyl group from 5-methyltetrahydrofolate, a reaction catalyzed by methionine synthase (MS) with vitamin $B_{12}$ as cofactor or by transfer of a methyl group by betaine (Fig. 42–10). An excess of homocysteine may occur as a result of (1) genetic deficiency in cystathione β-synthase, deficiency in 5,10-methyltetrahydrofolate reductase (MTHFR) or defective methionine synthase. The best-described genetic abnormality is cystathione β-synthase deficiency, an autosomal-recessive disorder characterized by connective tissue abnormalities—skeletal and ocular deformities that may be the consequence of homocysteine-induced alterations in matrix protein (e.g., collagen, fibrillin) cross linking. It bears clinical resemblance to Marfan syndrome but does not produce the joint laxity, aortic root enlargement, or mitral valve prolapse of Marfan. The principal cause of death is thromboembolic events, which occur in 50% of untreated patients by age 30 years. Although MTHFR deficiency is rare, a common polymorphism in the MTHFR gene (677C→ T) has been reported.[44] Findings of studies of CAD rates in subjects genetically homozygous for this polymorphism have been discordant. Recently, the Physicians' Health Study found that the most meaningful risk factor for CAD men homozygous for the MTHFR (677T) gene was concomitant low serum folate level.[45] Elevation of homocysteine can have acquired causes—systemic diseases such as renal failure (secondary to reduced catabolism of homocysteine), psoriasis or acute lymphoblastic leukemia (increased cell turnover), and hypothyroidism, among others. Transplant recipients also have elevated levels attributable to cyclosporine inhibition of folate-induced remethylation. Pharmaceuticals that affect homocysteine include those that interfere with folate-induced remethylation (e.g., methotrexate, anticonvulsants) or with folate absorption (bile acid sequestrants) and substances that block methionine synthase (nitric oxide) or increase S-adenosyl-methionine (niacin). Conditions that cause elevated homocysteine levels are shown in Fig. 42–11. Although levels in men are approximately 10% to 20% higher than those of premenopausal women, there are no significant gender differences after menopause. Observational studies have disclosed that, as homocysteine levels exceed 10 μmol/l, the risk of cardiovascular events increases. Similarly, in patients with preexisting CAD, the survival rates were highest in subjects with levels below 9 μmol/l (Fig. 42–12). The European Concerted Action Project is among the largest case-control studies to evaluate the relationships among plasma homocysteine, vitamins $B_6$ and $B_{12}$, folate levels, and vascular events. The investigators reported that elevated plasma homocysteine was as strong an independent risk factor for vascular disease as hyperlipidemia or cigarette smoking. Moreover,

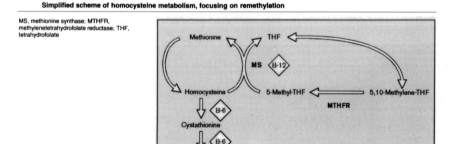

**Figure 42–10** ■ Simplified scheme of homocysteine. (Verhoef P, et al: Folate and coronary heart disease. *Curr Opin Lipidol* 1998;9:17–22.)

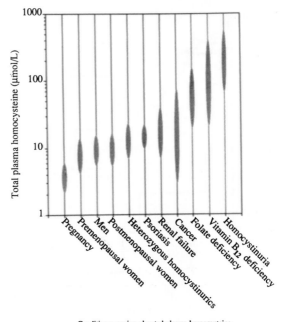

**Figure 42–11** ▪ Conditions causing elevated plasma homocysteine. (Ueland PM, Refsum H: Plasma homocysteine, a risk factor for vascular disease: Plasma levels in health, disease, and drug therapy. J Lab Clin Med 1989; 114:473–501.

Conditions causing elevated plasma homocysteine.

as compared with hypertensive patients with normal fasting homocysteine values, the combination of elevated homocysteine and hypertension nearly tripled the risk of CAD events.[46] The pathophysiologic mechanism that relates homocysteine to atherogenesis is believed to reflect a direct toxic effect on the endothelium and enhancing LDL uptake by macrophage. Enhanced thrombogenicity has also been reported, which is attributed to activation of tissue factor.[47] Post-mortem lesions in subjects afflicted with hyperhomocysteinemia have exhibited characteristic findings of atherosclerosis, which include intimal thickening and fibrotic changes in medium- and large-sized vessels.

## Treatment of Elevated Homocysteine Levels

The three main agents for lowering homocysteine are folate and vitamins $B_6$ and $B_{12}$. Before any therapeutic measures are initiated in patients with elevated homocysteine, however, serum $B_{12}$ levels should also be assessed, because administration of folate may obscure a clinical vitamin $B_{12}$ deficiency. Rich dietary sources of folate, $B_6$, and $B_{12}$ are listed in Table 42–10. Dietary sources can provide about 400 μg daily; higher doses (1 to 5 mg) are reserved for patients known to have hyperhomocysteinemia (>15 μmol/l). Patients receiving 1 mg or more of folate should also receive vitamin $B_{12}$, 200 to 1000 μg/day. Supplementation with vitamin $B_6$, 20 to 25 mg/day, may also be considered, in combination with a diet low in methionine. Methionine-rich foods include avocado, eggs, meats, seeds, and wheat germ. The critical question—whether lowering homocysteine reduces the cardiovascular event rate—awaits the results of ongoing randomized trials.

## Inflammatory Markers

In recent years, an infectious agent has been added to those implicated in atherothrombosis. Specific pathogens cited include *Chlamydia pneumoniae*, cytomeg-

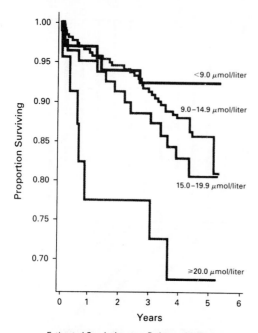

Estimated Survival among Patients with Coronary Artery Disease, According to Plasma Total Homocysteine Levels. The figure shows estimated survival for 55-year-old male former smokers with three-vessel disease, a left ventricular ejection fraction of 55 percent, a creatinine level of 1.5 mg per deciliter (130 μmol per liter), and a total cholesterol level of 241 mg per deciliter (6.24 mmol per liter) at four different total homocysteine levels. Survival curves have been estimated in a stratified Cox regression analysis.

**Figure 42–12** ■ Estimated survival. (Nygard O, Nordrehaug JE, Refsum H, et al: Plasma homocysteine levels and mortality in patients with coronary artery disease. N Engl J Med 1997;337:230–236.)

alovirus, and *Helicobacter pylori*. C-reactive protein has been studied as a marker of systemic inflammation, and elevated levels have been found to predict MI, stroke, and peripheral artery disease. The effectiveness of antiinflammatory agents such as aspirin and statin therapy in lowering CAD event rates may in part reflect reduction in CRP concentrations.[48–50] Moreover, short-term treatment with azithramycin recently was shown to reduce cardiovascular events in a small group of post-MI patients who had elevated antibody titers of *C. pneumoniae*.[51] These data await replication in ongoing randomized controlled trials. Until then, measurements of high sensitivity C-reactive protein or antibody titers to the aforementioned pathogens are generally reserved for research protocols.

## Mental Stress

The observation that MIs were more frequent after circadian release of catecholamines in the early morning and evening hours constituted the earliest documentation of mental stress as an important trigger of MI and sudden cardiac death. An example of how acute mental stress may lead to CAD events is shown in Figure 42–13. Indeed, reports of enhanced CAD rates have coincided with life crises such as earthquakes, war, and death of loved ones. A paradoxical vasoconstrictor response after administration of intracoronary acetylcholine was observed in patients

Table 42–10

## Common Food Sources of Folate, Vitamin B₆, and Vitamin B₁₂

| | Content |
|---|---|
| Folate | (μg) |
| ½ cup lentils | 179 |
| ½ cup chickpeas | 141 |
| ½ cup kidney beans | 115 |
| ½ cup frozen spinach | 102 |
| 1 cup Cheerios | 100 |
| 1 cup corn flakes | 100 |
| Vitamin B₆ | (mg) |
| 1 baked potato with skin | 0.7 |
| 1 banana | 0.7 |
| 1 cup raisin bran | 0.7 |
| 3 oz roasted chicken | 0.5 |
| Vitamin B₁₂ | (μg) |
| 1⅓ cups Total brand cereal | 6.2 |
| 3 oz tuna (in water) | 2.5 |
| 3 oz beef tenderloin | 2.2 |
| 2 Atlantic sardines | 2.0 |
| 3 fish sticks | 1.5 |
| 1 cup yogurt | 1.0 |
| 1 cup skim milk | 0.9 |

Modified from Tufts University Health & Nutrition Letter (3/98).

MENTAL STRESS AS A TRIGGER OF MYOCARDIAL ISCHEMIA AND INFARCTION

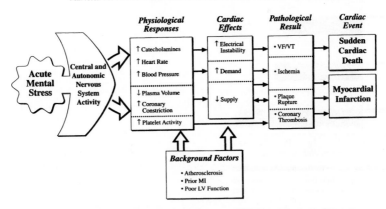

Pathophysiologic model of the actions of acute stress as a trigger of myocardial infarction and sudden death in vulnerable individuals. Via its actions on the central and autonomic nervous system, in patients with coronary artery disease stress can produce a cascade of physiologic responses that may lead to myocardial ischemia, ventricular fibrillation/tachycardia (VF/VT), plaque rupture, or coronary thrombosis. (MI = myocardial infarction; LV = left-ventricular.)

**Figure 42–13** ▪ Pathophysiologic model. (Krantz DS, Kop WJ, Santiago JT, Gottdiener JS: Mental stress as a trigger of myocardial ischemia and infarction. Cardiol Clin 1996;14:271–287.)

asked to perform mental arithmetic.[52] Other studies have extended these findings by demonstrating wall motion abnormalities, transient reductions in ventricular function, and silent ischemia in response to mental stress.[53] Most recently, these findings were extended to include a reduced likelihood of silent ischemia during periods of high positive stress (e.g., extreme happiness) as compared with negative stress such as tension, frustration, or sadness (Fig. 42–14).

# ▪ COMPREHENSIVE RISK REDUCTION THERAPIES

Recently, a guide to secondary prevention risk reduction therapies was designed by the AHA and ACC (Fig. 42–15). Some of these modalities (e.g., lipid management and blood pressure control) are discussed elsewhere in this book. In addition to quitting smoking, regular physical activity, and weight management (see earlier), other important considerations in maximizing secondary preventive efforts are antiplatelet agents, angiotensin-converting enzyme (ACE) inhibitors, beta-blockers, and, for postmenopausal women, estrogen replacement.

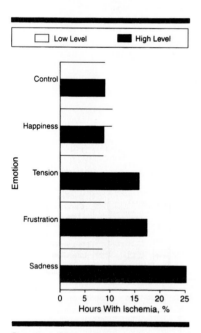

Percentage of hours with low and high ratings of feeling in control. happiness. tension. frustration, and sadness in which ischemia occurred during 2760 hours of monitoring. The percentage of ischemic hours was greater during higher levels of the negative emotions. ie. mental stress. Ischemic episodes associated with these emotions were distributed over several patients. There were 17 episodes of ischemia associated with high frustration ratings. representing 8 (31%) of those who endorsed high frustration ratings. Sixteen episodes of ischemia were attributable to high tension levels for 10 (43%) of those who endorsed high tension ratings. High sadness ratings were associated with 7 ischemic events in 4 (33%) of those endorsing high sadness ratings.

**Figure 42–14** ▪ Percentage of hours. (Gullette ECD, Blumenthal JA, Babyak M, et al: Effects of mental stress on myocardial ischemia during daily life. JAMA 1997;277:1521–1526. Copyrighted 1997, American Medical Association.)

| Risk Intervention | Recommendations |
|---|---|
| **Smoking:**<br>**Goal**<br>complete cessation | Strongly encourage patient and family to stop smoking.<br>Provide counseling, nicotine replacement, and formal cessation programs as appropriate. |
| **Lipid management:**<br>**Primary goal**<br>**LDL<100 mg/dL**<br>**Secondary goals**<br>**HDL>35 mg/dL;**<br>**TG<200 mg/dL** | Start AHA Step II Diet in all patients: ≤30% fat, <7% saturated fat, <200 mg/dL cholesterol.<br><br>Assess fasting lipid profile. In post-MI patients, lipid profile may take 4 to 6 weeks to stabilize. Add drug therapy according to the following guide: |

Lipid management sub-table:

| LDL<100 mg/dL | LDL 100 to 130 mg/dL | LDL >130 mg/dL | HDL<35 mg/dL |
|---|---|---|---|
| No drug therapy | Consider adding drug therapy to diet, as follows: | Add drug therapy to diet, as follows: | Emphasize weight management and physical activity.<br>Advise smoking cessation.<br>If needed to achieve LDL goals, consider niacin, statin, fibrate. |
| | ↘ Suggested drug therapy ↙ | | |
| | TG <200 mg/dL | TG 200 to 400 mg/dL | TG >400 mg/dL | |
| | Statin<br>Resin<br>Niacin | Statin<br>Niacin | Consider combined drug therapy (niacin, fibrate, statin) | |
| | If LDL goal not achieved, consider combination therapy. | | |

| Risk Intervention | Recommendations |
|---|---|
| **Physical activity:**<br>**Minimum goal**<br>**30 minutes 3 to 4**<br>**times per week** | Assess risk, preferably with exercise test, to guide prescription.<br>Encourage minimum of 30 to 60 minutes of moderate-intensity activity 3 or 4 times weekly (walking, jogging, cycling, or other aerobic activity) supplemented by an increase in daily lifestyle activities (eg, walking breaks at work, using stairs, gardening, household work). Maximum benefit 5 to 6 hours a week.<br>Advise medically supervised programs for moderate- to high-risk patients. |
| **Weight management:** | Start intensive diet and appropriate physical activity intervention, as outlined above, in patients >120% of ideal weight for height.<br>Particularly emphasize need for weight loss in patients with hypertension, elevated triglycerides, or elevated glucose levels. |
| **Antiplatelet agents/**<br>**anticoagulants:** | Start aspirin 80 to 325 mg/d if not contraindicated.<br>Manage warfarin to international normalized ratio=2 to 3.5 for post-MI patients not able to take aspirin. |
| **ACE inhibitors**<br>**post-MI:** | Start early post-MI in stable high-risk patients (anterior MI, previous MI, Killip class II [S₃ gallop, rales, radiographic CHF]).<br>Continue indefinitely for all with LV dysfunction (ejection fraction≤40) or symptoms of failure.<br>Use as needed to manage blood pressure or symptoms in all other patients. |
| **Beta-blockers:** | Start in high-risk post-MI patients (arrhythmia, LV dysfunction, inducible ischemia) at 5 to 28 days. Continue 6 months minimum. Observe usual contraindications.<br>Use as needed to manage angina rhythm or blood pressure in all other patients. |
| **Estrogens:** | Consider estrogen replacement in all postmenopausal women.<br>Individualize recommendation consistent with other health risks. |
| **Blood pressure**<br>**control:**<br>**Goal**<br>**≤140/90 mm Hg** | Initiate lifestyle modification—weight control, physical activity, alcohol moderation, and moderate sodium restriction—in all patients with blood pressure>140 mm Hg systolic or 90 mm Hg diastolic.<br>Add blood pressure medication, individualized to other patient requirements and characteristics (ie, age, race, need for drugs with specific benefits) if blood pressure is not less than 140 mm Hg systolic or 90 mm Hg diastolic in 3 months or if initial blood pressure is >160 mm Hg systolic or 100 mm Hg diastolic. |

Guide to comprehensive risk reduction for patients with coronary and other vascular disease. ACE = angiotensin-converting enzyme; AHA = American Heart Association; CHF = congestive heart failure; HDL = high density lipoprotein; LDL = low density lipoprotein; LV = left ventricular; MI = myocardial infarction; TG = triglycerides. Reprinted, with permission, from Smith SC, Blair SN, Criqui MH, et al. Preventing heart attack and death in patients with coronary disease. Circulation 1995;92:2–4.

**Figure 42–15** ▪ Guide to comprehensive risk reduction for patients with coronary and other vascular disease. (Smith SC, Blarr SM, Criqui MH, et al: Preventing heart attack and death in patients with coronary disease. Circulation 1995;92:2–4.)

## Antiplatelet Agents

The salutary effect of aspirin in secondary prevention of CAD is well-documented. In the Antiplatelet Therapy Trialists, significant reductions in recurrent MI (31%), nonfatal cerebrovascular accidents (42%), and mortality (12%) were observed among the nearly 20,000 participants surveyed. While the traditional dose of one adult aspirin (325 mg) daily has been shown to be effective, lower doses (e.g., baby aspirin, 160 mg) have also yielded favorable results in smaller-scale studies. Typically, aspirin provides 40% to 50% platelet inhibition. Fewer clinical outcome data are available for the phosphodiesterase inhibitor dipyridamole. Glycoprotein IIb/IIIa receptor antagonists, which prevent the binding of fibrinogen for subsequent conversion to fibrin, may provide up to 80% platelet inhibition. Intravenous administration has been shown to reduce the risk of death, MI, or revascularization in patients with unstable angina or non–Q wave MI or those treated with primary percutaneous transcatheter angioplasty for acute MI. Oral glycoprotein IIb/IIIa receptor antagonist compounds are currently under investigation. Ticlopidine inhibits platelet activity by impairing adenosine diphosphate P–mediated activation of the glycoprotein IIb/IIIa receptor. One report observed significant reductions in fatal and nonfatal MI during 6-month follow-up of patients with unstable angina. Another thienopyridine derivative, clopidogrel, was recently compared with aspirin in 19,185 patients at risk for ischemic events (CAPRIE). As compared with aspirin, 325 mg/day, clopidogrel, 75 mg/day, produced significant reductions in strokes, MI, and vascular deaths in aggregate over approximately 2 years' follow-up. Neutropenia, which may occur in 1% of ticlopidine-treated patients, has not been reported to be more frequent in patients who took clopidogrel. These agents appear to be effective for secondary prevention of CAD and, thus, may be particularly useful for aspirin-allergic or resistant patients.

## Angiotensin-Converting Enzyme Inhibitors

Randomized controlled trials in MI survivors have revealed significant reductions in recurrent cardiovascular events and mortality (20% to 25%) by ACE inhibitors. These results are most applicable to patients with reduced ventricular function (left ventricular ejection fraction <40%), although benefit has also been achieved in patients at high risk for cardiovascular disease even with normal LV function.[54] Mechanisms of reduction in ischemic events may include plaque stabilization and restoration of endothelial function. ACE inhibitor therapy should be instituted within 72 hours after an MI; contraindications include hypotension, renal insufficiency (creatinine >2 mg/dl), and bilateral renal artery stenosis.

## Beta-Blockers

Beta-blockers are very effective for reducing risk of recurrent MI (by 15% to 25%), sudden cardiac death (30% to 35%), and overall mortality (20%). In addition to their antiarrhythmic properties, these negative inotropic and chronotropic agents enhance coronary perfusion by increasing diastolic filling time. Despite unopposed α-adrenergic vasoconstriction, which may reduce lipoprotein lipase activity and lead to elevated triglycerides and reduced HDL-C, beta-blockers should not be withheld from post-MI patients. Hemodynamically stable post-MI patients with compromised ventricular function (>40%) may also benefit from beta-blockers.

## Estrogen Replacement Therapy

Observational studies have demonstrated that, for postmenopausal women, estrogen replacement with CAD was associated with reductions in cardiovascular events and death. Estrogen inhibits the potent endothelial vasoconstrictor endothelin and upregulates production of nitric oxide synthase. The Hormones Estrogen Replacement Study was the first randomized, placebo-controlled, double-blind study to investigate hormone replacement therapy (HRT) in women with CAD who had an intact uterus. Women were randomized to receive either placebo or conjugated equine estrogens, 0.625 mg, and medroxyprogesterone acetate, 2.5 mg (Prempro) daily. After an average of 4.1 years' follow-up, there were no significant differences in overall risk of MI or CHD-related death. An encouraging pattern of fewer CAD events among the HRT group began to emerge, however, during the fourth year of the study, and extended follow-up is planned for 2 more years to determine whether HRT significantly reduces CAD events in this high-risk subgroup. The Women's Health Initiative is currently investigating HRT in postmenopausal women. This study will also examine women who have had a hysterectomy to compare effects of estrogen therapy alone and of combination therapy on CAD event rates. Until these data resolve this issue, HRT cannot be recommended as routine first-line therapy for secondary prevention of CAD.

## ■ ORGANIZING A PREVENTIVE CARDIOLOGY PROGRAM

Recent findings indicate that proven secondary preventive strategies are not routinely employed: use of aspirin, ACE inhibitors, beta-blockers, and lipid-lowering agents are reportedly underutilized. In an effort to circumvent these critical shortcomings, preventive cardiology services should be offered by all hospitals and medical facilities that treat cardiovascular disease. The development and success of centralized preventive cardiology services is predicated on an organized and integrated multidisciplinary approach that bridges the gap between internal medicine, neurology, cardiothoracic surgery, and vascular surgery. Included in this continuity of care paradigm is a comprehensive outpatient clinic and an inpatient consultation division. Although a physician with a background or interest in preventive cardiology most often spearheads these efforts, day-to-day coordination is enhanced by the participation of other health care personnel, including nurses, dietitian, and physician assistants. Still, significant barriers remain (Table 42–11) that must be overcome to ensure successful implementation of these important services. All hospitalized patients evaluated for atherothrombotic disease should have complete risk factor assessment, including fasting lipid and lipoprotein measurements. Although lipid and lipoprotein alterations are common beyond the first 12 to 24 hours after an MI, lipid analysis may still be performed. An LDL-C obtained 24 hours following an acute MI is about 10% to 30% higher than baseline levels. While the vast majority of CAD patients exhibit LDL-C concentrations exceeding 100 mg/dl, approximately 10% have acceptable values, and they are likely to manifest elevated TG (>100 mg/dl) and/or low HDL-C. Thus, identifying lipid abnormalities in

Table 42–11

**Barriers to Successful Implementation of Preventive Services**

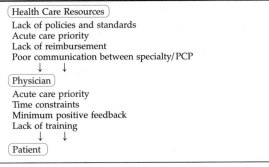

Health Care Resources
Lack of policies and standards
Acute care priority
Lack of reimbursement
Poor communication between specialty/PCP
↓     ↓
Physician
Acute care priority
Time constraints
Minimum positive feedback
Lack of training
↓     ↓
Patient

Modified from Pearson TA, McBride PE, Miller MH, Smith GC: 27th Bethesda Conference: Matching the intensity of risk factor management with the hazard for coronary disease events. Task Force 8. Organization of preventive cardiology service. J Am Coll Cardiol 1996;27:1039–1047.

hospitalized patients affords an exceptional opportunity to institute both hygienic and pharmacologic therapies. While such measures have gained increased acceptance in cardiovascular units, they may also be applicable to patients in surgical and neurologic units after CABG, femoropopliteal bypass surgery, or nonhemorrhagic cerebrovascular accidents. To facilitate transition between discharge instructions and follow-up appointments with the patient's primary care physician, it may be instructive to enclose a summary of the risk factors identified during the recent hospitalization and the therapies prescribed (Fig. 42–16). It would be useful to ensure that the 10 key measures are adopted and enforced (see Table 42–2). These measures may be instituted either during hospitalization or at preventive cardiology clinics for referred outpatients who have CAD or cardiovascular risk factors.

**UNIVERSITY OF MARYLAND SCHOOL OF MEDICINE**
**CENTER FOR PREVENTIVE CARDIOLOGY**
**22 SOUTH GREENE STREET, S3B06**
**BALTIMORE, MARYLAND 21201–1595**
**(410) 328-6299**

_____ ,1996

Dear Dr. _____ :

As you are aware, _____ was recently an inpatient in one of our cardiovascular units. On admission, the following risk factors were noted. The patient received the following cardioprotective medications upon discharge:

**RISK FACTORS**

| | |
| --- | --- |
| ____ | POSITIVE FAMILY HISTORY |
| ____ | HISTORY OF CIGARETTE SMOKING |
| ____ | ELEVATED LDL CHOLESTEROL |
| ____ | HIGH BOOD PRESSURE |
| ____ | DIABETES |
| ____ | LOW HDL |
| ____ | SEDENTARY LIFESTYLE |
| ____ | PREMATURE MENOPAUSE |

**MEDICATIONS**

____ ASA (CAD)
____ ACE INHIBITOR (CHF)
____ BETA-BLOCKER (POST-MI)
____ ESTROGEN REPLACEMENT THERAPY
____ LIPID-LOWERING THERAPY

(THESE VALUES ARE ___ /ARE NOT ___ POST MI. PLEASE RE-EVALUATE IN 8 WEEKS)

| | LDL | HDL | | TC:HDL | TG | AST | ALT | ALK.PHOS. |
| --- | --- | --- | --- | --- | --- | --- | --- | --- |
| | | Men | Women | | | | | |
| DESIRABLE | <100 | >45 | >50 | <4:1 | <200 | 10–59 | 21–72 | 38–126 |
| BORDERLINE | 101–130 | 40–45 | 45–50 | 4.1:5.4 | | | | |
| ABNORMAL | >130 | <40 | <45 | >5.5:1 | | | | |
| PATIENT'S VALUE | ____ | ____ | ____ | ____ | ____ | ____ | ____ | ____ |

The importance of risk factor modification was emphasized and the patient was informed that aggressive secondary preventive measures would be addressed in follow-up with you. We appreciate having had the opportunity to take care of this patient and if we can assist you in any way in the future regarding risk factor modification, please do not hesitate to contact us.

Sincerely,

Michael Miller, M.D., F.A.C.C.
Director, Preventive Cardiology
Assistant Professor of Medicine

**Figure 42–16** ■ Risk factor discharge form used at the University of Maryland Medical System.

Myriad manuals that cover a wide array of topics on cardiovascular prevention and that are endorsed by the AHA and ACC are now available to educate patients on cardiovascular disease and prevention. These will assuredly be enhanced by websites currently under development that are earmarked for informing allied-health professionals and the public of the continuing advances in this rapidly growing subspecialty.

# ■ REFERENCES

1. Connor WE, Hoak JC, Warner ED: The effects of fatty acids on blood coagulation and thrombosis. Thromb Diath Haemorrh Suppl 1965;17:89–102.
2. Dietschy JM: Dietary fatty acids and the regulation of plasma low density lipoprotein cholesterol concentrations. J Nutr 1998;128:444S–448S.
3. Mensink RP, Katan MB: Effect of dietary *trans* fatty acids on high-density and low-density lipoprotein cholesterol levels in healthy subjects. N Engl J Med 1990;323:439–445.
4. Zock PL, Mensink RP: dietary *trans*-fatty acids and serum lipoproteins in humans. Curr Opin Lipidol 1996;7:34–37.
5. Watts GF, Jackson P, Burke V, Lewis B: Dietary fatty acids and progression of coronary artery disease in men. Am J Clin Nutr 1996;64:202–209.
6. Willett WC, Stampfer MJ, Colditz GA: Intake of *trans* fatty acids and risk of coronary heart disease among women. Lancet 1993;341:581–585.
7. Lichtenstein AH: *Trans* fatty acids, plasma lipid levels and risk of developing cardiovascular disease. A statement for healthcare professionals from the American Heart Association. Circulation 1997;95:2588–2590.
8. Aviram M, Eias K: Dietary olive oil reduces low density lipoprotein uptake by macrophages and decreases the susceptibility of the lipoprotein to undergo lipid peroxidation. Ann Nutr Metab 1993;37:75–84.
9. de Lorgeril M, Renaud S, Marmelle N, et al: Mediterranean alpha-linolenic acid–rich diet in secondary prevention of coronary heart disease. Lancet 1994;343:1454–1459.
10. Garg A, Bantle JP, Henry RR, et al: Effects of varying carbohydrate content of diet in patients with non–insulin-dependent diabetes mellitus. JAMA 1994;271:1421–1428.
11. O'Byrne DJ, Knauft DA, Shireman RB: Low fat–monounsaturated rich diets containing high-oleic peanuts improve serum lipoprotein profiles. Lipids 1997;32:687–695.
12. Alderson LM, Hays KC, Nicolosi RJ: Peanut oil reduces diet-induced atherosclerosis in cynomolgus monkeys. Arteriosclerosis 1986;6:465–474.
13. Abbey M, Noakes M, Belling GB, Nestel P: Partial replacement of saturated fatty acids with almonds or walnuts lowers total plasma cholesterol and low density lipoprotein cholesterol. Am J Clin Nutr 1994;59:995–999.
14. Daviglus ML, Stamler J, Orencia AJ, et al: Fish consumption and the 30-year risk of fatal myocardial infarction. N Engl J Med 1997;336:1046–1053.
15. Albert CM, Hennekens CH, O'Donnell CH, et al: Fish consumption and risk of sudden cardiac death. JAMA 1998;279:23–28.
16. Hubbard JD, Inkeles S, Barnard RJ: Nathan Pritikin's heart. N Engl J Med 1985;313:52.
17. Ornish D, Brown SE, Scherwitz LW, et al: Can lifestyle changes reverse coronary heart disease? The Lifestyle Heart Trial. Lancet 1990;336:129–133.
18. Ornish D, Scherwitz LW, Billings JH, et al: Intensive lifestyle changes for reversal of coronary heart disease. JAMA 1998;280:2001–2007.
19. Watts GF, Lewis B, Brunt JNH, et al: Effects on coronary artery disease of lipid-lowering diet, or diet plus cholestyramine, in the St. Thomas' Atherosclerosis Regression Study (STARS). Lancet 1992;339:563–569.
20. Schuler G, Hambrecht R, Schlierf G, et al: Regular exercise and low-fat diet: Effects on progression of coronary artery disease. Circulation 1992;86:1–11.
21. Lichtenstein AH, Van Horn L: Very low fat diets. Circulation 1998;98:935–939.
22. Katan MB, Grundy SM, Willett WC: Should a low-fat, high carbohydrate diet be recommended for everyone? Beyond low fat diets. N Engl J Med 1997;337:563–566.
23. Kohlmeier L, Kark JD, Gomez-Gracia E, et al: Lycopene and myocardial infarction risk in the EURAMIC Study. Am J Epidemiol 1997;146(8):618–626.
24. Demrow HS, Slane PR, Folts JD: Administration of wine and grape juice inhibits in vivo platelet activity and thrombosis in stenosed canine coronary arteries. Circulation 1995;91:1182–1188.
25. Keli SO, Hertog MGL, Feskens EJM, Kromhout D: Dietary flavonoids, antioxidant vitamins and incidence of stroke. The Zutphen Study. Arch Intern Med 1996;154:637–642.
26. Anderson JW, Johnstone BM, Cook-Newell ME: Meta-analysis of the effects of soy protein intake on serum lipids. N Engl J Med 1995;333:276–282.

27. Hu FB, Stampfer MJ, Manson JE: Frequent nut consumption and risk of coronary heart disease in women: Prospective cohort study. Br Med J 1998;317:1341–1345.
28. Mosca L, Rubenfire M, Mandel C, et al: Antioxidant nutrient supplementation reduces the susceptibility of low-density lipoprotein to oxidation in patients with coronary artery disease. J Am Coll Cardiol 1997;30:392–399.
29. May J, Qu Z, Morrow J: Interaction of ascorbate and alpha-tocopherol in resealed human erythrocyte ghosts: Transmembrane electron transfer and protection from lipid peroxidation. J Biol Chem 1996;271:10577–10582.
30. Rodes J, Cote G, Lesperance J, et al: Prevention of restenosis after angioplasty in small coronary arteries with probucol. Circulation 1998;97:429–436.
31. Anonymous. Dietary supplementation with n-3 polyunsaturated fatty acids and vitamin E after myocardial infarction: Results of the GISSI-Prevenzione trial. Gruppo Italiano per lo Studio della Sopravvivenza nell'Infarto miocardico. Lancet 1999;354:447–455.
32. The Heart Outcomes Prevention Evaluation Study Investigators. Vitamin E supplementation and cardiovascular events in high-risk patients. N Engl J Med 2000;342:154–160.
33. Korpela H, Kumpulainen J, Jussila E, et al: Effect of selenium supplementation after acute myocardial infarction. Res Commun Chem Pathol Pharmacol 1989;65:249–252.
34. Roeback JR, Hla KM, Chambless LE, Fletcher RH: Effects of chromium supplementation on serum high-density lipoprotein cholesterol levels in men taking beta-blockers. A randomized, controlled trial. Ann Intern Med 1991;115:917–924.
35. Isaacsohn JL, Moser M, Stein EA, et al: Garlic powder and plasma lipids and lipoproteins. A multicenter, randomized, placebo-controlled trial. Arch Intern Med 1998;158:1189–1194.
36. Pietri S, Seguin JR, d'Arbigny P, et al: Ginkgo biloba extract (Egb 761) pretreatment limits free radical–induced oxidative stress in patients undergoing coronary bypass surgery. Cardiovasc Drugs Ther 1997;11(2):121–131.
37. Krieglstein J, Beck T, Seibert A: Influence of an extract of ginkgo biloba on cerebral blood flow and metabolism. Life Sci 1986;39(24):2327–2334.
38. Blume J, Kieser M, Holscher U: Placebo-controlled double-blind study of the effectiveness of *Ginkgo biloba* special extract Egb 761 in trained patients with intermittent claudication. Vasa 1996;25(3):265–274.
39. Chen X: Cardiovascular protection by ginsenosides and their nitric oxide releasing action. Clin Exp Pharmacol Physiol 1996;23(8):728–732.
40. Lee IM, Hsieh CC, Paffenbarger RS Jr: Exercise intensity and longevity in men: The Harvard Alumni Health Study. JAMA 1995;273(15):1179–1184.
41. Paffenberger RS Jr, Hyde RT, Wing AL, et al: The association of changes in physical activity level and other lifestyle characteristics with mortality among men. N Engl J Med 1993;328(8):538–545.
42. Byers T: Body weight and mortality. N Engl J Med 1995;333:723–724.
43. Leyva F, Godsland IF, Ghatei M, et al: Hyperleptinemia as a component of a metabolic syndrome of cardiovascular risk. Arterioscler Thromb Vasc Biol 1998;18:928–933.
44. Frosst P, Blom HJ, Milos R, et al: A candidate genetic risk factor for vascular disease: A common mutation in methylenetetrahydrofolate reductase. Nat Genet 1995;10:111–113.
45. Ma J, Stampfer MJ, Hennekens CH, et al: Methylenetetrahydrofolate reductase polymorphism, plasma folate, homocysteine and risk of myocardial infarction in U.S. physicians. Circulation 1996;94:2410–2416.
46. Graham IM, Daly LE, Refsum HM, et al: Plasma homocysteine as a risk factor for vascular disease: The European Concerted Action Project. JAMA 1997;277:1775–1781.
47. Fryer RH, Wilson BD, Gubler DB, et al: Homocysteine, a risk factor for premature vascular disease and thrombosis, induces tissue factor activity in endothelial cells. Arterioscler Thromb 1993;13:327–333.
48. Ridker PM, Cushman M, Stampfer MJ, et al: Inflammation, aspirin, and the risk of cardiovascular disease in apparently healthy men. N Engl J Med 1997;336:973–979.
49. Ridker PM, Cushman M, Stampfer MJ, et al: Plasma concentration of C-reactive protein and risk of developing peripheral vascular disease. Circulation 1998;97:425–428.
50. Ridker PM, Rifai N, Pfeffer MA, Sackie F, Braunwald E for the Cholesterol and Recurrent Events (CARE) Investigators. Long-term effects of pravastatin on plasma concentration of C-reative protein. Circulation 1999;100:230–235.
51. Gupta S, Leatham EW, Carrington D, et al: Elevated *Chlamydia pneumoniae* antibodies, cardiovascular events, and azithromycin in male survivors of myocardial infarction. Circulation 1997;96:404–407.
52. Yeung AC, Vekshtein VI, Krantz DS, et al: The effect of atherosclerosis on the vasomotor responses of coronary arteries to mental stress. N Engl J Med 1991;325:1551–1556.
53. Jain D, Shaker SM, Burg M, et al: Effects of mental stress on left ventricular and peripheral vascular performance in patients with coronary artery disease. J Am Coll Cardiol 1998;31:1314–1322.
54. The Heart Outcomes Prevention Evaluation Study Investigators. Effects of an angiotensin-converting-enzyme inhibitor, ramipril, on cardiovascular events in high-risk patients. N Engl J Med 2000;342:145–153.

# ▪ RECOMMENDED READING

Kris-Etherton PM, Krummel D, Russell ME, et al: National Cholesterol Education Program. The effect of diet on plasma lipids, lipoproteins, and coronary heart disease. J Am Diet Assoc 1988;88:1373–1400.

Ascherio A, Hennekens CH, Buring JE, et al: *Trans* fatty acid intake and risk of myocardial infarction. Circulation 1994;89:94–101.

Keys A, Menotti A, Aravanis C, et al: The Seven Countries Study; 2289 deaths in 15 years. J Prevent Med 1984;13:141–154.

Ferro-Luzzi A, Ghiselli A: Protective aspects of the Mediterranean diet. *In* Zappia V (ed): Advances in Nutrition and Cancer. New York: Plenum, 1993.

Harris WS: Fish oils and plasma lipid and lipoprotein metabolism in humans: A critical review. J Lipid Res 1989;30:785-N807.

Hertog MGL, Feskens EJM, Hollman PCH, et al: Dietary antioxidant flavonoids and risk of coronary heart disease: The Zutphen Elderly Study. Lancet 1993;342:1007–1011.

Gaziano JM: Antioxidants in cardiovascular disease. Randomized trials. Nutrition 1996;12:583–588.

Bijnen FCH, Caspersen CJ, Feskens EJM, et al: Physical activity and 10-year mortality from cardiovascular diseases and all causes. Arch Intern Med 1998;158:1499–1505.

Lee IM, Paffenbarger RS: Physical activity and stroke incidence: The Harvard Alumni Health Study. Stroke 1998;29:2049–2054.

Mayer EM, Jacobsen DW, Robinson K: Homocysteine and coronary atherosclerosis. J Am Coll Cardiol 1996;27:517–527.

Danesh J, Collins R, Peto R: Chronic infections and coronary heart disease: Is there a link? Lancet 1997;350:430–436.

Blumenthal JA, Jiang W, Waugh RA, et al: Mental stress–induced ischemia and ambulatory ischemia during daily life: Association and hemodynamic features. Circulation 1995;92:2102–2108.

Tisdale JE: Antiplatelet therapy in coronary artery disease: Review and update of efficacy studies. Am J Health Syst Pharm 1998;55:S8–S16.

Pfeffer MA, Braunwald E, Moye LA, et al: Effect of captopril on mortality and morbidity in patients with left ventricular dysfunction after myocardial infarction. Results of the Survival and Ventricular Enlargement Trial. N Engl J Med 1992;327:669–677.

Beta-blocker Heart Attack Trial Research Group: A randomized trial or propranolol in patients with acute myocardial infarction. JAMA 1982;247:1707–1714.

Hulley S, Grady D, Bush T, et al: Randomized trial of estrogen plus progestin for secondary prevention of coronary heart disease in postmenopausal women. Heart and Estrogen/Progestin Replacement Study (HERS) Research Group. JAMA 1998;280:605–613.

# Chapter 43

# Peripheral Vascular Disease

*Jonathan L. Halperin*

The most widely recognized peripheral vascular disease in adults *is obstructive atherosclerosis of the extremities.* The traditional term *arteriosclerosis obliterans* distinguishes the development of obstructive lesions from normal aging by which the arteries increase in diameter, rigidity, and calcium content.[1] The disease was defined in 1958 by the World Health Organization as a "variable combination of changes of the intima or arteries (as distinguished from arterioles) consisting of the focal accumulation of lipids, complex carbohydrates, blood and blood products, fibrous tissue and calcium deposits, and associated with medial changes."[2]

## ■ EPIDEMIOLOGY

By the time symptoms of obstructive arterial disease develop, at least 50% narrowing of the vascular lumen has occurred, with morbidity and mortality related to manifestations of coronary or cerebrovascular insufficiency. Based on 26-year longitudinal surveillance of the Framingham Heart Study cohort of 5209 subjects, the annual incidence of symptomatic ischemic arterial obstructive disease was 0.26% for men and 0.12% for women.[3] The incidence increased with age until age 75 years, with about a twofold male predominance at all ages (Fig. 43–1). The peak incidence of symptomatic limb arterial obstructive disease occurred in men in the sixth and seventh decades of life. Fewer than 10% of nondiabetic patients younger than 60 years were women; beyond menopause, the incidence in women rose quickly toward that in men. Lower extremity vascular disease causes considerable morbidity among women, particularly those post menopause. In a cross-sectional study enrolling 1601 healthy elderly women (mean age, 71 years; range, 65–93 years), the prevalence of lower extremity arterial disease assessed by ankle/brachial index ranged from 2.9% in those age 65 to 69 years to 15.5% in those age 80 years or older.[4] Approximately 20% of those with disease had symptoms of claudication.

The prevalence of pathophysiologic arterial obstructive disease exceeds that of symptomatic ischemia.[5] Using the ankle/arm pressure index for detection, unselected populations between ages 25 and 65 years demonstrated a 0.7% incidence of obstructive arterial disease in women and 1.3% in men, but prevalence depends on the threshold pressure index selected.[6] The prevalence of asymptomatic atherosclerosis is highest in elderly patients,[7] who frequently develop gangrene as the initial symptom because coexisting conditions limit ambulation. In an elderly nursing home population, severe obstructive arterial disease (ankle/arm index < 0.7) was present in approximately 50% and predicted increased mortality compared with patients without signs of this disease.[8] Among patients age 90 years or older, one of the most common surgical operations is lower extremity amputation for limb arterial disease or gangrene.

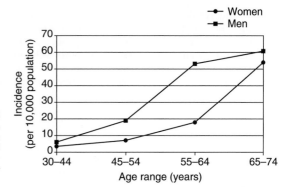

**Figure 43–1** ■ Age-specific annual incidence: intermittent claudication. (Adapted from Kannel WB, Skinner JJ, Schwartz MJ, Shuntleff D: Intermittent claudication, incidence in the Framingham Study. Circulation 1970;41:875–883.)

## Risk Factors

Like other manifestations of atherosclerosis, the prevalence of peripheral arterial disease is related to hypertension, hypercholesterolemia, diabetes mellitus, and tobacco smoking, which modify the effects of age, gender, and heredity. It is difficult to separate data pertaining to atherosclerotic disease in the peripheral circulation from observations of coronary artery disease, but there is little reason to suspect substantial difference on the basis of the anatomic site of involvement.[3] Specific risk factors appear additive, with some interaction, and better predict relative risk than absolute risk. Overall, a profile made up of the major cardiovascular risk factors correlates more closely with intermittent claudication than with clinical manifestations of coronary artery disease.

The incidence of claudication in patients with serum cholesterol levels exceeding 260 mg/dl averages more than twice that in those without lipid elevations. Conversely, the incidence of hyperlipoproteinemia in patients with limb arterial disease ranges in various studies from 31% to 57%.[9]

Peripheral atherosclerosis develops more commonly in diabetic patients, with a predilection for the tibial and peroneal arteries between the knees and ankles, for which revascularization procedures are more difficult. The incidence of femoropopliteal arterial obstructive disease is similar to that in the nondiabetic population, and aortoiliac occlusive disease may actually occur less frequently in diabetic persons. Diabetes raises the risk of ischemic gangrene 20-fold and that of surgical amputation 4-fold.[10] Coexisting sensory and autonomic neuropathy, lack of reflex hyperemia, loss of pain sensation, and arteriovenous shunting contribute to ischemic complications in diabetic individuals.

The incidence of atherosclerotic disease and its coronary and cerebral complications is increased in hypertensive patients. Autopsy studies demonstrate more extensive atherosclerosis of the aortoiliac arteries in hypertensive men than age-matched normotensive controls, and this difference is more widespread along the course of the arterial tree in women. Limb arterial obstructive disease occurs twice as frequently as coronary artery disease among hypertensive individuals.

The Framingham Heart Study found a relationship between the number of cigarettes smoked and the incidence of intermittent claudication,[11] and multivariate analysis finds tobacco smoking the strongest single risk factor for development of symptomatic obstructive arterial disease. Intermittent claudication is twice as common in smokers as nonsmokers, and in males with symptomatic atherosclerotic disease of the limb vessels, the majority report smoking cigarettes at the onset of the clinical phase of the disease. Seventy-three to 90% of patients with limb arterial disease are smokers, to the extent that it is distinctly rare to encounter a young woman who has the disease but who does not smoke cigarettes. Pathophysiologic mechanisms involve vasoconstriction, lipid metabolism, and thrombogenicity.[12]

Hereditary disorders associated with ischemic complications in the limbs include homocystinuria, oxalosis, inhibitors of von Willebrand factor, and inherited states associated with increased thrombogenicity, although the latter more often cause venous than arterial disease.

## ■ HISTOPATHOLOGY

Histopathologically, peripheral arteriosclerosis obliterans is identical to atherosclerosis that affects the aorta and its branches, including the coronary, visceral, cervical, and cerebral arteries. The basic lesion is the atherosclerotic plaque that produces *localized stenosis* of the lumen with or without areas of complete *arterial occlusion*. Deposition of thrombus and subsequently progressive fibrosis occur in eccentric layers. Fragmentation of the internal elastic lamina typically occurs, and areas of intraplaque hemorrhage and calcification characterize the advanced lesion.

Segmental lesions usually produce stenosis or occlusion of large and medium-sized arteries. After the thoracoabdominal aorta, the coronary arteries are most commonly affected, followed by the iliofemoral, carotid, renal, mesenteric, vertebrobasilar, tibial-peroneal, subclavian, brachial, radial, and ulnar arteries. Smaller arteries of the digits are generally spared even in advanced cases, although these may become obstructed by thrombus when there is proximal atherosclerotic disease. Patients with intermittent claudication may have disease at many arterial levels. In about 80% of cases, *femoropopliteal* disease is present; approximately 30% of symptomatic patients have lesions at the *aortoiliac* level, and as many as 40% have *tibial-peroneal* obstruction. Involvement of the distal vessels is most frequent in diabetic persons and the elderly.

## ■ NATURAL HISTORY AND PROGNOSIS

The clinical course of this disease varies markedly, with abrupt vascular occlusion in some cases and more favorable outcomes in others. In patients with aorto-iliac disease, symptoms evolve gradually, and a copious collateral circulation tends to develop with a generally favorable prognosis in terms of limb outcome. Patients with distal tibial-peroneal disease have a distinctly poorer outcome, undergoing amputation at annual rate of 1.4%.[13]

Followed without surgical intervention, yearly mortality averages more than 5%, with death usually due to coronary or cerebral vascular disease. In the Framingham Heart Study, the relative mortality risk imposed by symptomatic peripheral arterial disease without cardiovascular comorbidity was 1.3 for men and 2.1 for women; total mortality ratios were 2.2 and 4.1, respectively. The rate of coronary artery disease, defined angiographically in patients with severely symptomatic arterial obstructive disease as greater than 70% stenosis of at least one coronary vessel, was nearly 90%; about 50% had decreased left ventricular function,[14] raising the risk of myocardial infarction, ischemic stroke, and vascular death five- to sixfold (Fig. 43–2).[15]

Remissions of intermittent claudication are common. Among patients in the Framingham Study monitored for 4 or more years from onset of symptoms, 45% became asymptomatic.[16] In nondiabetic patients with obstructive disease of the superficial femoral artery at the Mayo Clinic, 24% improved and 69% had no progression of symptoms; clinical deterioration occurred in only 7%.[17, 18]

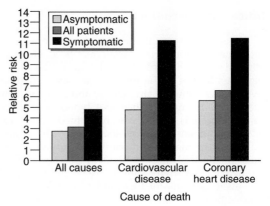

**Figure 43–2** ■ Relative risk of death in patients with peripheral arterial disease (PAD) compared with patients without PAD: All-cause mortality, cardiovascular, and coronary mortality are shown for asymptomatic, symptomatic, and all patients. (Adapted from Criqui MH, Langer RD, Fronck A, et al: Mortality over a period of 10 years in patients with peripheral arterial disease. N Engl J Med 1992;326:381–386.)

## ■ CLINICAL PRESENTATION

### Intermittent Claudication

The cardinal symptom of obstructive arterial disease in the lower extremities is *intermittent claudication.* Patients typically describe calf pain, because the gastrocnemius musculature has the greatest oxygen consumption of any muscle group in the leg during ambulation. Some patients report aching, heaviness, fatigue, or numbness when walking, but distress is usually relieved within a few minutes of rest. Ischemic claudication must be distinguished from other conditions producing exertional calf pain (Table 43–1). Diabetic patients with distal tibial or peroneal arterial obstruction may describe ankle or foot pain while walking; this may be difficult to distinguish from ischemic neuropathy. With proximal aortoiliac disease, thigh, hip, or buttock claudication or low back pain may develop while walking, usually preceded by calf pain. Bilateral high claudication accompanying impotence and global atrophy of the lower extremities characterizes the *Leriche syndrome.*

Many factors contribute to leg discomfort during exercise in patients with arterial occlusive disease. Hemodynamically significant arterial stenosis may reduce pressure and flow minimally at rest, but the pressure gradient across the stenosis increases during exercise. Extravascular compression by exercising muscle and lack of flow-mediated vasodilatation in atherosclerotic vessels may further blunt limb blood flow. Discomfort may be related to activation of local chemoreceptors due to accumulation of lactate or other metabolites.

Initial and absolute claudication thresholds are best expressed in terms of pace and incline. Ambient environmental conditions such as temperature and wind, training, and recruitment of muscle groups in less ischemic zones all influence walking capacity and have therapeutic implications in maintaining overall cardiovascular conditioning.

Table 43–1

**Differential Diagnosis of Exertional Calf Pain**

| | |
|---|---|
| Obstructive arterial disease | Venous claudication |
| Neurogenic pseudoclaudication | Muscular disorders |

## Critical Limb Ischemia

When the minimal nutritional requirements of resting skin, muscle, nerves, and bone are not met, *ischemic rest pain, ulceration,* and *gangrene* ensue and the prognosis is poor. Clinically, ischemia in the limb at rest is manifested first in the cutaneous tissues of the foot, where factors regulating perfusion differ from those governing calf muscle circulation, and reflexive sympathetically mediated vasoconstrictor activity may reduce foot blood flow even under conditions of ischemia. Tissue necrosis is typically accompanied by severe pain, worse at night with limb elevation and improved on standing. With advanced neuropathy, even ulceration and gangrene may occur painlessly, although patients may have a tendency to maintain the limb in a dependent position. Other symptoms of ischemia at rest include cold sensitivity, muscle weakness, joint stiffness, and contracture.

Severe ischemia of this kind usually demands angiographic examination and therapeutic intervention by percutaneous angioplasty or surgical revascularization. When these are not feasible, gangrene commonly ensues, leading to amputation, although remission has been described even at this advanced stage of disease. Critical limb ischemia results in some 150,000 amputations annually in the United States, with perioperative mortality rates of 5% to 10% for below-knee and up to 50% for above-knee amputation because of comorbid conditions.

## Acute Arterial Occlusion

The major causes of acute arterial occlusion are trauma, arterial thrombosis, and arterial embolism. Traumatic occlusion is usually associated with external compression, transection, or laceration. Increasingly, the clinical spectrum of traumatic arterial occlusive disease includes iatrogenic cases, most commonly associated with indwelling intravascular diagnostic or therapeutic cannulation. Atraumatic acute arterial occlusion includes systemic embolism, usually cardiogenic but occasionally derived from mural thrombi within aneurysms of the aorta, and thrombosis superimposed on chronic atherosclerosis or other intrinsic arterial disease. Systemic disorders of coagulation associated with arterial thrombosis include those associated with anticardiolipin antibodies, circulating lupus anticoagulants, and heparin-associated thrombocytopenia.

## Arterial Embolism

Nearly 85% of systemic arterial emboli arise from thrombi in the chambers of the left side of the heart. Atrial fibrillation accounts for about half the cases, and ventricular thrombi for most of the remainder. Infective endocarditis (particularly fungal), cardiac tumors, invasive lesions of the pulmonary venous system, mural thrombi within aortic aneurysms, ulcerated proximal atherosclerotic lesions, vascular grafts, arteritis, and traumatic arterial lesions represent additional sources.

Microembolism of atherosclerotic debris consisting of lipid and thrombotic material may originate in the aorta or more distal arteries, leading to occlusion of small distal limb arteries. The source may involve either aneurysmal disease or irregular ulceration of diffusely atherosclerotic vessels that are not dilated, and transesophageal echocardiography and magnetic resonance imaging (MRI) have identified such lesions.[19] The ischemic syndrome is often labeled the "blue toe syndrome," characterized by unilaterally or bilaterally painful, cyanotic toes in the presence of palpable pedal pulses. The lateral and plantar aspects of the feet are frequently involved, with livedo reticularis and petechiae on feet and legs. The violaceous parts generally blanch with pressure, and the surrounding skin may appear normally perfused. Calf pain and gastrocnemius muscle tenderness are often present as a result of embolic occlusion of small intramuscular vessels. Fever, eosinophilia, and acceleration of the erythrocyte sedimentation rate may signal an inflammatory reaction to microembolization, which may be difficult to distinguish from acute vasculitis.

*Atheroembolism* implies a physically unstable proximal atherosclerotic lesion and a risk of acute thrombotic arterial occlusion. Antithrombotic therapy should be given in the form of platelet inhibitor or anticoagulant medication. Although angioplasty has been reported effective, the intravascular catheterization may also provoke embolic phenomena, and the most definitive approach is to remove or exclude the source from the circulation. When the lower limbs are ischemic, this often requires aortobifemoral bypass, but an alternative is axillobifemoral extraanatomic bypass with ligation of the external iliac arteries proximal to the point of anastomosis. When renal emboli occur, more proximal aortic reconstruction may be necessary, the risks of which are considerable, particularly when severe atherosclerosis of the entire length of the aorta is accompanied by a malignant syndrome of cerebral, mesenteric, and limb ischemia.

# ■ DIFFERENTIAL DIAGNOSIS

Exertional calf pain may be produced by both nonatherosclerotic arterial obstructive diseases and conditions unrelated to the arterial circulation (Table 43–2). Among the latter are *neurogenic pseudoclaudication,* a form of lumbosacral radiculopathy in which ambulation provokes nerve root irritation with pain referred to the posterior aspect of the lower extremity. Pain when walking just a few steps without progression to ischemia at rest, relief on bending forward at the waist, and symptoms reproduced by straight leg raising point to this diagnosis whether or not there is an arterial pulse deficit.

*Venous claudication* illustrates the role of venous pressure as a factor in regional circulatory resistance. Exertional leg pain (especially near the medial aspect of the leg above the ankle) results from insufficiency of the musculovenous pumping mechanism that normally causes distal venous pressure to fall during ambulation. Venous hypertension contributes to local vascular resistance, resulting in exertional ischemia. Venous claudication is uncommon, and concomitant arterial insufficiency is usually present.

In patients with *McArdle syndrome,* skeletal muscle metabolites accumulate owing to phosphorylase deficiency, evoking exercise intolerance in the absence of an anatomic substrate producing ischemia. Similar metabolites, including but not limited to lactic acid, may be responsible for the pain of intermittent claudication due to obstructive arterial disease.

Obstructive arterial diseases other than atherosclerosis that may produce intermittent claudication include *thromboangiitis obliterans* (*Buerger disease*) and other arteritides, arterial entrapment syndromes (most commonly caused by the gastrocnemius muscles), fibromuscular hyperplasia, adventitial cysts and tumors, and

Table 43–2

**Differential Diagnosis of Obstructive Arterial Disease**

| | |
|---|---|
| Arteriosclerosis obliterans | Vasculitis |
| Thrombosis and embolism | Fibromuscular dysplasia |
| Vascular entrapment or compression | Adventitial cysts and tumors |

extravascular compressive lesions. The most prevalent of these is *fibromuscular dysplasia,* a hyperplastic disorder that primarily involves medium-sized and small arteries, usually affecting white females. The renal and carotid arteries are most frequently involved, but the disorder has also been observed in the mesenteric, coronary, subclavian, and iliac arteries. Three histologic varieties have been delineated on the basis of which layer of the arterial wall displays the predominant features of the process, with medial fibroplasia most common. Medial fibroplasia is characterized angiographically by a string-of-beads appearance, in which numerous thickened fibromuscular ridges alternate with areas in which the arterial wall is thin. The cause is unknown, but pathogenic concepts include influence of female sex hormones, vascular microtrauma, and genetic factors. The natural history in limb arteries is less well defined than in the renal and carotid arteries, where progression of stenosis occurs over 5 years in a third of cases but where regression has occasionally been observed. Clinical manifestations are similar to those of atherosclerosis, with intermittent claudication, rest pain, coldness and cyanosis of the limb, and even microembolism. In addition to surgical reconstruction, percutaneous angioplasty has been used for management of fibromuscular dysplasia. Balloon dilation with or without intravascular stenting has been successfully accomplished with relatively low inflation pressures.

Buerger disease (thromboangiitis obliterans) is a nonatherosclerotic segmental inflammatory obliterative disease that most commonly affects the small and medium-sized arteries and veins in both upper and lower extremities. Although in the past the disease was typically confined to young males, up to a third of cases in recently reported series occurred in women. Most patients are heavy users of tobacco products, usually cigarettes, and antigenic cross-reactivity between type III vascular collagen and a component of tobacco smoke has been considered etiologically important. The pathologic findings are distinctive and distinguish this disorder from other arterial occlusive diseases. Successful therapy is possible only with abstinence from tobacco.

## Physical Findings

*Trophic signs* of chronic limb ischemia include subcutaneous atrophy, brittle toenails, hair loss, pallor, coolness, or dependent rubor (Table 43–3). Other visible changes reflect sympathetic denervation and sensorimotor neuropathy. Severe ischemia produces petechiae, regional edema, tenderness, ulceration, or gangrene. The level of arterial obstruction may be judged by palpation of the femoral, popliteal, posterior tibial, and dorsalis pedis pulses. Vascular bruits denote turbulent flow but do not reflect the severity of stenosis.

Cutaneous perfusion may be estimated by the color and temperature of the feet during elevation above heart level at rest and after exercise. The rate of hyperemic color return in the foot and venous filling on dependence reflect collat-

Table 43–3

**Trophic Signs of Ischemia in Patients with
Peripheral Arterial Disease of the Extremities**

| Chronic arterial obstructive disease | Acute ischemia |
|---|---|
| Hair loss | Ulceration |
| Subcutaneous atrophy | Petechiae |
| Thickened nails | Calf tenderness |
| Dependent rubor | Dependent edema |

eral perfusion (Table 43–4). When this does not meet minimal tissue perfusion requirements, cutaneous ulceration is frequent. *Arterial ulcers* caused by arterial disease are often as small as 3 to 5 mm in diameter, with irregular borders and a pale base. They usually involve the tips of the toes or the heel of the foot and are typically painful on elevation and most bothersome at night. The clinical course of these ulcers is often one of rapid progression to more extensive gangrene. *Vasospasm* may produce cutaneous ischemia leading to ulceration of the digits in patients with *Raynaud phenomenon* or chronic *pernio*. Diabetic patients, who are prone to combined peripheral sensory neuropathy and ischemic disease, often develop deep *neurotrophic ulcers* due to trauma or pressure on the plantar surface. In patients with severe hypertension, painful *Hines ulcers* related to arteriolar obliteration tend to occur near the lateral malleoli. *Vasculitic ulcers* are also attributed to arteriolar thickening, with or without superimposed thrombosis. Hematologic disorders such as the hemoglobinopathies, hereditary spherocytosis, dysproteinemias, and myeloproliferative diseases may be associated with cutaneous infarction, venous thrombosis, and microvascular occlusion. *Chronic venous stasis* usually produces indolent or recurrent ulceration near the medial malleoli. These ulcers are more painful during dependence, which helps distinguish them from ulcers due to arterial disease. A host of systemic diseases may also be associated with cutaneous ulceration in the lower extremities, such as Kaposi sarcoma and other tumors, syphilitic chancre and gummas, tuberculous lupus vulgaris, and pyoderma gangrenosum. Factitious and traumatic ulcers may also mimic those induced by obstructive arterial disease.[20]

## Ancillary Diagnostic Modalities

*Doppler sphygmomanometry* has become part of the initial bedside vascular examination for determination of the ankle/brachial systolic blood pressure index. Normally, systolic arterial pressure at the ankle exceeds that over the brachial artery. An ankle/arm systolic pressure ratio (*ankle/brachial index*) less than unity (in practice, 0.95) at rest indicates hemodynamically significant arterial obstruction proximal to the pneumatic leg cuff. Advanced, calcific atherosclerosis of vessels beneath the cuff resists compression, producing overestimation of regional perfusion pressure. This constitutes the major limitation of sphygmomanometry and may lead to falsely elevated ankle/brachial pressure indices, in patients with diabetes mellitus or chronic renal failure.

Systolic pressure and ankle/brachial index may be normal at rest despite hemodynamically significant arterial stenosis yet may decline after calf muscle exercise. Postexercise systolic pressure readings less than 90 mm Hg are typical of patients with intermittent claudication, and values less than 60 mm Hg are typical of ulcerative ischemia at rest.[21]

Table 43–4

**Elevation and Dependence Tests in the Evaluation of Acral Ischemia**

|  | Color Return | Venous Filling |
|---|---|---|
|  | (seconds) |  |
| Normal | 10 | 10–15 |
| Adequate collaterals | 15–25 | 15–30 |
| Severe ischemia | >35 | >40 |

## ■ NONINVASIVE LABORATORY EVALUATION

### Segmental Pressure Measurement

To localize segmental arterial lesions, pneumatic cuffs are applied to determine systolic pressure at several levels, on the basis of the principle that obstruction is proximal to the level at which pressure drops. *Segmental pressure measurements* and *pulse volume recordings* are subject to the same limitations as Doppler sphygmomanometry. In general, ankle/arm systolic pressure indices exceeding 0.85 may occur in individuals with obstructive disease in the absence of symptoms; values between 0.5 and 0.8 are typical at rest in patients with intermittent claudication, and values less than 0.5 are frequently associated with ischemic rest pain, ulceration, and gangrene threatening the viability of the limb.

The amplitude of the pulse volume wave reflects local arterial pressure, vascular wall compliance, the number of arterial vessels beneath the cuff, and the severity of atherosclerotic disease. The normal pulse is characterized by a sharp systolic upstroke, which rises rapidly to a peak and then drops off more slowly toward the baseline. The downslope curves toward the baseline and usually contains a dicrotic notch and secondary wave about midway between the peak and the baseline. The pulse recorded distal to an arterial obstruction is more rounded, and the anacrotic slope is reduced. The crest is delayed, the catacrotic limb descends more gradually, and the dicrotic wave is lost.

Segmental compression cuffs combined with the Doppler ultrasound device, *photoplethysmograph,* or other flow detector are subject to error related to arterial rigidity, but the pulse volume recorder has the advantage of revealing distortions in pulse wave contour even in patients with vascular calcification. The pulse waveforms appear depressed and altered even when arteries are noncompressible. The *pulsatility index,* representing the ratio of pulse amplitude to mean volume obtained by integration of the deflection, is abnormally low even when systolic pressure readings are falsely elevated. The value of these observations is enhanced by exercise testing, which provides a quantitative estimate of functional capacity and distinguishes disorders producing similar symptoms, because the ankle/brachial pressure index declines after exercise in those with arterial obstructive disease.

### Ultrasound Velocity Spectroscopy and Imaging

*Doppler velocity analysis* of normal arteries reveals a triphasic signal. Rapid acceleration to peak systolic velocity occurs along a narrow frequency spectrum, end-systolic deceleration culminates in protodiastolic flow reversal, and antegrade flow resumes in mid-diastole. Peak systolic velocities diminish with advancing age. Arterial obstruction proximal to the probe transforms the waveform by loss of the reversed flow component and attenuation of all parts of the spectrum with delayed upstroke and decreased amplitude.

*Duplex ultrasound scanning* combines B-mode and pulsed Doppler ultrasound analysis to examine arterial configuration and localized velocity information at sites of stenosis. Flow through a stenosis is accelerated, and turbulence is detected as spectral broadening of the velocities instead of the narrow band seen with normal flow. Microprocessor-based systems for calculation of blood cell velocities allow accurate estimation of instantaneous pressure gradients and degrees of stenosis.[22] Duplex scanning is more sensitive and specific than segmental blood pressure measurements for detection of restenosis, even before pressure drops.

The clinical vascular noninvasive laboratory is subject to misconceptions that predispose to misuse. Among these are that findings can establish indications for specific therapeutic procedures, because clinical decisions are best based on symptoms and the physical appearance of the limb. Laboratory measures reflect the severity of ischemia, the contribution of obstructive arterial factors to symptoms, and the hemodynamic significance of lesions at various points, and have become important in clinical practice (Table 43–5).

## ■ VASCULAR IMAGING

### Nuclear Magnetic Resonance

*Magnetic resonance (MR) angiography* obviates arterial catheterization and iodinated contrast material and may identify runoff vessels not visualized by conventional angiography.[23] MRI methods are currently emerging to characterize the arterial wall and atherosclerotic lesions. In the magnetic field, water molecules are excited by a radiofrequency (RF) pulse generating a secondary RF signal that is detected and measured digitally by the MR device and displayed as images that distinguish fine details of tissue structure and composition. Plaque dimensions and composition are assessed using T1, proton density, and T2-weighted images, and techniques of real-time, cine MR angiography are under development.

### Contrast Angiography

The diagnosis of arterial obstructive disease does not generally require invasive techniques, and most patients with intermittent claudication do not need angiographic examination. *Contrast angiography* is usually indicated for mapping of the extent and location of arterial pathology before a revascularization procedure. Such testing should be reserved for patients in whom the diagnosis is in doubt or as a prelude to vascular intervention when conservative approaches are not satisfactory. Aortic injection of contrast material is indicated in patients with aortoiliac occlusive disease and can be accomplished either by the *retrograde transfemoral, translumbar,* or *transaxillary* approach. Aortic injection of contrast material provides visualization of the aorta and proximal limb vessels, but definition of the circulation distal to the popliteal trifurcations may be compromised by the dilution of proximally injected contrast. In patients with femoropopliteal obstructive disease, antegrade or retrograde transfemoral angiography often can be confined to the involved extremity with the definition of the distal vasculature.

Computer-enhanced *digital subtraction angiography* may be useful in patients with localized stenosis either to minimize the volume of contrast material injected or to improve image resolution. The technique may be used with either intravenous or intraarterial contrast injection, especially for postoperative examination of anastomotic segments, but is not effective as a means of visualizing large regions of the arterial tree.

Table 43–5

**Noninvasive Laboratory Evaluation of Peripheral Arterial Disease**

| | |
|---|---|
| Doppler sphygmomanometry | Venous-occlusion plethysmography |
| Segmental pressure measurement | Radionuclide mapping |
| Pulse volume recording | Duplex ultrasound imaging |

## Intravascular Angioscopy and Ultrasound

Fiberoptic *angioscopy* allows direct visualization of the arterial intima using a percutaneous catheter. The method has been coupled with other interventional devices to enhance the matching of therapeutic techniques with lesion morphology, but results are not yet sufficient to fully define the role of this form of indirect endoluminal vascular imaging. Catheter-mounted cardiovascular ultrasound transducer crystals have made possible *intravascular ultrasound imaging*. Areas of plaque narrowing and calcification are readily identified, and the technique is often used in conjunction with angioplasty, atherectomy, and intravascular stenting to assess the impact of these interventions on the arterial wall and associated atheromatous lesions.

## ■ MEDICAL THERAPY

The principles of patient care involve measures directed at protection of affected tissues, preservation of functional capacity, avoidance of disease progression or acute arterial thrombosis, and improvement of blood flow. These principles can be categorized as local measures, treatment of associated factors, exercise training, avoidance of vasoconstrictor stimuli, and drug therapy.

*Local measures* to reduce skin breakdown and infection are particularly important in diabetic persons and in patients with severe perfusion impairment. The feet should be kept clean. Moisturizing cream applied to prevent fissuring must be selected to avoid irritant effects. Well-fitted shoes reduce the risk of pressure-induced necrosis, and absorbent fiber stockings are recommended. The skin of the feet should be inspected frequently so minor abrasions may be promptly tended. Elastic support stockings may restrict cutaneous blood flow and should be avoided. In patients with ischemia at rest, conservative measures include positioning the affected limb below heart level to increase oxygen tension in ischemic tissues. To enhance healing, the limb should be kept horizontal when edema is present. The heels should be protected from pressure against the bed sheets with sheepskin padding. Blankets should be cradled over a footboard to reduce friction. Separation of the toes with cotton helps protect against intertriginous friction. Unless purulence is present, dryness is preferred to soaks except for intermittent cleansing. Gentle warmth is recommended to minimize vasoconstriction; excessive heat is to be avoided. Antimicrobial treatment of fungal onycholysis reduces skin breakdown and superinfection. Topical medicaments should be used cautiously to avoid inflammatory reactions. Open sores should be cultured; roentgenograms may detect osteomyelitis, but antibiotic medication is less effective when delivery to ischemic tissue is impaired. Passive physical therapy may proceed to progressive weight bearing and ambulation. Attention is given to foot care, and properly fitted, nonconstrictive shoes and soft cotton stockings should be worn.

## Risk Factor Modification

Modification of associated risk factors may reduce the likelihood of progression of atherosclerotic disease, as discussed earlier in this chapter. Accordingly, attention should be directed toward reduction of hyperlipidemia, control of hypertension, cessation of cigarette smoking, weight reduction in instances of obesity, and treatment of diabetes. Lipid-lowering therapy with hydroxymethylglutaryl coenzyme A reductase inhibitors has favorable effects in patients with intermittent claudication.[24] Aggressive control of blood glucose reduces the incidence of microvascular complications, but data related to the efficacy of this strategy on the progression and complications of peripheral atherosclerosis are insufficient.[25] Meta-analysis has shown approximately 40% reduction in the risk of stroke and 10% to 15% reduction in the risk of myocardial infarction with antihypertensive treatment, but specific effects of therapy on peripheral manifestations of atherosclerosis have not been quantified.[26] Clinical prognosis for those with arterial obstructive disease of the extremities also seems related to tobacco use. Observation of smokers with intermittent claudication found that 11% of those who continued to smoke required amputation, whereas this fate befell none of those who quit.[27] Over 10 years, smoking cessation also significantly reduced the risk of myocardial infarction. Hyperhomocystinemia is associated with peripheral atherosclerosis, and treatment with B-complex vitamins including folic acid, pyridoxine, and cyanocobalamin reduces homocysteine levels; however, no conclusive data define the efficacy of treatment on the clinical consequences of atherosclerosis.

*Exercise training* improves walking capacity among patients with obstructive arterial disease over a period of several months,[28] but most studies have not identified consistent improvement in measured indices of perfusion. Studies of animals subjected to the creation of arterial obstructions support the view that regular muscular exercise increased collateral development, but in the clinical setting, functional improvement may depend on other factors in muscle metabolism or ergonomics.

## Drug Therapy Aimed at Reducing Ischemia

### Vasodilator Drugs

In contrast to the usefulness of vasodilator drug therapy for treatment of angina pectoris, this approach has been disappointing for relief of intermittent claudication. In patients with limb ischemia, however, the goal is to increase the work capacity of exercising muscle. Blood supply is limited when an obstructive arterial lesion produces critical stenosis, and distal perfusion pressure is reduced. Intramuscular arterioles normally dilate in response to the metabolic demands of exercise, but flow augmentation is blunted in patients with proximal stenotic disease, and distal pressure falls during exercise, leading to accumulation of the ischemic metabolites thought to mediate claudication. The distal vasculature virtually collapses under the compressive force of exercising skeletal muscle, and this mechanism cannot be mitigated by arteriolar vasodilator therapy.

The history of limb arterial disease is replete with therapeutic agents that achieve popularity for a while before falling into disrepute and disuse when adequate studies confirm ineffectiveness. *β-Adrenergic agonists, α-adrenergic antagonists, nitrates,* and other vasodilator drugs have been evaluated in such clinical trials. None increases blood flow in exercising skeletal muscle subtended by significant arterial obstructive lesions, nor does any improve symptoms of intermittent claudication or objective measures of exercise capacity.[29]

### Pharmacologic Enhancement of Collateral Flow

An alternative tactic is to attempt augmentation of *collateral perfusion* in patients with obstructive disease of major limb arteries. This is the rationale behind the use of the selective serotonin antagonist *ketanserin,* which increased collateral blood flow in patients with obstructive lesions in one study. In a multicenter trial enrolling patients with intermittent claudication, however, treadmill exercise performance was no better 1 year after treatment with ketanserin than with placebo.[30]

### Hemorrheologic Agents

Abnormal rheologic findings are noted in many patients with atherosclerotic disease. Oral *pentoxifylline* is in clinical use to improve the walking capacity of patients with intermittent claudication related to obstructive arterial disease on the basis of beneficial results in several clinical trials.[31] In vitro, abnormally reduced erythrocyte flexibility of blood obtained from patients with claudication is partially corrected, and skeletal muscle oxygen tension has been reported to rise at rest after treatment with pentoxifylline, supporting a hemorrheologic mechanism of action. Improved blood fluidity in vivo has not been conclusively demonstrated, however, in patients with claudication during ischemia produced by leg exercise or arterial occlusion. Vascular resistance during reactive hyperemia showed no improvement after administration of pentoxifylline compared with placebo in a study of patients with stable intermittent claudication, suggesting that the hemorrheologic effects of this drug were not sufficient to reduce impedance to blood flow.

## Metabolic Agents

*Cilostazol,* an inhibitor of phosphodiesterase-III with vasodilator and platelet inhibitor actions, was approved by the U.S. Food and Drug Administration in 1999 for treatment of intermittent claudication. The mechanism of its effect is not well understood. Cilostazol has been compared with placebo in eight controlled trials involving more than 2000 patients and, in two studies, with pentoxifylline (the only other drug approved for intermittent claudication). Primary endpoints were the distances patients could walk on a treadmill before the onset of claudication pain (initial claudication distance, ICD) and before pain became intolerable (absolute claudication distance, ACD). In six of the eight studies, ICD and ACD were significantly improved on cilostazol compared with placebo. In one study, cilostazol was superior to pentoxifylline; in the other comparison with pentoxifylline, neither drug was superior to placebo. In general, 100 mg twice daily was superior to 50 mg twice daily. No data define longer-term aspects of treatment, such as limb preservation, rate of progression, and so on. Several other phosphodiesterase inhibitors have been associated with increased mortality when used as inotropic agents in patients with severe (New York Heart Association classes III and IV) heart failure, and cilostazol is currently contraindicated in any patient with a history of congestive heart failure.[32]

*Propionyl-L-carnitine* reportedly facilitates transfer of acetylated compounds and fatty acids across mitochondrial membranes, leading to enhanced energy storage. Accumulation of acylcarnitines in ischemic skeletal muscle correlates with impairment of exercise performance and may reflect abnormal oxidative metabolism.[33] Increased substrate availability has been suggested as the mechanism by which propionyl-L-carnitine supplementation may improve walking capacity in patients with intermittent claudication, as suggested by results from a European multicenter trial,[34] but results have been inconsistent in different populations and larger studies are needed.

The mechanism by which *prostaglandin $E_1$ (PGE$_1$)* and *prostacyclin (PGI$_2$)*, potent vasodilators and inhibitors of platelet aggregation, relieve ischemic rest pain and promote healing of ulcers remains controversial. Intravenous or intraarterial infusions of PGE$_1$ and PGI$_2$ have persisting effects on blood flow and exercise capacity for weeks to months after treatment, but intravenous administration has yielded inconsistent results.[35] The major drawback to this type of prostaglandin therapy is the short half-lives of these drugs, but oral analogues are under development. Overall, prostacyclins may provide temporary relief of ischemic rest pain in patients with severe arterial insufficiency, best when given intraarterially, but it is unknown whether this therapy will prevent amputation in patients not amenable to revascularization.

## Angiogenesis

Therapeutic angiogenesis involves administration of vascular growth factors, usually as recombinant protein or DNA to augment the collateral blood supply to ischemic tissues. Arterial gene transfer of plasmid DNA encoding for an isoform of human vascular endothelial growth factor in patients with critical limb ischemia effected relief of rest pain and improved limb blood flow at 1 year. At higher doses, histologic and angiographic neovascularization was apparent in these preliminary studies, and local intramuscular injection has shown promising early results.[36]

## Antithrombotic Therapy

Antithrombotic therapy may be considered for the management of peripheral arterial obstructive disease at various stages. In chronic disease, the goal is to prevent progression of the obliterative process leading to thrombotic occlusion of arteries. After revascularization procedures, the objective is to prevent thrombotic complications and preserve the patency of reconstruction. In acute arterial occlusion resulting from embolism or thrombosis, therapy is directed toward prevention of propagation of thrombi and recurrence of embolism. Available approaches include *anticoagulant medications, platelet inhibitor* agents, *thrombolytic* substances, and *direct inhibitors of thrombin.* A combination of approaches is warranted for high-risk patients.

No conclusive evidence shows that antithrombotic therapy alters the clinical course of vascular insufficiency related to arteriosclerosis obliterans, although occasional reports have suggested a benefit of anticoagulant or platelet inhibitor agents along these lines. Emerging data seem to confirm that antithrombotic therapy might actually delay the progression of atherosclerotic lesions. In double-blind studies of several hundred patients, serial angiography revealed less pronounced progression of arterial disease in patients randomly assigned to take platelet inhibitor medication (*aspirin* or the combination of aspirin plus *dipyridamole*) than in those given placebo.[37] The role of platelet inhibitor medication in retarding progression of the atherosclerotic plaque has been demonstrated for a longer period in patients with coronary artery disease.

Intermittent claudication carries important prognostic weight in terms of other atherothrombotic cardiovascular events. Aspirin therapy has been convincingly demonstrated to reduce the risks of myocardial infarction, ischemic stroke, and vascular death for many patients with apparent vascular disease. A meta-analysis of more than 100 randomized clinical trials involving about 70,000 participants concluded that aspirin reduces these vascular events by about 25%, regardless of the aspirin dose. Nonfatal myocardial infarctions and strokes were reduced by about one third, and vascular deaths were reduced by about one sixth.[38] The thienopyridine derivatives *ticlopidine* and *clopidogrel* antagonize the platelet adenosine diphosphate receptor. In a large multicenter trial (CAPRIE), clopidogrel (75 mg/day) was compared with aspirin (325 mg/day) for a mean follow-up of 1.5 years in 19,185 patients with clinical atherosclerosis.[39] Participants included survivors of myocardial infarction, nondisabling stroke, and symptomatic peripheral arterial disease; the primary endpoint was a composite of ischemic stroke, myocardial infarction, or vascular death. Patients treated with clopidogrel had a 5.32% annual risk of primary events, compared with 5.83% for those treated with aspirin (a statistically significant relative risk reduction of 8.7%). Most benefit was confined to the 6452 patients entered on the basis of peripheral arterial disease, in whom the relative risk reduction for occurrence of primary vascular events was 24% (p = 0.0028).

Insufficient data have been forthcoming to validate an advantage to long-term anticoagulation for patients with peripheral arterial disease. The incidence of ischemic events was lower, and survival was greater among selected anticoagulated patients after femoropopliteal bypass surgery than in a control group.[40] Ankle/

brachial systolic pressure indices declined more gradually in the anticoagulated patients, and graft patency was prolonged to 12 years, but this falls short of confirming delayed progression of atherosclerotic vascular disease.

## ▪ INTERVENTIONAL ANGIOGRAPHY

Considerable success has attended transluminal dilation for correction of iliac arterial stenoses, but patency rates are lower in the femoral and popliteal arteries. Initial and long-term success is related to the severity of ischemic symptoms as well as to the morphologic features of the atherosclerotic segment, particularly the length of obstruction, relation to anatomic branch points, and condition of the distal artery. Experience with obstructions distal to the popliteal trifurcation has been disappointing, but steerable devices drawn from coronary catheterization enhance outcome in selected cases. In view of the limitation of dilation techniques, various alternative recanalization tools have been developed.

Antithrombotic therapy before catheter intervention is advocated in conjunction with balloon angioplasty procedures to reduce thrombus formation and the associated risk of occlusion of the dilated site. Current practice tends toward preprocedural and postprocedural administration of aspirin plus ticlopidine, as well as intraprocedural administration of heparin, followed by maintenance therapy with aspirin or clopidogrel.

A simulation model suggested that angioplasty might be preferred as the initial approach to revascularization in patients with disabling claudication and femoropopliteal stenosis, whereas bypass surgery was superior for those with critical limb ischemia and femoropopliteal occlusion, but no randomized trials have compared balloon angioplasty with surgical revascularization in patients with peripheral arterial disease.

### Transcatheter Atherectomy and Endovascular Stents

Extraction of atherothrombotic material using the Simpson rotating blade device or abrasion and pulverization methods is intended to remove atheromatous material and leave the remaining surface smooth. Unlike other methods of angioplasty, atherectomy appears well suited to eccentric atherosclerotic lesions associated with calcification.[41] For stenoses at the femoropopliteal level, angiographic success has been reported in 87% to 93% of the lesions removed; symptoms recurred in 31% of patients during 6 months of clinical follow-up.[42]

Patency rates for angioplasty and endovascular stent deployment in iliac arterial stenosis were 92% at 9 months, and clinical benefit has been reported to extend for 2 years.[43] Results with infrainguinal endovascular stents, however, have been less successful, with restenosis or reocclusion rates of approximately 50% in the femoropopliteal segment.

### Intraarterial Thrombolysis

Catheter-directed intraarterial thrombolytic therapy has been used as an adjunct to revascularization for management of both acute and chronic critical limb ischemia, reducing the rates of mortality and amputation. Several studies have compared thrombolytic therapy with surgical revascularization in patients with acute peripheral arterial insufficiency, and though there have been some variations, when taken together these show comparable rates of mortality and limb salvage.[44] Although the rate of successful reperfusion (50% to 80%) is higher with local intraarterial than with systemic (intravenous) thrombolytic therapy, local infusions allow concurrent angiographic definition of effectiveness and define regional vascular disease so that angioplasty may be incorporated to prevent reocclusion. Bleeding or thromboembolism in up to 20% of cases may complicate prolonged periods of indwelling arterial catheterization. Thrombolytic therapy may be particularly useful in cases of thrombotic distal arterial occlusion in the forearm, hand, ankle, and foot, which may be surgically inaccessible.

## ■ SURGICAL THERAPY

Surgical intervention is not indicated in the majority of patients who have stable intermittent claudication with sufficient collateral blood supply to meet the nutritional requirement of resting limb tissue, unless functional limitation is severe and conservative measures have failed. The most pressing indication for surgical revascularization is ischemic rest pain, ulceration, or gangrene amenable to arterial reconstruction when more limited measures, including angioplasty, are insufficient, unsafe, or not feasible. Because the majority of patients with intermittent claudication remain stable or improve with time, this becomes an appropriate basis for surgical intervention only when severely debilitating or progressive.

Beyond the severity of ischemia and associated symptoms, the anatomic pathology becomes important in deciding whether surgery should be undertaken. In general, the syndromic approach to disease classification reflects the success of surgical bypass procedures. Revascularization for aortoiliac obstructive disease is associated with approximately 85% patency rates at 5 to 10 years; for patients undergoing femoropopliteal reconstruction, patency rates around 70% at 5 years are widely reported, whereas much poorer results, in the range of 40% to 60% after 2 years, are common in patients with distal anastomoses beyond the popliteal trifurcation. This aspect should be interpreted in the context of a patient's overall medical condition, with particular reference to risk imposed by associated coronary or cerebrovascular disease.

## ■ REFERENCES

1. Wilens SL: The nature of diffuse intimal thickening of arteries. Am J Pathol 1951;27:825–839.
2. World Health Organization Study Group: Classification of atherosclerotic lesions: Report of a study group. WHO Tech Rep Ser 1958;143:1–20.
3. Kannel WB, McGee DL: Update on some epidemiologic features of intermittent claudication: The Framingham Study. J Am Geriatr Soc 1985;33:13.
4. Vogt MT, Cauley JA, Kuller LH, Hulley SB: Prevalence and correlates of lower extremity arterial disease in elderly women. Am J Epidemiol 1993;137(5):559–568.
5. Criqui MH, Froner A, Barrett-Connor E, et al: The prevalence of peripheral arterial disease in a defined population. Circulation 1985;71:510–515.
6. Hiatt WR, Hoag S, Hamman RF: Effect of diagnostic criteria on the prevalence of peripheral arterial disease: The San Luis Valley Diabetes Study. Circulation 1995;91:1472–1479.
7. Mathiesen FR, Mune O: Arterial insufficiency in the lower extremities of elderly patients. Acta Chir Scand P [Suppl] 1966;357:78.
8. Paris BEC, Libow LS, Halperin JL, Mulvihill MN: The prevalence and one-year outcome of limb arterial obstructive disease in a nursing home population. J AM Geriatr Soc 1988;36:607–612.
9. Greenhalgh RM, Rosengarten DS, Mervart I, et al: Serum lipids and lipoproteins in peripheral vascular disease. Lancet 1971;3:947.
10. Strandness DE Jr, Priest RE, Gibbon GE: Combined clinical and pathologic study of diabetic and nondiabetic peripheral arterial disease. Diabetes 1964;13:366–372.
11. Kannel WB, McGee D, Gordon T: A general cardiovascular risk profile: The Framingham Study. Am J Cardiol 1976;38:46.
12. Coffman JD, Javett SL: Blood flow in the human calf during tobacco smoking. Circulation 1963;28:932.

13. Imparato AM, Kim G, Davidson T, et al: Intermittent claudication: Its natural course. Surgery 1975;78:795.
14. Hertzer NR, Young JR, Kramer JR, et al: Routine coronary angiography prior to elective aortic reconstruction. Arch Surg 1979;114:1336.
15. Criqui M, Langer RD, Fronek A, et al: Mortality over a period of 10 years in patients with peripheral arterial disease. N Engl J Med 1992;328:381–386.
16. The Framingham Study: An Epidemiologic Investigation of Cardiovascular Disease. Denver, Co: U. S. Government Printing Office, Section 25, 1970.
17. Schadt DC, Hines EA Jr, Juergens JL, et al: Chronic atherosclerotic occlusion of the femoral artery. JAMA 1961;175:937.
18. Coffman JD: Intermittent claudication: Be conservative. N Engl J Med 1991;325:577–578.
19. Montgomery DH, Ververis JJ, McGorisk G, et al: Natural history of severe atheromatous disease of the thoracic aorta: a transesophageal echocardiographic study. J Am Coll Cardiol 1996;27:95–101.
20. Thiele B: Evaluation of ulceration of the lower extremities. Vasc Diagn Ther 1980;1:33.
21. Karmody A, Wittmore AD, Baker JD, Ernst CB: Suggested standards for report dealing with lower extremity ischemia. J Vasc Surg 1986;4:80–94.
22. Halperin JL: Noninvasive vascular laboratory evaluation: Applications for laser angioplasty. In Sanborn TA (ed): Laser Angioplasty. New York: AR Liss, 1989.
23. Owen RS, Carpenter JP, Baum RA, et al: Magnetic resonance imaging of angiographically occult runoff vessels in peripheral arterial occlusive disease. N Engl J Med 1992;326:1577–1581.
24. Pedersen TR, Kjekshus J, Pyorala K, et al: Effect of simvastatin on ischemic signs and symptoms in the Scandinavian Simvastatin Survival Study (4S). Am J Cardiol 1998;81:333–338.
25. Diabetes Control and Complications Trial Research Group: The effect of intensive treatment of diabetes on the development and progression of long-term complications in insulin-dependent diabetes mellitus. N Engl J Med 1993;329:977–986.
26. Hansson L, Zanchetti A, Carruthers SG, et al: Effects of intensive blood-pressure lowering and low-dose aspirin in patients with hypertension: Principal results of the Hypertension Optimal Treatment (HOT) randomised trial. HOT Study Group. Lancet 1998;351:1755–1762.
27. Lassila R, Lepantalo M: Cigarette smoking and the outcome after lower limb arterial surgery. Acta Chir Scand 1988;154:635–640.
28. Skinner JS, Strandness DE Jr: Exercise and intermittent claudication: II. Effect of physical training. Circulation 1967;36:23.
29. Coffman JD, Mannick JA: Failure of vasodilator drugs in arterioclerosis obliterans. Ann Intern Med 1972;76:35–59.
30. PACK Claudication Substudy Investigators: Randomized placebo-controlled, double-blind trial of ketanserin in claudicants: Changes in claudication distance and ankle systolic pressure. Circulation 1989;80:1544–1548.
31. Porter JM, Cutler BS, Lee BY, et al: Pentoxifylline efficacy in the treatment of intermittent claudication: Multicenter controlled double-blind trial with objective assessment of chronic occlusive arterial disease patients. Am Heart J 1982;104:66–72.
32. Dawson DL, Cutler BS, Meissner MH, et al: Cilostazol has beneficial effects in treatment of intermittent claudication. Circulation 1998;98:678–686.
33. Hiatt WR, Nawaz D, Brass EP: Carnitine metabolism during exercise in patients with peripheral arterial disease. J Appl Physiol 1987;74:236–240.
34. Brevetti G, Chiariello M, Ferulano G, et al: Increases in walking distance in patients with peripheral vascular disease treated with L-carnitine: A double-blind, cross-over study. Circulation 1988;77:767–773.
35. The ICAI (Ischemia Cronica degli Arti Inferiore) Study Group: Prostanoids for chronic critical limb ischemia: A randomized, controlled, open-label trial with prostaglandin E₁. Ann Intern Med 1999;130:412–421.
36. Schainfeld RM, Isner JM: Critical limb ischemia: Nothing to give at the office? Ann Intern Med 1999;130:442–444.
37. Goldhaber SZ, Manson JE, Stampfer MJ, et al: Low-dose aspirin and subsequent arterial surgery in the Physicians' Health Study. Lancet 1992;340:143–145.
38. Antiplatelet Trialists Collaboration: Collaborative overview of randomised trials of antiplatelet therapy. Prevention of death, myocardial infarction, and stroke by prolonged antiplatelet therapy in various categories of patients. BMJ 1994;308:81–101.
39. CAPRIE steering committee: A randomised, blinded trial of clopidogrel versus aspirin in patients at risk of ischemic events (CAPRIE). Lancet 1996;348:1329–1339.
40. Kretschmer G, Herbst F, Prager M, et al: A decade of oral anticoagulant treatment to maintain autologous vein grafts for femoropopliteal atherosclerosis. Arch Surg 1992;127:1112–1115.
41. Zacca NM, Raizner AE, Noon GP, et al: Treatment of symptomatic peripheral atherosclerotic disease with a rotational atherectomy device. Am J Cardiol 1989;63:77–80.
42. vonPolnitz A, Nerlich A, Berger H, et al: Percutaneous peripheral atherectomy: Angiographic and clinical followup of 60 patients. J Am Coll Cardiol 1990;15:682–688.
43. Palmaz JC, Laborde JC, Rivera FJ, et al: Stenting of the iliac arteries with the Palmaz stent: Experience from a multicenter trial of cardiovascular intervention. Radiology 1992;15:291–297.
44. Ouriel K, Veith FJ, Sasahara AA: Comparison of recombinant urokinase with vascular surgery as initial treatment for acute arterial occlusion of the legs. N Engl J Med 1998;338:1105–1111.

# ■ RECOMMENDED READING

CAPRIE Steering Committee (on behalf of the CAPRIE Study Group): A randomised, blinded trial of clopidogrel versus aspirin in patients at risk of ischaemic events (CAPRIE). Lancet 1996;348:1329–1339.

Halperin JL, Creager MA: Arterial obstructive diseases of the extremities. *In* Vascular Medicine: A Textbook of Vascular Biology and Diseases, 2nd ed. Loscalzo J, Creager MA, Dzau VJ (eds): Boston: Little, Brown & Co, 1996:825–854.

Hirsch AT (ed): An Office-Based Approach to the Diagnosis and Treatment of Peripheral Arterial Disease, Parts I–III. American Journal of Medicine Continuing Education Series. Belle Mead, MD: Excerpta Medica, 1998–1999.

Jackson MR, Clagett GP: Antithrombotic therapy in peripheral arterial occlusive disease. Chest 1998;114:666S–682S.

Spittell JA (ed): Clinical Vascular Disease. Philadelphia: FA Davis, 1983.

# INDEX

Note: Page numbers in *italics* refer to illustrations; page numbers followed by t refer to tables.